Progress in Allergy and Clinical Immunology
Volume 2, Kyoto

Progress in Allergy and Clinical Immunology Volume 2, Kyoto

Proceedings of the XIVth International Congress of Allergology and Clinical Immunology, Kyoto, October 13–18, 1991

Edited by
Terumasa Miyamoto and Minoru Okuda

National Sagamihara Hospital, Kanagawa-ken, Japan
and
Nippon Medical School Hospital, Tokyo, Japan

Hogrefe & Huber Publishers
Seattle · Toronto · Bern · Göttingen

Section VI: Diagnosis and Monitoring of Allergic Diseases

Section VII: Epidemiology and Genetics of Allergic Diseases

Section VIII: Nasal Allergy: Pathophysiology and Management of Nasal Congestion

Section IX: The Role of PAF and the Importance of PAF Antagonists in Respiratory Diseases

Section X: Current Perspectives in Food Allergy

Section XI: Mediator Release and its Modulation

Section XII: New Concepts in Clinical Immunology

Section XIII: Inflammatory Cells and Cytokines in Allergy

Section XIV: Mast Cells and Basophils

Section XX: Pediatric Allergy

Section XXI: Physical Allergy

Preface

The XIVth International Congress of Allergology and Clinical Immunology (ICACI) was held in Kyoto, Japan, from October 13th through October 18th, 1991, with more than 3,000 participants from over 50 countries. The congress successfully achieved many of its goals, and has attained a high degree of renown.

Because of the ever rising numbers of allergic patients throughout the world, the community of allergists and clinical immunologists has been expanding as well and the IAACI has extended its work more than ever.

The field of allergy and clinical immunology has become all the more attractive to clinicians, scientists and researchers, and has also made significant and rapid progress. As a part of this growth in our knowledge, the papers presented at the congress reached a high standard of scientific material and clinical applicability.

The volume presents proceedings from 22 of the symposia by invited speakers to the congress, and they are being published here, partly as a pleasant memento to the delegates who attended, but also to convey the very exciting and meaningful results to those workers in the field who could not attend the meeting. We are convinced that the book is another milestone in our field. The editors would like to express their sincere appreciation to the contributors, and to the publishers, Hogrefe and Huber, for their cooperation. They also express their sincere gratitude to Janssen Pharmaceutical Co. for their generous support for this publication.

Terumasa Miyamoto, M.D.
Chairman

Organizing Committee of the XIVth ICACI

IL-4 Production by FcεRI$^+$ Cells

William E. Paul*

Interleukin-4 is produced constitutively by some transformed mast-cell lines and is induced in IL-3 dependent mast-cell lines by cross-linkage of FcεRI. Among mouse bone marrow and spleen cells, the capacity to produce IL-4 in response to immobilized IgE, immobilized IgG2a or to ionomycin is limited to cells that have high affinity FcεR. Morphologic analysis of such cells indicated that essentially all the granulated cells are basophils or basophilic myelocytes but that a substantial fraction of the FcεR+ cells were non-granulated. Short term cultures of such cells in IL-3 caused striking expansion of the percent of cells that are FcεRI$^+$. These cells could be subdivided based on the expression of *c-kit*. Cell sorting analysis indicated that the prinicipal IL-4 producing cells in this population were FcεRI$^+$, *c-kit*-, strongly suggesting that they were basophil lineage cells.

Cytokines are small proteins that play a powerful role in the regulation of immune responses and inflammatory reactions (1). Historically, a major subset of these, often designated as lymphokines, were believed to be exclusively produced by T lymphocytes in response to receptor-mediated cross-linkage, in the presence of accessory signals. For this reason, such molecules, including IL-2, IL-3, IL-4, IL-5, GM-CSF, lymphotoxin and interferon γ, were often referred to as T-cell derived lymphokines. However, evidence has amassed over the last several years that some of these molecules could be produced by other hematopoietic lineage cells, particularly in response to cross-linkage of the Fc receptors FcγRIII and FcεRI. A striking example of this is production of IL-4 by cells of the mast-cell and basophil lineages in response to the action of the *v-Abl* tyrosine kinase (2), treatment with ionomycin or cross-linkage of FcεRI or FcγRIII (3–7).

The capacity of cells bearing FcεRI to produce IL-4 was first appreciated as a result of studies that demonstrated that some, but not all, Abelson murine leukemia virus (Ab-MuLV)-transformed mast-cell produced IL-4 constitutively (2). This work was then extended by the demonstration that long term IL-3-dependent mast-cell lines could produce IL-4 and other lymphokines and cytokines in response to cross-linkage of FcεRI or to elevation of intracellular calcium concentration through the action of ionomycin (3). Indeed, it was demonstrated that such cells and short term cultures of bone marrow cells grown in IL-3 could produce a series of cytokines in response to receptor cross-linkage (3–5). These included IL-3, IL-4, IL-5, GM-CSF as well as IL-6, TNF, IL-1 and MIP-1a. Interestingly, the cells failed to produce IL-2, IFNγ or lymphotoxin. These results were particularly interesting because they suggested that mast-cells might participate in allergic type inflammatory responses at a regulatory as well as at an effector level.

Efforts were then undertaken to characterize cells present in normal mice and in mice that had elevated levels of IgE that could produce IL-4 in response to cross-linkage of FcεRI (6–8). It was observed that spleen cell suspensions depleted of both B and T-cells as well as bone marrow cell suspensions contained cells that produced IL-4 in response to immobilized IgE (6). Co-culture or pretreatment of these cells with IL-3 caused a striking increase in the IL-4 produced in response to cross-linkage of FcεR and also allowed these cells to produce IL-4 in response to immobilized IgG2a (6–7). The latter response was inhibited by the monoclonal antibody 2.4G2, implying that the receptor was either FcγRII or FcγRIII. The conclusion that the response to immobilized igE was mediated by FcεRI was based on the concentration of IgE needed to sensitize receptors and the capacity

* Laboratory of Immunology, National Institute of Allergy and Infectious Diseases, National Institutes of Health, Bethesda, MD 20892, USA.
Acknowledgments: I thank the colleagues who have made important contributions to the work described here, including S.Z. Ben-Sasson, Melissa Brown, Dan Conrad, Ann Dvorak, Fred Finkelman, Stephen Galli, Achsah Keegan, Graham Le Gros, Jacalyn Pierce, Marshall Plaut, Robert Seder and Joseph Urban, Jr.

of the receptor to retain this IgE for extended periods of time at 37C.

The capacity of bone marrow cells or splenic non-B, non-T-cells to produce IL-4 in response to FcR cross-linkage was found to be strikingly increased in spleen and bone marrow cell populations obtained from mice that had been infected with *Nippostrongylus brasiliensis* or treated with the *in vivo* polyclonal B cell activator anti-IgD (8). In these mice, the capacity of a fixed number of splenic non-B, non-T-cells to produce IL-4 increased 10 to 50-fold and the total number of these cells increased 3 to 10 fold, resulting in an increase in the IL-4-producing potentiality of this cell pool of 100-fold or more in some experiments. Analysis of the frequency of IL-4-producing cells in the non-B, non-T-cell population derived from spleens or from bone marrow of activated mice revealed that ~ 1/200 cells would produce IL-4 in response to immobilized IgE (9). For that reason, the characterization of these cells required a cell purification step. The initial strategy was to purify cells expressing FcεRI by cell sorting. Such cells usually comprised 1–2% of the starting population. However, all of the capacity to produce IL-4 in response to cross-linkage of FcεR or FcγR was in this small cell population (9). Transmission electron microscopic analysis, carried out by Ann Dvorak and Stephen Galli, indicated that 30–50% of these cells could be identified as basophils or basophilic myelocytes (10). The remainder of the FcεRI$^+$ population lacked distinguishing morphologic features. Analysis of the frequency of IL-4 producing cells in this purified population revealed that ~ 1/5 cells had this property. These results raised the possibility that the IL-4-producing cells might be in the basophil, in addition to or rather than in the mast-cell, lineage. However, because of the lack of total purity of the cell populations involved, the studies could not offer conclusive evidence as to the nature of the IL-4-producing cells.

In order to clarify this point, bone marrow cells were cultured for periods of 5 to 7 days in IL-3 alone or in IL-3 plus stem cell factor. The frequency of FcεRI$^+$ cells expanded strikingly during this period. When these cells were examined for expression of *c-kit*, it was observed that approximately 1/2 of the FcεRI$^+$ cells were *c-kit*$^+$. These cells were then sorted into the FcεRI$^+$,*c-kit*$^+$ and the FcεRI$^+$,*c-kit* populations and the resulting cells tested for their capacity to produce IL-4 in response to receptor cross-linkage. The FcεRI$^+$,*c-kit* proved to be very active producers of IL-4 while the FcεRI$^+$,*c-kit*$^+$ were quite poor producers (11). Light microscopic analysis indicated that the *c-kit*$^+$ population had large, Alcian-blue positive granules and monomorphic nuclei suggesting that they were mast-cells while the *c-kit* cells had smaller and sparser Alcian blue positive granules. Many of these cells had lobulated nuclei, suggesting that they were basophils or basophilic myelocytes. Studies of their morphology by electron microscopy are now in progress as are analyses of the frequency of cells that can produce IL-4 in response to cross-linkage of FcεRI.

The results described in this paper establish that mouse FcεRI$^+$ cells produce several lymphokines as a result of FcR-cross-linkage. Recent evidence indicates that-cells of the basophil lineage are particularly striking producers of IL-4. IL-4 production by these cells requires cross-linkage of FcR and is strikingly enhanced if the cells have been pretreated with IL-3. Indeed, recent work indicates that IL-3 enhances signalling through FcεRI by causing increased tyrosine phosphorylation of certain substrates (12). The capacity of these cells to produce IL-4 and the enhancing action of IL-3 suggests that these cells may act to strikingly amplify IL-4 production in thymus-dependent immune responses. However, such cells may also act to produce IL-4 in the absence of T-cells and may mediate important lymphokine related functions. In particular, they may produce lymphokines at sites of local immune complex deposition and may have powerful regulatory effects in allergic types of inflammatory responses.

References

1. Paul, W.E. 1989. Pleiotropy and redundancy: T-cell-derived lymphokines in the immune response. Cell 57:521.
2. Brown, M.A., Pierce, J.H., Watson, C.J., Falco, J., Ihle, J.N., and Paul, W.E. 1987. B cell stimulatory factor-1/interleukin-4 mRNA is expressed by normal and transformed mast-cells. Cell 50:809.
3. Plaut, M., Pierce, J.H., Watson, C.J., Hanley-Hyde, J., Nordan, R.P., and Paul, W.E. 1989. Mast-cell lines produce lymphokines in re-

sponse to cross linkage of FcεRI or to calcium ionophores. Nature 339:64.
4. Wodnar-Filopowicz, A., Heusser, C.H., and Moroni, C. 1989. Production of the haemopoietic growth factors GM-CSF and interleukin-3 by mast-cells in response to IgE receptor-mediated activation. Nature 339:150.
5. Burd, P.R., Rogers, H.W., Gordon, J.R., Martin, C.A., Jayaraman, S., Wilson, S., Dvorak, A.M., Galli, S., and Dorf, M.E. 1989. Interleukin 3-dependent and independent mast-cells stimulated with IgE and antigen express multiple cytokines. J. Exp. Med. 170:245.
6. Ben-Sasson, S., LeGros, G., Conrad, D.H., Finkelman, F.D., and Paul, W.E. 1990. Cross-linking Fc receptors stimulate splenic non-B, non-T-cells to secrete interleukin 4 and other lymphokines. Proc. Natl. Acad. Sci. USA 87:1421.
7. LeGros, G., Ben-Sasson, S.Z., Conrad, D.H., Clark-Lewis, I., Finkelman, F.D., Plaut, M., and Paul, W.E. 1990. Interleukin-3 promotes production of IL-4 by splenic non-B, non-T-cells in response to Fc receptor cross-linkage. J. Immunol. 145:2500.
8. Conrad, D.H., Ben-Sasson, S.Z., LeGros, G., Finkelman, F.D., and Paul, W.E. 1990. Infection with *Nippostrongylus brasiliensis* or injection of anti-IgD antibodies markedly enhances Fc-receptor-mediated interleukin 4 production by non-B, non-T-cells. J. Exp. Med. 171:1497.
9. Seder, R.A., Plaut, M., Barbieri, S., Urban, Jr. J., Finkelman, F.D., and Paul, W.E. 1991. Purified FcεR⁺ bone marrow and splenic non-B, non-T-cells are highly enriched in the capacity to produce IL-4 in response to immobilized IgE, IgG2a, or ionomycin. J. Immunol. 147:903.
10. Seder, R.A., Paul, W.E., Dvorak, A.M., Sharkis, S.J., Kagey-Sobotka, A., Niv, Y., Finkelman, F.D., Barbieri, S.A., Galli, S.J., and Plaut, M. 1991. Mouse splenic and bone marrow cell populations that express high affinity Fcε receptors and produce IL-4 are highly enriched in basophils. Proc. Natl. Acad. Sci. USA 88:2835.
11. Seder, R.A., Plaut, M., Dvorak, A.M., Galli, S.J., and Paul, W.E. 1991. The major IL-4-producing cells in short term bone marrow cultures are FcεRI+ and *c-kit⁻* with morphologic features of basophils. Manuscript in preparation.
12. Keegan, A.D., Pierce, J.H., Artip, J., Plaut, M., and Paul, W.E. 1991. Ligand stimulation of transfected and endogenous growth factor receptors enhances cytokine production by mast cells. EMBO J. 10: in press.

IgE Synthesis and Interleukins

Sergio Romagnani, Gianfranco Del Prete, Enrico Maggi, Paola Parronchi, Marco De Carli, Donatella Macchia, Marie-Pierre Piccinni, Cecilia Simonelli, Roberto Manetti, Francesco Santoni Rugiu, Maria-Grazia Giudizi, Roberta Biagiotti, Fabio Almerigogna, Mario Ricci*

It is well established that human IgE synthesis is dependent on the B-cell helper activity of T cells (T_H) capable of producing interleukin 4 (IL-4), but not, or only limited amounts of, gamma-interferon (IFN-γ). The selective activation of such a type of T_H cells may be responsible for the enhanced IgE antibody production in patients with allergic disorders or helminthic infestations. Virtually all human $CD4^+$ T cell clones specific for the excretory/secretory component of Toxocara canis, as well as the majority of $CD4^+$ T cell clones specific for Dermatophagoides group I (Der p I) or Lolium perenne Group I allergens produce IL-4 and IL-5 but not IFN-γ (T_H2-like), whereas the majority of T cell clones specific for the mycobacterial antigen PPD produce IL-2 and IFN-γ, but not IL-4 and IL-5 (T_H1-like). Human T_H2 clones provide B-cell help for IgE synthesis and are not cytolytic for antigen-presenting cells (APC), thus accounting for the chronicity of IgE antibody responses against common environmental allergens or helminthic components. In contrast, T_H1 clones do not provide help for IgE synthesis and most of them are cytolytic for APC, including B lymphocytes. The T_H1-like pattern of PPD-specific T cell clones can be changed by culturing PPD-specific T cells in the presence of IL-4. Likewise, the T_H2-like pattern of Der p I-specific T cell clones can be modified by culturing Der p I-specific T cells in the presence of IFN-γ or in the absence of IL-4. These data indicate that a better knowledge of factors that modulate the activation of T_H cells may provide a means for therapeutic interventions in IgE-mediated disorders through successful transformation of a T_H2-like into a T_H1-like response.

Factors Modulating the Activation of T_H Cells

Role of $CD4^+$T Helper (T_H) Cells and T_H Cell-Derived Cytokines in the Regulation of Human IgE Synthesis

In the last few years, a pathway of human IgE regulation, essentially based on the reciprocal activity of interleukin-4 (IL-4) and gamma-interferon (IFN-γ), has been discovered (reviewed in 1). The first demonstration that IL-4- or IFN-γ-producing $CD4^+$ T_H cell subsets play a reciprocal role in the regulation of human IgE synthesis was provided in our laboratory by assaying the activity of large numbers of phytohemagglutinin (PHA)-induced T cell clones (TCC) derived from different lymphoid organs. When PHA-induced TCC or their supernatants (SUP) were assayed for their ability to induce the synthesis of IgE and to produce IL-2, IL-4 and IFN-γ, a significant positive correlation between helper function for IgE and production of IL-4 was found (2). In contrast, there was a significant inverse correlation between the IgE helper activity of TCC (or SUP derived from them) and their ability to produce IFN-γ (2). The opposite regulatory role of IL-4 and IFN-γ in the synthesis of human IgE was confirmed by the observations that (a) human recombinant IL-4 can induce the synthesis of IgE in peripheral blood mononuclear cells (PBMNC), and that (b) this effect is inhibited by addition of recombinant IFN-γ (2,3). However, the activity of IL-4 alone is not sufficient for the induction of human IgE synthesis. Both recombinant IL-4 and IL-4-containing SUP are consistently ineffective in inducing IgE synthesis by highly purified B cells (2,3). IL-4-dependent IgE synthesis can be restored by the readdition to

* Division of Clinical Immunology and Allergology and of Internal Medicine, University of Florence, Istituto di Clinica Medica 3, Viale Morgagni, 85. Firenze 50134, Italy.
Acknowledgements: This work was supported by funds in part from CNR and in part from AIRC.

highly purified B cells of appropriate concentrations of autologous or allogeneic T cells or of CD4+ TCC (2). Subsequent experiments demonstrated that both noncognate and cognate interaction with CD4+ T cells may render B cells susceptible to the activity of IL-4 (1,4).

Altered Proportions of IL-4- and/or IFN-γ-Producing CD4+ T Cells in the Blood and/or Target Organs of Patients with Helminthic Infections or Allergic Disorders.

The findings reported above encouraged investigations into whether alterations of CD4+ T cell subsets (or of cytokines they produce) are involved in the genesis of human diseases characterized by hyperproduction of IgE. We first examined the ability of PHA-induced TCC from the PB of four children with the hyper-IgE syndrome to produce different cytokines. These children had significantly lower proportions of circulating T cells that can produce IFN-γ and tumor necrosis factor (TNF)-α (but not of T cells producing IL-2 or IL-4) in comparison with controls (5). Thus, the defective production of IFN-γ may account for hyperproduction of IgE and the combined defect of IFN-γ and TNF-α may contribute to the susceptibility to infections found in patients with the hyper-IgE syndrome (5). Patients with helminthic infections or atopic disorders usually exhibit both elevated IgE serum levels and eosinophilia. Based on the findings mentioned above, as well as on the knowledge that IL-5 (another T-cell derived cytokine) acts as a selective differentiation factor for eosinophils, it was reasonable to suggest that both atopic patients and patients with helminthic infections may harbor Th cells resembling the T_H2 subset described in mice (6) for their ability to produce IL-4 and IL-5, but not IFN-γ. To test this possibility, we first investigated the profile of cytokine production of PHA-induced TCC established from the PB of patients with helminthic infections or severe atopic diseases. Significantly higher proportions of IL-4-producing and significantly lower proportions of IFN-γ-producing TCC were recovered from the PB of both groups of patients in comparison with healthy controls (1). Furthermore, PHA-induced TCC derived from the conjunctival infiltrates of three patients suffering from vernal conjunctivitis (VC) were examined. The great majority of TCC obtained from VC infiltrates were CD4+ T cells inducible to the production of high concentrations of IL-4 and able to provide helper function for IgE synthesis by B cells (7). In contrast, even after maximal stimulation, such as that delivered by phorbol myristate acetate (PMA) plus anti-CD3 monoclonal antibody, a few TCC expressed IFN-γ mRNA and could produce IFN-γ (7). By using a different experimental approach, a strong IL-5, but poor IL-2 and no IFN-γ, message has recently been found in T cells present in the bronchial biopsies of patients with allergic asthma (8). Taken together, these data suggest that in patients with helminthic infections or atopic disorders both production of IgE and eosinophilia probably result from the expansion of T_H2-like cells and/or their accumulation in target organs.

Bacterial Antigens Activate T_H1-Like Cells, Whereas Helminthic Antigens and Allergens Preferentially Activate T_H2-Like Cells.

In an attempt to provide additional information on the nature of the T_H2-like cells found in patients with helminthic infections or allergic disorders, as well as on the mechanisms responsible for their development, our strategy has been to establish TCC specific for allergens including (a) the Dermatophagoides pteronyssinus group I (Der p I) and the Lolium perenne Group I (Lol p I9), (b) helminthic components: excretory/secretory antigen of Toxocara canis: TES, or (c) bacterial components: protein purified derivative (PPD) of Mycobacterium tuberculosis and tetanus toxoid (TT). This approach was based on the observation that Toxocariasis is quite rare, but there is frequent exposure to this helminth, as demonstrated by the high prevalence of anti-TES antibodies and of *in vitro* PB lymphoproliferative responses to TES in the general population. The choice of PPD was based on the observation that, unlike helminthic infection and allergy, infection with Mycobacterium tuberculosis usually results in delayed type hypersensitivity reactions, but not production of IgE and eosinophilia. When large series of PPD- or TES-specific TCC derived from two healthy individuals were compared, a clear- cut dichotomy in the profile of cytokine secretion was observed. Virtually all PPD-specific clones produced IL-2 and IFN-γ , but not IL-4 and IL-5 (T_H1), whereas the great majority of TES-specific clones produced IL-4 and IL-5, but not IL-2 and IFN-γ (T_H2). PPD2-specific TCC that failed to secrete IL-4 and IL-5, and TES-specific TCC that failed to secrete IL-2 and IFN-γ, were found to lack transcripts for IL-4 and IL-5 or for IL-2 and IFN-γ, respectively (9). As expected, T_H2-like TES-specific TCC consistently supported the synthesis of IgE by autologous B cells under MHC-restricted conditions, whereas T_H1-like PPD-specific TCC did not. These results demonstrate that PPD and TES antigens expand helper T cells with opposite (T_H1 or T_H2) phenotype of cytokine secretion. High numbers of Der p I- or Lol p I-specific TCC could be obtained from mite- or grass-sensitive atopic individuals and compared for their phenotype of cytokine secretion with PPD- or TT-specific TCC derived from the same donors. Virtually all the allergen-specific TCC produced IL-4 (and IL-5) in response to stimulation with PMA plus anti-CD3 antibody, and a proportion of them, too, failed to produce IFN-γ. When assessed with the specific antigen under MHC-restricted conditions, the great majority of allergen-specific TCC behave as T_H2-like helper T cells. While most TCC specific for TT produced both IL-4 and IFN-γ (particularly in response to PMA plus anti-CD3 antibody), all TCC specific for PPD produced high amounts of IFN-γ, but most of them did not produce IL-4 and IL-5 (10). These data are partially at variance with those recently reported by Wierenga et al. (11), who showed clear-cut T_H1 and T_H2 dichotomy between TT- and allergen-specific TCC derived from atopic donors. However, they support the view that the immune response to environmental allergens results in the preferential activation of T_H2-like clones. These cells are responsible for both the induction of IgE antibody production and increase of eosinophils via the release of IL-4 and IL-5, respectively.

Human T_H1 and T_H2 TCC Differ not Only in Their Profile of Cytokine Production, but Also in Their Cytolytic Potential and Mode of B-Cell Help.

With a large series of human T-cell clones exhibiting clearcut T_H1 or T_H2 phenotypes, we then determined other functional properties of the two subsets. T_H1, but not T_H2, clones produce TNF-β, whereas both types of clones can produce variable amounts of IL-3, IL-6, TNF-α, and Granulocyte Macrophage-Colony Stimulatory Factor (12). In addition, human T_H1 and T_H2 clones also differ in their cytolytic potential and mode of help for B-cell Ig synthesis. In fact, the majority of T_H1 (77%), but only a minority of T_H2 (18%) clones exhibit cytolytic activity in a 4h PHA-dependent assay (12,13). All T_H2 (noncytolytic) clones induced IgM, IgG, IgA, and IgE synthesis by autologous B cells in the presence of the specific antigen, and the degree of response was proportional to the number of T_H2 cells added to B cells. Under the same experimental conditions, T_H1 (cytolytic) clones provided B-cell help for IgM, IgG and IgA, but not IgE, synthesis with a peak response at a T-cell:B-cell ratio of 1:1. At higher T-cell:B-cell ratios, a decline in B-cell help was observed (13). Interestingly, all these T_H1 clones lysed Epstein-Barr virus (EBV)-transformed autologous B cells pulsed with the specific antigen and the decrease of Ig production correlated with the lytic activity of T_H1 clones against autologous antigen-presenting B-cell targets (14). This may represent an important mechanism for the down-regulation of antibody responses *in vivo* (14,15). Interestingly enough, none of the 13 allergen (Der p I or Lol p I)-specific T_H2-like TCC tested exhibited cytolytic activity against EBV-transformed autologous B cells, whereas 6 out of 7 PPD-specific TCC established from the same donor did (unpublished results). Thus, the ability of T_H2-like cells to produce IL-4 (but no or only limited IFN-γ) together with their inability to kill the antigen-presenting cell, may explain, at least in part, the chronicity of IgE antibody responses to common environmental allergens. Taken together, these data clear up all doubt about the existence of human $CD4^+$ T-cell susbsets secreting different patterns of cytokines similar to those described in mice and support the view that these T-cell subsets are of major importance in determining the class of immune effector function.

Enhanced Capacity of T_H Cells from Atopics to Produce IL-4

Additional elements of complexity emerged when the phenotype of cytokine secretion of a total number of 158 PPD- and 202 TT-specific

TCC obtained from 3 atopic and 3 nonatopic donors was compared. The proportions of TT-specific TCC with T_H2-like profile of cytokine production were significantly higher in atopics than in nonatopics. More importantly, even if all PPD-specific clones from both atopic and nonatopic donors were able to produce elevated concentrations of IFN-γ, a clear difference emerged with regard to their ability to produce IL-4. Indeed, 37% of PPD-specific TCC derived from atopic patients, but only 4% of those obtained from nonatopic individuals, produced IL-4 in response to stimulation with the specific antigen (16). These data suggest that atopic patients have enhanced ability to produce IL-4 even in response to antigens other than common environmental allergens or helminthic components. The molecular alteration(s) responsible for the enhanced ability of helper T cells from atopic patients to produce IL-4 are at present unknown.

IFN-γ and IL-4 Reciprocally Regulate the Development of PPD-Specific T Cells into T_H1 TCC and of Der p I-Specific T Cells into T_H2

More recently the effects exerted on the *in vitro* development of PPD-specific or Der p I-specific T cell lines (TCL) and TCC by IL-4 or IFN-γ addition or neutralization in human peripheral blood PBMNC cultures were examined. As expected, PBMNC from normal individuals, which were stimulated with PPD and then cultured in IL-2 alone, developed into PPD-specific TCL and TCC able to produce IFN-γ and IL-2, but not IL-4 and IL-5 (T_H1-like). IFN-γ or anti-IL-4 antibody addition in bulk cultures before cloning did not influence the PPD-specific TCL profile of cytokine production. In contrast, the addition of IL-4 resulted in the development of PPD-specific TCL and TCC able to produce not only IFN-γ and IL-2 but also IL-4 and IL-5. PBMNC from one atopic Dermatophagoides pteronyssinus Group I (Der p I)-sensitive patient, which were stimulated with Der p I and then cultured in IL-2 alone, developed into Der p I-specific TCL and TCC capable of producing IL-5 and high amounts of IL-4 but no, or only limited amounts of, IFN-γ (T_H2-like). The development of Der p I-specific T cells into IL-4 (and IL-5)- producing TCL and into T_H2-like TCC was markedly inhibited by the addition in bulk cultures before cloning of either IFN-γ or anti-IL-4 antibody (17). These data suggest that the presence or the absence of IL-4 and IFN-γ in bulk cultures of PBMNC before cloning may have strong regulatory effects on the *in vitro* development of human $CD4^+$ T cells into T_H1 or T_H2 clones.

Possible Pathophysiological Implications

The most important question to be solved, however, is why circulating PPD-specific memory T cells are apparently conditioned to produce IFN-γ, but no IL-4, whereas Der p I-specific memory T cells usually produce IL-4 and IL-5, but no IFN-γ upon *in vitro* re-stimulation with the specific antigen. This question involves both the origin of T_H1 and T_H2 cells and the factors influencing their development *in vivo*. So far, the most clear cut requirements for the generation of murine T_H1 or T_H2 effector cells *in vivo* also include lymphokines. IL-2 promotes effector cell development in general regardless of other lymphokines (18). Studies with the murine leishmaniasis model have provided significant evidence that IFN-γ can strongly influence T_H cell precursors to differentiate into cells that produce the T_H1 set of cytokines and that IL-4 may be the counterpart that promotes T_H2 differentiation of the same precursors (19). These findings suggest that the endogenous levels of IFN-γ and/or IL-4 may regulate the differentiation process of naive T_H cells *in vivo*. If IL-4 is responsible for *in vivo* generation of human TH2 cells, we can wonder what kind of cells produce IL-4. It has been reported that fresh cells from some mouse strains produce much higher levels of IL-4 (18). Another possibility is that IL-4 is provided by cells other than T lymphocytes. It is known that mouse mast cell lines, as well as splenic and bone marrow non-B, non-T cells can secrete IL-4 (20,21). The IL-4-producing capacity of non-B, non-T cells expands dramatically in Nippostrongylus brasiliensis infection and in association with anti-IgD injection (22), suggesting that these cells play an important role in lymphokine production in helminthic infections and other situations marked by striking elevations of serum IgE levels. More recently, we have demonstrated the existence of human bone marrow non-B, non-T cells, probably belonging to mast cell/basophil lineage, capable of producing IL-4 in response to FcE receptor cross-linkage (23). Thus, IL-4 production by cells of the mast cell/basophil lineage might very well reflect a means through which T_H2 cells could be strikingly amplified *in vivo* during allergic reactions and parasitic infestations. The results of our studies indicate that a better knowledge of factors that modulate the activation of T_H2 cells may provide a means for therapeutic interventions in IgE-mediated disorders through successful transformation of a T_H2-like response into a T_H1-like response. For instance, a bias toward T_H1 activation could be achieved *in vitro* either by addition of IFN-γ or neutralization of IL-4 in the microenvironment where the T_H cell-allergen interaction occurs. A further characterization of the events required for selective activation of T_H1 or T_H2 clones might offer potential sites for pharmacological manipulation of T_H1 and T_H2 activation, leading to the development of drugs that selectively activate or inhibit specific T_H subsets *in vivo*.

References

1. Romagnani, S. 1990. Regulation and deregulation of human IgE synthesis. Immunol. Today 1:316.
2. Del Prete, G.F., Maggi, E., Parronchi, P., Chretien, I., Tiri, A., Macchia, D., Ricci, M., Banchereau, J., de Vries, J. E., and Romagnani S. 1988. IL-4 is an essential factor for the IgE synthesis induced in vitro by human T cell clones and their supernatants. J. Immunol. 140:4193.
3. Pene, J.F., Rousset, F., Briere, F., Chretien, I., Bonnefoy, J.Y., Spits, H., Yokota, T., Arai, N., Arai, K.-I., Banchereau, J., and de Vries, J.E. 1988. IgE production by normal human lymphocytes is induced by interleukin 4 and suppressed by interferons γ and α and prostaglandin E2. Proc. Natl. Acad. Sci. USA 85:6880.
4. Vercelli, D.H., Jabara, H., Arai, K., and Geha, R.S. 1989. Induction of human IgE synthesis requires interleukin 4 and T/B interactions involving the T cell receptor/CD3 complex and MHC class II antigens. J. Exp. Med. 169:1295.
5. Parronchi, P., Tiri, A., Macchia, D., Biswas, P., Simonelli, C., Maggi, E., Del Prete, G.F., Ricci, M., and Romagnani, S. 1990. Noncognate contact-dependent B cell activation can promote IL-4-dependent in vitro human IgE synthesis. J. Immunol. 144:2102.
6 Del Prete, G.F., Tiri, A., Maggi, E., De Carli, M., Macchia, D., Parronchi, P., Ross, M.E., Pietrogrande, M.C., Ricci, M., and Romagnani, S. 1989. Defective in vitro production of γ-interferon and tumor necrosis factor-α circulating T cells from patients with the hyperimmunoglobulin E syndrome. J. Clin. Invest. 84:1830.
7. Mosmann, T.R., Cherwinski, H., Bond, M.W., Giedlin, M.A., and Coffman, R.L. 1986. Two types of murine helper T cell clone. I. Definition according to profiles of lymphokine activities and secreted proteins. J. Immunol. 136:2348.
8. Maggi, E., Biswas, P., Del Prete, G.F., Parronchi, P., Macchia, D., Simonelli, C., Emmi, L., De Carli, M., Tiri, A., Ricci, M., and Romagnani, S. 1991. Accumulation of T_H2-like helper T cells in the conjunctiva of patients with vernal conjunctivitis. J. Immunol. 146:1169.
9. Hamid, Q., Azzawi, M., King, S., Moqbel, R., Wardlaw, A.J., Corrigan, C.J., Bradle, B., Durham, S.R., Collins, J.V., Jeffery, P.K., Quint, D.J., and Kay, A.B. 1991. Expression of mRNA for interleukin-5 in mucosal bronchial biopsies from asthma. J. Clin. Invest. 87:1541
10. Del Prete, G.F., De Carli, M., Mastromauro, C., Biagiotti, R., Macchia, D., Falagiani, P., Ricci, M., and Romagnani, S. 1991. Purified protein derivative (PPD) of Mycobacterium tuberculosis and excretory-secretory antigen(s) (TES) of Toxocara canis expand in vitro human T cells with stable and opposite (T_H1 or T_H2) profile of cytokine production. J. Clin. Invest. 88:346.
11. Parronchi, P., Macchia, D., Piccinni, M-P., Biswas, P., Simonelli, C., Maggi, E., Ricci, M., Ansari, A.A., and Romagnani, S. Allergen and bacterial antigen-specific T cell clones established from atopic donors show a different profile of cytokine production. Proc. Natl. Acad. Sci. USA 88:4538
12. Wierenga, E.A., Snoek, M., de Groot, C., Chretien, I., Bos, J.D., Jansen, H.M., and Kapsenberg, M. 1990. Evidence for compartmentalization of functional subsets of $CD4^+$ T lymphocytes in atopic patients. J. Immunol. 144:4651.
13. Romagnani, S. 1991. Type 1 T helper and type 2 T helper cells: Functions, regulation and role in protection and disease. Int. J. Clin. Lab. Res. 21:152.

14. Del Prete, G.F., De Carli, M., Ricci, M., and Romagnani, S. 1991. Helper activity for immunoglobulin synthesis of T_H1 and T_H2 human T cell clones: The help of T_H1 clones is limited by their cytolytic capacity. J. Exp. Med. 174:809.
15. Romagnani, S. 1991. Human T_H1 and T_H2 subsets: Doubt no more. Immunol. Today 12:256.
16. Parronchi, P., De Carli, M., Manetti, R., Simonelli, C., Piccinni, M.-P., Macchia, D., Maggi, E., Del Preten, G.F., Ricci, M., and Romagnani, S. 1992. Aberrant IL-4 and IL-5 production in vitro by CD4 helper T cells from atopic subjects. Eur. J. Immunol. (in press).
17. Maggi, E., Parronchi, P., Manetti, R., Simonelli, C., Piccinni, M-P., Santoni Rugiu, F., De Carli, M., Ricci, M., and Romagnani, S. 1992. Reciprocal regulatory effects of gamma-interferon (IFN-γ) and interleukin 4 (IL-4) on the in vitro development of human T helper 1 (T_H1) and T_H2 clones. J. Immunol. 198 (in press).
18. Swain, S.L. 1991. Regulation of the development of distinct subsets of $CD4^+$ T cells. Res. Immunol. 142:14.
19. Coffman, R.L., Chatelain, R., Leal, L.M.C.C., and Varkila, K. 1991. Leishmania major infection in mice: A model system for the study of $CD4^+$ T cell subset differentiation. Res. Immunol. 142:36.
20. Plaut, M., Pierce, J.H., Watson, C.J., Hanley-Hyde, J., Nordan, R.P., and Paul, W.E. 1989. Mast cell lines produce lymphokines in response to cross-linkage of FcERI or to calcium ionophores. Nature (London) 339:64.
21. Ben Sasson, S.Z., Le Gros, G., Conrad, D.H., Finkelman, F. , and Pau, W.E. 1990. Cross-linking Fc receptors stimulate splenic non-B, non-T cells to secrete interleukin 4 and other lymphokines. Proc. Natl. Acad. Sci. USA 87:1421.
22. Conrad, D.H., Ben-Sasson, S.Z., LeGros, G., Finkelman, F.D., and Paul, W.E. 1990. Infection with Nyppostrongylus brasiliensis or injection of anti-IgD antibodies markedly enhances Fc-receptor-mediated interleukin-4 production by non-B, non-T cells. J. Exp. Med. 171:1497.
23 Piccinni, M-P., Macchia, D., Parronchi, P., Giudizi, M.G., Bellesi, G., Grossi, A., Maggi, E., and Romagnani, S. 1991. Human bone marrow non-B, non-T cells produce IL-4 in response to cross-linkage of FcE and Fcγ receptors. Proc. Natl. Acad. Sci. USA 88:8656.

Molecular Aspects of IgE Synthesis

Jan E. de Vries, Gregorio G. Aversa, Juha Punnonen, Hugues Gascan, Jean-François Gauchat*

IgE production by normal B cells is specifically induced by IL-4, but requires additional signals that are provided by activated CD4$^+$ T cells. This induction of IgE synthesis reflects directed isotype switching and is not a stochastic process, since single sIgM$^+$ B cells could be induced to proliferate and switch to IgG4 and IgE producing cells in the presence of CD4$^+$ T cells and IL-4. Although IL-4 is the sole inducer of IgE synthesis, many cytokines have been shown to modulate IL-4 induced IgE synthesis *in vitro*. IFN-γ, IFN-α, TGF-β and IL-10 were inhibitory, whereas IL-5, IL-6 and TNF-α acted synergistically with IL-4. Switching to ε and IgE synthesis is preceded by the induction of germline ε transcripts. These germline ε transcripts are specifically induced by IL-4. None of the other recombinant cytokines known today were found to induce germline ε mRNA expression. Interestingly, germline ε transcripts were also induced via a contact mediated signal provided by a non-IL-4 producing CD4$^+$ T cell clone. However, each of these signals were insufficient to induce IgE synthesis, indicating that germline ε mRNA expression, as such, is an insufficient condition for IgE production, which required both signals. The role of germline ε transcription in IgE regulation was further investigated. It was shown that sIgM$^+$ B cell clones that were induced to switch to IgE production, all first expressed germline ε mRNA. IgE production was never observed in the absence of germline ε RNA synthesis. In addition, TGF-β and TNF-α, which block or enhance IL-4 induced IgE synthesis, respectively, also inhibited and enhanced IL-4 induced germline ε mRNA synthesis. Collectively, these results indicate that modulation of IgE production by TGF-β or TNF-α is regulated through modulation of germline ε mRNA synthesis and that there is a close functional relationship between germline ε mRNA synthesis and subsequent IgE production. Therefore, inhibition of germline ε mRNA synthesis may provide a novel and efficient way to prevent IgE switching, IgE production and IgE mediated hypersensitivity reactions.

The effector function of antibody molecules is determined by the constant region of the immunoglobulin (Ig) heavy chain (C_H). Antibodies retain their specificity while their effector functions are changed by isotype switching at the DNA level. In virgin mature B cells that synthesize IgM, the VDJ gene segment is situated 5′ to the Cμ gene, whereas in B cells that produce the other Ig isotypes, VDJ is relocated just 5′ to the C_H gene encoding the secreted isotype, with deletion of the intervening C_H genes (1). *In vitro* studies in murine B cell lines have indicated that Ig class switching is preceded by expression of the corresponding germline C_H gene. Murine germline C_H transcripts initiate upstream of the corresponding switch (S) regions. Transcription transverses the S regions and it has been proposed that isotype switching may occur through modulation of accessibility of the specific switch regions to a common recombinase system (2). Alternatively, germline C_H gene transcripts may play a direct regulatory role in promoting switch processes (3). IgE antibodies have the property to bind to high affinity IgE receptors on mast cells and basophils. Crosslinking of these receptors by allergens causes these cells to degranulate and to release mediators that induce hypersensitivity reactions. Significant progress has been made in understanding the cellular and molecular mechanisms underlying regulation of human IgE synthesis. Determination of the regulatory pathways resulting in IgE switching in normal B cells is of importance for defining (a) aberrant regulatory processes associated with enhanced production of IgE in allergy, and (b) ways to intervene in overproduction of IgE and IgE mediated allergic responses. In the present report the role of T cells and cytokines in regulation of germline ε transcription and IgE switching is summarized.

* DNAX Research Institute, 901 California Avenue, Palo Alto, California, USA.

IL-4 Induces IgG4 and IgE Synthesis

Early studies have demonstrated that the IgE response in mice was T cell dependent (4). Only recently has it become clear that cytokines play an important role in determining isotype switching (5). IFN-γ directs B cells activated by bacterial lipopolysaccharide to switch to IgG2a production, whereas IL-4 induces these cells to switch to IgG1 and IgE synthesis. Furthermore, TGF-β determines B cells to switch to IgA production (5). Human IL-4 added to cultures of mononuclear cells (MNC) derived from peripheral blood, tonsils or spleens induced IgG4 and IgE synthesis in the absence of any polyclonal B cell activators (6,7). IL-4 was also found to induce IgE synthesis in cultures of MNC from cord blood, indicating that cord blood B cells are mature in their capacity to switch to IgE production (8). In contrast to adult MNC, cord blood MNC failed to produce measurable quantities of IL-4 following activation (8). This lack, or suppression, of IL-4 production by activated cord blood T cells may account for the absence of detectable amounts of IgE in cord- or neonatal blood. In addition to IL-4, costimulatory signals provided by $CD4^+$ T cells were required for induction of IgE synthesis. $CD8^+$ T cells were ineffective (7,9). The nature of this signal remains to be determined, but it is clear that it required T-B cell contact, and activation of the $CD4^+$ T cells. The fact that intact $CD4^+$ T cells could be replaced by plasma membranes prepared from these cells furthermore indicates that the T cell signal is mediated through a membrane associated molecule, which is induced by or undergoes conformational changes, following activation of the $CD4^+$ T cells (10; Gascan *et al.*, submitted). IL-4 induced IgE synthesis reflects IgE switching since single $sIgM^+$ B cells could be induced with high frequencies to proliferate and to switch to IgE production (7). Multiple isotypes (IgM, IgG4 and IgE) were produced in these cultures, suggesting that switching to IgE proceeds in successive steps, from IgM to IgG4 and from IgG4 to IgE. This notion is compatible with recent murine studies in which analysis of switch circular DNA excised by Ig class switching of murine B cells induced by IL-4 occurred in successive steps from IgM to IgG1 (the murine homologue of human IgG4) and from IgG1 to IgE (11).

Modulation of IL-4 Induced IgE Synthesis by Cytokines

Induction of IgE synthesis is a specific property of IL-4. All other recombinant cytokines known to date were ineffective. However, many cytokines can modulate IL-4 induced IgE synthesis. Both IFN-γ and IFN-α strongly block IL-4 induced IgE synthesis *in vitro* (6) and the enhanced serum IgE levels in patients with the hyper IgE syndrome (12,13). More recently, it was demonstrated that induction of IgE synthesis was also blocked by TGF-β and IL-10 (de Waal Malefyt et al., submitted). Other cytokines augmented IL-4 induced IgE synthesis. IL-5 enhanced IgE synthesis, but only when IL-4 was present at suboptimal concentrations, whereas IL-6 and TNF-α augmented IgE production in the presence of saturating concentrations of IL-4 (14,15; Gauchat et al., submitted). Although inhibition of IgE synthesis by IFN-γ, IFN-α, TGF-β and IL-10 occurred at early stages of the cultures, little is known about the mechanisms of their antagonistic effects. Recently we demonstrated that TGF-β blocks IL-4 induced IgE synthesis through inhibition of germline ε transcription, which precedes ε switching, whereas the enhancing effects of TNF-α on IL-4 induced IgE synthesis could be explained by its synergistic effects on germline ε mRNA synthesis (see below). IL-10 blocked IgE production in cultures of MNC by preventing activation of $CD4^+$ T cells (de Waal Malefyt, submitted).

Molecular Cloning of the Exon Encoding the Human Germline ε Transcript

To gain more knowledge about the molecular mechanisms underlying ε switching in human B cells, the expression of ε mRNA in B cells was investigated. Two major mRNA species were induced. A 1.7kB truncated ε mRNA was already induced after 2 hr, whereas induction of a 2.2kB ε mRNA was first observed at day 6 or 7 of the cultures. Both the truncated and 2.2kB ε transcripts were maximally expressed at day 11–12 of the culture (16). Molecular cloning and sequencing of the exon encoding the 1.7kB truncated transcript indicated that it represented the germline ε transcript, whereas the 2.2kB species represented the productive ε mRNA. The exon encoding germline ε transcripts was mapped 3.5kB 5′ from ε, just upstream of the switch ε region. The germline ε gene did not contain an initiation codon in frame with the Cε region, and stop codons were present in all three reading frames. In addition, it contained no TATA boxes. Together these data indicate that the germline ε gene is not capable of encoding large proteins.

Regulation of Germline ε Transcription by Cytokines

IL-4 was the only cytokine inducing germline ε transcripts in purified B cells. None of the other known recombinant cytokines were effective. The only other signal inducing germline ε transcripts was a contact mediated signal provided by a non-IL-4 producing CD4⁺ T cell clone. However, each of these signals was insufficient for subsequent induction of productive ε transcripts and IgE synthesis. IL-4 and the non-IL-4 producing CD4⁺ T cell clone added together had synergistic effects on germline ε expression and induced subsequent expression of productive ε transcripts and IgE synthesis (16). If the hypothesis that germline ε transcripts play a regulatory role in ε switching and IgE production is correct, the prediction is that ε switching always should be preceded by expression of germline ε transcripts, and that modulation of germline ε transcript synthesis should reflect modulation of IgE synthesis. Although germline ε transcripts can be induced in the absence of subsequent IgE synthesis in cultures of cloned B cells, ε switching and IgE synthesis was always preceded by germline ε mRNA expression. IgE production was never observed in the absence of germline ε transcription (Gauchat et al., submitted). These data indicate that induction of germline ε mRNA synthesis indeed seems to be required for subsequent switching to ε. This implies that inhibition of germline ε transcription could result in inhibition of IgE synthesis. IFN-γ, IFN-α, IL-10 and TGF-β all inhibit IL-4 induced IgE synthesis, but only TGF-β blocked IL-4 induced germline ε transcription, suggesting that inhibition of IgE synthesis by TGF-β may occur through inhibition of germline ε mRNA. In contrast, IFN-γ, IFN-α and IL-10 had no effect on germline ε transcription, indicating that these cytokines inhibited IgE synthesis at other stages of the regulatory process (Gauchat et al., submitted). The observation that IFN-γ and IFN-α failed to block IL-4 dependent IgE synthesis induced by anti-CD40 mAbs, i.e. in the absence of CD4⁺ T cells (17), indicates that IFN-γ and IFN-α may act on the CD4⁺ T cell signal which in addition to IL-4 is required for IgE synthesis. Interestingly, TNF-α, which has synergistic effects on IL-4 induced IgE synthesis, also enhanced IL-4 induced germline ε mRNA synthesis (Gauchat et al., submitted), confirming the notion that there is a strong functional relationship between germline ε transcription and induction of IgE switching and IgE synthesis.

Concluding Remarks

It is clear that novel approaches to block IgE synthesis in an early stage should be aimed at inhibition or neutralization of IL-4 production *in vivo* by using IL-4 antagonists such as soluble IL-4 receptor, inhibitors of IL-4 synthesis, or compounds that interact with productive IL-4/IL-4 receptor interactions. It is of interest to note that the first experiments carried out with "natural" IL-4 antagonists like IFN-γ and IFN-α seem to be promising in lowering serum IgE levels in patients with the hyper IgE syndrome. B cells undergoing ε switching are other suitable targets for novel therapeutic approaches. Inhibition of germline ε transcription would prevent productive IgE synthesis. Therefore, availability of compounds that block germline ε transcription in B cells would allow us to intervene in a very precise and harmless way in overproduction of IgE in allergic disease, and IgE mediated hyper sensitivity reactions.

References

1. Shimizu, A., Takahashi, N., Yaoita, Y., and Honjo, T. 1982. Organization of the constant region gene family of the mouse immunoglobulin heavy chain. Cell 28:499.
2. Stavnezer-Nordgren, J., and Sirlin, J. 1986. Specificity of immunoglobulin heavy chain switch correlates with activity of germline heavy chain genes prior to switching. EMBO J. 5:95.
3. Collier, D.A., Griffin, J.A., and Wells, R.D. 1988. Non-B right-handed DNA conformations of homoporine homopyrimidine sequences in the murine immunoglobulin Ca switch region. J. Biol. Chem. 263:7397.
4. Ishizaka, K. 1976. Cellular events in the IgE antibody response. Adv. Immunol. 23:1.
5. Coffman, R.L., Lee, F., Yokota, T., Arai, K.-I., and Mosmann, T.R. 1987. The effect of BSF1 and IFN-γ upon mouse immunoglobulin isotype expression. In: UCLA Symposium: Immune regulation by characterized polypeptides. G. Goldstein, J. Bach, and H. Wigzell, eds. New York: Alan Liss, p. 523.
6. Pène, J., Rousset, F., Brière, F., Chrétien, I., Bonnefoy, J.Y., Spits, H., Yokota, T., Arai, N., Arai, K.-I., Banchereau, J., and de Vries, J.E. 1988. IgE production by normal human lymphocytes is induced by interleukin 4 and suppressed by interferons γ and α and prostaglandin E2. Proc. Natl. Acad. Sci. USA 85:6880.
7. Gascan, H., Gauchat, J.-F., Roncarolo, M.-G., Yssel, H., Spits, H., and de Vries, J.E. 1991. Human B cell clones can be induced to proliferate and to switch to IgE and IgG4 synthesis by IL-4 and a signal provided by activated $CD4^+$ T cells. J. Exp. Med. 173:747.
8. Pastorelli, G., Rousset, F., Pène, J., Peronne, C., Roncarolo, M.-G., Tovo, P.A., and de Vries, J.E. 1990. Cord blood B cells are mature in their capacity to switch to IgE producing cells in response to interleukin 4 *in vitro*. Clin. Exp. Immunol. 82:114.
9. Pène, J., Chrétien, I., Rousset, F., Brière, F., Bonnefoy, J.Y., and de Vries, J.E. 1989. Modulation of IL-4 induced human IgE production *in vitro* by IFN-γ and IL-5: The role of soluble CD23 (s-CD23). J. Biol. Chem. 39:253.
10. Hodgkin, P.D., Yamashita, L.C., Coffman, R.L., and Kehry, M.R. 1990. Separation of events mediating B cell proliferation and Ig production by using T cell membranes and lymphokines. J. Immunol. 145:2025.
11. Matsuoka, M., Yoshida, K., Maeda, T., Usuda, S., and Sakano, H. 1990. Switch circular DNA formed in cytokine-treated mouse splenocytes: Evidence for intramolecular DNA deletion in immunoglobulin class switching. Cell 62:135.
12. King, C.L., Gallin, J.I., Malech, H.L., Abramson, S.L., and Nutman, T.B. 1989. Regulation of immunoglobulin production in hyperimmunoglobulin E recurrent-infection syndrome by interferon-γ. Proc. Natl. Acad. Sci. USA 86:10085.
13. Souillet, G., Rousset, F., and de Vries, J.E. 1989. Alpha-interferon treatment of patient with hyper IgE syndrome. Lancet (letters) 1:1384.
14. Pène, J., Rousset, F., Brière, F., Chrétien, I., Wideman, J., Bonnefoy, J.Y., and de Vries, J.E. 1988. Interleukin 5 enhances interleukin 4 induced IgE production by normal human B cells. The role of soluble CD23 antigen. Eur. J. Immunol. 18:929.
15. Vercelli, D., Jabara, H.H., Arai, K.-I., Yokota, T., and Geha, R.S. 1989. Endogenous interleukin 6 plays an obligatory role in interleukin 4-dependent human IgE synthesis. Eur. J. Immunol. 19:1419.
16. Gauchat, J.-F., Lebman, D.A., Coffman, R.L., Gascan, H., and de Vries, J.E. 1990. Structure and expression of germline ε transcripts in human B cells induced by IL-4 to switch to IgE production. J. Exp. Med. 172:463.
17. Gascan, H., Gauchat, J.-F., Van Vlasselaer, P., Aversa, G.G., and de Vries, J.E. 1991. Anti-CD40 mAbs or $CD4^+$ T cell clones and IL-4 induce IgG4 and IgE switching via different signalling pathways. J. Immunol. 147:8.

Antigen-Specific Regulation of IgE Antibody Production

Yutaka Tagaya*, Peter Thomas*, Hideho Gomi*, Akio Mori*/**, Makoto Iwata**, Kimishige Ishizaka*/**

An immunological maneuver was devised to construct antigen-specific suppressor T cell hybridomas from the antigen-primed mouse spleen cells. Upon stimulation with antigen-pulsed macrophages or by cross-linking of TcR or CD3 on the cells, the hybridomas produced antigen-binding glycosylation inhibiting factor (GIF), which suppressed the in vivo antibody response of the donor of T cells in carrier (antigen)-specific manner. The same principle was applied to peripheral blood mononuclear cells of patients allergic to honey bee venom, and human Ts hybridomas specific for bee venom phospholipase A_2 were constructed. Some of the hybridomas produced the antigen-binding GIF upon cross-linking of CD3 on the cells. The murine antigen-binding GIF shares many immunological properties with antigen-specific suppressor T cell factor (TsF) and consists of antigen-binding polypeptide chain and nonspecific GIF. The nonspecific GIF from murine hybridoma was isolated to biochemical homogeneity. Both murine and human GIF represent a single polypeptide chain of 14 kDa. Although this cytokine reacts with monoclonal antibodies against lipomodulin, evidence was obtained that GIF does not belong to the anexin family. The antigen-binding GIF shares the same epitope specificity with TcR on the cell source of the factor, and cross reacts with monoclonal antibodies against TcR. The results suggest that the antigen-binding GIF and antigen-specific TsF consist of nonspecific GIF and a soluble form or a derivative of TcR chain.

In many atopic patients, the concentration of total IgE in their serum is only slightly higher than normal levels. However, these patients have substantial amounts of both IgE and IgG antibodies against allergens, to which they are sensitve. In contrast, normal individuals, who live in the same environment, do not have a detectable amount of either IgE or IgG antibodies to the allergen. These findings suggest the possibility that regulation of the antibody response to specific allergen would be one of the approaches to control the IgE-mediated diseases. In our experiments on the regulation of IgE antibody response in the mouse, we described a unique cytokine, glycosylation inhibiting factor (GIF), which facilitated the generation of antigen-specific suppressor T (Ts) cells, and reproduced the findings obtained with murine lymphocytes with peripheral blood lymphocytes of allergic patients. Based on the findings, we will discuss possible approaches for antigen specific regulation of the IgE antibody response in allergic patients.

GIF-Producing T Cell Hybridomas

Construction from Peripheral Blood Lymphocytes of Allergic Patients

Before the last International Congress of Allergology, we reported an immunological maneuver to generate antigen-specific suppressor T cells from antigen-primed spleen cells, and to obtain antigen-specific suppressor T cell factors which suppress both IgE and IgG antibody responses in a carrier-specific manner (1). This method is based on the fact that GIF facilitates the generation of antigen-specific suppressor T cells in vivo (2). Considering the possible application of such a method to lymphocytes of allergic patients, we immunized BDF1 mice

* La Jolla Institute for Allergy and Immunology, La Jolla, CA 92037 USA;
** The Johns Hopkins University, School of Medicine, Baltimore, MD 21239, USA.
Acknowledgements: This work was supported by Research Grants AI-11202 and AI-14784 from the U.S. Health and Human Services. This is publication number 24 from the La Jolla Institute for Allergy and Immunology.

with alum-absorbed ovalbumin (OVA) for persistent IgE antibody formation, and their spleen cells were cultured with antigen to activate antigen-specific T cells. The activated T cells were then propagated by IL-2 in the presence or absence of GIF. T cells obtained in the cultures were then stimulated with OVA-pulsed syngeneic macrophages. The T cells propagated by IL-2 alone produced glycosylation enhancing factor (GEF) having affinity for OVA, while those propagated in the presence of GIF produced GIF having affinity for OVA (3). Since our previous experiments provided evidence that the antigen-binding GIF has immunosuppressive effects (4), we constructed T cell hybridomas from the latter T cell population, and selected T cell hybridomas which produce OVA-binding GIF upon antigenic stimulation. The OVA-binding GIF obtained from a representative hybridoma suppressed anti-DNP IgE antibody response of BDF1 mice to DNP-OVA, but failed to suppress the anti-hapten antibody response to DNP-KLH (3). The results show that the antigen-binding GIF obtained by the method is effective in suppressing the antibody response to specific antigen in the donor of T cells. Since the series of experiments in the mouse provided a maneuver to obtain antigen-specific TsF from antigen-primed T cells, we applied a similar protocol to obtain antigen-binding GIF (or TsF) from lymphocytes of allergic patients (5). As an experimental model, we chose patients allergic to honey bee venom. As the major allergen in honey bee venom is phospholipase A_2 (6), peripheral blood mononuclear cells of allergic patients were cultured with chemically modified bee venom PLA_2, and activated T cells were propagated by IL-2 in the presence of recombinant human lipocortin I. The reason for using lipocortin I in the system was that phospholipase inhibitory activity of GIF has proved to be responsible for the generation of suppressor T cells in the murine system (7). As expected, human T cells propagated in the presence of lipocortin produced GIF (5). Therefore, these

TABLE I. Formation of antigen-binding GIF by anti-CD3-treated human hybridoma clones

Clone	unstimulated cells GIF[b)]	Cells stimulated by cross-linking of CD3 [a)] IgE-BF[c)] %	GIF activity in PLA_2-Sepharose [b)] effluent	eluate
CL3	30/0	23	34/0 (+)	0/24 (-)
AC5	28/0	40	0/21 (-)	31/0 (+)
AF10	24/0	36	19/0 (+)	0/21 (-)
BA6	28/0	8	29/0 (+)	0/24 (-)
BE12	24/0	65	0/31 (-)	25/0 (+)
BF5	20/0	65	0/27 (-)	20/0 (+)
CB7	23/0	64	0/28 (-)	17/0 (+)
CE5	32/0	58	0/28 (-)	35/0 (+)
medium control	0/29		0/32	

a) 1.2 x 10^7 cells were treated with OKT3 and seeded in an anti-mIg-coated flask. Culture supernatants were concentrated 4 fold and absorbed with IgE-Sepharose. Effluents from IgE-Sepharose were then fractionated on PLA_2-Sepharose and GIF activity in the effluent and eluate fraction was determined.

b) GIF activity was determined by using the 12H5 cells, which produce glycosylated IgE-BF upon incubation with murine IgE. When the cells were cultured with IgE in the presence of GIF, essentially all IgE-BF formed by the cells was unglycosylated and failed to bind to lentil lectin Sepharose. In the presence of GIF, however, the same cells produce unglycosylated IgE-BF which failed to be retained in lentil lectin Sepharose. Numbers in the column represent the percent rosette inhibition by the effluent/eluate fractions from lentil lectin Sepharose. (+) (-) indicate the presence or absence of GIF.

c) Acid eluate fractions from IgE-Sepharose were assessed for the presence of IgE-BF. Numbers represent the percentage of rosette inhibition by IgE-binding factor.

T cells were fused with a HAT-sensitive CEM line to construct T cell hybridomas. As the results of two sets of experiments, we obtained 8 GIF-producing hybridomas (Table I). Thus, we stimulated the hybridomas by cross-linking of CD3. Upon stimulation, 7 out of 8 hybridomas produced IgE-binding factors. The culture supernatants were absorbed with IgE-Sepharose and the effluent was further fractionated on immunosorbent coupled with bee venom PLA_2. As shown in Table I, GIF in the culture supernatant of 5 hybridomas bound to antigen-coupled Sepharose and was recovered by elution at acid pH, indicating that these hybridomas produce antigen-binding GIF. As we do not have an appropriate *in vitro* system, we cannot evaluate immunosuppressive activity of human antigen-specific GIF. However, if one considers that antigen-specific GIF from mouse T cell hybridomas could suppress the *in vivo* antibody response of syngeneic mice in carrrier-specific manner, we suspect that allergen-specific GIF from human T cell hybridomas will suppress the antibody response of the donor of parent T cells to the specific allergen.

Biochemical Characterization of GIF

We realized that the antigen-binding GIF shares many immunological properties with antigen-specific, effector type TsF. Both factors bind to the native antigen, and exert carrier-specific suppressive effects. Evidence has been presented that both antigen-binding GIF and antigen-specific TsF are composed of antigen-binding polypeptide chain and a polypeptide chain carrying so-called I-J determinant (4,8,9). The antigen-binding GIF contains an antigenic determinant recognized by the monoclonal antibody 14–12, which was believed to be specific for the antigen-binding chain of effector type TsF (10). A unique property of GIF is that this lymphokine reacts with monoclonal antibodies against lipomodulin, a phospholipase inhibitory protein, and exerts phospholipase inhibitory activity upon dephosphorylation (11). However, collaboration with Dr. Martin Dorf from Harvard and Douglas Green in our Institute revealed that our anti-lipomodulin antibody bound not only GIF but also all of the five different hapten-specific TsF and a peptide-specific TsF, and these TsF could be purified by using anti-lipomodulin-coupled immunosorbent (12). Furthermore, these TsF actually have GIF-bioactivity and could switch our T cell hybridomas from the formation of IgE-PF (potentiating factors) to the formation of IgE-suppressive factors. These findings collectively suggest that the antigen-binding GIF is identical to an effector type, antigen-specific TsF described by previous investigators.

We have obtained evidence that the antigen-binding GIF consists of antigen-binding chain and nonspecific GIF (13). Thus, we tried to biochemically characterize the nonspecific GIF chain. GIF-producing murine hybridoma cells were cultured in serum-free medium, and GIF in the culture supernatant was purified by using anti-lipomodulin-coupled immunosorbent. The purified GIF gave a single spot of 14 kDa with an isoelectric point of approximately 5.5 in 2D gel (Fig. 1) (14). In order to confirm the homogeneity of isolated GIF, affinity purified GIF was labeled with ^{125}I, and a mixture of ^{125}I-labeled GIF and crude culture supernatant was fractionated by HPLC. The radio-labeled 14 kDa protein gave a single peak in DEAE chromatography, and GIF bioactivity was detected only in the peak fraction. We have also set up an ELISA assay for GIF using monoclonal anti-GIF antibody (15). As shown in Figure 2, the distribution of GIF antigen was in agreement with the distribution of ^{125}I-labeled 14 kDa protein. Comigration of GIF with the 14 kDa protein was also observed when the

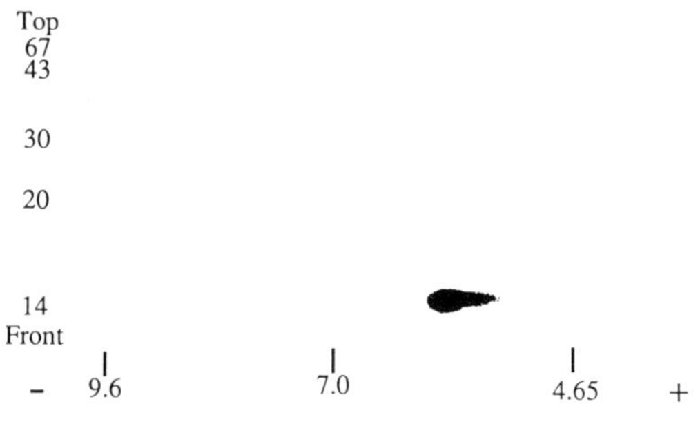

Figure 1. Two dimensional electrophoresis of affinity-purified GIF. First dimension was separated in the pH gradient between 3 and 10 by NEPHEGE method. PI markers: phycocyanine (4.65), equine myoglobin (7.0) and cytochome C (9.6). Second dimension was conventional SDS/PAGE with the molecular weight markers BSA (67 kDa), ovalbumin (43 kDa), carbonic anhydrase (30 kDa), soybean trypsin inhibitor (20.1 kDa) and ribonuclease A (14.4 kDa).

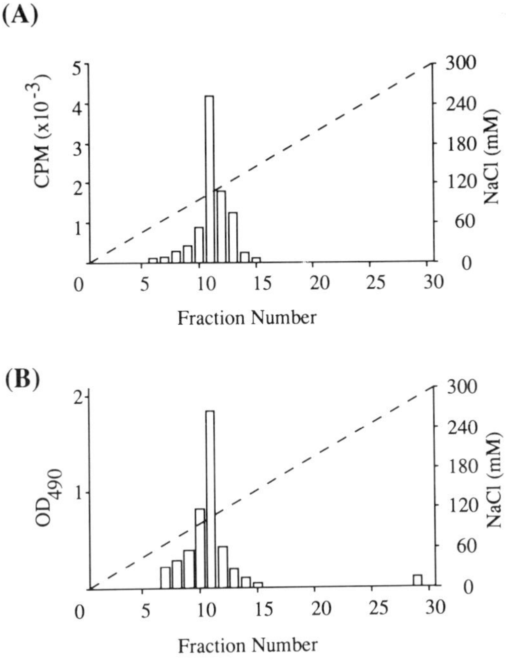

Figure 2. Co-migration of GIF activity and GIF antigen with the 14 kDa protein in ion-exchange chromatography. A mixture of ^{125}I-labeled 14 kDa protein (10,000 cpm) and crude GIF was applied to a TSK-3SW column and analyzed by HPLC with a linear gradient of NaCl (- - - -) in 10 mM Tris-HCl (pH 8.1). Distributions of radioactivity (A) and GIF antigen, determined by ELISA (B) are shown. Fractions were also assessed for GIF-bioactivity by using the 12H5 cells. Distributions of IgE-BF between the effluent and eluate fractions from lentil lectin Sepharose were 22/19 for Fr. 10, 27/8 for Fr. 11, 32/33 for Fr. 12 and 0/24 for control. The results of the bioassay indicated that the peak fraction of GIF bioactivity was Fr. 11.

mixture of ^{125}I-GIF and culture supernatant was fractionated on reverse phase column and by gel filtration. The results show the biochemical homogeneity of the 14 kDa protein and indicate that the bioactivity and antigenic determinant recognized by anti-GIF are associated with the 14 kDa protein (14).

Another important finding obtained with the purified GIF was that this cytokine is distinct from lipocortin (14). It is well known that lipocortin belongs to Ca^{2+}-dependent, phospholipid binding protein (16). Indeed, ^{125}I-labeled human lipocortin bound to phosphatidylserine vesicles, and the binding

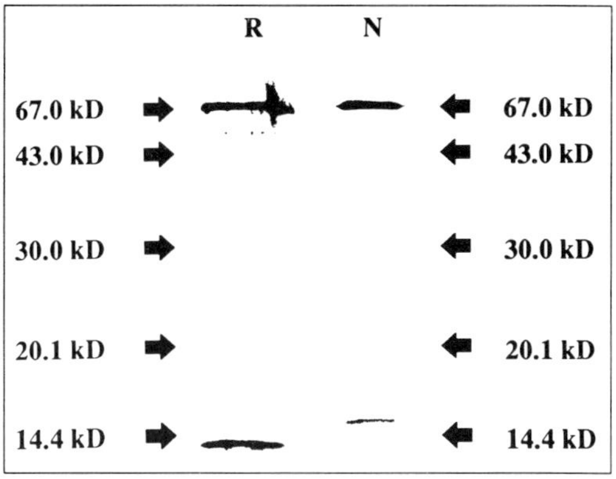

Figure 3. SDS-PAGE analysis of affinity-purified human GIF. Culture supernatants of the AC5 clone were fractionated on a DEAE-Sepharose, and GIF in a DEAE fraction was affinity-purified by using affigel coupled with the monoclonal anti-human GIF. Affinity purified preparation was analyzed by SDS-PAGE under reducing (R) and non-reducing (N) conditions. Position of molecular weight markers are shown by arrows.

was inhibited by unlabeled lipocortin. In contrast, ^{125}I-labeled GIF failed to bind to any of the phosphatidylserine, phosphatidylinositol or phosphatidylcholine. We have obtained partial amino acid sequence of the 14 kDa GIF and initiated gene cloning of this cytokine. Therefore, we expect that recombinant GIF will be obtained in the near future. We have also purified human GIF by adjusting human hybridomas to serum-free medium, and fractionated the culture supernatant on DEAE-Sepharose followed by affinity chromatography on anti-human GIF-immunosorbent. Analysis of the purified GIF by SDS-PAGE and silver staining gave two bands; however, we have additional evidence that the 14 kDa band represents human GIF (Fig. 3). The mobility of this protein was almost the same under reducing and non-reducing conditions, indicating that the human GIF is also a single polypeptide chain.

Relationship Between Antigen-Binding Chain of TsF and T Cell Receptor (TCR)

Since T helper cells recognize processed antigen in the context of class II molecules, but do not respond to nominal antigen (18), many immunologists are suspicious of the presence of a T cell-derived soluble factor which has affinity for nominal antigen. Therefore, we determined the epitope specificity of OVA-specific T cell hybridomas that produce OVA-binding factors upon antigenic stimulation. The results clearly showed that all of the hybridomas recognize the epitope representing amino acid 307 to 317 in the original OVA molecule (19). This epitope is distinct from those recognized by OVA-specific helper T cells. The peptide does not stimulate the proliferative response of OVA-primed lymph node cells. An important finding was that this peptide has affinity for OVA-binding GIF (10). Thus, the binding of OVA-binding GIF to ovalbumin-coupled Sepharose was prevented by the peptide 307-317, but not by the peptide 323-339, which represents the major immunogenic epitope in OVA. It was also found that OVA-binding GIF binds to an immunosorbent coupled with the peptide 307-317 and can be recovered by elution at acid pH. The results collectively indicate that TcR on the suppressor T cells, which form OVA-binding GIF, has a unique epitope specificity, and that the antigen-binding GIF formed by the cells recognize the same epitope. It was also found that monoclonal antibody specific for α chain of TcR binds OVA-binding GIF as well as antigen-specific TsF from various suppressor T cell hybridomas (19-21), but does not bind nonspecific GIF (11). Furthermore, experiments by Green and his coworkers provided evidence that Va gene for TcRα chain is utilized for the formation of antigen-specific TsF (21). All of these findings collectively indicate that antigen-binding chains of TsF share common structures with TcR. It appears that the antigen-binding chain is a soluble form of TcRα chain or the α chain-like molecule. Some immunologists may argue against this idea, because TcR on helper and cytotoxic T cells do not recognize nominal antigen. Apparently, binding of antigen-binding GIF to nominal antigen is due to unique epitope specificity of TcR on suppressor T cells. The amino acid sequence of the peptide 307-317 in OVA molecules strongly suggests that this peptide represents an external structure in the OVA molecule whereas the major immunogenic epitope includes an internal structure of the antigen. It appears that antigen-binding GIF binds nominal antigen, because the factor is specific for an external structure of the antigen (10).

Summary

Many controversial issues existed on antigen-specific suppressor factors. However, it became clear that the factors are derived from T cells, and share common structures with T cell receptors. The reason why the factor can bind nominal antigen could be explained by the epitope specificity of the T cells from which the TsF are derived. TsF and T cell receptors on their cell sources appear to be specific for a common epitope, representing an external structure of antigen molecule. We propose that the functional subunit of TsF is a unique cytokine, GIF. We have described a maneuver to generate antigen-specific suppressor T cells from the peripheral blood mononuclear cells of allergic patients, and to obtain antigen-specific TsF. We expect that application of recombinant gene technology to the system may provide a chance to control allergen-specific IgE antibody response in allergic patients.

References

1. Ishizaka, K., Iwata, M., Carini, C., and Takeuchi, T. 1989. A new approach to suppressing the IgE antibody response to allergen. In: Progress in allergy and clinical immunology. W.J. Picheler, B.M. Stadler, C.A. Dahinden, A.R. Pecoud, P. Frei, C.H. Schneider, and A.L. de Weck, eds. Toronto: Hogrefe and Huber, p. 129.
2. Akasaki, M., Jardieu, P., and Ishizaka, K. 1986. Immunosuppressive effects of glycosylation inhibiting factor on the IgE and IgG antibody response. J. Immunol. 136:3172.
3. Iwata, M., and Ishizaka, K. 1988. Construction of antigen-specific suppressor T cell hybridomas from spleen cells of mice primed for the persistent IgE antibody formation. J. Immunol. 141:3270.
4. Jardieu, P., Akasaki, M., and Ishizaka, K. 1987. Carrier-specific suppression of antibody response by antigen-specific glycosylation inhibiting factors. J. Immunol. 138:1494.
5. Carini, C., Iwata, M., Warner, J., and Ishizaka, K. 1990. A method to generate antigen-specific suppressor T cells in vitro from peripheral blood T cells of honey bee venom-sensitive allergic patients. J. Immunol. Method 127:221.

6. King, T.P., Sobotka, A.K., Kochoumain, A.L., and Lichtenstein, L.M. 1976. Allergens of honey bee venom. Arch. Biochem. Biophys. 172:661.
7. Ohno, H., Iwata, M., Nakamura, T., and Ishizaka, K. 1989. Effect of phospholipase A_2 inhibitors on mouse T lymphocytes I. Phospholipase A_2 inhibitors exert similar immunological activities as glycosylation inhibiting factor. Int. Immunol. 1:425.
8. Saito, T., and Taniguchi, M. 1984. Chemical features of an antigen-specific suppressor T cell factor composed of two polypeptide chains. J. Mol. Cell Immunol. 1:137.
9. Turck, C.W., Kapp, J.A., and Webb, D.R. 1986. Structural analysis of a monoclonal heterodimeric suppressor factor specific for L-glutarmic acid-L-alanine-L tyrosine. J. Immunol. 137:1904.
10. Iwata, M., Katamura, K., Kubo, R.T., Grey, H.M., and Ishizaka, K. 1989. Relationship between T cell receptors and antigen-binding factors II. Common antigenic determinants and epitope recognition shared by T cell receptors and antigen-binding factors. J. Immunol. 143:3917.
11. Uede, T., Hirata, F., Hiroshima, M., and Ishizaka, K. 1983. Modulation of the biologic activities of IgE-binding factors I. Identification of glycosylation inhibiting factor as a fragment of lipomodulin. J. Immunol. 130:878.
12. Steele, J.K., Kuchroo, V.K., Kawasaki, H., Jayaraman, S., Iwata, M., Ishizaka, K., and Dorf, M.E. 1989. A monoclonal antibody raised to lipomodulin recognizes factors in two-independent hapten-specific suppressor networks. J. Immunol. 142:2213.
13. Jardieu, P., and Ishizaka, K. 1987. Possible relationship of an antigen-specific suppressor factor to phospholipase inhibitory protein. In: Immune regulation by characterized polypeptides. G. Goldstein, J.F. Bach, and H. Wigzell, eds. New York: Alan R. Liss, p. 595.
14. Tagaya, Y., Mori, A., and Ishizaka, K. 1991. Biochemical characterization of murine glycosylation inhibiting factor. Proc. Natl. Acad. Sci., USA, 88:9117.
15. Katamura, K., Iwata, M., Mori, A., and Ishizaka, K. 1990. Biochemical identification of glycosylation inhibiting factor. Proc. Natl. Acad. Sci., USA 87:1903.
16. Schlaepfer, D.D., and Haigler, H.T. 1987. Characterization of Ca^{2+}-dependent phospholipid binding and phosphorylation of lipocortin I. J. Biol. Chem. 262:6931.
17. Shimonkevitz, R., Kappler, J., Marrack, P., and Grey, H. 1983. Antigen recognition by H-2 restricted T cell. Cell free antigen processing. J. Exp. Med. 158:303.
18. Marrack, P., and Kappler, J. 1986. The antigen-specific, major histocompatibility complex-restricted receptor on T cells. Adv. Immunol. 38:1.
19. Iwata, M., Katamura, K., Kubo, R.T., and Ishizaka, K. 1989. Relationship between T cell receptors and antigen-binding factors I. Specificity of functional T cell receptors on mouse T cell hybridomas that produce antigen-binding T cell factors. J. Immunol. 143:3909.
20. Fairchild, R.L., Kubo, R.T., and Moorhead, J.W. 1988. Soluble factors in tolerance and contact sensitivity to 2, 4 dinitrofluorobenzene in mice IX. A monoclonal T cell suppressor molecule is structurally and serologically related to the α/β cell receptor. J. Immunol. 141:3342.
21. Zheng, H., Beni, M., Kilgannon, P., Fotedar, A., and Green, D.R. 1989. Specific inhibition of cell surface T cell receptor expression by antisense oligonucleotides and its effect on the production of an antigen-specific regulatory T cell factor. Proc. Natl. Acad. Sci., USA 86:3758.

Recent Progress in the Analysis of the Structure and Function of the High Affinity Receptor for IgE

Henry Metzger, Gottfried Alber, Su-Yau Mao, Larry Miller, Nadine Varin-Blank*

The genes for the subunits of the receptor for IgE have been isolated, so it is now possible to analyze the structure and function of the receptor by genetically engineering structural changes in selective portions of the receptor. We have prepared variant subunits of the receptor and have studied the effect of these alterations in transfected COS cells. We found that substantial changes in the cytoplasmic domains (CD) of the receptor do not critically affect the assembly and surface expression of the receptors, but the COS cells do not become activated when the wild-type receptors with which they have been transfected are stimulated. Thus the COS cells appear to lack critical "post-receptor" molecules. Nevertheless, upon aggregation, the receptors on these cells exhibit many of the characteristics observed on mast cells: They become immobile, are internalized, and are no longer soluble in detergent. Each of these phenomena is thought to result from interactions between the receptor and cytoskeletal or other cellular structures. We find that these phenomena are surprisingly little affected by removal of one or another of the CD. Receptors have also been transfected into the mast cell-like tumor P815. When transfected with wild-type receptors, such cells exhibit some of the early events typical of mast cells, when the receptors are aggregated. Some of the altered receptors stimulated normal responses in the P815 cells transfectants, whereas other receptor variants did not. Together these results indicate that mutational analysis will provide a powerful new tool for exploring structure/function relationships of the IgE receptor.

When our laboratory reported at the last Congress 3 years ago, we had just isolated the genes that code for each of the subunits for the receptor with high affinity for IgE (FcεRI) (1,2). We indicated at that time that this would allow us to use genetic engineering as an additional tool with which to probe structural/functional relationships in this important molecule through which allergens and the allergen-specific IgE mediate some of the responses that are associated with the allergic state. Before summarizing what progress we have made in this respect, a few remarks about the conceptual basis of our work are appropriate.

As noted in a still earlier report at the time of the XII International Congress in 1985 (3), one can envision two general therapeutic approaches focussed on inhibiting the action of the receptor.

The most obvious one is to interfere with the binding of IgE to the receptor. Attempts to inhibit this interaction using either specific peptides based on the known sequences of IgE, or totally unrelated molecules that might have been identified in a drug-screening approach, do not necessarily require knowledge about the IgE-binding site on the receptor. However, this approach had been hampered by the lack of a suitable source of human FcεRI which could be used in simple *in vitro* assays. The cloning of the human analogue of the IgE-binding α chain of the receptor (4,5) and its successful expression, first in conjunction with the other subunits of the rodent receptor (6) and, more recently, alone (7,8), now makes a search for such inhibitors much more practical.

A second approach, which is the principal focus of our laboratory, is to interfere with the early steps in the biochemical cascade(s) in-

Table I. Assembly and Surface Expression of Mutated FcεRI[a]

Modification	Relative Percent Expression
None	"100"
One CD truncated	80–100
Two CD truncated	30–100
Three CD truncated	3–40
Four CD truncated	7–50
Five CD truncated	10

[a]: The data are sumarized from Fig. 2 in Ref. 16.

* Section on Chemical Immunology, Arthritis and Rheumatism Branch, National Institute of Arthritis and Musculoskeletal and Skin Diseases, National Institutes of Health, Bethesda, MD 20892, USA.

itiated by aggregation of the receptor. Again one can approach this empirically or analytically. Using the insights gained from functional studies on mast cells and related systems, one can attempt to find inhibitors of the receptor-initiated perturbations, and see whether one or more could conceivably be transformed into a therapeutically useful drug. Alternatively, more complete knowledge about the normal mechanism, gained by analysis of the system, should suggest a variety of alternative ways by which one can intervene.

We are working principally on this latter strategy. As noted previously (9), one can distinguish between two principal alternative mechanisms by which aggregation of the receptor might initiate the biochemical cascades that eventuate in degranulation. One mechanism posits that the receptor itself becomes activated as the primary event. Such an "intrinsic" mechanism appears to be the one utilized by the receptors for growth factors such as insulin (10) and EGF (11). Alternatively, the aggregated receptor may initially activate a "post receptor" molecule; such an "extrinsic" mechanism is utilized by a family of receptors that stimulate the adenyl cyclase system using GTP-binding proteins as go-betweens (12).

Although there is still a paucity of hard data, most data suggest that FcεRI does not utilize an intrinsic mechanism. First, the sequences of the protein have failed to reveal any consensus sequences (2), i.e. sequences that in other proteins have been correlated with intrinsic activities. Second, we have not observed receptor-initiated biochemical cascades when wild-type receptors were transfected either into COS cells (13), or more recently, into CHO cells (unpublished observations). Thus these cells appear to lack some necessary "post-receptor" component(s).

Overall Strategy

In order to identify such components we have employed the following approach: (A) We identified cells that lacked functional receptors, but that responded normally when transfected with wild-type receptors. (B) These cells were transfected with modified receptors and functionally assessed. By identifying one or more parts of the receptor as being functionally critical, one should be in a much better position to identify proximal "post-receptor" component(s) and to study rigorously their interaction with the receptor.

Assembly and Expression of Mutant Receptors

A fundamental requirement for this strategy to be successful is that the mutant receptors must be expressible on the surface of the transfected cells. This was of particular concern with respect to the FcεRI because of its demanding requirements for expression (2) and its intrinsic instability (14). Since in many other receptor systems the cytoplasmic domains (CD) are critical, we focussed our initial manipulations of the receptor principally on these regions. We first examined COS cells but subsequent stable transfections of P815 cells have yielded similar results. The details of our findings have been published (15,16). The results from studies in which one or more CDs were genetically truncated (16) are summarized in Table I. It is apparent that one can modify the CDs of the receptor considerably and still obtain adequate surface expression of the altered protein.

Studies on Transiently Transfected COS Cells

In COS cells, the transfected wild-type receptors do not stimulate a variety of cellular responses that have been observed when the endogenous receptors on mast cells are aggregated. However, the receptors do exhibit some of the characteristics observed with many other plasma membrane proteins. Thus like other membrane proteins the receptors diffuse more slowly than proteins studied in simple lipid bilayers even when unaggregated. When aggregated they become largely immobile, are internalized, and with sufficient aggregation can no longer be extracted when the cells' membrane lipids are dissolved with mild detergents (17,18). It has been thought that these phenomena reflect interactions between a membrane protein and various cytoplasmic or plasma membrane components loosely referred to as "cytoskeletal" elements. The functional significance of these interactions (other than those related to internalization where the biological significance could have several plausible explanations) is unclear. However, some data on mast cells and other cells suggest that these phenomena are associated with receptor "desensitization" (19). The results of our mutational analyses with FcεRI are summarized in Table II, and have been published (17,18). Although our results are unambiguous, two particular observations illustrate that the results of mutational analysis are not always simple to rationalize. Almost without exception, receptors containing α β subunit whose COOH-terminal CD has been truncated behave abnormally (Table II). Nevertheless, chimeric receptors containing only human α and rodent γ chains behave quite normally. The latter result clearly indicates that there are no specific sites on the β subunit that are required to mediate the phenomena we have examined. How then can we explain that a mutated β chain can interfere with the aggregation-induced responses of the receptor? We have no simple answer, but possibly the mutant subunit affects the appropriate approximation of the receptors and we are currently exploring this possibility. Taken together, our data provide no evidence for site-specific interactions between the receptor and the cytoskeletal structures. Instead, they suggest that the changes in the disposition of the receptors result more from non-specific physical phenomenon (18). Although our findings do not necessarily preclude that these receptor:cytoskeletal interactions are functionally significant, it complicates further analysis.

Signal Transduction in P815 Transfectants

The tumor line, P815, derived from a murine mast cell-like neoplasm (20), is well known to immunologists because it is a sensitive target cell for those interested in cell-mediated cytotoxicity. We first studied these cells as a possible source to study FcεRI but failed to detect any IgE binding (21). Ironically, these cells now turn out to be valuable just because of this deficiency. Using molecular probes one can show that the cells fail to express mRNA for either the FcεRI's α or β subunits but do express γ chains (13,22). They also express two isoforms of FcγR (23): FcγRII, thought to consist of a single α-like subunit, and FcγRIII, consisting of an α-like subunit combined with γ chains (24). When these cells were transfected with cDNA for each of the FcεRI subunits as well as with a selectable antibiotic marker, clones could be isolated that expressed IgE-binding. Northern blots demonstrated that the cells were express-

Table II. Functional Characteristics of Wild-type and Modified FcεRI

Modification	Receptor mobility[a]		Internalization[b]	Insolubilization[c]	Signal transduction[d]
	Unaggregated	Aggregated			
None	restricted	immobile	rapid	substantial	yes
α-CD	restricted	immobile	rapid	substantial	yes
β-(NH_2)CD	restricted	immobile	rapid	substantial	yes
β-(COOH)CD	restricted	partially mobile	reduced	substantial (COS) reduced (P815)	no
γ-CD	restricted	immobile	rapid	substantial	no
α(hum)γ(mouse)[e]	restricted	immobile	rapid	substantial	yes

[a]: Data from Ref. 17. Mobility was assessed by fluorescence photobleaching and recovery. All data from COS transfectants.
[b]: Data from Ref. 17 (COS cells) and unpublished data (P815 cells). Internalization was assessed by acid stripping.
[c]: Data from Ref. 18. Transfected receptors on COS and P815 cells were aggregated and the cells were then treated with non-ionic detergent.
[d]: Data from Ref. 15. The signals measured were protein tyrosine phosphorylation, increase in cytoplasmic Ca^{2+}, and phosphoinositide hydrolysis.
[e]: Receptors consisting of only the human α chain and rat or mouse γ chains, i.e. without β chains.

ing α, β and γ mRNA, the latter in amounts four- to five-fold more than the endogenous γmRNA in the untransfected controls (13).

The cells transfected with wild-type receptors exhibited some of the early biochemical perturbations associated with aggregation of FcεRI on mast cells (13). Cells transfected with modified subunits were then assessed and the results, summarized in Table II, have recently been published (15). It is apparent that the functional data in the P815 cells transfected with modified receptors resemble the topological data obtained in COS cells. Again the β subunit with a modified COOH-terminus interferes with function even though the β-less chimeric receptor consisting of the human α and rodent γ chains shows activity. The cells transfected with truncated γ chains are the principal exception, i. e. although the receptors on such cells had normal topological responses when aggregated, they failed to initiate the normal biochemical cascade. On further study of these transfectants, we found a curious paradox. It will be recalled that the P815 cells have endogenous γ chains. We had assumed that in the cells transfected with the mutated γ, the loss of function was due to the mutant chains being preferentially assembled into the receptor. This proved not to be the case, and the receptors in these cells were found to be completely normal. (Of course this is not true in the COS transfectants because these cells have no endogenous γ chains.) Nevertheless, transfection with the mutated γ chains had interfered with the receptor-initiated cascade. We are currently exploring this interesting phenomenon.

Concluding Remarks

It is apparent that mutational analysis of the receptor is proving be a useful tool for analyzing FcεRI. Initial studies from our own laboratory have strongly implicated the CD of the γ chains as a critical region and complementary studies by others on the same region, and on the corresponding CD of the γ-like ζ and η chains (25,26) suggest that this domain alone may initiate some of the early biochemical events triggered by the receptor. The role of the β chains is more problematic. Earlier studies from our own group suggested that the β chain was particularly susceptible to specific phosphorylations (27) and recent studies from other laboratories suggest that some of these accompany receptor aggregation. Possibly this reflects some regulatory functions which our functional data on the P815 cells also suggest. Others have reported that the receptor associates with specific kinases (28) and we are aware of data that similarly implicate an association of the receptor with phospholipase C after aggregation. There is now a burst of activity in this area, and there is reason to be optimistic that the initial molecular interactions that follow aggregation of the receptor will soon be considerably clarified. This will then set the stage for attempts to develop receptor-specific inhibitors that may foreseeably lead to exciting new therapeutic approaches.

References

1. Metzger, H., Kinet, J.-P., Blank, U., et al. 1989. The mast cell receptor for immunoglobulin E.: Prospects for therapy. Allergy and Clin. Immunol. 1:43.
2. Blank, U., Ra, C., Miller, L., Metzger, H., and Kinet, J.-P. 1989. Complete structure and expression in transfected cells of high affinity IgE receptor. Nature 337:187.
3. Metzger, H. 1986. The mast cell receptor for immunoglobulin E: Prospects for therapy. In: Proceedings XII Int. Con. Allerg. Clin. Immunol. C.E. Reed, ed. St. Louis: C.V. Mosby, 1986, p. 308.
4. Kochan, J., Pettine, L.F., Hakimi, J., Kishi, K., and Kinet, J.-P. 1988. Isolation of the gene coding for the alpha subunit of the human high affinity IgE receptor. Nucleic Acids Res. 16:3584.
5. Shimizu, A., Tepler, I., Benfey, P.N., Berenstein, E.H., Siraganian, R.P., and Leder, P. 1988. Human and rat mast cell high-affinity immunoglobulin E receptors: Characterization of putative alpha-chain gene products. Proc. Natl. Acad. Sci. USA 85:1907.
6. Miller, L., Blank, U., Metzger, H., and Kinet, J.-P. 1989. Expression of high-affinity binding of human immunoglobulin E by transfected cells. Science 244:334.
7. Blank, U., Ra, C., and Kinet, J.-P. 1991. Characterization of truncated α chain products from human, rat, and mouse high affinity receptor for immunoglobulin E. J. Biol. Chem. 266:2639.

8. Hakimi, J., Seals, C., Kondas, J.A., Pettine, L., Danho, W., and Kochan, J. 1990. The α subunit of the human IgE receptor (FcεRI) is sufficient for high affinity IgE binding. J. Biol. Chem. 265:22079.
9. Metzger, H. 1983. The receptor on mast cells and related cells with high affinity for IgE. Contemp. Top. Mol. Immunol. 9:115.
10. Maegawa, H., Olefsky, J.M., Thies, S., Boyd, D., Ullrich, A., and McClain, D.A. 1988. Insulin receptors with defective tyrosine kinase inhibit normal receptor function at the level of substrate phosphorylation. J. Biol. Chem. 263:12629.
11. Margolis, B., Li, N., Koch, A., et al. 1990. The tyrosine phosphorylated carboxyterminus of the EGF receptor is a binding site for GAP and PLC-gamma. EMBO J. 9:4375.
12. Gilman, A.G. 1987. G Proteins: Transducers of receptor-generated signals. Ann. Rev. Biochem. 56:615.
13. Miller, L., Alber, G., Varin-Blank, N., Ludowyke, R., and Metzger, H. 1990. Transmembrane signalling in P815 mastocytoma cells by transfected IgE receptors. J. Biol. Chem. 265:12444.
14. Rivnay, B., Wank, S.A., Poy, G., and Metzger, H. 1982. Phospholipids stabilize the interaction between the alpha and beta subunits of the solubilized receptor for immunoglobulin E. Biochemistry 21:6922.
15. Alber, G., Miller, L., Jelsema, C., Varin-Blank, N., and Metzger, H. 1991. Structure/function relationships in the mast cell high-affinity receptor for IgE (FcεRI): Role of cytoplasmic domains. J. Biol. Chem., in press.
16. Varin-Blank, N., and Metzger, H. 1990. Surface expression of mutated subunits of the high affinity mast cell receptor for IgE. J. Biol. Chem. 265:15685.
17. Mao, S.-Y., Varin-Blank, N., Edidin, M., and Metzger, H. 1991. Immobilization and internalization of mutated IgE receptors in transfected cells. J. Immunol. 146:958.
18. Mao, S.-Y., Rivera, J., Kochan, J., and Metzger, H. 1991. Interaction of aggregated native and mutatant IgE receptors with the cellular skeleton. Proc. Natl. Acad. Sci. USA, in press.
19. Seagrave, J., and Oliver, J.M. 1990. Antigen-dependent transition of IgE to a detergent-insoluble form is associated with reduced IgE receptor-dependent secretion from RBL-2H3 mast cells. J. Cell. Physiol. 144:128.
20. Dunn, T., and Potter, M. 1957. A transplantable mast-cell neoplasm in the mouse. J. Natl. Cancer Inst. 18:587.
21. Kulczycki, A., Jr., Isersky, C., and Metzger, H. 1974. The interaction of IgE with rat basophilic leukemia cells. I Evidence for specific binding of IgE. J. Exp. Med. 139:600.
22. Ra, C., Jouvin, M.-H.E., Blank, U., and Kinet, J.-P. 1989. A macrophage Fcγ receptor and the mast cell receptor for IgE share an identical subunit. Nature 341:752.
23. Benhamou, M., Bonnerot, C., Fridman, W.H., and Daëron, M. 1990. Molecular heterogeneity of murine mast cell Fcgamma receptors. J. Immunol. 144:3071.
24. Ravetch, J.V., and Kinet, J.-P. 1991. Fc receptors. Annu. Rev. Immunol. 9:457.
25. Irving, B.A., and Weiss, A. 1991. The cytoplasmic domain of the T cell receptor ζ chain is sufficient to couple to receptor-associated signal transduction pathways. Cell 64:891.
26. Romeo, C., and Seed, B. 1991. Cellular immunity to HIV activated CD4 fused to T cell or Fc receptor polypeptides. Cell 64:1037.
27. Quarto, R., and Metzger, H. 1986. The receptor for immunoglobulin E: Examination for kinase activity and as a substrate for kinases. Mol Immunol. 23:1215.
28. Eiseman, E., and Bolen, J.B. 1990. src-related tyrosine protein kinases as signaling components in hematopoietic cells. Cancer Cells 2:303.

The Low Affinity Receptor for IgE

G. Delespesse, M. Sarfati*

FcεRII, also known as CD23, belongs to a novel superfamily of type II integral membrane proteins displaying a lectin motif at their carboxy terminal end. There is strong evidence that FcεRII has other ligands than IgE, however these remain to be identified. FcεRII binds IgE via its lectin-like domain by interacting with the protein and probably also with the carbohydrate moiety of IgE. The FcεRII gene encodes two proteins differing by a few amino acids in their intracytoplasmic domain; these isoforms, named A and B, differ by their cellular expression, their function and probably by their signalling pathways. The expression of FcεRII is regulated by several cytokines in a tissue-specific manner. Functionally, FcεRII should be viewed not only as an IgE receptor but also as the membrane bound precursor of a multifunctional cytokine (soluble FcεRII). All the well characterized functions of membrane FcεRII are IgE-dependent and vary according to the cell types on which it is expressed; most of the activities ascribed to sFcεRII are IgE-independent.

The low affinity receptor for IgE (FcεRII or CD23) differs from the other Fc receptors by its structure and by its function. Unlike FcεRII or the Fc-Rs for IgG and IgA, FcεRII does not belong to the Ig gene superfamily. FcεRII is a member of a novel gene superfamily encoding type II integral membrane proteins displaying a lectin motif at their extracellular carboxy terminal end. Other members of this superfamily include: (a) the liver and macrophage asialoglycoprotein receptors (1); (b) CD72, the ligand of CD5 (2,3); (c) the family of Ly-49 antigens, preferentially expressed on NK cells (4); (d) the signal transducing molecule NKR-P1 specifically found on NK cells (5); and (e) the T-cell antigen A1 (6). The lectin-like domain of FcεRII also displays a striking homology with several calcium-dependent (C-type) animal lectins (7) including a recently described family of adhesion molecules, the selectins (ELAM-1, CD62 or GMP-140and LECAM-1 or Mel-14) (8). The IgE-binding domain of FcεRII is identical to its lectin-like domain and spans from cysteine 163 to cysteine 282 (9,10). By means of homolog scanning mutagenesis, two discontinuous stretches of amino acids located in that domain were recently shown to be involved in the IgE binding (10). Similar to the interactions of C-type lectins with their specific carbohydrates, the binding of IgE to FcεRII is calcium-dependent (11). These structural and functional features strongly suggest that FcεRII binds to the carbohydrate moiety of IgE, which is known to be heavily glycosylated. This prediction was however not confirmed experimentally inasmuch as unglycosylated native or recombinant IgE or IgE peptides were shown to bind to FcεRII (12). By means of a solid-phase radioimmunoassay allowing the measurement of the binding of IgE to immobilized soluble FcεRII, we have confirmed that indeed the binding of IgE is calcium-dependent. However and most interestingly, it is specifically suppressed by Fucose-1-phosphate but not by several other mono- or disaccharides. These results suggest that the binding of IgE to FcεRII involves both protein-protein interactions and carbohydrate-protein interactions. Such dual interactions have been reported for other C-type lectins (13).

The transcription of human FcεRII gene may start at two different sites, resulting in the expression of two distinct proteins differing only by the last 6–7 amino acids in the intracellular N terminal domain (14). These two isoforms named A and B differ by their cellular expression, their function and perhaps also by their signal transduction pathways. The expression of FcεRIIA is strictly restricted to B cells, whereas FcεRIIB has been found on monocytes, T cell eosinophils and on nasopharyngeal carcinoma cells harboring the Epstein-Barr virus (15). IL4-treated normal B cells coexpress type A and B FcεRII. The isoform of FcεRII

* Notre-Dame Hospital Research Center, University of Montreal, Canada.
Acknowledgements: Supported by a grant from MRC and by the financial and scientific help from CIBA-GEIGY Pharmaceutical, Basel, Switzerland.

expressed on platelets, on epidermal Langerhans cells and on thymic epithelial cells has not yet been determined. According to a recent study, mouse FcεRII gene may also encode two transcripts differing in their 5' untranslated sequence and in their intracytoplasmic region (16). Of these two murine FcεRII isoforms, one is similar to the human type A while the other is very different from the human type B FcεRII. This explains why in the mouse the expression of FcεRII is restricted to B cells (17).

On B cells, FcεRII is a differentiation marker which is selectively expressed on mature sIgM/sIgD double bearing B cells. FcεRII is lost after isotype switching as well as during the differentiation of B cells into Ig secreting cells, regardless of isotype-switching (18,19). Interestingly, FcεRII may still be transiently expressed on the surface of B cells which have recently switched (19). This may account for the presence of FcεRII on single IgG bearing B cell clones isolated from some patients with chronic lymphocytic leukemia (CLL). Incidently, these sIgG CD23 B cell clones may be induced to secrete monoclonal IgE following stimulation with IL-4 and hydrocortisone, indicating that the switching to IgE may be sequential. FcεRII is cleaved from the cell surface by an autocatalytic mechanism (15). This results in the formation of soluble FcεRII (sFcεRII) that are still capable of binding IgE. Soluble FcεRII are first released as unstable 37- and 33-kDa fragments that are subsequently transformed into a more stable 25 kDa molecule (15). The rate of FcεRII cleavage is reduced by IgE, resulting in an apparent upregulation of FcεRII expression (15).

The regulation of FcεRII varies according to the cell type on which it is expressed. On B cells FcεRII is induced by IL4 and suppressed by IFN-γ, IFN-α, TGF-β and glucocorticoids. B cell stimulatory signals like those provided by contact-dependent interactions with T cells or by the engagement of either sIg, CD40 or CD72 significantly enhance the IL4-induced FcεRII expression (15). Interestingly, engagement of CD40 renders the B cells refractory to the suppressive effect of the IFNs and of TGF-β (10). On monocytes, FcεRII may be induced by IL4, IL3 and GM-CSF; it is not suppressed by IFN-γ but it is inhibited by glucocorticoids, TGF -β and by 1,25 dihydroxy-vitamin D3 (15). These observations and others (15) indicate that the regulation of FcεRII expression is tissue-specific. To date, there is no evidence that the expression of the two FcεRII isoforms on the same cell, i.e. on B cells, is regulated by different mechanisms. On the contrary, 1, 25 (OH)2 vitamin D3 inhibits type B FcεRII on monocytes but does not affect the expression of the two isoforms A and B by B cells, as shown by RNAse protection assay (21). The expression and the regulation of FcεRII on CLL-B cells are profoundly abnormal suggesting that this molecule is not an innocent bystander and that it may play a role in some aspect of the malignant process. Freshly isolated CLL-B cells not only overexpress FcεRII on their surface but they also contain type A and B FcεRII mRNAs (22). Note that freshly isolated normal B cells express only FcεRIIA. Most strikingly, the induction of FcεRII expression on CLL-B cells by IL4 is abnormally low (23) and it is dramatically increased by cytokines that either suppress (IFN-γ, IFN-α) or do not influence (TNF-α) the effect of IL4 on normal B cells (Fournier & Sarfati, unpublished observation). A possible role of FcεRII in CLL disease is further suggested by the potent inhibitory effect of anti-FcεRII mAbs on the *in vitro* proliferative response of the leukemic cells to several stimuli.

Function of FcεRII

There is mounting evidence suggesting that FcεRII is not only an IgE-receptor but also the membrane bound precursor of a multi-functional lymphokine (sFcεRII or sCD23) whose activities are largely IgE-independent. Although all the well characterized activities of FcεRII/CD23 are IgE-dependent, it is felt that this molecule has other functions that are thought to be mediated by its lectin-like domain. For example, Kishimoto provided preliminary but suggestive evidence that FcεRII may function as an adhesion molecule (24). The IgE-dependent functions of FcεRII vary according to the cell type on which it is expressed. On inflammatory cells (monocytes, eosinophils and platelets) FcεRII may trigger several IgE-dependent activities including: (a) the killing of some parasites; (b) the phagocytosis of IgE-coated particles; (c) the release of IL-1 and TNF-α; and (d) the release of inflammatory mediators (25). Although the exact role of

FcεRII on the surface of B cells remains to be clarified, there is mounting evidence that it may be involved in the two major functions of the B cells, namely the presentation of antigen to T cells and their differentiation into Ig secreting cells.

Specific IgE antibodies, either cell bound or complexed to antigen, confer to non-antigen-specific B cells the capacity of presenting the corresponding antigen to T cells. This very efficient IgE-dependent presentation of antigen to T cells is mediated by the FcεRII expressed on the B cell surface (26,27). An interesting implication of these findings is that specific IgE antibodies and B cell FcεRII may amplify the T cell response to the corresponding antigen by expanding the pool of antigen-specific T cells. The role of FcεRII in antigen-presentation must be related to its physical but non-covalent association with Class II MHC molecules on the B cell surface (28).

Signalling via CD23 may alter the progression of B cells into the cell cycle (from late G1 to S) and their subsequent differentiation into Ig secreting cells. However, depending upon the experimental condition, this signal may either enhance or inhibit the B cell proliferation (29–32). It is possible that in human B cells the outcome of the FcεRII-mediated signal depends on the selective engagement of one of its two isoforms; our laboratory is currently examining the relative role of type A and B FcεRII in the regulation of B cell proliferation and differentiation. Regardless of the outcome of these experiments it was clearly shown that the cross-linking of FcεRII on the surface of IL4-treated B cells prevents both their proliferation and differentiation into cells secreting Ig, including the IgE isotype. These observations indicate that FcεRII may be involved in a negative feedback mechanism regulating the synthesis of IgE.

Functions of Soluble FcεRII (sCD23)

The concept emerging from a very fast growing number of publications is that sFcεRII is a multi-functional molecule capable of controlling the differentiation or the activity of several cell types. Most of these functions are clearly IgE-independent and great efforts are being made to identify the counter structure of sFcεRII on its target cells. In synergy with IL-1, sFcεRII promotes the differentiation of early thymocytes (33), of myeloid cell precursors (34) and of a subset of germinal center B cells, named centrocytes (35). Most interestingly, sFcεRII was shown to induce the expression of bcl-2 protein in the centrocytes and to rescue these cells from apoptosis (36). It is possible that this mechanism may also account for the effect of sFcεRII not only on the differentiation of thymocytes and myelocytes but also for its IgE enhancing activity. Indeed, apoptosis is a common homeostatic mechanism involved in the process of cellular differentiation and selection (37). Moreover, the expression of bcl-2 protein is required from the *in vivo* generation of long-lived Ig secreting cells and of memory B cells (38).

The ability of sFcεRII to regulate the synthesis of IgE was suggested several years ago by the observation that the IgE-binding factors released in the culture supernatants of FcεRII B cell lines were capable of enhancing the spontaneous *in vitro* synthesis of IgE by lymphocytes of atopic donors (39). The possible role of FcεRII or its soluble fragments in the regulation of human IgE synthesis was subsequently supported by the observations made in several laboratories that anti-FcεRII mAbs inhibit both the ongoing and the IL4-stimulated synthesis of IgE. Given that Ig secreting cells do not express FcεRII, the suppressive effect of these antibodies on the ongoing IgE synthesis cannot be explained by the cross-linking of FcεRII on the surface of IgE producing cells. Two alternatives were considered to explain the effect of anti-FcεRII mAbs on the *in vitro* ongoing synthesis of IgE by the lymphocytes of allergic donors: (a) the antibodies cross-link FcεRII on the surface of accessory cells and induce the release of inhibitors from these cells; or (b) the antibodies neutralize the IgE potentiating activity of sFcεRII. The observation that monovalent Fab fragments are as active as the intact mAb strongly supports the second possibility. The anti-FcεRII mAbs or their fragments display the same suppressive effect on the synthesis of IgE by normal lymphocytes which have been preactivated *in vitro* by IL4. Note that in each of these two *in vitro* models, the ongoing synthesis of IgE is IL4-independent inasmuch as it cannot be blocked by neutralizing anti-IL4 mAb. Taken collectively, the data strongly suggest that sFcεRII act on IgE preactivated B cells. This view was confirmed by the observations that highly purified native or recombinant sFcεRII significantly enhance the ongoing synthesis of IgE in the above models. The effect of exogenous sFcεRII is best observed when the endogenous production of these molecules is minimized. In the case of IL4 prestimulated normal PBMC, this is easily achieved by prestimulating the cells with a suboptimal concentration of IL4 in the presence of hydrocortisone.

Further analysis of the mode of action of sFcεRII indicates that the IgE-potentiating activity does not require the presence of T cells and that it is not accompanied by an increased proliferation of B cells. We suggest as a working hypothesis that sFcεRII enhance the synthesis of IgE by a mechanism similar to that explaining its effect on centrocytes, i. e., by preventing the apoptosis of activated IgE B cells.

Conclusion

At this stage it is virtually impossible to integrate the current knowledge about FcεRII/CD23 in a unified concept. As a surface molecule, FcεRII exists in two forms differing by their cellular distribution, their function and probably also by their signal transduction pathway. There is no doubt that FcεRII is involved in protective immunity against parasites and in IgE-mediated inflammatory responses. The role of FcεRII on human B cells is most difficult to evaluate not only because these cells may express the two isoforms in a variable proportion but also because they may respond, at some stage of their differentiation, to the soluble FcεRII. In spite of these difficulties, it is reasonable to propose that FcεRII may regulate two major aspects of the B cell function; (a) the presentation of antigen to T cells, and (b) their differentiation into Ig secreting cells. The multiple activities ascribed to sFcεRII confer to this molecule the profile of acytokine. Given that most of these activities are IgE-independent it will be most informative to identify the counter structure of sFcεRII on the surface of the responding cells. At this stage, it is tempting to speculate that the main mode of action of sFcεRII might be to activate the bcl-2 gene, a process allowing the responding cell to escape from apoptosis.

References

1. Li, M., Kurata, H., Itoh, N., Yamashina, I., and Kawasaki, T. 1990. Molecular cloning and sequence analysis of cDNA encoding the macrophage lectin specific for galactose and N-acetylgalactoramine. J. Biol. Chem. 265:11295.
2. Van de Velde, H., Von Hoegen, I., Luo, W., Parnes, J.R., and Thielemans, K. 1991. The B-cell surface protein CD72/Lyb-2 is the ligand for CD5. Nature 351:662.
3. Von Hoegen, I., Hsieh, C.L., Scharting, R., Francke, U., and Parnes, J.R. 1991. Identity of human Lyb-2 and CD72 and localization of the gene to chromosome 9. Eur. J. Immunol. 21:1425.
4. Wong, S., Freeman, J.D., Kelleher, C., Mager, D., and Takei, F. 1991. Ly-49 multigene family. J. Immunol. 147:1417.
5. Giorda, R., Rudert, W.A., Vavassori, C., Chamber, W.H., Hiserodt, J.C., and Trucco, M. 1990. NKR-P1, a signal transduction molecule on natural killer cells. Science 249:1298.
6. Yokoyama, W.M., Jacobs, L.B., Kanagawa, O., and Shevach, E.M. 1989. A murine T lymphocyte antigen belongs to a novel T cell surface disulfide-bonded dimer distinct from the α/β antigen receptor. J. Immunol. 143:1379.
7. Ludin, C., Hofstetter, H., Sarfati, M., Levy, C.A., Suter, U., Alaimo, D., Kilchherr, E., Frost, H., and Delespesse, G. 1987. Cloning and expression of the cDNA coding for a human lymphocyte IgE receptor. EMBO J. 6:109.
8. Stoolman, L.M. 1989. Adhesion molecules controlling lymphocyte migration. Cell 56:907.
9. Bettler, B., Maier, R., Ruegg, D., and Hofstetter, H. 1989. Binding site for IgE of the human lymphocyte low-affinity FcεRII receptor (FcεRII/CD23) is confined to the domain homologous with animal lectins. Proc. Natl. Acad. Sci. USA 86:7118.
10. Bettler, B., Texido, G., Raggini, S., Ruegg, D., and Hofstetter, H. 1991. Immunoglobulin E binding-site in FcεRII receptor (FcεRII-/CD23) identified by homolog-scanning mutagenesis. Proc. Natl. Acad. Sci., in press.
11. Richards, M.L., and Katz, D.H. 1990. The binding of IgE to murine FcεRII is calcium-dependent but not inhibited by carbohydrate. J. Immunol. 144:2638.

12. Vercelli, D., Helm, B., Marsh, P., Padlan, E., Geha, R.S., and Gould, H. 1989. The B-cell binding site on human immunoglobulin E. Nature 338:649.
13. Drickamer, K. 1988. Two distinct classes of carbohydrate-recognition domains in animal lectins. J. Biol. Chem. 263:9557.
14. Yokota A., Kikutani, H., Tanaka, T., Sato, R., Barsumian, E.L., Suemura, M., and Kishimoto, T. 1988. Two species of human FcεRII epsilon receptor II (FcεRII epsilon /CD23): Tissue-specific and IL-4-specific regulation of gene expression. Cell. 55:611.
15. Delespesse, G., Suter, U., Mossalayi, D., Bettler, B., Sarfati, M., Hofstetter, H., Kilcherr, E., Debre, P., and Dalloul, A. 1991. Expression, structure and function of the CD23 antigen. Advances in Immunology 49:149.
16. Richards, M.L., Katz, D.H., and Liu, F.T. 1991. Complete genomic sequence of the murine low affinity FcεRII receptor for IgE. J. Immunol. 147:1067.
17. Conrad, D.H. 1990. FcεRII /CD23: The low affinity receptor for IgE. Ann. Rev. Immunol. 8:623.
18. Kikutani H., Suemura, M., Owaki, H., Nakamura, H., Sato, R., Yamasaki, K., Barsumian, E.L., Hardy, R.R., and Kishimoto, T. 1986. FcεRII epsilon receptor, a specific differentiation marker transiently expressed on mature B cells before isotype switching. J. Exp. Med. 164:1455.
19. Snapper, C.M., Hooley, J.J., Urban Jr., J.F., and Finkelman, F.D. 1991. Lack of FcεRII expression by murine B cells after *in vivo* immunization is directly associated with Ig secretion and not Ig isotype switching. J. Immunol. 146:2161.
20. Gordon, J., Katira, A., Strain, A.J., and Gillis, S. 1991. Inhibition of interleukin 4-promoted CD23 production in human B lymphocytes by transforming growth factor-β interferons or anti-CD19 antibody is overriden on engaging CD40. Eur. J. Immunol. 21:1917.
21. Fargeas, C., Wu, C., Luo, H., Sarfati, M., Delespesse, G., and Wu, J.. 1990. 1, 25 (OH)2 Vitamin D3 inhibits the CD23 gene expression by human peripheral blood monocytes. J. Immunol. 145:4053.
22. Fournier, S., Trans, I.D., Suter, U., Biron, G., Delespesse, G., and Sarfati, M. 1991. The *in vivo* expression of type B CD23 mRNA in B-chronic lymphocytic leukemic cells is associated with an abnormally low CD23 upregulation by IL-4: comparison with their normal cellular counterparts. Leukemia Research 15:609.
23. Sarfati M., Fournier, S., Christoffersen, M., and Biron, G. 1990. Expression of CD23 antigen and its regulation by IL-4 in chronic lymphocytic leukemia. Leuk. Res. 14:47.
24. Kikutani, H., Yokota, A., Uchibayashi, N., Yukawa, K., Tanaka, T., Sugiyama, K., Barsumian, E.L., Suemura, M., and Kishimoto, T. 1989. Structure and function of FcεRII epsilon receptor II (FcεRII epsilon /CD23): A point of contact between the effector phase of allergy and B cell differentiation. CIBA Found. Symp. 147:23.
25. Capron, A., Dessaint, J.P., Capron, M., Joseph, M., Ameisen, J.C., and Tonnel, A.B. 1986. From parasites to allergy: the second receptor for IgE (FcεRII). Immunol. Today 7:15.
26. Kehry, M.R., and Yamashita, L.C. 1989. Low-affinity IgE receptor (CD23) function on mouse B cells: role in IgE-dependent antigen focusing. Proc. Natl. Acad. Sci. USA 86:7556.
27. Pirron, U., Schlunch, T., Prinz, J.C., and Rieber, E.P. 1990. IgE-dependent antigen focusing by human B lymphocytes is mediated by the low-affinity receptor for IgE. Eur. J. Immunol. 20:1547.
28. Bonnefoy, J.Y., Guillot, O., Spits, H., Blanchard, D., Ishizaka, K., and Banchereau, J. 1988. The low-affinity receptor for IgE (CD23) on B lymphocytes is spatially associated with HLA-DR antigens. J. Exp. Med. 167:57.
29. Luo, H., Hofstetter, H., Banchereau, J., and Delespesse, G. 1991. Cross-linking of CD23 antigen by its natural ligand (IgE) or by anti-CD23 antibody prevents B lymphocyte proliferation and differentiation. J. Immunol. 146:2122.
30. Waldschmidt, T.J., and Tygrett, L. 1991. Crosslinking surface Ig and the low affinity IgE FcεRII receptor induces B cells to enter cell cycle. FASEB J. 5:1389A.
31. Gordon J., Webb, A.J., Guy, G.R., and Walker, L. 1987. Triggering of B lymphocytes through CD23: Epitope mapping and studies using antibody derivatives indicate an allosteric mechanism of signalling. Immunology 60:517.
32. Campbell, K.A., Lees, A., Finkelman, F.D., and Conrad, D.H. 1991. Crosslinking FcεRII and surface IgD enhances anti-IgD mediated B cell activation. FASEB J. 5:1384A.
33. Mossalayi, M. D., Lecron, J.C., Dalloul, A.H., Sarfati, M., Bertho, J.M., Hofstetter, H., Delespesse, G., and Debre, P. 1990. Soluble CD23 (FcεRII epsilon) and interleukin 1 synergistically induce early human thymocyte maturation. J. Exp. Med. 171:959.

34. Mossalayi, M.D., Arock, M., Bertho, J.M., Blanc, C., Dalloul, A.H., Hofstetter, H., Sarfati, M., Delespesse, G., and Debre, P. 1990. Proliferation of early human myeloid precursors induced by interleukin-1 and recombinant soluble CD23. Blood 75:1924.
35. Liu, Y.J., Cairns, J.A., Holder, M.J., Abbot, S.D., Jansen, K.U., Bonnefoy, J.Y., Gordon, J., and MacLennan, I.C.M. 1991. Recombinant 25-kDa CD23 and interleukin 1α promote the survival of germinal center B cells: Evidence for bifurcation in the development of centrocytes rescued from apoptosis. Eur. J. Immunol. 21:1107.
36. Liu, Y.J., Mason, D.Y., Johnson, G.D., Abbot, S., Gregory, C.D., Hardie, D.L.,Gordon, J., and MacLennan, I.C.M. 1991. Germinal center cells express bcl-2 protein after activation by signals which prevent their entry into apoptosis. Eur. J. Immunol. 21:1905.
37. Collins, M. 1991. Death by a thousand cuts. Current Biology 3:140.
38. Nunez, G., Hockenbery, D., McDonnell, T.J., Sorensen, C.M., and Korsmeyer, S.J. 1991. Bcl-2 maintains B cell memory. Nature 35:71.
39. Sarfati M., Rector, E., Wong, K., Rubio-Trujillo, M., Sehon, A.H., and Delespesse, G. 1984. In vitro synthesis of IgE by human lymphocytes. II. Enhancement of the spontaneous IgE synthesis by IgE-binding factors secreted by RPMI 8866 lymphoblastoid B cells. Immunology 53:197.

Immunobiology of IgE and IgE Receptor

André R. Capron, Jean-Paul Dessaint, Michel Joseph, Monique Capron*

Extensive studies of the basic mechanisms of defense against helminth parasite, and in particular schistosomes, have underlined the preeminent role played by antibody-dependent cellular cytotoxicity mechanisms in *in vitro* and *in vivo* parasite killing. IgE antibodies have been shown to be one of the major humoral components of ADCC through their interaction with macrophages, eosinophils and platelets revealing the existence of unsuspected IgE-binding sites on these cell populations. Evidence for the protective role of IgE against helminth parasites, initially based on *in vitro* experiments, and passive transfer of monoclonal IgE antibody in rats, have recently been conclusively supported by epidemiological studies in human populations. Three independent surveys, performed in Gambia, Kenya and Brazil, have led to the demonstration of a highly significant correlation between IgE antibody levels to schistosomes and immunity to reinfection in man. These findings confirm the relevance of our experimental results in rats, and support our research strategy which has recently led to the development of a potential vaccine against schistosomiasis. These findings also bring additional support to the primary role of IgE during evolution in immune defense against parasites. Following IgE-dependent triggering of inflammatory cells, macrophages, platelets and eosinophils, a large array of cytocidal mediators and cytokines has been characterized which may account both for protective immunity and for the inflammatory components of allergic reactions. Although the molecular structure of FcεRII (low affinity receptor for IgE) on inflammatory cells is not entirely elucidated, its identity with CD23 appears well documented on monocytes and macrophages. There is accumulating evidence that besides CD23 other IgE binding proteins might be involved in IgE-dependent triggering of eosinophils. These results indicate that in parasitic infections as well as in allergic disorders IgE is an essential humoral partner of cell effector functions through its interaction with multiple cell populations.

Since the early days of the basic studies on immediate type hypersensitivity and of parasitic diseases, emphasis was given to the existence in both situations of so-called reaginic antibodies, which was exemplified by the description of anaphylaxis by Richet and Portier on the one hand and the Casoni's reaction on the other hand. For many years we have lived with the concept of a proverbial association of most helminthic infections with elevated IgE antibody response and hypereosinophilia, both of which are also observed in allergic diseases (although often at lower levels), but we did this without knowing their biological significance and the reasons for their emergence late in phylogeny. It is striking that many of the most significant biological observations leading to our present basic knowledge of the molecular and cellular mechanisms of allergy have been in fact provided by the extensive study of parasitic models in which allergic symptoms are not a predominant feature (1–4). This has naturally led to the concept of a dual function of IgE in immunopathology and immune defense against helminths and possibly other parasites, raising the question of the real biological significance of IgE during evolution (5–6). This brief review will attempt to illustrate from recent epidemiological and experimental data some new dimensions regarding the role of IgE in immune defense and to analyze common mechanisms in the effector or regulatory phases of both allergic manifestations and parasitic infections.

Immunobiology of IgE

Extensive studies performed during the last 15 years, mainly in our laboratory, concerning the basic mechanisms of defense against a major

---

* Centre d'Immunologie et de Biologie Parasitaire, Unité Mixte INSERM U167-CNRS 624, Institut Pasteur, rue du Pr Calmette, B.P. 245, 59019 Lille, France.
Acknowledgements: The work summarized in this manuscript was supported by INSERM, CNRS and the Institut Pasteur de Lille.

human parasitic disease, schistosomiasis, have led to the demonstration of IgE antibody-dependent cytotoxicity (ADCC) mediated *in vitro* by monocytes/macrophages, eosinophils, and platelets both in experimental rat infection and in human schistosomiasis. Multiple experiments using polyclonal and monoclonal IgE antibodies to the parasite, supported by specific immunoabsorption of immune rat serum or competition protocols, have clearly indicated the prominent participation of IgE in cellular cytotoxicity against schistosomes (6). At the same time, evidence was brought for the existence of specific receptors for IgE on subsets of monocytes/macrophages, eosinophils and platelets in man and rodents. These receptors differ from the classical mast cell or basophil receptors (FcεRI) by exhibiting a hundred-fold lower affinity for IgE (7–10). The production of polyclonal and monoclonal antibodies to inflammatory cell receptors has indicated that they bind similarly to macrophages, eosinophils and platelets, do not express any cross-reactivity with the FcεRI α-chain of mast cells and basophils, justifying the characterization of a second class of receptor for IgE (FcεRII) (11), which is expressed by subsets of inflammatory cells. Accordingly, such anti-FcεRII antibodies were found to block IgE antibody-dependent killing by macrophages, eosinophils, and platelets (12). In contrast with these experimental demonstrations of *in vitro* activation by IgE of FcεRII bearing cells to kill parasite targets, we have for a long time lived with only circumstantial evidence for the involvement of this cooperation *in vivo*.

Pioneering observations made by Sadun and Gore (13) and by Ogilvie, Smithers and Terry (14) regarding the production of reaginic antibodies during experimental schistosome infections had indicated a possible association of anaphylactic antibodies with resistance to infection. A close chronological relationship was also observed during our studies between the development of protective immunity in rats infected by schistosomes and the evolution both of their levels of IgE and of the ability of their cells and serum to cooperate in killing parasites *in vitro* (6). Moreover, passive transfer experiments using selectively IgE-depleted immune rat serum indicated the potential role of IgE in protection. More conclusively, administration of anti-schistosome monoclonal IgE antibody conferred to rats a significant protection to a challenge schistosome infection (15). These observations were also supported by a significant decrease of resistance in selectively IgE immunosuppressed neonate rats (16). Since all these experiments were based on the use of the experimental rat model, the relevance of these findings to protective mechanisms in human populations has been debated for a long time. In fact, a clear demonstration of the role of IgE antibodies in immune defense against helminth parasites *in vivo* has only recently been gained through a series of convergent epidemiological studies performed in human populations exposed to schistosomiasis following their rate of reinfection after treatment. In Gambia, Paul Hagan and co-workers (17) convincingly demonstrated that resistance to reinfection by *Schistosoma haematobium* was positively correlated with the presence of anti-schistosome IgE antibodies. Multiple logistic regression showed that individuals with high IgE antibody levels were ten times more resistant to reinfection, whereas individuals with high IgG4 levels but no IgE antibody were ten times more susceptible. Similarly, in Kenya, in collaboration with David Dunn and Anthony Butterworth, it was shown that acquired resistance to *Schistosoma mansoni* infection was significantly correlated with the level of anti-schistosome antibodies of the IgE class. Similar correlations have recently been observed by Alain Dessein in Brazil, who showed moreover that the association of low IgE levels with high IgG4 antibodies to schistosome antigens led to an increase in susceptibility to infection of more than one hundred-fold (18).

From these recent epidemiological studies, it appears therefore that IgE antibody response is an important if not essential component in the expression of protective immunity in human populations exposed to a major helminthic infection. These observations clearly support the views which we have published in recent years on the basis of our experimental findings regarding the role of IgE in immune defense and the biological significance of this immunoglobulin class during evolution. They also bring additional support to the research strategy that we have followed towards the development of a potential vaccine against schistosomiasis, which has now led to the molecular cloning and expression of a protective antigen of *Schistosoma mansoni*, the Sm28 glutathione S-transferase (19–20).

Immunobiology of IgE Receptors

The participation of IgE both in immune defense against parasites and in allergic manifestations naturally raises the question of the various cell populations which can be triggered into effector cells after IgE-binding. Although FcεRII is of lower affinity than the mast cell or basophil receptors, the increased extrinsic affinity of FcεRII for IgE dimers or complexes (21–22) gives this class of receptors a particular significance in all situations where IgE complexes are produced. This is the case not only in parasitic infections (1) but also in various allergic diseases (23). In addition, the number of FcεRII bearing cells increases in all pathological or experimental situations associated with elevated IgE levels. Furthermore, *ex vivo* studies of parasitised or allergic individuals have indicated the existence of surface bound (cytophilic) IgE on a large proportion of monocytes, alveolar macrophages, peripheral blood or tissue eosinophils, and platelets (24,25,26). One can therefore accept the general view that both *in vitro* and *in vivo* subsets of monocytes, macrophages, eosinophils and platelets can, like mast cells or basophils, selectively bind IgE molecules. The important question is thus the possible participation of these cells in IgE-dependent reactions through mediators released after their activation. Another essential issue is the real nature of the IgE receptor involved, and in particular its identity with the CD23 molecule, recognized and characterized as the low affinity receptor for IgE on B cell populations. As in the case of mast cells or basophils, the initial step in the stimulation of cells through IgE bound to FcεRII receptors is the aggregation of the receptors. It has been shown, particularly for macrophages, that dimers of IgE constitute the unit signal for cell stimulation which can be detected 10–15 minutes after IgE-dependent FcεRII aggregation (27).

Monocytes/macrophages respond to IgE by releasing lysosomal enzymes, neutral proteases, interleukin-1, reactive oxygen metabolites, and also such potent mediators of anaphylaxis as sulfidopeptide leukotrienes (LTC4, LTD4, LTB4), prostaglandins, and platelet activating factor (PAF-acether). Recent experiments have provided evidence that in addition to IL-1 and IL-1 inhibitory factor, alveolar macrophages harvested from the lung of allergic asthmatics release large amounts of TNF-α as well as IL-6 after addition of anti-human IgE antibodies or of the specific allergen. It is noticeable that this increase in TNF-α and IL-6 production, which is correlated with the messenger RNA expression, was only observed for the patients developing a late asthmatic reaction, while asthmatics with only an early response did not differ from controls (28). Therefore it seems clearly established that, following IgE-dependent triggering, mononuclear phagocytes release a large variety of inflammatory mediators and cytokines which can be potentially involved both in parasite killing mechanisms and in allergic reactions.

Regarding the structural identity of the monocyte/macrophage IgE receptors, clear evidence has been brought that mRNA encoding CD23 was expressed in human monocytes. Moreover, the FcεRIIb gene was detected in U937 cell lines as well as in human monocytes

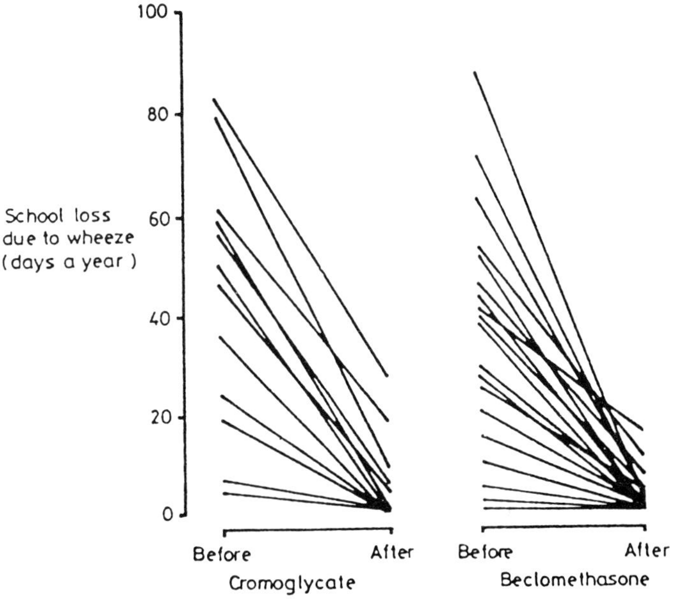

Fig. 1

following IL-4 dependent activation (29). The gene was also shown to be spontaneously expressed in monocytes from atopic patients.

Platelets under IgE-dependent triggering mainly produce reactive oxygen metabolites and cytotoxic mediators that kill schistosomula *in vitro*. They also release a granule-stored mediator (histamine) but no serotonin and do not aggregate on triggering via their FcεRII. For some years, the possible existence of two distinct pathways of platelet stimulation leading either to the expression of a killing activity or to aggregation has remained debated. Recent experiments performed in our laboratory, using PAF induced or thrombin induced activation (30), show that the same ligand can, in a dose-dependent manner, lead first to platelet-mediated killing expression and at higher doses to platelet aggregation. The expression of the IgE receptor on platelets can be enhanced by various cytokines among which INF-γ, TNF-α and TNF-β appear to play a major role in synergising IgE-dependent killing. Although the precise molecular structure of the platelet IgE receptor has not been elucidated, it has recently been shown that various monoclonal antibodies to the CD23 molecule can significantly inhibit IgE-dependent cytotoxicity, indicating at least the existence of common epitopes to CD23.

Eosinophils are now recognized as playing a major role both in immune defense and in various allergic manifestations (10,31). In parasitic infections, such as schistosomiasis, eosinophils mediate highly effective antibody-dependent cellular cytotoxicity against schistosome larvae in various animal models and in man. Although several isotypes can participate in eosinophil triggering, IgE appears to be the more potent immunoglobulin, for inducing eosinophil-mediated cytotoxicity. It is noteworthy that IgE-dependent eosinophil cytotoxicity is increased in subjects presenting the highest levels of resistance to reinfection by schistosomes, whereas isotypes exerting a blocking activity on eosinophils, such as IgG4, are detected in patients with the lowest resistance (17). IgE can trigger the release by eosinophils of many potentially cytocidal molecules including proinflammatory granule components (basic proteins), mainly Eosinophil Peroxidase (EPO) and Major Basic Protein (MBP) as well as lipidic mediators such as PAF-acether. An interesting phenomenon of selective mediator release has been evidenced in this context. Whereas IgE preferentially induces the release of EPO and PAF but not the release of Eosinophil Cationic Protein (ECP), IgG triggers the secretion of ECP but not EPO (31). This apparent selectivity in mediator release may be related to the heterogeneity of eosinophil populations, i.e., the existence of "hypodense" versus "normodense" subsets, or to the induction of a piecemeal degranulation process, as documented in recent experiments. Although messenger RNA encoding the CD23 molecule has been shown to be expressed in the so-called eosinophilic cell line EoL-1, the exact molecular structure of the IgE receptors on human eosinophils remains unclear and its identity with the CD23 molecule still debated.

All the evidence favoring the existence of a specific IgE receptor on human eosinophils has been reviewed recently (32). We will only summarize here some of the recent information available:

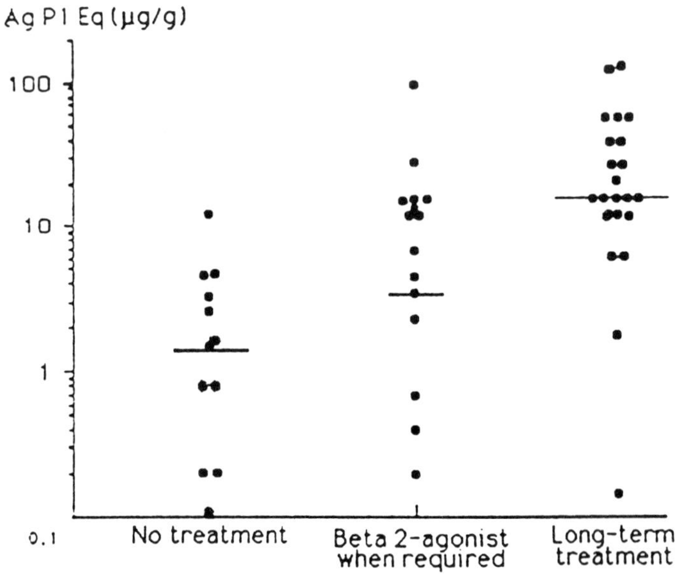

Fig.2

(A) Three different monoclonal antibodies to CD23, designated 135, 3-5 and 8-30 inhibit in a dose-dependent manner IgE binding to human eosinophils and IgE-dependent cytotoxicity mediated by eosinophils, illustrating a novel aspect of the functions of the CD23 molecule in parasitic infections. (B) Northern blot analysis with the cDNA probe of CD23 reveals a weak band in 3 patients out of 6 who were shown to express membrane CD23 by flow cytometry. Evidence has been gained of a variable expression of mRNA encoding various eosinophil molecules (33). Comparison of mRNA expression between cord blood derived eosinophils and mature blood eosinophils indicates the lability of the expression of some of these messages following differentiation (34). It is therefore possible that the variability in expression of CD23 by eosinophils, known to be a very heterogeneous population, may rely on a decreased expression of CD23 mRNA in mature blood eosinophils. (C) IgE binding proteins distinct from CD23 have now been identified in eosinophils. The binding to eosinophils of monoclonal antibodies against Mac2, a galactose specific lectin that binds IgE, as well as the detection of mRNA hybridizing to the cDNA probe encoding human Mac2, provide preliminary evidence that eosinophils might express IgE binding proteins belonging to the family of carbohydrate binding proteins. The cloning of the molecule(s) involved in IgE binding to eosinophils and platelets, currently in progress, will certainly help clarify these debated questions.

Through its interaction with one or the other of its receptors, IgE can thus trigger multiple cell populations and play a key role in many biological reactions, either in immune defense against helminth parasites, or as direct effector cells in allergic disorders. In both cases, the network of cells responsive to IgE appears to be highly complex and interconnected through IgE itself, cytokines, and so-called factors of anaphylaxis. Thus it is perhaps not surprising that common IgE-dependent mechanisms might appear to diverge in their functional consequences in parasitized and parasite-free individuals.

References

1. Dessaint, J.P. 1982. Anaphylactic antibodies and their significance. Clin. Imm. Allergy 2:621.
2. Capron, A., Dessaint, J.P., and Capron, M. Allergy and immune defense: Common IgE-dependent mechanisms or divergent pathways. In: Allergy and parasitism. R. Moqbel, ed., in press.
3. Jarrett, E.E.E., and Miller, H.R.P. 1982. Production and activities of IgE in helminth infection. Prog. Allergy 31:178.
4. Ishizaka, K. 1984. Regulation of IgE synthesis. Ann. Rev. Immunol. 2:159.
5. Holgate, S.T., Hardy, C., Robinson, C., Agius, R.M., and Howarth, P.R. 1986. The mast cell as a primary effector cell in the pathogenesis of asthma. J. Allergy Clin. Immunol. 77:274.
6. Capron, A., Dessaint, J.P., Capron, M., Ouma, A., and Butterworth, A.E. 1987. Immunity to schistosomes: Progress toward vaccine. Science 238:1065.
7. Capron, A., Dessaint, J.P., Capron, M., and Bazin, H. 1975. Specific IgE antibodies in immune adherence of normal macrophages to *Schistosoma mansoni* schistosomules. Nature 253:474.
8. Joseph, M., Auriault, C., Capron, A., Vorng, H., and Viens, P. 1983. A role for platelets in IgE dependent killing of schistosomes. Nature 303:810.
9. Capron, M., Spiegelberg, H.L., Prin, L., Bennich, H., Butterworth, A.E., Pierce, R.J., Ouaissi, M.A., and Capron, A. 1984. Role of IgE receptors in effector function of human eosinophils. J. Immunol. 232:462.
10. Capron, M., Grangette, C., Torpier, G., and Capron, A. 1989. The second receptor for IgE in eosinophil effector function. Chem. Immunol. 47:128.
11. Capron, A., Dessaint, J.P., Capron, M., Joseph, M., Ameisen, J.C., and Tonnel, A.B. 1986. From parasites to allergy: The second receptor for IgE (FcεRII). Immunol. Today 7:15.
12. Capron, M., Jouault, T., Prin, L., Ameisen, J.C., Butterworth, A.E., Papin, J.P., Kusnierz, J.P., and Capron, A. 1986. Functional study of a monoclonal antibody to IgE Fc receptor (FcεRII) of eosinophils, platelets, and macrophages. J. Exp. Med. 164:72.
13. Sadun, E.H, and Gore, R.W. 1970. *Schistosoma mansoni* and *Schistosoma haematobium*: Homocytotropic reagin like antibodies in infections of man and experimental animal. Exp. Parasit. 28:435.
14. Ogilvie, B.M., Smithers, S.R., and Terry, R.J.

1966. Reagin-like antibodies in experimental infection of *Schistosoma mansoni* and the passive transfer of resistance. Nature 209:1221.
15. Verwaerde, C., Joseph, M., Capron, M., Pierce, R.J., Damonneville, M., Velge, F., Auriault, C., and Capron, A. 1987. Functional properties of a rat monoclonal IgE antibody specific for *Schistosoma mansoni*. J. Immunol. 138:4441.
16. Kigoni, E., Elsas, P., Lenzi, H., and Dessein, A.J. 1986. IgE antibody and resistance to infection. II. Effect of IgE suppression on the early and late skin reaction and resistance of rats to *Schistosoma mansoni* infection. Eur. J. Immunol. 16:589.
17. Hagan, P., Blumenthal, U.J., Dunn, D., Simpson, A.J.G., and Wilkins, H.A. 1991. Human IgE, IgG4 and resistance to reinfection with *Schistosoma haematobium*. Nature 349:243.
18. Rihet, P., Demeure, C.E., Bourgois, A., Prata, A., and Dessein, A.J. 1991. Evidences for an association between human resistance to *Schistosoma mansoni* and high anti-larval IgE levels. Eur. J. Immunol. 21:2679.
19. Balloul, J.M., Sondermeyer, P., Dreyer, D., Capron, M., Grzych, J.M., Pierce, R.J., Carvallo, D., Lecocq, J.P., and Capron, A. 1987. Molecular cloning of a protective antigen against schistosomiasis. Nature 326:149.
20. Taylor, J.B., Vidal, A., Torpier, G., Meyer, D.J., Roitsch, C., Balloul, J.M., Southan, C., Sondermeyer, P., Pemble, S., Lecocq, J.P., Capron, A., and Ketterer, B. 1988. The glutathione transferase activity and tissue distribution of a cloned Mr27K protective antigen of *Schistosoma mansoni*. Embo Journal 7:465.
21. Dessaint, J.P., Waksman, B.H., Metzger, H., and Capron, A. 1980. Cytophilic binding of IgE to the macrophage. III. Involvement of cyclic GMP and calcium in macrophage activation by dimeric or aggregated rat myeloma IgE. Cell. Immunol. 51:280.
22. Finbloom, D.S., and Metzger, H. 1982. Binding of immunoglobulin E to the receptor on rat peritoneal macrophages. J. Immunol. 129:2004.
23. Brostoff, J., Johns, P., and Stanworth, D.R. 1977. Immune complexed IgE in atopy. Lancet II:741.
24. Joseph, M., Tonnel, A.B., Torpier, G., Capron, A., Arnoux, A., and Benveniste, J. 1983. Involvement of immunoglobulin E in the secretory processes of alveolar macrophages from asthmatic patients. J. Clin. Invest. 71:221.
25. Joseph, M., Capron, A., Ameisen, J.C., Capron, M., Vorng, H., Pancré, V., Kusnierz, J.P., and Auriault, C. 1986. The receptor for IgE on blood platelets. Eur. J. Immunol. 16:396.
26. Capron, M., Kusnierz, J.P., Prin, L., Spiegelberg, H.L., Ovlaque, G., Gosset, P., Tonnel, A.B., and Capron, A. 1985. Cytophilic IgE on human blood and tissue eosinophils: Detection by flow microfluorometry. J. Immunol. 134:3013.
27. Dessaint, J.P., Capron, M.,and Capron, A. 1990. Immunoglobulin E-stimulated release of mediators from mononuclear phagocytes, eosinophils, and platelets. In: Fc receptors and the action of antibodies. H. Metzger, ed., p. 260.
28. Gosset, P., Tsicopoulos, A., Wallaert, B., Vannimenuss, C., Joseph, M., Tonnel, A.B., and Capron, A. 1991. Increased secretion of tumor necrosis factor α and interleukin-6 by alveolar macrophages consecutive to the development of the late asthmatic reaction. J. Allergy. Clin. Invest. 88:561.
29. Yokota, A., Kikutani, H., Tanaka, T., Sato, S., Barsumian, E.L., Suemura, M., and Kishimoto, T. 1988. Two species of human Fcε receptor II (FcεRII/CD23): Tissue-specific and IL-4 specific regulation of the gene expression. Cell 55:611.
30. Tran, A., Vanhee, D., Capron, A., Vorng, H., Braquet, P., and Joseph, M. Separate induction of human blood platelet aggregation or cytotoxicity by different concentrations of PAF-acether and thrombin. Agents and Action, in press.
31. Capron, M., Grangette, C., Torpier, G., and Capron, A. 1989. The second receptor for IgE in eosinophil effector function. Chemical Immunol. 47:128.
32. Capron, M., and Joseph, M. 1991. The low affinity receptor for IgE on eosinophils and platelets. Monographs in Allergy 29:63.
33. Gruart, V., Truong, M.J., Plumas, J., Zandecki, M., Kusnierz, J.P., Prin, L., Capron, A., and Capron, M. Decreased expression of eosinophil peroxidase and major basic protein mRNAs during eosinophil maturation. Blood, in press.
34. Capron, M., Coffman, R.L., Papin, J.P., Ajana, F., and Capron, A. 1991. Fc epsilon receptor II expression in parasitic diseases: Effects of cytokines on IgE-dependent activation of eosinophils. Advances in Prostaglandin, Thromboxane and Leukotriene Research 21:975.

Sektion II

Recently Developed Anti-Allergic and Related Drugs

Modulation of IgE Synthesis by a New Drug, IPD-1151T

Akihide Koda*, Yukiyoshi Yanagihara**, Naosuke Matsuura*

IPD-1151T, a dimethylsulfonium derivative, inhibits not only IgE antibody formation but also antigen-induced histamine release from mast cells. The present paper describes the inhibitory effect of IPD-1151T on the IgE antibody formation. The IgE antibody formation in BALB/c mice which had been immunized with dinitrophenylated ascaris extract (DNP • As) plus alum was inhibited dose-dependently by IPD-1151T given p.o. Anti-DNP • IgM and IgG antibodies, however, were unaffected by the agent. Ongoing IgE antibody formation was also inhibited by this agent. The total IgE in sera of atopic patients showed a tendency to decrease when IPD-1151T was given p.o. for 6 to 12 weeks, though the titer of specific IgE antibody against *Dermatophagoides pteronyssinus* or *D. farinae* clearly decreased. In these cases, the ratio of B cells expressing FcεRII also decreased. Antigen-induced production of IL-4 from a helper T-cell line (TCL) prepared from peripheral blood lymphocytes of an allergic patient sensitive to Japanese cedar pollen was reduced with the addition of IPD-1151T. This agent also decreased antigen-inducd IgE synthesis by autologous B cell concomitant with the TCL and antigen presenting cell.

Drugs specifically inhibiting IgE antibody formation would be most desirable for the therapy of atopic diseases. However, such drugs are not available. It is well known that reactions involving the transfer of methyl radical (transmethylation) play a great variety of roles in the expression and regulation of various physiological functions (1–5). We have studied the immunopharmacology of a series of dimethylsulfonium compounds and found interesting properties in IPD-1151T{()-[2-[4-(3-ethoxy-2-hydroxypropoxy) phenylcarbamoyl]ethyl] dimethylsulfonium p-toluenesulfonate shown in Figure 1 (6). This agent inhibits not only IgE antibody formation, but also antigen-induced histamine release from mast cells and has a low toxicity. Clinical trials on the efficacy of IPD-1151T on asthma, atopic dermatitis and allergic rhinitis are now underway and have been producing excellent results. The present paper describes the effects of IPD-1151T on the IgE antibody formation in mice and humans. Furthermore the effect on the production of human helper T cell-derived IL-4 which has been established as an essential cytokine for IgE synthesis (7,8) elucidates the mechanism regarding the inhibition of IgE antibody formation by the agent.

Methods and Results

The Effect on IgE Antibody Formation in Mice

Female BALB/c mice, 9 to 10 weeks of age, were immunized by an i.p. injection of 5 mg of dinitrophenylated ascaris extract (DNP • As) (9) concomitant with 1 mg of alum, and boosted with the same dose of antigen each after 30 and 60 days (10). The blood was drawn on the days shown in Figure 2, and the IgE antibody titer was measured by 24-hr heterologous PCA in rats. The titers of anti-DNP • IgM and IgG antibodies were also assayed by an enzyme-linked immunosorbent assay (ELISA). IPD-1151T was given p.o. to mice in doses of 10 to 100 mg/kg/day for 5 days from the first immunization. As shown in Figure 2, the IgE antibody formation was distinctly decreased with IPD-1151T, and such an inhibitory effect was observed even after the tertiary immunization. However, formations of IgM and IgG antibod-

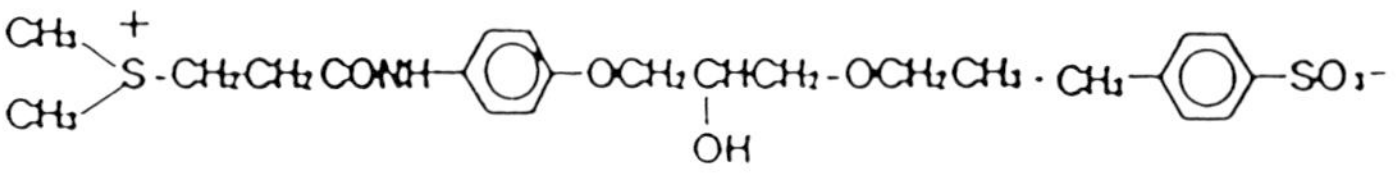

Fig. 1. The chemical structure of IPD-1151T.

* Department of Pharmacology, Gifu Pharmaceutical University, Gifu 502, Japan.
** Clinical Research Center for Rheumato-Allergology, National Sagamihara Hospital, Kanagawa 228, Japan.

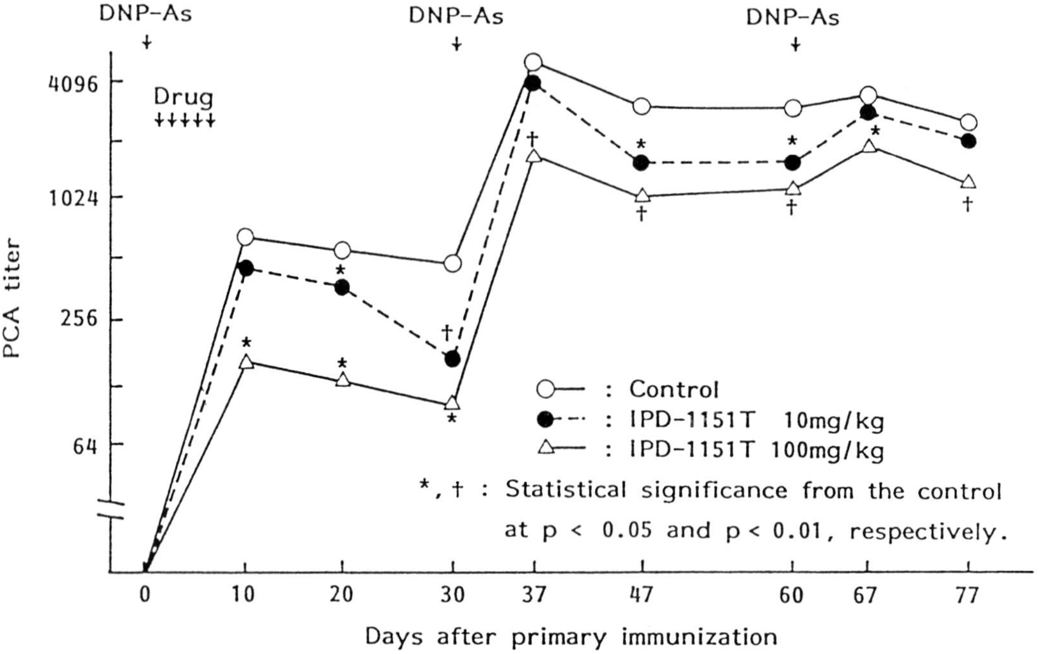

Fig. 2. Effect of IPD-1151T on IgE antibody formation in female BALB/c mice. Mice were immunized with DNP • As and alum on day 0, day 30 and day 60. IPD-1151T was given p. o. for 5 days from the primary immunization. Each group included 5 to 6 animals. Data of 20 mg/Kg and 50 mg/Kg were omitted to avoid complexity.

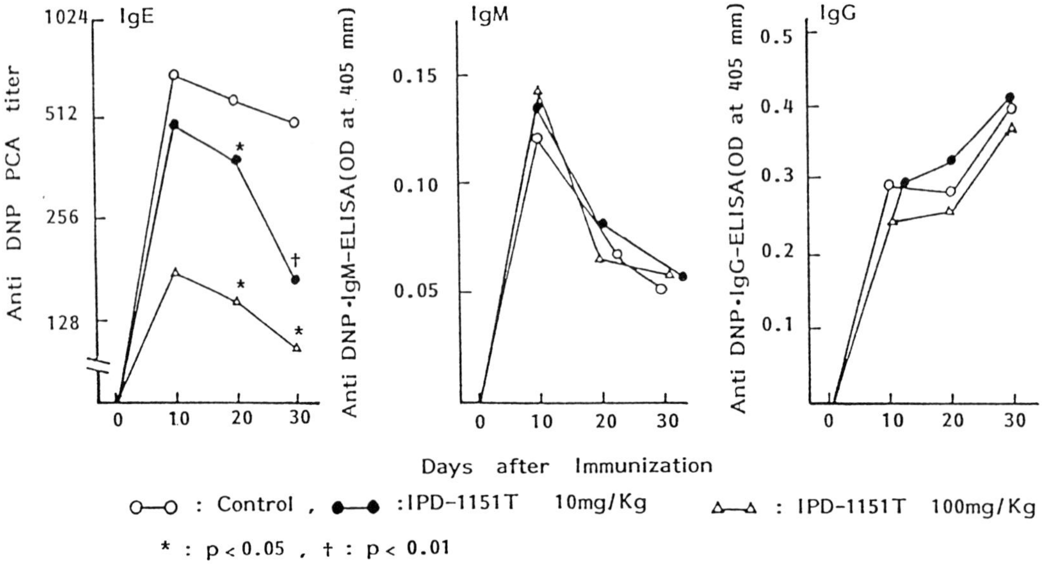

Fig. 3. Effect of IPD-1151T on formations of anti DNP • IgE, IgG and IgM antibodies in mice. Mice were immunized with DNP • As and alum. IPD-1151T was given p. o. for 5 days after the immunization. Each group included 5 to 6 animals.

Table 1. IgE decreased cases and its typical subjects after administration of IPD-1151T in patients of atopic dermatitis.

Total IgE ↓ : 30/59	Specific IgE ↓ : DP ; 29/43 , DF ; 31/43

Case No.	Admini.	Total IgE(IU/ml)		DP (PRU/ml)		DF (PRU/ml)		Clinical efficacy
		Pre	Post	Pre	Post	Pre	Post	
13	10wk	4700	3500	190	110	130	97	+++
28	7wk	5000	4800	30	24	46	24	+++
35	8wk	1300	960	15.0	9.1	1.9	1.9	++
41	10wk	15000	10000	590	550	260	230	+
53	13wk	2300	1400	200	140	130	99	+
56	13wk	7000	5000	290	280	150	130	+
59	12wk	8400	3300	340	140	210	130	+

ies were hardly affected with this agent (Fig. 3). For the experiment on ongoing IgE antibody formation, only the primary immunization was performed with 0.3 mg of DNP • As and 1 mg of alum in the same manner. IPD-1151T was given to mice in a dose of 10 mg/kg/day for 30 days after the immunization when the IgE antibody formation had become nearly constant. Ongoing formation of IgE antibody was inhibited by IPD1151T, whereby a robust statistical significance was found 40 and 50 days after the immunization.

The Effect on Serum IgE Levels and FcεRII⁺ B cell in Atopic Patients with Asthma or Atopic Dermatitis

Table I shows the effect of IPD-1151T on the levels of total and specific IgE in the sera of patients suffering from atopic dermatitis who have received p. o. 300 mg/day of this agent for 6 to 12 weeks. As shown in the upper part of the table, a decrease in the total IgE level assayed by a radioimmunosorbent test (RIST) was found in 30 of 59 cases, and the specific IgE level against *Dermatophagoides pteronyssinus* and *D. farinae* which had been assayed by a radioallergosorbent test (RAST) was decreased in 29 of 43 cases and in 31 of 43 cases, respectively. Representative cases are shown below. Clinical efficacy was observed in close proportion to the decrease of IgE antibody level. Similar results were obtained in asthmatic patients. In addition, the expression of FcεRII on peripheral B cells from such patients was analyzed with a fluorescene-activated cell sorter (FACS 440), and the ratio of $FcεRII^+$ B cell, assayed by two-color FACS analysis with the anti-CD20 and anti-CD23 monoclonal antibodies as previously described (11), was decreased by the administration of IPD-1151T.

The Effect on Human IgE Synthesis and IL-4 Production In Vitro

We have tried to elucidate the mechanism regarding the inhibition of IgE antibody formation by IPD-1151T using a helper T cell line (TCL) responding specifically to sugi (Japanese cedar) basic protein (SBP: Cry J1) (12). This TCL was prepared from peripheral blood lymphocytes of an atopic patient sensitive to Japanese cedar pollen as previously described (13). Since the surface phenotype of this TCL (given the name of SN-4) is $CD3^+$, $CD4^+$, $CD29^+$ and $CD8^-$ as determined by single color FACS analysis, it is a typical helper/helper inducer type of TCL. Autologous B cell suspension containing SN-4 and antigen presenting cell (APC) was incubated with SBP, mite antigen or ovalbumin (OA) for 7 days, and IgE and IgG were assayed in the culture supernatant by

Histamine and Histamine Antagonists in Asthma

Stephen T. Holgate*

Following from the pioneer observations of Dale and Laidlaw in 1919 histamine has been associated with allergen-induced bronchoconstriction and asthma (1). With the recognition that the majority of histamines in human airways are mast cell-derived it is difficult to consider the role of histamine as a mediator without first considering mast cells in asthma.

Mast Cells and Asthma

Mast cells are found throughout the respiratory tract both in the alveolar walls and bronchi. In the latter situation their numbers increase progressively down the respiratory tract with mast cells being located within, or just beneath the bronchial epithelium. The ability of being able to obtain lavage and biopsy samples from the airways has enabled a comparison of the relative number of mast cells in different situations. In mucosal biopsies mast cells identified by the presence of the granule protease tryptase, are present in similar numbers in the submucosa, but are increased in the epithelium of atopic asthmatic compared to non asthmatic subjects. This is in clear contrast to eosinophils whose numbers in asthma are markedly increased in both the epithelium and submucosa (2).

Bronchoalveolar lavage studies have repeatedly shown increased numbers of mast cells in asthma, the number of these cells correlating closely with the mast cell content of the epithelium but not the submucosa. While the number of mast cells and the cell-associated histamine in lavage may be increased 2–4-fold in atopic asthma, histamine measured in the fluid phase is 10–15-fold higher in asthma indicating the increased level of mast cell activation in this disease (Table 1).

Although mast cell numbers may not be increased in the airway submucosa in asthma, transmission electron microscopy shows widespread activation of these cells with both classical degranulation via channel formation and piecemeal secretion compatible with ongoing mediator release (3). That this contributes to air flow limitation in asthma is suggested by showing an increased correlation between mast cell numbers in both BAL and in the epithelium of biopsies ($r = 0.82$, $p < 0.004$).

Bronchial Provocation

In atopic subjects challenge of asthmatic airways with a specific allergen causes both early and late phases of bronchoconstriction (EAR, LAR). Following local allergen challenge via the fibreoptic bronchoscope, the caliber of the airway becomes severely compromised within 3–5 mins with preservation of the definition of the airway wall and subcarina and concentric narrowing of the wall compatible with smooth muscle contraction. The recovery of histamine, PGD_2, tryptase and LTC_4 in increased concentrations from the airway surface by lavage strongly supports the view that the EAR is mast cell dependent, an observation that aligns with

Table 1. Cell-Associated and Cell Free Histamine in BAL of Normal and Asthmatic Subjects.

	Cell-Associated Histamine (ng/ml)	Cell-Free Histamine, ng/ml
Normals (n=13)	1.90 ± 0.61	0.47 ± 0.22
Atopic Asthma (n=21)	6.09 ± 1.29	5.31 ± 1.49
Intrinsic Asthma (n=6)	3.42 ± 0.86	2.60 ± 1.51

* Medicine 1, Level D, Centre Block, Southampton General Hospital, Southampton, and University of Southampton, UK.

the ability of drugs such as sodium cromoglycate and nedocromil sodium to inhibit the response. By contrast the LAR reaches maximum 6–8 hrs after challenge; and being largely composed of an oedematous response, it is likely to be eosinophil dependent with release of such mediators as PGI_2, PGE_2, LTC_4, PAF and the arginine-rich granule proteins.

Exercise is another stimulus which is mast cell dependent and therefore attenuated by sodium cromoglycate and related drugs. Anderson argued that exercise-induced asthma (EIA) occurs secondarily to an increase in the osmolality of the airway lining fluid with mast cells on the airway surface becoming activated by a hyperosmolar stimulus (4). Such a mechanism explains why EIA can be largely reproduced by isocapnic hyperventilation (ICH) and aerosol challenge with hypertonic solution. McFadden suggested that at least a component of EIA results from rebound vasodilation and oedema secondary to hyperventilation-induced cooling of reactive bronchial blood vessels (5). A third possibility which applied more particularly to cold air challenge is involvement of local and vagal reflexes.

Histamine Receptors and Antihistamines

From the foregoing discussion mast cell-derived histamine is likely to be a contributary mediator to allergen and exercise-induced asthma. Since both smooth muscle contraction and increased microvascular permeability are mediated through stimulation of H_1-Receptors, H_1-receptor antagonists should be highly active in attenuating responses involving these processes. It has been shown that the new "selective" non-sedative H_1-antagonists such as terfenadine, azelastine, astemizole and cetirizine are highly effective at protecting asthmatic airways against the constrictor effects of inhaled histamine, especially when compared with the older preparations such as chlorpheniramine and bronpheniramine, 20-fold potency differences being observed (6).

In single doses the newer antihistamines exert a small but consistent bronchodilator action in asthma, supporting the view of ongoing mast cell activation in this disease (7). In addition most of these drugs attenuate the EAR following allergen challenge adding to evidence supporting the mast cell as the primary effector cell of this response (8). However, no matter how high the antihistamine dose, this level of attenuation cannot be exceeded due to the contribution of other mast cell products to the EAR, particularly LTC_4, LTD_4 and prostaglandin D_2 (10,11). Several studies have also shown a protective effect of antihistamines against the LAR (12,13), but with repeated dosing this is lost and is, therefore, likely to be accounted for by the protection afforded by prolonged bronchodilation.

In support of the mast cells' role in EIA, blockade of H_1 receptors attenuates the response, but as with allergen this is limited to 30–50%. The reason for this is the contribution of other mediators, particularly LTC_4 and LTD_4 and probably also from mast cells (14). Antihistamines are more effective at inhibiting the constrictor response to ICH and hypertonic saline (15,16) suggesting that while being mast cell dependent, these stimuli differ slightly from the situation in EIA, and therefore cannot be considered as exact substitutes.

Antihistamines in the Treatment of Asthma

Although a number of clinical studies have suggested therapeutic benefit of antihistamines in asthma the effects are relatively small and limited to mild disease (17,18,19). Although a number of anti-asthma properties other than H_1-receptor blockade have been attributed to some anti-histamines such as mast cell stabilization (azelastine, terfenadine), PAF blockade (ketotifen) and interference with eosinophil functions (azelastine, cetirizine) it is difficult to be certain how these contribute to any observed clinical benefit since most have been studied in organs other than the lung. In the author's opinion the marginal benefit afforded by anti-histamines in the treatment of asthma can largely be accounted for by their H_1 receptor blocking capacity. However, what is clearly needed is a more thorough evaluation of the role of these drugs in asthma treatment both in terms of efficacy and non-H_1-blocking pharmacological actions that may be pertinent to this.

References

1. Dale, H.H., and Laidlaw, P.P. 1910. The physiological action of imidazolethylamine. J. Physiol. (Lond) 41:318.
2. Djukanovic, R., Wilson, J.W., Britten, K.M., Wilson, J.J., Walls, A.F., Roche, W.R., Howarth, P.H., and Holgate, S.T. 1990. Quantitation of mast cells and eosinophils in the bronchial mucosa of symptomatic atopic asthmatics and healthy controls using immunohistochemistry. Am. Rev. Respir. Dis. 142:863.
3. Djukanovic, R., Lai, C.W.K., Wilson, J.W., Britten, K.M., Wilson, S.J., Roche, W.R., Howarth, P.H., and Holgate, S.T. 1992. Bronchial mucosal manifestations of atopy: A comparison of markers of inflammation between atopic asthmatics, atopic non-asthmatics and healthy controls. Eur. Respir. Dis., in press.
4. Smith, C.M., and Anderson, S.D. 1989. A comparison between the airway response to isocapnic hyperventilation and hypertonic saline in subjects with asthma. Eur. Respir. J. 2:36.
5. McFadden, E.R., Lenner, K.A.M., and Strohl, K.P. 1986. Post exertional airway rewarming and thermally induced asthma. New insights into pathophysiology and possible pathogenesis. J. Clin. Invest. 78:18.
6. Wood-Baker, R., and Holgate, S.T. The comparative efficacy and adverse effect profile of single doses of H_1-receptor antagonists in the airways and skin of asthmatic subjects. J. Allergy Clin. Immunol., in press.
7. Ollier, S., Gould, C.L., and Davies, R.J. 1986. The effect of single and multiple dose therapy with azelastine on the immediate asthmatic response to allergen provocation testing. J. Allergy Clin. Immunol. 78:358.
8. Rafferty, P., Beasley, C.R.W., and Holgate, S.T. 1987. The contribution of histamine to immediate bronchoconstriction provoked by inhaled allergen and adenosine 5'-monophosphate in atopic asthma. Am. Rev. Respir. Dis. 136:369.
9. Rafferty, P., and Holgate, S.T. 1989. The inhibitory effect of azelastine hydrochloride on histamine-and allergen-induced bronchoconstriction in atopic asthma. Clin. Exp. Allergy 19:315.
10. Beasley, C.R.W., Featherstone, R.L., Church, M.K., Rafferty, P., Varley, J.G., Harris, A., Robinson, C., and Holgate S.T. 1989. The effect of the thromboxane receptor antagonist–GR32191 on PGD2 and allergen-induced bronchoconstriction. J. Appl. Physiol. 66:1685.
11. Taylor, I.K., O'Shaughnessy, K.M., Fuller, R.W., and Dollery, C.T. 1991. Effect of cysteinyl leukotriene receptor antagonist ICI 204,219 on allergen-induced bronchoconstriction and airway hyperreactivity in atopic subjects. Lancet 337:690.
12. Hamid, M., Rafferty, P., and Holgate, S.T. 1990. The inhibitory effect of terfenadine on early and late-phase bronchoconstriction following allergen challenge in atopic asthma. Clin. Exp. Allergy 20:261.
13. Rafferty, P., Ng, W.H., Phillips, G., Ollier, S., Aurich, G., and Holgate, S.T. 1989. The inhibitory actions of azelastine hydrochloride on early and late bronchoconstriction response to inhaled allergen in atopic asthma. J. Allergy Clin. Immunol. 84:649.
14. Finnerty, J.P., and Holgate, S.T. 1990. The inhibitory effect of terfenadine and flurbiprofen alone and in combination on exercise-induced asthma: Evidence for the roles of histamine and prostaglandins as mediators of the response. Eur. Respir. J. 3:540.
15. Finnerty, J.P., Harvey, A., and Holgate, S.T. 1992 . The relative contributions of histamine and prostanoids to bronchoconstriction provoked by isocapnic hyperventilation in asthma. Eur. Respir. Dis., in press.
16. Finnerty, J.P., Wilmot, J., and Holgate, S.T. 1989. Inhibition of hypertonic saline-induced bronchoconstriction by terfenadine and flurbiprofen: Evidence for the predominant role of histamine. Am. Rev. Respir. Dis. 140:593.
17. Dijkma, J.H., Hekking, P.R.M., Molkenboer, J.F., Nierop, G., et al. 1990. Prophylactic treatment of grass pollen-induced asthma with cetirizine. Clin. Exp. Allergy 20:483.
18. Rafferty, P., Jackson, L., Smith, R., and Holgate, S.T. 1990. Terfenadine, a potent histamine H_1-receptor antagonist in the treatment of grass pollen sensitive asthma. Br. J. Clin. Pharmacol. 30:229.
19. Tinkelman, D.G., Bucholtz, G.A., Kemp, J.P., Koepe, J.W., Repsher, L.H., Spector, S.L., Storms, W.W., and Van As, A. 1990. Evaluation of the safety and efficacy of multiple doses of azelastine to adult patients with bronchial asthma. Am. Rev. Respir. Dis.141:569.

Leukotriene Antagonists and Inhibitors

Anthony W. Ford-Hutchinson*

Leukotrienes are products of arachidonic acid metabolism derived through the action of 5-lipoxygenase in association with 5-lipoxygenase activating protein (FLAP), a novel 18–kD leukocyte membrane protein. Leukotriene B_4 initiates leukocyte and lymphocyte–activation and hence is a potential mediator of inflammation. Leukotriene D_4 receptor activation causes a number of effects, including contraction of smooth muscle, and has been implicated in the pathology of immediate hypersensitivity reactions. Therapeutic approaches to manipulating the leukotriene pathway include leukotriene D_4 receptor antagonists (MK-571 and ICI 204,219), direct 5-lipoxygenase inhibitors (Zileuton) and indirect leukotriene biosynthesis inhibitors (MK-886). The latter class of agents bind to FLAP and hence prevent the activation of 5-lipoxygenase. Leukotriene D_4 receptor antagonists have been shown to inhibit antigen and exercise induced bronchoconstriction, bronchodilate moderate asthmatics and cause improvements in multiple disease parameters during chronic asthma therapy, indicating that leukotrienes may have an important role in the disease. Leukotriene biosynthesis inhibitors, such as Zileuton and MK-886, have shown evidence of biochemical and clinical efficacy. However, a final evaluation of the therapeutic efficacy of inhibitors awaits the development of more potent agents.

Leukotrienes are products of the metabolism of arachidonic acid formed via the 5-lipoxygenase enzyme pathway (Fig. 1) (1). The enzyme, 5-lipoxygenase, differs from other lipoxygenases (12- and 15-lipoxygenase) in two important ways. First, 5-lipoxygenase appears to be present only in cells of the myeloid lineage, including inflammatory cells such as polymorphonuclear leukocytes, mast cells, eosinophils, basophils and macrophages. Secondly, the enzyme has an apparently unique mechanism of activation. Following stimulation of the cell, a rise in intracellular calcium occurs leading to the activation and translocation from the cytosol to the membrane fraction of both phospholipase A_2 and 5-lipoxygenase (2,3). The activation of 5-lipoxygenase occurs in the presence of a novel 18 kD membrane protein which has been termed 5-lipoxygenase activating protein (FLAP) (Fig. 2) (4,5). The 5-lipoxygenase enzyme catalyses a two step catalytic process involving oxygenation to produce the intermediate, 5-hydroperoxyeicosatetraenoic acid, fol-

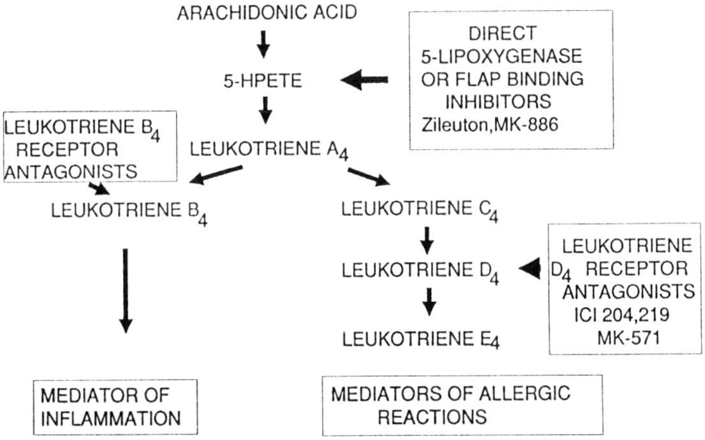

Figure 1. Metabolism of arachidonic acid to leukotrienes.

* Department of Pharmacology, Merck Frosst Centre for Therapeutic Research, P.O. Box 1005, Pointe Claire Dorval, Quebec H9R 4P8 Canada.

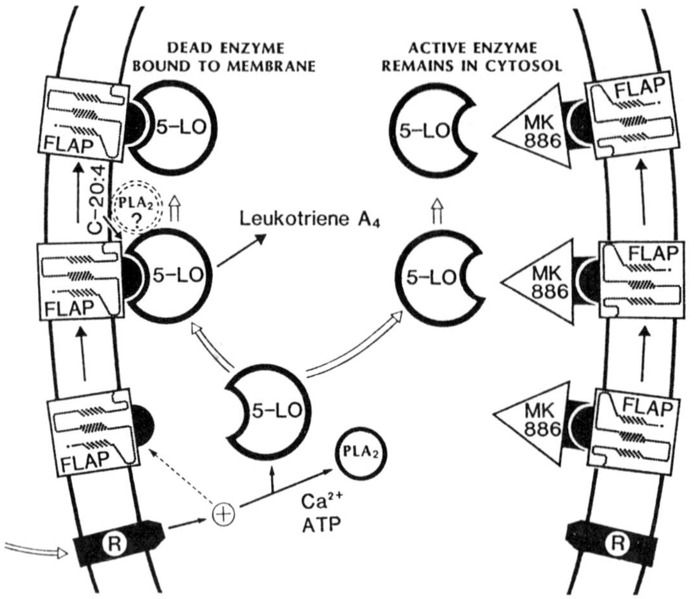

Figure 2. Hypothetical scheme for the involvement of 5-lipoxygenase (5-LO),–5-lipoxygenase activating protein (FLAP) and phospholipase A_2 (PLA_2) in-cellular leukotriene biosynthesis and inhibition of leukotriene biosynthesis by MK-886 (from Ford-Hutchinson et al., Drug News & Perspectives, 1991, 4:271).

lowed by a dehydrase step to produce the epoxide intermediate, leukotriene A_4 (1). There are two distinct enzymes which catalyse the further metabolism of leukotriene A_4 to biologically active products. Leukotriene A_4 hydrolase catalyses the insertion of water into the epoxide to produce the dihydroxyeicosatetraenoic acid, leukotriene B_4. Leukotriene C_4 synthase catalyses a conjugation with glutathione to produce the peptidolipid conjugate, leukotriene C_4. Leukotriene C_4 is in turn converted to leukotriene D_4 by loss of L-glutamic acid through the action of γ-glutamyl transpeptidase. Leukotriene D_4 can then be further metabolised by dipeptidases through loss of glycine to produce leukotriene E_4.

Leukotriene D_4 exerts its biological effects through interactions with a high affinity, structurally specific, G protein coupled receptor present in a variety of smooth muscle preparations (6). In human airway smooth muscle, leukotrienes C_4 and E_4 interact with the same receptor to produce contractile effects. In various animal preparations there is evidence for additional peptidolipid leukotriene receptors (e.g. LTC_4 receptors) although as yet no evidence for these receptors exists in man. Activation of the leukotriene D_4 receptor has been proposed to be an important event in the initiation of various allergic diseases, in particular human bronchial asthma (7,8). The reason why this receptor may be important in human asthma is as follows. First, activation of the receptor results in potent bronchoconstrictor actions in both animals and man and when compared to other vasoactive mast cell derived mediators, such as histamine, leukotriene D_4 is approximately 1000 times more potent and causes more prolonged bronchoconstriction in man (7). Peptidolipid leukotrienes may also be involved in mediating other aspects of decreased airway function, including vascular permeability changes, mucous production and changes in mucocillary clearance. Evidence for leukotriene involvement in the induction of bronchial hyperreactivity is as follows. Administration of a single aerosol dose of leukotriene D_4 to normal subjects caused an increase in the degree of airway narrowing when compared with methacholine as well as a heightening of the level of maximal response to methacholine for a prolonged period of time without affecting the position of the dose response curve (9). Administration of aerosols of leukotriene E_4 to asthmatic subjects, but not to normal individuals, induced not only a bronchoconstriction but also a subsequent increase in responsiveness to methacholine and histamine which persisted for up to 1 week up to challenge (10). There is also evidence for leukotriene production in human bronchial asthma as determined through increased levels of excretion of leukotriene E4 in urine following provocation of sensitive subjects with either antigen or aspirin (11,12).

Leukotriene B4 also has high affinity, structurally specific, G protein coupled receptors which have been most extensively characterized on leukocyte cell surfaces (13). Leukotriene B_4 is a potent stimulator of leukocyte activation and can stimulate a number of leukocyte functions including chemotaxis, chemokinesis, aggregation, adhesion, expression of surface receptors and lysosomal enzyme release (13,14). In addition, leukotriene B_4 may modulate lymphocyte functions, including augmentation of suppressor and natural killer cell activity and potentiation of the production and action of cytokines. Because of these biological properties, the major therapeutic interest in modulating the action of leukotriene B_4 has been in its potential role as a mediator of inflammatory conditions (13). In man considerable attention has focussed on the role of leukotriene B_4 as a possible mediator of inflammatory bowel disease (15).

Therapeutic Approaches to Inhibiting Either the Action or Production of Leukotrienes

Therapeutic interventions in the 5-lipoxygenase enzyme pathway have concentrated on either the antagonism of G protein coupled receptors involved in the transduction of leukotriene actions or in the prevention of synthesis through interference with either the 5-lipoxygenase enzyme directly or with its activation step. Although some medicinal chemistry effort has focussed on the leukotriene B_4 receptor, the majority of work on receptor antagonists has been carried out with the leukotriene D_4 receptor. As a result of this, potent, orally active leukotriene D_4 receptor antagonists have been developed and studied in clinical trials, including compounds such as MK-571 (16) and ICI 204,219 (17).

Blockade of leukotriene biosynthesis can either be carried out by enzymes which directly inhibit the 5-lipoxygenase enzyme or through compounds that interfere with 5-lipoxygenase activation. Direct 5-lipoxygenase inhibitors generally fall into two groups. The first group has been classified as redox compounds and examples of these are the hydroxyurea compound, Zileuton (18), which may act in part by reducing the iron at the active site of the enzyme. A second group of compounds, as exemplified by ICI 211,965, do not possess redox activity and have properties similar to those that would be expected of a fully competitive, reversible inhibitor. Inhibitors of 5-lipoxygenase activation include compounds such as MK-886 (19). MK-886 is a potent inhibitor of leukotriene biosynthesis in a variety of intact leukocyte preparations exposed to a variety of stimuli. However, MK-886 has no effect on either crude or highly purified 5-lipoxygenase enzyme preparations. Evidence for an activation step for 5-lipoxygenase was obtained by Rouzer and Kargman (2) who showed that following cellular activation, 5-lipoxygenase translocated from the cytosol to the cell membrane where it could be detected as "dead" enzyme having undergone suicide inactivation. MK-886 was shown to prevent this translocation and destruction of 5-lipoxygenase, providing the first evidence that the compound might inhibit an activation process (20). MK-886 was also shown, through the use of photoaffinity labels, to bind with high affinity to a novel 18 kD, leukocyte membrane protein (4). The rat protein was isolated through the use of affinity columns and the rat and human proteins cloned and expressed (5). Expression studies in osteosarcoma cells have demonstrated that expression of both 5-lipoxygenase and the 18 kD protein, FLAP, are necessary for both cellular leukotriene biosynthesis and inhibition of this biosynthesis by MK-886 (5). More recently it has been shown that other classes of inhibitors may also work through this mechanism, including quinoline based inhibitors (21).

Leukotriene D_4 Receptor Antagonist: Clinical Result

Results obtained in early clinical trials with leukotriene D_4 receptor antagonists in human bronchial asthma were disappointing reflecting the relatively low potency of these compounds. However, more recently potent leukotriene D_4 receptor antagonists, active in the nM range, have been developed, such as MK-571 (16) and ICI 204,219 (17). Unlike early compounds both these structures have been shown to be potent antagonists of leukotriene D_4 induced bronchoconstriction in either normal volunteers or asthmatic subjects (22,23). In addition, both compounds have been shown to inhibit the early and late phase bronchoconstriction associated with antigen provocation of allergic asthmatic individuals (24,25). In patients with moderate asthma (baseline FEV_1 50–80% predicted), MK-571 has been shown to cause a clinically significant bronchodilatation (~20% increase in FEV_1) within 20 min of initiation of an infusion of the drug, this bronchodilatation being maintained throughout the study period. This bronchodilatation induced by MK-571 appeared to be additive with that produced by inhaled albuterol (26). In these studies the baseline airway obstruction could be correlated with the degree of bronchodilatation achieved with MK-571, suggesting that leukotriene D_4 receptor activation may be proportional to the severity of airway obstruction in asthmatic subjects. ICI 204,219 has also been shown to cause a modest bronchodilatation in asthmatic individuals (27). In addition, MK-571 has shown significant activity against exercise induced bronchoconstriction in asthmatic man (28). MK-571 has been studied in a chronic asthma study at doses of up to 150 mg TID for 4 weeks. During this study, improvements in multiple disease parameters were observed, including increases in FEV_1 and decreases in daytime and nocturnal symptoms as well as agonist inhaler usage (29). These results are consistent with leukotriene D_4 receptor activation being a central event in human bronchial asthma and indicate that potent leukotriene D_4 receptor antagonists should find a place in the therapy and management of human bronchial asthma as well as other allergic diseases.

Leukotriene Biosynthesis Inhibitors: Clinical Trial Results

In man only two leukotriene synthesis inhibitors have shown evidence of biochemical and clinical efficacy. These are the direct 5-lipoxygenase inhibitors, Zileuton (A60477) (18) and the leukotriene biosynthesis inhibitor, MK-886 (19). In terms of biochemical activity in man, both compounds have been shown to inhibit ionophore A23187 induced leukotriene B4 synthesis in whole blood *ex vivo* (30,31). MK-886 has been shown to cause some modest inhibition of the early and late phase asthmatic response to antigen challenge, this being associated with a partial inhibition of the urinary excretion of leukotriene E_4 (32). Zileuton, in addition, has been shown to inhibit bronchoconstriction induced by eucapnic hyperpnea of cold air (31). The compound has also been shown to reduce the amount of leukotriene B_4 present in nasal secretions following antigen challenge, this reduction being associated with some improvement in nasal congestion (33). Finally, Zileuton has been tested in patients with inflammatory bowel disease, where it has been found to decrease the levels of leukotriene B_4 in colonic dialysates (34). There is considerable interest in the potential clinical indications of compounds such as this in this human disease (15).

Conclusions

The biological activities of the peptidolipid leukotrienes are consistent with their playing a role in diseases such as human bronchial asthma. The initial clinical trial results with potent leukotriene D_4 receptor antagonists, such as MK-571 and ICI 204,219, are consistent with leukotriene D_4 receptor activation being an important event in this disease. However, a number of questions remain to be answered with leukotriene D_4 receptor antagonists. These include: (A) Are the results obtained with MK-571 and ICI 204,219 typical of the maximal effects to be seen with a leukotriene D_4 receptor antagonist? (B) What are the effects of prolonged leukotriene D_4 receptor blockade on the etiology of the disease? With regard to the latter point it will be important to investigate the effects of receptor antagonists on bronchial hyperreactivity. This is because leukotrienes have been shown to induce bronchial hyperreactivity in asthmatic subjects, and in animal models leukotriene D_4 receptor activation has been shown to be an important event in antigen induced eosinophil accumulation. It will also be of interest to determine the clinical effects of leukotriene D_4 receptor antagonists in other diseases including allergic rhinitis and allergic conjunctivitis.

For leukotriene biosynthesis inhibitors there remains the key question of what the role of leukotriene B_4 is in the pathology of inflammatory diseases. With regard to inhibitors the field is in a similar situation to that seen following the clinical trials with early leukotriene D_4 receptor antagonists. This is because Zileuton and MK-886 have shown some evidence of clinical efficacy, but in biochemical studies in man have been shown to be incomplete inhibitors of leukotriene biosynthesis. Accordingly it will be necessary to wait for the development of more potent leukotriene biosynthesis inhibitors, which can ensure > 95% blockade of the systemic production of leukotrienes, to fully investigate their potential in various disease states.

References

1. Ford-Hutchinson, A.W. 1990a. Arachidonic acid metabolism enzymatic pathways. In: Eicosanoids and the skin. T. Ruzicka, ed. Boca Raton, Florida: CRC Press, p. 322.
2. Rouzer, C.A., and Kargman, S. 1988. Translocation of 5-lipoxygenase to the membrane in human leukocytes challenged with ionophore A23187. J. Biol. Chem. 263:10980.
3. Clark, J.D., Lin LL, Kriz, R.W., Ramesha, C.S., Sultzman, L.A., Lin, A.Y., Milona, and Knopf, J.L. 1991. A novel arachidonic acid selective cytosolic PLA_2 contains Ca^{2+}-dependent translocation domain with homology to PKC and GAP. Cell 65:1043.
4. Miller, D.K., Gillard, J.W., Vickers, P.J., Sadowski, S., Léveillé, C., Mancini, J.A., Charleson, P., Dixon, R.A.F., Ford-Hutchinson, A.W., Fortin, R., Gauthier, JY., Rodkey, J., Rosen, R., Rouzer, C., Sigal, I.S., Strader, C.D., and Evans, J.F. 1990. Identification and isolation of a membrane protein necessary for leukotriene production. Nature 343:278.
5. Dixon, R.A.F., Diehl, R.E., Opas, E., Rands, E., Vickers, P.J., Evans, J.F., Gillard,J.W., and Miller, D.K. 1990. Requirement of a 5-lipoxygenase activating protein for leukotriene synthesis. Nature 343:282.
6. Lewis, M.A., Mong, S., Vessella, R.L., and Crooke, S.T. 1985. Identification and characterization of leukotriene D_4 receptors in adult and fetal human lung. Biochem. Pharmacol. 34:4311.
7. Piper, P.J. 1985. Leukotrienes: Potent mediators of airway constriction. Int. Arch. Allergy Appl.Immun. 76(Suppl.1):4348.
8. Samuelsson, B. 1983. Leukotrienes: Mediators of immediate hypersensitivity reactions and inflammation. Science 220:568.
9. Bel, E.H., Tanaka, W., Spector, R., Friedman, B., v.d. Veen, H., Dijkman, J.H., and Sterk, P.J. 1990. MK-886, an effective oral leukotriene biosynthesis inhibitor on antigen-induced early and late asthmatic reactions in man. Am. Rev. Respir. Dis. 141:A31.
10. Arm, J.P., Spur, B.W., and Lee, T.H. 1988. The effects of inhaled leukotriene E_4 on the airway responsiveness to histamine in subjects with asthma and normal subjects. J. Allergy Clin. Immunol. 82:654.
11. Taylor, G.W., Taylor, I., Black, P., Maltby, N.H., Turner, N., Fuller, R.W., and Dollery, C.T. 1989. Urinary leukotriene E_4 after antigen challenge in acute asthma and allergic rhinitis. Lancet I:584588.
12. Christie, P.E., Tagari, P., Ford-Hutchinson, A.W., Charleson, S., Chee, P., Arm, J.P., and Lee, T.H. 1991. Urinary leukotriene E_4 concentrations increase after aspirin challenge in aspirin sensitive asthmatic subjects. Am. Rev. Respir. Dis. 143:1025.
13. Ford-Hutchinson, A.W. 1990b. Leukotriene B_4 in inflammation. Crit. Rev. Immunol. 10:112.
14. Ford-Hutchinson, A.W., Bray, M.A., Doig, M.V., Shipley, M.E., and Smith, M.J.H. 1980. Leukotriene B, a potent chemokinetic and aggregating substance released from polymorphonuclear leukocytes. Nature 286:264.
15. Fretland, D.J., Djuric, S.W., and Gaginella, T.S. 1990. Eicosanoids and inflammatory bowel disease: Regulation and prospects for therapy. Prostaglandins Leukot. Essent. Fatty Acids 41:215.
16. Jones, T.R., Zamboni, R., Belley, M., Champion, E., Charette, L., Ford-Hutchinson, A.W., Frenette, R., Gauthier, JY., Leger, S., Masson, P., McFarlane, C.S., Piechuta, H., Rokach, J., Williams, H., Young, R.N., DeHaven, R.N., and Pong, S.S. 1989. Pharmacology of L-660,711 (MK-571): A novel, potent and selective leukotriene D_4 receptor antagonist. Can. J. Physiol. Pharmacol. 67:1728.
17. Krell, R.D., Aharony, D., Buckner, C.K., Keith, R.A., Kesner, E.J., Snyder, D.W., Bernstein, P.R., Matassa, V.G., Yee, Y.K., Brown, F.J., Hesp, B., and Giles, R.E. 1990. The preclinical pharmacology of ICI 204,219. A pep-

tide leukotriene antagonist. Am. Rev. Respir. Dis. 141:978.

18. Carter, G.W., Young, P.R., Albert, D.H., Bouska, J., Dyer, R., Bell, R.L., Summers, J.B., and Brooks, D.W. 1991. 5-lipoxygenase inhibitory activity of Zileuton. J. Pharm. Exp. Therap. 256:929.
19. Gillard, J., Ford-Hutchinson, A.W., Chan, C., Charleson, S., Denis, D., Foster, A., Fortin, R, Leger, S., McFarlane, C.S., Morton, H., Piechuta, H., Riendeau, D., Rouzer, C.A., Rokach, J., Young, R., MacIntyre, D.E., Peterson, L., Bach, T., Eiermann, G., Hopple, S., Humes, J., Hupe, L., Luell, S., Metzger, J., Meurer, R., Miller, D.K., Opas, E., and Pacholok, S. 1989. L-663,536 (MK-886) (3-[1-(4-chlorobenzyl)-3-t-butyl-thio-5-isopropylindol-2-yl]-2,2-dimethylpropanoic acid), a novel, orally active leukotriene biosynthesis inhibitor. Can. J. Physiol. Pharmacol. 67:456.
20. Rouzer, C.A., Ford-Hutchinson, A.W., Morton, H.E., and Gillard, J.W. 1990. MK-886, a potent and specific leukotriene biosynthesis inhibitor blocks and reverses the membrane association of 5-lipoxygenase in ionophore challenged leukocytes. J. Biol. Chem. 265:1436.
21. Evans, J.F., Léveillé, C. Mancini, J.A., Prasit, P., Thérien, M. Zamboni, R., Gauthier, J.Y., Fortin, R., Charleson, P., MacIntyre, D.E., Luell, S., Bach, T.J., Meurer, R., Guay, J., Vickers, P.J., Rouzer, C.A., Gillard, J.W., and Miller, D.K. 1991. 5-lipoxygenase-activating protein is the target of a quinoline class of leukotriene synthesis inhibitors. Mol. Pharmacol. 40:22.
22. Kips, J., Joos, G., DeLepeleire, I., Margolskee, D., Buntinx, A., Pauwels, R., and Van-der Straeten, M. 1991. MK-571: A potent antagonist of LTD_4 induced bronchoconstriction in man. Am. Rev. Respir. Dis. 144:617.
23. Smith, L.J., Geller, S., Ebright, L., Glass, M., and Thyrum, P.T. 1990. Inhibition of leukotriene (LT) D_4 induced bronchoconstriction in asthmatic subjects by the oral LTD_4 receptor antagonist ICI 204,219. Am. Rev. Respir. Dis. 141:A33.
24. Hendeles, L., Davison, D., Blake, K., Harman, E., Cooper, R., and Margolskee, D. 1990. Leukotriene D_4 is an important mediator of antigen induced bronchoconstriction: Attenuation of dual response with MK-571, a specific LTD_4 receptor antagonist. J. Allergy Clin. Immunol. 85:197 (Abstr.).
25. Taylor, I.K., O'Shaughnessy, K.M., Fuller, R.W., and Dollery, C.T. 1991. Effect of cysteinyl-leukotriene receptor antagonist ICI 204,219 on allergen induced bronchoconstriction and airway hyperreactivity in atopic subjects. Lancet 337:690.
26. Gaddy, J., Bush, R.K., Margolskee, D., Williams, V.C., and Busse, W. 1990. The effects of a leukotriene D_4 (LTD_4) antagonist (MK-571) in mild to moderate asthma. J. Allergy Clin Immunol. 85:197 (Abstr.).
27. Hui, K.P., and Barnes, N.C. 1991. Lung function improvement in asthma with acysteinyl-leukotriene receptor antagonist. Lancet 337:1062.
28. Manning, P.J., Watson, R.M., Margolskee, D.J., Williams, V.C., Schwartz, J.I., and O'Byrne, P.M. 1990. Inhibition of exercise induced bronchoconstriction by MK-571, a potent leukotriene D_4 receptor antagonist. N. Engl. J. Med. 323:1736.
29. Margolskee, D., Bodman, S., Dockhorn, R., Israel, E., Kemp, J., Mansmann, H., Minotti, D.A., Spector, S., Stricker, W., Tinkelman, D., Townley, R., Winder, J., and Williams, V. 1991. The therapeutic effects of MK-571, a potent and selective leukotriene (LT) D_4 receptor antagonist, in patients with chronic asthma. J. Allergy Clin. Immunol. 87:309 (Abstr).
30. Tanaka, W., Dallob, A., Winchell, G., Kline, W., Spector, R., Bjornsson, T., and DeSchepper, P. 1990. Safety, pharmacokinetics and leukotriene B_4 (LTB4) inhibition after MK-886 administration in normal male volunteers. Am. Rev. Respir. Dis. 141:A32.
31. Israel, E., Dermarkarian, R., Rosenberg, M., Sperling, R., Taylor, G., Rubin, P., and Drazen, J.M. 1990. The effects of 5-lipoxygenase inhibitor on asthma induced by cold, dry air. N. Engl. J. Med. 323:1740.
32. Bel, E.H., van der Veen, H., Kramps, J.A., Dijkman, J.H., and Sterk, P.J. 1987. Maximal airway narrowing to inhaled leukotriene D_4 in normal subjects. Comparison and interaction with methacholine. Am. Rev. Respir. Dis. 136:979.
33. Knapp, H.R. 1990. Reduced allergen induced nasal congestion and leukotriene synthesis with an orally active 5-lipoxygenase inhibitor. N. Engl. J. Med. 323:1745.
34. Laursen, L.S., Naesdal, J., Bukhave, K., Lauritsen, K., and Raskmadsen, J. 1990. Selective 5-lipoxygenase inhibition in ulcerative colitis. Lancet 335:683.

New Antiasthmatic Drugs of Plant Origin

W. Dorsch*, H. Wagner**

Several plants and plant extracts which are used in traditional medicine have been investigated in order to identify antiasthmatic or antiinflammatory compound(s) and their mode of action. As active compounds in onion extracts (Allium cepa), thiosulfinates and cepaenes have been identified. They exert a wide spectrum of pharmacologic activities, both *in vitro* and *in vivo*. Tetragalloyl quinic acid and other gallic acid derivatives from Galphimia glauca suppressed allergen- and PAF-induced bronchial obstruction, PAF-induced bronchial hyperreactivity (5 mg/kg orally, 0.5 mg as aerosol) *in vivo* and thromboxane biosynthesis *in vitro*. Hitherto unknown alkaloids from Adhatoda vasica showed pronounced protection against allergen-induced bronchial obstruction in guinea pigs (10 mg/ml aerosol). Androsin from Picrorhiza kurroa prevented allergen- and PAF-induced bronchial obstruction in guinea pigs (10 mg/kg, orally). Chemical modification of Androsin and its aglykon increased markedly their pharmacological activity. We are now proceeding to test for the pharmacological effects in man.

There are many plants and plant extracts which are used for the treatment of bronchial asthma and other inflammatory diseases in the traditional medicine of various countries. In most of the cases, however, detailed pharmacological investigations and clinical trials which could confirm these claims, are lacking. Furthermore the active principles are either totally unknown or identified only in part. Therefore we have started a systematic screening program in order to identify active components of these plants and their mode of action. As chemical methods different chromatographic procedures, HPLC, MPLC, UV-, mass-, 1H and 13C-NMR-spectroscopy have been used. Whole plant extracts, fractionated extracts and pure compounds were tested by the following pharmacological test systems: cyclooxygenase and 5-lipoxygenase pathway of arachidonic acid metabolism, bronchial obstruction of guinea pigs after inhalation of allergens, PAF, histamine or acetylcholine, PAF-induced bronchial hyperreactivity of guinea pigs, histamine release, chemoluminescence and chemotaxis of human polymorphonuclear leukocytes as well as thromboxane biosynthesis of human platelets (1). This paper gives a short review of our actual results: (A) Onions (Allium cepa) were cultivated 6,000 years ago in the Middle East. The Egyptian Papyros Ebers describes the use of onions in a number of major and minor disorders. In 1983 we reported on antiasthmatic and antiinflammatory properties of onion extracts. (B) Galphimia glauca (Thyrallis glauca), abundant in Middle and South America, is prescribed from *curanderos* of some tribes in the rain forest of Brasil against allergies. (C) Picrorrhiza kurroa grows in the Himalayan mountains at altitudes of 3,000-5,000 meters. The Ayurvedic medicine uses extracts of its roots mainly for the treatment of liver and lung diseases, but also for chronic dysentery and other complaints. Controlled trials in different arthritic conditions showed marked improvement of clinical symptoms. (D) Extracts from Adhatoda vasica are widely used in India against cough, bronchitis and bronchial asthma. The active principle is unknown. A broncholytic activity of vasicinon has been reported, but this alkaloid becomes rapidly converted into the bronchoconstrictive alkaloidvasicin.

Material and Methods

Plant Material

The plant material was purchased from German, Indian and Mexican drug companies. Specimens of all plants are deposited in the herbarium of the Institute of Pharmaceutical Biology, Munich.

* Childrens Hospital of the Johannes Gutenberg University, D-6500 Mainz, Germany;
** Institute of Pharmaceutic Biology, Ludwig Maximilian University, Munich, Germany.

Chemical Methods

The fractionation of the extracts was performed partly by classical solvent extraction and silicagel or sephadex column chromatography using various solvent systems or by application of middle and high pressure liquid chromatographic procedures. The structure of the isolated compounds were elucidated by ultraviolet-, infrared, proton-, carbon- and mass-spectroscopy with all modern variants, i. e., 2D-NMR, COSY and NOE-experiments. In some cases X-ray spectroscopy was used.

Inhalation Challenge in Guinea Pigs

Male Pirbright guinea pigs were sensitized by intraperitoneal and intramuscular injection of ovalbumin as described previously (2). Inhalation challenge tests were performed 4 to 6 weeks later according to a randomized cross-over protocol on groups of at least ten animals. Ovalbumin, histamine hydrochloride and acetylcholine were dissolved in saline (1:99, 1:999, 1:99: w/v), while platelet activating factor (PAF) was first dissolved in ethanol and then in saline containing 0.25% bovine serum albumin yielding a final concentration of 1 μg PAF/ml. All solutions were nebulized ultrasonically (Heyer USE 77, size of droplets 3–5 μm). Ovalbumin was given twice (at time 0 and 10 min) for 20 or 40 secs., while PAF, histamine and acetylcholine were administered only once for 90, 20 or 20 secs, respectively. Lung function measurements were performed by whole body plethysmography on spontaneously breathing animals (2,3). The degree of bronchial obstruction was estimated by the parameter "compressed air". This highly sensitive parameter (3) reflects the air volume by which intrathoracic gas volume has to be compressed in order to overcome an acute bronchoconstriction. The results of other pharmacological tests have been or will be published elsewhere.

Statistics

All figures and tables in this paper show mean values and standard deviations (SD). The statistic significance of differences was estimated using Student's t-test for unpaired data. The degree of "percent inhibition" was calculated by comparing maximal values after control (solvent) treatment (100%) with maximal values after active treatment (x%). The statistical significance of percent inhibition was estimated by Student's t-test and the Wilcoxon test for paired data.

Results and Discussion

Allium Cepa (Onions)

Cepaenes and thiosulfinates have been identified as biologically active compounds in onion juice (4–7). These compounds are not present in the intact bulb. They are generated enzymatically from genuine sulfur containing amino acids upon violation of the plant by, e.g., squeezing or slicing. Zwiebelanes seem to be a luxury product of onion chemistry without pronounced pharmacological properties. Cepaenes, hitherto unknown compounds, are by far the most active known inhibitors of the lipoxygenase pathway of arachidonic acid metabolism found in plants or plant extracts (5). The effects on cyclooxygenase are less pronounced. Platelet function and thromboxane biosynthesis have been shown to be reduced (4). Both compounds are highly active in inhibiting the chemotaxis of human polymorphonuclear cells (8). In experimental animals onion extracts, onion derived and synthetic thiosulphinates are able to counteract allergen- and PAF-induced bronchial obstruction as well as PAF-induced bronchial hyperreactivity (9,10). In man, topical onion extracts are able to depress immediate and late allergic skin reactions (11). Similarly, immediate and late bronchial obstruction after allergen inhalation challenges were markedly suppressed in volunteers after the oral intake of ethanolic onion extract prepared from 200 grams of onions (7). Pharmacological data on pure, i.e., synthetic compounds are not available as yet. A good deal of work including toxicology has to be done in this field. Ethanolic onion extracts can hardly be used in the treatmet of asthmatics. The specific smell would render the patient a social outcast. We are trying to improve onion extracts with regard to smell, stability and reproducibility of their pharmacologic effects. We are now in possession of onion capsules which might be suitable for the use in patients (Fig. 1).

Figure 1. Pharmacology of onions.

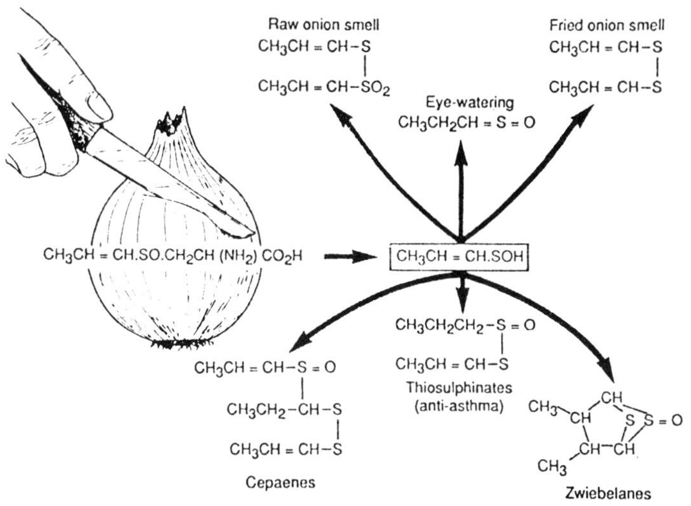

Galphimia glauca

Guinea pigs pretreated with a methanolic extract from Galphimia glauca (320 mg/kg, orally) are protected almost totally against bronchial obstruction due to the inhalation of ovalbumin or PAF. This was observed not only 1 or 12 hours after one single dose as shown here, but even after 4 days (12). A stepwise fractionation of the extract led to the discovery of gallic acid derivatives as active compounds (13). Tetragalloyl quinic acid showed the highest activity: the oral dose of 5 mg/kg reduced bronchial reactions of guinea pigs to allergen by 86 ± 24% (n = 12), $p < 0.01$, (Figs. 2 and 3) and to PAF by 60 ± 24% (n = 12, $p < 0.01$). Methyl gallate, gallic acid and quercetin demonstrated approximately the same activity in preventing the allergen induced bronchial obstruction. Methyl gallate was more effective on the PAF-induced bronchial obstruction. Its antiasthmatic property was superior to a mixture of quercetin and gallic and protocatechic acid (Table II). Extracts and/or active compounds from Galphimia glauca achieve their full antiasthmatic activity with time: PAF and ovalbumin dependent bronchial reactions of animals receiving 2 mg/kg, three times a day for each of 3 days, of

Figure 2. Inhibition of allergen-induced bronchial obstruction in 12 guinea pigs by the oral pretreatment with 5 mg/kg tetragalloyl quinic acid 2 hours prior to the sequential inhalation of 1% ovalbumin aerosol (time 0 and 10 min, 30 and 60 secs); x: $p < 0.05$, xx: $p < 0.01$; xxx: $p < 0.001$; t-test for unpaired data, percent inhibition of bronchial obstruction: 86% ± 24%, $p < 0.01$, 60% ± 43%, $p > 0.05$); control: broken line; tetragalloyl quinic acid: solid line.

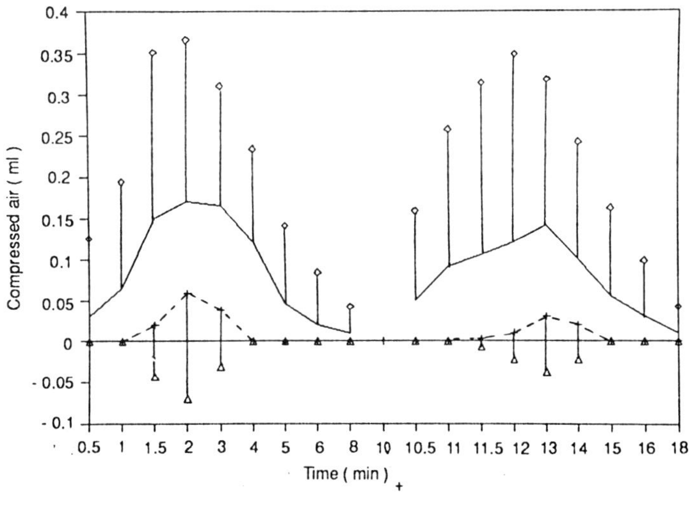

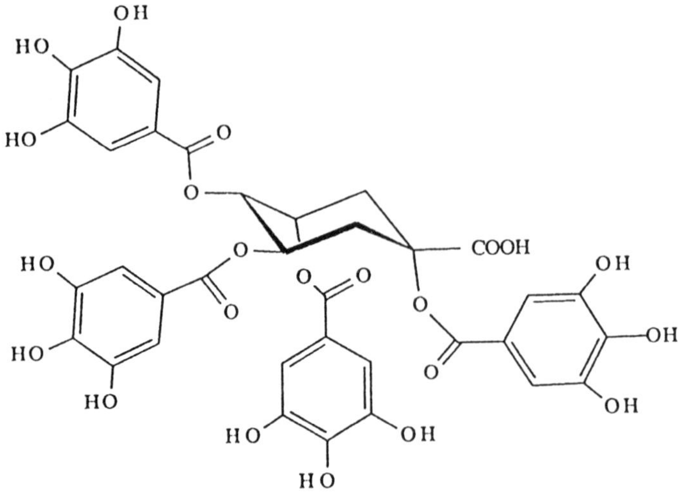

Figure 3. Chemical structure of tetra-galloyl quinic acid.

fraction GG II containing tetragalloyl quinic acid as main constituent (10%) and other gallic acid derivatives were reduced by more than 70% (Table I, and Fig. 4). As with acute PAF-induced bronchial obstruction, the PAF-induced bronchial hyperreactivity was markedly depressed by both the methanolic whole plant extract and by methyl gallate. Bronchial reactions to inhalation challenges with histamine or acetylcholine were altered neither by the methanolic whole plant extract nor by methyl gallate.

Picrorrhiza kurroa

Roots of the plant were extracted by complete Soxhlet extraction using the following solvents: hexane, chloroform, ethyl-acetate and metha-

Table I: Galphimia Glauca

Fractions/ Compunds (dose)		Percent Inhibition of Bronchial Obstruction after Allergen Inhalation 1st challenge	2nd challenge	PAF Inhalation
Fraction II	(30 mg/kg)	55% ± 52%#	54% ± 28%$^{+}$	51% ± 32%*
Fraction I	(30 mg/kg)			–12% ± 35%^{ns}
Fraction III	(30 mg/kg)	–19% ± 68%^{ns}	–22% ± 65%^{ns}	18% ± 24%^{ns}
SubfractionII/1	(30 mg/kg)	59% ± 32%*	43% ± 46%#	57% ± 29%#
SubfractionII/2	(30 mg/kg)	28% ± 69%^{ns}	25% ± 51%^{ns}	22% ± 45%^{ns}
Methyl gallate	(45 mg/kg)	43% ± 34%*	41% ± 24%$^{+}$	65% ± 24%+
Gallic acid	(45 mg/kg)	37% ± 35%#	40% ± 31%*	
Quercetin	(45 mg/kg)	53% ± 23%*	34% ± 33%#	
Mixture 1	(45 mg/kg)			36% ± 45%#
Tetragalloyl quinic acid	(5 mg/kg)	86% ± 24%§	60% ± 43%^{ns}	60% ± 43%§
Fraction GG II (3 days, 2 mg/kg T.I.D)		75% ± 63%§		71% ± 38%

Effect of fractions and pure compounds from Galphimia glauca on bronchial reactions of at least 12 guinea pigs in each group to inhalation challenges with allergen (oval bumin) and platelet activating factor. The test material or adequate control solutions were given orally 1 hour, in the case of tetragalloyl quinic acid 2 hours, prior to the inhalation test. Fraction GG II was given three times a day for 3 days each at a dosage of 2 mg/kg. Finally, 1 hour after the last dose the inhalation challenges were performed. #: $p < 0.05$; *: $p < 0.02$; +: $p < 0.001$; ns: not significant (t-test for paired data).

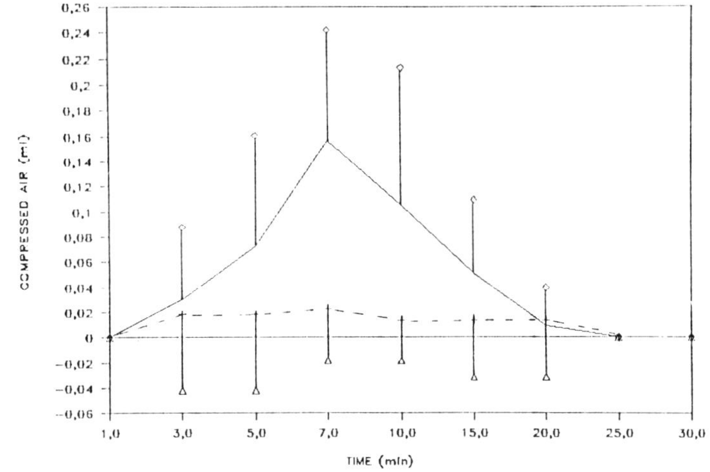

Figure 4. Prevention of PAF-induced bronchial obstruction in ten guinea pigs by repeated treatment with three daily dosages of 2 mg/kg fraction GGII from Galphimia glauca over 3 days prior to the inhalation of PAF-aerosol (1 µg/ml, 90 secs, percent inhibition of bronchial obstruction: 71% ± 38%, $p < 0.01$); control: broken line; fraction GGII: solid line.

nol. The methanol-extract was divided into a water soluble and a butanol soluble subfraction. Both failed to alter histamine release from human peripheral leukocytes and PAF-induced bronchial obstruction in guinea pigs. The chloroform and ethyl acetate fractions in contrast demonstrated significant effects on histamine release. Both fractions showed almost identical chromatographic characteristics. Using the ethyl acetate fraction we observed marked inhibitory effects on PAF- and allergen-induced bronchial obstruction of sensitized guinea pigs. The ethyl acetate fraction was divided by sephadex chromatography into two subfractions. The former contained cucurbitacin glycosides and was found to be inactive. Similarly, the major component of this fraction, the cucurbitacinglycosid Cuc3 (25-Acetoxy-2-beta-D-glucosyloxy- 3,16,20- trihydroxy-19-norlanosta-5,23-diene-22-one) showed no significant effect. The active fraction was divided into the inactive subfraction PIC containing Pikrosid II, minecosids, veronicosid and 6-trans- feruloylctalpol and the active subfraction containing picroside 1 (Pic 1) and androsin as major compounds. Pic 1 did not affect the allergen-induced bronchial obstruction. Androsin in contrast demonstrated significant inhibitory effects on bronchial reactions to the inhalation of allergen and PAF. The inhalation of androsin was much more effective than the oral route (Fig. 5). Chemical modifications of androsin

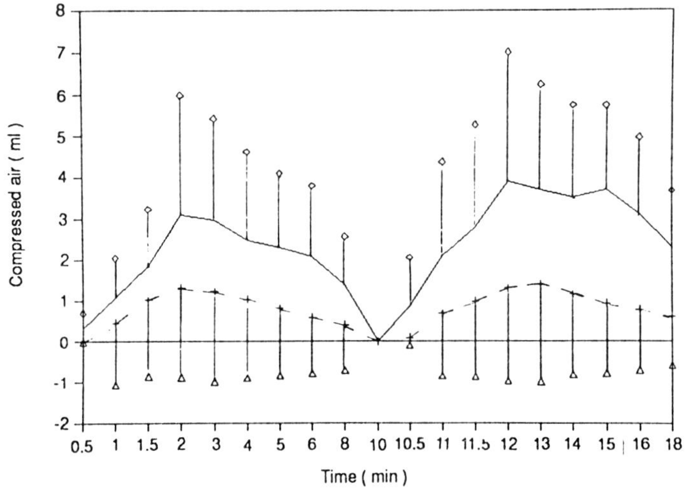

Figure 5. Prevention of allergen-induced bronchial obstruction in ten guinea pigs by the oral intake of 10 mg/kg androsin 1 hour prior to the inhalation of ovalbumin (percent inhibition of bronchial obstruction: 57% ± 50%, $\pi < 0.05$, 71 ± 38%, $p < 0.01\%$, respectively); control: broken line; Androsin: solid line.

Table II: Picrorrhiza kurroa

Fractions/ Compounds (dose)		Percent Inhibition of Bronchial Obstruction after Allergen Inhalation 1st challenge	2nd challenge	PAF Inhalation
Androsin	(0,6 mg)	67% ± 34%~	34% ± ns	72% ± 39%#
Apocynine	(0,5 mg)	76% ± 48%~	64% ± 59%*	
	(0,34 mg)			65% ± 42%#
DMHA	(0,5 mg)	83% ± 27%#	86% ± 24%~	44% ± 67%*
Methoxy-Androsin	(0,5 mg)	71% ± 61%*	75% ± 21%#	79% ± 35%~
Picein	(0,6 mg)	ns		ns
HMHAG	(0,5 mg)	ns	38% ± 34%*	
HHAG	(0,5 mg)	33% ± 43%*	42% ± 17%#	
VG	(0,5 mg)	64% ± 44%*	ns	

Effect of Androsin and related compounds on bronchial reactions of at least 12 guinea pigs in each group to inhalation challenges with allergen (1% ovalbumin aerosol, twice at times 0 and 10 min, and at 30 and 60 secs.) and platelet activating factor (1 µg/ml aerosol, once at 90 secs.).The test material or adequate control solutions were given by inhalation 30 min. prior to the inhalation test. #: $p < 0.05$; *: $p < 0.02$; +: $p < 0.001$; ns: not significant (t-test for paired data). Abbreviations:
DMHA: 3,5-dimethoxy-4-hydroxy-acetophenon;
HMHAG: 2-hydroxy-3-methyl-4-hydroxy-acetophenon-4-O-glycoside;
HHAG: 2-hydroxy-4-hydroxy-acetophenon-4-O-glycoside;
VG: Vanillin-O-glycoside.

or its aglykon, apocynine, markedly improved the pharmacologic activity (Table II, and Figs. 6 and 7). Bronchial reactions of the animals to histamine and acetylcholine were not altered by androsin. Androsin did not affect hista mine release of human peripheral leukocytes (14,15).

Adhatoda vasica

Extracts from Adhatoda vasica leaves are widely used in India to treat cough, bronchitis, and bronchial asthma. There are some data on the broncholytic activity of vasicinon, but this alkaloid rapidly becomes converted into the bron-

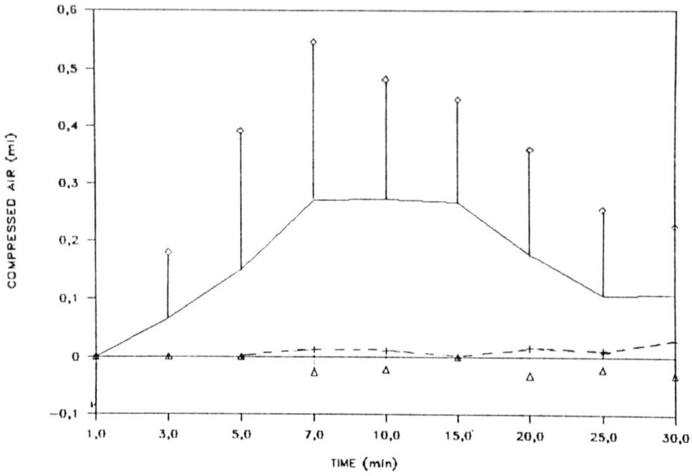

Figure 6. Prevention of PAF-induced bronchial obstruction in 10 guinea pigs by the oral intake of 10 mg/kg 3-5 dimethoxy-4-hydroxy-acetophenon 30 min. prior to the inhalation of PAF-aerosol (1 µg/ml, 90 secs, percent inhibition of bronchial obstruction: 90 ± 21 %, $p < 0.01$); control: broken line; acetophenon: solid line.

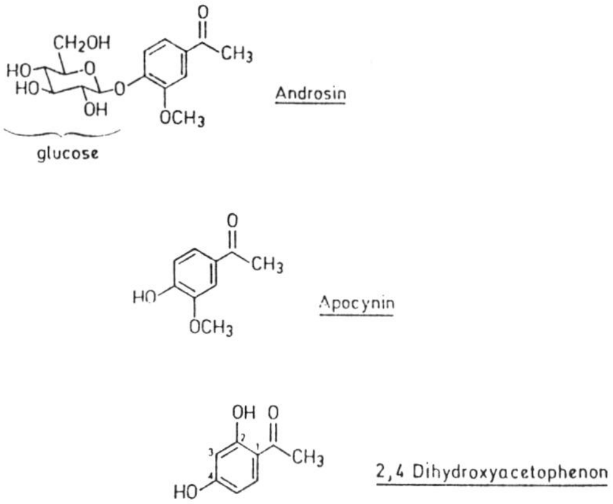

Figure 7. Chemical structure of Androsin and its derivatives.

choconstrictive vasicin. We were able to demonstrate marked protection of guinea pigs against allergen induced bronchoconstriction. Sequential fractionation of this extract led to the discovery of other alkaloids than vasicinon/vasicin (Fig. 8, and references 16,17).

Conclusions

Most of the antiasthmatic drugs used today are related to plants or plant extracts used in traditional medicine. Attempts at treating asthma have already been documented from early historical times, and we have useful findings from their experience as in many fields of medicine. Five thousand years ago in China, extracts from Ma Huang (Ephedra vulgaris) were used for the treatment of asthmatics. Instead of Ephedrin, we now use synthetic betasympathicomimetics which act directly and are highly bronchoselective. Tea, the source of theophyllin, comes from China, too. 500 years ago in Europe the smoke of Atropa belladonna leaves and related plants were inhaled by asthmatics, while today we use synthetic anticholinergics. The development of disodium cromoglycate was initiated by the discovery of antiasthmatic properties of Khellin, the active agent of an old Egyptian plant named Ammi visnaga. By following this old tradition, we have in fact been able to detect new antiasthmatic acting constituents in plants or plant extracts.

References

1. Dorsch, W., and Wagner, H. Development of new antiasthmatic drugs from traditional medicine? Int. Arch. Allergy Appl. Immunol., in press.
2. Dorsch, W., Waldherr, U., and Rosmanith, J. 1981. Continuous recording of intrapulmonary "compressed air" as a sensitive noninvasive method of measuring bronchial obstruction in guinea pigs. Pflrs. Arch. 391:236.
3. Dorsch, W., and Hess, V. 1991. Computerized lung function analysis in small animals: The Labtec Lung Function System, -XIV. International Congress of Allergology and Clinical Immunology, Kyoto, 1991, Abstract Nr. 0136.

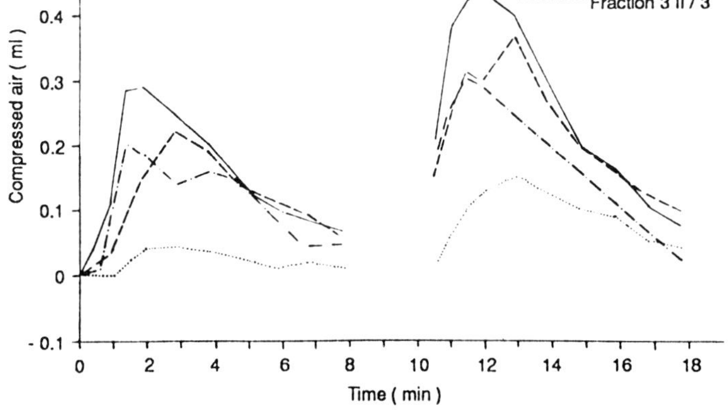

Figure 8. Prevention of allergen-induced bronchial obstruction in 10 guinea pigs by the inhalation of different fractions from Adhatoda vasica 1 hour prior to the inhalation of 1% ovalbumin aerosol (time 0 and 10 min, 30 and 60 secs), fraction 3 II/1 contains new alkaloids yet to be identified.

4. Dorsch, W., Wagner, H., Bayer, Th., Fessler, B., Hein, G., Ring, J., Scheftner, P., Sieber, W., Strasser, Th., and Weiss, E. 1988. Antiasthmatic effects of onions: Alk(en)ylsulfinothioic acid alk(en)ylesters inhibit histamine release, leukotriene and thromboxane biosynthesis *in vitro* and counteract PAF-and allergen-induced bronchial obstruction *in vivo*. Biochem. Pharmacol. 37:4479.
5. Bayer, Th.H., Wagner, H., Wray, V., and Dorsch, W. 1988. New inhibitors of cyclooxygenase and 5-lipoxygenase from lipophilic onion extracts. The Lancet Oct. 15:906.
6. Wagner, H., Dorsch, W., Bayer, Th., Breu, W., and Willer, F. 1990. Antiasthmatic effects of onions: Inhibition of 5-lipoxygenase and cycloxygenase *in vitro* by thiosulfinates and "cepaenes". Prostaglandins, Leukotrienes and Essential Fatty Acids 39:59.
7. Dorsch, W., Adelmann-Grill, B., Bayer, T., Ettl, M., Hein,. G, Jaggy, H., Ring, J., Scheftner, P., Schneider, T., and Wagner, H. 1987. Zwiebelextrakte als Asthma-Therapeutika? Allergologie 10:316.
8. Dorsch, W., Schneider, E., Bayer, Th., Breu, W., Wagner, H. 1990. Antiinflammatory effects of onions: Inhibition of chemotaxis of human polymorphonuclear cells by thiosulfinates and cepaenes. Int. Arch. Allergy Appl. Immunol. 92:39.
9. Dorsch, W., and Weber, J. 1984. Prevention of allergen-induced bronchial obstruction by crude alcoholic onion extract. Agents & Actions 14:626.
10. Dorsch, W., Scharff J., Bayer, T., and Wagner, H. 1988. Antiasthmatic effects of onions: prevention of PAF-induced bronchial hyperreactivity to histamine in guinea pigs by diphenylthiosulfinate. Int. Arch. Allergy Appl. Immunol. 88:228.
11. Dorsch, W., and Ring, J. 1984. Suppression of immediate and late cutaneous allergic skin reactions by alcoholic onion extrakt applied topically. Allergy 39:43.
12. Wagner, H., Dorsch, W., Bittinger, M., and Koch, S. 1989. Long lasting antiasthmatic effects of extracts from galphimia glauca. Allergologie 12:139.
13. Dorsch, W., Bittinger, M., Kaas, A., Meer, A., Kreher, B., and Wagner, H. Antiasthmatic effects of Galphimia Glauca: Gallic acid and related compounds prevent allergen- and PAF-induced bronchial obstruction as well as bronchial hyperreactivity in guinea pigs. Int. Archs. Allergy Appl. Immunol., in press.
14. Dorsch, W. Stuppner, H., Wagner, H., Gropp, M., Demoulin, S., and Ring, J. Antasthmatic effects of Picrorrhiza Kurroa: Androsin prevents allergen- and PAF-induced bronchial obstruction in guinea pigs. Int. Archs. Allergy Appl. Immunol., in press.
15. Kepler, P., Stuppner, H., Wagner, H., Gropp, M., and Dorsch, W. 1991. Asthmaschutzwirkung von Picrorhiza kurroa: Androsin, Apocynin und verwandte Substanzen behindern das allergische und das PAF-induzierte Asthma bronchiale von Meerschweinchen. Allergologie 14:85.
16. Grampp, M., Koch, S., Wagner, H., and Dorsch, W. 1989. New antiasthmatic alcaloids from Adhatoda vasica. Allergologie 12:125.
17. Dorsch, W., Dumoulin, S., Stuppner, H., and Wagner, H. 1990. Screening of drugs of traditional medicine for new @TAB-

Recent Insights into the Mechanisms of Anti-Inflammatory Steroid Action

Robert P. Schleimer, Bruce S. Bochner*

The clinical efficacy of glucocorticoids in allergic diseases such as asthma, hayfever, etc., is widely accepted. In fact, most clinical practitioners believe that steroids are the most effective anti-allergic drugs available. Clinical experimentation reveals that glucocorticoids inhibit the delayed response to experimental challenge with allergen in allergic individuals (the so-called late phase response: LPR) (1). Although brief administration of topically applied or oral steroids fails to inhibit the acute anaphylactic response to antigen challenge in a local site such as the skin or lungs, prolonged application of topical steroids in the nose or the lungs can dampen the acute response somewhat. The purpose of this review is to discuss recent insights into the mechanisms of anti-inflammatory steroid action that are of relevance to their therapeutic efficacy in allergic diseases. This is not a comprehensive review but consists of a brief overview of general steroid actions followed by a discussion of the mechanisms by which steroids inhibit the recruitment of inflammatory cells to a local site of exposure to allergen, an effect which is felt to be among the most important of steroid actions in this context. For more extensive discussions of the mechanisms of steroid action, the reader is referred to other sources (2–5).

Overview of Anti-Inflammatory Steroid Actions In Vivo

Effects of Steroids on Neuromuscular Responses

Very little literature is available discussing the direct actions of glucocorticoids on the function of either muscle or nerve cells. However, *in vivo* it is clear that glucocorticoids can influence airway and vascular smooth muscle responses to β-adrenergic modulating systems. Potentiation of the ability of β-adrenergic agonists to relax airway smooth muscle by glucocorticoids can improve the efficacy of administered β-agonists and may help prevent the development of resistance to β-adrenergic agonists (6). A variety of *in vitro* studies suggest that glucocorticoids potentiate β-adrenergic effects by increasing β-adrenergic receptors, increasing receptor-cyclase coupling, and inducing G-protein synthesis (7). Considerable interest is now being focussed on the role of neuropeptides in the control of airway smooth muscle function. Recent studies have indicated that glucocorticoids can upregulate neutral endopeptidase and other peptidases, modifying neuropeptide responses by hastening the degradation of neuropeptides (8).

Effects of Glucocorticoids on Vascular Responses

Recent physiologic studies suggest that edema in the airways, either between the muscular layer and the mucosa or outside the smooth muscle, can have a profound effect on bronchial reactivity by diminishing the resting diameter of conducting airways (9). The same degree of smooth muscle constriction in an edematous airway can lead to much greater increases in airways resistance than in a normal airway. A well-established effect of glucocorticoids is their ability to inhibit the increases in vascular permeability induced by a variety of agents which cause vascular leak, including prostaglandins, histamine, bradykinin, serotonin, leukotrienes, etc. (10–11). Although little is known about the mechanisms by which steroids prevent vascular leakage, the possibilities include inhibition of the release of permeability-inducing agents (e.g., arachidonic acid

* The Johns Hopkins Asthma and Allergy Center, 5501 Bayview Circle, Unit Office 3A.62, Baltimore, Maryland 21224 USA.
Acknowledgements: This work was supported by National Institutes of Health grants AR31891, AI20136, and AI27429. The authors thank Ms. Bonnie Hebden for assistance in the preparation of the manuscript.

metabolites, kinins, etc.), induction of the synthesis of permeability-inhibiting substances (e.g., vasocortin, etc.), or induction of direct structural or functional changes in endothelial cells which dampen the endothelial response.

Effects of Steroids on Secretory Responses

Secretion of excess quantities of mucous and/or failure to eliminate secretions in the airways is an important pathologic observation in asthma. Although no studies have been performed to quantitate the effects of steroids on mucous secretion in asthmatics, several *in vitro* studies suggest that glucocorticoids can inhibit mucous secretion by two mechanisms: indirectly, by preventing the appearance of mucous secretagogues, and directly as an effect on mucous-secreting cells (12).

Effects of Glucocorticoids on Immune and Inflammatory Cell Recruitment

Associated with the LPR in allergic subjects is a dramatic influx of immune and inflammatory cells to the site of local antigen challenge. Concomitant with the influx of inflammatory cells is a second wave of appearance of inflammatory mediators. Glucocorticoids inhibit this response regardless of whether they are administered before or immediately after the acute phase response has occurred. Inhibition of the influx of inflammatory cells by glucocorticoids leads to inhibition of the appearance of inflammatory mediators during the late phase (13–14). Both topical and oral glucocorticoids inhibit cell recruitment in nasal challenge models suggesting that the effects of glucocorticoids are exerted locally (15–17). Discussion of the mechanisms of glucocorticoid inhibition of the recruitment of immune and inflammatory cells in the late phase in allergic reactions is the focus of the next section of this review.

Effects of Steroids on Leukocyte Recruitment Mechanisms

Inhibition of leukocyte recruitment is an important effect of glucocorticoids in all inflammatory diseases, not just those of allergic etiology. There are a number of special considerations in allergic diseases, however. In particular, this section will focus upon the mechanisms of recruitment of eosinophils and basophils to allergic reaction sites, a prominent characteristic which distinguishes allergic reactions from many other types of inflammatory cellular infiltrates. It is now clear that both leukocytes and endothelium play active roles in the process by which the leukocyte adheres to and spreads over the endothelial surface and emigrates across the vessel wall (18). Leukocytes become activated in this process either initially by the presence of a chemoattractant or by the presence of endothelial adhesion molecules with which it comes in contact during the blood flow-dependent process of rolling along the luminal surface of the vessel wall. Endothelial cells, following activation by a variety of cytokines (see below), can express adherence molecules de novo which will cause leukocyte rolling and activate leukocyte adherence and transendothelial migration. The latter event may be facilitated by endothelial cell-produced chemoattractants such as IL-8 or PAF which can help direct leukocyte migration across the vessel wall.

Leukocyte Activation: Adherence

A large number of leukocyte surface molecules are involved in adherence to endothelium prior into emigration into a tissue. Prominent among the adherence molecules are the β_1 and β_2 integrins (19–21). The β_2 integrin family includes the complement receptor (CR3) known as Mo1/Mac-1 which goes by the CD designation of CD11b/CD18. The β_2 chain (CD18) is also found in LFA-1 (CD11a/CD18) and p150,95 (CD11c/CD18). Patients whose cells lack the CD11/CD18 β_2 integrins have peripheral blood neutrophils which are deficient in both adherence and chemotaxis and which do not emigrate out of the circulation. Interestingly, eosinophils and lymphocytes from these patients do migrate into tissues (22). It is, therefore, believed that the CD11/CD18 complex is critical for neutrophil emigration but may not be absolutely essential for migration of eosinophils or lymphocytes. The β_1 or VLA family of integrins include at least six separate members, each having a distinct α-chain (19–21,23). Among these, VLA-4 (in which the α-chain is CD49d) is of particular interest. The recent demonstration that VLA-4 can be detected on the surface of eosinophils, basophils and lymphocytes, but not neutrophils, has led to the suggestion that VLA-4, by virtue of its interaction with a known endothelial counter-receptor, VCAM-1, may be responsible for recruitment of these cell types in allergic reactions (24–25). A third family of adhesion molecules, the selectins or LEC-CAMS, includes two on endothelium (see below) and one, LECAM-1 (also known as LAM-1 or Leu-8, etc.), on circulating leukocytes (26). These molecules contain an N-terminus lectin-like domain which interacts with specific carbohydrate moieties on the target cell. Present concepts of the dynamics of leukocyte binding and recruitment in a blood vessel maintain that LECAM-1 is an anchor which allows the leukocyte to roll along the vessel wall rather than to travel freely through the lumen of the vessel as do red cells (27–28). By maintaining a "sticky" surface, LECAM-1 permits the leukocyte to feel its way along the surface of endothelium and to travel much more slowly than if it were not anchored. Both of these effects permit an adherence response of the leukocyte should it come into contact with either a chemoattractant or an area of the endothelial surface which also expresses other adhesion molecules, such as discussed below. Following the initial adhesion event, the LECAM-1 "anchor" is rapidly shed as it is apparently no longer necessary and the leukocyte then can transmigrate (28).

As far as glucocorticoids are concerned, adherence of human neutrophils or basophils to vascular endothelial cells following stimulation with leukocyte activators such as PAF or fmet-peptide is not inhibited by prior incubation with glucocorticoids (29–31). In accordance with this, glucocorticoids also do not inhibit the upregulation of expression and function of β_2 integrins on neutrophils. Other studies established that chemotaxis of neutrophils or eosinophils, another β_2 integrin-dependent process, is not inhibited by treatment with glucocorticoids (29). It seems unlikely, then, that glucocorticoids directly inhibit activation of leukocyte adherence and migration responses.

Leukocyte Activation: Priming

Leukocyte priming refers to an exaggerated response of leukocytes to their normal activating stimuli; priming is typically induced following exposure to certain cytokines. The relevance of leukocyte priming to recruitment is not completely known. However, a number of studies *in vivo* and *in vitro* suggest that priming of eosinophils can potentiate their adherence and recruitment to tissue sites (32–34). This may occur by increasing the expression of β_2 integrins on eosinophils and by a global potentiation of eosinophil signal transduction and cellular responses. A limited number of studies have determined the effects of glucocorticoids on leukocyte priming in the context of cellular recruitment. Dexamethasone failed to inhibit the potentiation of fmet-peptide-induced CD11b expression or adherence of eosinophils to either plastic or endothelial cells following culture with GM-CSF (35). It should be noted that these *in vitro* studies were performed in the presence of exogenously added cytokine. *In vivo* studies suggest that the potent inhibitory effects of steroids on cytokine production effectively inhibit eosinophil priming. For example, circulating eosinophils were found to show enhanced CD11b responses in a patient with episodic hypereosinophilia (i.e., they were "primed"). Oral steroids reversed this priming, reduced eosinophil numbers, and dramatically reduced circulating cytokine levels (GM-CSF and others) in this patient (36).

Leukocyte Activation: Eosinophil Survival

Associated with priming of eosinophils by cytokines such as IL-3, IL-5 or GM-CSF, is a marked prolongation of their survival *in vitro* (37–39). The apparent selective eosinophil recruitment during allergic reactions *in vivo* may, in part, be related to selective survival of eosinophils in target tissues which contain the relevant cytokines. Glucocorticoids show a remarkable ability to inhibit this prolongation of eosinophil survival by cytokines *in vitro*, although the glucocorticoid effect can be overcome by excess cytokine in the culture systems used (40,41). Associated with inhibition of eosinophil survival by glucocorticoids is an inhibition of the change of eosinophil density phenotype to the "hypodense" form. In addition to a direct effect of glucocorticoids on eosinophil survival, the glucocorticoids are anticipated to indirectly inhibit this same process by diminishing the concentration of cytokine in the tissue. Thus, studies *in vitro* clearly demonstrate that steroids are potent inhibitors of the release of cytokines such as IL-3, GM-CSF, and IL-5 (3). By increasing the requirement of the eosinophils for cytokines and by decreasing the availability of cytokine, the glucocorticoids are expected to have a profound suppressive effect on the longevity of eosinophils at an allergic reaction site.

Endothelial Activation

The endothelium is now recognized to play an important role in recruitment of leukocytes by expressing a variety of specific adherence molecules on its surface. Two of these molecules, ELAM-1 and GMP-140 (CD62), are members of the LEC-CAM or selectin gene family while others, including VCAM-1, ICAM-1 (CD54) and 2, and PECAM-1 (CD31), are members of the immunoglobulin supergene family (21). ICAM-1, ICAM-2 and PECAM-1 are expressed on endothelium at rest; ICAM-1, ELAM-1, and VCAM-1 are induced following activation of endothelial cells by cytokines such as IL-1 and TNF, or by bacterial endotoxins. Concordantly with the expression of these adhesion molecules the endothelium functionally displays increased adhesive properties for circulating leukocytes. The ability of a given leukocyte subtype to bind to activated endothelium depends to a great degree on the counter-ligands which are expressed on the leukocyte surface. For example, LFA-1 or Mac-1 are required for binding to ICAM-1 (21). As far as allergic cell recruitment is concerned, the expression of VCAM-1 by endothelial cells can render them adhesive for eosinophils, basophils, and lymphocytes, (but not neutrophils), the cell types commonly seen at allergic reaction sites (24,42,44). Interestingly, activation of endothelium by IL-4 selectively increases VCAM-1 expression without inducing the other adhesion molecules (43,44). IL-4 activated endothelial cells are adhesive for eosinophils and basophils, but not neutrophils (44). Interestingly, production of IL-4 *in vivo* by transfected tumor cells or in transgenic animals elicits an eosinophil-rich inflammatory response reminiscent of allergic reactions (45). In vitro glucocorticoids do not inhibit the expression of ICAM-1, ELAM-1, or VCAM-1 induced by either IL-1 or IL-4, nor do they inhibit the acquisition of adhesive properties for eosinophils, basophils or neutrophils (29,30, and unpublished observations). Once again, this is in a model system in which the cytokine is supplied exogenously. Although the effects of glucocorticoids on IL-4 production are not known, glucocorticoids have been demonstrated to be potent inhibitors of the production of IL-1 and TNF and thus are expected to block endothelial activation and the consequent leukocyte adhesion and recruitment by diminishing the expression of endothelial adhesion molecules secondary to a reduction of the production of the cytokines which activate endothelium (3,30).

Production of Inflammatory Factors which Induce Leukocyte Recruitment

Numerous *in vitro* studies suggest that the main site of glucocorticoid action with regard to leukocyte recruitment is the inhibition of the release of those factors which induce the recruitment processes. While glucocorticoid actions are dependent upon the cell type and the stimulus, they have been demonstrated to inhibit the release of a range of recruitment-inducing factors including simple lipid-derived chemoattractants such as PAF and LTB_4, oligopeptide chemoattractants such as IL-3 and complement fragments (via a reduction of plasma leakage), and endothelial-activating cytokines such as IL-1 and TNF (3,18,46).

Possible Relationships Between the Steroid Regulation of Gene Expression and Anti-Inflammatory Effects

Steroid-Induced Proteins

Some glucocorticoid anti-inflammatory effects (e.g., in animal skin) have been shown to be inhibited by pretreatment with protein synthesis inhibitors and thus may depend upon induction of anti-inflammatory proteins by glucocorticoids (47). Glucocorticoid-induced proteins which may contribute to their anti-inflammatory effects include lipocortins and vasocortin. Discussion of these proteins is beyond the scope of this review and can be found elsewhere (48).

New Insights into Inhibition of Gene Expression by Steroids

Recent studies from several laboratories have led to novel models of glucocorticoid action. These models complement the classical model of steroid action in which the steroid-receptor complex induces gene expression directly by association with specific sequences in the promoter region of the genes of interest. Glucocorticoid receptor-steroid complexes have now been shown to interact directly with the AP-1 (*jun fos*) transcription-activating factor and, by so doing, inhibit the ability of AP-1 to induce those genes which it activates (49,50). AP-1-induced genes include collagenase, stromolysin, IL-2 and others. Thus, in some cases where glucocorticoids *inhibit* the expression of selected genes, they may do so by removing the presence of an activator of those genes rather than by directly inhibiting transcription of the relevant genes. Whether this mechanism of action is important in regulation of cytokine gene production has not been determined. However, analogous glucocorticoid effects, with transcription factors other than AP-1, may well explain some of the inhibitory effects of steroids on cytokine gene expression.

Summary and Conclusions

It seems certain at this point that one of the reasons that glucocorticoids are so widely effective and potent in inflammatory diseases in general, as well as in allergic diseases in particular, results from their diverse mechanisms of action on numerous components of inflammatory and immune responses. It seems unlikely that selective disruption of individual biochemical pathways or hormone-receptor/autacoid-receptor interactions by designed drugs will achieve an anti-inflammatory efficacy equivalent to that of glucocorticoids. Thus, future developments of improved anti-inflammatory and anti-allergic compounds may well be most likely to succeed if they are focussed upon improvement of the design of glucocorticoids to eliminate systemic effects and maximize local effects in the tissue of interest. As more is learned about the effects of steroids on selected gene regulation, as well as the importance of selected genes (e.g., cytokines such as IL-4, IL-5, adhesion molecules, etc.), the possibilities for targeted therapies may expand.

References

1. Gleich, G.J. 1982. The late phase of the immunoglobulin E-mediated reaction: A link between anaphylaxis and common allergic disease? J. Allergy Clin. Immunol. 70:160.
2. Schleimer, R.P. 1988. Glucocorticosteroids: Their mechanisms of action and use in allergic diseases. In: Allergy: Principles and practice. E. Middleton, Jr., C.E. Reed, E.F. Ellis, N.F. Adkinson Jr., and J.W. Yunginger, eds. St. Louis, MO: C.V. Mosby, p. 739.
3. Schleimer, R.P. 1990. Effects of glucocorticoids on inflammatory cells relevant to their therapeutic applications in asthma. Am. Rev. Respir. Dis. 141:59.
4. Barnes, P. 1989. Drug therapy: A new approach to the treatment of asthma. N. Engl. J. Med. 321:1517.
5. Brattsand, R., and U. Pipkorn. 1990. Glucocorticoids: Experimental approaches. In: Asthma: Its pathogenesis and treatment. M. Kaliner, P. Barnes, and C. Persson, eds. New York: Marcel Dekker, p. 667.
6. Ellul-Micallef, R., and Fenech, F.F. 1975. Effect of intravenous prednisolone in asthmatics with diminished adrenergic responsiveness. Lancet 2:7948.
7. Davies, A.O. 1989. Steroid hormone-induced regulation of adrenergic receptors. In: Anti-inflammatory steroid action. Basic and clinical aspects. R.P. Schleimer, H.N. Claman, and A. Oronsky, editors. San Diego: Academic Press, p. 96.
8. Borson, D.B., and D.C. Gruenert. 1991. Glucocorticoids induce neutral endopeptidase in transformed human tracheal epithelial cells. Am. J. Physiol. 260:L83.
9. James, A.L., Pare, P.D., and Hogg, J.C. 1989. The mechanisms of airway narrowing in asthma. Am. Rev. Respir. Dis. 139:242.
10. Svensjö, E., and Roempke, K. 1985. Time-dependent inhibition of bradykinin and histamine-induced increase in microvasular permeability by local glucocorticosteroid treatment. In: Glucocorticosteroids, inflammation and

bronchial hyperreactivity. J.C. Hogg, R. Ellul-Micallef, and R. Brattsand, eds. Excerpta Medica, p. 136.

11. Inagaki, N., Miura, T., Nagai, H., Ono, Y., and Koda, A. 1988. Inhibition of vascular permeability increase in mice. Int. Arch. Allergy Appl. Immunol. 87:254.

12. Lundgren, J.D., Hirata, F., Marom, Z., Logun, C., Steel, L., Kaliner, M., and Shelhamer, J. 1988. Dexamethasone inhibits respiratory glycoconjugate secretion from feline airways *in vitro* by the induction of lipocortin (lipomodulin) synthesis. Am. Rev. Respir. Dis. 137:353.

13. Dunsky, E.H., Atkins, P.C., and Zweiman, B. 1977. Histologic responses in human skin test reactions to ragweed. IV. Effects of a single intravenous injection of steroids. J. Allergy Clin. immunol. 59:142.

14. Charlesworth, E.N., Kagey-Sobotka, A., Schleimer, R.P., Norman, P.S., and Lichtenstein, L.M. 1991. Prednisone inhibits the appearance of inflammatory mediators and the influx of eosinophils and basophils associated with the cutaneous late-phase response to allergen. J. Immunol. 146:671.

15. Pipkorn, U., Proud, D., Lichtenstein, L.M., Kagey-Sobotka, A., Norman, P.S., and Naclerio, R.M. 1987. Inhibition of mediator release in allergic rhinitis by pretreatment with topical glucocorticosteroids. N. Engl. J. Med. 316:1506.

16. Pipkorn, U., Proud, D., Lichtenstein, L.M., Schleimer, R.P., Peters, S.P., Adkinson, N.F., Jr., Kagey-Sobotka, A., Norman, P.S. and Naclerio, R.M. 1987. Effect of short-term systemic glucocorticoid treatment on human nasal mediator release after antigen challenge. J. Clin. Invest. 80:957.

17. Bascom, R., Wachs, M., Naclerio, R.M., Pipkorn, U., Galli, S.J., and Lichtenstein, L.M. 1988. Basophil influx occurs after nasal antigen challenge: Effects of topical corticosteroid pretreatment. J. Allergy Clin. Immunol. 81:580.

18. Bochner, B.S., Lamas, A.M., Benenati, S.V., and Schleimer, R.P. 1990. On the central role of vascular endothelium in allergic reactions. In: Late phase allergic reactions. R. Dorsch, ed. Boca Raton: CRC Press, p. 221.

19. Albelda, S.M., and Buck, C.A. 1990. Integrins and other cell adhesion molecules. FASEB J. 4:2868.

20. Kishimoto, T.K., Larson, R.S., Corbi, A.L., Dustin, M.L., Staunton, D.E., and Springer, T.A. 1989. The leukocyte integrins. Adv. Immunol. 46:149.

21. Springer, T.A. 1990. Adhesion receptors of the immune system. Nature 346:425.

22. Anderson, D.C., Schmalstieg, F.C., Finegold, M.J., Hughes, B.J., Rothlein, R., Miller, L.J., Kohl, S., Tosi, M.F., Jacobs, R.L., Waldrop, T.C., Goldman, A.S., Shearer, W.T., and Springer, T.A. 1985. The severe and moderate phenotypes of heritable Mac-1, LFA-1, p150,95 deficiency: their quantitative definition and relation to leukocyte dysfunction and clinical features. J. Infect. Dis. 152:668.

23. Hemler, M.E. 1990. VLA proteins in the integrin family: Structures, functions, and their role on leukocytes. Annu. Rev. Immunol. 8:365.

24. Walsh, G.M., Mermod, J., Hartnell, A., Kay, A.B., and Wardlaw, A.J. 1991. Human eosinophil, but not neutrophil, adherence to IL-1-stimulated human umbilical vascular endothelial cells is $\alpha4\beta1$ (very late antigen-4) dependent. J. Immunol. 146:3419.

25. Bochner, B.S., Luscinskas, F.W., Gimbrone, M.A., Jr., Newman, W., Sterbinsky, S.A., Derse-Anthony, C., Klunk, D., and Schleimer, R.P. 1991. Adhesion of human basophils, eosinophils, and neutrophils to IL-1-activated human vascular endothelial cells: Contributions of endothelial cell adhesion molecules. J. Exp. Med. 173:1553.

26. Rosen, S.D. 1990. The LEC-CAMs: An emerging family of cell-cell adhesion receptors based upon carbohydrate recognition. Am. J. Respir. Cell Mol. Biol. 3:397.

27. Butcher, E.C. 1990. Cellular and molecular mechanisms that direct leukocyte traffic. Am. J. Pathol. 136:3.

28. Kishimoto, T.K., Warnock, R.A., Jutila, M.A., Butcher, E.C., Lane, C., Anderson, D.C., and Smith, C.W. 1991. Antibodies against human neutrophil LECAM-1 (LAM-1/Leu-8/DREG-56 antigen) and endothelial cell ELAM-1 inhibit a common CD18-independent adhesion pathway *in vitro*. Blood 78:805.

29. Schleimer, R.P., Freeland, H.S., Peters, S.P., Brown, K.E., and Derse, C.P. 1989. An assessment of the effects of glucocorticoids on degranulation, chemotaxis, binding to vascular endothelial cells and formation of leukotriene B4 by purified human neutrophils. J. Pharmacol. Exp. Therap. 250:598.

30. Bochner, B.S., Rutledge, B.K., and Schleimer, R.P. 1987. Interleukin 1 production by human lung tissue. II. Inhibition by antiinflammatory steroids. J. Immunol. 139:2303.

31. Bochner, B. S., Peachell, P.T., Brown, K.E., and Schleimer, R.P. 1988. Adherence of human basophils to cultured umbilical vein vascular endothelial cells. J. Clin. Invest. 81:1355.
32. Henocq, E., and Vargaftig, B.B. 1988. Skin eosinophilia in atopic patients. J. Allergy Clin. Immunol. 81:691.
33. Venge, P., Hakansson, L., and Peterson, C.G.B. 1987. Eosinophil activation in allergic disease. Int. Archs Allergy appl. Immun. 82:333.
34. Bousquet, J.B., Chanez, P., Lacoste, J.Y., Barneon, G., Ghavanian, N., Enander, I., Venge, P., Ahlstedt, S., Lafontaine, J.S., Godard, P., and Michel, F.B. 1990. Eosinophilic inflammation in asthma. N. Engl. J. Med. 323:1033.
35. Tomioka, K., Bochner, B.S., Derse-Anthony, C., Lichtenstein, L.M., MacGlashan, D.W., Jr., and Schleimer, R.P., 1991. GM-CSF enhances PAF- and FMLP-induced eosinophil expression of adherence molecules (CD11b) and increases FMLP-induced elevations of intracellular calcium. FASEB J. 5:A640 (Abstr.).
36. Bochner, B.S., Friedman, B., Krishnaswami, G., Schleimer, R.P., Lichtenstein, L.M., and Kroegel, C. 1991. Episodic eosinophilia-myalgia-like syndrome in a patient without L-tryptophan use: Association with eosinophil activation and increased serum levels of granulocyte-macrophage colony-stimulating factor. J. Allergy Clin. Immunol. 88:629.
37. Silberstein, D.S., and David, J.R. 1987. The regulation of human eosinophil function by cytokines. Immunol. Today 8:380.
38. Owen, W.F., Jr., Rothenberg, M.E., Silberstein, D.S., Gasson, J.C., Stevens, R.L., and Austen, K.F. 1987. Regulation of human eosinophil viability, density, and function by granulocyte/macrophage colony-stimulating factor in the presence of 3T3 fibroblasts. J. Exp. Med. 166:129.
39. Rothenberg, M.E., Owen, W.F., Jr., Silberstein, D.S., Soberman, R.J., Austen, K.F., and Stevens, R.L. 1987. Eosinophils cocultured with endothelial cells have increased survival and functional properties. Science 237:645.
40. Lamas, A.M., Marcotte, G.V., and Schleimer, R.P. 1989. Human endothelial cells prolong eosinophil survival. Regulation by cytokines and glucocorticoids. J. Immunol. 142:3978.
41. Lamas, A.M., Leon, O.G., and Schleimer, R.P. 1991. Glucocorticoids inhibit eosinophil responses to granulocyte-macrophage colony-stimulating factor. J. Immunol. 147:254.
42. Weller, P.F., Rand, T.H., Goelz, S E., Chi-Rosso, G., and Lobb, R.R. 1991. Human eosinophil adherence to vascular endothelium mediated by binding to vascular cell adhesion molecule 1 and endothelial leukocyte adhesion molecule 1. Proc. Natl. Acad. Sci. USA 88:7430.
43. Thornhill, M.H., Kyan-Aung, U., and Haskard, D.O. 1990. IL-4 increases human endothelial cell adhesiveness for T cells but not for neutrophils. J. Immunol. 144:3060.
44. Schleimer, R.P., Sterbinsky, S.A., Kaiser, J., Klunk, D.A., Tomioka, K., Newman, W., Luscinskas, F.W., Gimbrone, M.A.J., McIntyre, B.W., and Bochner, B.S. 1992. Interleukin-4 induces adherence of human eosinophils and basophils but not neutrophils to endothelium: Association with expression of VCAM-1. J. Immunol. 148:1086.
45. Tepper, R.I., Levinson, D.A., Stanger, B.Z., Campos-Torres, J., Abbas, A.K., and Leder, P. 1990. IL-4 induces allergic-like inflammatory disease and alters T cell development in transgenic mice. Cell 62:457.
46. Guyre, P.M., Girard, M.T., Morganelli, P.M., and Manganiello, P.D. 1988. Glucocorticoid effects on the production and actions of immune cytokines. J. Ster. Biochem. 30:89.
47. Tsurufuji, S., Sugio, K., and Takemasa, F. 1979. The role of glucocorticoid receptor and gene expression in the anti-inflammatory action of dexamethasone. Nature 280:408.
48. Flower, R.J. 1989. Glucocorticoids and the inhibition of phospholipase A_2. In: Anti-inflammatory steroid action. Basic and clinical aspects. R.P. Schleimer, H.N. Claman, and A. Oronsky, eds. San Diego: Academic Press, p. 48.
49. Schule, R., Rangarajan, P., Kliewer, S., Ransome, L.J., Bolado, J., Yang, N., Verma, I.M., and Evans, R.M. 1990. Functional antagonism between oncoprotein c-Jun and the glucocorticoid receptor. Cell 62:1217.
50. Yang-Yen, H.-F., Chambard, J.-C., Sun, Y.-L., Smeal, T., Schmidt, T.J., Drouin, J., and Karin, M. 1990. Transcriptional interference between c-Jun and the glucocorticoid receptor: Mutual inhibition of DNA binding due to direct protein-protein interaction. Cell 62:1205.

Sektion III

Ophthalmic Allergy

HLA and Ocular Inflammation

Shigeaki Ohno*

It has long been suspected that a genetically determined susceptibility to certain diseases may exist, and this may play an important role in the development of the disease. Among various genetic loci which limit or modify the strength and character of the immune response to a variety of antigens, immune response genes associated with the major histocompatibility complex (MHC) have been most extensively investigated (1). Each vertebrate species studied so far has been shown to have a very similar genetic system. The major histocompatibility complex of the mouse, for example, is located on the 17th chromosome and is called the H-2 system. Multiple tightly linked genes which are essential for the immune response and immune surveillance exist in a cluster within the H-2 complex. The human major histocompatibility complex is called the HLA system, and this was discovered in the late 1950s.

HLA and Disease

In the mouse, it has become apparent in recent years that a significant correlation exists between the H-2 system and susceptibility to some oncogenic viruses. In Gross virus leukaemia, for example, strains carrying the H-2b allele were shown to be resistant, and strains carrying the H-2k allele were susceptible. These experimental data from animal models impelled many investigators to search for associations between HLA antigens and certain diseases. More than 530 diseases have been studied so far.

In the field of ophthalmology, more than 20 diseases have been shown to be closely associated with certain HLA antigens (1). One of the first diseases studied was Beh's disease, which is known to occur most frequently among the Japanese and Mediterranean populations. However, there was no satisfactory explanation for this biased geographic distribution. It was shown that the frequency of HLA-B51, a split antigen of HLA-B5, is significantly increased in patients with Beh's disease as compared to the normal controls. The relative risk for HLA-B51 is 10.7, and an individual with HLA-B51 is considered to have a risk of developing Beh's disease 10.7 times more than an individual without it. This association has been confirmed not only in Japan, but also in Korea, Taiwan, Kuwait, Israel, Turkey, Greece, Italy, Tunisia, France, England and Mexico. Therefore, Beh's disease is one of the few diseases which have the same HLA association, even in different ethnic groups (2). In addition to HLA-B51, we have also found that the frequency of HLA-DRw52 is significantly increased in these patients. Etiologic fraction of exposed individuals (EFe) is 0.91 for HLA-B51 and 0.82 for HLA-DRw52. This means that if HLA-B51 or HLA-DRw52 per se is one of the causes of this disease, 91% of the HLA-B51 positive cases or 82% of the HLA-DRw52 positive cases will be caused by these HLA phenotypes.

In contrast to the disease susceptibility factors, HLA-DR1 and HLA-DQW1 were shown to be significantly decreased in the patients. This means that those who are positive for HLA-DR1 or HLA-DQW1 are resistant to the development of Beh's disease, and so it is reasonable to presume that not only disease susceptibility genes but also disease resistance genes are closely associated with the immunogenetic mechanism of this disease.

It is interesting to note that the frequency of HLA-B51 and HLA-DRw52 is also increased in the parents and the siblings of the patients, but they have a higher frequency of HLA-DQW1, and this may account for the fact that familial occurrence is rather rare in this disease, although they live in the same or a similar environment.

It is noteworthy that this disease seems to occur most frequently between the latitudes of 30 and 45 degrees north in Asian and Eurasian populations. This area coincides with the Silk Route, and Beh's disease may have spread from a certain area within this zone, both to the East

* Department of Ophthalmology, Yokohama City University School of Medicine, Yokohama, Japan

and West, along with the migration and mixture of various populations via the Silk Route (2). This disease may therefore be called a "Silk Route Disease".

At any rate, it seems clear that there are two major immunogenetic factors, disease susceptibility genes and disease resistance genes which are closely associated with this disease, and they may play an important role in its etiopathogenesis, in addition to unknown exogenous agents.

Molecular Immunogenetics

It has now become evident that the number of HLA alleles which serological reagents can define is quite limited and the serologically defined alleles have been further split into several suballeles at the DNA level, which can be assigned by polymerase chain reaction (PCR)-DNA typing techniques such as PCR-SSO (sequence specific oligonucleotide) and PCR-RFLP (polymerase chain reaction-restriction fragment length polymorphism). These PCR-based DNA typing techniques have revolutionised the characterisation of HLA-DR, DQ and DP allelic polymorphisms at the nucleotide level and are expected to facilitate molecular analysis of the relationship between HLA and diseases.

As many as 67 genes so far have been identified in the HLA gene region which is about 3,500 kb in size. Furthermore, HLA has a multigene family, with 17 class I genes, 7 class II α chain genes, and 9 class II chain β genes. Interestingly enough, HSP, or heat shock protein 70 genes, and TNF or tumor necrosis factor genes were also found to be present in the HLA gene region. These newly found genes may also be involved in the immunogenetic backgrounds of various ocular diseases. The genetic polymorphisms in the HLA class II gene products which are usually HLA*B1 genes, are localised in the N terminal domains of these molecules, particularly in the discrete regions termed allelic hypervariable regions (AHVRs). The considerable influence of AHVRs on peptide binding and T-cell recognition suggests that the genetic polymorphisms in these molecules regulate the extent of immune response, varying among individuals with different HLA allele.

Examination of the nucleotide sequences using molecular techniques (such as PCR-RFLP DNA typing) enables us to identify the exact residues within the HLA amino acid sequences responsible for disease susceptibility. Recently it was revealed that foreign antigen peptide can bind only to the open form of the MHC molecule. All three molecules, the T-cell receptor, the antigenic peptide, and the MHC molecule interact in a trimolecular complex to initiate T-lymphocyte activation. Therefore, amino acid sequences of each HLA antigen seem very important in the antigen presentation. In insulin-dependent diabetes mellitus, for example, non-aspartic acid in the 57th amino acid of HLA-DQ β chain is known to be an important genetic susceptibility factor (3). Similarly, arginine in the 69th DQ β chain and arginine in the 71st DR β chain work as genetic susceptibility factors, in myasthenia gravis and rheumatoid arthritis, respectively.

Our preliminary data in Beh's disease also suggests that both the 63rd and 67th amino acids of the α1 domain of the HLA class I molecule seem to be important in the immunomolecular susceptibility to it. The reason for this is that all 313 amino acid sequences of HLA-B51 and Bw52 were analysed and only the 63rd and 67th amino acids were different, although close association with Beh's disease was solely found in HLA-B51, and not in HLA-Bw52. Resistant genetic factors, B44.1 or B44.2 also showed amino acid sequences different from B51. Our recent data on HLA-DNA typing in Beh's disease using the PCR-RFLP method showed that the frequency of HLA-DRB1*0802 was significantly increased, whereas DRB1*1502 was significantly decreased in the patients. As for the HLA-DQA1 genotyping, HLA-DQA1*0301 was significantly higher, and DQA1*0103 and DQA1*0101 significantly lower in the patients than healthy controls. Similarly, HLA-DQB1*0303 was significantly increased and DQB1*0601 and DQB1*0501 significantly decreased in the patients. Although HLA-DPB1*0201 was slightly increased in the patients HLA-DPB1 allelic frequencies showed no significant difference between the two groups.

In our next study, we investigated polymorphism of tumor necrosis factor (TNF) β gene by RFLP analysis, as TNF α and TNF β genes were found to be located between the HLA class III region and the HLA-B locus on chromosome 6. Although the TNF α gene did not show any polymorphism, the TNF β gene was shown to have a double allelic restriction fragment length polymorphism, that is, a 5.5 kb fragment and a 10.5 kb fragment, by means of restriction enzyme NcoI. The TNF β NcoI 5.5 kb allele is known to represent a trait of high TNF production, and the TNF β NcoI 10.5 kb allele a trait of low TNF production. TNF genes are tightly linked to HLA alleles. Southern hybridisation analysis showed that 53.3% of normal Japanese controls had monozygous 10.5 kb NcoI fragments, 10.7% had monozygous 5.5 kb fragments, and the remaining 36% were heterozygous for 10.5 kb and 5.5 kb fragments. As compared with the theoretical frequency, which was calculated from the frequencies of HLA-B alleles carried by the patients, the 10.5 kb NcoI fragment was more frequently seen in the patients. Moreover allelic distribution at the TNF β locus in the patient deviated considerably from a linkage disequilibrium with the HLA-B locus.

Therefore, the disease susceptibility gene to Beh's disease, or Beh gene, may probably be located around the TNF gene region centromic ofthe HLA-B gene, and strongly associated with a TNF β NcoI 10.5 kb allele. Our hypothesis is that an ancestral or primordial haplotype of Beh's disease in the HLA gene region was HLA-DPB1*0201-DQB1*0303-DQA1*0301 -DRB1*0901-TNF β 10.5 kb and B51 haplotype. This original HLA haplotype was spread from somewhere in the Eurasian Continent, both to the East and West via the Silk Route.

HLA and Allergy

In recent years there have been several reports discussing allergic disorders and HLA. For example, Sasazuki (4) reported the association of Japanese cedar pollenosis with HLA-DQw3, and IgE production against a certain antigen was shown to be genetically regulated. Sadanaga et al. (5) also reported that HLA-A 26 and DQw3 were significantly increased in the patients, and an individual with HLA-DQw3 was shown to have a risk of developing Japanese cedar pollenosis 3.3 times more than an individual without it. HLA-A26 and DQw3 were again significantly higher in patients with orchard grass pollenosis than the normal controls (5). Kitao et al. (6) reported that nasal allergy to mite antigen, Dermatophagoides farinae was significantly associated with HLA-DQw3. Conversely, HLA-A2 was significantly lower in the patients, and thus may be a resistant genetic factor in mite allergy. Further molecular genetic studies revealed that HLA-DQB1*0303 which corresponds to HLA specificity HLA-DQw9, was significantly increased in patients with mite allergy. Therefore, allelic hypervariable regions associated with the HLA-B1*0303 gene may considerably influence the extent of immune response to mite antigen. In a HLA family study, the correlation between nasal allergy to Dermatophagoides farinae and the HLA haplotype was calculated by the affected sib-pair method. A X2 test on 16 sib-pairs of 12 families reached a value of 6.375 with a degree of freedom of 2. The probability of error was reported to be less than 0.05 (5). The linkage of mite allergy to HLA haplotype was calculated by Morton's sequential test in 20 families (5). The sum of lod scores was 4.16, and the recombination fraction represented by θ was 0.00, suggesting that genes conferring allergy to mites are linked to HLA haplotypes.

Conclusion

From these HLA analyses, it can be concluded that the genes which control allergic disposition to various antigens are linked to the HLA haplotypes, and are transmitted hereditarily. However, the exact association of HLA and allergy is still obscure. For example, it is still unknown whether IgE production, mast cell releasability, migration of inflammatory cells to the eye, and expression of receptors of inflammatory cells, are all regulated by HLA genes or not. Further immunogenetic and molecular genetic studies will clarify the true nature of disease susceptibility and resistance in ocular allergy and ocular inflammation in the near future.

References

1. Ohno, S. 1987. Immunogenetic studies on ocular diseases. In: Acta XXV Concilium Ophthalmologicum. F. Blodi et al., eds. Amsterdam, Berkeley, Milano: Kugler & Ghedini, p. 144.

2. Ohno, S., et al. 1982. Close association of HLA-Bw51 with Beh's disease. Arch. Ophthalmol. 100:1455
3. Todd, J.A., et al. 1987. HLA-DQ gene contributes to susceptibility and resistance to insulin-dependent diabetes mellitus. Nature 329:599.
4. Sasazuki, T., et al. 1983. HLA-linked genes controlling immune response and disease susceptibility. Immunol. Rev. 70:51.
5. Sadanaga, Y., et al. 1990. Allergy and genetics. Jpn. J. Clin. Immun. 13:448.
6. Kitao, Y., et al. 1987. Genetic regulation of allergic rhinitis. Acta Paediatr. Jpn. 29:654.

Early and Late Conjunctival Reactions

Sergio Bonini*, Stefano Bonini**, Massimo G. Bucci**, Francesco Balsano*

Allergic diseases of the conjunctiva include different clinical pictures which are at present grouped together under the term of "allergic conjunctivitis" because of the assumption that a common IgE-mediated Type I hypersensitivity mechanism is responsible for their pathophysiology and symptoms (Fig. 1). Recently, however, extensive evidence has become available for several allergic diseases, such as asthma, rhinitis and allergic skin diseases, indicating that their pathogenesis cannot be confined to the mast cell and basophil mediator release triggered by IgE-allergen interaction, but must be extended to several other mechanisms such as the involvement of secondary effector cells and mediators, the allergic inflammation underlying late-phase reactions, and the hyperresponsiveness of target organs (1–3). Accordingly, it is conceivable that the pathogenesis of many forms of "allergic conjunctivitis" is also more complex than the typical IgE-mediated immediate hypersensitivity reaction. In fact, from a clinical point of view, many patients with "allergic conjunctivitis" have a family and personal history which is negative for atopic diseases, do not show sign of sensitization

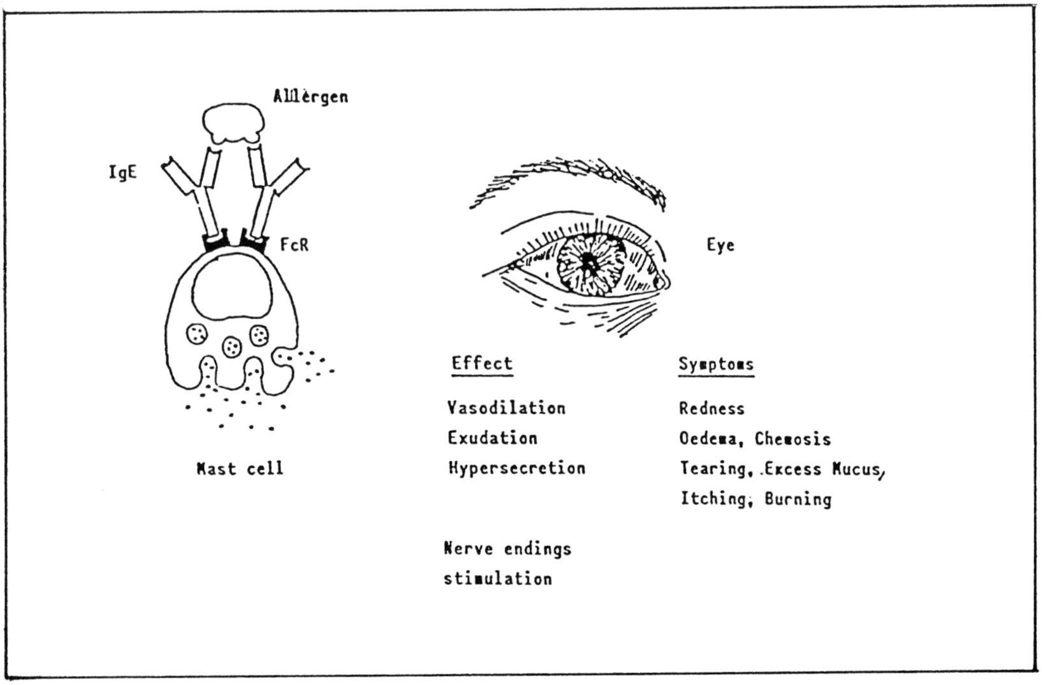

Figure 1. Type I hypersensitivity reaction and "allergic conjunctivitis".

* Andrea Cesalpino Foundation, I Clinica Medica, University "La Sapienza" Rome, Italy.
** Department of Ophthalmology, University "Tor Vergata", G.B. Bietti Foundation, Rome, Italy.
Acknowledgements: This paper reviews a series of studies performed with the collaboration of E. Adriani, M. Tomassini, E. Ciafre', L. Magrini, M. Centofanti and M. Schiavone. Immunohistochemical staining of conjunctival biopsies was performed by S.T. Holgate, S. Lightman, A. Bacon, D. Metz and S. Baddeley (Southampton and London, U.K.). Animal data were obtained by St. Bonini in collaboration with M.R. Allansmith, (Boston, USA). Research was supported by grants of the Italian Research Council (CNR) and Ministry of Public Education (MPI 40%).

to common allergens by skin tests and/or immunoassays for IgE antibody, and do not respond to conventional "anti-allergic" treatment but rather to topical or systemic steroids (4). Moreover, the inflammatory and productive pictures observed in some forms of "allergic conjunctivitis", such as vernal keratoconjunctivitis (VKC), atopic keratoconjunctivitis (AKC) or contact-lens conjunctivitis (CLC), cannot be explained by an immediate hypersensitivity reaction alone. This paper will review personal research, mainly based on the study of early and late conjunctival reactions to specific (allergen) and non-specific (histamine) stimuli, showing that a polyfactorial pathophysiology can be invoked in allergic eye diseases too. In particular, using VKC as a model, we shall focus on the following three aspects: (a) the cells and mediators involved in allergic eye diseases, (b) the effects of conjunctival allergen challenge, and (c) the effects of conjunctival histamine challenge.

Cells and Mediators in Allergic Eye Diseases

Mast cells (MCs) are largely represented in the conjunctiva of rats in comparison to other ocular tissues (5). MCs are also present in human conjunctiva, and their number is increased in both seasonal allergic conjunctivitis (SAC) and VKC. Irani and co-workers (6) and Morgan and co-workers (7) showed that conjunctival mast cells in allergic subjects are resistent to formalin and contain both tryptase and chymase, being therefore very similar to the connective-tissue type MCs present in the skin and other organs.

Preliminary experiments, performed in collaboration with S. Holgate's and S. Lightman's groups, using avidin-biotin immunohistochemical staining with a monoclonal anti-tryptase antibody (AA1), seem to confirm in VKC previous findings of Morgan et al. (6) in SAC that MCs in allergic eye patients are not only increased in number, but also show a different distribution. In fact, in normal subjects MCs are mainly present in the stroma while in allergic conjunctivitis patients several intra-epithelial MCs are found. This can have relevant implications with reference to the availability of MCs to interact with allergen and other cells and cytokines.

In VKC, MCs not only are present, but also appear to be activated and to degranulate following challenge. In fact, we measured significantly ($p < .02$) increased levels of tryptase in tears of VKC patients (36 ± 45.1 µg/l; $n = 12$) when compared to those found in controls (6.6 ± 9.1 µg/l; $n = 8$). In hay fever conjunctivitis, where we were not able to detect significant amounts of tryptase in basal conditions and out of pollen season (0.4 ± 0.3 µg/l; $n = 9$), allergen provocation induced the appearance of tryptase in tears 20 minutes after challenge (29 ± 72.1 µg/l; $n = 9$) but not 6 hours later (0.5 ± 0.7 µg/l; $n = 9$). Therefore, as shown by Butrus et al. (8), tryptase can represent a useful marker of MCs activation and degranulation in patients with allergic conjunctivitis.

Eosinophils represent a common finding in conjunctival scrapings and tears of patients with VKC, being present both in IgE-mediated cases (19/39 = 48% of our series) and in cases where no sensitization is detectable with skin tests and RAST (20/39 = 52%). For these last cases of VKC, very similar to NARES, we propose the term of NACES (non-allergic conjunctivitis with eosinophilia). Recently, we were able to show by immunohistochemical staining using EG2 antibody that eosinophils in VKC are activated (unpublished observations) and release peroxidase (EPO) and cationic protein (ECP) after allergen *in vitro* and *in vivo* challenge (9). Therefore, we suggest that the eosinophil has a central role in VKC and possibly in other forms of allergic conjunctivitis with eosinophil recruitment.

T cells are present in the lymphoid tissue of the normal conjunctiva. Their number, phenotype and distribution seem to be different in patients with VKC. Th2 like cell clones were in fact produced from biopsies of VKC patients (10). These cells not only contribute to an exaggerated IgE production through IL4, but also influence inflammatory processes through the modulatory effects on MCs and eosinophils of IL3 and IL5.

Fibroblast proliferation and collagen production are modulated by several cells and cytokines. Excess collagen production is a feature of the giant papillae observed in VKC. Therefore, adequate investigations should be strongly recommended for a better understanding of fibroblast activation and collagen deposition in VKC. We tested tears of VKC patients for their content of hyaluronic acid, a collagen marker used successfully in other disturbances of collagen turn-over. Hyaluronic acid was shown to be significantly higher in tears of patients with VKC (1080 ± 1510 µg/l; n = 14) when compared to the amount found in tears of patients with SAC (58±27 µg/l; n = 5).

Summarizing, the above reported data indicate that several inflammatory cells and mediators are present in VKC and possibly play a role in the pathophysiology of this disease and of other inflammatory allergic eye disorders.

Effects of Allergen Challenge

Recently we were able to show (11) that allergen challenge of human conjunctiva causes persisting inflammatory changes of ocular tissues similar to those previously described in rats (12). Therefore, the concept of late-phase allergic reaction can be applied to the eye too, as previously to the skin, nose and bronchi. In the eye, LPR is characterized, at the clinical level, by redness (with minor itching and tearing) persisting long after allergen provocation, accompanied by a sensation of foreign body (13). At the cytological level, the analysis of conjunctival scrapings or tears shows an early accumulation of neutrophils (mainly) during the immediate phase, followed by a prevalent recruitment of eosinophils 6–10 hours after provocation and of lymphocytes and monocytes later on, with persistent inflammatory changes up to 24 hours after challenge (11,13).

The recruitment of inflammatory cells during LPR is associated with the detection in tears of mediators released by primary and secondary effector cells (14). For instance, we were able to detect significant amounts of LTC4, EPO, ECP and histamine (but not tryptase) during ocular LPR (15). This last finding is in agreement with the hypothesis of the Baltimore group, based on the different pattern of mediators found in nasal washing at different time periods after allergen challenge, that basophils but not MCs have a role in LPR (16). Interestingly enough, mediators present in tears (6 hours after allergen challenge) can passively transfer the ocular LPR (Bonini et al., JACI, submitted for publication).

Clinical and cytological changes of conjunctival LPR appear to be a continuous dose-dependent process (17). When low allergen doses are used for challenge, or when the sensitivity of the patients is low, only cytological changes are observed during the early phase of conjunctival reaction, not associated with clinical symptoms. Increasing the dose of allergen results in a more intense cellular reaction and in typical clinical immediate response of the conjunctiva. When the dose of allergen is further increased, or when patients with higher sensitivity are challenged, a more intense and prolonged cell recruitment is induced, with a clinical LPR when consistent allergen doses are used. Therefore, from our studies in the eye it appears that LPR is a constant outcome of the immediate reaction, provided that large allergen doses are administered to highly sensitized patients.

Summarizing, our studies of conjunctival allergen challenge indicate that persisting inflammatory changes with participation of several cells and mediators are induced by the mast cell activation after IgE-allergen interaction. We can also speculate that similar changes might occur in non IgE-mediated mast cell and basophil activation, thus suggesting a common inflammatory pathway for IgE-dependent and non-IgE dependent reactions. Finally, we suggest that, since the conjunctival changes can be easily and repeatedly monitored with the advantage of having the contralateral eye as an internal control, conjunctival provocation can represent a very useful model for the study of the mechanisms involved in persisting allergic inflammation and clinical disease as well as of their pharmacologic control.

Effects of Histamine Challenge

Extensive evidence in target organs other than the eye indicates that allergic patients are hyperreactive to various non-specific substances in addition to the sensitizing allergen (18). Although close relationships exist between reactivity to allergens and to non-allergic substances, specific and non-specific kinds of hyperreactivity represent distinct concurrent mechanisms in the pathogenesis of several allergic diseases such as bronchial asthma (19). We compared the conjunctival responsiveness to histamine diphosphate (0.1–1.0 mg/ml) in patients with VKC and in healthy controls (20). Both VKC patients and controls reacted to histamine with a dose-dependent conjunctival redness 2 to 5 minutes after allergen challenge. However, at low histamine doses (0.01, 0.5 mg/ml) VKC had a significantly ($p < .05$) more intense reaction than controls. Moreover, the concentration of histamine diphosphate causing a threshold conjunctival redness (provoking concentration of histamine, PC) was significantly lower ($p < .02$) in patients with VKC than in controls.

The existence of a conjunctival hyperresponsiveness to histamine in VKC might be relevant for a better understanding of the pathogenesis and some clinical features of this disease. For instance, non-specific conjunctival hyperreactivity may play a role in causing the variable course of the disease not correlating with environmental changes of the sensitizing allergen. In fact, sun, wind, dust or other natural agents may represent only triggers of a non-specific abnormal reactivity of the conjunctiva. We can also speculate that non-specific conjunctival hyperreactivity has a primary pathogenetic role in forms of "allergic" conjunctivitis where no clinical sensitization is detectable, as in many cases of VKC and CLC.

Summarizing, our studies of histamine challenge in VKC patients indicate that hyperreactivity to non-specific substances can be documented for human conjunctiva as it is for other target organs of allergic diseases. Only the extensive use of well-standardized conjunctival provocation tests with non-specific agents can prove the hypothesis that this novel concept in ocular allergic diseases can be of pathogenetic relevance and clinical utility.

Concluding Remarks

The above reported data strongly suggest that the pathogenesis of "allergic conjunctivitis" cannot be confined to the classic type I hypersensitivity reaction. Several mechanisms other than the IgE-dependent mast cell mediator release can be operating in different forms of "allergic conjunctivitis", including the participation of a complex network of inflammatory cells and mediators, the occurrence of late-phase persistent inflammatory changes, and the presence of an enhanced reactivity of the conjunctiva, shown in Figure 2. As this figure indicates, allergen exposure causes, in sensitized subjects, not only mast cell and basophil activation and mediator release, but also activation of other cells with FcεRII such as macrophages, lymphocytes, eosinophils and platelets. It is also possible that non-IgE mediated triggering of the process occurs. Th2 like lymphocytes are responsible both for hyperproduction of IgE (IL-4) and for differentiation and activation of mast cells (IL-3) and eosinophils (IL-5). Mast cell (and basophil) mediators do cause the immediate reaction (represented in Fig. 1), but also the recruitment of other inflammatory cells observed during the late-phase reaction, such as eosinophils, basophils, lymphocytes and platelets. This recruitment (favored, at tissue site, by the endothelial expression of adhesion molecules induced by mononuclear cell products) results in the release of other mediators and epithelial damage. Moreover, several inflammatory cell products can induce fibroblast proliferation and collagen production. Finally the complexity of the entire network is increased by the fact that most of the cell interactions are bi-directional: for example, epithelial cells and fibroblasts can act not only as targets but also as modulators of the inflammatory process; mast cells can release ILs regulating T cell function and inflammation, etc. Selective or preferential pathways might be involved in different forms of "allergic conjunctivitis" or depending on the intensity of the triggering stimuli and/or the patient sensitivity.

This polyfactorial pathophysiology possibly explains the heterogeneity of "allergic conjunctivitis" and should prompt us to develop a new classification, a more articulated diagnostic approach and a more selective therapeutic control of allergic eye diseases.

References

1. Gleich, G.J. 1982. The late phase of the immunoglobulin E-mediated reaction:A link between anaphylaxis and common allergic disease? J. Allergy Clin. Immunol. 70:160.
2. Magnussen, H., and Nowak, D. 1989. Roles of hyperresponsiveness and airway inflammation in bronchial asthma. Respiration 55:65.
3. Kay, A.B. 1991. Asthma and inflammation. J. Allergy Clin. Immunol. 87:893.
4. Bonini, St., and Bonini, Se. 1987. Studies of allergic conjunctivitis. Chibret Int. J. 5:12.

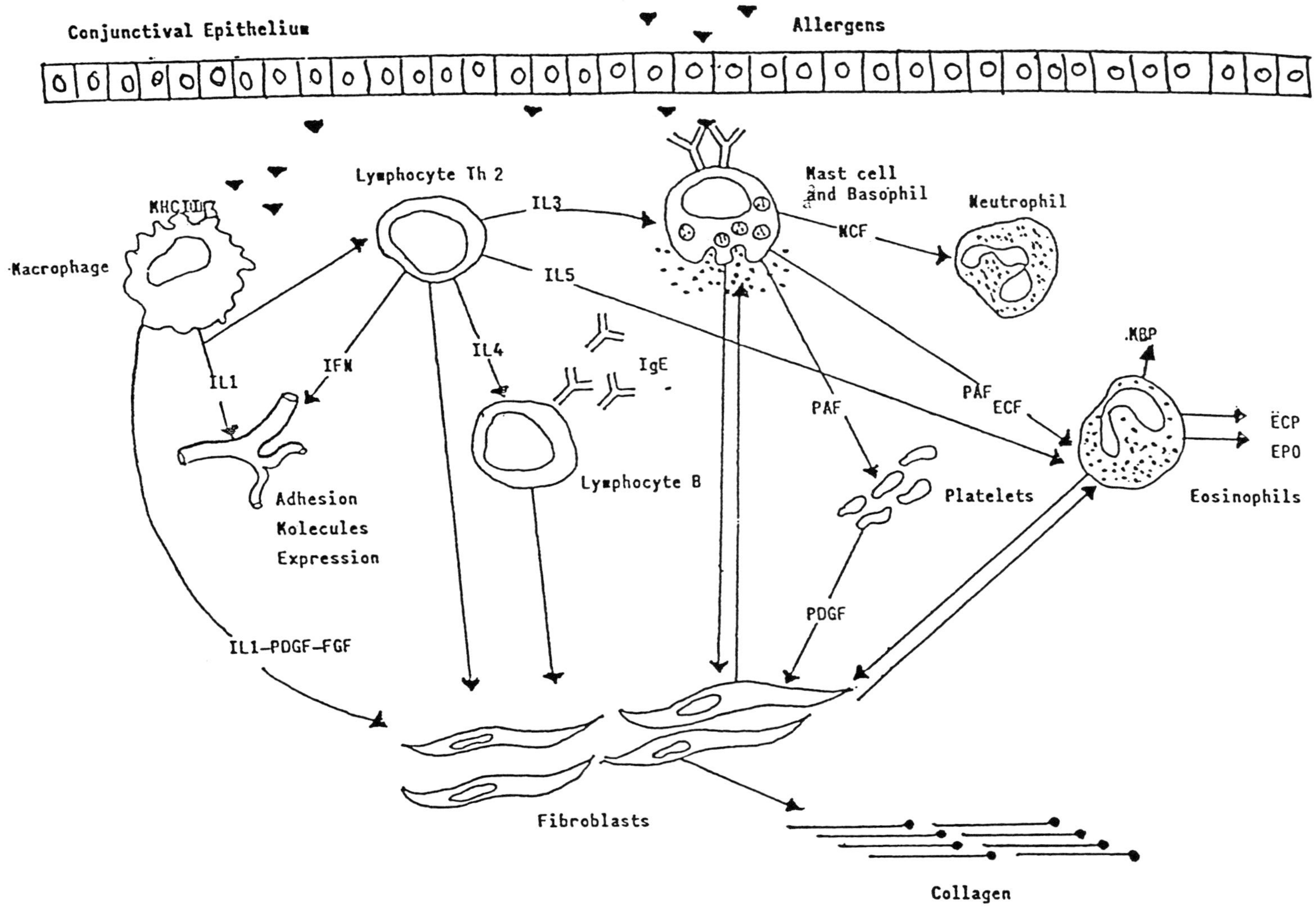

Figure 2. A simplified schematic representation of the complex and polyfactorial pathophysiology of allergic eye diseases based on some data reviewed in the paper (some networks are hypothetical in allergic eye diseases).

5. Allansmith, M.R. 1982. The eye and immunology. St. Louis: Mosby.
6. Irani, A.A., Butrus, S.I., Tabbara, K.A., and Schwartz, L.P. 1990. Mast cell subtypes in vernal and giant papillary conjunctivitis. J. Allergy Clin. Immunol. 86:34.
7. Morgan, S.J., Williams, J.H., Walls, A.F., Church, M.K., Holgate, S.T., and McGill, J.I. 1991. Mast cell numbers and staining characteristics in the normal and allergic human conjunctiva. J. Allergy Clin. Immunol. 87:111.
8. Butrus, S.I., Ochsner, K.I., Abelson, M.B., and Schwartz, L.B. 1990. The level of tryptase in human tears. An indicator of activation of conjunctival mast cells. Ophthalmology 97:1678.
9. Tomassini, M., Capron, M., Bonini, S., and Balsano, F. 1991. Meccanismi di attivazione in vitro degli eosinofili umani. Proc. XX Congr. It. Soc. Allergol. Clin. Immunol. Firenze: OIC Medical Press Srl, p. 397.
10. Maggi, E., Biswas, P., Del Prete, G., Parronchi, P., Macchia, D., Simonelli, C., Emmi, L., De Carli, M., Tiri, A., Ricci, M., and Romagnani, S. 1991. Accumulation of Th-2 like helper T cells in the conjunctiva of patients with vernal conjunctivitis. J.Immunol. 146:1169.
11. Bonini, Se., Bonini, St., Vecchione, A., Naim, D.M., Allansmith, M.R., and Balsano, F. 1988. Inflammatory changes in conjunctival scrapings after challenge provocation in humans. J. Allergy Clin. Immunol. 82:462.
12. Bonini, St., Trocme', S.D., Barney, N.P., Brash, P.C., Block, K.J., and Allansmith, M.R. 1987. Late-phase reaction and tear fluid cytology in the rat ocular anaphylaxis. Curr. Eye Res. 6:659.
13. Bonini, Se., Bonini, St., Bucci, M.G., and Balsano, F. 1989. Allergic mechanisms of the eye. Allergologie 12:158.
14. Proud, D., Sweet, J., Stein, P., Settipane, R.A., Kagey-Sobotka, A., Friedlander, M.H., and Lichtenstein, L.M. 1991. Inflammatory mediator release on conjunctival provocation of allergic subjects with allergen. J. Allergy Clin. Immunol. 85:896.
15. Bonini, Se., Bonini, St., Berruto, A., Tomassini, M., Carlesimo, S., Bucci, M.G., and Balsano, F. 1989. Conjunctival provocation test as a model for the study of allergy and inflammation in humans. Int. Archs. Allergy Appl. Immunol. 88:144.
16. Naclerio, R.M., Proud, D., Togias, A.G., Adkinson, N.F., Jr, Meyers, D.A., Kagey-Sobotka, A., Plaut, M., Norman, P.S., and Lichtenstein, L.M. 1985. Inflammatory mediators in late antigen-induced rhinitis. N. Engl. J. Med. 313:65.
17. Bonini, St., Bonini, Se., Bucci, M.G., Berruto, A., Adriani, E., Balsano, F., and Allansmith, M.R. 1990. Allergen dose response and late symptoms in a human model of ocular allergy. J. Allergy Clin. Immunol. 86:869.
18. Cockroft, D.W. 1985. Bronchial inhalation tests. I. Measurement of nonallergic bronchial responsiveness. Ann. Allergy 55:527.
19. Pauwels, R. 1987. Relationship between bronchial responsiveness and immunological hypersensitivity. In: Bronchial hyperresponsiveness. J.A. Nadel, R. Pauwels, P.D. Nashall, eds. Oxford: Blackwell., p. 342.
20. Bonini, St., Bonini, Se., Schiavone, M., Centofanti, M., Allansmith, M.R., and Bucci, M.G. 1992. Conjunctival hyperresponsiveness to ocular histamine challenge in patients with vernal conjunctivitis. J. Allergy Clin. Immunol. 89:103.

Contact Lens Allergic Disease

Roger J. Buckley*

Allergic disease related to the use of contact lenses is a relatively new concept, probably dating back no more than 17 years. Though it is likely that a large number of distinct clinical manifestations exist that could be placed under this heading, just three syndromes, the best known, will be described here. These are Contact Lens-Associated Papillary Conjunctivitis, Thiomersal Keratoconjunctivitis and Contact Lens-Associated Sterile Keratitis.

Contact Lens-Associated Papillary Conjunctivitis

The condition was first reported by Spring (1) in 1974 in soft contact lens wearers. In 1977 Allansmith et al. (2) described the condition also in wearers of rigid lenses and named it Giant Papillary Conjunctivitis (GPC). A similar clinical manifestation was described in ocular prosthesis (artificial eye) wearers by Srinivasan et al. (3) in 1979, and in the presence of sutures on the ocular surface by Sugar et al. (4) in 1981. The tarsal conjunctival surface which lines the inside of the eyelids is normally smooth or covered by *micropapillae* whose diameter is less than 0.3 mm. *Macropapillae,* which are not within the range of normality, have diameters between 0.3 and 1.0 mm, while *giant papillae* are defined as those of 1.0 mm or more in diameter.

Signs of CLAPC

In CLAPC the chief area of abnormality is the upper tarsal surface, which is characterized by papillary hypertrophy (macropapillae, giant papillae, or both); the lower may be affected also, though this is less usual, and in severe cases there may be inflammation of the corneoscleral limbus, resembling that seen in Vernal Keratoconjunctivitis (VKC), a primary ocular allergic disease. Corneal changes (which are characteristic VKC) do not occur, however.

Symptoms of CLAPC

The symptoms of CLAPC are as follows: itching, especially on removing lenses; discomfort (awareness of lenses); reduced lens wearing time; redness; mucous discharge; and, displacement of the lenses under the upper lid.

Management of CLAPC

CLAPC is managed in the following ways:

Careful attention to lens hygiene: Contact lenses of all types become coated with organic and inorganic deposits derived from the tear film, the ocular surface and the environment. Some types are much more prone to deposition than others. Daily-worn lenses should be cleaned daily using a surfactant cleaner and digital friction. The cleaner should then be rinsed off and the lenses placed in a disinfecting system (types include cold dilute antiseptic solutions, weak hydrogen peroxide, and Pasteurisation). It is estimated that around a half of all lens wearers do not follow these simple guidelines, because of ignorance or neglect. Since the presence of deposits on the lens surface is implicated in the pathogenesis of CLAPC, it follows that a clean lens will be less offensive to the ocular mucous membrane.

Attention to the fit and the surface qualities of the lens: Lenses that fit poorly, so that their edges stand off excessively from the ocular surface, or that move excessively, or are unnecessarily large, are more likely than well-fitting lenses to cause CLAPC. The inherent surface qualities of some materials renders them more challenging than others to the conjunctiva: for example, soft (hydrogel) lenses tend to produce the condition more frequently than do rigid (acrylic or gas-permeable) lenses.

Minimizing the wearing time: CLAPC is "dose dependent"; shortening the wearing time reduces the challenge. Many lens users wear their lenses for 16 or more hours per day who could manage perfectly well with, say, 12 hours

* Moorfields Eye Hospital, 57 A Wimpole St., London W1M 7DF, U.K.

per day, a reduction of 25%. Others can wear their glasses except, perhaps, for sports and certain occupations. Most contact lens wearers have the capacity to reduce their wearing times, and the final sanction is of course to discontinue lens wear altogether.

Use of drugs such as sodium cromoglycate: When the conservative measures already outlined have failed or proved inadequate, sodium cromoglycate (Opticrom, Fisons plc) in 2% ophthalmic solution can be used four times daily to provide relief from the symptoms, and often to reduce the signs, of CLAPC. The 4% ointment preparation can also be used at night, when the lenses are not being worn. In a double-blind trial (5), 37 patients with GPC were treated with either unpreserved sodium cromoglycate (SCG) 2% drops or placebo, four times daily for six weeks, while lens wear continued. At the end of the study, 78% of the patients given SCG and 50% of those receiving placebo rated treatment as moderately successful or very successful. The clinician assessed treatment as moderately successful or very successful in 72% of patients treated with SCG, compared with only 22% of those given placebo. Independently analysed photographs of the tarsal surfaces taken before and after treatment indicated moderate or great improvement in 13 of the 19 patients in the SCG group but in only one of the 18 patients assigned to the placebo group.

Topical steroid preparations are to be avoided, because of the high risk of serious unwanted effects, including steroid glaucoma, cataract and the enhancement of infection. In prosthesis wearers these considerations do not apply. When the condition is due to a projection from the ocular surface, such as a suture, the condition is simply relieved by removing the projection.

Thiomersal Keratoconjunctivitis

Many, but not all ophthalmologists are familiar with the condition of thiomersal keratoconjunctivitis (first described in 1978 by Pedersen [6], a Danish dermatologist) seen in the wearers of hydrogel contact lenses. This reaction, which is basically a superior limbic keratitis, has the characteristics of a type 4, delayed hypersensitivity response. Leukotriene C4 and prostaglandin E2 appear in the tears in thiomersal keratopathy: this finding may be further evidence in favour of a hypersensitive, rather than a toxic, aetiology.

Thiomersal in Contact Lens Fluid

Thiomersal (thimerosal, merthiolate) is used as a disinfecting agent in some soft contact lens solutions, in low concentrations such as 0.0025% or less. The compound is unstable and readily breaks down to thiosalicylic acid and ethylmercuric hydrochloride; the latter (which may be an "active principle" of thiomersal solutions) readily liberates elemental mercury.

Signs

The condition presents as a "superior limbic keratitis" and often features tongues of abnormal epithelial cells which grow across the corneal surface, sometimes as far as the visual axis where they can affect vision, and vascular ingrowth at the limbus. There are minimal conjunctival signs.

Symptoms

The symptoms include lens intolerance and redness of the eyes; they are produced and perpetuated even by rare intermittent wear of the contaminated lenses. In severe cases, the vision is affected.

Conjunctival Challenge Test

The diagnosis may be established by a challenge test, in which a positive result is an acutely inflamed eye surface following the instillation of normal saline drops preserved with thiomersal 0.005%, applied twice daily. The reaction is usually seen within 24 hours.

Skin Patch-Testing

On the subject of skin patch-testing in thiomersal keratoconjunctivitis, experiences differ. In a 1981 paper by Wilson et al. (7) from the United States, 27 of 31 patients patch-tested to thiomersal showed positive results; a hypersensitivity (Type IV) reaction was postulated. Wright and Mackie (8) in Great Britain showed a positive result in only one of 21 patients patch-tested; the existence of a locally-produced, high-affinity antibody was postulated. (In the same study, ten out of 10 patients tested showed a positive conjunctival challenge.) The contradictory results seen in different parts of the world may reflect the practice of immunisation with thiomersal-preserved preparations, which occurs in some countries and not in others.

Management

Once the diagnosis is made, the patient must permanently avoid thiomersal-containing solutions. Lens wear should be discontinued until the epithelium returns to normal, a process that may take weeks or months. If lens wear is resumed, the lenses should be renewed, as it is usually impossible to remove all traces of thiomersal after contamination. For disinfection, the patient should change to a non-thiomersal-containing disinfecting system, such as hydrogen peroxide, or Pasteurisation.

Chronic Thiomersal Keratoconjunctivitis

Much less common, and certainly less likely to be attributed by the ophthalmologist to thiomersal hypersensitivity, is a chronic and irreversible corneal epitheliopathy in which the entire population of epithelial cells becomes replaced by conjunctivally-derived cells. Such cells are semi-opaque and have abnormal wetting characteristics. Eventually, a fibrovascular pannus develops which may cover the entire cornea. This, and the irregularity of the surface of the cornea, can produce a severe reduction of visual acuity. The picture resembles, in fact, a chemical injury such as then produced by ammonia, in which there is limbal ischaemia and loss of the normal population of corneal epithelial cells. The feature that unites these patients, however, is a history of exposure to thiomersal in contact lens solutions.

This condition does not resolve spontaneously, nor does it respond to drug treatment. A logical initial approach is to establish a population of more normal epithelial cells on the eye surface. The concept of *conjunctival transplantation* was introduced in a classic paper published in 1977 by Thoft (9). He used islands of bulbar conjunctiva from the fellow eye, arranged around the limbus, to establish a new population of epithelial cells on the surface of the injured eye, following removal of the entire corneal epithelium and a 5 mm band of adjacent conjunctival epithelium. A new approach to this problem, however, makes use of the stem cell concept introduced in 1986 in another classic paper by Schermer et al. (10). These authors concluded, from the pattern of expression of a cornea-specific 65 kilo dalton keratin, that the stem cells which give rise to the corneal epithelium are located at the limbus. Utilizing the new stem cell concept, Kenyon and Tseng (11) introduced in 1989 the surgical procedure known as *limbal autograft transplantation*. In this, islands of limbal tissue are transplanted to the injured eye from the less involved fellow eye.

Prevention of Thiomersal Keratoconjunctivitis

The condition will not occur if thiomersal-containing contact lens solutions are avoided. The solution manufacturers have responded over time, by withdrawing thiomersal-containing formulations from their ranges and introducing new solution entities. It is clear that this compound should no longer be included in contact lens care solutions.

Contact Lens-Associated Sterile Keratitis

This condition must be carefully distinguished from infective keratitis, a severe sight-threatening condition which requires immediate treatment; this is not always easy. Contact lens-associated sterile keratitis is probably a delayed hypersensitivity reaction to microbial protein adherent to the lens. It is known to be related to poor lens hygiene, microbial contamination of the lens case, and contact lens type. A paper by Bates et al. (12) established that the condition is rare, accounting for 0.49% of all casualties. The relative risk is 2.3 times for hydrogel lenses worn overnight, and 1.6 times for hydrogel lenses worn during the waking hours only: these figures compare to a referent, the gas-permeable rigid lens, of unity.

Symptoms of CLA Sterile Keratitis

Discomfort or pain; redness; epiphora; photophobia; intolerance of the contact lens; "white spot" on the cornea.

Signs of CLA Sterile Keratitis

Corneal stromal infiltrate, conjunctival hyperaemia and oedema.

Differential Diagnosis

If a corneal infiltrate is less than 1 mm in diameter, and there is no epithelial defect, and no anterior chamber inflammation; also if pain and discharge are absent, the diagnosis is probably sterile infiltration. If, however, the infiltrate is more than 2 mm in diameter, if there is an epithelial defect, if anterior chamber activity is present, and there is pain and discharge, the lesion is probably infected.

Management of CLA Sterile Keratitis

Once a confident diagnosis has been made, the cause (microbial products on the contact lens) can be eliminated by the cessation of lens wear. No specific drug treatment may be required, but topical steroid is often employed to suppress the inflammatory response, with or without topical antibiotic prophylaxis. Because of possible confusion with infective microbial keratitis, which is a sight-threatening ocular emergency, only an ophthalmologist should attempt to diagnose and manage this condition.

References

1. Spring, T.F. 1974. Reaction to hydrophilic lenses. Med. J. Aust. 1:449.
2. Allansmith, M.R., Korb, D.R., Greiner, J.V., Henriquez, A.S., Simon, M.A., and Finnemore, V.M. 1977. Giant papillary conjunctivitis in contact lens wearers. Am. J. Ophthalmol. 83:697.
3. Srinivasan, B.D., Jacobiec, F.A., Iwamoto, T., and DeVoe, G. 1979. Giant papillary conjunctivitis with ocular prostheses. Arch. Ophthalmol. 97:892.
4. Sugar, A., and Meyer, R.F. 1981. Giant papillary conjunctivitis after keratoplasty. Am. J. Ophthalmol. 91:239.
5. Matter, M., Rahi, A.H.S., and Buckley, R.J. 1985. Sodium cromoglycate in the treatment of contact lens-associated giant papillary conjunctivitis. Proc. 7th Congr. Europ. Soc. of Ophthalmol. (Helsinki) p. 383.
6. Pedersen, N.B. 1978. Allergic contact conjunctivitis from merthiolate in soft contact lenses. Contact Dermatitis 4:165.
7. Wilson, L.A., McNatt, J., and Reitschel, R. 1981. Delayed hypersensitivity to thimerosal in soft contact lens wearers. Ophthalmology 88:804.
8. Wright, P., and Mackie, I.A. 1982. Preservative related problems in soft contact lens wearers. Trans. ophthalmol. soc. UK 102:3.
9. Thoft, R.A. 1977. Conjunctival transplantation. Arch. Ophthalmol. 95:1425.
10. Schermer, A., Galvin, S., and Sun, T.-T. 1986. Differentiation-related expression of a major 64K corneal keratin in vivo and in culture suggests limbal location of corneal epithelial stem cells. J. Cell Biol. 103:49.
11. Kenyon, K.R., and Tseng, S.C.G. 1989. Limbal autograft transplantation for ocular surface disorders. Ophthalmology 96:709.
12. Bates, A.K., Morris, R.J., Stapleton, F., Minassian, D.C., and Dart, J.K.G. 1989. "Sterile" corneal infiltrates in contact lens wearers. Eye 3:803.

Immunopathogenesis of Vernal Keratoconjunctivitis

Khalid F. Tabbara*

Vernal Keratoconjunctivitis (VKC) is a disabling allergic disease of children and young adults. The disease can be mild or severe and may lead to visual disability. Several immunopathologic mechanisms have been implicated. The conjunctiva of VKC patients may show hyperplasia, with eosinophilic, lymphocytic and plasma cell infiltration. In addition, there may be fibrous hyperplasia of the substantia propria. Mast cells play an important role in the pathogenesis of VKC. These have been described according to their neutral protease composition, T lymphocyte dependency, and ultrastructural characteristics. Mast cell containing tryptase but no chymase is known as MC_T and mast cells containing both tryptase and chymase are known as MC_{TC}. We studied the distribution of the two mast cell subtypes in the conjunctival tissue of patients with VKC and normal subjects. There were no mast cells in the conjunctival epithelium of normal subjects. In contrast, there was a marked increase in the number of mast cells in the conjunctival epithelium of VKC patients with a mean of 7,994(±5,192) mast cells/mm^3. Mast cells containing both tryptase and chymase are the predominant cell type in the conjunctiva. A significant increase in the number of mast cells containing tryptase is seen in the conjunctival epithelium and substantia propria of VKC subjects but not in normal subjects. In conclusion, the pathogenesis of VKC involves an intricate complex immunologic network involving various inflammatory cells and numerous mediators. Recent advances and research work on these cells contributed immensely to our understanding of these mechanisms and have elucidated the pathogenesis of VKC. Search for drugs that target and selectively interfere with these mechanisms is highly desirable.

Vernal Keratoconjunctivitis (VKC) is an immune-mediated disorder of children and young adults. The disease may vary from one individual to another ranging from mild and self-limiting disorder to severe and vision-threatening disease. Unlike hay fever and other forms of type I hypersensitivity reactions, major corneal and conjunctival structural changes may occur. VKC may lead to visual loss either due to corneal changes or as a complication of steroid therapy.

Clinical Findings

The disease leads to major suffering in the afflicted individual. VKC patients complain of redness, itching, tearing, photophobia, mucus discharge and blurring of vision. Pseudoptosis of the upper eyelids may occur. The eyelids may become floppy and the upper eyelid is everted with great ease. Initially, the conjunctiva shows mild papillary hypertrophy, and as the disease progresses there is evidence of tissue growth and proliferation leading to hyperplasia of the substantia propria of the conjunctiva with formation of giant papillae. The giant papillae are formed due to the polygonal septate attachment of the upper palpebral conjunctiva to the upper tarsus. Progressive hyperplasia in severe forms of VKC may eventuate in pedunculated polypoid conjunctival tissue. The bulbar conjunctiva shows hyperemia and edema. Conjunctival hypertrophy is not remarkable but may occur close to the limbus. The limbus displays a wide variety of signs including tissue hyperplasia, Trantas' dots, pannus, limbal giant papillae, thinning, and Herbert-like pits which are seen in trachoma. Although Trantas are seen more frequently at the limbus and indicate disease activity, I have seen Trantas dots in the center of the cornea, and over the bulbar and palpebral conjunctiva. Diffuse dust-like intraepithelial white-grey microdots are seen sprayed throughout the corneal epithelium which shows punctate staining with fluorescein and Rose Bengal indicating epithelial cell damage. The damage may become severe leading to localized single, or multiple round or oval persistent epithelial defect. In some patients

* Professor and Chairman, Department of Ophthalmology, College of Medicine, King Saud University, P.O. Box 55307, Riyadh 11534, Saudi Arabia.

the epithelial defects become covered with a plaque consisting of PAS positive material. The basement membrane may be damaged during this process.

Immunopathogenesis

Recent advances in the field of immunology and molecular biology have greatly influenced our understanding of immune-mediated disorders. Although the disease has been referred to as an IgE-mediated hypersensitivity disorder of the conjunctiva, VKC appears to have a more diverse and intricate network of immunological pathways leading to the clinical findings mentioned earlier. There are several possible important pillars that lead to the immunopathogenesis of the disease including genetic predisposition, hormonal factors, environmental factors, and local ocular factors. I have noticed that symptoms and signs of vernal keratoconjunctivitis become more severe when the patients develop infectious conjunctivitis such as trachoma. Whether VKC patients are more susceptible to infections due to bacteria such as Hemophilus remains to be elucidated. We performed stool microscopy on 20 patients with VKC and found that seven out of 20 patients with severe VKC had parasitic infestation and elevated serum IgE levels. It is proposed that patients with genetic susceptibility to develop allergy, may be influenced by exogenous factors that augment antigen non-specific stimulation of IgE synthesis. The total number of mast cells may show dramatic increase by certain triggers, and the mast cell functions can be later induced by immune or non-immune stimuli. The association of VKC with the hyper-IgE syndrome (1), which is characterized by a deficiency in T-suppressor cells, suggests a regulatory role for T lymphocytes in VKC. The tissue hyperplasia of lymphocytic and plasma cell infiltration indicates a chronic self perpetuating mechanism leading to the clinical picture of tissue growth and proliferation. VKC, therefore, appears to have a unique immune-mediated network of events leading to the pathogenesis of this disorder and cannot be regarded as an isolated IgE mediated reaction (1,2).

Several cells and mediators play a role in the immunopathogenesis of VKC, and a cascade of chemical mediators and reactions are involved. Conjunctival biopsy specimens of patients with active VKC demonstrate infiltration by lymphocytes, plasma cells, eosinophils, basophils and mast cells. In addition, we have found that limbal conjunctival biopsy specimens obtained from patients with severe VKC show a marked increase in the number of epithelial and intestinal mast cells, Langerhans cells, and T-lymphocytes when compared to normal control specimens. Mast cells play a crucial role in the pathogenesis of VKC. Recent studies have shown that the mast cells have structural and functional heterogeneity. Different regulatory mechanisms exist in the mast cell mRNA transcription of various groups of cytokines. Different types of mast cells respond differently to physiologic, immunologic or pathologic stimuli. IgE mediated activation of mast cells leads to mobilization of intracellular calcium and activation of protein kinase C. Phenotypically distinct mast cell populations may express different functions in health and disease.

Furthermore, immunological studies have shown that the mast cell participates in a broader spectrum of biochemical and immunological process than those involving IgE. Mast cells appear to participate in a variety of mechanisms including persistent chronic inflammation, tissue remodeling, pathologic fibrosis, and tissue hyperplasia. Bacterial lipopolysaccharide (LPS), neuropeptides, products of complement activation, insect venoms, and certain antigens may nonspecifically stimulate the release of bioactive mediators from the mast cell. This is supported by clinical observation that bacterial conjunctivitis may precipitate or aggravate the symptoms of VKC.

Mast cells also elaborate tumor necrosis factor α (TNFα) and transforming growth factors (TGF) β. TGFα is a multifunctional cytokine that can augment fibrosis and angiogenesis. This may explain the tissue hyperplasia that occurs in many patients with VKC. Many important questions remain concerning the mechanisms that regulate production of these mast cell factors.

Morphologic and immunohistochemical characteristics of mast cells have been studied. Mast cells have been described according to their T-lymphocyte dependency, neutral protease composition, and ultrastructural characteristics (3–8). Mast cells containing tryptase but no chymase are known as T mast cells

Table 1. Conjunctival Mast Cell Distribution.

Group	Epithelium Total No. of Mast Cells	Substantia Propia Total No. of Mast Cells
VKC	7,994 (±2,120)	24,689 ± 7,748
ΓΠΧ	3,814 (±2,052)	17,313 ± 3,801
ΣΧΛ	0	13,168 ± 2,095
Αλλεργιχ		
Χονφυνχτιϖιτισ	0	15,380 ± 2,830
Νορμαλ	0	11,054 ± 1,491

VKC = Vernal Keratoconjunctivitis, GPC = Giant Papillary Conjunctivitis, SCL = Soft Contact Lens wearers (Reference 9)

(MC_T) while those containing both tryptase and chymase are known as TC mast cells (MC_{TC}). We studied the distribution of these two mast cell types in the conjunctival tissue of patients with VKC, giant papillary conjunctivitis (GPC), and normal subjects (9). There were no mast cells in the epithelium of normal conjunctiva. In contrast, there was a marked increase in the number of mast cells in the conjunctival epithelium of patients with VKC with a mean of 7,994 (±5192) mast cells mm^3 (Table 1). Ninety percent of the mast cells were MC_T and 10% were MC_{TC} in the conjunctiva of patients with VKC. The number of mast cells in the conjunctival substantia propria of VKC patients was 24,689 (±7,784). In GPC on the other hand, all mast cells observed were MC_{TC} and no MC_T were seen in either the epithelium or substantia propria. Mast cell subtypes may react differently to exogenous or endogenous stimuli which may have important clinical implications. Further search for therapeutic targets should take into consideration the factors that lead to mast cell proliferation and predominant trigger stimuli. Mast cell subtypes and different physiologic, pathologic or immunologic stimuli may lead to the release of different types of mediators and may display variability in response to topical medication.

The biochemical events that trigger the release of biologically active mediators by the mast cells are determined by several factors. The initiation of the process is important but the propagation and perpetuation of the events leading to the chronicity of VKC are determined by the number of mast cells, by their ability to induce the perpetuation of the reaction, and exposure to specific triggers. T helper cells also play an important role in the initiation and stimulation of MC_T in the epithelium and substantia propria of patients with VKC.

We are currently studying the effects of topical medications on conjunctival mast cell subtypes and distribution in VKC.

References

1. Butrus, S.I., Leung, D.Y.M., Gellis, S., Baum, J., Kenyon, K., and Abelson, M.B. 1984. Vernal conjunctivitis in the hyperimmunoglobulinemia E syndrome. Ophthalmology 91:1213.
2. Ballow, M., Donshik, P.C., and Mendelson, L. 1985. Complement proteins and C3 anaphylatoxin in the tears of patients with conjunctivitis. J. Allergy Clin. Immunol. 76:544.
3. Schwartz, L.B., Irani, A.A., Roller, K., Castells, M.C., and Schechter, N.M. 1987. Quantitation of histamine, tryptase, and chymase in dispersed human T and TC mast cells. J. Immunol. 138:2611.
4. Craig, S.S., Schechter, N.M., and Schwartz, L.B. 1988. Ultrastructural analysis of human T and TC mast cells identified by immunoelectronmicroscopy. Lab. Invest. 59:682.
5. Irani, A.A., Craig, S.S., DeBlois, G., Elson, C.O., Schechter, N.M., and Schwartz, L.B. 1987. Deficiency of tryptase-positive, chymase-negative mast cell type in gastrointestinal mucosa of patients with defective T lymphocyte function. J. Immunol. 138:4381.
6. Irani, A.A., Bradford, T.R., Kepley, C.L., Schechter, N.M., and Schwartz, L.B. 1989. Detection of MC_T and MC_{TC} types of human mast cells by immunohistochemistry using new

monoclonal anti-tryptase and anti-chymase antibodies. J. Histochem. Cytochem. 37:1509.
7. Craig, S.S., DeBlois, G., and Schwartz, L.B. 1986. Mast cells in human keloid, small intestine, and lung by immunoperoxidase technique using a murine monoclonal antibody against tryptase. Am. J. Pathol. 124:427.
8. Benyon, R.C., Lowman, M.A., and Church, M.K. 1987. Human skin mast cells: Their dispersion, purification, and secretory characterization. J. Immunol. 138:861.
9. Irani, A.A., Butrus, S., Tabbara, K.F., and Schwartz, L.B. 1990. Human conjunctival mast cells: distribution of MC_T and MC_{TC} in vernal keratoconjunctivitis. J. Allergy Clin. Immunol. 86:34.

Management of Ocular Allergic Diseases

L. M. T. Collum*

Ocular allergic diseases are a potent cause of ocular morbidity. Many drugs, such as corticosteroids, are too toxic for continuous use in these conditions; and other drugs, such as the antihistamines do not have sufficient effect. Mast cell stabilisation is the main treatment of most of these allergic conditions, as degranulation of the mast cell with the release of vasoactive substances is the cause of the symptoms. There is a range of allergies, varying from mild conjunctivitis to severe atopic keratoconjunctivitis. The milder conditions respond readily to mast cell stabilisation alone, though the severe allergic conditions require the addition of adjunctive therapy, in some instances corticosteroids. The principle of treatment is to keep the use of corticosteroids to a minimum and this is achieved by the use of mast cell stabilisers, such as Sodium Cromoglycate. The great advantage of Sodium Cromoglycate is that it is non-toxic and can thus be used all the year round. The role of mast cell stabilisation and other forms of treatment are discussed in the different types of ocular allergy.

The general expression, "immunologically mediated ocular disease", is a good umbrella to cover the wide spectrum of conditions produced in the eye, either by humoral or cellular activity. This term covers, therefore, a full range of conditions including IgE mediated disorders, the effects of generalised systemic diseases, such as rheumatoid arthritis, systemic lupus and various forms of vasculitis, together with pemphigus and other related entities, uveitis, corneal graft rejection and other reactions such as conjunctivitis medicamentosa. The term "ocular allergy" is used almost synonymously with external eye disease inflammation, though this is not entirely correct. However, for the purpose of this paper, the term "ocular allergic disease" will be confined to inflammation of the external eye. These inflammations have a number of methods of production, though mast cell degranulation forms the basis for most of them. It is, however, inaccurate to consider the mast cell as the sole mediator in the conditions to be discussed, but the role of other cells has not been accurately established. In addition, it is also likely that the genetic profile, external and environmental factors and HLA type are also relevant in determining the severity and pattern of diseases and probably the response to therapy. Ocular allergic disease can be classified as follows: (a) acute allergic conjunctivitis; (b) hay fever conjunctivitis; (c) chronic allergic conjunctivitis; (d) vernal keratoconjunctivitis; (e) giant papillary conjunctivitis; and (f) eczematous keratoconjunctivitis.

Acute Allergic Conjunctivitis

Acute allergic conjunctivitis may be unilateral and is an explosive oedema of the lids and conjunctiva. It generally tends to occur in later life as distinct from some of the other allergic conditions which tend to occur at an early age. It is a 24 hour phenomenon which will usually clear spontaneously. The exact mechanism has not been fully established, though the large number of mast cells in the normal conjunctiva are undoubtedly an instigating factor. At a recent symposium in Sardinia (1) it was felt that acute allergy did not fit readily into the general classification of ocular allergy, although there is some uncertainty about this. Very often, treatment is not required, as by the time the patient presents at the Accident/Emergency Department the condition has settled. If the patient is having recurring attacks, treatment should consist of prophylactic Sodium Cromoglycate. Anti-histamines are helpful in the acute stage.

Hay Fever Conjunctivitis

This term is used to cover such conditions as seasonal, perennial, rag-weed, pollenosis and sensitivities to allergen, all of which have a common clinical presentation. There is no

* Royal College of Surgeons in Ireland and Royal Victoria Eye and Ear Hospital, Dublin, Ireland.

doubt that this is an IgE mediated disease (2). It is usually bilateral, often asymmetrical and affects young adults. The diagnosis is based on clinical signs and symptoms and may be confirmed by laboratory tests. There is usually itching, though this may be mild, and also a burning sensation in the eye, with watering. The eyes tend to be red, with mild conjunctival oedema and some conjunctival hyperplasia. Laboratory tests that are useful consist of conjunctival scrapings and skin tests with RAST. A positive personal history of other allergy is present in 94% of patients (3), rhinitis being the most common. Because the rhinitis is frequently more severe than the ocular condition, the patient often ignores the eye symptoms and presents to his family practitioner with his nasal problems. The management of the ocular symptoms should be the use of mast cell stabilisers, particularly Sodium Cromoglycate (4,5,6,7). The use of Sodium Cromoglycate on a prophylactic basis is also indicated in this condition. Ideally, Sodium Cromoglycate should be introduced prior to the identified season and continued for some time thereafter. This use of Sodium Cromoglycate on a prophylactic basis insures that symptoms are minimised; and because of the absence of side effects the drug may be continued for as long as is thought necessary. It is likely that Nedocromil Sodium will have a role to play in hay fever conjunctivitis (8), though this has not been, as yet, fully established. Antihistamines have only a limited role, while local corticosteroids are never indicated. These patients present problems if they wish to wear contact lenses and, while hay fever conjunctivitis is not an absolute contraindication, a warning should be given that the use of lenses may aggravate the pre-existing condition.

Chronic Allergic Conjunctivitis

Chronic allergic conjunctivitis is a difficult diagnosis to make (9). Patients present with chronic ocular irritation which they describe as burning and grittiness. Itchiness may be a feature, though the condition is so chronic and the complaints so variable that there is no absolute characteristic symptom. The eyes tend to be slightly hyperaemic, with a watery discharge and there is mild papillary hyperplasia. The problem in chronic allergic conjunctivitis is to identify the cases. The symptoms described occur in many conditions, such as tear film disorders, chronic blepharitis and chronic lid margin disease. It is therefore important to outrule other possible causes of the symptoms before making a diagnosis of chronic allergy. Eosinophils in conjunctival scrapings may be helpful, though they are not as numerous as in hay fever disease. Once a diagnosis is established, the treatment of choice is mast cell stabilisation. The use of other drugs, such as antibiotics is contraindicated as they often aggravate the condition. The problem with these patients is that they are frequently inaccurately diagnosed initially and the use of varying medications so confuses the clinical picture that it becomes difficult at a later stage to establish a proper diagnosis. Therefore, full investigation of patients, who present with these non-specific symptoms, is mandatory, first withdrawing any local medications that they may be using.

Vernal Keratoconjunctivitis

Vernal keratoconjunctivitis is a severe chronic bilateral inflammatory disease with periodic exacerbations. Its geographic distribution is variable (10), being most common in the Mediterranean area. It has a number of forms, limbal, palbebral, or combined. Between the ages of 4 and 14 years there is a 2:1 male preponderance (11) but this ratio reverses at puberty. Symptoms of itching, watering, photophobia, foreign body sensation and grittiness are the main complaints while examination of the conjunctiva and cornea will show changes varying from mild papillary hyperplasia to severe corneal ulceration with the possible presence of pseudo-gerontoxon. There is a positive personal or family history of other associated allergic diseases, varying in different studies from 15 to 65% (12,13), rhinitis being the most common. The management of vernal keratoconjunctivitis requires great care and attention. It is a sight threatening disorder and the object of treatment is to minimise damage to the cornea. Vernal keratoconjunctivitis can be divided into three types, mild, moderate or severe, the severe type occurring in the young male, while the mild form occurs in the older age group. Eighty per cent of patients with vernal disease can be controlled with Sodium Cromoglycate alone or at most with the occasional addition of low dose corticosteroid drops (14). The disease in some cases requires maintenance all the year round, but is sometimes punctuated by exacerbations when treatment may have to be increased. In 20% of patients, the use of corticosteroids is necessary. The disease wanes as the patient gets older allowing treatment to be withdrawn and the sequalae, if the proper regime is carried out, will be minimal. Associated atopic phenomena, such as rhinitis and asthma, should be treated concurrently.

Giant Papillary Conjunctivitis

Giant papillary conjunctivitis is a multifactorial inflammation of the external eye, mainly associated with contact lens wear, protruding sutures and ocular prostheses. Factors that aggravate the problem are atmospheric pollution, bacterial infection and tear film disorders, as well as iatrogenic agents. Contact lens type and fitting are relevant, and pre-existing atopy is also important (15,16). The development and severity of the disease is also related to the length of lens wear, the type of maintenance system used and the frequency with which lenses are replaced. The classical symptom is intolerance to lens wear, with irritation, grittiness, ocular discharge and soreness. The clinical signs consist of a mucus discharge, ocular hyperaemia and papillary hyperplasia on the tarsal conjunctiva. This papillary hyperplasia can be quite subtle and is best demonstrated in the early stages by fluorescein. There is considerable geographic variation in the incidence and type of the disease, which may also be related to the HLA profile of the patient. Mild papillary disease can be treated with Sodium Cromoglycate. In severe giant papillary conjunctivitis, it may be necessary to withdraw the lenses at least on a temporary basis with their reintroduction at a later stage, combined with mast cell stabilisers. A change of lens material and size is sometimes helpful and a change in the solutions used may also be beneficial. There is no contraindication to using Sodium Cromoglycate drops even with soft contact lenses. With proper follow-up, frequent change of lenses, atmospheric modifications and the use of mast cell stabilisers, it is possible for over 80% of patients with GPC to use lenses at least part of the time (17).

Eczematous Keratoconjunctivitis

Eczematous keratoconjunctivitis is a chronic condition associated with eczema (18). The childhood variety is fairly benign but the adult form has significant complications, including cataract (19), keratoconus (20) and conjunctival fibrosis (21). Symptoms can be extremely severe and the clinical signs include thickening and keratinisation of lid edges, together with conjunctival fibrosis, punctate keratopathy and corneal neovascularization. Seventy percent of these patients have associated personal or familial atopic conditions (22). Mild eczematous keratoconjunctivitis in childhood is managed with mast cell stabilisers, with the addition of low-dose corticosteroid. These patients have to be monitored carefully. Adult eczematous keratoconjunctivitis, however, is a severe debilitating condition and almost always requires systemic corticosteroids. The use of local Sodium Cromoglycate is useful in reducing the amount of corticosteroids necessary.

Discussion

Though many factors are involved in the production of allergic eye diseases, as defined in this paper, there is no doubt that mast cell degranulation, with the release of vaso-active substances, is the main mechanism. Mast cell stabilisers, such as Sodium Cromoglycate and possibly Nedocromil Sodium, therefore, play a major role in the control of these conditions. The use of these drugs substantially reduces the need for cortico-steroids and their associated toxicity. The fact that Sodium Cromoglycate is non-toxic means it can be used longterm, without any threat to sight.

References

1. Collum, L.M.T., Bonini, S., Secchi, A.G. et al. Guidelines for the study of allergic conjunctivitis. In preparation.
2. Allensmith, M.R. 1982. The eye and immunology. St. Louis: Mosby.

3. Bonini, S., and Bonini, S. 1987. Studies on allergic conjunctivitis. Chibret Int. J. Ophthalmol. 5:12.
4. Collum, L.M.T., Cassidy, H.P., and Benedict-Smith, A. 1981. Disodium Cromoglycate in vernal and allergic kerato-conjunctivitis. Ir. Med. J. 74:1:14.
5. Ostler, H.B., Martin, R.G., and Dawson C.R. 1977. Symposium of ocular therapy 10:99.
6. Kazdan, J.J., Crawford, J.S., Langer, H., and MacDonald, A.L. 1976. Sodium Cromoglycate in the treatment of vernal keratoconjunctivitis and allergic conjunctivitis. Can. J. Ophthalmol. 11:300.
7. Engstrom, I., Obergerm, E., Blyckert A., and Kraepelein S. 1971. Disodium Cromoglycate in the treatment of seasonal allergic rhinoconjunctivitis in children. Ann. Allergy 29:505.
8. Collum, L.M.T. Clinical experience with Nedocromil Sodium, ongoing research.
9. Collum, L.M.T. Diagnostic problems in conjunctivitis. 1981. The current role of Opticrom in the management of allergic conjunctivitis – Proceedings of Workshop. Pubs. Medical Education Services Ltd., 8.
10. Beigelman, M.N. 1950. Vernal conjunctivitis. Los Angeles: University of Southern California Press.
11. Bonini, S. 1990. Le congiuntiviti allergiche. Milano: Ghedini Editore.
12. Neumann, E., Guttmann, M.J., and Blumenkrantz, N.A. 1959. Review of 400 cases of vernal conjunctivitis. Am. J. Ophthalmol. 47:166.
13. Allansmith, M.R. 1989. Vernal conjunctivitis. In: Duane System of Ophthalmology – Clin. Ophthal. 4,9:1.
14. Collum, L.M.T. 1989. Clinical experience with Opticrom. In: The Second Fisons International Workshop proceedings. E. Bloch Michel, ed. Pubs. Br. Library Cataloguing in Publication Data, 90.
15. Allensmith, M.R., Korb, D.R., Greiner, J.V., Henriquez, A.S., Simon, M.A., and Finnemore, V.N. 1977. Giant papillary conjunctivitis in contact lens wearers. Am. J. Ophthalmol. 83: 697.
16. Allensmith, M.R. 1987. Giant papillary conjunctivitis. In: Duane System of Ophthalmology – Clinical Ophthalmology 4,9A:1.
17. Donshik, P.C., Ballow, M., Luistro, A., and Samartino, L. 1984. Treatment of contact lens-induced giant papillary conjunctivitis. The CLAO Journal 10,4:3460.
18. Friedlander, M.H. 1985. Ocular allergy. J. All. Clin. Immun. 76:645.
19. Ingram, R.M. 1965. Retinal detachment associated with atopic dermatitis and cataract. Br.J. Ophthalmol 49:96.
20. Brunsting, L.A., Reed, W.B., and Bair, H.L. 1955. Occurence of cataracts and keratoconus with atopic dermatitis. Arch. Derm. Symph. (Chicago). 72:237.
21. Bloch-Michel, E. 1988. Oeil et allergie. Acta Soc. Franc. d'Ophthalmol. 5:147–172.
22. Hanifin, J.M. 1987. Epidemiology of atopic dermatitis. Allergy 21:116.

SECTION IV

House Dust and Mite Allergy

The Importance of Dust Mites in Environmental Allergy: Asthma and Atopic Dermatitis

T. A. E. Platts-Mills, L. Gelber, B. Deuell, M. D. Chapman, R. Sporik*

In 1964 Dr. Voorhorst and Spieksma demonstrated that mites were an important source of allergens in mattress and furniture dust and also succeeded in culturing pyroglyphid mites. Within a few years extracts of Dermatophagoides pteronyssinus became widely available and it became clear that a large proportion of patients with asthma had positive skin tests to mite allergens (see reference 1). In particular Dr. Morrisson-Smith demonstrated that mite sensitivity was strongly correlated with asthma among school children in Birmingham England (2). As early as 1967 it was suggested that there was a specific level of mites in house dust (500/g) that would increase the risk of symptoms. However, at that time the widely held view was that bronchial hyper-reactivity (BHR) was a "physiological" abnormality of the lung and that allergens were just one, of many, trigger factors for acute attacks. This led (a) to the assumption that triggering effects would be obvious to the patient, and thus (b) to the often cited opinion that the role of allergens should be considered when the patient gave a history of exacerbation on exposure to specific allergen.

Over the past twenty years our understanding of the significance of BHR, the pathology of asthma, and the role of allergens has changed completely. This process started in 1970 when Roger Altounyan reported that some patients with hay fever developed nonspecific reactivity to histamine during the pollen season, which was associated with symptomatic asthma. He also reported that this increase could be blocked by treatment with cromolyn sodium (3). The significance of those observations was not widely understood at the time and in the same year Kerrebijn reported clear evidence for reversibility of BHR among mite allergic children who spent a year in Davos (i.e., at 6000 feet elevation), but that report failed to recognize the significance of the data (4). It had been known for years that asthmatics often improved when they were moved from their houses to Davos in Switzerland (Thomas Mann's magic mountain). It had also been shown that the same improvement could occur in a "climate chamber" at sea level in the Netherlands (see 1). Altounyan's results formed the intellectual basis of two experiments that reinforced the view that allergen exposure is a primary cause of nonspecific BHR. Hargreave and his colleagues demonstrated that bronchial provocation with allergen could increase nonspecific reactivity for days or weeks (5). Working from the opposite angle we took mite allergic patients from houses with high mite exposure and allowed them to live in a research unit in London with very low exposure for 3 to 9 months and observed progressive decrease in BHR in 5 of 7 patients (6). Interestingly most of these patients had no awareness that house dust caused their attacks and in some cases no history suggestive of allergy. This led to the hypothesis that chronic low dose exposure to allergens and particularly to the dust mite could lead to progressive increases in nonspecific BHR (1,7). Inherent in this view was that the impact of allergens must create some form of "inflammatory" focus which in turn leads to nonspecific reactivity to cold air histamine or other irritants.

The fact that the lungs of some asthmatics were inflamed has been known for many years from post mortems and from the presence of curls of shed epithelium (creola bodies) in sputum. In addition, it was well known that eosinophils and Charcot Leyden crystals were present in asthmatic sputum as well as in the post mortem specimens. Nonetheless as late as 1985 many physicians were still unconvinced that mild or moderate asthma was an inflammatory disease. However, this was in large part

* University of Virginia, Health Sciences Center, Department of Medicine, Charlottesville, VA 22908, USA.

due to the absence of biopsy evidence. Between 1985 and 1991 a series of biopsy studies showed unequivocally that the lungs of even mild asthmatics are inflamed as judged by epithelial damage, eosinophil and lymphocyte infiltration. This has been followed by evidence that late reactions following segmental challenge of the lung involve production of mediators and an influx of eosinophils. Furthermore the Hamilton group demonstrated that saline provocation of mild asthmatics can induce the production of sputum containing both eosinophils and metachromatic cells. Thus it is now clear that the lungs of most asthmatics are inflamed, and that allergen provocation can induce this form of eosinophil rich inflammation. Given the extensive evidence for an association between sensitization to mite allergens and asthma it is clearly a reasonable hypothesis that exposure of the lungs of allergic patients to dust mite allergens is a major cause of asthma.

Dust Mite Immunochemistry

Successful purification of dust mite allergens was difficult before large quantities of mite culture were available (i. e., 400 g). Purification of the 24,000 allergen *Der p I* in 1980 allowed the development of inhibition assays to measure allergen in extracts of house and airborne dust in houses of asthmatic patients (8,9). These studies showed that mite fecal pellets contained *Der p I* and were probably the main form in which the allergen accumulated and became airborne (9,10). In 1984 high affinity IgG monoclonal antibodies to*Der p I* were developed and have since been used to characterize these allergens and for two site monoclonal antibody assays (11). It was clear from early on that there was one or more other important allergens. In 1985 Lind reported the purification of an allergen Dpx and Aalberse obtained a monoclonal antibody against this antigen which led to full definition of a second major allergen *Der p I*I (MW 14,000) (12,13). In fact by this time homologous allergens of *D. farinae* were also described and new terms were adopted: Group I (*Der p I* and *Der f I*) and Group II (*Der p I*I and *Der f* II (14). The next major development was the cloning of mite allergens which was carried out by Dr. Thomas and his colleagues in Perth, Australia (15). Because antisera and sequence data were already available it was possible to identify that the clones were producing *Der p I* and *Der p* II. Subsequently the D. farinae allergens have been successfully cloned in Japan (16). There is also evidence for Group III allergen MW 29,000 and Group IV allergens MW 60,000. Analysis of sequence data strongly suggested that the Group I and Group III allergens were enzymes, and Stewart directly demonstrated this activity. The presence of a digestive enzyme (*Der p I*) in feces is not surprising. The function of the Group II allergens remains unclear and they probably accumulate in dust and become airborne as some other part of the mite. Several studies have shown that both Group I and Group II mite allergens become airborne during disturbance but fall rapidly afterwards (9,17,18). In keeping with this rapid falling neither Group I nor Group II of mite allergens are measurable in a still room and the majority of airborne allergen appears to be carried on particles > 10 µm in diameter.

The Relevance of "Threshold" Levels of Exposure to Mite Allergens

Measurements of dust mite allergen in dust from a series of houses found levels ranging from < 0.2 to > 200 µg p *Der p I*/g of dust. From several different studies it was estimated that 2 µm *Der p I*/g of dust was equivalent to 100 mites/g (14). It is easy to assume that there is a direct quantitative relationship between the level of allergen and the risk of sensitization. However, this information is not easy to use either in discussing risk or particularly in advising individual patients. For this reason threshold levels proposed for several studies were adopted by an International Workshop in 1989 (14). Two separate thresholds were proposed: 2 µg and 10 µg Group I mite allergen/g dust. Exposure to the lower level was considered to increase the risk of sensitization and development of BHR while the higher level (equivalent to the 500 mites/g proposed originally by Spieksma) was considered to increase the risk of symptomatic or acute asthma. Since then at least 4 studies have directly confirmed the relevance of these thresholds. In Berlin, Baltimore and Marseilles exposure to 2 μg Group I mite allergen/g dust has been associated with sensitization and asthma (19,20,21). Previous studies from Denmark and Sydney had also suggested that patients living in houses with > 100 mites/g dust were more likely to present with the combination of mite sensitivity and asthma (22,23). Taken together it now seems clear that > 2 μg Group I/g dust is a useful threshold, above which the risk of sensitization is increased. The study in Marseilles demonstrated another result which is of great importance: that children raised in Briancon with low levels of exposure to mite allergens had a lower prevalence of asthma (24). In a prospective study in Poole, UK, we found that not only was mite sensitivity strongly correlated with asthma (Relative Risk 19.8) but that exposure to > 10 μg Group I allergen/g in early childhood increased the risk of developing asthma by four fold (25). If this conclusion can be confirmed it is of great importance because it implies that measures should be directed at housing design to prevent children developing asthma, rather than waiting until they present with symptoms.

Avoidance Measures as a Treatment for Asthma

Mite cultures require a relative humidity of ≥ 60% to flourish and a temperature of > 65°F. In keeping with this, houses in dry areas are regularly found to have no or very few mites. Clearly keeping humidity down is an important aspect of mite control which may be achieved simply by increasing ventilation (22). However, in many parts ofthe world controlling humidity is difficult or expensive. In these areas it is essential to control the sites in which mites can grow. The primary measures are physical, i.e., barriers, washing or removal. Indeed the successful studies on mite avoidance in the home have focussed on bedrooms: all mattresses and pillows were covered with impermeable covers, all bedding washed in hot water weekly, curtains were washable, clutter removed and carpets either removed or treated (1,26). Some issues remain to be solved but the most difficult are the management of sofas and carpets. Carpets or sofas kept in humid warm conditions will grow high levels of dust mites and will become both a source of exposure and a site for reinfestation of other sites in the house. If control of humidity or replacement is not possible, carpets can be treated with either acaricides or tannic acid. Several different acaricides have shown potential, e.g., benzylbenzoate, pyrethroids or pirimiphos methyl. Benzyl benzoate powder can achieve major reductions in mite allergen levels if applied aggressively (i.e., for 12 hours brushed in twice). Similarly tannic acid can denature mite antigens by 90–95%. However, in some studies benzyl benzoate has not proved effective and tannic acid can only have a temporary effect, i.e., 6 weeks to 2 months. It appears that if a carpet or sofa is maintained damp, no chemical treatment is routinely effective. However, this is because of the inability to penetrate the material not because the chemicals don't kill mites.

What Role do Allergens Play in Asthma?

One of the problems in accepting the role of house dust in asthma is that many or most of the patients do not appreciate that dust exposure causes their attacks and indeed many of them are not aware that they are allergic. As long as mite allergens were considered to be a trigger factor this was a major stumbling block. However, it now appears much more likely that chronic low dose exposure to mites (and other indoor allergens) contributes to reactivity imperceptibly, presumably by creating foci of inflammation which take time to heal. Indeed it may be that the mite fecal pellet is the ideal form of exposure to increase BHR *without* the patient being aware of symptoms at the time of exposure (1,7,14). Some results have suggested that early exposure to allergens is essential in the development of allergy and asthma (25), and it may be that in some cases once BHR is established it is irreversible. However, the evidence that avoidance measures can produce reductions in BHR suggests that continued exposure is necessary. Thus there are multiple different roles that allergen plays: (a) sensitization, (b) induction of BHR, (c) maintenance of chronic BHR and (d) triggering acute attacks. Although we have suggested that mite exposure is not an important "trigger" it seems likely that cat or rat allergens commonly "trigger" attacks in allergic individuals. Further it is likely that high level exposure to pollen can trigger acute attacks even without marked increases in BHR.

In most areas that have been studied cat allergy is associated with 10–20% of cases of asthma. In urban areas of the United States cockroach sensitivity is also very common and replaces cat sensitivity (27,28). Indeed there is a striking inverse correlation between cat and cockroach sensitivity and exposure. This is important because it allows us to make estimates of the threshold level for cat and cockroach allergens. In a recent study (in Wilmington, Delaware) cat, cockroach and mite sensitivity were each associated with asthma and overall 35 of the 42 individuals, who were both sensitized and had relevant exposure, presented with asthma (odds ratio 7.4) (29). In very dry areas such as northern Sweden or central Canada animal sensitivity dominates. By contrast in urban America and probably elsewhere in subtropical regions cockroaches may be as important as the mites. While some progress has been made in understanding techniques for controlling cat allergen we have only limited understanding of mold or cockroach avoidance (30). However, what is increasingly obvious is that avoidance measures should be explored specifically for different allergens and that making any recommendation about avoidance depends on knowing the patient's specific sensitivity.

Mite Sensitivity and Mite Exposure of Patients with Atopic Dermatitis

As with asthma, the proposal that house dust was causally related to AD was made in the 1930's; in 1947 Tuft reported that ~ 80% of adults and older children with AD were skin test positive to house dust. He also demonstrated that in some cases they improved when their houses were cleaned. More recently, it has been confirmed that patients with AD over the age of 7 years have a very high prevalence of sensitivity to mites and very high levels of IgE antibodies to mites (31). The correlation between mite sensitivity and AD is very strong indeed. Evidence has also been obtained that application of mite allergen to the skin of patients with AD can produce a delayed eczematous response (32,33). This response includes basophils and increased mast cells, but is particularly rich in eosinophils and T cells. Recently a new hypothesis has been developed that the primary triggering cell in the skin is the Langerhans cell with IgE on the surface (34). Whatever the mechanism, there is now a wide range of evidence that exposure of the skin to mite allergens is an important cause of AD. There is also anecdotal evidence that avoidance measures are beneficial; what remains to be shown is that avoidance is effective in a controlled trial (35).

Conclusion

Following the discovery of dust mites in 1964, it rapidly became obvious that there was a strong association between sensitivity to mites and asthma. By some authors and physicians this was already considered to imply a causal relationship between exposure to mites and asthma. However, there were many missing pieces to the argument. Over the last 10 years the evidence that mite allergen exposure is an important cause of asthma has been strengthened by a series of different experiments: (a) The association has been confirmed repeatedly; (b) many studies have shown a quantitative relationship between exposure to mite allergens and asthma; (c) there is now very good evidence that asthma is an inflammatory disease and that inhalation of allergens including dust mite can induce this form of inflammation; and (d) following some early failures, three controlled studies have demonstrated that allergen avoidance is helpful in the management of asthma.

If pharmacological management of asthma had controlled the disease (as was and is still promised), then it might be appropriate to restrict allergen specific management to patients with moderately severe disease. However, it is now clear that beta-two-agonists and inhaled steroids alone cannot control asthma in patients who have continued exposure to high levels of allergen. Thus, we conclude that diagnosis of specific sensitivity and advice on avoidance of the relevant indoor allergens should be routine for any patient who requires more than occasional beta-two-agonist treatment. Indeed, it is reasonable to propose that allergen avoidance should be the primary "anti-inflammatory" treatment for asthma.

References

1. Platts-Mills, T.A.E., and Chapman, M.D. 1987. Dust mites: immunology, allergic disease, and environmental control. J. Allergy Clin. Immunol. 80:755.
2. Smith, J.M., Disney, M.E., Williams, J.D., and Goels, Z.A. 1969. Clinical significance of skin reactions to mite extracts in children with asthma. Brit. Med. J. 1:723.
3. Altounyan, R.E. 1970. Changes in histamine and atropine responsiveness as a guide to diagnosis and evaluation of therapy in obstructive airways disease. In: Disodium chromoglycate in allergic airways disease. J. Pepys, and A.W. Frankland, eds. London: Butterworth, 47–53.
4. Kerrebijn, K.F. 1970. Endogenous factors in childhood CNSLD: methodological aspects in population studies. In: Bronchitis III. N.G.M. Orie, and R. van der Lende. The Netherlands: Royal Vangorcum Assen, 38–48.
5. Cockcroft, D.W., Ruffin, R.E., Dolovich, J., and Hargreave, F.E. 1977. Allergen-induced increase in non-allergic bronchial reactivity. Clin. Allergy. 7:503.
6. Platts-Mills, T.A.E., Tovey, E.R., Mitchell, E.B., Moszoro, H., Nock, P., and Wilkins, S.R. 1982. Reduction of bronchial hyperreactivity during prolonged allergen avoidance. Lancet 2:675.
7. Cockcroft, D.W. 1983. Mechanism of perennial allergic asthma. Lancet 2:253.
8. Chapman, M.D., and Platts-Mills, T.A.E. 1980. Purification and characterization of the major allergen from *Dermatophagoides pteronyssinus*-antigen P1. J. Immunol. 125:587.
9 Tovey, E.R., Chapman, M.D., Wells, C.W., and Platts-Mills, T.A.E. 1981. The distribution of dust mite allergen in the houses of patients with asthma. Amer. Rev. Resp. Dis. 124:630.
10. Tovey, E.R., Chapman, M.D., and Platts-Mills, T.A.E. 1981. Mite faeces are a major source of house dust allergens. Nature 289:592.
11. Chapman, M.D., Sutherland, W.M., and Platts-Mills, T.A.E. 1984. Recognition of two *Dermatophagoides pteronyssinus*-specific epitopes on antigen P1 by using monoclonal antibodies. J. Immunol. 133:2488.
12. Lind, P. 1985. Purification and partial characterization of two major allergens from the house dust mite *Dermatophagoides pteronyssinus*. J. Allergy Clin. Immunol. 76:753.
13. Heymann, P.W., Chapman, M.D., Aalberse, R.C., Fox, J.W., and Platts-Mills, T.A.E. 1989. Antigenic and structural analysis of Group II allergens (*Der f II* and *Der p II*) from house dust mites (Dermatophagoides spp). J. Allergy Clin. Immunol. 83:1055.
14. Platts-Mills, T.A.E., and De Weck, A. 1989. Dust mite allergens and asthma: A worldwide problem. Bull. W.H.O. 66:769; and J. Allergy Clin. Immunol. 83:416.
15. Chua, K.Y., Stewart, G.A., Thomas, W.R., Simpson, R.J., Dilworth, R.J., Plozza, T.M., and Turner, K.J. 1988. Sequence analysis of cDNA coding for a major house dust mite allergen, *Der p I*. J. Exp. Med. 167:175.
16. Yuuki, T., Okumura, Y., Ando, T., Yamakawa, H., Suko, M., Haida, M. Okudaira, H. 1990. Cloning and sequencing of cDNAs corresponding to mite major allergen, *Der f II*. Jap. J. Allergol. 39:557.
17. De Blay, F., Heymann, P.W., Chapman, M.D., and Platts-Mills, T.A.E. 1991. Airborne dust mite allergens: Comparison of Group II allergens with Group I mite allergen and cat allergen *Fel d* I. J. Allergy Clin. Immunol. (in press).
18. Swanson, M.A., Agarwal, M.K., and Reed, C.E. 1985. An immunochemical approach to indoor aeroallergen quantitation. J. Allergy Clin. Immunol. 76:724.
19. Lau, S., Falkenhorst, G., Weber, A., Werthman, I., Lind, P., Bucttner-Goetz, P., and Wahn, U. 1989. High mite-allergen exposure increases the risk of sensitization in atopic children and young adults. J. Allergy Clin. Immunol. 84:718.
20. Charpin, D., Birnbaum, J. Haddi, E., Genard, G., Lanteaume, A., Toumi, M., Faraj, F., Van der Brempt, X., Vervloet, D. 1991. Altitude and allergy to house dust mites: A paradigm of the influence of environmental exposure on allergic sensitization. Amer. Rev. Respir. Dis. 143:983.
21. Wood, R.A., Eggleston, P.A., Mudd, K.E., and Adkinson, N.F. Jr. 1989. Indoor allergen levels as a risk factor for allergic sensitization. J. Allergy Clin. Immunol. 83:1:199.
22. Korsgaard, J. 1983. Mite asthma and residency. A case-control study on the impact of expo-

sure to house-dust mites in dwellings. Amer. Rev. Resp. Dis. 128:231.

23. Peat, J.K., Britton, W.J., Salome, C.M., and Woolcock, A.J. 1987. Bronchial hyperresponsiveness in two populations of Australian schoolchildren. III. Effect of exposure to environmental allergens. Clin. Allergy. 17:297.
24. Vervloet, D., Penaud, A., Razzouk, H., Senft, M., Arnaud, A., Boutin, C., and Charpin, J. 1982. Altitude and house dust mites. J. Allergy Clin. Immunol. 69:290.
25. Sporik, R., Holgate, S.T., Platts-Mills, T.A.E., and Cogswell, J. 1990. Exposure to housedust mite allergen (*Der p I*) and the development of asthma in childhood: A prospective study. N. Eng. J. Med. 323:502.
26. Hayden, M.L., Rose, G., Diduch, K.B., Domson, P., Chapman, M.D., Heymann, P.W., and Platts-Mills, T.A.E. 1991. Reduction of dust mite allergens in carpets using Benzyl benzoate in the form of a wet powder. J. Allergy Clin. Immunol. (in press).
27. Pollart, S.M., Chapman, M.D., Fiocco, G.P., Rose, G., and Platts-Mills, T.A.E. 1989. Epidemiology of acute asthma: IgE antibodies to common inhalant allergens as a risk factor for emergency room visits. J. Allergy Clin. Immunol. 83:875.
28. Kang, B., Vellody, D., Homburger, H., and Yunginger, J.W. 1979. Cockroach cause of allergic asthma. J. Allergy & Clin. Immunol. 63:80.
29. Gelber, L.E., Seltzer, L.H., Bouzoukis, J.K., Pollart, S.M., Chapman, M.D., and Platts-Mills, T.A.E. 1991. Sensitization and exposure to indoor biological pollutants (dust mite, cat and cockroach) as risk factors for acute asthma. (Submitted).
30. De Blay, F., Chapman, M.D., and Platts-Mills, T.A.E. 1991. Airborne cat allergen (*Fel d* I): Environmental control with the cat in situ. Am. Rev. Resp. Dis. 143:1334.
31. Chapman, M.D., Rowntree, S., Mitchell, E.B., Di Prisco de Fuenmajor, M.C., and Platts-Mills, T.A.E. 1983. Quantitative assessments of IgG and IgE antibodies to inhalant allergens in patients with atopic dermatitis. J. Allergy Clin. Immunol. 72:27.
32. Mitchell, E.B., Crow, J., Chapman, M.D., Jouhal, S.S., Pope, F.M., and Platts-Mills, T.A.E. 1982. Basophils in allergen-induced patch test sites in atopic dermatitis. Lancet 1:127.
33. Mitchell, E.B., Crow, J., Rowntree, S., Webster, A.D., and Platts-Mills, T.A.E. 1984. Cutaneous basophil hypersensitivity to inhalant allergens in atopic dermatitis patients. J. Invest. Derm. 83:290.
34. Bruinzeel-Koomen, C.A., Fokkens, W.J., Mudde, G.C., and Bruinzeel, P.L. 1989. Role of Langerhans cells in atopic disease. Int. Arch. All. Appl. Imm. 90(1):51.
35. Deuell, B.L., Wilson, B., Heymann, P.W., and Platts-Mills, T.A.E. 1991. Atopic dermatitis (AD): The role of dust mite allergy and monitoring of disease activity by assay of IgG in skin scales. J. Allergy Clin. Immunol. 87:237.

The Airborne Mite Antigens

Mario Sánchez-Medina*, Enrique Fernández-Caldas**

In recent years there has been increasing interest in determining the concentrations of specific antigens in the air. New technologies and more sensitive immunoassays have been developed to detect minimal concentrations of airborne allergens in the indoor and outdoor environment. Using these methods, investigators have demonstrated that mite antigens become airborne during domestic activities and remain in the air during short periods of time. Inhibition tests using radioimmunoassays (RIA), enzyme linked immunoassays (ELISA) or two-site immunometric assays are used to quantitate mite aeroallergens. Mite allergens have been detected in particles larger than 10 μ and in particles smaller than 1 μ. The larger particles are associated with mite faecal pellets and have been measured using monoclonal antibodies against *Der p I*. *Der p II* and *Der f II* have also been detected in air samples.

Immunochemical Quantitation of Mite Aeroallergens

Several methods have been used to estimate the quantity of airborne allergens (Table I). These methods have helped in the understanding of the natural distribution of allergenic particles. None of these methods measures amorphous nonviable airborne allergens, such as mite faeces, mammalian allergens and insect debris. Therefore, an immunochemical method to quantitate airborne allergens present in amorphous and morphologically identifiable particles was developed. It has been successfully used to quantitate indoor, outdoor and occupational allergens (1–21). This method involves the collection of airborne particles from a measured volume of air onto a special filter and the extraction of the soluble allergens. Quantitation is done immunochemically by inhibition tests using radioimmunoassays (RIA), enzyme linked immunoassays (ELISA) or two-site immunometric assays with capture and detecting antibodies that recognize different epitopes on the allergen molecules. Either polyclonal (rabbit or human) or monoclonal antibodies can be used. The tracer antibody can be radiolabeled or tagged with an enzyme (16). The use of plastic microtiter plates as solid phase adsorption media for the immunochemical assays has many advantages as well as some possible disadvantages. The advantages include rapid assay turn around time, good overall sensitivity and low cost. The disadvantages might be questionable adsorption of some important allergens, quantitative differences in the quality of the plates and poor presentation of immunobinding sites for some allergenic molecules. Coating conditions vary from allergen to allergen and must be determined experimentally. Usually, 1 mg of allergen is adsorbed to the surface of each well using sodium carbonate/bicarbonate buffer, pH 9.2–9.6. Either human IgE or human or rabbit IgG polyclonal antibodies or mouse monoclonal antibodies can then be added, depending on the purpose of the study. The main advantage of using IgE antibody and standardized whole extracts, rather than monospecific antibodies to purified allergens, is that it assures detection of all the allergens to which allergic patients have developed antibodies. The main advantage of using monoclonal antibodies, especially with a double antibody or sandwich technique, is a

Table I. Traditional methods used to estimate the concentration of airborne allergens

1. Counting identifiable allergenic particles, such as pollen grains and mold spores
2. Culturing bacteria and fungi
3. Assaying chemicals, such as diisocyanate, by sensitive specific chemical analysis

* Colombia National University, Carrera 9, 117-20 Suite 508, Santa Fe de Bogotá, Colombia, S. A.
** University of South Florida College of Medicine, Division of Allergy and Immunology, c/o VA Hospital (VAR III D), 13,000 Bruce B. Downs Blvd., Tampa, FL 33612, U.S.A.

greater specificity and sensitivity of these assays. Another important advantage is that monoclonal antibodies allow more accurate comparison of results from time to time and laboratory to laboratory (22). The limit of sensitivity of some of the assays requires sampling a large volume of air to measure the low allergen levels sometimes encountered. Indoors, the volume of air is finite and high volume samplers may clean air as it is sampled and result in underestimation of allergen concentrations if air is recirculated through the sampler. High volume samplers are also too noisy for occupants to tolerate for more than a few minutes. For these reasons, special sampling equipment and filters are available for indoor studies. The sampling pumps have a moderate flow (2 L/min) and are equipped with built-in timers for sample initiation and termination. The filters allow efficient collection of particle and complete extraction in small volumes of buffer. Cascade impactors sample the air at a rate of 20 L/min and high volume samplers at approximately 10 m^3/per hour.

Mite Aeroallergens

Mite allergens settle more rapidly than cat allergens. Particle size is an important variable that determines the site in the body where the particle deposits. Most particles of more than 10 μm mean mass aerodynamic diameter are filtered in the nose. Only smaller particles penetrate to the bronchi and about 10% actually deposit in the lungs. However, it has been suggested that mite fecal pellets may occasionally enter the lung and cause local inflammation and bronchoconstriction (23). Volumetric samples equipped with sizing devices have been used to estimate the particle size of indoor allergens. These studies have shown that mite allergens remain airborne for a short period of time and that allergenic activity can be detected in fractions larger than 10 μ and in smaller than 1 μ (12,13,14). Cat allergens seem to remain airborne for longer periods and can be detected in air samples collected in homes under disturbed and undisturbed conditions (17). Sakaguchi et al. (19) demonstrated that Group I (*Der p I* and *Der f I*) and Group II (*Der p II* and *Der f II*) aeroallergen levels were very low in 10 homes during normal domestic

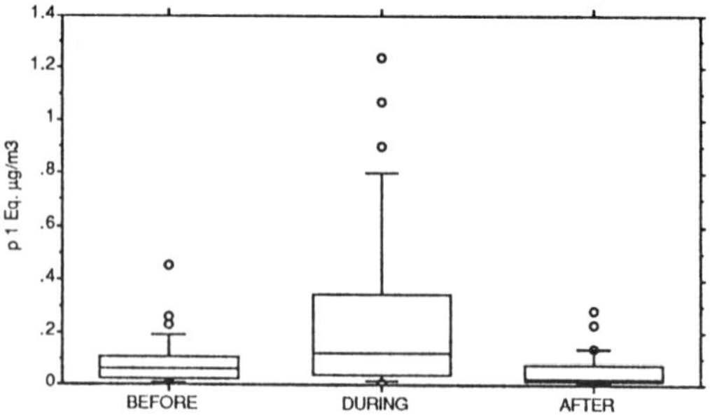

Figure 1. Box plot view of aeroallergen levels before, during and after vacuum cleaning in Tampa, Florida (n=13). Air samples collected on teflon filters with the Air Sentinel™ (QUAN-TEC-AIR) Rochester, MN). Results expressed in mg Antigen p 1 equivalents/m^3.

activities (29.5 and 6.3 pg/m^3, respectively) with a Group I/Group II ratio of 4.7:1. However, samples collected during bedmaking revealed a 1,000 fold increase in Group I and Group II aeroallergen concentrations with a Group I/Group II ratio of 2.5:1. They concluded that Group I allergens are more prone to become airborne than Group II allergens. Mite allergens also become airborne during vacuum cleaning activities (Figure 1) (24). A better correlation between mite airborne allergens and mite allergens in settled dust is obtained when air samples are collected during vacuum cleaning (Figure 2). Other authors have described a poor correlation between mite allergen concentrations in the air and mite allergen concentrations in the dust. They suggested that mite aeroallergen concentrations

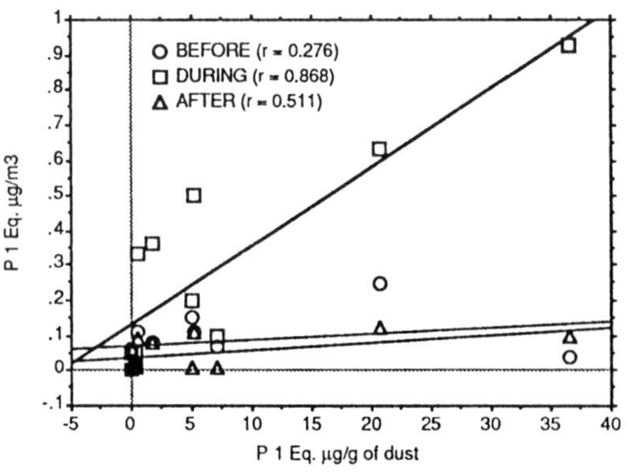

Figure 2. Regression analysis of the allergen concentrations in the air and in settled dust.

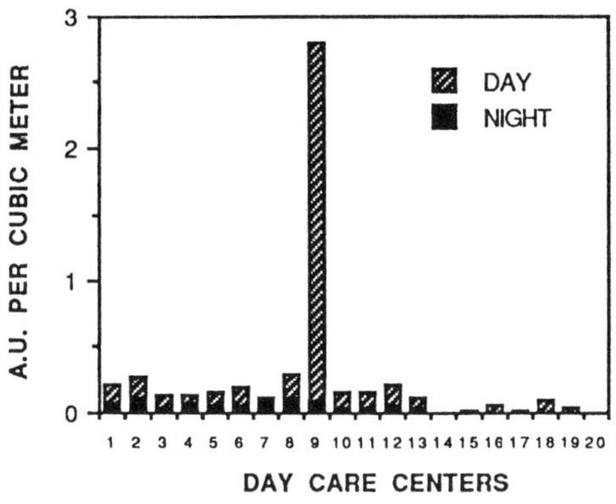

Figure 3. Mite aeroallergen levels in 20 day care centers in Tampa, FL. Airborne allergen quantitated using RAST inhibition and human mite-specific IgE (1 Allergy Unit is equivalent to 200 ng of protein of *Dermatophagoides ptronyssinus*).

are more important for sensitization than mite allergen concentrations in the house dust (15). Air samples have also been used to quantitate mite aeroallergen exposure in day care centers in Tampa, Florida. Mite aeroallergen concentrations, expressed in standardized allergy units (AU) (one AU is equivalent to approximately 200 ng of mite protein), were higher during the day when the children were playing than during the night (Figure 3) (25). The highest mite aeroallergen concentration was detected in the day care center with the highest *Der p I* concentration in the dust (21.8 mg/g of dust). Mite allergens have also been detected in air samples collected in barns in Cooperstown, NY, and Rochester, MN (10). A high concentration of p 1 equivalents and allergens of the storage mite *Lepidoglyphus destructor* was measured.

Conclusions

The immunochemical quantitation of mite aeroallergens is a useful tool to determine mite allergen exposure and allergen levels that produce symptoms and/or sensitization. More research is needed to identify other allergens besides *Der p I* and *Der p II* in air samples. The advantage of using IgE antibody and standardized whole extracts in RAST inhibition assays instead of monoclonal antibodies and purified allergens is that they assure detection of all the allergens to which allergic patients are sensitized. The advantage of monoclonal antibodies and purified allergens is a greater specificity and sensitivity of these assays. Mite airborne allergens have been detected in quantities ranging from a few nanograms to approximately 1 μg per cubic meter of air.

References

1. Agarwal M.K., Yunginger, J.W., Swanson, M.C., and Reed, C.E. 1981. An immunochemical method to measure atmospheric allergens. J. Allergy Clin. Immunol. 68:194.
2. Agarwal, M.K., Reed, C.E., Swanson, M.C., and Yunginger, J.W. 1983. Immunochemical quantitation of airborne short ragweed. *Alternaria*, Antigen E and Alt-1 allergens: A two year prospective study. J. Allergy Clin. Immunol. 72:40.
3. Reed, C.E., Swanson, M.C., López, M., Ford, A.M., Major, J., Witmer, W.B., and Valdes, T.B. 1983. Measurement of IgE antibody and airborne antigen to control an industrial outbreak of hypersensitivity pneumonitis. J. Occup. Med. 25:207.
4. Agarwal, M.K., Reed, C.E., Swanson, M.C., and Yunginger, J.W. 1984. Airborne ragweed allergens: Association with various particle sizes and short ragweed plant parts. J. Allergy Clin. Immunol. 73:137.
5. Fernández-Caldas, E., Swanson, M.C., Yunginger, J.W., and Reed, C.E. 1989. Immunochemical demonstration of red oak aeroallergens outside the oak pollination season. Grana. 28:205.
6. Ostrom, N.K., Swanson, M.C., Agarwal, M.K., and Yunginger, J.W. 1986. Occupational allergy to honey bee body dust in a honey processing plant. J. Allergy Clin. Immunol. 77:736.
7. Twiggs, J.T., Agarwal, M.K., Dahlberg, M.J.E., and Yunginger, J.W. 1982. Immunochemical measurement of airborne mouse allergens in a laboratory facility. .J Allergy Clin. Immunol. 69:522-527.
8. Swanson, M.C., Agarwal, M.K., Reed, C.E., and Yunginger, J.W. 1984. Guinea pig derived allergens: Clinico-immunologic studies, characterization, airborne quantitations and size distribution. Am. Rev. Respir. Dis. 129:844.

9. Wynn, S.R., Swanson, M.C., Reed, C.E., Penny, N.D., Showers, W.B., and Smith, J.M. 1988. Immunochemical quantitation, size distribution, and crossreactivity of Lepidoptera (moth) aeroallergens in southeastern Minnesota. J. Allergy Clin. Immunol. 82:47.
10. Campbell, A.R., Swanson, M.C., Fernández-Caldas, E., Reed, C.E., May, J. J., and Pratt, D.S. 1989. Aeroallergens in Dairy Barns near Cooperstown, New York and Rochester, Minnesota. Am. Rev. Respir. Dis. 140:317.
11. Swanson, M.C., Campbell, A.R., Klauck, M.J., and Reed, C.E. 1988. Correlations between levels of mite and cat allergens in settled and airborne dust. J. Allergy Clin. Immunol. 83:776.
12. Swanson, M.C., Agarwal, M.K., and Reed, C.E. 1985. An immunochemical approach to indoor aeroallergen quantitation with a new volumetric air sampler: Studies with mite, roach, cat, mouse, and guinea pig antigens. J. Allergy Clin. Immunol. 76:724.
13. Platts-Mills, T.A.E., Heymann, P.W., Longbottom, J.L., and Wilkins, S.R. 1986. Airborne allergens associated with asthma: Particle sizes carrying dust mite and rat allergens measured with a cascade impactor. J. Allergy Clin. Immunol. 77:850.
14. Tovey, E.R., Chapman, M.D., Wells, C.W., and Platts-Mills, T.A.E. 1981. The distribution of dust mite allergen in the house of patients with asthma. Am. Rev. Respir. Dis. 124:630.
15. Price J.A., Pollock, I., Little, S.A., Longbottom, J.L., and Warner, J.O. 1990. Measurement of airborne mite antigen in homes of asthmatic children. Lancet 336:895.
16. Platts-Mills, T.A.E., Chapman, M.D., Heymann, P.W., and Luczynska, C.M. 1989. Measurements of airborne allergen using immunoassays. Immunology and Allergy Clinics of North America 9(2):269.
17. Luczynska, C.M., Li, Y., Chapman, M.D., and Platts-Mills, T.A.E. 1990. Airborne concentrations and particle size distribution of allergen derived from domestic cats (*Felis domesticus*). Measurement using cascade impactor, liquid impinger, and a two-site monoclonal antibody assay for *Fel d* I. Am. Rev. Respir. Dis. 141:361.
18. Spieksma, F.Th.M., Kramps, J.A., Van Der Linden, A.C., Nikkels, B.H., Plomp, A., Koerten, H.K., and Dijkman, J.H. 1990. Evidence of grass-pollen allergenic activity in the smaller micronic atmospheric aerosol fraction. Clinical Experimental Allergy 20:271.
19. Sakaguchi, M., Inouye, H., Yasueda, H., Irie, T., Yoshizawa, S., and Shida, T. 1989. Measurement of allergens associated with dust mite allergy. II. Concentrations of airborne mite allergens (*Der* I and *Der* II) in the house. Int. Arch. Allergy Appl. Immunol. 90:190.
20. Jensen, J., Poulsen, L.K., Mygind, K., Weeke, E.R., and Weeke, B. 1989. Immunochemical estimations of allergenic activities from outdoor aeroallergens, collected by a high-volume air sampler. Allergy 44:52.
21. Kino, T., Chihara, J., Fukuda, K., Sasaki, Y., Shogaki, Y., and Oshima, S. 1987. Allergy to insects in Japan. III. High frequency of IgE responses to insects (moth, butterfly, caddis fly, and chironomid) in patients with bronchial asthma and immunochemical quantitation of the insect-related airborne particles smaller than 10 mm in diameter. J. Allergy Clin. Immunol. 79:857.
22. Fernández-Caldas, E., Reed, C.E., and Lockey, R.F. 1991. Distribution of indoor allergens. In: Allergen immunotherapy. R.F. Lockey, and S.C. Bukantz, eds. New York: Marcel Dekker, p.69.
23. Platts-Mills, T.A.E., and Chapman, M.D. 1987. Dust mites: Immunology, allergic disease and environmental control. J. Allergy Immunol. 80:755.
24. Trudeau, W., Fernández-Caldas, E., Fox, R.W., and Lockey, R.F. 1989. Mite aeroallergen concentrations before, during and after vacuum cleaning. J. Allergy Clin. Immunol. [Abstract]. 83(1):264.
25. Aronoff D., Ledford, D.K., Schou, C., Fernández-Caldas, E., Trudeau, W.L., and Lockey, R.F. 1989. House dust mite and cockroach allergen concentrations in daycare centers. J. Allergy Clin.. Immunol. [Abstract] 83(1):197.

Mites in Amazonia

Júlio Croce*

Covering one-third of the South American territory, the Amazon region occupies an area of 6,500,000 sq.km., 60% of which are within Brazilian boundaries, the remaining 40% being divided among eight other countries. The Brazilian Amazon Forest, with an extension of 3,912,000 sq.km., i.e. 45% of the Brazilian territory, is the largest humid tropical forest in the world (1). Acknowledging the fact that studies on bronchial asthma in that area are very scarce, we decided to carry out surveys in order to assess the prevalence of this condition, as well as the significance of its most important allergenic triggers, such as house dust mites and airborne fungi.

Research Locales

The areas chosen for examination were: Macapá (Amapá Territory), Icoaraci (Pará State), and Castanhal (Pará State). Additionally, nine asthmatic individuals were investigated in Belém, the capital of Pará State, with house dust being collected from their houses for the purpose of mite population analysis.

Methods

According to the method adopted for the investigation, at first a detailed map was drawn and subdivided into a number of blocks equivalent in area. Next, lots were chosen at random, in order to determine which blocks were to be visited. All individuals with variable intensity dyspnea, either paroxistic or continuous, and improving under the action of bronchodilators, were considered to be asthmatic. These asthmatic patients were then submitted to skin tests according to the prick test method, using lancets with an antigen fixed on the top (Phazet-Pharmacia Laboratory, Sweden). The antigens used were *Dermatophagoides pteronyssinus, Cladosporium herbarum, Alternaria alternata,* as well as positive and negative controls. Blood was drawn from all patients aged 8 years and more, in order to have specific antibodies analyzed by the immunoenzimatic method ELISA (Pharmacia). Finally, house dust was collected from and under the patients' beds, in order to study the existing mite population of all houses visited.

Macapá

Macapá is the capital of Amapá Territory, located near the Amazon river mouth, on its left bank, with the Equator line crossing a little to the South of its urban concentration. The town population is estimated at 180,000 inhabitants. Its climate is humid tropical, with relative humidity rates ranging between 70 and 90%. A total of 1,100 individuals were interviewed in 317 houses visited, and 34 people were found to be asthmatics (2,4), indicating a 3% prevalence. Only 22 of the 34 asthmatic patients were submitted to skin tests, as the remaining 12 were under 8 years of age. From the 22 patients tested, 13 (59%) were strongly reactive to mite extracts, three (13.6%) presented mild reaction and six were negative. Specific antibodies tested by ELISA revealed only seven positive (31.8%) to *D. pteronyssinus,* two being Class III, and three being Class II. On the other hand, three people (13.6%) had positive skin tests (one strong, one moderate and one mild reaction to mold extract). The ELISA test, using ten species of airborne fungi on 18 individuals, revealed ten positive cases (45%) to one or more extracts, although their titers were of low to moderate intensity, and only three sera presented Class II values. The mite species in the house dust samples collected were: *Blomia tropicalis* (Bronswijck, Cook and Oshima,

---

* Allergy Department, Faculdad de Medicina da Universidade S. Paolo, Brazil.
Acknowledgements: The author kindly acknowledges the help of Prof. Domingos Baggio, Dr. Laércio J. Zuppi, Dr. José Ferreira Mello, Dr. Fábio F. M. Castro, Dr. Martti A. Antila, Dr. Leonai R. Garcia, and AC. Clio B. Croce.

1975): 55.5%; *Dermatophagoides pteronyssinus* (Trouessart, 1877): 16.0%; *Cheyletus malaccensis* (Oudemans, 1903): 10.0%; *Euroglyphus maynei* (Cooreman, 1950): 5.5%; *Tarsonemus granarius* (Lindquist, 1972): 3.0%; other mites: 9.0%. The total of positive samples was 36 (83.7%) and of negative samples was 7 (16.3%).

Icoaraci

The town is located in the State of Pará, on the right bank of the Amazon river mouth, and has a relative humidity rate of 90%. Its population is estimated at 110,000 inhabitants (3). From a total of 808 individuals interviewed at random, 41 were asthmatics (5.07%) and 15 of these were further investigated. Skin tests to *D. pteronyssinus* revealed 5 strongly positive skin tests (33%) and one slightly positive reaction; specific IgE tests were found in four (26.6%) with three moderate (Class III) and one mildly positive (Class II) by ELISA. As to molds, all the individuals had negative skin tests and low positivity titres in five sera (Class I or II) to 13 molds of specific antibodies tests by ELISA. The analysis of house dust samples revealed: *Blomia tropicalis:* 4,400 mites/g, 57.9%; *Dermatophagoides pteronyssinus:* 2,500 mites/g, 32.9%; *Euroglyphus maynei:* 4,006, 5.26%; *Cheyletus sp:* 300 mites/g, 3.9%; this makes a total of 7,600 mites/g 100.00%, for a total of 1,000 samples, with 300 negative samples.

Castanhal

The town is located close to the Belém-Brasília highway, in the State of Pará, with relative humidity rates of approximately 80%. Its population is estimated at 130,000 inhabitants (3). Sixteen of the 667 individuals interviewed at random were asthmatics (2.39%) and, from this total, eight people were further investigated. The mite tests revealed three positive (two strong and one mild) skin tests to *D. pteronyssinus* (18.7%), and three positive (2 strong and 1 mild) specific antibody tests by ELISA. As to molds, all skin tests were negative, while specific IgE antibodies to 16 species of molds presented two mildly positive cases (12.5%). Analyses of house dust samples revealed: *Dermatophagoides pteronyssinus:* 60%; *Blomia tropicalis:* 33.3%; *Cheyletus sp.*: 6.7%. The total of samples collected was 500, with 200 (40%) negative.

Belém

Belém is located to the left of the Negro river, close to the Amazon river mouth. It is the capital of the State of Pará, and the most important city in the region. The temperature is constant, around 27/28°C, and relative humidity rates range in the neighborhood of 90% (3). Only nine asthmatic patients were interviewed in that city, from one private clinic. Skin tests to *D. pteronyssinus* revealed six strongly positive and 2 mildly positive; specific antibodies to *D. pteronyssinus* (ELISA) revealed three positives in Class IV, two in Class II and three negative; and the skin test to molds revealed all negative. Specific antibodies to molds (ELISA) showed two positives in Class II and six positives in Class I. House dust analyses revealed: *D. pteronyssinus*, 58.62%; *Blomia tropicalis*, 34.49%; *Suidasia pontificia*, 6.89%. The total of samples collected was 800, with 500 (62.5%) negative samples.

Discussion

House dust mites were found in the four localities surveyed in the Amazon region: Macapá, Icoaraci, Castanhal and Belém. The species of mites most frequently found were *Blomia tropicalis* and *Dermatophagoides pteronyssinus*, with the remainder appearing only in small percentages (5). The predominance of the two species in the towns studied varied according to weather conditions: *Blomia tropicalis* lives under relative humidity rates above 70% and temperatures between 14 and 25°C, while *Dermatophagoides pteronyssinus* lives under relative humidity rates below 70% and temperatures between 18 and 21°C. *Dermatophagoides farinae* was not found in the Amazon region, as it lives in conditions of relative air humidity below 65%. The temperature in the Amazon region is normally around 25 to 28°C, with very small variations during the whole year. The four seasons do not exist as they occur in the temperate zones. There are only two seasons: the rainy season and the dry season. In spite of high relative humidity rates in the Amazon region, microclimates found indoors may not correspond to the outdoors weather, thus offering appropriate conditions for the growth of different species of mites. Generally, the houses are ventilated by keeping doors and windows open and by the frequent use of fans and air conditioning. Usually, the houses are not equipped with carpets, rugs or upholstered furniture. It was expected that environmental factors leading to asthma and rhinitis, such as mites and molds, would be frequent in the Amazon region, with high numbers of sensitized people. However, this supposition was not proved by the surveys. In those places close to the Amazon river, such as Belém and Macapá where the amount of mites was significant, the prevalence of bronchial asthma was generally found to be 3 to 5%, i.e. relatively low for Brazilian standards (5,6,7). The sensitization of the people with asthma, measured by ELISA, is found specially in Classes I and II, and very rarely in classes III and IV. The same fact was observed with the airborne molds. The skin tests were generally of low positivity, and the occurrence of sensitized persons was low, as were their titers. The predominant house dust mites in the surveyed areas (Macapá, Icoaraci, Castanhal and Belém) were *Dermatophagoides pteronyssinus* and *Blomia tropicalis*. The number of individuals sensitized to mites and molds is relatively small and generally with low titres of specific IgE. The presence of mites from the samples of house dust collected revealed: in Macapá 83.7% positivity, in Icoaraci 81.25% positivity, in Castanhal 60% and in Belém 37.5%. The prevalence of bronchial asthma in the researched areas (Macapá, Icoaraci, Castanhal and Belém) varied from 2.39 to 5.00%.

References

1. Teixeira Guerra, A. 1969. Geografia do Brasil. A Regiao Norte, Vol. 1 Série A, Rio de Janeiro.
2. Garcia, L.R.F., Baggio, D., Croce, J., and Espto Santo, M.N.A.I. Acaros do pó domiciliar em Macapá, Amapá. (Mites of house dust in Macapá [State of Amapá]. XXI Congresso Brasileiro de Alergia e Imunopatologia. Florianópolis, Brasil.
3. Mello, J.F., Baggio, D., Zuppi, L., Bellesi, N., and Croce, J. Acaros do pó domiciliar em Belém, Icoaraci e Castanhal no Pará (Mites in house dust in Belém, Icoaraci and Castanhal, in the State of Pará) Paper presented in the XXI Congresso Brasileiro de Alergia e Imunopatologia. Florianópolis, Brasil.
4. Croce, J. 1988. The epidemiology of bronchial asthma in the Brazilian Amazon. Paper presented in the symposium "Epedimiologia y repercursion medico-social del asma bronchial". In: XVI Reunion Internacional de Asmologia (Interasma) Havana, Cuba.
5. Croce, J. Nueva flora de acaros en la etiopatogenia del asma. Symposium on "Asthma Physiopathology." International Association Asthmology (INTERASMA), Buenos Aires.

Mite-Group I Allergens and Symptoms

D. Vervloet, D. Charpin*

In the general population, the percentage of positive results to intracutaneous testing with mites ranges from 5 to 30% (1), but only a fraction of sensitized subjects have a frank allergic disorder. Owing to the possibility of quantifying the amount of major mite allergens in the domestic environment, epidemiological studies have led to proposals for threshold values above which there is an increased risk for (a) the occurrence of mite sensitization, (b) the development of asthma and (c) the occurrence of symptoms. These three major points will be analyzed below in relation to the level of group I allergens in the environment, especially in mattress dust. A better knowledge of these threshold values has obvious relevance in management of mite-allergic patients.

Group I Allergens and Occurrence of Sensitization

In a prospective study of 92 children with at least one atopic parent, the development of the specific antibody responses to food and inhalant allergens during the first 5 years of life was assessed (2). Samples of dust were collected from the houses of 66 patients. All children with positive RAST to mites (46 out of 66) had group I allergen levels in bedroom floor dust higher than 2 µg/g. More recently it was demonstrated that a level of group I allergen higher than 2 µg/g increased by 7 the risk of mite sensitization, and a level higher than 10 µg/g increased this risk 11-fold (3). Price et al. (4) showed a significant association between mite sensitization in atopic children and group I allergens 0.5 µg/g house dust or with a detectable airborne group I allergen. Very recently, our group showed (5) that in school children from the fourth and fifth grades, the prevalence of positive skin tests to mites was strikingly different in the group living at sea level (Martigues) and in altitude (Briançon). Only 4.1% of the children born in Briançon (mean group I allergens in mattress dust = 0.36 µg/g) were sensitized to mites versus 16.7% of the children living in Martigues (mean group I allergens in mattress dust = 15.8 µg/g) (Table I, and Figure 1).

Group I Allergens and Development of Asthma

Sporik et al. (6) performed a prospective study including 67 children born to atopic parents. At age 11, 17 children had active asthma. Among them, all but one were exposed at 1 year of age to more than 10 µg of group I allergen per g of dust. This indicates that in addition to genetic factors, exposure in early childhood to house dust mite allergens is an important determinant of subsequent development of asthma. Our

Table I Percentage of Skin Reactions to common Aero-Allergens in Martigues Schoolchildren and in native and non-native Briançon Schoolchildren

	Martigues	p Value	Briançon Natives	p Value	Briançon Non-natives
Cat danders	5.6	NS	3.3	NS	4.5
House dust	13.9	$p < 0.001$	2.0	$p = 0.10$	8.0
House dust mites	16.7	$p < 0.02$	4.1	$p = 0.17$	10.2
Grass pollens	8.5	$p < 0.001$	21.7	NS	16.9

from D. Charpin et al. Am. Rev. Respir. Dis. 1991, 143:983–986 (ref. 5)

* Service de Pneumo-Allergologie, Département des Maladies Respiratoires, Hôpital Sainte-Marguerite, Marseille, France.

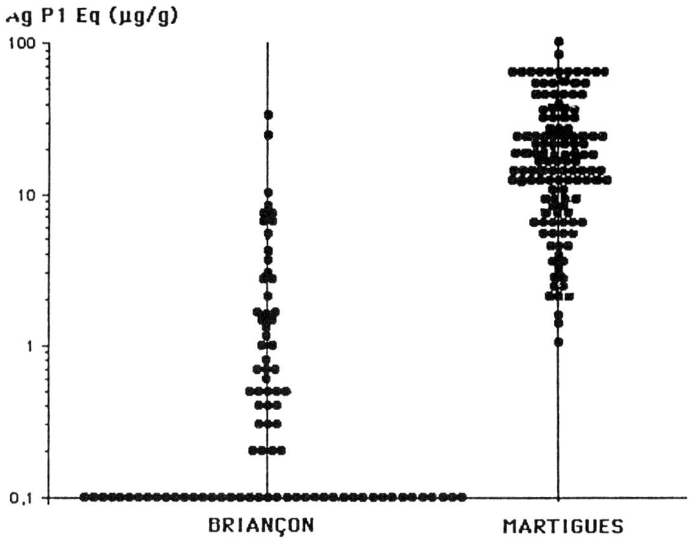

Figure 1. Distribution of individual Group I antigen levels on mattresses at high altitude (Briançon) and at sea level (Martigues) (from Ref. 5).

group showed that the prevalence of asthma with positive skin test to mites was significantly higher (3%) in children living at sea level than in children of Briançon at a higher altitude (0%) (5) (Table II).

Group I Allergens and Occurrence of Symptoms

A team headed by Platts-Mills in the USA conducted several investigations both in children and adults and concluded that levels of group I allergens above 10 µg could lead to onset of frank symptoms of asthma. For instance, 12/20 mite allergic children with asthma (7) and 16/23 mite allergic patients with asthma (8) had a level of group I allergens above 10 µg/g dust. The same group also showed that 16/18 mite allergic patients admitted in emergency room for asthma have high group I allergens higher than10 µg/g (9).

A group of 20 mite allergic children with moderate to severe asthma was studied by Arruda et al. (10) in São Paulo, Brazil. In 18 out of 20 houses, at least one dust sample contained group I allergens level higher than 10 µg/g dust. In another study from our group, we observed that group I allergen levels in the mattresses of mite allergic asthmatic patients who had asthma attacks during the previous 3 months were on average 5 times higher than in asthmatics who did not have attacks (11). We studied 49 out patients. In the 12 patients reporting no attack in the last 3 months (score 0), the geometric mean of group I allergens was 1.4 µg/g. In 15 patients reporting occasional

Table II Percentage of combined Symptoms and Skin Reactions to common Aeroallergens in Martigues Schoolchildren and native and non-native Briançon Schoolchildren

	Martigues	p Value	Briançon Natives	p Value	Briançon Non-natives
Asthma attacks and positive skin test to HDM	3.0	$p < 0.01$	0	$p = 0.18$	2.6
Perennial rhinitis and positive skin test to HDM	3.8	NS	1.0	NS	4.7
Hay fever and positive skin test	1.6	$p < 0.001$	6.9	NS	2.4

from D. Charpin et al. Am. Rev. Respir. Dis. 1991; 143:983–986

Table III Relationship between symptoms and P1 Eq level (sum of Der p I and Der f I) in mattresses

Symptoms score	Ag P1 Eq (μg/g house dust) Geometric means (95 % confidence interval)
0 (n = 12)	1.4 (0.58-3.39)**
1 (n = 15)	9.06 (4.06-20.4)**
2 (n = 12)	14.9 (5.9-33.11)NS
3 (n = 10)	13.49 (4.3-45.6)

(** P 0.01)
from D. Vervloet et al. 1991. Allergy 46:554 (from Ref. 5).

asthma, i.e. less than one attack/month, the mean level was 9 μg/g. In the 22 patients reporting more than one attack per month (scores 2 and 3) the mean level of group I allergens was high, over 10 μg/g house dust. The difference in mean group I allergens level between score 0 and score 1 and between score 1 and score 2 was significant ($p < 0.01$) (Table III). The season during which the dust mite samples were obtained was comparable in the four groups. Similarly, we could classify asthma patients into three groups according to the treatment required for symptoms. Those three groups had different mean group I allergens levels in their mattresses. In particular, 11 out of the 12 untreated asthmatics had group I allergen levels lower than 10 μg/g mattress dust while 18 out of the 22 patients who were on maintenance therapy, had levels higher than 10 μg/g (Fig. 2). This finding is not conflicting with those of Arruda et al. (10) and Quoix et al. (12) who showed similar group I allergen levels in mite atopic asthmatics and non-atopic controls. Actually, active asthmatics have high group I allergen levels, while antigenic levels in control subjects are dependent upon mite-infestation in the areas where the study has been performed. Indeed, in São Paulo, Brazil and Strasbourg, France, mites are numerous.

Conclusions

All our studies and some others dealing with the number of mites in house dust (13,14,15) support the hypothesis that exposure to house dust mites may have a major influence on developing allergic diseases, and, as was summarized in a recent international workshop (16), more work is needed for a better understanding of the relationship between asthma and mite allergy but also atopic dermatitis and mite allergy.

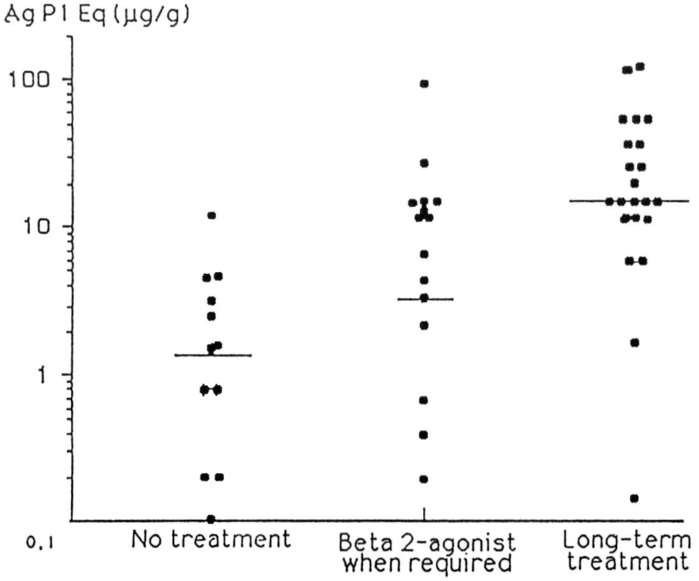

Figure 2. Distribution of individual Group I antigen levels on mattresses of asthmatic patients according to the treatment required for symptoms. Each patient is represented by a simple dot. The horizontal bars represent the mean level computed in each group (from Ref. 11).

References

1. Platts-Mills, T., and Chapman, M. 1987. Dust mite: Immunology, allergic diseases and environmental control. J. Allergy Clin. Immunol. 80:755.
2. Rowntree, S., Cogswell, J.J., Platts-Mills, T.A.E., and Mitchell, E.B. 1985. Development of IgE and IgG antibodies to food and inhalant allergens in children at risk of allergic diseases. Arch. Dis. Child. 60:727.
3. Lau, S., Falkenhorst, G., Weber, A., Werthmann, I., Lind, P., Buettner-Goetz, P, and Wahn, U. 1989. High mite-allergen exposure increases the risk of sensitization in atopic children and young adults. J. Allergy Clin. Immunol. 84:718.
4. Price, J.A., Pollock, I., Little S.A., Longbottom, J.L., and Warner J.O. 1990. Measurement of airborne mite antigen in homes of asthmatic children. Lancet 336:895.
5. Charpin, D., Birnbaum, J., Haddi, E., Genard, G., Toumi, M., Faraj, F., Lanteaume, A., and Vervloet, D. 1991. Altitude and allergy to house dust mites: A paradigm of the influence of environmental exposure on allergic sensitization. Am. Rev. Respir. Dis. 143:983.
6. Sporik, R., Holgate, S.T., Platts-Mills, T.A.E., and Cogswell, J.J. 1990. Exposure to house-dust mite allergen (Der p I) and the development of asthma in childhood. A prospective study. N. Engl. J. Med. 323,8:502.
7. Smith, T.F., Kelly, L.B., Heymann, P.W., Wilkins, S.R., Tech, B., and Platts-Mills, T.A.E. 1985. Natural exposure and serum antibodies to house dust mite of mite-allergic children with asthma in Atlanta. J. Allergy Clin. Immunol. 76:782.
8. Platts-Mills, T.A.E., Heymann, P.W., Chapman, M.D., Hayden, M.L., and Wilkins, S.R. 1986. Cross-reacting and species-specific determinant on a major allergen from *Dermatophagoides pteronyssinus* and *D. farinae*: Development of a radioimmunoassay for antigen P1 equivalent in house dust and dust mite extracts. J. Allergy Clin. Immunol. 78:398.
9. Platts-Mills, T.A.E., Hayden, M.L., Chapman, M.D., and Wilkins, S.R. 1987. Seasonal variation in dust mite and grass pollen allergens in dust from the house of parents with asthma. J. Allergy Clin. Immunol. 79:781.
10. Arruda, L.K., Rizzo, M.C., Chapman, M.D., Fernandez-Caldas, E., Baggio, D., and Naspitz, C.K. 1991. Exposure and sensitization to house dust mite allergens among asthmatic children in São Paulo, Brazil. Clin. Exp. Allergy 21:433.
11. Vervloet, D., Charpin, D., Haddi, E., N'Guyen, A., Birnbaum, J., Soler, M., and Van Der Brempt, X. 1991. Medication requirements and house dust mites exposure in mite-sensitive asthmatics. Allergy 46:554.
12. Quoix, E., Hedelin, G., Verot, A., Dietemann A., Bessot, J.C., and Pauli, G. 1991. Occurrence of mite-allergens in the home of Dpt-allergic patients and matched control subjects. J. Allergy Clin. Immunol. 87:A318.
13. Korsgaard, J. 1983. Mite asthma and residency: A case control study on the impact of exposure to house dust mites in dwellings. Am. Rev. Respir. Dis. 128:231.
14. Dowse, G.K., Turner, K.J., Stewart, G.A., Alpers, M.P., and Woolcock, A.J. 1985. The association between *Dermatophagoides* mites and the increasing prevalence of asthma in village communities within the Papua New Guinea highlands. J. Allergy Clin. Immunol. 75:75.
15. Woolcock, A.J., Peat, J.K., Keena, V., Smith, D., Molloy, C., Simpson, A., Middleton, P., Vallance, P., Alpers, M., and Green, W. 1989. Asthma and chronic airflow limitation in the highlands of Papua New Guinea: Low prevalence of asthma in the Asaro Valley. Eur. Resp. J. 2:822.
16. Platts-Mills, T.A.E., Thomas, N.R., Aalberse, R.C., Vervloet, D., and Chapman, M.D. 1991. Dust mite allergens and asthma: Report of a second international workshop. Minster Lovell, England, Sept. 19–21, The UCB Institute of Allergy.

Immunogenicity and Immunotherapy with Polymeric Antigen from the House Dust Mite *Dermatophagoides Pteronyssinus*

Manuel Asrilant*, Silvia Hajos**, Claudia Waldner**, Elida Alvarez**, Norma Gutiez*

We have shown that PDP has a higher MW and maintained its immunogenic capacity in rabbits immunized I.P. weekly or in Freund's adjuvant, inducing similar titers of Ab. Conformation changes may occur during polymerization leading to (a) the expression of new epitopes or (b) hiding some of them, which might be responsible for the I.G. The first possibility should be considered, since Anti-PDP sera reacted strongly with PDP but it bound only weakly to the MDP Ags. The latter possibility seems improbable since anti-MDP strongly reacted with PDP, which is able to partially inhibit the interaction between anti-MDP serum and MDP Ag indicating that A.D. responsible for the I.G. could be preserved. On the other hand, skin testing in humans showed that reactions with the PDP extract were, in general, less intense than the MDP reaction, which might be related to the hiding of some epitopes. Three randomly selected groups of patients suffering from mite induced type I.A.R.D. (rhinitis, bronchial asthma and rhinitis plus asthma) were treated either with an MDP or with a glutaraldehyde polymer (PDP). Remarkable symptomatic improvement was observed progressively during a year in treatment in both groups, but no significant differences were observed between them. Nasal and bronchial symptoms scores as well as the number of days with symptoms and medication consumption scores were also significantly reduced. Respiration function tests performed in 36 asthmatics also showed no significant differences between the M.D.P. and P.D.P. treated patientes, but FEV 1 and FEF (25–75%) improved significantly in both groups. No significant changes were observed with either nasal or bronchial provocation tests, or with the skin tests' size evolution. Adverse reactions (local, symptomatic or systemic) were more frequently observed with the MDP extract.

Immunotherapy (I. T.) with polymerized allergenic extract (P. A. E.) has been used in order to reduce allergenicity (IgE mediated response) while retaining immunogenicity (I. G.) (IgE mediated response). Patterson et al. stated that classical I. T. might be improved using P. A. E. of the same antigens with the same efficacy, higher safety but with fewer injections and costs as well. Polymerization can reduce allergenicity by concealing certain antigenic (Ag) determinants and/or decreasing its capacity to bridge IgE antibody (Ab) molecules on mast cell surfaces, and because of its slower diffusion through tissues. I.G. might be retained because epitopes could still be available for processing by macrophages, initiating an immune response(1). In order to assess whether the advantages mentioned in several papers with some P.A.E. pollen Ags (in relation to the aqueous extract of the same allergens) could be extended to house dust mites (HDM) Ags, we polymerized a dermatophagoides pteronyssinus (DP) extract and tried to evaluate its I. G. in rabbits and its activity and tolerance in human I. T. (2,3).

Experimental Trial

Isolated D.P. (Biopol) were extracted in glycero-coca, called: monomeric Ag (MDP). The polymerized Ag (PDP) was obtained by a method modified from that described by Patterson et al. (4) for 1 hr. at room temperature and for 24 hrs. at 4°C. Polymerization was stopped with glycine, and Ags were separated in a Sephacryl column. Fraction protein content was evaluated, and both Ags were dialized and sterilized (5). The elution profiles showed that the pattern of MDP correspond to a MW=69 Kd and that of PDP to a MW=135 Kd. (Fig. 1).

* Cedenal: Centro de Enfermedades Alicas e Inmunolcas, Buenos Aires, Argentina;
** Immunology Department, Biochemistry Faculty, University of Buenos Aires, Argentina.

Figure 1. Sephacryl S-300 column chromat fractionation. Profiles of DPD, MDP and Dextran Bluc. Arrows localization of MW markers: TG = 600 Kd, IgG 150 Kd and human albumin 69 Kd.

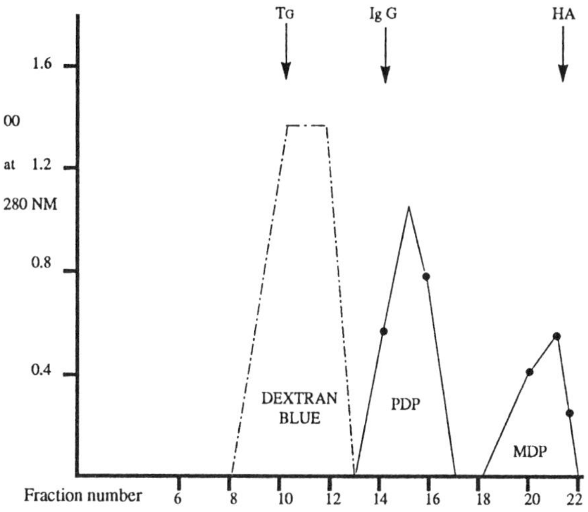

Figure 2: Antibody response to MDP and to PDP in rabbits. Arrows show the immunization schedule wit and without adjuvant (dotted line).

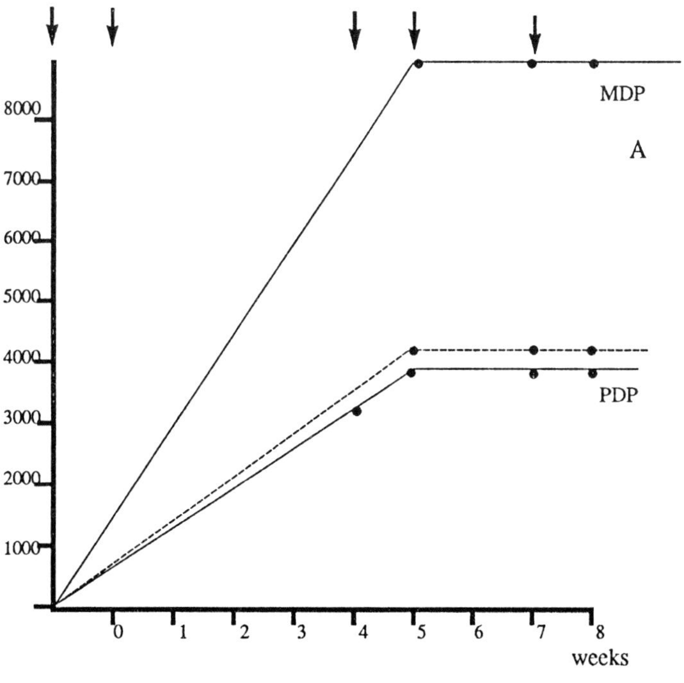

Six rabbits were injected with MDP or PDP in Freund's adjuvant (days 1, 8 and 28). Others were inoculated by an I.P. route weekly. The Ab response was evaluated by a dot immunoenzymobinding test method (DIB) (Hawkes et al., Ref. 6). The Ags, placed in nitrocelulose paper strips and, later, in microtiter plates, were incubated with different dilutions of rabbit antisera and, afterwards, with an anti-rabbit Ig-peroxidase conjugate. Positive reactions, when developed with naphtol/hidrogen-peroxide, show blue dots, which are graded from 1 to 4 +. The titer of Abs induced by both Ags were similar. Antisera reacted up to 1/8000 dilution with MDP and up to 1/4000 with PDP (1 dilution difference) (Fig. 2). Inhibition studies, performed to see if PDP changes the immunoreactivity (I.R.) to MDP as a consequence of the hiding of some epitopes, showed that, after absorption with PDP, anti-MDP sera reduced its titer to 1/2000, when reacting with MDP, while the reaction with PDP was completely inhibited. Other inhibition tests showed that anti-PDP sera reduced its titer from 1/4000 to 1/500 after absorption with the PDP Ag. (Fig. 3).

Clinical Trial

The effectiveness of I. T. with house dust (H.D.) extract is supported by a long, but somewhat controversial clinical experience. I. T. with H.D.M. has been widely used in most countries, since Voorhorst et al. discovered the importance of H.D. Mites (1964, Ref. 7). In our experience of more than 20 years, I. T. with H.D.M. Ags has shown clearly better clinical results than those observed with the whole H.D. This therapeutic tool seems to be the most reliable one in H.D. allergy because of the enormous ubiquity of pyrogliphidae mites, while the "home control measures" present only partial usefulness (8). However, because of the possibility of strong local or systemic reactions, certain very sensitive patients are sometimes unable to tolerate high doses of aqueous extracts in long I. T. schedules. As mentioned above, a number of authors showed that p.a.e. was superior to the classical I. T. with aqueous extracts of ragweed, grasses and trees, due to its reducing the frequency and intensity of untoward reactions and its still achieving similar effectiveness. (9,10).

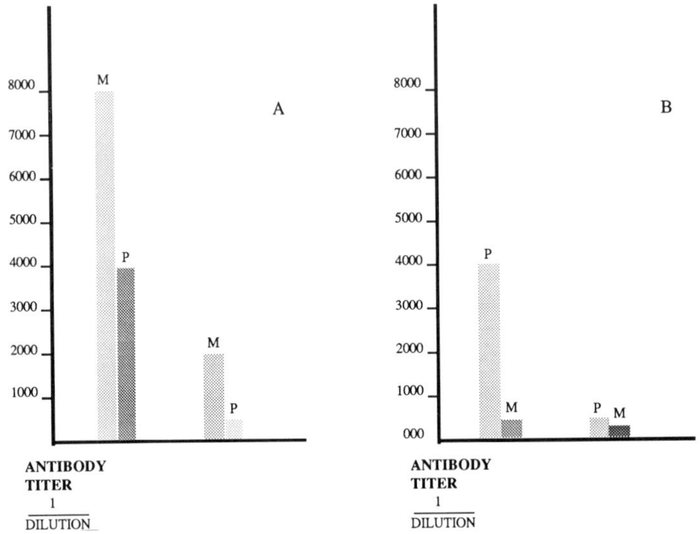

Figure 3

A = Inhibition of rabbit anti-MDP sera by both antigens (MDP and PDP) before (left) and after (right) absorption.
B = Inhibition of rabbit anti-PDP sera by both antigens (MDP and PDP) before (left) and after (right) absorption.

Patients

We evaluated the response to I.T. with PDP and MDP in 59 patients with allergic respiratory diseases (A.R.D.): 20 with perennial rhinitis, 18 with asthma and 21 with both conditions. 96 patients started with this trial, and 37 drop outs were registered. Criteria for inclusion were: (a) presence of chronic and/or recurrent symptoms; (b) mite related seasonal exacerbations (that is, the spring and fall in Buenos Aires); (c) diagnosed upon the presence of positive family and personal histories of atopy condition I or diseases; and (d) mean high level of total serum IgE. Hypersensitivity to DP was determined by the presence of: (a) positive skin testing to DP and (b) specific serum IgE positive for DP (Rast or Elisa). No corticosteroids had been administered in the past 12 months or I.T. in the past 3 years. The study was carried out by a "single blind" method evaluating four parameters: (I) symptom scores, (II) respiratory function testing, (III) provocation tests, and (IV) skin testing.

(I) The patients completed daily symptom scores on cards and, later, on weekly sheets, alloting 4 points of value: 3, 2, 1 and 0 (=no symptoms). Each patient was carefully instructed in order to give each symptom score according to precise standards for: I.1: Bronchial-asthma: wheezing, cough, physical signs, etc.; I.2: Rhinitis: sneezing, nasal dischange, blockage, itching, etc.; I.3: Medications used: type, number and frequency of symptomatic drugs consumed; I.4: Number of days with symptoms in a certain period of time.

(II) Respiratory function testing included: evaluation of FVC, FEV, and FEF (25–75%), development and control of the seasonal variations.

(III) Provocation tests included nasal and bronchial challenge with progressive doses of Ags and evaluated by rhinomanometry and spirometry respectively.

(IV) Skin testing involved comparing MDP and PDP Ags by prick test vs. five to tenfold dilutions of DP titrated in B.U. The 1/20 dilution of our extracts were equivalent to the titer of 10 B.U. On the other hand, PDP and MDP showed similar wheal and erythema sizes in many cases, but, in one of the patients, PDP showed less intense reactions than MDP and those of DP mite extracts produced in other labs. Late reactions (24/48 hs.) were somewhat more frequent with PDP.

Treatment

The patients were randomly assigned to one of two groups: one treated with PDP and the other one with the MDP extract. Three tenfold dilutions from the original 1/5000 N.U. were employed. The 1:1.000 and the 1:100 dilutions were injected weekly during 3 months (0.1, 0.3 and 0.6 ml. doses), the 1:10 dilution fortnightly and the same dilution or (when possible) the full strength, monthly (0.2 / 0.6 ml.).

Results

(I): The symptom scores recorded by each patient were evaluated periodically (after 15 or 30 days) during the trial; mean values were calculated in each case and each time. The development of the individual and the mean values of the recorded scores were analyzed separately for each group. Mean values registered previously and after 4–5 months (m=6) and after 11-13 months (m=12) were compared (Fig. 4). Group 1 (20 rhinitis patients) showed the following mean values: 2.1, 1.68 and 1.01 with MDP, and 2.02, 1.68 and 0.96 with PDP. Group 2 (with 18 bronchial asthma patients) had values of 2.09, 1.1 and 1.12 for MDP and 2.15, 1.22 and 1.04 for PDP. Group 3 (with 21 rhinitis/asthma patients) scored with 2.07, 1.3 and 0.88 for MDP and 1.95, 1.02 and 0.87. Significant falls in the mean scores were observed during and after 1 year: for I.T. with both (PDP and MPP) extracts; but no significant differences were found between them (Fig. 4). The number of days with allergic symptoms during a certain period (registered before and at 3, 6, 9 and 12 months) showed a significant reduction, especially after 9 and 12 months after the begining of the trial; nonetheless, even in this case, no significant differences were observed between the PDP and the MDP treated groups (Fig. 5).

(II): Pulmonary functional tests showed a significant rise in the FEV 1 and FEF (25–75%) values, after 6/9 months of treatment, but not with FVC and, just as in the case of the symp-

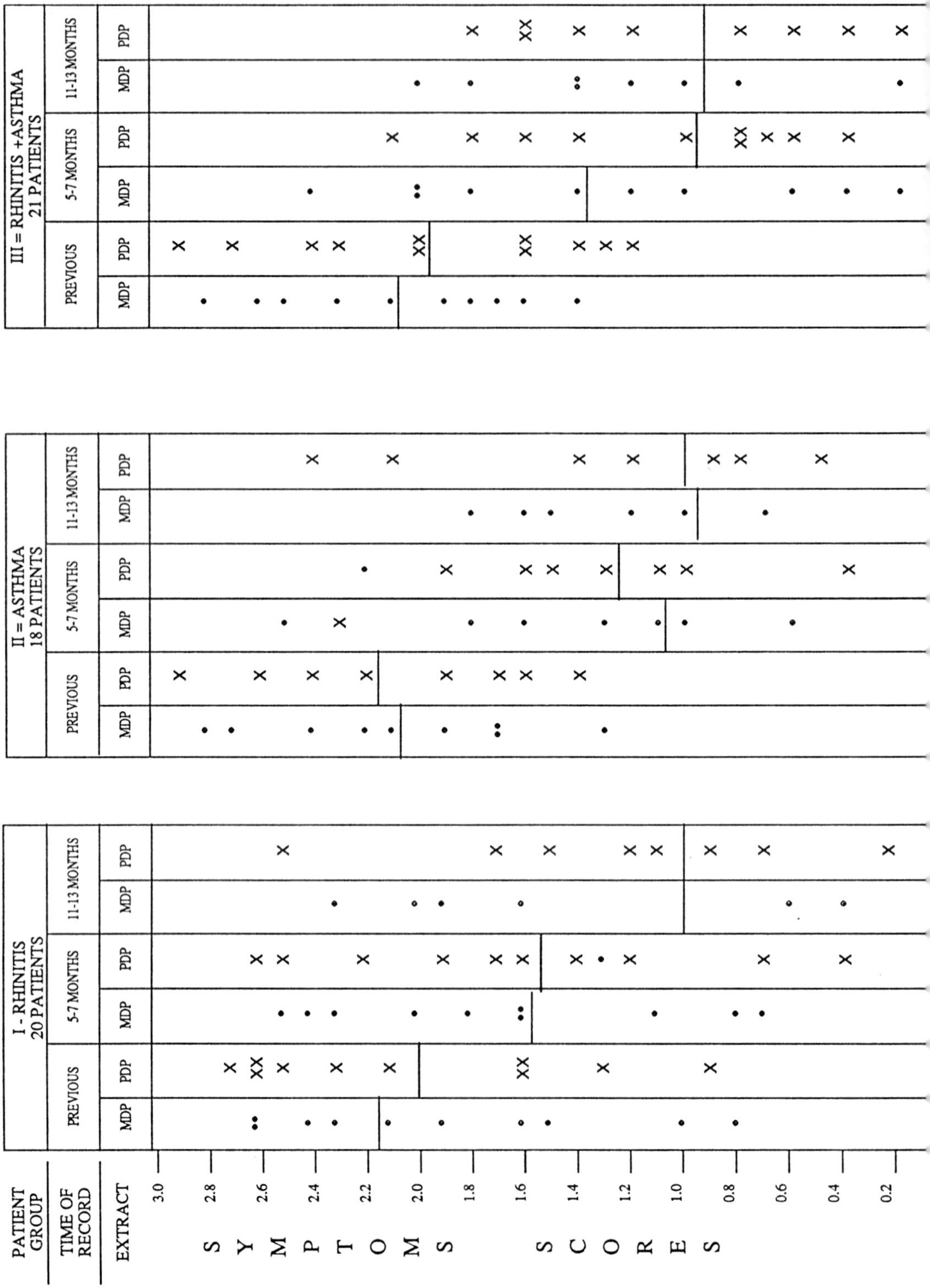

Figure 4. Evolution of symptoms scores in the 3 Groups of Patientes with immunotherapy with M.D.P. and P.D.P.

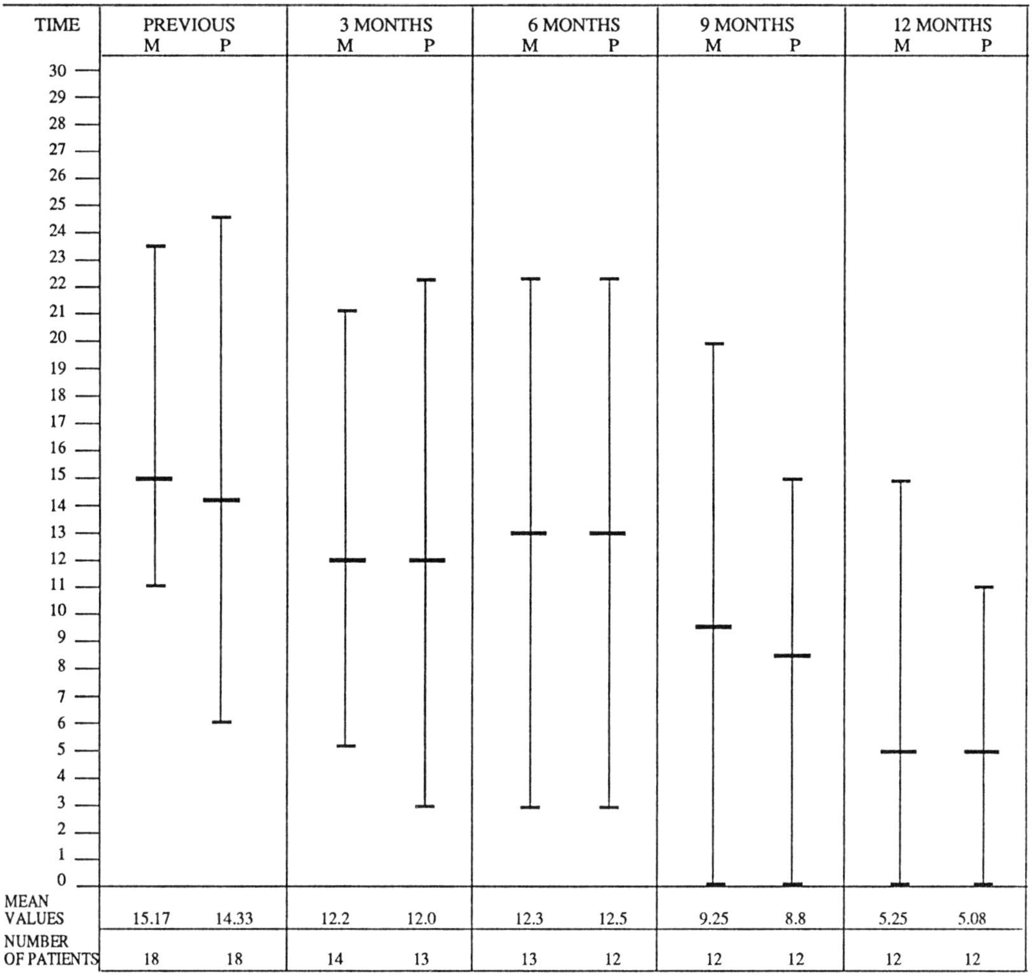

Figure 5. Evolution of Number of Days symptoms in Rhinitis and/or Asthma Patientes treated with MDP (M) or PDP (P)

tom development, no differences were detected in the 36 asthmatic patients studied (18 with MDP I.T. and 18 with PDP) in either group (Fig. 6). The statistical analysis (performed with the student T test) showed no significant differences between the MDP and the PDP groups for symptoms scores, number of days with symptoms or functional tests (Fig. 4, 5 and 6). As can be seen in Fig. 4, there is a clear decrease in scores from the previous values to the 12 month values and for the three classes of pathology ($P < 0.001$ to $P < 0.0001$, using an Anova and Newman-Keuls test for multiple comparisons). The fall is approximately 50% of the FEV 1 and the FEF (25–75 %) and showed a significant increase with a gradient of more than 2.0 ($P < 0.01$) and ($P < 0.05$). FVC showed no significant differences between the successive data (previous, during and after treatment).

(III and IV): In 12 provocation tests and 19 skin testing series carried out up to the present moment with both antigens, no significant differences have yet been detected.

Adverse Reactions

Patients were instructed to record carefully any reaction only if they followed an injection or were I.T. related. Side effects were observed

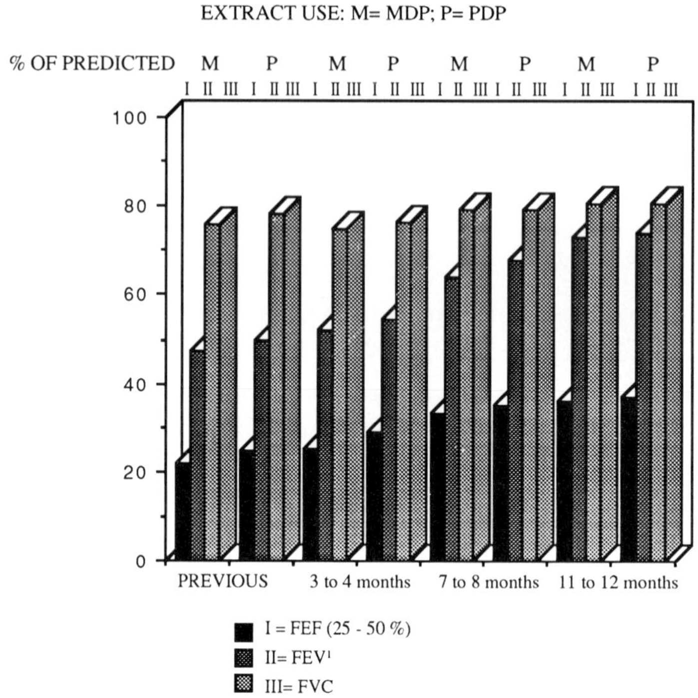

Figure 6. Evolution of mean Values of Pulmonary Tests in 25 Asthmatic Patients (before, during and a Year i.t. with MDP or PDP). 13 Patients were treated with PDP and 12 with MDP.

especially with high doses or in high concentrations, and much more frequently with MDP than with PDP. More than 600 injections have been administrated with each Ag extract up to the present (altogether 1,200). During the nearly 18 months duration of this trial, the following reactions have been observed: Local reactions in the MDP-treated group were mild in 64 and severe in 24. In the PDP-treated group the reactions were mild in 31 and severe in 7. Focal (symptomatic) reactions in the MDP's were mild in 21 and severe in 4. In the PDP's they were mild in 9 and severe in 1. Systemic (generalized) reactions were observed as well: In the MDP group there were 4 (3 "drop outs"), and in the PDP there was just 1. (These are to date unpublished data.)

References

1. Patterson, R. 1981. Allergy immunotherapy with modified allergens. Journal Allergy Clin. Immunol. 68:85.
2. Grammer, L.C., Shaugnessy, M.A., Silvestry, L., and Patterson, R. 1985. Allergenicity, immunogenicity and safety of immunotherapy with various molecular weight ranges of polymerized ragweed. Journal Allergy Clin. Immunol. 76:195.
3. Metzger, J.W., Patterson, R., Zeiss, C.R., Irons, J.S., Pruzansky, J.J., Suszko, I.M, and Levits, D. 1976. Comparison of immune reactivity to polyvalent monomeric and polymeric ragweed antigens. New Engl. J. Med. 295:1160.
4. Patterson, R., Suszko, I.M., Raymond-Zeiss, C., Pruzansky, J.J., and Bacal, E. 1978. Comparison of polymerized and unpolymerized antigen E for immunotherapy of ragweed allergy. Journal Allergy Clin. Immunol. 61:28.
5. Lowry, O.H., Rosebrough, N.J., Farr, A.L., and Randall, R.J. 1951. Protein measurement with the Folin phenol reagent. J. Biol. Chem. 193:268.
6. Hawkes, R., and Niday Gordon, J. 1982. A dot-immunobinding assay for monoclonal and other antibodies. Anal. Bioch. 119:142.
7. Voorhorst, R., Spjieksma, F.T.M., Varekamp, H., Leupen, M.G., and Lyklema, A.M. 1967.

The house dust white (D.P.) and the allergens it produces: Identity with the house dust allergens. J. Allergy 39:325.

8. Platts-Mills, T.A.E., and Chapman, M.D. 1987. The house dust mite (DP) and allergens it produces: Immunology, allergic disease and environmental control. J. Allergy Clin. Immunol. 80:755.
9. Patterson, R., Suszko, I.M., Hendrix, S.G., and Zeiss, C.R. 1982. Polymerized tree pollen antigens. Journal Allergy Clin. Immunol. 67/2:162.
10. Grammer, L.C., Shaugnessy, M.A., Suszko, I.M., and Patterson, R. 1983. A double-blind histamine placebo-controled trial of polymerized whole grass for immunotherapy of grass allergy. Journal Allergy Clin. Immunol. 72:448.
11. Chapman, M.D., Platts-Mills, T.A.E. 1980. Purification and characterization of the major allergen from Dermatophagoides pteronyssinus-Antigen P1. Journal Immmunol. 125:587.

Identification of *Der f* I as a Cystein Protease and Production of Biologically Active Recombinant *Der f* II

Hirokazu Okudaira*, Matsunobu Suko*, Tohru Ando**, Yoshitaka Into**, Toshifumi Yuuki***, Namiko Iwamoto***, Toshiro Takai***, Yasushi Okumura***

A cystein protease in the crude *Dermatophagoides farinae* mite extract was detected and purified using various column chromatographies. Both the potent cysteine protease activity and the allergenic activity were detected in the same fractions by anion exchange chromatography on a DEAE-Sephacel, gel chromatographies, and Chelating Sepharose 6B chromatography. In the double immunodiffusion test, the highly purified cysteine protease and rabbit anti-*Der f I* sera reacted to give a single precipitin line which fused completely with a precipitin line formed by *Der f I* and anti-*Der f I* sera. Sequences of the first 10 N-terminal amino acids from the cysteine protease and *Der f I* were identical. Based on the results above, we concluded that the mite cystein protease and *Der f I* are the same molecule. A cDNA library corresponding to mite protein was screened using anti-*Der f II* antibody. Three possible clones were obtained that contained cDNA fragments coding for *Der f II*, and the nucleotide sequences of the fragments were determined. There were minor differences observed affecting the deduced amino acid sequence among the three cDNA fragments. The amino acid sequence of the purified native *Der f II* protein could be analyzed to 45 residues from the N-terminus. As a result of comparison, all the three cDNA fragments code for a mature protein with a derived molecular weight of about 14,000. The amino acid sequence was not homologous to any known protein sequences and it contained six cysteine residues and no N-glycosylation sites.

Identification of *Der f* I as a Cysteine Protease

In 1988, Chua and coworkers reported the sequence analyses of the *Der p I* cDNA clone and the homology (about 20%) between its inferred amino acid sequence and the group of cystein proteases such as papain, actinidin or cathepsin B (1). Based on their finding, we tried to detect, purify and characterize a cystein protease in the crude extract of *Dermatophagoides farinae* (2,3).

Purification of a Cystein Protease in the Crude Mite Extract (CME)

One point five grams of CME was dissolved in 50 ml of 0.01 M PBS, pH 7.0, and stirred for 1 hr at 4°C, followed by centrifugation at 9,500 rpm for 1 h at 4°C. The supernatant was collected, and saturated ammonium sulfate was added to 60% saturation. The precipitate was separated from the supernatant by centrifugation at 9,500 rpm for 1 h at 4°C. The precipitate was dissolved in 10 ml of 0.02 M phosphate buffer (PB), pH 6.0, then dialyzed against the same buffer and applied to a DEAE-Sephacel (Pharmacia) column equilibrated with the same PB. The column was then eluted with a linear sodium chloride gradient from 0 to 0.03 M, and aliquots of 5 ml were collected. The fractions containing high cysteine protease activity were pooled (Fr. 1) and dialyzed against 0.05 M Tris-HC1 buffer, pH 8.0, and applied to a DEAE-Sephacel column equilibrated with the same Tris buffer. The stepwise elution was then performed with 0.05 M Tris-HC1, pH 8.0, 0.05 M Tris-HC1 containing 0.2 M sodium chloride, pH 7.4, and 0.05 M Tris-HC1 containing 0.5 M sodium chloride, pH 7.4. Aliquots of 5 ml were collected. The fraction eluted with 0.05 M Tris-HC1 containing 0.2 M sodium chloride, pH 7.4 (Fr. 2), was concentrated from 45 ml to 6.5 ml by ultrafiltration through a PM-10 membrane

* Department of Medicine and Physical Therapy, Faculty of Medicine, University of Tokyo, 7-3-1, Hongo, Bunkyo-ku, Tokyo 113, Japan;
** Research Laboratories, Torii & Co., Ltd., 14–3, Minamiyawata 3-chome, Ichikawa, Chiba 272, Japan;
*** Central Research Laboratories, Asahi Breweries, Ltd., 2–13–1, Ohmori-kita, Ohta-ku, Tokyo 143, Japan.

(Amicon), and fractionated on a Sephacryl S-200 (Pharmacia) column equilibrated with 0.02 M PBS, pH 6.0. The fractions containing cysteine protease (Fr. 3) were concentrated in volumes from 90 ml to 20 ml, dialyzed against 0.05 M Tris-acetate containing 0.5 M sodium chloride, pH 7.5, and subjected to chelate chromatography on Chelating Sepharose 6B (Pharmacia) which was previously chelated with Zinc ion and equilibrated with the Tris-acetate buffer. The sample was applied to the column and the stepwise elution was performed by decreasing the pH of 0.05 M Tris-acetate buffer from 7.5 to 6.5, 5.5 and 4.5. Five ml of each eluate was collected. The fraction with cysteine protease activity, eluted with 0.05 M Tris-acetate containing 0.5 M sodium chloride at pH 5.5 (Fr. 4), was concentrated to 3 ml and applied to a Sephadex G-75 (Pharmacia) column equilibrated with 0.02 M PBS, pH 6.0. In all isolation procedures, protein content of each fraction was monitored by measuring absorbance at 280 nm. Both the cystein protease activity and allergenic activity were checked in each step. The Sephadex G-75 gel filtration profile is shown in Fig. 1. The cystein protease activity, the allergenic activity and the protein concentration were detected in a single peak. The peak fractions were collected and reprecipitated with ammonium sulfate at 55% saturation, and regarded as a highly purified cystein protease. The cystein potease activity of the final preparation (153 nml/min/mg protein) was increased about 6.5 times in comparison with that of CME (24 nml min/mg protein).

Comparison of D. farinae Cystein Protease with Der f I

Subsequently, comparison of the purified cystein protease from *D. farinae* extract with purified *Der f I* (kind gift of Dr. Hiroshi Yasueda, National Sagamihara Hospital) (4) was carried out. Our results revealed: (A) There was complete agreement in the retention times of the cystein protease and *Der f I* in HPLC [Model 130 A, Applied Biosystems Co.; Column, C8 300A (2.1 ID × 30 mm); Buffer A, 0.1% trifluoroacetic acid (TFA) in H_2O; Buffer B, 0.1% TFA in 70% acetonitrile; Gradient, 0% buffer B to 100% buffer B at 2.2% per minutes; flow rate, 2μl/min]. (B) The amino acid composition of the purified cystein protease was very simlar with that reported for *Der f I* (4). (C) N-terminal amino acid sequence of the purified cystein protease was examined to prove that the first 10-amino acid-sequence was just the same as that of *Der f I* reported by Heyman et al. (5). (D) An immunological identification experiment was carried out by double immunodiffusion test. The purified cystein protease and hyper-immune rabbit anti-*Der f I* serum reacted to give a single precipitin line which fused completely with a single band formed between the authentic *Der f I* and the hyper immune

Figure 1. Sephadex G-75 Column Chromatography.

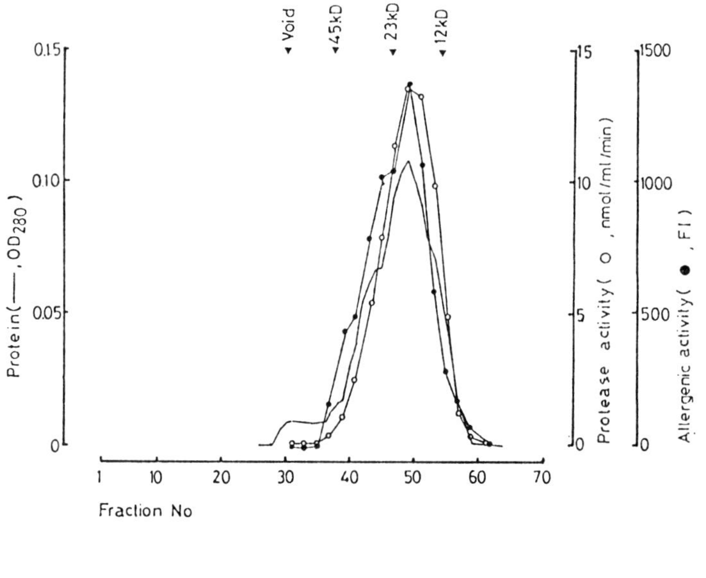

serum. Based on the experimental results above we concluded that *Der f I* is actually the same molecule as a cystein protease itself (3). After identification of *Der f I* as a cystein protease, we employed cystein protease activity as a marker of *Der f I*. It shortened the time required for the *Der f I* assay to improve the purification procedures.

Cloning and Expression of cDNA Coding for *Der f* II in *Escherichia Coli* (7,8)

Preparation of cDNA Library to D. farinae.

Five grams of live mites were rapidly frozen with liquid nitrogen and 10 ml of guanidine isothiocyanate solution (RNA extraction kit, RPN. 1264; Amersham International plc.) were added. The suspension was immediately homogenized. After the insoluble mite materials were separated by centrifugation, the RNA fraction was precipitated with LiCl solution. The pelleted RNA was fractionated on an oligo (dT) cellulose column (mRNA Purification Kit, 27-9258-01; Pharmacia LKB Biotechnology AB) and bound RNA [poly (A)$^+$] was isolated. The cDNA was synthesized by the method of Gubler and Hoffman (6) using a kit (cDNA synthesizing system plus, RPN 1256Y; Amersham International plc.).

Selection of the Clone Containing Der f II gene.

cDNA prepared from *D. farinae* was inserted to an expression vector pUEX1, and then *E. coli* MC1061 was transformed by the recombinant plasmids. Among 1,600 transformants, three clones, No. 1, No. 2 and No. 11, appeared to be the desired clones using a colony immunoassay with anti-*Der f II* antibody. Each plasmid was recovered from the clones and analyzed by agarose gel electrophoresis. All plasmids had approximately 500 base-pair insertions at the end of the β-galactosidase gene. Therefore, the foreign proteins were concluded to be fused to β-galactosidase, and the plasmids of the clones were named pFL1, pFL2 and pFL11, respectively.

Western Blot Analysis of Fused Der f II Protein

It was possible to make the inclusion bodies visible using phase-contract light microscopy in the recombinant *E. Coli*, the transformants were grown in broth culture, and the proteins were detected by Western Blotting using anti-*Der f II* antibody. As shown in Figure 2, clones No. 1 (pFL1) and No. 11 (pFL11) did not produce 116-kilodalton β-galactosidase bands but instead produced antibody-binding components with molecular weights about 130 kilodalton. They were consistent with fusion proteins with *Der f II* contributing a 14-kilodalton moiety. On the other hand, clone No. 2 (pFL2) did not produce such a protein.

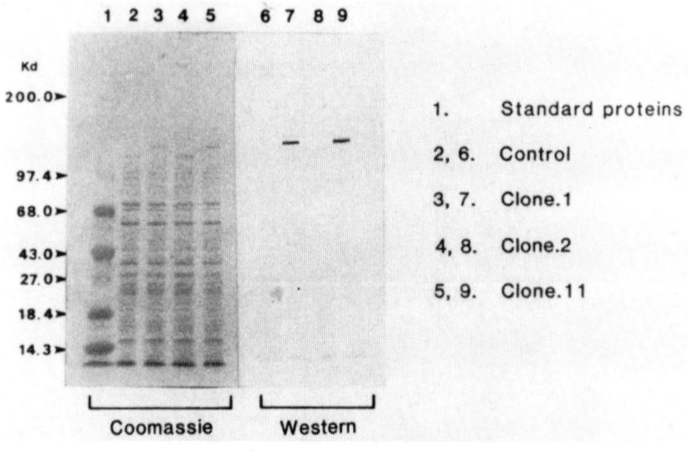

Figure 2. Western Blotting Analysis of Recombinant *Der f II* protein. Total cellular proteins of *E. coli* JM105 transformed by recombinant plasmids pFL1 (lanes 2 and 6). pFL2 (lanes 3 and 7), and pFL11 (lanes 4 and 8) were analyzed on SDS-polyacrylamide gel. *E. coli* containing vector plasmids, pUEX1 was analyzed in the same manner (lanes 1 and 5). Molecular weight markers (BRL) were run in lane M. Proteins blotted on the membrane were stained with Coomassie Brilliant Blue (lanes M, 1, 2, 3 and 4) or by immunostaining (lanes 5, 6, 7 and 8).

Sequencing of cDNA

Plasmid DNA was prepared from the selected anti-*Der f II* binding plasmid clone and characterized using restriction endonuclease. The subcloning was done using the plasmids pUC118 and pUC119 (9) for sequence analysis. The cDNA insert was excised by *Bam*HI. *Bam*HI-cDNA fragments were digested with various restriction endonucleases such as *Nco* I and subcloned into the appropriate sites of the vector. After transformation of the *E. coli* JM105, the isolated transformed colonies were infected by the helper phage M13K07. Single-strand DNAs were extracted from the resulting phage particles. DNA sequencing was done by the method of Sanger (10) using a 7-DEAZA sequencing kit (Takara). The sequence was analyzed using the sequence analysis software DNASIS (Hitachi Software Service). The cDNA inserts of the three clones were about the same length. To confirm their identity, the cDNA inserts of the clones were characterized using restriction endonucleases (Fig. 3). The common restriction sites (up-stream *Nco* I and *Cla* I) were observed in all of the inserts, while inserts of pFL11 lacked the *Eco*RV and downstream *Nco*I sites. The nucleotide sequence analyses were done on these clones.

The cDNA sequence and the deduced amino acid sequence from the cDNA insert of pFL1 is shown in Figure 4. It consists of 501 nucleotides including a 17-nucleotide-long poly (A) tail. A putative polyadenylation signal, AATAAC, was located at position 474-479, 15 bp upstream from the poly (A) tail. An open reading frame consisting of 416 nucleotides was found to code for a polypeptide of 139 amino acids in the same frame as β-galactosidase.

The amino acids of native *Der f II* purified by HPLC were sequenced. Forty-five amino acid residues from the N-terminus could be identified and the sequence was completely the same as that deduced from the cDNA indicated by the underline in Fig. 4. The mature *Der f II* protein is coded for by a single open reading frame ending at the TAA stop codon at nucleotide position 427-429 and consists of 129 amino acids containing six cysteine residues with a derived molecular weight of 14,043. The predicted *Der f II* amino acid sequence has no potential *N*-glycosylation sites. No significant similarities were found between this sequence and other DNA and protein sequence in the EMBL/GENBANK and NBRF/SWISSPROT data banks. We compared nucleotide sequences of cDNA inserts of pFL1 with pFL2 and pFL11. As shown in Fig. 5, several base substitutions were found among the different clones. It was confirmed that the differences of the restriction cleavage sites resulted from base substitutions. Among them, some of the substitutions caused amino acid changes as shown in Fig. 6. These base substitutions might be due to polymorphisms among gene sequences.

All the sequences included 5' proximal end sequences. That is, cDNA of the *Der f II* has a pre-sequence. Inspection of the amino acid se-

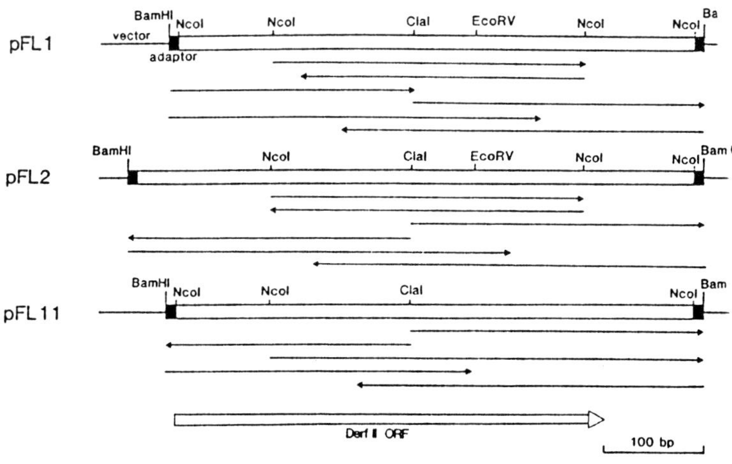

Figure 3. Restriction Map and Sequencing Strategy for the Three cDNAs Encoding *Der f II*. The open boxes indicate cloned fragments, and the closed boxes indicate the "adaptor". The sequencing strategy is indicated by arrows showing the direction and extent of DNA sequencing.

leukocytes from atopic individuals sensitized to *Dermatophagoides* mites. The data show that the recombinant *Der f II* we prepared is biologically active. Recently, we have succeeded in direct expression of recombinant *Der f II* in *Escherichia coli* in relatively large quantity (about 10 mg/l). The recombinant *Der f II* directly expressed showed clear biological activity. Recombinant *Der f II* contained six cysteins (amino acid numbers 8, 21, 27, 78 and 119 from N-terminus). In order to explore the epitope of *Der f II* which reacts with human antimite IgE antibody, deletion mutants of recombinant *Der f II* which lack N-terminal or C-terminal portions were prepared. Removal of 31 amino acids from N-terminus and 17 amino acids from C-terminus resulted in the loss of IgE antibody binding capacity, which may mean that an S-S bond between cysteins numbers 27 and 119 is essential to keep the tertiary structure of *Der f II* reactive with atopic anti-*Der f II* IgE antibody.

References

1. Chua, K.Y. Stewart, G.A., Thomas, W.R., Simpson, R.J., Dilworth, R.J., Plozza, T.M., and Turner, K.J. 1988. Sequence analysis of cDNA cording for a major house dust mite allergen, *Der f I*. Homology with cysteine protease. J. Exp. Med. 167:175.
2. Ino, Y., Ando, T., Haida, M., Nakamura, K., Iwaki, M., Okudaira, H., and Miyamoto, T. 1989. Characterization of the proteases in the crude mite extract. Int. Arch. Allergy. Appl. Immunol. 89:321.
3. Ando, T., Ino, Y., Haida, M., Honma, R., Maeda, H., Yamakawa, H., Iwaki, M., and Okudaira. H. 1991. Isolation of cystein protease in the crude mite extract, *Dermatophagoides farinae.* Int. Arch. Allergy Appl. Immunol., in press.
4. Yasueda, H., Mita, H., Yui, Y., and Shida, T. 1986. Isolation and characterization of two allergens from *Dermatophagoides farinae.* Int. Arch. Allergy Appl. Immunol. 81:214.
5. Heymann, P.W., Chapman, M.D., Platts-Mills, T.A.E. 1986. Antigen *Der f I* from the house dust mite *Dermatophagoides farinae:* Structual comparison with *Der p I* from *Dermatophagoides pteronyssinus* and epitope specificity of murine IgG and human IgE antibodies. J. Immunol. 137:2841.
6. Gubler, U., and Hoffman, B. 1983. A simple and very efficient method for generating cDNA libraries. Gene 25:263.
7. Yuuki, T., Okumura, Y., Ando, T., Yamakawa, H., Suko, M., Haida, M., and Okudaira, H. 1990. Cloning and sequencing of cDNA corresponding to mite major allergen *Der f II*. Jpn. J. Allergol. 39:557.
8. Yuuki, T., Okumura, Y., Ando, T., Yamakawa, H., Suko, M., Haida, M., and Okudaira, H. 1991. Cloning and expression of cDNA coding for the major house dust mite allergen *Der f II* in *Escherichia coli.* Agric. Bio. Chem. 55:1233.
9. Vieira, J., and Messing, J. 1987. Production of single-stranded plasmid DNA. In: Methods in enzymology, Vol. 153. R. Wu, ed. New York: Academic Press, p.3.
10. Sanger, F. 1981. Determination of nucleotide sequences in DNA. Science 214:1205.
11. Kozak, M. 1984. Computation and analysis of sequences upstream from the translational start site in eukaryotic mRNAs. Nucl Acids Res. 12:857.

Mite Allergens, Monoclonal Antibodies and the Immune Response

Martin D. Chapman*, L. Karla Arruda*, Frederique DeBlay**, Moeness M. Al-Shistawy*, Lisa D. Vailes*, Peter W. Heymann*, Thomas A. E. Platts-Mills*

The development of sensitive and specific immunoassays for dust mite (Dermatophagoides spp.) allergens has applications in four research areas: (a) epidemiology; (b) aerobiology; (c) avoidance; and (d) standardization. There has been significant progress in each of these areas over the past 3 years. Allergen measurements in dust samples have become established as a primary method of assessing mite exposure and used in epidemiologic studies to assess risk levels for sensitization and exacerbation of allergic symptoms. For Dermatophagoides spp., measurements of the Group I and/or Group II allergens are sufficient for most purposes. However, other mite species are associated with allergic disease and can comprise a significant part of the acarofauna in houses. Recent studies have focussed on analysis of Euroglyphus maynei, Blomia sp., and Lepidoglyphus destructor allergens, including cross reactivity with Dermatophagoides allergens, the immunochemical properties of allergens from different species, and the production of monoclonal antibodies. Together, these studies provide further evidence that exposure to mite allergens is an important cause of asthma.

Over the past 3 years, there have been significant advances in our understanding of the role of house dust mite allergens in the etiology of allergic disease, especially asthma. Much of this progress (outlined in Table 1) has relied on immunochemical studies, which have led to better definition of mite allergens (i. e., allergen purification, sequencing and the production of monoclonal antibodies [mAb]); on assays for serum IgE antibodies, to assess sensitization; and on the development of sensitive immunoassays for assessing mite allergen exposure (reviewed in 1). Most studies have focussed on the importance of allergens produced by Dermatophagoides spp. (D. pteronyssinus and D. farinae), which usually account for > 90% of the mite fauna in houses. However, there have been several recent studies on other domestic mites, e. g., Blomia spp, Euroglyphus maynei, and L. destructor, which can become the predominant species in house dust under certain environmental conditions, and which also cause allergic respiratory disease.

Dermatophagoides spp.: Allergens and Antibodies

Four groups of mite allergens were recognized at the 2nd International Mite Workshop (Minster Lovell, U.K., September 1990): Group I, 25kd cysteine proteases; Group II, 14kd proteins; Group III, ~ 30kd serine proteases; and, provisionally, "Group IV", ~ 60kd, amylase from D. pteronyssinus (1). Both the Group I and II allergens from D. pteronyssinus and

Table 1. Mite allergen measurements in the evaluation of allergic disease: progress from 1988–91.

1. Development of proposed threshold values for indoor exposure, as risk factors for:
   i) sensitization;
   ii) exacerbations of allergic disease (asthma).
2. Comparison of the forms in which mite allergens become airborne and enter the lung.
3. Objective monitoring of mite avoidance procedures and their use in the management of allergic patients.
4. Improved standardization of allergen extracts.

---

* Division of Allergy and Clinical Immunology, Department of Medicine, University of Virginia, Charlottesville, VA 22908, U.S.A.;

** Hospices Civils de Strasbourg, Strasbourg, France.

Acknowledgements: Supported by NIH grants AI 24687, AI 24261 and AI 20565; by a Fullbright Scholarship and a UCB Institute of Allergy Fellowship to Dr. DeBlay; and by a Peace Fellowship of the Egyptian Embassy and U.S. Agency for International Development to Dr. Al-Shistawy.

D. farinae have been cloned and partial amino acid sequence data has been obtained for the other allergens. The immunochemistry of the Group I and II allergens has been extensively studied and panels of murine mAb have been raised against these allergens for use in allergen purification, immunoassay development and epitope mapping. The use of mAb in allergen measurement has been predicated by the specificity of the murine IgG antibody responses under the various conditions used for immunization. The mAb to the Group I allergens are almost exclusively species specific and enzyme immunoassays (ELISA) for these allergens measure either Der p I or Der f I (2,3). In contrast, IgG antibody responses to Group II allergens are weak in BALB/c mice and the responses in "high responder" mouse strains (A/J, BALB/b, BALB/k, BALB/A10) are strongly cross reactive. Recent studies of 17 anti-Group II mAb derived from A/J, BALB/b or BALB/c mice showed that 15/17 bound to both Group II allergens. Radioimmunoassays (RIA) have been developed using monoclonal or polyclonal antibodies to Group II allergens and have the advantage that a single assay can be used to measure Der p II and Der f II (4,5). The RIA format has limited the widespread use of these assays; however, with the larger number of anti-Group II mAb that have recently been produced, there are better prospects for the development of an ELISA.

Monitoring Allergen Exposure in Dust Samples and in the Air

Because of their sensitivity and reproducibility, ELISA assays for Der p I and Der f I have been widely used in epidemiologic studies to assess levels of mite allergen exposure that constitute risk factors for allergic disease. These studies have now been carried out in several parts of the world, e.g., U.S.A., Europe, the Far East and South America, and, in general, support the proposed threshold values for sensitization (2 µg Group I allergen/g dust) and symptom exacerbations (> 10 µg/g dust) proposed in the International Workshops (1). A full account of these studies is given in the chapter by Platts-Mills et al. in this volume. There are several potential sources of variability associated with reservoir measurements of allergens in floor, carpets, furnishing and bedding samples, including the gross composition of the dust (and whether or not it is sieved); the area to be sampled; the power of the vacuum cleaner and duration of cleaning, etc. While these variables make absolute standardization very difficult, consistent results have been obtained using a modified hand held vacuum cleaner and sampling 1 square meter for 2 minutes. For example, two separate studies have compared Group I and Group II allergen levels in dust samples: In each case there was a good quantitative correlation between Group I and II allergen levels and the mean ratio of Group I:Group II in the extracts was very similar (0.8:1 and 0.96:1) (5,6). Reservoir measurements of allergens in dust are also being used to monitor the efficacy of allergen avoidance regimes, using either physical or chemical methods to reduce mite growth and allergen levels. Some of these treatments can affect allergen measurements, e.g., chemicals or acaricides can affect the weight of dust sampled and might also have inhibitory effects on allergen assays. Nonetheless, reservoir measurements have proved effective in monitoring changes in allergen levels following treatment of houses with either benzyl benzoate or tannic acid (7–9). It may be necessary to measure both Group I and Group II allergens following chemical treatments because these allergens have different susceptibility to denaturation.

Although it has been suggested that airborne measurements provide a more realistic assessment of mite allergen exposure, these methods have not been widely adopted. There is a poor temporal relationship between exposure to mite allergens and the onset of respiratory symptoms (which is not fully understood) and current evidence suggests that Group I and Group II allergens only become airborne following "disturbance" of the dust (Table 2). Furthermore, mite feces (the major source of Group I allergens) are large particles (10–40µ dia.), which do not usually remain airborne for more than 30 minutes, and similarly large particles are also associated with Group II allergens (10). Sakaguchi, Yasueda and colleagues could detect between 5–110 pg/m^3 airborne Group I and II allergens under "undisturbed" conditions ("of normal domestic life") using very sensitive RIA's (10pg/ml detection limit)

Table 2. Comparison of airborne Group I & Group II allergen levels.

Allergen	Mean airborne allergen (ng/m³) in rooms: Undisturbed	Disturbed (20–40 min)	20 min Post Disturbance
Group I			
De Blay et al. (10)	< 0.2	68	< 0.2
Sakaguchi et al. (11)	< 0.05 (30 pg/m³)	31	n.d.
Warner et al. (12)		(< 5–85)	n.d.
Group II			
De Blay et al. (10)	< 0.3	26	< 0.3
Sakaguchi et al. (11)	< 0.05 (6 pg/m³)	13	n.d.

n.d.: no data

(11). Using Casella personal samplers, Warner and colleagues reported airborne levels of 5–80 ng/m³ during normal domestic activity, not involving excessive disturbance, and suggested that airborne levels were a more suitable measure of exposure (12). In comparing airborne studies, it is difficult to define a particular level of "disturbance", to standardize air sampling methods, and to make reproducible measurements. Of the studies that have been reported, the most consistent data has been obtained following some form of disturbance, resulting in airborne allergen levels of ~ 10–100 ng/m³ (Table 2). At present it is not clear whether air sampling would be useful for epidemiologic studies, though further work in this area is clearly necessary to understand the process of sensitization for IgE antibody responses.

Standardization

Examples of Group I and II allergen levels in Dermatophagoides extracts marketed in the U.S. and in Europe are shown in Table 3. In the U. S., all commercial mite extracts are prepared from crushed mite bodies and the ratio of Group I:Group is ~ 1:1, whereas in Europe, several companies market extracts of whole mite culture and the Group I:II ratio ranges from 5–20:1. The table illustrates the diversity of units that are currently recommended by different standardization agencies (International Units, IU; Allergy Units, AU; and Biologic Units, BU), most of which are based on skin testing as the primary method of standardization (reviewed in 13). Specific allergen measurements provide a simpler and more con-

Table 3. Group I & Group II allergen levels in commercial mite extracts.

Manufacturer	Potency (per ml)	Group I (μg/ml)	Group II (μg/ml)	GpI : GpII*
D. pteronyssinus				
(NIBSC 82/518)+	100,000 IU	12.5	0.4	31.2
Abello	100 BU	67.0	12.0	5.6
Bencard	1.2%	102.0	16.0	6.4
Hollister Stier	30,000 AU	120.0	87.0	1.4
D. farinae				
Abello	100 BU	59.0	4.0	14.3
Hollister Stier	30,000 AU	110.0	24.0	4.6
Greer	10,000	39.0	60.0	0.7

*See also Yasueda et al. (5).
+WHO/IUIS International Reference Preparation (13).

sistent method of standardization that could readily be used by manufacturers to monitor extraction procedures and improve quality control (13).

Other Domestic Mites

Over the past 2 years, there has been renewed interest in the role of other mite species, principally Euroglyphus maynei, Blomia tropicalis, B. kulagini and Lepidoglyphus destructor, in causing allergic disease. E. maynei, a pyroglyphid mite related to Dermatophagoides sp., has previously been associated with asthma symptoms in damp housing, e. g. in Europe, where it can become the predominant species (14–16). Blomia spp. and L. destructor are examples of "storage mites", which usually infest stored food products, but can also occur in large numbers in house dust samples (17,18). Blomia sp. are widely distributed in tropical and subtropical areas of the world (e. g. Southern U.S., Brazil, Japan, Taiwan) and have been found in large numbers in house dust (up to 3,000 mites/g) (19,20). IgE antibodies to Blomia allergens have been demonstrated by skin testing and RAST and high levels of serum IgE antibodies have been found in Brazilian patients with asthma (6,19–22). Studies of other domestic mites are complicated by the fact that patients are almost always concordantly exposed to Dermatophagoides allergens. However, recently there has been significant progress in defining some of the allergens involved, and in the production of mAb, in large part because improved culture methods for these species have been developed (6,15,19,20). A Group I cross reacting allergen from E. maynei has been purified and sequenced by Hart and colleagues, and 39kd and 14kd L. destructor allergens have been identified using mAb (23–25). Immunoabsorption and RAST inhibition experiments have shown that Blomia spp. allergens do not show extensive cross reactivity with Dermatophagoides allergens and that mAb to B. tropicalis are species specific (6,22). The implications of these studies are that mites other than Dermatophagoides should be evaluated as a cause of asthma in houses or geographic areas where they form a significant part of the acarofauna.

Conclusions

Current evidence suggests that measurements of Group I and/or Group II allergens are sufficient for assessing exposure to Dermatophagoides spp. allergens and that allergen levels in reservoir dust samples provide the most consistent measure of exposure. In areas of the world where other mite species can predominate, assessments of exposure may require the development of separate immunoassays for those species (e. g. Blomia). The present assays are being routinely used in epidemiologic and clinical studies and a major emphasis over the next few years will be their application to monitor avoidance regimes. In order to achieve maximum patient compliance with avoidance procedures, it will be necessary to develop assays that can be used by physicians or in the home. This should enable better methods of reducing mite allergen exposure to be developed and should make avoidance a more effective treatment for the management of patients with asthma.

References

1. Platts-Mills, T.A.E., Thomas, W.R., Aalberse, R.C., Vervloet, D., and Chapman, M.D. 1992. Dust mite allergens and asthma: Report of a 2nd international workshop, Minster Lovell, England, September 19–21, 1990. J. Allergy Clin. Immunol., in press.
2. Luczynska, C.M., Arruda, L.K., Platts-Mills, T.A.E., Miller, J.D., Lopez, M., and Chapman, M.D., 1989. A two site monoclonal antibody Eliza for the quantitation of the major Dermatophagoides spp. allergens, Der p I and Der f I. J. Immunol. Meth. 118:227.
3. Lind, P., 1986. Enzyme linked immunosorbent assay for determination of major excrement allergens of house dust mite species D. pteronyssinus, D. farinae and D. microceras. Allergy 41:442.
4. Heymann, P.W., Chapman, M.D., Aalberse, R.C., Fox, J.W., and Platts-Mills, T.A.E., 1989. Antigenic and structural analysis of Group II allergens (Der f II and Der p II) from house dust mites (Dermatophagoides spp.). J. Allergy Clin. Immunol. 83:1055.
5. Yasueda, H., Mita, H., Yui, Y., and Shida, T.,

1989. Comparative analysis of physicochemical and immunochemical properties of the two major allergens from Dermatophagoides pteronyssinus and the corresponding allergens from Dermatophagoides farinae. Int. Arch. Allergy Appl. Immunol. 88:402.
6. Arruda, K., Rizzo, M.C., Chapman, M.D., Fernandez-Caldas, E., Baggio, D., Platts-Mills, T.A.E., and Naspitz, C.K., 1991. Exposure and sensitization to dust mite allergens among asthmatic children in Sao Paulo, Brazil. Clin. Exp. Allergy 21:433.
7. Ehnert, B., Lau Schadendorf, S., Weber, A., and Wahn, U., 1991. Reduction of mite allergen exposure and bronchial hyperreactivity. J.Allergy Clin. Immunol. 87:321.
8. Pauli, G., Dietemann, A., Ott, M., Hoyet, C., and Bessot, J.C., 1991. Levels of mite allergen and guanine after use of an acaricidal solution in highly infested mattresses and dwellings. J. Allergy Clin. Immunol. 87:321.
9. Hayden, M.L., Rose, G., Diduch, K.B., Domson, P., Chapman, M.D., Heymann, P.W. and Platts-Mills, T.A.E., 1992. Benzyl benzoate wet powder: investigation of acaricidal activity in cultures and reduction of mite allergens in carpets. J. Allergy Clin. Immunol. 89:536.
10. De Blay, F., Heymann, P.W., Chapman, M.D., and Platts-Mills, T.A.E., 1992. Airborne dust mite allergens: Comparison of Group II allergens with Group I mite allergen and cat allergen Fel d I. J. Allergy Clin. Immunol. 88:919.
11. Sakaguchi, M., Inouye, S., Yasueda, H., Irie, T., Yoshizawa, S., and Shida, T., 1989. Measurements of allergens associated with dust mite allergy. II. Concentrations of airborne mite allergens (Der I and Der II) in the house. Int. Arch. Allergy Appl. Immunol. 90:190.
12. Price, J.A., Pollock, J., Little, S.A., Longbottom, J.L., and Warner, J.O., 1990. Measurements of airborne mite allergen in houses of asthmatic children. Lancet 336:895.
13. Platts-Mills, T.A.E. and Chapman, M.D., 1991. Allergen standardization. J. Allergy Clin. Immunol. 87:621.
14. Arlian, L.G., 1989. Biology and ecology of house dust mites, Dermatophagoides spp. and Euroglyphus spp. Immunol. Allergy Clin. N. Am. 9(2):339.
15. Colloff, M.J., 1991. A review of biology and allergenicity of the house dust mite Euroglyphus maynei (Acari: Pyroglyphidae). Exp. Appl. Acarol. 11:177.
16. Colloff, M.J., Stewart, G.A., and Thompson, P.J., 1991. House dust acarofauna and Der p I equivalent in Australia: the relative importance of Dermatophagoides pteronyssinus and Euroglyphus maynei. Clin. Exp. Allergy 21:225.
17. Van Hage Hamsten, M., and Johansson, S.G.O., 1989. Clinical significance and allergenic cross reactivity of Euroglyphus maynei and other non-pyroglyphid and pyroglyphid mites. J. Allergy Clin. Immunol. 83:581.
18. Luczynska, C.M., Griffin, P., Davies, R.J., and Topping, M.D., 1990. Prevalence of specific IgE to storage mites (A. siro , L. destructor, and T. longior) in an urban population and crossreactivity with the house dust mite (D. pteronyssinus). Clin. Exp. Allergy 20:403.
19. Fernandez-Caldas, E., Fox, R.W., Bucholtz, G.A., Trudeau, W.L., Ledford, D.K., and Lockey, R.F., 1990. House dust mite allergy in Florida. Mite survey in households of mite sensitive individuals in Tampa, Florida. Allergy Proceedings 11:263 267.
20. Arruda, L.K. and Chapman, M.D., 1992. A review of recent immunochemical studies of Blomia tropicalis and Euroglyphus maynei allergens. Exp. Appl. Acarol. in Press.
21. Fernandez-Caldas, E., Fox, R.W., Trudeau, W., and Lockey, R.F., 1988. Allergenicity of the mite, Blomia tropicalis . J. Allergy Clin. Immunol. 88:270.
22. Van Hage Hamsten, M., Machado, L., Barros, M.T., and Johansson, S.G.O., 1990. Immune response to Blomia kulagini and Dermatophagoides pteronyssinus in Sweden and Brazil. Int. Arch. Allergy Appl. Immunol., 91:186.
23. Hill, M.A., Kent, N.A., Holland, P.W.H., and Hart, B.J., 1991. Characterisation of Euroglyphus maynei allergens. In: "Dust mite allergens and asthma: Report of a second international workshop", UCB Institute of Allergy, Brussels, Belgium.
24. Ansotegui, I.J., Harfast, B., Jeddi-Tehrani, M., Johansson, E., Johansson, S.G.O., van Hage-Hamsten, M., and Wigzell, H. 1991. Identification of a new major allergen of 39 kilodaltons of the storage mite Lepidoglyphus destructor. Immunol. Lett. 27:127.
25. Ventas, P., Carreira, J., and Polo, F., 1991. Identification of IgE binding proteins from Lepidoglyphus destructor and production of monoclonal antibodies to a major allergen. Immunol. Lett. 29:229.

Mite Allergen Elimination and Prevention of Mite Allergy

U. Wahn, S. Lau-Schadendorf, B. Ehnert*

During the last years epidemiological studies have provided strong evidence that early exposure to inhaled allergens plays an important role in the development of both bronchial hyperreactivity and acute attacks of asthma. Among indoor allergens, beside those produced from cats, others produced by house dust mites seem to be of special clinical significance. A number of indoor and outdoor climate factors have been demonstrated to influence mite growth: From studies of Wharton (1) and van Bronswijk (2) we know that house dust mites grow best at 25°C and 70–80% relative humidity. Guatemala City, with average minimal and maximal temperatures ranging between 11°C and 28°C and a relative humidity ranging between 65 and 88%, offers ideal conditions for Dermatophagoides pteronyssinus growth. Mite allergen concentrations in dust samples from Guatemala City have been found to be 50-fold higher than in Central Europe. In this region IgE mediated hypersensitivity to house dust mite allergens is most common (3). Among indoor climate factors coal heating is demonstrably a significant risk factor facilitating mite growth (4).

Dose-Response-Relationship Between Exposure and Sensitization

In a study of 133 atopic children in Berlin (5) we were able to demonstrate a clear dose-response-relationship between major mite allergen exposure and the degree of sensitization to Dermatophagoides (Fig. 1). Patients were grouped according to their mite allergen exposure, forming four "dust mite exposure classes" as suggested by Platts-Mills. Atopic children with significant (2 µg/g < 10 µg/g) or high (> 10 µg/g) amounts of Der p I and Der f I had significantly higher serum-IgE-antibodies to Dpt than children with low (< 0.4 µg/g) concentrations of Der p I and Der f I. Similar results were observed on investigating cell bound IgE in histamine release experiments: Patients' leukocytes were incubated with serial dilutions of Der p I, and histamine release was measured. 86% of highly exposed children (sum of Der p I and Der f I > 10 µg/g) and 64% of significantly exposed children (sum of Der p I and Der f I > 2 µg/g) demonstrated positive histamine release to Der p I compared with 17% in the group with low exposure. We calculated an odds ratio for the relative risk, in order to assess a significant threshold concentration of mite allergen exposure, above which the risk for sensitization in atopics is increased. For those exposed to 2 µg Der p I and Der f I/g dust the risk of sensitization is 7- to 19-fold increased, for those exposed to 10 µg/g the risk is 11- to 32-fold increased compared with patients with low exposure. From our data we conclude that 2 µg of major mite allergen/g of mattress dust can be considered a threshold concentration for sensitization. Similar thereshold concentrations have been suggested by other authors, e.g. 10 µg/g, 2-5 µg/g or 100 mites/g (6,7,8).

The question of a possible correlation between mite allergen exposure and the natural course of atopic disease has been addressed in only few studies up to now. In the UK between 1978 and 1989 the relationship between house dust mite exposure and the development of sensitization and asthma was studied prospectively in 67 children with a family history of allergic disease (9). The age at onset of wheezing was demonstrated to be inversely related to the level of exposure at the age of one year. In a longitudinal study a cohort of 714 children was followed up to the age of 13 in New Zealand. Sensitization to house dust mite, beside other allergens, was a significant risk factor for the development of bronchial hyperreactivity and asthma (10).

* Department of Pediatric Pneumology and Immunology, University Children's Hospital, Free University, Heubnerweg 6, D-1000 Berlin 19.

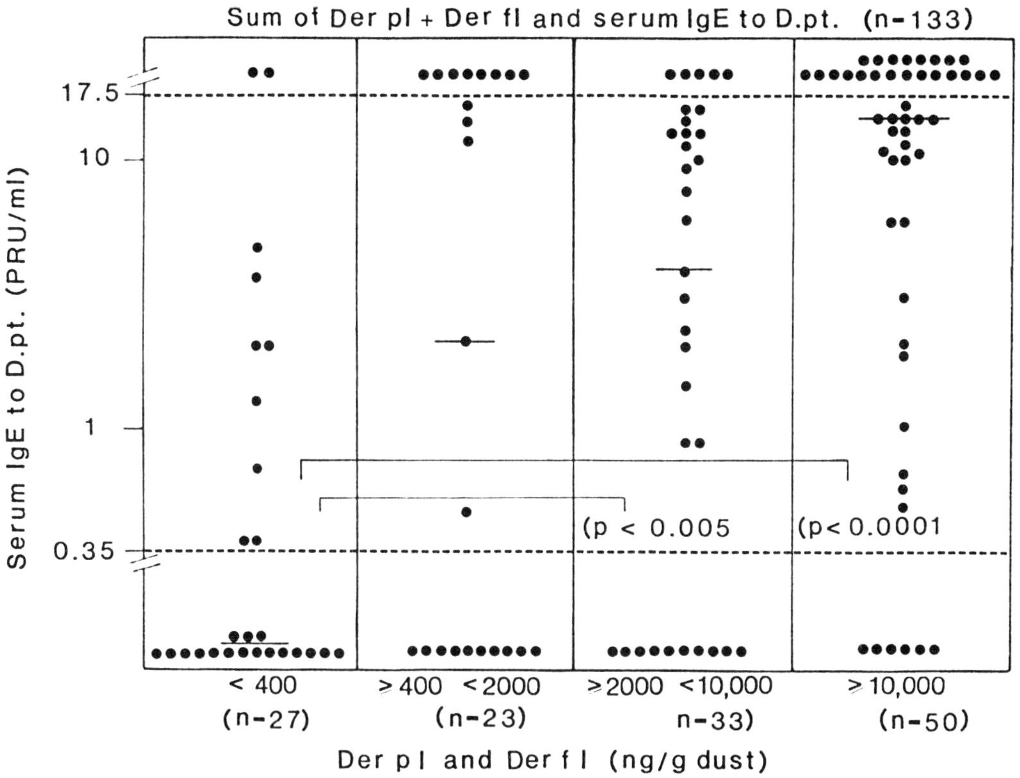

Figure 1. Mite allergen exposure (sum of Der p I and Der f I) and serum IgE antibody concentration to Dermatophagoides pteronyssinus (D. pt). (Reproduced with kind permission of the Journal of Allergy and Clinical Immunology, Saint Louis (USA): Mosby).

Strategies for Elimination

If the domestic exposure to mite allergens higher than 2 µg/g over a period of time is confirmed to be a significant threshold concentration for sensitization and bronchial hyperreactivity, the reduction of mite allergens below this level has to be the first line of treatment. As has been demonstrated by Platts-Mills, bronchial hyperreactivity in mite allergic children may be significantly reduced if children are transferred to hospitals with no mite allergens (11). Similar observations were made after mite sensitive patients were removed from a mite infested house to a high altitude sanatorium (12). A number of studies have addressed the question of the most effective mite elimination procedure in households (Table 1). The degree of mite or mite allergen reduction in these trials ranges from 20–90%. Unfortunately, some of the studies were not performed in a double blind placebo controlled fashion (for a review see ref. 12). In order to investigate the short term effect of solidified benzyl benzoate, we treated mattresses and carpets in 22 households in a placebo controlled study. Compared to placebo, the effect of benzyl benzoate was significantly stronger only on carpets. Mite allergen reduction on mattresses with acaricides or chemicals seems difficult to achieve because mattresses appear to be too thick and the chemicals cannot penetrate properly (14). Therefore other strategies have been developed like mattress encasings, covered with vinyl or polyurethane.

Allergen Reduction and Bronchial Hyperreactivity

In a recent study, we investigated 24 children with mild and moderate asthma and mono-

Table 1. Mite reducing measures in households

Procedure	Authors
Removal of soft furnishings, carpets; Vacuuming (effective)	Murray (1983) Whalshaw (1986) Sarsfield (1974)
Removal of soft furnishings, carpets; Vacuuming (not effective)	Burr (1980) Korsgaard (1983) Carswell (1982)
Pirimiphos methyl (effective)	Heller-Haupt (1974) Mitchell (1985)
Liquid nitrogen (effective)	Dorward (1988) Colloff (1986)
Benzyl benzoate impregnated sheets (effective)	Burr (1988)
Allersearch DMS (benzyl derivate polyphenols) (effective)	Green (1989) Price (1990)
Benzyl benzoate (partly effective)	Elixman (1988) Dietemann (1989) Lau-Schadendorf (1991)
Tannic acid 3% (effective)	Miller (1989)

specific sensitivity to house dust mites. All children were exposed to high mite allergen concentrations on their mattrasses (sum of Der p I and Der f I 2 μg/g). Patients were randomly allocated into three treatment groups. In group 1, mattresses, pillows and comforts were covered with polyurethane encasings, and in addition the carpets were treated with 3% tannic acid solution. In group 2 and 3, mattresses were treated with either benzyl benzoate or placebo foam and carpets with powder in a double blind fashion. Before as well as 4, 8 and 12 months after the beginning of the study parameters of sensitization (skin test, specific serum-IgE) as well as bronchial hyperreactivity (titrated histamine challenge test) were sought. While neither placebo nor benzyl benzoate treatment resulted in a significant decrease in mattress allergen concentrations and BHR, the encasing regime led to a reduction in mite allergen concentrations on mattresses of more than 90% (see Fig. 2). This allergen elimination was as-

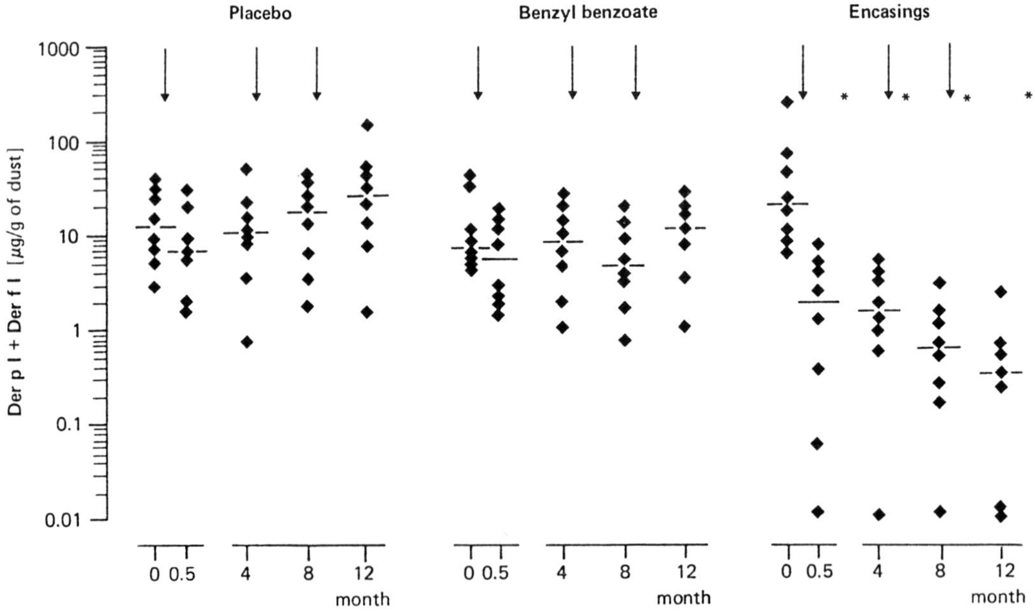

Figure 2. Mite allergen concentrations on mattresses after treatment with benzyl benzoate, placebo or covering with polyurethane covered encasings.

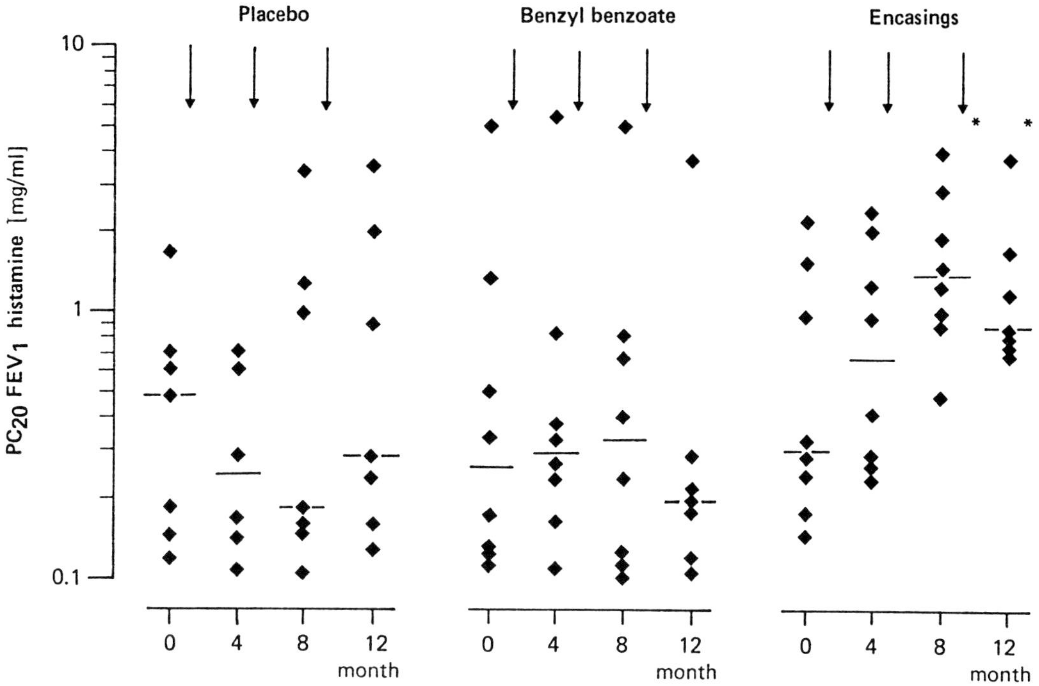

Figure 3. Bronchial hyperreactivity (expressed as $PC_{20}FEV_1$ histamine) of house dust mite sensitive asthmatic children after allergen reduction with benzyl benzoate, placebo or polyurethane covered mattress encasings.

sociated with a statistically significant decrease of bronchial hyperreactivity with a $PC_{20}FEV_1$ for histamine increasing 4.5-fold after 8 months (see Fig. 3). Similar improvements of bronchial hyperreactivity were reported when patients were sent to the mite free environment in a hospital, where the $PC_{20}FEV_1$ for histamine increased 8-fold or more after 5 months. Walshaw et al. (15) observed only a 2-fold increase of $PC_{20}FEV_1$ for histamine after introduction of cleaning measures and plastic covers for pillows and mattresses in 21 adult asthmatic patients.

Allergen Elimination and the Prevention of Atopic Symptoms

It appears reasonable to suppose that a prophylactic elimination of mite allergens before birth is likely to influence the age at onset of allergic symptoms as well as the natural course of atopic disease in infancy and childhood. However, there are no prospective studies in defined high risk populations confirming this hypothesis.

Conclusion

In atopic individuals there appears to be a dose-response-relationship between allergen exposure and sensitization as well as bronchial hyperreactivity. For house dust mites 2 μg major allergen/g of mattress dust appear to be a threshold concentration of clinical relevance. Elimination procedures should aim at a reduction of mite allergens below this level. Among different elimination strategies, the encasing/tannic acid procedure seems to be a rational approach eliminating mite allergens below this threshold level. First obervations indicate that such an elimination is associated by a decrease of bronchial hyperreactivity in mite sensitive asthmatic individuals.

References

1. Wharton, G.W. 1976. House dust mites. J. Med. Entomol. 12:557.
2. van Bronswijk, J.E.M.H., and Sinha, R.N.

1971. Pyroglyphid mites (Acar) and house dust mite allergy: A review. J. Allergy 47:31.
3. Chur, V., Lau, S., and Wahn, U. 1989. Dermatophagoides pteronyssinun: An important allergen source in Guatemala. J. Allergy Clin. Immunol. 83:198 (abstract).
4. Lau, S., Weber, A., Spelzberg, A., Winkler, S., Rau, S., and Wahn, U. 1989. Housing conditions and mite allergen exposure. Allergologie 12:141 (Kongreβband).
5. Lau, S., Falkenhorst, G., Weber, A., et al. 1989. High mite-allergen exposure increases the risk of sensitization in atopic children and young adults. J. Allergy Clin. Immunol. 84:718.
6. Rowntree, S., Cogswell, J.J., Platts-Mills, T.A.E., and Mitchell, E.B. 1985. Development of IgE and IgG antibodies to food and inhalant allergens in children at risk of allergic disease. Arch. Dis. Child. 60:727.
7. Platts-Mills, T.A.E., and Chapmann, M.D. 1987. Dust mites: Immonology, allergic disease and environmetal control. J. Allergy Clin. Immunol.80:755.
8. Korsgaard, J. 1983. Mite asthma and residency: A case-control study on the impact of exposure to house dust mites in dwellings. Am. Rev. Respir. Dis. 128:231.
9. Sorik, R., Holgate, S.T., Platts-Mills, T.A.E., and Cogswell, J.J. 1990. Exposure to housedust mite allergen (Der p I) and the development of asthma in childhood. N. Engl. J. Med. 323:502.
10. Sears, M.R., Herbison, G.P., Holdaway, M.D., Hewitt, C.J., Flannery, E.M., and Silva, P.A. 1989. The relative risks of sensitivity to grass pollen, house dust mite and cat dander in the development of childhood asthma. Clin. Exp. Allergy 19:419.
11. Platts-Mills, T.A.E., Tovey, E.R., Mitchell, E.B., Moszoro, H., Nock, P., and Wilkins, S.R. 1982. Reduction of bronchial hyperreactivity during prolonged allergen avoidance. Lancet ii:675.
12. Kerrebijn, K.F. 1970. Endogenous factors in childhood CNSLD: Methodological studies. In: N.G.M. Orie, and R. van der Lende, eds. Bronchitis III. The Netherlands: Royal Vangorcum Assen, p.38.
13. Lau-Schadendorf, S., and Wahn, U. 1991. Exposure to indoor allergens and development of allergy. Pediatr. Allergy Immunol. 2:63.
14. Lau-Schadendorf, S., Rusche, A.F., Weber, A-K., Buettner-Goetz, P., Wahn, U. 1991. Short-term effect of solified benzyl benzoate on mite-allergen concentrations in house dust. J. Allergy Clin. Immunol. 87:41.
15. Whalshaw, M.J., and Evans, C.C. 1986. Allergen avoidance in house dust mite sensitive adult asthma. J. Med. 226:199.

Section V

Occupational and Environmental Allergy

Occupational Immunologic Lung Disease Especially Characteristic of Japan

Setsuo Kobayashi*

Occupational bronchial asthma and hypersensitivity pueumonitis in Japan are reviewed here, with special emphasis on allergens unique to Japan, where there are more than 120 kinds of occupational allergens. The incidence of occupational asthma is around 5% of the workers, but it ranges from 0.05 to 10% depending on the nature of the allergens and exposure conditions. The hypersensitivity pneumonitis unique to Japan is due to mushroom spores. Bronchial asthma and hypersensitivity pneumonitis are the representative diseases in OILD (for all abbreviations, see footnote below). They are caused by gases, vapors, organic or inorganic dusts. Some enhancing factors are smoking and air pollution. Industrial workers are exposed to many natural or artificial substances; especially since World War II, the workers have been exposed to many artificial simple chemicals or organic compounds. Most of them are sensitizers which are active at concentrations lower than that of TLV.

Occupational Asthma

Occupational asthma is induced by (a) irritants or by (b) pharmacologic or (c) allergic mechanisms. (A) We have examined a case of asthma which developed after exposure to alkylcyanoacrylate during work, presumably induced by a minute amount of SO_2 contained in it. (B) An anticholinesterase effect of organic insecticides can induce an asthmatic symptom in farmers. The allergic and β-blocking effect of TDI, the histamine liberating effects of various plants, and the complement activating effect in red cedar allergy are well known. (C) The most important mechanism is of course the allergic one; there are about 120 kinds of occupational allergens reported in Japan, and these will be treated here under the following headings: (a) vegetable origins; (b) animal origins; (c) drugs, inorganic and synthetic substances; (d) epidemiology; and (e) allergic mechanisms.

Vegetable Origins

"Maiko" is an allergen which is active in the form of floating dust which arises while pounding the dried slices of the tuberous root of "devil's tongue" in the preparation of the Japanese food "Konnyaku". The allergen is a glycoprotein of around 30,000 molecular weight. Pyrethrum pollen induces asthma during cultivation work. Strawberry is usually insect pollinated, but recently it has been cultivated in a vinyl house, with the result that pollen from the flower may be floating in the house and thus cause asthma in workers. Pollen from Boronia imported from Australia can also induce asthma in workers. Pollen from peaches, pears and apples are inhaled by workers during the work of artificial pollination. Pollen from ragweed or rose rarely induces asthma in academic employees. Pollen from chrysanthemum, cosmos, grapes, corn, plum blossom, orchard grass, Italian rye grass and sugar beet can also be inhaled by cultivators, resulting in allergy. Many wood dusts, such as from western red cedar, lauan and Nara (Pterocarpus indicus Willd), are imported species. In others (such as mulberry, magnolia obovata, clethra barbinervis, red or black sandalwood, pseudocydomia sinensis Shneid, white birch and zelkova tree) dust induces asthma during several phases of processing (sawing, engraving, etc.). Spores from mushrooms sometimes induce hypersensitivity pneumonitis, but rarely do they cause asthma when the worker is atopic. However, spores from lycopodium and malt are reported as an asthma

* Gunma University School of Medicine, Japan.
Abbreviations: DLCO: Diffusing capacity for carbon monoxide; HDI: Hexamethylene diisocyanate; MDI: Diphenylmethane diisocyanate; OILD: Occupational Immunologic Lung Disease; TDI: Toluene diisocyanate; TLV: Threshold Limit Value; TMA: Trimellitic anhydride.

Hypersensitivity Pneumonitis and Environmental Factors

Jordan N. Fink*

Hypersensitivity pneumonitis is an environmentally-induced immune inflammation of the lung resulting from sensitization and repeated inhalation of orgnic dusts. Bacteria, fungi, proteins and chemicals are common offending antigens and various occupations or contaminated forced air heating or cooling systems are common sources of antigens. Retention in the lung of offending antigen may also be important in pathogenesis. Symptoms of the illness include both respiratory and systemic types occurring four to six hours after exposure. Clinical abnormalities are related to the inflammation, alveolitis and immune responses of the affected individual. Corticosteroids are used for acute control of symptoms but avoidance of inhalation remains curative in most cases. However, with prolonged exposure permanent pulmonary parenchymal damage may occur.

Hypersensitivity pneumonitis is a syndrome resulting from repeated inhalation and sensitization to any of a wide and ever expanding variety of organic dusts. This results in an immune inflammation of the lung characterized by cellular and granulomatous involvement of the alveolar spaces and interstitium. The disease was first recognized in ill grain workers by Ramazzini in 1713 (1) and described as farmer's lung by Campbell in 1932 (2). Clinical and pathologic correlates were evaluated by Dickie and Rankin (3) and Emanuel and his associates (4) and the thermophilic actinomycetes were identified as the offending antigen involved in the immune response by American and British investigators (5,6). While the clinical and laboratory features of the disease have been clearly defined, the immune mechanisms involved in the disease pathogenesis remain undefined. Although there is widespread exposure to the antigens inducing the disease, the attack rate is relatively low, ranging from 7 to 15 percent. It has become clear, however, that immunogenicity of the organic dust, exposure levels and host factors are important in the induction of the disease.

Clinical Features

Hypersensitivity pneumonitis presents with respiratory and with/without systemic symptoms. The symptoms are similar whatever the offending agent, suggesting that the mechanism(s) involved and the pulmonary responses are the same. Acute, subacute and chronic forms of the disease have been defined when large patient populations are studied (3,4,7). The form the disease presents clinically is the result of the characteristics of the organic dust inhaled, the intensity and frequency of exposure, and the severity and sequelae of the inflammatory response induced. The acute form of hypersensitivity pneumonitis is the most common form seen, with explosive episodes resembling a flu-like syndrome, and occurring at 4 to 6 hours following exposure. Acute cough, dyspnea and fever to 104°F, chills, myalgia and malaise occur and may persist for up to 18 hours. With repeated episodes, weight loss due to anorexia and progressive dyspnea may be prominent. Physical examination during the acute episode reveals an ill appearing, dyspneic patient, with prominent bibasilar and inspiratory rales. Cyanosis and nail clubbing are rarely found. Leukocytosis with a left shift and eosinophilia is common. IgE levels are normal but the other immunoglobulin isotypes are elevated. Chest x-ray demonstrates fine sharp nodulations and reticulations in most lung fields, frequently sparing the apices. Localized patchy infiltrates may also be noted and on occasion hilar adenopathy has been detected. These features usually resolve over sufficient time after avoidance. Pulmonary function abnormalities most often parallel the acute episodes (3,5,7). A decrease in forced vital capacity and one-second forced expiratory volume occurs between 4 and 6 hours, and there is little change in expiratory flow, but a decrease in compliance, diffusion capacity and arterial oxy-

* Medical College of Wisconsin, Milwaukee, Wisconsin, USA.

gen content can be detected. These features subside spontaneously, recurring with each episode. Lung biopsy of patients with hypersensitivity pneumonitis has usually demonstrated an alveolar and interstitial inflammatory response involving lymphocytes, plasma cells, and macrophages (4,8). The alveolar spaces and small airways may be occluded by this process. Langhans giant cells and granulomas with or without central necrosis may be found in the lymphocytic infiltrations. In very early cases vasculitis and bronchiolitis with neutrophilic, eosinophilic and mononuclear infiltration can be found. In chronic cases fibrosis may develop.

The subacute form of hypersensitivity pneumonitis is a more insidious disease with features of chronic bronchitis. Patients present with cough and sputum production, anorexia and weight loss. Physical examination and laboratory features are as in the acute form. Chest x-ray may demonstrate nodular infiltrates or early fibrosis and pulmonary function abnormalities are restrictive. The chronic form of the disease occurs in few patients and is characterized by irreversible pulmonary damage (4,7). Progressive dyspnea without acute episodes or systemic features, chronic cough, weight loss and weakness are common. A restrictive impairment and diffusion defect with hypoxemia may be seen, though some individuals develop high grade obstruction. Chest x-rays often demonstrate diffuse fibrosis. Such patients have permanent changes as they do not respond to avoidance or corticosteroids.

Immunologic Features

Characteristic of hypersensitivity pneumonitis is the demonstration of serum precipitating antibodies to the offending antigen (3,7). The precipitins are of the IgG isotype, but antibodies of IgA and IgM isotypes have also been detected (9). However, as many as 50 percent of exposed but well individuals may also have similar titers of serum precipitating antibody exposure, not disease. Evaluation of bronchoalveolar lavage has demonstrated marked increases in T-cell populations in both exposed but well individuals and patients (10,11). The T-cells are predominately CD8 or suppressor cells and are generally more abundant in patients than their well counterparts (10). The T-cells and macrophages are activated, and mast cell populations are increased, and increases in cytotoxic and natural killer cells are found as well as IgG, IgA and IgM antibodies to specific antigens. Functional studies of the cellular populations in the lavage fluids point to an immunoregulatory imbalance in ill patients, since the lavage suppressor T-cells of patients could not reduce the effect of mitogen or specific antigen stimulation of peripheral lymphocytes as the lavage T-cells of exposed but well individuals (12,13) could.

Environmental Factors

Inhalation of antigen is necessary for sensitization and induction of the episodes. Antigens inducing the disease range from bacteria such as thermophilic actinomycetes, amebae, a variety of fungi encountered in certain occupational situations, to avian proteins from aerosolized bird dander and excreta, and reactive chemical mists. Since many of the antigens are particulate, retention in the lung may be prolonged, allowing immune responses to occur. Most environments associated with the disease are occupational, where there is continuous and/or frequent exposure to antigen which is often used in the work process. In some cases, forced air heating, cooling and humidification systems in which stagnant water is present and maintenance is shoddy, may be conducive to the growth of a variety of antigenic micro-organisms including fungi and amebae. Inhalation of these particulates by the workers may then lead to disease.

The majority of antigens are of a size that penetrates the alveoli, but some, such as spores of *Alternaria* may deposit in the airways and be solublized. Chemicals may be inhaled as fine mists or dust particles with antigen or antigenic determinants absorbed. The most frequent causative antigens are the thermophilic actinomycetes which have been implicated in farmer's lung, bagassosis, mushroom worker's lung and ventilation pneumonitis (14,15). They are vegetable composting organisms and have been isolated from hay, compost piles, soil, manure, grain and forced air systems. Workers contacting hay, compost or sugar cane (bagasse) piles or living or working in environments served by contaminated ventilation systems are susceptible. The thermophilic organisms associated with hypersensitivity pneumonitis thrive best at 56 to 60°C and include *Faeni rectivergula* (formerly *Micropolyspora faeni*), *Thermoactinomyces vulgaris*, *T. viridis*, *T. vulgaris*, *T. sacharii* and *T. candidus*. These organisms function in nature by secreting multiple enzymes which cause decay of vegetable matter. The organisms require moisture content of over 28 percent to thrive, and are abundant in wet hay and are dispersed into the air when the hay pile is disturbed, such as by a pitchfork (25). Similar conditions exist in sugar cane piles and in mushroom compost which consists of hay and horse manure.

Hypersensitivity pneumonitis induced by avian proteins was first described by Plessner (16) in individuals working with geese and ducks and by Pearsall (17) in a parakeet breeder. Reed et al. described the disease in pigeon breeders (18), and other avian species have also been implicated (1). Avian antigens involved in hypersensitivity pneumonitis have been demonstrated in serum, droppings and feathers (19,20).

Highly reactive chemicals used in the plastics industry have been identified as causative agents in hypersensitivity pneumonitis. The isocyanates and phthalic anhydrides (21) may react with airway proteins, altering their structure and resulting in antigenicity. In Japan a particular pneumonitis associated with home dust contamination with Trichoderma has been described only in the summer months (22). Its characteristics are similar to the other types of alveolitis.

Thus particulate antigens, if retained in the lung or if present in antigen presenting cells, may enhance their immunogenicity by fixation of complement and by action as adjuvants. This may result in immune activation and inflammation and release of soluble mediators inducing symptoms.

Diagnosis

The diagnosis of hypersensitivity pneumonitis should be considered in patients exposed to particular environments who develop recurrent episodes of a flu-like syndrome with characteristic physical examination, laboratory, pulmonary function and x-ray features. Immunologic studies are confirmatory and inhalation challenge under controlled situations may offer a clue to the diagnosis by reproducing the acute episode.

Treatment

In the treatment of hypersensitivity pneumonitis, environmental avoidance of antigen remains paramount and environmental changes may be necessary. Corticosteroids remain the only proven effective drug, but should be used only where environmental controls and/or avoidance cannot be carried out. Inhaled corticosteroids are of little benefit; systemic therapy is necessary. Since the disease may be associated with permanent pulmonary parenchymal changes, it is essential to make an early diagnosis and undertake whatever measures are necessary to reduce the ongoing or recurrent pulmonary inflammatory process.

References

1. Ramazzini, B. 1940. De morbus artificum diatriba. 1713. Translation. Chicago: University of Chicago Press.
2. Campbell, J.M. 1932. Acute symptoms following work with hay. Br. Med. J. 2:114.
3. Dickie, H.A., and Rankin, J. 1958. Farmer's lung: An acute granulomatous interstitial pneumonitis occurring in agricultural workers. JAMA. 167:1067.
4. Emanuel, D.A., Wenzel, F.J., Bowerman, C.I., et al. 1964. Farmer's lung; clinical pathological and immunologic study of twenty-four patients. Am. J. Med. 37:392.
5. Gregory, P.M., and Lacey, M.E. 1963. Mycological examination of the dust from mouldy hay associated with farmer's lung disease. J. Gen. Microbiol. 30:75.
6. LaBerge, D.E., and Stahmann, M.A. 1966. Antigens from moldy hay involved in farmer's lung. Proc. Soc. Exp. Biol. Med. 121:458.
7. Fink, J.N., Sosman, A.J., Barboriak, J.J., et al. 1968. Pigeon breeder's disease: A clinical study of a hypersensitivity pneumonitis. Ann. Inter. Med. 68:1205.
8. Kawassami, O., Basset, F., Barrios, R., et al.

1983. Hypersensitivity pneumonitis in man. Light and electron microscopic studies of 18 lung biopsies. Am. J. Pathol. 110:275.
9. Kawassami, O., Basset, F., Barrios, R., et al. 1974. Hypersensitivity pneumonitis in man. Light and electron microscopic studies of 18 lung biopsies. Am. J. Pathol. 110:275.
10. Kawassami, O., Basset, F., Barrios, R., et al. 1980. Hypersensitivity pneumonitis in man. Light and electron microscopic studies of 18 lung biopsies. Am. J. Pathol. 110:275.
11. Leatherman, J.W., Michael, A.F., Schwartz, B.A., et al. 1984. Lung T-cells in hypersensitivity pneumonitis. Ann. Intern. Med 100:390.
12. Keller, R.H., Schwartz, S., Schlueter, D.P., et al. 1984. Immunoregulation in hypersensitivity pneumonitis: Phenotypic and functional studies of bronchoalveolar lavage lymphocytes. Am. Rev. Resp. Dis. 130:766.
13. Barquin, N., Sansores, R., and Chapela, R. 1990. Immunoregulatory abnormalities in patients with pigeon breeder's disease. Lung. 168:103.
14. Banaszak, E.F., Thiede, W.H., and Fink, J.N. 1970. Hypersensitivity pneumonitis due to contamination of an air conditioner. N. Engl. J. Med. 283:271.
15. Grant, I.W., Blyth, W., Wardrop, V.E., et al. 1972. Prevalence of farmer's lung in Scotland. A pilot survey. Br. Med. J. 1:530.
16. Plessner, M.M. 1960. Une maladie des trieurs de plumes: La fievre de canard. Arch. Mal. Prof. 21:67.
17. Pearsall, H.R., Morgan, E.H., Tesluk, H., et al. 1960. Parakeet dander pneumonitis: Acute psittaco-kerato-pneumoconiosis. Bull. Mason. Clin. 14:127.
18. Reed, C.E., Sosman, A.J., and Barbee, R.A. 1965. Pigeon breeder's lung. JAMA 193:26119.
19. Edwards, J.H., Barboriak, J.J., and Fink, J.N. 1970. Antigens in pigieon breeder's disease. Immunology 19:729.
20. Edwards, J.H., Fink, J.N., and Barboriak, J.J. 1969. Excretion of pigeon serum proteins in pigeon droppings. Proc. Soc. Exp. Biol. Med. 132:907.
21. Fink, J.N., and Schlueter, D.P. 1978. Bathtub refinisher's lung: An unusual response to toluene diisocyanate. Am. Rev. Resp. Dis. 118:955.
22. Kawai, T., Tamura, M,. and Murao, M. 1984. Summer type hypersensitivity pneumonitis. A unique disease in Japan. Chest 85:311.

Agricultural Allergy

C. Molina*

Agricultural allergy (A. A.) includes a wide variety of diseases (mainly respiratory and skin changes) due to a number of allergens. Even if the farming population is regularly decreasing, farmworkers are exposed to higher concentrations of the offending substances, among which the role of chemicals is increasing. A list of these allergens would include: *organic* (animals, vegetables, mites, moulds, bacteria, antibiotics) and *chemicals* (pesticides [insecticides, fungicides], inorganic metals). They induce either respiratory reactions which are often severe (asthma) or cutaneous reactions (contact dermatitis). Food allergy is rare. Prevention by removal of the allergen is difficult. Masks are not always easy to wear during work. The creation of centers for education, prevention and research in A. A. must be encouraged.

Agricultural allergy may be defined as rural occupational allergy. It is a very large field because many occupations are involved, depending upon climatic, seasonal or geographical conditions and local habits (Europe, USA, Japan). Many substances acting as allergens during farm work may provoke allergic diseases. The target organs are the *lungs* and *skin.* Among *respiratory* diseases, we must emphasize the frequency of *rhinitis* and mainly *asthma* (allergic alveolitis is discussed in a special lecture). *Skin* diseases include atopic dermatitis and contact dermatitis.

Nowadays A. A. is marked by new trends: The *decrease* in the number of exposed persons is apparent. In our industrial Westernized countries and due to the hard work and poor income of farmers, the rural population is regularly decreasing. Conversely, and in order to improve the yield of their cultures, the farmers are frequently exposed to higher concentrations of various allergens. Among these allergens, organic dusts which are themselves very aggressive are more and more associated with *chemicals*, which act as irritants or toxic substances and may influence the immune system.

Frequency of Agricultural Allergy

The first point to discuss is the comparison between rural and urban environments. According to several studies (1,2,3) there appears to be no difference in the prevalence of allergic diseases in urban and rural populations. In an epidemiological study we carried out on 1,200 adults suffering from asthma and who had visited their doctor for over 18 months in a French rural department (Puy de Dôme – Auvergne), no difference was observed in the prevalence of asthma between agricultural workers and industrial workers nor between country and city inhabitants. In terms of *incidence*, we were able to confirm that age has a significant influence on the severity of the disease.

Organic Allergens

All these organic allergens are high molecular weight (HMW) substances, and often provoke *respiratory* diseases. They usually act in atopic patients, giving immediate positive reaction on skin test, such as specific IgE in serum. There is a good correlation between these tests and bronchial provocation challenge, which may be mandatory for medico-legal purposes.

Concerning farm animals, the highest-risk occupations according to the literature and personal experience are: pig farming (4), poultry farming (5), dairy farming (cow danders) (6), but all animals including especially horses, birds, rodents, cats, rabbits, may be the source of allergens by their feathers, urine, saliva or droppings. In Japan sericulture is also regarded as a high-risk occupation (5).

Vegetable sources (including dusts such as flour, wheat, barley, oats, rye, corn and mainly

* Comité National contre les Maladies Respiratoires et la Tuberculose, 66 Boulevard Saint-Michel, F-75006 Paris, France.

soya, but also wood, coffee, tobacco, tea, and alfalfa) may be offending agents for the lungs. On the other hand a wide range of vegetable sources may elicit contact dermatitis: tulip, onion, chrysanthemum, poison ivy, colophony, devil's tongue root (7), garlic (6, 13), and Frullania. More precise etiological diagnosis has been made possible by recent developments on the role of mites or moulds which infest these vegetable dusts.

Mites and insects are incriminated as well. Storage mites (8) (Acarus siro, Lepidoglyphus destructor, Tyrophagus putrescentiae and others) are the most important parasites of these dusts and potent allergens. There is a frequent but variable cross-reaction with domestic mites (Dermatophagoides species). Other mites such as Ornithonissus sylvarum may be responsible, in bird breeders, for rhinitis and asthma (9). It is the fecal excreta of these mites which are the main sources of allergens.

Insects such as Chironomides are frequently the cause of allergic manifestations with positive skin tests, especially among dairy farmers (10). Euroglyphus Maynéi, Ephestia, Sitophilus granarius are other parasites are of importance in grain, straw or hay.

Among moulds, it is well known that Aspergillus plays an important role in A.A. but also Penicillium (for cheese workers), Rhizopus, Paecilomyces, and Botrytis (frequent on garlic dust). Exposure to these moulds results in the production of IgE and in the case of heavy inhalation, precipitating antibodies (IgG). Thus, differential diagnosis from allergic alveolitis is often difficult and all the more so as in this disease about 30% of patients show alveolar inflammation associated with bronchial involvement. Bronchoalveolar lavage with its specific cellular and biochemical profile can be decisive.

In some cases, microbial sources (by way of their endotoxins from gram negative bacteria) may account for the febrile reactions experienced by the farmers, a few hours after inhalation of dusts. These reactions cause bronchial inflammatory changes and bronchial hyperreactivity. There is no clear evidence that an immune mechanism is involved in these reactions, and in fact some authors evoke a toxic phenomenon (mycotoxicosis).

Finally, antibiotics, used in cattle food, such as Penicillin or Oleandomycin, may induce allergic respiratory or skin reactions. Furthermore, we must emphasize the frequent polysensitization of farm workers bearing in mind that smoking is another predisposing factor (11).

The course of these respiratory disorders is favorable if the patient avoids contact with the allergens. Otherwise there is a worsening of the disease leading to chronic respiratory insufficiency.

We must mention that atopic *dermatitis* due to these organic dusts may be observed after inhalation. Evidence has been provided (12) that mites can induce eczematous lesions in atopic patients. In other cases contact dermatitis is caused by: avian proteins (13), mites such as panonychus ulmi among apple-tree gardeners (14), Acarus siro (cheese mite dermatitis) among cheese workers (15), and vegetable dust (garlic) (6,13). Food allergy may be associated with respiratory allergy in cases of the so-called bird egg syndrome (16).

Chemical Agents

The influence of chemicals in agriculture is increasing. These are usually substances of low molecular weight (LMW) acting either by a *pharmacologic* mechanism (plicatic acid in red cedar asthma, abietic acid in pine resin asthma) or by an *irritant* (inducing bronchial inflammation and hyperreactivity). But all these chemicals influence sensitization. They act as haptens which by reaction with a carrier (protein) lead to the formation of antigen. The specificity of recognition of a given hapten lies in the T cell receptor (17). Chemicals more often account for *skin diseases* (contact dermatitis) but all chemical products which induce eczema may cause *asthma*. The most offending chemical agents are: pesticides including insecticides such as pyrethroids, herbicides such as carbamates, fungicides (such as Amprolium chloride, used in poultry feed, and coccidomycosis, inhalation of which induces asthma) (18), and thiurame (a cause of eczema).

Inorganic chemicals include metals (nickel, chromium), and halogens (chlorides). We must remember the role of chlorine molecules in an allergy to platinum, and the allergenic power of chlorhexdine by dilution in chlorinated water with induction of IgE antibody. Some other products like isocyanates may be used in agriculture as in industrial works.

Immunotoxicology is a new and exciting concept, evaluating the suppressive or stimulating effects of drugs, chemicals or toxic environmental substances on the immune system, the same product being able to induce allergic or toxic reaction, auto-immunity or even cancer.

Prevention and Medico-Legal Aspects

From a clinical point of view and according to French statistics on A.A., we must remember that skin diseases are usually benign and rarely lead to disability whereas asthma or alveolitis are often the cause of hospitalization, cessation of work, or attempts at indemnification. But the relationship between these diseases and occupation is difficult to prove. The occupational history must be detailed. Skin tests are useful when the allergens are known, but provocation tests are not easy to perform either by inhalation or by patch tests (in skin diseases). However, improvement after avoidance of exposure and recurrence after reexposure are important indices of prevention and legal aspects. A wide supply of legal tables in France recognizes allergic diseases in agriculture. The most important is related to asthma and allergic alveolitis. The tasks liable to provoke these diseases are mentioned as follows: handling or habitual use, during work hours, of all products essential to the occupation.

In young patients the major problem is that of occupational reorientation. In older farmers there is a question of compensation, according to the severity of the disease, and the degree of disability to work.

Prevention should consist mainly of the removal of allergens, which is exceedingly difficult, as the farmer is exposed to a variety of allergens in his working and domestic environment. So the use of masks is strongly recommended, particularly during hard and heavily exposing work. The *efficacy* and duration of protection has been analyzed for some types of masks. Simple cardboard disposable masks are usually sufficient, but only for a short time. Others (Air Stream type) are efficient for a long time (average 16 h) but difficult to wear in spite of breathing equipment (19, 20, 21). Other measures for decreasing allergen exposure are equally important. The creation of Centers for Agricultural Education Diseases with prevention and research, such as in the USA (Iowa), must be encouraged in all countries in order to set up programs on agricultural health and safety for workers and their families.

Bibliography

1. Jessen, M., and Janzon, L. 1989. Prevalence of non-allergic nasal complaints in an urban and a rural population in Sweden. Allergy 44:582.
2. Pepys, J. 1981. Asthma in rural environment: Proceedings of 10th Congress of InterAsthma. Vol. 1. Paris. Abstract number 108, 83.
3. Molina, Cl., Cheminat, J. C., Maillet, J., Gourgand, A.J., and Collin A. 1979. Asthme de l'adulte: Enquête de prévalence et retentissement socio-économique. Rev. Fr. Mal. Resp. 7:181.
4. Malmberg, R.A., Andersen, L., and Palmgren. 1985. Respiratory allergy among farmers. Proceedings of Annual Meeting of E.A.A.C.I. Stockholm. Vol. 1, 29. Pharmacia.
5. Kobayashi, S. 1974. Occupational asthma due to inhalation of pharmacological dusts and other chemical agents with some reference to other occupational asthmas in Japan. Proceedings of the VIIIth International Congress of Allergology. Tokyo, 1973, October 14–20. Amsterdam-Oxford: Excerpta Medica, p. 124.
6. Molina, Cl., Passemard, N., Cheminat, J.C., Petit, R., and le Chapelain, M. 1968. L'asthme en milieu agricole. Rev. Fr. Allerg. 1:1.
7. Matsumura, T. 1974. Bronchial asthma in children in rural districts of Japan with particular reference to occupational asthma in adults. Proceedings of the VIIIth International Congress of Allergology. Tokyo 1973, October 14–20. Amsterdam-Oxford: Excerpta Medica 139.
8. Terho, E.O., Husman, K., Vohlonen, I., Rautalahti, M., and Tukiainen, H. 1985. Allergy to storage mites or cow dander as a cause of rhinitis among Finnish dairy farmers. Allergy 40:23.
9. Lutsky, I., Teichtal, H., and Bar-Sela, S. 1984. Occupational asthma due to poultry mites. J. Clin. Immunol. 73:56.
10. Erikson, N.E., Peterson, I., Vedal., S., Hogsteddt, B., Belin, L., and Johansson, S.G.O. 1985. Allergy among farmers. Proceedings of

Annual Meeting of the E.A.A.C.I. June 25, Vol. 1, Pharmacia.
11. Warren, P. 1977. Lung disease in farmers. Canada Med. Ass. J. 116:391.
12. Mitchell, C., 1970. Occupational asthma due to Western or Canadian red cedar (Thuya plicata). Med. J. Aust. 2:233.
13. Couturier, P., Mathieu, G., and Castelain , P.Y. 1989. La dermite de contact aux protéïnes, à propos de trois observations d'employés manipulant des volailles dans leur entreprise. Rev. Fr. Allergol. 29(2):67.
14. Michel, F.B. 1978. Allergie à Panonychus ulkmi (Koch). Rev. Fr. Allerg. 17:93.
15. Fields, J.P., Moke, A.W., and Cronce, P.C. 1969. Cheese mite dermatitis. Arch. Derm. 98:669.
16. Mandallaz, M., de Weck, A.L., and Dahinden, C.A. 1988. Bird-egg syndrome. Int. Arch. Allergy Appl. Immunol. 87:143.
17. Benezra, C. 1973. Allergènes végétaux. Méthodes chimiques d'isolement et d'identification. Rev. Fr. Allerg. 13:51.
18. Pepys, J. 1991. Extrapolation de l'asthme professionnel à l'asthme en général. Sem. Hôp. Paris 67 (no. 26–27):1266.
19. Muller, Wening, D., and Repp, H. 1989. Investigation on the protective value of breathing masks in farmer's lung using an inhalation provocation test. Chest 95:100.
20. Nuutinen, J., Terho, E.O., Husman, K., Kotimaa, M., Harkonen, R., and Nousiaienen, H. 1987. Protective value of powered dust respirator helmet for farmers with farmer's lung. J. R. D. (Suppl) 152.
21. Dalphin, J.C., Pernet, D., Roux, C., Reboux, G., Martinez, J., Laplante, J.J. Barale, Th., and Depierre, A. 1991. Etude de l'efficacité des masque de protection respiratoire sur les actinomycètes thermophiles. Rev. Fr. Mal. Resp. Abstract 101.

Isocyanates and Asthma

G. Pauli, M.-C. Kopferschmitt-Kubler*

Isocyanates are highly reactive chemical compounds which may cause several pulmonary diseases in exposed workers. Chemical bronchitis usually occurs after heavy exposures and can lead to the persistence of symptoms and nonspecific bronchial hyperreactivity. Long-term effects on lung function in asymptomatic workers are minimized when exposures are well controlled. Hypersensitivity pneumonitis can be accompanied by variable degrees of airflow obstruction. However, classic asthma is the most frequent pulmonary disease in patients exposed to isocyanates. The possibility of underlying hypersensitivity mechanisms is suggested by the insidious onset of symptoms, a latency period of months to years, the elicitation of symptoms after exposure to small levels (5 to 20 ppb) both at work and in laboratory tests, and the evidence of immunoreactivity to isocyanates in several animal models and in a small subset of patients. However, the pathogenesis of isocyanate asthma remains uncertain; immunological mechanisms other than IgE-mediated ones and pharmacological actions of isocyanate could also be involved. Despite the controversy that still surrounds the pathogenesis, new data derived from clinical studies of sensitized workers suggest that there is a high risk of persistence of symptoms; all available methods should therefore be used to diagnose the illness as early as possible.

Since the first observation by Fuchs and Valade (1951), there have been numerous reports of isocyanate-related asthma. There is also good evidence that isocyanates cause chemical bronchitis, nonspecific airway disease (including chronic bronchitis), and hypersensitivity pneumonitis. The mechanisms involved are still not completely understood; this is partly due to the difficulty in reproducing effects in experimental animals. Isocyanates are highly reactive chemical compounds because they contain NCO groups attached to an organic radical and react exothermically with compounds containing active hydrogen atoms to form a polymer (polyurethane), resulting in rigid or flexible foams. Toluene diisocyanates (TDI) are the most commonly used commercial isocyanates. Two isomers are available from commercial sources: 2-4 toluene diisocyanate and 2-6 toluene diisocyanate. TDI is used for flexible foams, but because of its volatility it has largely been replaced by less volatile compounds such as methylene diphenyl diisocyanate (MDI) for producing rigid polyurethane foams. Other diisocyanates such as hexamethylene diisocyanate (HDI) which is almost as volatile as TDI, naphtylene diisocyanate (NDI), isophorone diisocyanate (IPDI) and hydrogenated MDI (HMDI) also have commercial uses. Isocyanate products were first available in Germany in 1947. Flexible foams are widely used for cushioning in automobiles and furniture, mattresses and packaging materials. The rigid foams (mainly MDI) are used for packaging materials and insulation. Polyurethanes are of great value as paints where their hardness and durability offer special advantages. They are also used as adhesives and binders and as elastomers in automobile bumpers, printing rolls, liners for mine and grain elevator chutes, shoe soles, etc. (1). They thus have a wide variety of industrial and domestic uses. Occupations with potential exposure risks include: diisocyanate workers, polyurethane foam makers, upholstery workers, spray painters, wire coating workers, plastic foam makers, plastic molders and rubber workers. Proper atmospheric control of TDI can be achieved by modern engineering techniques; however, air concentrations of isocyanates are often high in small furniture firms and car repair shops. Domestic exposure may occur from the use of polyurethane paints and varnishes and "do-it-yourself" polyurethane foams (2).

---

* Service de Pneumologie, Pavillon Laennec, Hôpitaux Universitaires de Strasbourg, Hôpital Civil, B.P.426, 67091 Strasbourg Cedex.

Measurements of Exposure Levels to Isocyanates

Accurate knowledge of an individual's exposure level to the different isocyanates is vital for understanding their effects or for developing industry standards.

Methods

Marcali (1957) devised a simple colorimetric procedure based on bubbling workplace air samples through an acid absorption medium in which TDI is hydrolyzed to its toluene diamine derivative. This amine is then diatomized and coupled with 1-naphthylethylene-diamine to produce a reddish blue color, the intensity of which is measured spectrophotometrically. This method is only able to detect aromatic amines and does not detect aliphatic isocyanates such as HDI.

Paper tape monitors are presently the only practical instantaneous and continuous detectors for isocyanates available on the market. A recent technique for measuring aliphatic isocyanates involves reactions between isocyanate groups and a reactive group of a chromophore-bearing compound. Presently, paper tape monitors such as the MD 7100 can be calibrated for TDI, HDI, MDI, IPDI and others. MDI aerosols can also be measured with a certain accuracy but the measured values should be confirmed with a parallel method since abnormally low results may be found.

Chromatographic methods (especially HPLC) are the most sensitive for measuring and distinguishing between isocyanates, especially aliphatic isocyanates, but are technically difficult, expensive, and discontinuous. Personal sampling strategies in the workplace give better estimates of exposure than those made by area sampling. Comparisons between different band tape monitors and the HPLC reference method showed that under identical conditions variations greater than 100% could be observed, especially at low humidity, where band tape values were lower (3).

Permissible Exposure Levels

The threshold limit committee of the American Conference of Governmental Industrial Hygienists reduced the exposure limit from 100 ppb in 1956 to 20 ppb for TDI in 1968; the National Institute for Occupational Safety and Health recommended in 1978 a time-weighted average concentration of TDI less than 5 ppb for 8 hours, or less than 20 ppb for a 20 minute period. In diisocyanate manufactures 8-hour time-weighted average levels of TDI ranged from 0.1 ppb to 25 ppb from 1973 to 1978 (1). The introduction of exhaust ventilation in polyurethane production plants led to reductions in TDI concentrations.

Animal Studies

Rats inhaling TDI at high concentrations (4–13.5 ppm) showed severe epithelial damage consistent with a corrosive irritant effect (4); repeated exposures at lower concentrations (0.1 ppm) caused fibrous tissue proliferation. All these inhalation studies used concentrations much higher than those likely to occur in ordinary industrial exposures. Animal models of sensitization to isocyanates include the injection of TDI-protein conjugates into rabbits (5). Guinea pigs were also sensitized to monofunctional and/or bifunctional isocyanate compounds by inhalation (6). It has been shown that the immune response mounted by guinea pigs immunized with diisocyanate-haptened protein conjugates (7) was heterogeneous and involved multiple specificities for hapten, carrier protein and new antigen determinants.

Human Respiratory Effects (Except "Isocyanate Asthma")

Chemical Bronchitis

Accidental heavy exposure to TDI fumes in a group of 35 firemen (8) demonstrated that both immediate and delayed respiratory symptoms can occur: Chest tightness, breathlessness and cough were more pronounced 3 days after the accident. Follow-up showed that 14 out of 31 patients had persistent respiratory symptoms present 4 years later in some cases. Observed deteriorations in lung function appeared to improve over 1–2 years. Some subjects submitted to high exposure levels of isocyanates may have symptoms for years and persistent non-specific bronchial hyperreactivity, presenting like an "asthmatic illness" (9).

Acute and Long-Term Effects on Lung Function

Several studies have shown that TDI workers may have asymptomatic airway obstruction during the course of a workshift; the degree of obstruction is thought to depend on the amount of exposure. Especially important are long-term effects on pulmonary function in asymptomatic workers. Peters et al. (10) examined a group of 38 polyurethane-foam workers at 6-month intervals over 3 years (i. e., concentrations of TDI during the study period from 1965–1968 ranged up to 0.014 ppm) and found an excessive average annual decline in FEV_1. Wegman et al. (11) made serial pulmonary function measurements in workers exposed to variable TDI concentrations. A dose-response relationship was demonstrable: Subjects exposed to levels greater than 0.0035 ppm had an annual decline in FEV_1 of 0.103 l, whereas those exposed to levels below 0.0015 had no significant changes in FEV_1. In a 5-year prospective study, Diem et al. (12) showed that among nonsmokers, subjects exposed to higher TDI concentrations (i. e., 15% of the time spent above 5 ppb) had a decline of 42 ml/year, compared to subjects exposed to lower TDI concentrations (i. e., 2% of the time above 5 ppb) who had a decline of 24 ml/year. Pham (13) observed significantly reduced values for FEV_1, VC and DLCO among workers exposed to MDI concentrations ranging from 0.02 ppm to 0.005 ppm. According to Musk (14), who reexamined at 5-year intervals 94 subjects from an initial cohort of 259, exposed to between 0.0010 and 0.0015 ppm of TDI and between 0.0003 and 0.0006 ppm of MDI, a normal age- and smoking-related rate of decline in FEV_1 was observed, which was not related to isocyanate exposure; this seems to demonstrate that controlling isocyanate exposure is sufficient for protecting industrial workers against measurable deterioration in lung function. It should be pointed out that the interpretation of many longitudinal studies suffers from attrition of subjects, sometimes related to a contraction of the work force but also to worker turnover.

Hypersensitivity Pneumonitis/Allergic Alveolitis

Hypersensitivity pneumonitis was first reported by Charles et al. (15). There have been subsequent reports implicating MDI and HDI in similar reactions, often accompanied by variable air flow obstruction. Specific serum antibodies of the IgG class against involved diisocyanates have been found in some instances but not in others.

"Isocyanate Asthma"

There may be an insidious onset of asthmatic symptoms in isocyanate-exposed workers. The diagnosis of isocyanate hypersensitivity is based on improvement after removal of exposure and prompt recurrence of symptoms after exposure to slight concentrations (< 0.020 ppm). Recognition of isocyanate asthma is essential, because sudden death from acute severe asthma has been reported in sensitized subjects (16). Sensitization occurs with a variable delay (i. e., from several weeks to over 10 years).

Prevalence

Various estimates of the prevalence of isocyanate asthma have been reported: 5 to 25% in isocyanate production plants and 25 to 30% in polyurethane manufacturing plants. For some authors, isocyanate-induced asthma is dose-dependent (17), whereas for others high sensitization rates of up to 30% can be observed even when workers have reduced exposures varying from 0.3 to 3 ppb (18). Environmental data are not always available and symptoms of isocyanate asthma can be the consequence of intermittent high exposures, or of continuous exposure. TDI and HDI are volatile at room temperature, whereas MDI and NDI become volatile when heated; however, the latter isocyanates may be inhaled as an aerosol, especially by painters.

Clinical Features

Atopy does not seem to influence the development of TDI asthma: The percentage of atopics was 37% in a study of 113 workers with isocyanate-induced asthma (19), 21.5% in another study of 93 workers (20) and 33.4% in a personal study of 27 car painters with isocyanate-asthma (21). A low proportion of smokers has been reported: 7.5% by C. Mapp (20), and 5.4% by Moscato (19). The severity of isocyanate-asthma is variable: Patients can develop symptoms during the exposure period or in the evening and/or night. Cough is often associated with shortness of breath; chest tightness is found in 1/3 of patients (22). Pulmonary function may not be notably impaired at the time of diagnosis. A significantly increased reactivity to metacholine is found in most patients (78.3% of 113 workers for Moscato; 90% in our personal series of painters), but hyperreactivity may be absent in some cases, despite a typical history of occupational asthma to TDI (23). Increases in airway hyperresponsiveness to metacholine can appear during the workweek.

Evolution

Early diagnosis and early removal from exposure to isocyanates may lead to complete recovery in some cases (24). However, studies concerning the long-term follow-up of patients with isocyanate asthma report that over 50% of subjects who had left the workplace continued to have respiratory symptoms and airway hyperresponsiveness to nonspecific stimuli (25,26). In a recent study, only 22.9% of patients lost sensitivity to isocyanates and airway hyperresponsiveness to metacholine after exposure removal (22). More longitudinal studies are needed to understand the factors predictive of persistent asthma months and years after cessation of exposure: It has been suggested that a longer duration of both exposure and symptoms and late isolated asthmatic reactions after inhalation challenge are of great significance (22).

Diagnosis of IgE-Mediated Isocyanate-Asthma

IgE-mediated sensitization has been demonstrated in some workers by direct skin testing or radioallergosorbent tests (RAST) using isocyanate-human serum albumin compounds (27,28,29). The percentage of all workers with respiratory isocyanate-induced symptoms who showed positive indices for IgE to isocyanate-HSA was less than 20% in the different studies. The large number of cases of isocyanate asthma in which no immunological mechanisms can be demonstrated raises several questions: Are the methods used reliable in identifying specific IgE in cases of isocyanate-asthma? Are conjugates characterized and standardized with respect to the degree of haptenization? It has been demonstrated in a recent study (30) that specific IgE from selected workers reacted optimally to conjugates with ≤10 isocyanate molecules bound per molecule of human serum albumin. Is there a role for cell-mediated mechanisms? Immune cross-reactivity between TDI, HDI and MDI protein conjugates due to new antigenic sites created by isocyanate-protein interactions may exist (31). In a personal study we demonstrated that 7 painters with isocyanate-asthma who were mainly exposed to HDI had significant IgE antibody levels not only to HDI-HSA, but also to TDI-HSA and MDI-HSA (21). RAST and ELISA inhibition studies demonstrated that the magnitude of cross-reactivities differs from one patient to the next (31,32). Recent determinations of specific IgG antibodies against isocyanates in workers with occupational asthma showed a close association with positive bronchial inhalation tests (33) but more prospective studies are needed.

Inhalation Challenge Testing in the Diagnosis of Isocyanate-Induced Asthma

The information provided by clinical examination is usually inadequate for establishing the diagnosis of isocyanate asthma; only in a small subgroup of symptomatic workers are RAST with HSA-bound isocyanate helpful for diagnosis. In some cases, the development of respiratory symptoms with a decline in FEV_1 during a workday or an increase in airway hyperresponsiveness to metacholine after a workweek can substantiate the diagnosis of isocyanate-induced asthma. In other cases, a laboratory-based isocyanate challenge is necessary. Prior assessment of bronchial hyperresponsiveness to metacholine may help determine the initial challenge dose and duration. Several groups performed the tests in dynamic flow chambers, the airborne concentration of isocyanate being continuously measured with an MDA monitor. Hospitalization is necessary to document and treat late asthmatic reactions. After a placebo day, specific challenges are performed on several days, beginning with an isocyanate exposure of 5 ppb for 30 minutes. In the absence of a positive reaction, an exposure of 10 and 20 ppb is delivered on successive days for as little as 15 minutes or more according to the authors. A positive challenge test is defined by the development of asthma symptoms and/or a decline in FEV_1 greater than 20%. Different types of bronchial reactions can be observed: immediate isolated late reactions, dual reactions and progressive delayed reactions. According to Fabbri (34), late-asthmatic responses and dual responses are associated with increased neutrophilia in bronchoalveolar lavage fluid and increased bronchial hyperreactivity. The outcome of the inhalation challenge test cannot be predicted from the nonspecific bronchial hyperreactivity: A proportion of TDI reactors have normal responses to metacholine: 21.7% for Moscato (19), 9% for Banks (35), 10% for Kopferschmitt (21). Only 43% of the results from laboratory challenge testing had the same temporal pattern of asthma as that resulting from workplace reactions according to Banks (35). These results point out the limits of inhalation challenge tests, which have been considered the gold standard for proving isocyanate-induced asthma. Several studies reported a similar percentage of positive isocyanate challenge tests among patients referred with respiratory symptoms in isocyanate-exposed workplaces: 56% for Mapp (20), 48% for Banks (35) and 52% in our painter group (21). It is especially difficult to assess the degree of confidence of a negative inhalation challenge test when the test is performed after the patient has been unexposed for an extended period. A negative test does not rule out occupational asthma related to another chemical such as non-cross-reacting isocyanates or amines present at the workplace; it can also be suggested that the duration of laboratory exposure is too small and that the incidence of positive inhalation tests could be increased by lengthening the exposure time. Control studies to exclude false positive diagnoses have also been performed: Vogelmeier et al. (36) showed that one out of 10 healthy volunteers and 3 out of 14 patients with asthma unrelated to isocyanate reacted to exposure levels of 10-30 ppb for 1-2 hours.

Pathogenesis of Isocyanate Asthma

The pathogenesis of isocyanate asthma remains uncertain. Both immunologic and nonimmunologic mechanisms appear to be involved (37). Humoral (i.e., IgE-mediated) immunoreactivity can be demonstrated only in a small subset of workers. It is not clear at present if this small number of proven examples of sensitization to isocyanates is the consequence of inadequate methods for reliably identifying specific IgE in cases of asthma due to isocyanates, or if it is related to other immunological or non-specific mechanisms. In the absence of IgE antibodies, IgG involvment, the formation of immune complexes generated by a pulmonary IgG or IgA response and complement activation by chemically modified self proteins have been proposed. These latter immunological reactions, as well as strong IgE reactions could be responsible for late or dual reactions observed both after workplace and laboratory exposures. Different pharmacological actions of isocyanates have also been demonstrated by *in vitro* studies: inhibition of erythrocyte acetylcholinesterase activity (38), and inhibition of the formation of intracellular c-AMP (39). Experimental studies in guinea pigs have shown that inhalation of TDI can inhibit neutral endopeptidases which break down tachykinins released by nerve endings supplying the airways (40); this may induce airway reactivity by potentiating tachykinin effects. These experimental data collectively suggest that isocyanates may cause nonspecific inhibition of various enzyme systems; this effect is consistent with the high reactivity of these substances. Studies of bronchoalveolar lavage fluid after isocyanate inhalation challenge tests suggest that an acute inflammatory reaction occurs which is responsible for hyperresponsiveness and late asthmatic reactions (34). Despite numerous new data derived from experimental and clinical investigations, there is no agreement concerning the possible mechanisms involved in isocyanate asthma. It can be suggested that the cause of occupational asthma to isocyanates is multifactorial and that we are far from a unitarian model of TDI asthma.

Although there are many unresolved questions concerning the pathogenesis of isocyanate asthma, the results of follow-up studies of TDI asthmatics clearly indicate that there is a high risk of persistence. Thus, occupational isocyanate-induced asthma should be diagnosed as early as possible; all available methods should be used, keeping in mind their limits, which have been better defined for biological and inhalation tests. Isocyanate air concentrations at workplaces should be as low as possible and significant transient increases in isocyanate air concentration should be entirely avoided. Serious prospective studies are still needed to evaluate workers forced to retire because of isocyanate-induced asthma.

References

1. Musk, A.W., Peters, J.M., and Wegman, D.H. 1988. Isocyanates and respiratory disease: Current status. Am. J. Ind. Med 13:331.
2. Peters, J.M., and Murphy, R.L.H., Jr. 1971. Hazards to health: do it yourself polyurethane foam. Am. Rev. Respir. Dis. 104:432.
3. Mazur, G., Baur, X., Pfaller, A., and Römmelt, H. 1986. Determination of toluene diisocyanate in air by HPLC and band-tape monitors. Int. Arch. Occup. Environ. Health 58:269.
4. Duncan, B., Scheel, L.D., Fairchild, E.J., Killens, R., and Graham, S. 1962. Toluene diisocyanate inhalation toxicity: Pathology and mortality. Am. Ind. Hyg. Assoc. J. 23:447.
5. Scheel, L.D., Killens, R., and Josephson, A. 1964. Immunochemical aspects of toluene diisocyanate (TDI) toxicity. Am. Ind. Hyg. J., 25:179.
6. Karol, M.H., Dixon, C., Brady, M., and Alary, Y. 1980. Immunologic sensitization and pulmonary hypersensitivity by repeated inhalation of aromatic isocyanates. Toxicol. Appl. Pharmacol. 53:260.
7. Chen, S.E., and Bernstein, I.L. 1982. The guinea pig model of diisocyanate sensitization. I. Immunologic studies. J. Allergy Clin. Immunol. 70:383.
8. Axford, A.T., McKerrow, C.B., Jones, A.P., and Le Quesne, P.M. 1976. Accidental exposure to isocyanate fumes in a group of firemen. Br. J. Ind. Med. 33:65.
9. Luo, J.C.J., Nelsen, K.G., and Fischbein, A. 1990. Persistent reactive airway dysfunction syndrome after exposure to toluene diisocyanate. Br. J. Ind. Med. 47:239.
10. Peters, J.M., Murphy, R.L.H., and Ferris, B.G., Jr. 1969. Ventilatory function in workers exposed to low levels of toluene diisocyanate: A six-month follow-up. Br. J. Ind. Med. 26:115.
11. Wegman, D.H., Musk, A.W., Main, D.M., and Pagnotto, L.D. 1982. Accelerated loss of FEV_1 in polyurethane production workers: A four-year prospective study. Am. J. Ind. Med. 3:209.
12. Diem, J.E., Jones, R.N., Hendrick, D.J., Glindmeyer, H.W., Dharmarajan, V., and Butcher, B.T. 1982. Five-year longitudinal study of workers employed in a new toluene diisocyanate manufacturing plant. Am. Rev.Respir.Dis. 126:420.
13. Pham, Q.T., Meyer-Bisch, C., Mur, J.M., Teculescu, D., Gaertner, M., St-Eve, P., and Massin, M. 1986. Etude de l'évolution clinique et fonctionnelle respiratoire sur 5 ans d'ouvriers exposés à de faibles teneurs d'isocyanate de diphenylmethane (MDI). Arch. Mal. Prof. 47:311.
14. Musk, A.W., Peters, J.M., DiBerardinis, L., and Murphy, R.L.H. 1982. Absence of respiratory effects in subjects exposed to low concentrations of TDI and MDI. J. Occup. Med. 24:746.
15. Charles, J., Bernstein, A., Jones, B., Jones, D.J., Edwards, J.H., Seal, R.M.E., and Seaton, A. 1976. Hypersensitivy pneumonitis after exposure to isocyanates. Thorax 31:127.
16. Fabbri, L.M., Danieli, D., Crescioli, S., Bevilacqua, P., Meli, S., Saetta, M., and Mapp, C.E. 1988. Fatal asthma in a subject sensitized to toluene diisocyanate. Am. Rev. Respir. Dis. 137:1494.
17. Baur, X. 1990. New aspects of isocyanate asthma. Lung (suppl.):606.
18. White, W.G., Sugden, E., Morris, M.J., and Zapata, E., 1980. Isocyanate-induced asthma in a car factory. Lancet i:756.
19. Moscato, G., Dellabianca, A., Vinci, G., Candura, S.M., and Bossi, M.C. 1991. Toluene diisocyanate-induced asthma: clinical findings and bronchial responsiveness studies in 113 exposed subjects with work-related respiratory symptoms. J. Occup. Med., 33:720.
20. Mapp, C.E., Boschetto, P., Dal Vecchio, L., Maestrelli, P., and Fabbri, L.M. 1988. Occupational asthma due to isocyanates. Eur. Respir. J. 1:273.
21. Kopferschmitt-Kubler, M.C., Rought-Rought, S., Dietemann, A., Bessot, J.C., and Pauli, G. 1991. Etude de 27 cas d'asthme aux isocyanates lié aux peintures de carrosserie. Rev. Fr. Mal. Resp. 8:R47.
22. Mapp, C.E., Chiesura Corona, P., De Marzo, N., and Fabbri, L.M. 1988. Persistent asthma due to isocyanates. Am. Rev. Respir. Dis. 137:1326.
23. Mapp, C.E., Dal Vecchio, L., Boschetto, P., et al. 1986. Toluene diisocyanate-induced asth-

ma without airway hyperresponsiveness. Eur. J. Respir. Dis. 68:89.
24. Paggiaro, P.L., Loi, A.M., Rossi, O., Ferrante, B., Pardi, F. Roselli, M.G., and Baschieri, L. 1984. Follow-up study of patients with respiratory disease due to toluene diisocyanate (TDI). Clin. Allergy 14:463.
25. Moller, D.R., McKay, R.T., Bernstein, I.L., and Brooks, S.M. 1986. Persistent airway disease caused by toluene diisocyanate. Am. Rev. Respir. Dis. 134:175.
26. Cockcroft, D.W. 1982. Acquired persistent increase in nonspecific bronchial reactivity associated to isocyanate exposure. Ann. Allergy 48: 93.
27. Butcher, B.T., O'Neil, C.E., Reed, M.A., and Salvaggio, J.E. 1980. Radioallergosorbent testing of toluene diisocyanate reactive individuals using p-tolyl isocyanate antigen. J. Allergy Clin. Immunol. 66:213.
28. Baur, X., Dewair, M., and Fruhmann, G. 1984. Detection of immunologically sensitized isocyanate workers by RAST and intracutaneous skin tests. J. Allergy Clin. Immunol. 73:610.
29. Keskinen, H., Tupasela, O., Tiikkainen, U., and Nordman, H. 1988. Experiences of specific IgE in asthma due to isocyanates. Clinical Allergy 18:597.
30. Wass, U., and Belin, L., 1989. Immunologic specificity of isocyanate induced IgE-antibodies in serum from 10 sensitized workers. J. Allergy Clin. Immunol. 83:126.
31. Baur, X. 1983. Immunologic cross-reactivity between different albumin-bound isocyanates. J. Allergy Clin. Immunol. 71:197.
32. Grammer, L.C., Harris, K.E., Malo, J.L., Cartier, A., and Patterson, R. 1990. The use of an immunoassay index for antibodies against isocyanate human protein conjugates and application to human isocyanate disease. J. Allergy Clin.Immunol. 86:94.
33. Cartier, A., Grammer, L., Malo, J.L., Lagier, F., Ghezzo, H., Harris, K., and Patterson, R. 1989. Specific serum antibodies against isocyanates: association with occupational asthma. J. Allergy Clin. Immunol. 83:507.
34. Fabbri, L.M., Boschetto, P., Zocca, E., Milani, G., Pivirotto, F., Plebani, M., Burlina, A., Licata, B., and Mapp, C.E. 1987. Bronchoalveolar neutrophilia during late asthmatic reactions induced by toluene diisocyanate. Am. Rev. Respir. Dis. 136:36.
35. Banks, D.E., Sastre, J., Butcher, B.T., and Ellis, E. 1989. Role of inhalation challenge testing in the diagnosis of isocyanate-induced asthma. Chest 95:414.
36. Vogelmeier, C., Baur, X., and Fruhmann, G. 1991. Isocyanate induced asthma: results of inhalation tests with TDI, MDI and metacholine. Int. Arch. Occup. Environ. Health 63:9.
37. Bernstein, I.L. 1982. Isocyanate-induced pulmonary diseases: a current perspective. J. Allergy Clin. Immunol. 70:24.
38. Dewair, M., Baur, X., and Fruhmann, G. 1983. Inhibition of erythrocyte acetylcholinesterase by diisocyanates. J. Occup. Med. 25:279.
39. Davies, R.J., Butcher, B.T., O'Neil, C.E., and Salvaggio, J.E., 1977. The in vitro effect of toluene diisocyanate on lymphocyte cyclic adenosine monophosphate production by isoproterenol, prostaglandin and histamine. A possible mode of action. J. Allergy Clin. Immunol. 60:223.
40. Sheppard, D., Thompson, J.E., Scypinski, L., Dusser, D., Nadel, J.A., and Borson, D.B. 1988. Toluene diisocyanate increases airway responsiveness to substance P and decreases airway neutral endopeptidase. J. Clin. Invest. 81:1111.

New Aspects in Occupational Asthma

Jean-Luc Malo*

Occupational asthma is now the most common occupational respiratory condition. Surveys conducted in the United Kingdom have shown that it is more frequently seen than standard pneumoconiosis and mesotheliomas. Cross-sectional epidemiologic surveys have estimated the frequency of occupational asthma to vary between 2 and 5% for high-molecular weight agents and between 5 and 10% for low-molecular weight agents. Efforts have been made recently to quantify the degree of exposure, especially to high-molecular weight agents. An association was found between degree of exposure and the risk of sensitization. Diagnosis still depends on the precision of the objective testing. Specific inhalation challenges in the laboratory, the methodology for which has recently been improved, are still regarded as the gold standard. As subjects with occupational asthma can be left with permanent impairment even after they are removed from exposure, it has been suggested that scales be set for determining the degree of impairment in terms of a percentage. Occupational asthma is a good model for asthma as subjects can be seen before, during and after they are affected by the condition, and experimental tools such as bronchoalveolar lavage and bronchial biopsies can be performed.

Increasing Frequency of Occupational Asthma

Occupational asthma is now the most common of the occupational respiratory conditions. In a U.S. national survey of 6,000 subjects, Blanc found that nearly 8% identified asthma as a medical condition they suffered from and 15% of those with asthma attributed it to the workplace (1). Medicolegal data points out that it is the most commonly reported condition, outnumbering standard pneumoconiosis (silicosis and asbestosis). Physician based surveys have been carried out in several American states (2) and in Great Britain (3). In Great Britain, 554 cases were identified in 1989, representing the leading type (26%) of occupational respiratory ailment. Occupational asthma bears several features which are different from standard pneumoconiosis and should be kept in mind in epidemiological surveys and clinical investigation. Lung fibrosis, which is the result of pneumoconiosis, is a rare occurrence in a general population, just as mining or being exposed to silica or asbestos dust in significant quantity are rare. When a worker presents with radiological shadows suggestive of lung fibrosis and a history of exposure to minal dust, the diagnosis of pneumoconiosis is usually obvious and there is no need to prove it with more objective testing such as lung biopsy, which in any case will be too agressive and would not necessarily distinguish between fibrosis induced by mineral dusts and fibrosis from another cause. The situation with occupational asthma is completely different. Asthma is a common condition, 5 to 10% of a random population being affected by it at one time or another. Accepting a diagnosis of occupational asthma on the grounds of proven asthma and a history of exacerbated symptoms at work would have a major impact on the number of cases diagnosed. Occupational asthma has the advantage over standard pneumoconiosis of being reproducible experimentally; the functional abnormalities can be reproduced either at work or in the laboratory without harming the worker.

Population Surveys

In recent years, increasing numbers of cross-sectional type surveys have been carried out. All studies are weakened by a bias inherent in this type of epidemiological survey, i.e. the healthy worker effect. It is expected that longitudinal studies will be carried out although they are very difficult to plan for several reasons: the

* Department of Chest Medicine, Hopital du Sacre-Coeur, 5400 West Gouin, Montreal, Canada H4J 1C5.
Acknowledgements: The author wants to thank Katherine Tallman for reviewing the mansucript.

cost, the need to follow subjects who leave the company, rapid changes in the way products are handled at work, and so on. By and large, the frequency of occupational asthma due to high-molecular-weight agents has been found to vary between 2 and 5% and to low-molecular-weight agents between 5 and 10%, as shown by some studies from our group (4–8).

Quantification of Sensitizers: Relationship with Sensitization

It is now possible to obtain information on the concentration of occupational sensitizers. This has been done for high-molecular (9) and low-molecular-weight sensitizers. Some association can be detected between the quantity of an antigen and the risk of sensitization in some workplaces like bakeries (10), soldering manufacturers (11) and sawmills processing Western red cedar (12). It is likely that the coming years will see new developments in this interesting field of research. New methods of airborne-allergen quantification will be found, and studies to examine the association between degree of exposure and the risk of sensitization and development of occupational asthma will be carried out.

Diagnosis

Questionnaire

A questionnaire is a basic, essential tool used in most epidemiological surveys and all individual assessments. The most commonly used questionnaire for respiratory diseases is the ATS questionnaire. The problem with this questionnaire is that it was originally designed for assessing non-specific chronic obstructive lung disease. Typical features of asthma such as awakenings at night due to respiratory symptoms are not included. The International Union against Tuberculosis (IUAT) recently designed and validated a questionnaire available in different languages. The association between airway responsiveness to pharmacological agents and answers to an administered "closed" respiratory questionnaire has been explored in some studies, but has not generally been satisfactory. Open clinical questionnaires are not reliable tools in predicting the presence or absence of bronchial hyperresponsiveness either. Because occupational asthma is a condition that can lead to permanent disability, a questionnaire should be a sensitive tool. The validity of survey questionnaires in assessing work-related asthma is summarized in Table 1. It is clear that the questionnaire used in these studies, which was derived from the IUAT questionnaire, is sensitive. Biases could affect questionnaires; these are related primarily to the compensation of occupational asthma, which depends on what part of the world the surveys are carried out in. If occupational asthma is well compensated, workers may tend to exaggerate their symptoms; they may minimize them if the reverse is true. Open clinical questionnaires are also sensitive in picking up cases of occupational asthma. We showed recently that the positive predictive value of an open questionnaire was 63% in 162 subjects referred for possible work-related asthma (13). This means that in more than one third of the cases, subjects whose initial questionnaires were suggestive of occupational asthma, did not have a positive diagnosis with objective testing (Table 2). The questionnaire we used incorporated the typical symptomatology of occupational asthma: symptoms that worsen at work or shortly after a workshift and improve at weekends and on vacation.

Spirometry

Just as normal spirometry does not exclude asthma, a normal FEV 1 value at work does not imply that the diagnosis should be excluded. Comparison of pre- and post-shift FEV 1 has not been found to be a satisfactory tool either (4,5,14).

Immunological Testing

Immediate skin reactivity or increased specific IgE or IgG antibodies may reflect exposure and/or sensitization but they do not imply that the target organ (the bronchi in this case) is involved. This has been shown for common allergens and occupational sensitizers. Nineteen percent of pharmaceutical workers exposed to psyllium demonstrated immediate skin reactivity to the agent but only 4% had

Table 1. Validity of questionaire in various epidemiological surveys

Agent/work place	number of workers participating/ total number of workers	number of workers with a suggestive history	number of workers with occupational asthma (%) *	reference
snow-crab processors	303/313	64	33(52%)	(34)
isocyanates/paint-shops	48/ 48	14	6(43%)	(7)
psyllium/pharmaceutical company	130/140	39	5(13%)	(5)
spiramycin/pharmaceutical company	51/ 51	12	3(25%)	(6)
guar gum/carpet manufacture	162/177	37	3(8%)	(9)
psyllium/chronic care nurses	197/252	79	8(10%)	(8)

* % of those with a suggestive history of occupational asthma; diagnosis confirmed with objective means (specific inhalation challenges and/or serial peak expiratory flow rates monitoring).

occupational asthma (4). Furthermore, evidence of immunological sensitization of the IgE or IgG type has been shown for only a proportion of occupational sensitizers, principally the high-molecular-weight agents.

Bronchial Responsiveness

Bronchial responsiveness is the hallmark of asthma but it is also present in other conditions such as rhinitis and chronic obstructive and restrictive lung diseases. The presence of increased bronchial responsiveness may suggest that the subject has occupational asthma, common asthma or one or the other of the conditions listed above. However, the absence of bronchial hyperresponsiveness as assessed shortly (minutes, hours) after a workshift virtually excludes occupational asthma. The fact that bronchial hyperresponsiveness can persist for months and even years after removal from exposure to the offending agent points to the fact that this tool can be used in assessing subjects even if they have been away from work for long intervals, and even if it is not completely sensitive.

Peak Expiratory Flow Rate Monitoring

The availability of portable, inexpensive devices has contributed considerably to our understanding of the functional behavior of asthma, identifying specific patterns that mean asthmatic subjects are at greater risk (15). This approach was first used in the investigation of work-related asthma by Sherwood Burge and colleagues (16). Coupling peak expiratory flow rate monitoring with changes in bronchial re-

Table 2. Physician's Global Assessment in Relation to Final Diagnosis*

Physician Assessment from Questionaire on Occupational Asthma Final diagnosis	Very likely	Likely	Uncertain	Unlikely	Absent	Total
Occupational Asthma	54	11	6	3	1	75
Asthma	16	9	19	6	4	54
No Asthma and no Occupational Asthma	8	6	10	3	6	33
Total	78	26	35	12	11	162

Prospective evidence in 162 subjects referred for investigation of work-releted asthma-like symptoms of the likelihood of occupational asthma according to the physician's initial assessment based on a medical questionnaire as compared with the final diagnosis obtained through objective testing (specific inhalations tests in 72 subjects, serial monitoring of peak expiratory flow rates for periods at work and off-work (n = 29) or both (n = 61). Modified from reference 13.

sponsiveness for periods at work and away from work has been proposed (17).The specificity and sensitivity of this means of confirming occupational asthma was assessed prospectively in two studies using specific inhalation challenges as the gold standard (18,19). Figures for sensitivity and specificity are greater than 75%. This mean value is satisfactory for individual investigations but not for epidemiological surveys, as it requires close supervision from the personnel. It also depends on the honesty and collaboration of the subject. The interpretation of results cannot be quantified, and "eye balling" the graphs is still the most satisfactory index.

Specific Inhalation Challenges

These tests still represent the gold standard for confirming a diagnosis of occupational asthma. They were developed by Jack Pepys and his team (20). The tests have to be done in specialized centers with expertise in the field. There are pitfalls. With particles that the subjects tip from one tray to another in dust or powder form, the concentrations of particles are not assessed and can be high at times, above the recommended so-called Threshold-Limit-Value-Short-Term-Exposure-Levels (TLV-STEL). This exposure can result in immediate non-specific irritant reactions. The temporal pattern of these reactions cannot be distinguished from the ones that occur after exposure to non-sensitizing agents such as pharmacological substances or hyperventilation of unconditioned air. High exposure can also result in severe bronchospastic reactions (21). In the case of isocyanates, it is difficult to obtain steady concentrations, particularly for the new types such as hexamethylene diisocyanate (HDI), which should be aerosolized, and diphenylmethane diisocyanate (MDI), which has to be heated. Using challenge rooms can also result in exposing medical personnel to the offending agent with the risk of sensitizing them.

Models of closed-circuit small challenge rooms for exposing subjects to isocyanates have been constructed (22). We initially proposed a closed-circuit inhalation challenge room for exposing subjects to particles (23). We estimate that one third of our challenges used products in particle-form. The methodology has been thoroughly described elsewhere (23). The advantage of our challenge room is that subjects are exposed to steady concentrations of particles well below the TLV-STEL of 10 mg/m3. The generator was recently modified slightly and a new automated version of the apparatus was developed: Pre-set concentrations can be generated automatically with less need for supervision on the part of the technician in charge of the test. We have shown that dose-response curves can be generated in a safe way. Changes in FEV 1 close to 20% can be obtained progressively by increasing the concentration and/or duration of exposure. We have now validated the use of the device on more than 50 subjects referred for investigation of occupational asthma due to agents in powder form (flour and grains, red cedar, psyllium, guar gum, persulfate, miscellaneous) in whom specific inhalation challenges were required to confirm the diagnosis. The duration of exposure was progressive and varied from one breath to a maximum of 180 minutes depending on the reaction. When no significant fall in FEV 1 occurred after exposure with the new aerosolization device, the standard approach of tipping powder from one tray to another (20) was used. Eighteen subjects experienced isolated immediate bronchospastic reactions, and four had dual (immediate and late) reactions. In 18/22 instances (82%), the fall in FEV 1 did not exceed 30%, thus showing that dose-response curves can generally be generated in a safe way. In all instances except one (26/27), subsequent exposure using the traditional method of tipping powder from one tray to another did not result in significant falls in FEV 1. The only exception was a subject who had been exposed for one hour using the new device; more prolonged exposure might have been required. The new procedure for exposing subjects to occupational sensitizers in powder form generally results in safe tests in terms of the % change in FEV 1 during immediate reactions (generally between 20 and 30%) and very rare false negative challenges (only one).

We recently extended this approach to isocyanates, developing a closed-circuit exposure chamber that ensures that subjects are exposed to concentrations below the threshold limit of 20 ppb (24). This closed-circuit inhalation challenge apparatus consists of two main components: an isocyanate generating system and an exposure chamber, each of them having regulating and monitoring equipment. Isocyanates are generated in gaseous form by blowing air onto the surface of pure isocyanate monomers deposited in a stoppered glass flask. The airflow rate passing through the flask is adjusted by a valve rotameter. We have prospectively assessed 20 subjects, exposing them in random fashion to isocyanates either in the new exposure device or with the traditional room proposed by Pepys and Hutchcroft (20). Isocyanate concentrations are more stable with the closed-circuit apparatus than with the traditional challenge-room method. The total exposure time during which concentrations were above 20 ppb was reduced from 11.3% to 4.5%. The duration of exposure had to be longer with the new closed-circuit approach, preventing brisk falls in FEV 1 and making it possible to generate dose-response curves.

Medicolegal Aspects

Occupational asthma is accepted as a pulmonary ailment for compensation by most medicolegal agencies. However, several aspects of the compensation process are highly variable from one place to the other. Moreover, agencies have so far delt primarily with pneumoconiosis; physicians sitting on workers' compensation boards seldom have expertise in the new and rapidly increasing number of conditions that fall under the categories of occupational asthma and industrial bronchitis.

In countries like the U.K. and France, the diagnosis can be accepted based on a suggestive history and on indications that the subject is exposed to a recognized sensitizer. There are several pitfalls to this approach: (a) there is no proof that the subject really has occupational asthma for the reasons mentioned above; and (b) a subject may well have occupational asthma but the condition will not be accepted as such if he or she is exposed to an agent that is not on the list. It is also essential that the compensation process work efficiently and quickly. If claims take a long time to be processed, subjects may have left the workplace on the advice of their physician or spontaneously because of severe symptoms. It can be difficult to prove the diagnosis if the workplace investigation is carried out too long after the subject left. Working conditions could have changed completely and offending agents may no longer be used. Exposing the subject in a laboratory may also result in false negative tests if the subject has not been exposed for a while, and returning the subject to the workplace is useless if the sensitizer is no longer present.

Temporary disability status is usually granted, although the duration of the disability may vary greatly from one country to another. If temporary disability leave is short, claimants will not have enough time to find a new job or to retrain. This point is crucial as, unlike standard pneumoconiosis, occupational asthma often affects young workers. In 40% of the cases of occupational asthma due to Western red cedar and isocyanates, the onset of symptoms was within one year of the beginning of exposure. It is therefore essential that these workers be retrained quickly and efficiently.

It is now well known that occupational asthma leads to permanent disability. Only a minority of subjects will continue to have airway obstruction after leaving the workplace, but most of them will continue to have both asthmatic symptoms requiring medication and increased bronchial responsiveness. This has been documented in more than ten retrospective studies published so far, the original ones of which were carried out on cedar mill workers (25). The results cover a variety of occupational sensitizers (26,27). In the case of snow-crab workers, it has also been shown that a plateau of improvement generally occurs approximately two years after exposure ends (28). The problem is that the criteria to be used in compensating these subjects have not been set. It is clear that the criteria used for standard pneumoconiosis are useless because the characteristics of the condition are very different from occupational asthma in terms of pattern of physiological abnormalities (Table 3). The American Thoracic Society recently asked a special committee to come up with guidelines. A scaling system has been used in Quebec since 1985. Claimants are examined two years after they stop work. Disability compensation is determined taking into account three main factors: airway caliber, bronchial hyperresponsiveness and the need for medication; it is well known that the three factors taken together are a good reflection of the clinical severity of asthma.

Table 3. Features differentiating occupational asthma standard pneumoconiosis

	Occupational asthma	Standard pneumoconiosis (asbestosis, silicosis)
Functional abnormalities	obstructive response to bronchodilator bronchial hyperresponsiveness	restrictive abnormalities of gas exchange
Response to therapy	present	none
Behaviour	improvement and plateau	plateau or deterioration
Radiological changes	absent	present
Influence of the degree of exposure	questionable	present

Occupational Asthma as an Experimental Model for Asthma

Occupational asthma can be used as a model for asthma from the epidemiological and physiopathological point of view. A proposed scheme of the possible natural history of occupational asthma is illustrated in Figure 1. Studying the natural history of occupational asthma can tell us more about the natural history of asthma per se. This is because in some instances it is possible to get information on predisposing host factors before exposure starts, which is not possible for asthma. We can now get information, too, on the degree of exposure to the offending agent. This is difficult in the case of asthma as several allergens can be present at the time of sensitization and at the onset of symptoms. Moreover, the behavior of the condition can be studied after exposure ends, which is again not possible with asthma as one is never sure an asthmatic subject has been entirely isolated from exposure to possible sensitizers. With occupational asthma, we can get information on the predisposing factors before sensitization or before the onset of symptoms and follow a subject after exposure ends. Occupational asthma is also an interesting model for studying the physiopathology of asthma. Animal models of asthma are not generally satisfactory. With the availability of techniques such as bronchoalveolar lavage and bronchial biopsies, it is now possible to assess subjects with occupational asthma during challenges. Interesting information on the pathophysiology of immediate and late bronchospastic reactions can be obtained in this way, for both low- and high-molecular-weight agents, which are assumed to be similar to common allergens that cause sensitization through an IgE mechanism (29–31). The effect of medication can also be studied (32,33), as can the physiopathology of occupational asthma when subjects are symptomatic, or after removal from exposure to the offending agent.

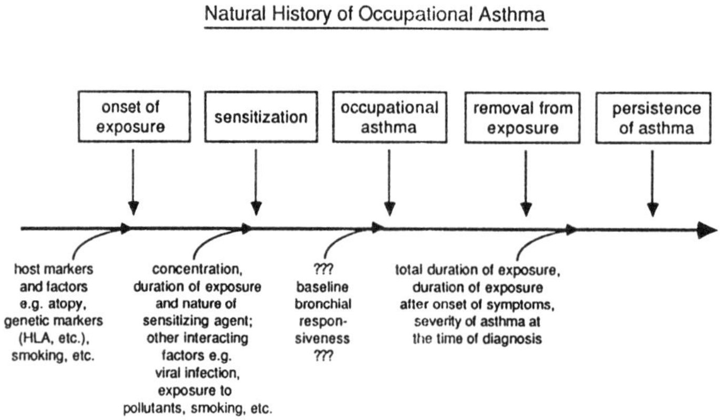

Figure 1. Proposed scheme for the interaction of factors that may play a role in the development of sensitization and asthma to an occupational sensitizer. From discussions with Moira Chan-Yeung.

Conclusion

Figures clearly show that occupational asthma is now the most common of the respiratory ailments. It is hoped that these figures will lead to the improvements in the clinical tools to confirm the diagnosis, in epidemiological investigations aimed at identifying risk factors, in instituting adequate medicolegal compensation so that patients can find another job without being affected by permanent sequelae, and in using the ailment as a model in the study of asthma.

References

1. Blanc, P. 1987. Occupational asthma in a national disability survey. Chest 92:613.
2. Matte, T.D., Hoffman, R.E., Rosenman, K.D., and Stanbury, M. 1990. Surveillance of occupational asthma under the SENSOR model. Chest 98:173S.
3. Meredith, S.K., Taylor, V.M., and McDonald, J.C. 1991. Occupational respiratory disease in the United Kingdom 1989: A report to the British Thoracic Society and the Society of Occupational Medicine by the SWORD project group. Br. J. Ind. Med. 48:292.
4. Bardy, J.D., Malo, J.L., Seguin, P., Ghezzo, H., Desjardins, J., Dolovich, J., and Cartier, A. 1987. Occupational asthma and IgE sensitization in a pharmaceutical company processing psyllium. Am. Rev. Respir. Dis. 135:1033.
5. Malo, J.L., and Cartier, A. 1988. Occupational asthma in workers of a pharmaceutical company processing spiramycin. Thorax 43:371.
6. Séguin, P., Allard, A., Cartier, A., and Malo, J.L. 1987. Prevalence of occupational asthma in spray painters exposed to several types of isocyanates, including polymethylene polyphenylisocyanates. J.O.M. 29:340.
7. Malo, J.L., Cartier, A., L'Archevêque, J., Ghezzo, H., Lagier, F., Trudeau, C., and Dolovich, J. 1990. Prevalence of occupational asthma and immunologic sensitization to psyllium among health personnel in chronic care hospitals. Am. Rev. Respir. Dis. 142:1359.
8. Malo, J.L., Cartier, A., L'Archevêque, J., Ghezzo, H., Soucy, F., Somers, J., and Dolovich, J. 1990. Prevalence of occupational asthma and immunological sensitization to guar gum among employees at a carpet-manufacturing plant. J. Allergy Clin. Immunol. 86:562.
9. Reed, C.E., Swanson, M.C., Agarwal, M.K., and Yunginger, J.W. 1985. Allergens that cause asthma. Identification and quantification. Chest 87:40S.
10. Musk, A.W., Venables, K.M., Crook, B., Nunn, A.J., Hawkins, R., Crook, G.D.W., Graneek, B.J., Tee, R.D., Farrer, N., Johnson, D.A., Gordon D.J., Darbyshire, J.H., and Newman-Taylor, A.J. 1989. Respiratory symptoms, lung function, and sensitisation to flour in a British bakery. Br. J. Ind. Med. 46:636.
11. Burge, P.S., Edge, G., Hawkins, R., White, V., Newman-and Taylor, A.. 1981. Occupational asthma in a factory making flux-cored solder containing colophony. Thorax 36:828.
12. Vedal, S., Chan-Yeung, M., Enarson, D., Fera, T., Maclean, L., Tse, K.S., and Langille, R. 1986. Symptoms and pulmonary function in Western red cedar workers related to duration of employment and dust exposure. Arch. Environ. Health 41:179.
13. Malo, J.L., Ghezzo, H., L'Archevêque, J., Lagier, F.., Perrin, B., and Cartier, A. 1991. Is the clinical history a satisfactory means of diagnosing occupational asthma. Am. Rev. Respir. Dis. 143:528.
14. Burge, P.S. 1982. Single and serial measurements of lung function in the diagnosis of occupational asthma. Eur. J. Respir. Dis. 63 (suppl 123):47.
15. Turner-Warwick, M. 1977. On observing patterns of airflow obstruction in chronic asthma. Br. J. Dis. Chest 71:73.
16. Burge, P.S., O'Brien, I.M., and Harries, M.G. 1979. Peak flow rate records in the diagnosis of occupational asthma due to isocyanates. Thorax 34:317.
17. Cartier, A., Pineau, L., and Malo, J.L. 1984. Monitoring of maximum expiratory peak flow rates and histamine inhalation tests in the investigation of occupational asthma. Clin. Allergy 14:193.
18. Coté, J., Kennedy, S., and Chan-Yeung, M. 1990. Sensitivity and specificity of PC20 and peak expiratory flow rate in cedar asthma. J. Allergy Clin. Immunol. 85:592.
19. Perrin, B., Malo, J.L., L'Archevêque, J., Ghezzo, H., Lagier, F., and Cartier, A. 1990. Comparison of peak expiratory flow rates and bronchial responsiveness with specific inhalation challenges in occupational asthma. Eur. Respir. J., in press.
20. Pepys, J., and Hutchcroft, B.J. 1975. Bronchial provocation tests in etiologic diagnosis and

analysis of asthma. Am. Rev. Respir. Dis. 112:829.

21. Cartier, A., Malo, J.L., and Dolovich, J. 1987. Occupational asthma in nurses handling psyllium. Clin. Allergy 17:1.
22. Butcher, B.T., Karr, R.M., O'Neil, C.E., Wilson, M.R., Dharmarajan, V., Salvaggio, J.E., and Sweill, H. 1979. Inhalation challenge and pharmacologic studies of toluene diisocyanate (TDI) sensitive workers. J. Allergy Clin. Immunol. 64:146.
23. Cloutier, Y., Lagier, F., Lemieux, R., Blais, M.C., St-Arnaud, C., Cartier, A., and Malo, J.L. 1989. New methodology for specific inhalation challenges with occupational agents in powder form. Eur. Respir. J. 2:769.
24. Cloutier, Y., Cartier, A., Vandenplas, 0., Perrin, B., Trudeau, C, and Malo, J.L. 1991. New methodology for inhalation challenges with isocyanates. J. Allergy Clin. Immunol. 87:300 (abstract).
25. Chan-Yeung, M., Lam, S., and Koener, S. 1982. Clinical features and natural history of occupational asthma due to western red cedar (Thuja plicata). Am. J. Med. 72:411 .
26. Hudson, P., Cartier, A., Pineau, L., Lafrance, M., St-Aubin, J.J., Dubois, J.Y., and Malo, J.L. 1985. Follow-up of occupational asthma caused by crab and various agents. J. Allergy Clin. Immunol. 76:682.
27. Allard, C., Cartier, A., Ghezzo, H., and Malo, J.L. 1989. Occupational asthma due to various agents. Absence of clinical and functional improvement at an interval of four or more years after cessation of exposure. Chest 96:1046.
28. Malo, J.L., Cartier, A., Ghezzo, H., Lafrance, M., Mccants, M., and Lehrer, S.B. 1988. Patterns of improvement on spirometry, bronchial hyperresponsiveness, and specific IgE antibody levels after cessation of exposure in occupational asthma caused by snow-crab processing. Am. Rev. Respir. Dis. 138:807.
29. Lam, S., LeRiche, J., Phillips, D., and Chan-Yeung, M. 1987. Cellular and protein changes in bronchial lavage fluid after late asthmatic reaction in patients with red cedar asthma. J. Allergy Clin. Immunol. 80:44.
30. Chan-Yeung, M., Chan, H., Salari, H., and Lam, S. 1989. Histamine, leukotrienes and prostaglandins release in bronchial fluid during plicatic acid-induced bronchoconstriction. J. Allergy Clin. Immunol. 84:762.
31. Chan-Yeung, M., and Lam, S. 1990. Evidence for mucosal inflammation in occupational asthma. Clin. Exper. Allergy 20:1.
32. Boschetto, P., Fabbri, L.M., Zocca, E., Milani, G., Pivirotto, F., Dal Vecchio, A.,Plebani, M., and Mapp, C.E. 1987. Prednisone inhibits late asthmatic reactions and airway inflammation induced by toluene diisocyanate in sensitized subjects. J. Allergy Clin. Immunol. 80:261.
33. Mapp, C., Boschetto, P., Dal Vecchio L., Crescioli, S., De Marzo, N., Paleari, D., and Fabbri, L.M. 1987. Protective effect of anti-asthma drugs on late asthmatic reactions and increased airway responsiveness induced by toluene diisocyanate in sensitized subjects. Am. Rev. Respir. Dis 136:1403.
34. Cartier, A., Malo, J.L., Forest, F., Lafrance, M., Pineau, L., and St-Aubin, J.J. 1984. Occupational asthma in snow crab-processing workers. J. Allergy Clin. Immunol. 74 :261.

Childhood Asthma in The Occupational Environment

Shimpei Torii*

Occupational asthma is defined as reversible airways obstruction induced by inhaled dusts, vapors, fumes and gases encountered in the workplace and should be distinguished from preexisting asthma that is exacerbated by exposure to industrial irritants. Overall prevalence of occupational asthma is difficult to determine, because the diagnosis of occupational asthma and identification of the putative agent are often difficult. The diagnostic value of careful in-depth personal, medical, and occupational history cannot be overemphasized. Occupational asthma has generally involved an occupational disease of the working man, but his family members or his neighbors who themselves are not engaged in the job many occasionally be exposed to occupational allergens carried by the working men or polluted air, and have asthma. Occupational asthma in childhood may be equivalent to asthma of non-working men provoked by occupational allergens. The diagnosis of this childhood asthma may often be more difficult than that of occupational diseases of workers by occupational allergens. We shall present several cases of this type who consulted our clinic, and report a summary of these patients from a questionnaire filled out by doctors of 10 allergy clinics, and the importance of occupational allergens in childhood asthma will be stressed.

Case Y. S., 7-Year-Old-Girl; Diagnosis: Allergic Bronchopulmonary Aspergillossis and Bronchial Asthma

She consulted N C Hospital in 1987 with a history of recurrent episodes of nocturnal cough of a 4-year duration. The cough episodes were not accompanied by any wheezing, dyspnea or febrility. Because pulmonary infiltrations on her bilateral chest roentgenogram were observed June 7, 1987, she was brought to our clinics. Peripheral blood revealed eosinophilia. Candida albicans was detected by sputum culture but no other molds. Hyper-IgE was observed, and Aspergillus fumigatus, Aspergillus orizae, Alternaria alternata, Cladosporium herbarum, Penicillium notatum and Candida albicans were strongly positive in either RAST or skin tests. Precipitating antibodies were detected to both Aspergillus fumigatus and Sapergillus orizae (A. orizae). During the period that pulmonary infiltrations and persistent cough were observed, serum IgE levels and peripheral blood eosinophil counts were elevated, and high levels of specific IgE antibody and positive precipitating antibodies to Aspergillus orizae were observed. Cough usually aggravated when she stayed at home. On August 12, the administration of predonisolone was started, and hyper-IgE and eosinophilia remarkably improved as well as her cough and chest X-ray findings. Middle of September, during reduction of the dose, her first attack of asthma occurred. Afterwards, whenever she went home, the episodes of cough, wheezing, and febrility were usually observed. She lived in the room adjacent to the bean paste manufactory. In the manufactory, steamed soybeans are mixed with rice fermented with A. orizae and, furthermore, are fermented. Since she has lived in a new house remote from the factory, the frequency of attacks has decreased. In the survey of fungi collected by the use of an air sampler, most of the colonies on the culture plate were Aspergillus orizae and 150 colonies in 54 liters of air were detected in her bedroom, as many as in the manufactory.

Case A. T., 10-Year-Old Boy; Diagnosis: Bronchial Asthma

At the age of 1 year, 6 months, he had a first attack of asthma. At the age of 9, asthma had gradually aggravated, and a poor response to

* Nagoya University, College of Medical Technology, 1-20 Daikominami-1-Chome, Higashi-Ku, Nagoya, 461, Japan.

Table 1 Occupational Allergens in Childhood Asthma

offending allergens	No. patients	related occupations
buckwheat flour	8	buckwheat noodle maker
silk	6	silk mill, or sericultural industrie
Aspergillus orizae	5	miso or soy maker
animal hair	5	writing brush maker
animal danders, or fowl droppings	3	veterinary business, or management of riding ground
rice flour	3	rice mill
hoya	3	business of shelling oysters or oyster farming
wheat flour	2	bakery
konjak flour	2	konjak industry
chips of lauan	1	sawmill
laver	1	laver processing industry

symptomatic treatment was more frequently observed. At the age of 10, we were informed that his father worked in a buckwheat noodle manufactory, and often had severe asthma attacks when he visited the manufactory. Because the indirect exposure of the buckwheat flour through the contaminated clothes or body of his father was suspected as the cause of asthma in the boy, we recommended that his father change his working uniform for different clothes and take a shower before coming home. Since this trial, the asthma remarkably improved. A RAST score revealed 3 for house dust, 3 for mites, 2 for cat, 4 for orchard grass, and 4 for buckwheat. Buckwheat noodle called "Soba" has been a very popular food for the Japanese, therefore buckwheat flour is an important inhalant as well as food allergen in Japan.

Case T. S., 2-Year, 6-Month-Old Boy; Diagnosis: Bronchial Asthma and Atopic Dermatitis

The patient has suffered from atopic dermatitis since infancy and his first attack of asthma was at the age of 1 year, 6 months. His father has worked in a horse riding club which is managed by his grandfather. He had attacks of asthma whenever he visited his grandfather's house, and one day he had a severe attack when riding a horse with his grandfather. The frequency of asthma attacks remarkably decreased when his father had a shower and changed the working uniform, which was contaminated by horse dust. Hyper-IgE and eosinophilia were observed. A RAST score revealed 4 for mites, 2 for house dust, 4 for cat, 4 for horse danders.

Table 1 shows the results on the effects of occupational allergens on children, derived from work in our clinic and from a questionnaire sent to physicians in ten allergy clinics as well as from Japanese medical literature. Twenty percent of the allergens come from buckwheat flour, and 15 percent from silk. A. orizae and animal hair, that are materials of the writing brush, account for 13 percent respectively. Buckwheat noodle is a very popular food for the Japanese and A. orizae is a fermented fungus used to make bean paste or soy that is a basic flavoring of the Japanese kitchen. Animal hairs are materials of the writing brush. These hairs come from sheep, cat, goat, horse, deer, weasel, badger, flying squirrel, pig, and skunk, and are frequently offending allergens of asthma. The work environment is not only polluted by hair dust allergen, but also stimulant gases are exhaled from the paints, the solvent, or the adhesives. Animal danders or fowl droppings are found extensively in the working environment of veterinarians or riding grounds. Table 2 shows the classification of 39 asthmatic children according to the exposure of occupational allergens. Most of the patients (72%) live near a small manufactory in their own houses. In such an environment, the exposure

Table 2 Occupational Allergy in Childhood Asthma

Patients living in a small manufactory in their own houses	28
Patients living around industrial areas	2
Patients in worker's families	9

Table 3 Allergic diathesis

atopic diaseases in their family histories or in their past histories	13
atopic diseases in their family histories and in their past histories	16
atopic diseases neither in their family histories nor in their past histories	10

of non-working persons is naturally very similar to that of the workers themselves. Twenty-three percent of the asthmatic children were family members of working men. These patients may be exposed to the allergens carried by the worker's uniform or his body, contaminated by the allergens. Most of them have atopic diathesis (Table 3). The avoidance of indirect exposure through the working uniform or working man's body and stopping the patient's access to the manufactory were sufficiently effective treatment (Table 4). These methods were only possible for children who do not make their living by working.

Conclusion

Summarizing these results, the treatment of childhood asthma in occupational environments is as follows: the first is that the patients should not live in the house adjacent to the manufactory and their access to the working place should be forbidden. Second, they should avoid indirect exposure to occupational allergens as carried by the workers. Information on the occupation(s) of a patient's other family members or his or her immediate environs certainly affords the pediatrician important clues on the offending allergens which are often overlooked while treating otherwise intractable childhood asthma.

Table 4 Effective Avoidance of Offending Allergens

effective treatment	No. patients	related occupation
changing their working uniform	4	buckwheat noodle maker
into different clothes and taking a shower before coming home	1	management of riding ground
forbidding their access to the	1	miso or soy maker
manufactory	3	silk mill or sericultural maker
	4	writing brush maker
	1	veterinary business, or oyster farming
transferring their residence far away from the manufactory	1	miso or soy maker
specific hyposensitizaton	1	distilling industry
	1	writing brush maker

Industrial Asthma

C. Raymond Zeiss*

Many fine reviews have appeared in the recent literature that document the extensive number of allergens that can cause asthma in the industrial setting (1–6). The usual focus is centered upon the worker related to a particular occupation. This presentation will focus on specific large industries in which industrial asthma has been recognized. The agents that can cause industrial asthma divide themselves into the high molecular weight (HMW) antigens and the low molecular weight/reactive chemicals that can sensitize workers in the industrial setting. The high molecular weight antigens and low molecular weight reactive chemicals that induce industrial asthma are delineated in Tables I and II. The spectrum of disease that can be induced by these agents is broad.

Table I. Occupational Asthma – High Molecular Weight Allergens

Agents	Occupation/Industry	No. of Subjects	Prevalence
Animal products, insects, others (rats, mice, rabbits, guinea pigs)	Laboratory workers Veterinarians	1487	3.1%
	Animal handlers	399	7.5%
Insects			
Locust	Research laboratory	119	26%
River fly	Power plant along rivers	1284	3.1%
Wood dust			
Western red cedar (Thuja plicata)	Carpenter, construction, cabinet maker, sawmill worker	1320 22 185	3.4%
Biologic enzymes			
B. subtilis	Detergent industry	98	50%
Trypsin	Plastics, pharmaceutical	14	29%
Vegetables			
Gums			
Gum Acacia	Printers	63	51%
Others			
Crab	Crab processing	303	16%
Prawns	Prawn processing	50	36%
Hoya	Oyster farm	1413	29%
Larva of silkworm	Sericulture	5519	0.2%

* Adapted from Cahn-Yeung M, et al., Am. Rev. Respir. Dis., 1986, 137:686.

* Department of Veterans Affairs, Lakeside Medical Center, 400 East Ontario Street, and the Department of Medicine, Section of Allergy and Immunology, Northwestern University Medical School, Chicago, Illinois USA
Acknowledgements: Supported by the Department of Veterans Affairs (Medical Research Service) and the Ernest S. Bazley Grant.

Table II. Reactive Chemical in Industrial Asthma

Class	Lung Response Chemical	Occupational Exposure	Asthma* I L R	Hyper-sensitivity Pneumonitis	Immunologic Response
Anhydrides	Phthalic anhydride	Plasticizers	+ +		IgE, ST
	Trimellitic anhydride paints, coatings	Epoxy resins, plasticizers,	+ + +		IgG, A, E, ST
	Hexahydro-phthalic anhydride	Electrical transformer production	+ +		IgE, IgG
	Tetrachloro-phthalic anhydride	Epoxy resin	+ + +		IgE
	Himic anhydride	Fire retardant	+ +		IgE, G
Diisocyanates	Toluene diisocyanate	Polyurethane foam TDI manufacture	+ + +	+	No IgE
	Diphenylmethanne diisocyanate	Foundry core-workers, polyurethane foam	+ + +	+	IgE, G
	Hexamethylene diisocyanate	Auto paint	+ +	+	IgG
Pharmaceuticals	Ampicillin	Pharmaceutical	+ +		
	Sulfonechlor-amide cotton,	Pharmaceutical, brewery	+ +		IgE
Metallic Salts					
Nickel Salts	Nickel sulfate	Metal plating	+ +		IgE
Platinum salts	Ammonium tetrachloro-platinate	Platinum refining	+ +		IgE

* I = Immediate; L = Late; R = Repititive Immunoglobulin class of antibody to anhydride (A, G, E)
ST: Skin test positive

This review will focus on the asthmatic syndromes which can be immediate, late, dual, and repetitive. In addition, these antigens can cause hypersensitivity pneumonitis and pulmonary hemorrhage (7).

Immunologic Mechanisms

The high molecular allergens can cause classic IgE mediated hypersensitivity. An intense IgE mediated reaction can lead to a dual response with the late phase reaction postulated to be secondary to the release of mediators from lung mast cells in the early phase. An IgG immune response in the lung to high molecular weight antigens can result in immune complex disease which, when accompanied by a T-cell inflammatory response, can lead to hypersensitivity pneumonitis. The reactive chemicals are not complete allergens in themselves unless they react with self-proteins to become antigenic. The reactive chemical can act as a classic hapten with the antibody response directed against the reactive chemical as hapten, or the reactive chemical can induce a confirmational change in the self-protein resulting in new antigenic determinants (NADS) to which the antibody response is directed (8). These chemicals can cause a classic IgE mediated hypersensitivity and, with an intense IgE mediated reaction in the lung, result in a late phase reaction and a dual response. The interaction of reactive

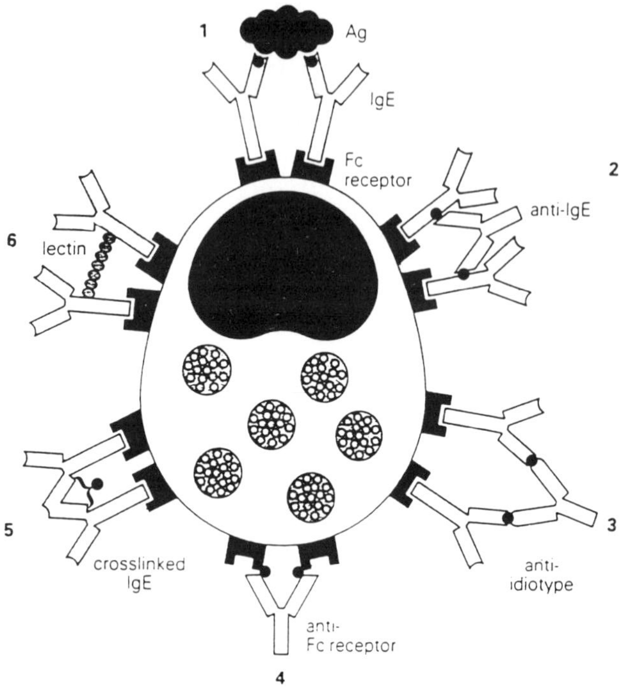

Figure 1. The possible complex interaction of a reactive chemical (●) with mast cell IgE or Fc receptor that could trigger mediator release.

chemicals with mast cell surface proteins can lead to the haptenization of IgE on the surface of the mast cell (Figure 1) with a second antibody (IgG) cross-linking haptenized IgE molecules resulting in mediator release. This is similar to mediated release induced by anti-IgE (9,10). In addition, the reactive chemical could haptenize the Fcε1 receptor with antibody directed against the modified IgE receptor and the cross-linking of these molecules by a second antibody would result in mediator release. Lastly, bifunctional reactive chemicals could cross-link IgE in respiratory secretions resulting in dimers and trimers of IgE. Dimers and trimers of IgE have been found to be potent stimuli for the release of mediators from basophils (11). In addition, reactive chemicals can modify respiratory secretion immunoglobulin, IgG and IgA, to which a self antibody response is generated resulting in immune complexes in the airway. This could lead to the syndrome that we recognize as late asthma (12) or to hypersensitivity pneumonitis if accompanied by a T-cell response to altered self antigens in the airway.

Examples of Industrial Asthma

The acid anhydrides are characteristic of a class of reactive chemicals that can cause sensitization of workers in the plastics industry. Some of the reactive anhydrides that cause significant industrial problems are listed in Table II.

Trimellitic Anhydride (TMA)

This well characterized reactive chemical has been studied by a number of investigators since the appearance of early reports of asthma due to this compound (13,14,15,16). The spectrum of lung disease that can be induced by TMA inhalation is broad (Table III) (12). TMA can cause classic immediate-onset asthma/rhinitis mediated by IgE antibody. This syndrome requires a latent period of exposure before the onset of symptoms; however, once sensitized, symptoms will occur immediately with exposure. The syndrome has been found to be mediated by IgE antibody directed against a variety of trimellityl (TM)-modified human protein conjugates. The IgE antibody is directed not only against TM acting as a hapten, but against new antigenic determinants that arise when TMA couples with self-proteins. A second immunologic syndrome, the late respiratory systemic syndrome, is characterized by cough, occasional wheezing dyspnea, mucus production, and systemic symptoms of malaise, chills, myalgias, and arthralgias occurring 4 to 12 hours after TMA inhalation exposure. The syndrome clinically resembles hypersensitivity pneumonitis and requires a latent period following exposure before the onset of symptoms. The syndrome is accompanied by elevated levels of IgG, IgA, and IgM antibody directed against TM-modified human serum albumin. Workers in several plants in Canada and United States have developed a pulmonary presentation characterized by hemoptysis, dyspnea, pulmonary infiltrates, restrictive lung disease, and anemia; it has been termed the pulmonary disease-anemia syndrome. This illness develops with high-dose TMA fume exposure, which occurs when heated metal surfaces are sprayed with TMA-containing materials. Again, the syndrome requires a latent period of exposure, with a range of clinical severity from mild to severe. High levels of IgG, IgA, and IgM antibody to TM-coupled protein and TM-conjugated erythocytes have been identified in these patients (17). In addition, several cases of isolated late asthma have been described (16). The pathogenesis of this syndrome is not clear.

The immunology of antibody directed at a variety of self-proteins has been illustrated by work with TMA. IgA and human leukemia lysozyme were reacted with TMA to give TM-modified proteins. IgA represents a major respiratory tract secretory protein, whereas lysozyme is found in trace amounts. Both IgE and IgG antibody to TM-modified human serum albumin, TM-IgA, and TM-modified human leukemia lysozyme were identified by radioimmunoassay. The antibody activity was greatest for the modified human serum albumin, next for the modified IgA, and lowest for the modified human lysozyme (2), which would be expected based on the relative amounts of these proteins found in respiratory tract secretions. In humans, the antibody specificity directed against TMA-modified proteins is directed primarily against new antigenic determinants that arise with the interaction between TMA and self-proteins such as human serum albumin. That antibody specificity was not directed against a particular amino acid-TM configuration was shown by the fact that a variety of amino acids including TM-lysine and TM-polylysine were poor inhibitors of the reaction between TM-modified human serum albumin and

Table III. Trimellitic Anhydride Pulmonary Reactions

Type	Terminology	Mechanism	TMA Reactions In Vitro or In Vivo Tests	Diseases
I	Anaphylactic, immediate type, IgE antibody mediated	IgE antibody-sensitized mast cell react with TM-protein and bioactive mediators are released	Immediate-type skin test In vitro histamine release	Asthma, rhinitis, conjunctivities
II	Cytotoxic	Antibody against hapten-cell results in cell damage or destruction	Antibodies against TM-E lyse cells in presence of complement	Anemia of pulmonary disease; anemia syndrome? Other?
III	Toxic antigen-antibody complex reaction	Immune complexes fix complement, attract polymorphonuclear leukocytes, which results in tissue damage	Experimental skin reaction	Probable cause of LRSS associated with increase in total antibody and IgG and IgA antibodies against TM proteins. Late asthma?
IV	Lymphoocyte-mediated delayed, tuberculin-type	Sensitized T lymphocytes stimulated by antigen, resulting in tissue damage	In vitro lymphocyte transformation	Uncertain; possible component of LRSS and pulmonary disease anemia syndrome

Adapted (12.)

antibody. These observations have been confirmed by other workers examining the fine specificity of IgE antibody to a variety of inhaled reactive anhydrides. NAD specificity has been shown for TMA, PA and TCPA (18,19).

Epidemiologic Studies on TMA

Zeiss and co-workers have followed workers involved in the manufacture of TMA since 1976 (13,14,15,16). These studies have been based on a voluntary surveillance program evaluating workers presenting for evaluation of TMA related respiratory symptoms. In a recent cross-sectional study (20) of the entire work force at this facility, 474 employees were surveyed in 1 year related to the presence of TMA immunologic lung disease. This study included 153 employees who had joined the previous voluntary surveillance program and 321 who had not. The prevalence of TMA immunologic lung disease was 6.8% in the total population (Table IV). In the 321 employees who had not previously been surveyed only 1.3% had a TMA related immunologic syndrome. This indicated that the voluntary surveillance program had worked well and had not missed a significant number of cases. In addition, the development of total and IgE antibody to TM-HSA was related to one of five exposure classes determined for each employee. There was a marked fall-off in mean total and IgE antibody levels with decreasing exposure. This result will allow the targeting of further environmental control measures to job classifications in the groups with the highest potential TMA exposure. Environmental control procedures have been shown to decrease the number of workers sensitized to TMA in a plant mixing TMA with resins to make coating materials (21).

TCPA

One of the largest epidemiologic surveys has been done in TCPA workers (22). In this survey of 276 workers, IgE antibody to TCPA was found in 12% of atopic subjects and 6% of non-atopics. There was a strong association of IgE to TCPA and asthma with smoking with a six-fold excess of IgE antibody to TCPA in current smokers. IgE antibody levels to TCPA have been shown to fall after removal from exposure with a half life of 1 year. Skin test reactivity persisted for over 4 years (23).

Laboratory Animal Allergens

In the health and scientific investigation industries animal allergen sensitization poses a major problem for exposed workers. This is indeed a large scale industrial problem with thousands of individuals becoming sensitized to animal allergens (Table V). In this area much has been learned about molecular characteris-

Table IV. Populations, Syndrome Classification And Antibody Levels

Syndrome	All Surveyed Employees	New Enrollees	Mean* Total Antibody	Mean* IgE Antibody
Asthma/Rhinitis	12	2	13225	3.70
LRSS	10	1	15400	0.40
LRSS (OLD HX)	5	1	0	0.00
Late Asthma	4			
LAMS	1			
Total Immunologic	32 (6.8%)	4 (1.3%)		
Irritant	150 (31.6%)	59 (18.4%)	88	0.02
None	292 (61.6%)	258 (80.3%)	91	0.01
Total Non Immunologic	442 (93.2%)	317 (98.7%)		
Total	474	321		

*IgE and total antibody levels in ng TM-HSA bound/ml of serum
LRSS: The late respiratory systemic syndrome
LRSS (OLD HX): A distant history of LRSS without current symptoms
LAMS: The late arthralgia myalgia syndrome

Table V. Prevalence Of Laboratory Animal Allergy

Number of animal workers surveyed	% Symptoms	% Asthma	% Asthma in those with symptoms
258	11.3	5	48
1293	14.7	10.4	71
474	23	9	39
625	14.5	7.4	51
399	15	7.5	50
585	19.5	3	15.3
179	27	12	44
146	30	8	26.6
144	19	7.5	39.4
121$^{\alpha}$	32.2	4	12
Mean$^{\beta}$ 455.8	19.3	7.75	42.7

$^{\alpha}$ Exposure to mice; $^{\beta}$ excluding mice only survey (Adapted from 24.)

tics of the allergens involved and in the science of the aerobiology of laboratory animal allergens (6,24).

Summary

This short review could only touch on a few examples of agents that cause industrial asthma and some progress that has been made in the study of this important area. It is clear that asthma in the industrial setting will continue to provide challenges and opportunities for internal investigation for years to come.

References

1. Pepys, J. 1984. Occupational respiratory allergy. Clin. Immunol. Allergy 4:3.
2. Zeiss, C.R. 1985. Occupational lung disease induced by reactive chemicals. Clin. Rev. Allergy. 3:217.
3. Salvaggio, J.E., Butcher, B.T., and O'Neil, C.E. 1986. Occupational asthma due to chemical agents. J. Allergy Clin. Immunol. 78:1053.
4. Chan-Yeung, M., and Lam, S. 1986. Occupational asthma. Am. Rev. Respir. Dis. 133:686.
5. Zeiss, C.R. 1989. Reactive chemicals as inhalent allergens. Immunol. Allergy Clin. N. Amer. 9:235.
6. Chan-Yeung, M. 1990. Occupational asthma. Chest 98:148.
7. Zeiss, C.R. 1991. Reactive chemicals in industrial asthma. In: Update (10): Allergy principles and practice. E. Middleton, C.E. Reed, E.F. Ellis, N.F. Adkinson, J.W. Yunginger, eds. St. Louis, MO: C.V. Mosby, p. 1.
8. Zeiss, C.R., Levitz, D., and Chacon, R. 1980. Quantitation and new antigenic determinant specificity of antibodies induced by inhalation of trimellitic anhydride in man. Int. Arch. Allergy Appl. Immunol. 61:380.
9. Akiyama, K., Pruzansky, J.J., and Patterson, R. 1984. Hapten-modified basophils: A model of human immediate hypersensitivity that can be elicited by IgG antibody. J. Immunol. 133:3286.
10. Ishizaka, T. 1981. Analysis of triggering events in mast cells for immunoglobulin E-mediated histamine release. J. Allergy Cln. Immunol. 67:90.
11. Kagey-Sobotka, A., Dembo, M., and Goldstein, G. 1981. Qualitative characteristics of histamine release from basophils by covalently cross-linked IgE. J. Immunol. 127:2285.
12. Patterson, R., Zeiss, C.R., and Pruzansky, J.J. 1982. Immunology and immunopathology of trimellitic anhydride pulmonary reactions. J. Allergy Clin. Immunol. 70:19.
13. Zeiss, C.R., Patterson, R., and Pruzansky, J.J. 1977. Trimellitic anhydride-induced airway syndromes: Clinical and immunologic studies. J. Allergy Clin. Immunol. 60:96.
14. Zeiss, C.R., Wolkonsky, P., and Chacon, R. 1983. Syndromes in workers exposed to

trimellitic anhydride. A longitudinal clinical and immunologic study. Ann. Intern. Med. 98:18.
15. Zeiss, C.R., Wolkonsky, P., Pruzansky, J.J., and Patterson, R. 1982. Clinical and immunologic evaluation of trimellitic anhydride workers in multiple industrial settings (Symposium NIH). J. Allergy Clin. Imunol. 70:15.
16. Zeiss, C.R., Mitchell, J.H., and Van Peenen, P.F.D. 1990. A twelve year clinical and immunologic evaluation of workers involved in the manufacture of trimellitic anhydride (TMA). Allergy Proc. 11:71.
17. Patterson, R., Addington, W., Banner, A.S., Byron, G.E., Franco, M., Herbert, F.A., Nicotra, M.B., Pruzansky, J.J., Rivera, M., Roberts, M., and Zeiss, C.R. 1979. Antihapten antibodies in workers exposed to trimellityl anhydride fumes: A potential immunopathogenetic mechanism for the trimellitic anhydride pulmonary disease-anemia syndrome. Am. Rev. Respir. Dis. 120:1259.
18. Topping, M.P., Venables, K.M., and Luczynska, C.M. 1986. Specificity of the human IgE response to inhaled acid anhydrides. J. Allergy Clin. Immunol. 77:834.
19. Bernstein, D.I., Gallagher, J.S., D'Souza, L., and Bernstein, I.L. 1984. Heterogeneity of specific IgE responses in workers sensitized to acid anhydride compounds. J. Allergy Clin. Immuno. 74:794.
20. Zeiss, C.R., Mitchell, J., Van Peenen, P.F.D., Grammer, L., Kavich, D., Shaughnessy, M., and Patterson, R. 1990. Evaluation of an entire chemical plant related to trimellitic anhydride (TMA) exposure. J. Allergy Clin. Immunol. 85:190.
21. Bernstein, D.I., Roach, D.E., McGrath, K., Zeiss, C.R., and Patterson, R. 1983. The relationship of airborne trimellitic anhydride concentrations to trimellitic anhydride induced symptoms and immune responses. J. Allergy Clin. Immunol. 72:709.
22. Venables, K.M., Topping, M.D., Howe, W., Lucznska, C.M., Hawkins, R., and Newman Taylor, A.J. 1985. Interaction of smoking and atopy in producing specific IgE antibody against a hapten protein conjugate. Br. Med. J. 290:201.
23. Venables, K.M., Topping, M.D., Nunn, A.J., Howe, W., and Newman Taylor, A.J. 1987. Immunological and functional consequences of clinical tetrachlorophthalic anhydride induced asthma after four years of avoidance of exposure. J. Allergy Clin. Immunol. 80:212.
24. Longbottom, J.L. 1984. Occupational allergy due to animal allergens. Clin Immunol. Allergy. 4:19.

Section VI

Diagnosis and Monitoring of Allergic Diseases

Serological Diagnosis of Allergy

S. G. O. Johansson, Marianne van Hage-Hamsten*

In 1921 Prausnitz and Küstner demonstrated that atopic allergy was mediated by a serum factor, later called reagin. In the late 1960's it was shown that reagins belonged to a unique immunoglobulin class, IgE (1). Access to IgE and antibodies to IgE made it possible to develop the first sensitive immunoassays for *in vitro* diagnosis of allergy based on determination of IgE and IgE antibodies to allergens (2). The classical approach to the diagnosis of atopic allergy was based on case history and skin tests, performed by extracts of material eliciting allergic symptoms. However, due to difficulties in measuring allergen potency accurately by *in vivo* systems, essentially non-standardized and non-characterized allergen preparations were used for diagnosis and treatment for well over 100 years. Thus, access to *in vitro* assays allowing both allergy diagnosis and allergen extract standardization had a significant impact on the clinical practice of allergology. Hypersensitivity symptoms from the mucosal membranes and the skin are very common in industrialized countries. Epidemiological studies indicate prevalences in the order of 40–50%. Almost half of this figure is due to true allergy, that is, disorders mediated by immunological mechanisms. By far the most common type of allergy is classical allergy, usually referred to as atopic allergy which by itself has a prevalence in the order of 20–30%.

The problem we are facing when trying to identify the population at risk for atopic allergy is that, although a rather small number of allergens is responsible for the great majority of allergic reactions, the total number of allergens involved is probably in the order of 300–400. Information about which allergen to suspect can sometimes be obtained from the case history, but quite often the case history is difficult to interpret. There are several reasons why the case history provides insufficient information to allow for proper diagnosis: the symptoms of allergy and non-allergic hypersensitivity are essentially identical; in cases of chronic exposure it is almost impossible to detect an exacerbation of symptoms upon contact with the allergen; many patients are sensitive to multiple allergens of varying clinical importance, and for rare allergens it is very difficult for the clinician to have gathered enough experience to evaluate the information obtained from the patient. Because of the very high number of individuals with symptoms, it is also difficult to create a medical organization which enables every patient to contact a specialist. Many countries have developed procedures that include a primary screening performed by non-allergy-specialists such as general practitioners and family doctors who will then, whenever necessary, refer the patient to an allergy specialist. Serological tests based on IgE are useful for that purpose. We describe here one approach with which we have had satisfying experience.

Screening for Atopy

The first step in the identification of a patient with hypersensitivity symptoms that can be considered allergic is to establish whether the patient has an atopic constitution and therefore whether symptoms are likely to be due to IgE-mediated allergy. Such a differential diagnosis can be made *in vitro* by determining the total IgE serum concentration, or by detecting the presence of IgE antibodies to any common inhalant allergen. Since atopy is defined as IgE sensitization to at least one common allergen, a test based on the detection of IgE antibodies to common allergens should have a very high correlation to atopic allergy. The recently introduced multiallergen mix RAST disc or CAP

* Department of Clinical Immunology, Karolinska Hospital, S-104 01 Stockholm, Sweden.
Acknowledgements: This work was supported in part by grants from the Swedish Medical Research Council (16X-105), the Swedish Heart-Lung Foundation, the Swedish Work Environment Fund (project no. 83-1182, 89-0506) and the Karolinska Institute.

(Phadiatop®, Pharmacia Diagnostics, Uppsala, Sweden) contains 10–15 common inhalant allergens. Thus, in one single immunoassay test it is possible to detect a sensitization to one or several common allergens and then to classify the individual as atopic or non-atopic. A suitable combination of several allergen mixes, each containing a lesser number of allergens, could serve the same purpose. Since the test is designed on the basis of the definition of atopy it is not surprising that clinical trials have shown excellent correlations to the final diagnosis of atopic allergy (Table I). Both sensitivity and specificity figures are usually higher than 90% (3). The Phadiatop® can be used not only to single out allergic individuals among those with hypersensitivity symptoms but also to exclude a possible IgE-mediated mechanism underlying the symptoms of a patient undergoing an allergy investigation.

When the very first IgE quantitations were performed it was already noticed that patients with allergic asthma and rhinitis had an increased IgE concentration in serum (4). These findings have since been confirmed and extended, and today it is well established that a significant proportion of patients with atopic diseases have an increased IgE-level. The serum IgE concentration is related to the degree of allergen exposure, since the more the immune system is stimulated by allergens, the more IgE is produced. Accordingly, the highest IgE levels in a case of hayfever are usually found some weeks after the peak of the pollen season. In contrast, atopic patients sensitized to one single allergen to which they are only rarely exposed quite often have normal IgE levels. Other complications are the high concentrations of IgE found in helminth infestations and the modulating effects of certain viral infections as well as smoking (5). Thus, the sensitivity of a total IgE determination is rather low while the specificity is fairly good. On the other hand, this is the only test available which can discriminate atopic allergy from non-allergic hypersensitivity that is not dependent on the specificity of the sensitization. This fact should be taken advantage of in cases where less common allergens are suspected or when atypical symptoms occur. A total IgE determination is especially useful in the diagnosis of occupational allergy and food allergy, or in other similar circumstances.

IgE Antibodies

The presence in serum of IgE antibodies specific to an allergen can be quantitatively determined by the RAST test (2). A well standardized RAST test has an excellent sensitivity, and the result shows a strong correlation with the final allergy diagnosis. Technically false positive or negative results are rare and mainly due to inadequately standardized allergen preparations or non-specific trapping of IgE when sera with several thousand kU/l of IgE are tested. Recently the CAP test (Pharmacia CAP System, Pharmacia Diagnostics, Uppsala) was introduced. In CAP a solid phase with a highly increased allergen capacity is used which leads to less interference of non-IgE antibodies and a higher sensitivity (7% more patients with IgE antibodies are detected) without loss of specificity (6).

Because of the very large number of possible allergens it is sometimes difficult for the physician to ask the appropriate question when requesting a RAST test. Therefore, mixed allergen preparations have been developed. They can have a composition typical for a geographic region or they might mirror the occurrence of the most common allergens in a particular microenvironment such as a particular occupational setting. Carefully selected and well

Table I. Atopic individuals can be identified from an increased serum IgE level or the presence of IgE antibodies to common allergens.

	Total IgE[1]	Specific IgE[2]
Sensitivity	Low (20%)	Very high (> 90%)
Specificity	Good (60%)	Very High (> 90%)
Efficiency	Moderate (40%)	Very high (90%)

1) Independent of allergen specificity
2) Inhalation allergy to common allergens (Phadiatop®)

characterized allergen mixes will not only simplify the diagnostic procedure but also increase the accuracy, since in the case of a negative RAST test one could exclude not only a specific sensitization, but also an atopic constitution, of the patient. The final step in the allergy diagnosis is to determine the allergen specificity of the IgE-sensitization. This information is of course necessary (a) for allergen specific immunotherapy but also (b) for initiation of more specific preventive measures in families with an allergic child or (c) for motivating an allergic patient to invest time and money in extensive allergen avoidance programs. A patient who is concerned about his allergic disease has the right to know which allergens he is sensitized to, and this information will increase his willingness to participate in treatment regimens.

However, although the occurrence of IgE antibodies is an indication of a specific sensitization, it is not necessarily the same as the presence of clinically relevant symptoms. There are so many biological and psychological reasons for the presence or absence of symptoms in a particular environment that one should not expect a single immunological factor to provide the complete pattern. As with all other *in vitro* test procedures, it is the conclusion of the experienced physician considering all available information that represents the final diagnosis. In contrast to many other immunological tests, there is, however, a remarkably good correlation between the presence of IgE antibodies in serum and clinically relevant disease. The several hundred allergens available today for RAST testing not only represent classical inhalation and food allergens but also drugs, chemicals and occupational allergens. Thousands of scientific articles have been published on this issue since the very first report of the radioallergosorbent test, RAST (2), in 1967. We will give just a few examples of allergens that we have been working with recently without any ambition for giving a representative review of the field.

For several years now our group has studied the importance of IgE-mediated allergy in occupational settings. Occupational allergens are found among plant and animal materials, chemicals, metals and pharmaceuticals (Table II). Examples of potent allergens are green coffee bean, castor bean, experimental animals, storage mites, silk work, fish feed, diisocyanates, phthalic anhydrides, formaldehyde, psyllium

Table II. Some occupational allergens available in RAST

Animal material	*Plant Material*
Mouse	Sesame seed
Rat	Cotton seed
Rabbit	Castor bean
Feathers	Green coffee
	Silk
Mites and Insects	Latex
Storage mites	Ficus Benjamina
A. siro	
L. destructor	*Chemicals*
T. putrescentiae	Isocyanates
G. domesticus	TDI
Insects	MDI
Cockroach	HDI
Mosquitos	Anhydrides
Chironomi	PA
	TMA
Drugs	Ethylene oxide
Penicillin	Chloramine T
Isphagula	Formaldehyde
Moulds	

(ispaghula) and antibiotics. Allergy to all these allergens can be detected by RAST. Allergic and hypersensitive reactions to metals such as nickel and chromium are cell mediated, while the mechanisms behind reactions to platinum salts are still unclear.

In northern Europe it has become very popular to keep green plants indoors during the winter. Professional plant keeping companies take care of the plants. Among those plant keepers a large proportion were found to have developed IgE mediated allergy to weeping fig (Ficus Benjamina), a non-pollinating ficus plant (7). Our hypothesis is that dust which has settled on the leaves gets impregnated by sap proteins from the tree and when the dust is airborne and inhaled, the sensitization to proteins from the sap might occur.

Occupational allergy to latex is another example of IgE antibody production to proteins from the sap of trees (8), in this case not a ficus but the rubber tree Hevea braziliensis. Despite the rather rough treatment involved in the production of latex gloves, which includes heating to over 100°C, there is enough protein contamination from the original sap to induce an IgE-mediated allergy usually presenting as contact urticaria. Although allergy to latex can be considered as an occupational allergy among medical personnel, many cases have also been reported among other people with intimate, irregular contact with latex, such as patients developing shock when undergoing dentistry or reacting during surgical and gynecological investigations, and children reacting when playing with balloons. Recently, the FDA in the USA issued a Medical Alert warning physicians and health care personnel to be on the look out for latex-allergic patients.

Farming is an occupation involving hundreds of millions of people in the world. At a farm, one is exposed not only to common inhalant allergens in large amounts, but also to special allergens such as cattle-dander, grain flour and insects. Apparently allergy to pollens and other common allergens is not frequent among farmers (9). Instead, a very large proportion is allergic to storage mites. In our investigations storage mites were the most common allergens, responsible for more than 1/3 of all allergic reactions (10). In addition to the classic house dust mite, there are about 40,000 other species of mites known, few of which have been studied so far. Since storage mites have been detected not only in farms but also in ordinary homes (11), they are also likely to be of general importance.

Another area in which serological investigations of IgE are of value is in the definition of clinical entities. Studies of IgE levels in patients with "atopic dermatitis" indicated that this diagnosis, like asthma, included multiple disease entities with different mechanisms but similar symptoms (12). The majority of the cases seem to be IgE-mediated and thus constitute cases of true atopic dermatitis, while the others may resemble a form of "intrinsic atopic dermatitis". A change of the eczema nomenclature would be useful. Patients with true atopic eczema, especially chronic cases with high IgE levels, are often sensitized to Pityrosporum orbiculare (also called P. ovale) (13), a yeast present on the skin of most adults. The eczema may possibly be initiated by IgE antibodies to classical inhalation and food allergens, becoming chronic by IgE sensitization to P. orbiculare allergens penetrating the damaged skin.

Future Aspects

Some recent technical developments are likely to improve the diagnostic value of IgE antibody determination in serum. The introduction of modified RAST procedures such as the CAP system (which, compared to classical RAST, have an increased amount of allergen in each test) will allow a more accurate quantitative determination of the IgE antibody concentration. Some studies indicate that such an assay can detect a quantitative relationship between the sum of a patient's IgE antibodies and the severity of his allergic disease (14). Further studies are necessary to confirm and extend this hypothesis.

Using monoclonal antibodies to individual allergens as capture antibodies in a modified RAST (15), it is possible to specify the sensitization to the presence or absence of IgE antibodies to defined major and minor allergens. As an example, allergy to house dust mites can now be described in terms of concentrations of IgE antibodies to defined allergens like Der pI, Der pII and Der fI. This will certainly lead to an improved resolution of the serologic characterization of allergy, but whether it will strengthen the impact of clinical diagnostics is not yet known.

References

1. Bennich, H., Ishizaka, K., Johansson, S.G.O., Rowe, D.S., Stanworth, D.R., and Terry, W.D. 1968. Immunoglobulin E, a new class of human immunoglobulin. Bull. WHO. 38:151.
2. Wide, L., Bennich, H., and Johansson, S.G.O. 1967. Diagnosis of allergy by an in-vitro test for allergen antibodies. Lancet ii:1105.
3. Duc, J., Peitrequin, R., and Pécoud, A. 1988. Value of a new screening test for respiratory allergy. Allergy 43:332.
4. Johansson, S.G.O. 1967. Raised levels of a new immunoglobulin class (IgND) in asthma. Lancet ii:951.
5. Johansson, S.G.O. 1981. The clinical significance of IgE. In: Clinical immunology update. Reviews for physicians. E.C. Franklin, ed. New York: Elsevier, p 123.
6. Ewan, P.W., and Coote, D. 1990. Evaluation of a capsulated hydrophilic carrier polymer (the ImmunoCAP) for measurement of specific IgE antibodies. Allergy 45:22.
7. Axelsson, I.G.K., Johansson, S.G.O., and Zetterström, O. 1987. Occupational allergy to weeping fig in plant keepers. Allergy 42:161.
8. Axelsson, I.G.K., Johansson, S.G.O., and

Wrangsjö, K. 1987. IgE-mediated anaphylactoid reactions to rubber. Allergy 42:46.
9. Van Hage-Hamsten, M., Johansson, S.G.O., and Zetterström, O. 1987. Predominance of mite allergy over allergy to pollens and animal danders in a farming population. Clinical Allergy 17:417.
10. Van Hage-Hamsten, M., Johansson, S.G.O., Höglund, S., Tüll, P., Wirén, A., and Zetterström, O. 1985. Storage mite allergy is common in a farming population. Clinical Allergy 15:555.
11. Korsgaard, J., Dahl, R., Iversen, M., and Hallas, T. 1985. Storage mites as a cause of bronchial asthma in Denmark. Allergol. et Immunopathol. 13:143.
12. Öhman, S., and Johansson, S.G.O. 1974. Immunoglobulins in atopic dermatitis with special reference to IgE. Acta Dermatovener. 54:193.
13. Nordvall, S.L., and Johansson S. 1990. IgE Antibodies to Pityrosporum orbiculare in children with atopic diseases. Acta Paediatr. Scand. 79:343.
14. Zimmerman, B. 1988. Atopic burden (specific IgE) and severity of allergic disease in children. In: Clinical workshop IgE antibodies and the Pharmacia CAP System in allergy diagnosis. S.G.O. Johansson, ed. Uppsala: Pharmacia Diagnostics AB, p. 29.
15. Ansotegui, I.J., Härfast, B., Jeddi-Tehrani, M., Johansson, E., Johansson, S.G.O., van Hage-Hamsten, M., and Wigzell, H. 1991. Identification of a new major allergen of 39 kilodaltons of the storage mite Lepidoglyphus destructor. Immunology Letters 27:127.

Mast Cell Products in the Monitoring of Allergic Inflammation

Ilkka T. Harvima, Lawrence B. Schwartz*

Mast cells and basophils are the two principal cell types that initiate immediate-type allergic reactions. These cells are also capable of generating and regulating tissue inflammation. Mast cells are most abundant in tissues near the interface between host and external environment such as skin, lung and intestine. IgE-dependent activation of mast cells results in secretion of preformed mediators that reside in secretory granules, and of newly generated mediators including those that are derived from arachidonic acid and those that fall under the rubric of cytokines, as shown in Figure 1 (1). Degranulation is the primary manifestation of mast cell activation; production of selected lipid and cytokine mediators might not occur with non-IgE-dependent forms of activation or because of various pharmacologic interventions. Histamine is the primary mediator of the immediate humoral response to mast cell activation; but lipids such as PGD_2 and LTC_4 also may participate. These lipids, cytokines and possibly granule proteases may initiate the late cellular response. The phlogistic capability of mast cells may be particularly relevant to diseases such as chronic eczema, psoriasis, scleroderma, rheumatoid arthritis, and atopic asthma where mast cell activation, hyperplasia or both have been observed.

Indicators of Mast Cell Activation

A clinically practical test to evaluate mast cell activation depends on the specificity and sensitivity of the assay. Both newly-generated lipids and granule-derived mediators of mast cells have been used to monitor mast cell activation (Table I). Maximal production of LTC_4 and PGD_2 normally occurs within the first 5 to 15 minutes after mast cell activation. But LTC_4 also is synthesized by monocytes, eosinophils, and basophils, and therefore lacks cell speci-

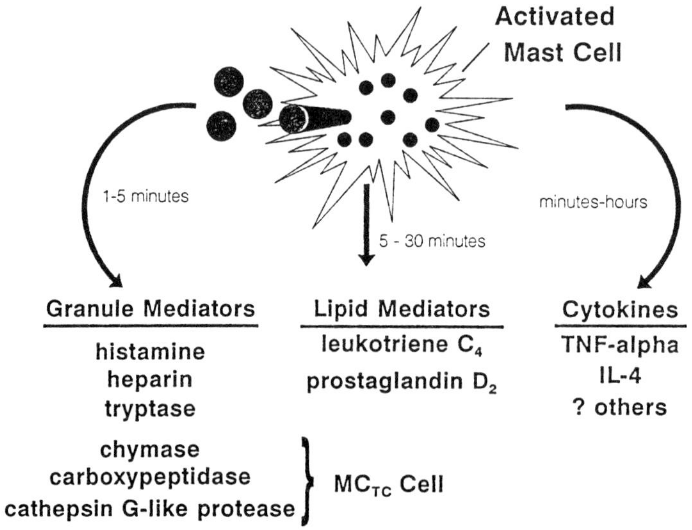

Figure 1: The major mediators produced by activated human mast cells.

* Department of Internal Medicine, Medical College of Virginia, Virginia Commonwealth University, Richmond, Virginia 23298, USA.

Table I Potential Mediators for Measuring Mast Cell Activation *In Vivo*

Mediator	Properties
HISTAMINE	Stored preformed in granules of all mast cells & basophils Half-life of minutes in the circulation Bacterial and food sources Sensitive immunoassay
TRYPTASE	Stored preformed in granules of all mast cells Half-life of about 2 hours in the circulation Immunoassay
HEPARIN	Stored preformed in granules of all mast cells Concentration half-life of minutes in the circulation Lacking satisfactory assay
PROSTAGLANDIN D_2	Newly-generated by mast cells and antigen processing cells Half-life of minutes in the circulation Immunoassay
LEUKOTRIENE C_4	Newly-generated by mast cells, basophils, eosinophils and macrophages Half-life of minutes in the circulation Immunoassay for sulfidopeptide leukotrienes or GC/mass spectrophotmeter

ficity. Normal basophils synthesize LTC_4 but not PGD_2 (2); absent PGD_2 in the presence of elevated levels of histamine and LTC_4 thereby suggesting basophil activation (Table I). Elevated levels of histamine and PGD_2 have been detected in the venous blood after induced urticarial reactions (3), in nasal lavage fluid after allergen challenge (4), and in bronchoalveolar lavage fluid after allergen challenge (5). The half-life of PGD_2 in the blood circulation is short, about 2 min (3), restricting its practical clinical use. Also, PGD_2 may be blocked by acetylsalicylates without affecting degranulation, and activation of mast cells by nonimmunologic secretogogues such as C3a cause degranulation without lipid mediator production. Finally, antigen-processing cells such as Langerhans' cells exhibit high levels of PGD synthase (5) suggesting these cells are the source for PGD_2 released during hypersensitivity reactions. Thus, ambiguity as to the cell source of PGD_2 and its sensitivity are problematic for routine clinical use.

Histamine is a widely used indicator of immediate-type hypersensitivity reactions. Normal concentrations of histamine are $\leq 5\,nM$ in plasma, 6 to 24 μg/cc of human dermis and 15 to 40 μg/cc of lung (6). In lavage fluids from the nose, lung and other sites, normal levels of histamine depend on dilution as well as local rates of production and removal. Elevated levels of histamine are detected in plasma of cold urticaria subjects after cold challenge (5,7), after anaphylaxis (8), and in subjects with systemic mastocytosis (9,10). Elevated levels of histamine are also detected during the late phase of cutaneous allergic reactions (11) and in bronchoalveolar lavage fluid taken from subjects with chronic asthma (12). However, several factors impede the use of histamine levels as a practical test for allergic reactions. Histamine is present in basophils as well as mast cells, and it can be released from both cell types by similar mechanisms. During blood clotting, small amounts of histamine released from basophils result in marked elevations in levels of extracellular histamine. Histamine turnover is rapid, with a half-life of minutes in the circulation due to diffusion, degradation, and renal excretion. Histamine also can be produced and secreted by other cell types (13). Thus, in complex biologic fluids, the cell source of histamine is ambiguous; carefully collected specimens are necessary to prevent artifactual elevations in detected levels and there is a narrow window of time for collecting samples. Heparin proteoglycan is present predominantly in mast cells, and it could serve as a specific indicator of mast cell activation. However, a suitably specific and sensitive assay is not available.

Neutral Proteinases of Mast Cells

Neutral proteinases of mast cells have the greatest potential utility for indicating mast cell involvement in clinical events because of their abundant and selective presence in mast cell secretory granules. Several neutral proteases have been localized to human mast cells (14). These include the serine proteinases, tryptase, chymase, and cathepsin G-like protease, and the Zn-dependent exopeptidase, carboxypeptidase. Human mast cells have been subclassified into two types based on the presence of neutral proteases. MC_T cells contain only tryptase, whereas MC_{TC} cells contain both chymase, carboxypeptidase, cathepsin G-like protease and tryptase. Ultrastructurally, the distinguishing features of mast cell subtypes are granules rich in scrolls in MC_T cells and granules with gratings or lattices in MC_{TC} cells (15,16). The tissue distribution of each type of mast cell is also characteristic. Mast cells in the skin and intestinal submucosa are predominantly of the MC_{TC} type, whereas those of lung and intestinal mucosa are mostly of the MC_T type.

High tryptase levels have been measured in cutaneous MC_{TC} cells (35 pg/cell) and pulmonary MC_T cells (10 pg/cell). Tryptase is selectively localized to mast cells; peripheral blood basophils contain negligible amounts of tryptase (0.04 pg/cell) (17). The content of chymase in cutaneous MC_{TC} cells is 4.5 pg/cell, whereas levels of carboxypeptidase and cathepsin G-like protease are estimated to be in a range of 3 to 20 pg/MC_{TC} cell.

At least two genes, called α and β, for tryptase have been identified on human chromosome 16. Several highly homologous cDNA molecules corresponding to β-tryptase have been cloned and sequenced (18–20), but their cellular distribution among different mast cell types, translation into functional protein, and the heteromeric nature of catalytically active enzyme molecules are not known. The different gene organization, chromosomal localization and cDNA sequences between tryptase, chymase (21) and carboxypeptidase (22) indicate that these major mast cell proteinases are distant by evolutionary criteria although they all are packaged in mast cell secretory granules.

Tryptase as an Indicator of Mast-Cell Activation

The utility of measuring levels of tryptase as a clinical indicator of mast cell involvement has been evaluated in several studies. Such measurements do not distinguish between different mast cell types, but do distinguish mast cells from basophils and other cell types. The immunoassay used currently to measure levels of tryptase employs one murine monoclonal antibody for capture and another for detection, each antibody recognizing a different epitope (23). The epitopes recognized by these antibodies appear to be present in both α and β tryptase molecules, because these antibodies bind to the corresponding recombinant α and β proteins. The sensitivity of this assay in serum is 1 ng/ml, and it also is applicable to plasma, tears, bronchoalveolar lavage fluid, nasal lavage fluid, tears, saliva, blister fluid, and skin chamber lavage fluid. Immunoreactive tryptase in serum is stable to freeze-thawing and to incubation at room temperature for at least 4 days.

Tryptase in the Circulation

Tryptase is released together with histamine from activated mast cells (24), but it diffuses more slowly through tissues from the activation site than histamine, presumably because it resides in association with heparin and chondroitin sulfate E proteoglycans in a macromolecular complex. This is the probable reason that the appearance of tryptase in plasma is delayed in relation to histamine during systemic anaphylaxis. For example, histamine levels are maximal at 5 minutes, whereas tryptase levels are maximal at 60–120 minutes after bee sting-induced anaphylaxis (8). Reactions induced by intravenous introduction of the secretogogue, such as those seen during induction of anesthesia, may result in peak levels of tryptase occurring within 30 minutes of exposure. Tryptase levels then decline with a half-life of 1.5 to 2.5 hours. Thus, blood samples for determination of tryptase levels for the diagnosis of allergic reactions can be collected over a relatively wide time range (15 minutes to at least 4 hours after onset of clinical response), whereas samples for histamine and PGD_2 assays should be obtained within 10 to 15 minutes.

Elevated levels of plasma tryptase have

been observed in about 50% of systemic mastocytosis patients during asymptomatic periods (25), and in a higher percentage during disease exacerbations. Serum tryptase levels higher than 5 ng/ml distinguish systemic anaphylaxis from non-allergic and mild or local allergic reactions in live subjects and those higher than 10 ng/ml in post-mortem samples (26). For example, tryptase levels in serum in suspected cases of anaphylaxis during hypotensive episodes induced by general anaesthesia are a more precise diagnostic test than clinical presentation (27). Also the tryptase levels in post-mortem sera examined in possible cases of fatal anaphylaxis appear to accurately indicate whether ante-mortem mast-cell activation had occurred.

Tryptase in Airways

The involvement of mast cells in diseases of the airways has been evaluated by measurements of tryptase levels in bronchoalveolar lavage fluid. Increased tryptase levels are found in lavage fluids after endobronchial allergen challenge of atopic subjects with and without asthma, but not in fluids of non-atopic subjects (28). Furthermore, tryptase levels were elevated at baseline in atopic subjects with asthma, indicating ongoing mast cell activation. In another study, tryptase levels in bronchoalveolar lavage fluid 12 minutes and 48 hours after single endobronchial challenge of atopic subjects without asthma at different doses of allergen were examined (12). Tryptase levels increased in a dose-response fashion at the 12 minute time point, but had returned to baseline by 48 hours. Histamine levels also increased at the 12 minute time point, but then remained above baseline at 48 hours. Levels of eosinophils and eosinophil mediators were elevated only at 48 hours. Thus, mast cells, but not basophils and eosinophils, are activated in the early response to allergen, whereas the reverse is true for the late response. The evidence for persistent degranulating activity in the airways of subjects with atopic asthma, in contrast to the lack of such activity during the late phase response to allergen challenge, suggests that the inflammatory state of the airway in asthma is special.

In contrast to allergen-induced asthma of atopic subjects, evidence for mast cell involvement in exercise-induced asthma of atopic subjects is lacking. Levels of tryptase, histamine, PGD_2 and LTC_4 in bronchoalveolar lavage fluid after exercise were not elevated above prechallenge baseline levels (29). As for allergen, aspirin-induced upper respiratory reactions involve mast cells, because elevated levels of tryptase have been detected in sera after aspirin challenge (30). However, only those patients with reactions that extended beyond the respiratory tract to include skin and intestine showed increased tryptase levels. In addition, rhinovirus infection in atopic rhinitis patients results in increased amounts of tryptase and histamine being released after bronchial allergen challenge and the appearance of a late phase airway response, suggesting that virus infection augments the mast cell response to allergen (31). In nasal lavage fluid tryptase has also been found to be released in atopic patients with allergic rhinitis after allergen challenge. Here the advantage of tryptase over histamine is that tryptase levels in lavage fluids show less variability at baseline and correlate better than histamine with the clinical response to allergen challenge (32).

Tryptase in Skin

Tryptase is released together with histamine into skin chamber fluid after local challenge of sensitive subjects with allergen for 1 hour (11). Levels of both mediators are maximal within the first hour and then decline to baseline. Rechallenge of the skin site with allergen 5 hours later results in release of histamine but not tryptase. When the skin is challenged continuously with allergen for several hours tryptase levels peak at 1 hour and then progressively decline to baseline by 5 hours. In contrast, histamine levels fall from their initial peak level to a plateau that remains above baseline for at least 5 hours with continuous antigen exposure (14,39). Both the release of histamine upon rechallenge with allergen and during the plateau phase with continuous exposure to allergen are inhibited by pretreatment with glucocorticosteroids, whereas the immediate release of histamine and of tryptase are unaffected (33). The steroid sensitive histamine appears to be derived from basophils that are recruited to the site where they are then activated by allergen. Although the predominant type of mast cell in human skin is the MC_{TC} cell, variable numbers of MC_T cells may be found in atopic dermatitis, scleroderma and keloids.

Conclusion

Among the indicators of mast cell activation of potential use to clinicians, only tryptase provides the specificity needed. Tryptase levels clearly reflect mast cell involvement, not that of other cell types, including basophils. Although current levels of sensitivity are adequate for detecting systemic reactions due to mast cell activation, local or mild systemic reactions are likely to yield levels of tryptase that are undetectable. High levels of circulating tryptase also are detected in a portion of patients with systemic mastocytosis during asymptomatic periods, presumably due to the turnover of increased numbers of mast cells. The current immunoassay measures levels of immunoreactive tryptase in physiologic salt solutions and in complex biological samples. Drugs, protease inhibitors and heparin do not interfere with the assay. Because tryptase is stored in all mast cell subtypes, it cannot be used to distinguish between MC_{TC} and MC_T cells. Rather, an assay for chymase or mast cell carboxypeptidase would be useful for assessing MC_{TC} involvement. An analogous potential marker for MC_T cells has not yet been identified. Basophil involvement also is difficult to assess. Histamine levels, when elevated in the absence of detectable tryptase or PGD_2, suggest basophil involvement. But proof requires demonstration of basophils at the site of inflammation, as performed in the skin (11,34) and nose (35). Unfortunately, no one mediator has been found to date that can serve as a specific indicator of basophil activation.

Based on measurements of tryptase levels near tissue sites of allergen challenge, mast cell degranulation occurs during the immediate response to allergen challenge, but not during the late response. Whether mast cells become dormant, enter into a recovery phase or persist in an activated state involving cytokine or lipid mediator production during the late phase response is not clear. In summary, tryptase measurements provide a valuable and practical indication of mast cell degranulation for the precise diagnosis of systemic anaphylaxis and for revealing involvement of mast cells in various forms of inflammation.

References

1. Schwartz, L.B., and Huff, T.F. 1991. Mast cells. In: The lung: Scientific foundations. R.G. Crystal, J.B. West, P.J. Barmes, N.S. Cherniack, and E.R. Weibel, eds. New York: Raven Press, p. 601.
2. MacGlashan, D.W., Jr., Peters, S.P., Warner, J., and Lichtenstein, L.M. 1986. Characteristics of human basophil sulfidopeptide leukotreine release: Releasability defined as the ability of basophils to respond to dimeric cross-links. J. Immunol. 136:2231.
3. Heavey, D.J., Kobza-Black, A., Barrow, S.E., Chappell, G.C., Greaves, M.W., and Dollery, C.T. 1986. Prostaglandin D2 and histamine release in cold urticaria. J. Allergy Clin. Immunol. 78:458.
4. Pipkorn, U., Proud, D., Lichtenstein, L.M., Schleimer, R.P., Peters, S.P., Adkinson, N.F., Jr., Kagey-Sobotka, A., Norman, P.S., and Naclerio, R.M. 1987. Effect of short-term systemic glucocorticoid treatment on human nasal mediator release after antigen challenge. J. Clin. Invest. 80:957.
5. Murray, J.J., Tonel, A.B., Brash, A.R., Roberts, L.J., Gosset, P., Workman, R., Capron, A., and Oates, J.A. 1986. Release of prostaglandin D2 into human airways during acute antigen challenge. N. Engl. J. Med. 315:800.
6. Harvima, R.J., Harvima, I.T., and Fraki, J.E. 1988. Optimization of histamine radio enzyme assay with purified histamine-N-methyltransferase. Clin. Chim. Acta 171:247.
7. Wasserman, S.I., Soter, N.A., Center, D.M., and Austen, K.F. 1977. Cold urticaria. Recognition and characterization of a neutrophil chemotactic factor which appears in serum during experimental cold challenge. J. Clin. Invest. 60:189.
8. Schwartz, L.B., Yunginger, J.W., Miller, J.S., Bokhari, R., and Dull, D. 1989. The time course of appearance and disappearance of human mast cell tryptase in the circulation after anaphylaxis. J. Clin. Invest. 83:1551.
9. Kettelhut, B.V., and Metcalfe, D.D. 1987. Plasma histamine concentrations in evaluation of pediatric mastocytosis. J. Pediatr. 111:419.

10. Rosenbaum, R.C., Frieri, M., and Metcalfe, D.D. 1984. Patterns of skeletal scintigraphy and their relationship to plasma and urinary histamine levels in systemic mastocytosis. J. Nuc. Med. 25:859.
11. Shalit, M., Schwartz, L.B., Golzar, N., von Allman, C., Valenzano, M., Fleekop, P., Atkins, P.C., and Zweiman, B. 1988. Release of histamine and tryptase *in vivo* after prolonged cutaneous challenge with allergen in humans. J. Immunol. 141:821.
12. Sedgwick, J.B., Calhoun, W.J., Gleich, G.J., Kita, H., Abrams, J.S., Schwartz, L.B., Volovitz, B., Ben-Yaakov, M., and Busse, W.W. 1991. Immediate and late airway response of allergic rhinitis patients to segmental antigen challenge: Characterization of eosinophil and mast cell mediators. Am. Rev. Respir. Dis. 144:1274.
13. Oh, C., Suzuki, S., Nakashima, I., Yamashita, K., and Nakano, K. 1988. Histamine synthesis by non-mast cells through mitogen-dependent induction of histidine decarboxylase. Immunology 65:143.
14. Irani, A.A., and Schwartz, L.B. 1990. Neutral proteases as indicators of human mast cell heterogeneity. In: Neutral proteases of mast cells. L.B. Schwartz, ed. Basel: Karger, p. 146.
15. Craig, S.S., Schechter, N.M., and Schwartz, L.B. 1988. Ultrastructural analysis of human T and TC mast cells identified by immunoelectron microscopy. Lab. Invest. 58:682.
16. Craig, S.S., and Schwartz, L.B. 1990. Human MC_{TC} type of mast cell granule: The uncommon occurrence of discrete scrolls associated with focal absence of chymase. Lab. Invest. 63:581.
17. Castells, M.C., Irani, A.M., and Schwartz, L.B. 1987. Evaluation of human peripheral blood leukocytes for mast cell tryptase. J. Immunol. 138:2184.
18. Miller, J.S., Westin, E.H., and Schwartz, L.B. 1989. Cloning and characterization of complementary DNA for human tryptase. J. Clin. Invest. 84:1188.
19. Miller, J.S., Moxley, G., and Schwartz, L.B. 1990. Cloning and characterization of a second complementary DNA for human tryptase. J. Clin. Invest. 86:864.
20. Vanderslice, P., Ballinger, S.M., Tam, E.K., Goldstein, S.M., Craik, C.S., and Caughey, G.H. 1990. Human mast cell tryptase: Multiple cDNAs and genes reveal a multigene serine protease family. Proc. Natl. Acad. Sci. USA 87:3811.
21. Caughey, G.H., Zerweck, E.H., and Vanderslice, P. 1991. Structure, chromosomal assignment, and deduced amino acid sequence of a human gene for mast cell chymase. J. Biol. Chem. 266:12956.
22. Reynolds, D.S., Gurley, D.S., Stevens, R.L., Sugarbaker, D.J., Austen, K.F., and Serafin, W.E. 1989. Cloning of cDNAs that encode human mast cell carboxypeptidase A, and comparison of the protein with mouse mast cell carboxypeptidase A and rat pancreatic carboxypeptidases. Proc. Natl. Acad. Sci. USA 86:9480.
23. Enander, I., Matsson, P., Nystrand, J., Andersson, A.-S., Eklund, E., Bradford, T.R., and Schwartz, L.B. 1991. A new radioimmunoassay for human mast cell tryptase using monoclonal antibodies. J. Immunol. Methods 138:39.
24. Schwartz, L.B., Lewis, R.A., Seldin, D., and Austen, K.F. 1981. Acid hydrolases and tryptase from secretory granules of dispersed human lung mast cells. J. Immunol. 126:1290.
25. Schwartz, L.B., Metcalfe, D.D., Miller, J.S., Earl, H., and Sullivan, T. 1987. Tryptase levels as an indicator of mast-cell activation in systemic anaphylaxis and mastocytosis. N. Engl. J. Med. 316:1622.
26. Yunginger, J.W., Nelson, D.R., Squillace, D.L., Jones, R.T., Holley, K.E., Hyma, B.A., Biedrzycki, L., Sweeney, K.G., Sturner, W.Q., and Schwartz, L.B. 1991. Laboratory investigation of deaths due to anaphylaxis. J. Forensic Sci. 36:857.
27. Matsson, P., Enander, I., Andersson, A.-S., Nystrand, J., Schwartz, L., and Watkins, J. 1991. Evaluation of mast cell activation (tryptase) in two patients suffering from drug-induced hypotensoid reactions. Agents Actions 33:218.
28. Wenzel, S.E., Fowler, A.A., 3d., and Schwartz, L.B. 1988. Activation of pulmonary mast cells by bronchoalveolar allergen challenge. *In vivo* release of histamine and tryptase in atopic subjects with and without asthma. Am. Rev. Respir. Dis. 137:1002.
29. Broide, D.H., Eisman, S., Ramsdell, J.W., Ferguson, P., Schwartz, L.B., and Wasserman, S.I. 1990. Airway levels of mast cell-derived mediators in exercise-induced asthma. Am. Rev. Respir. Dis. 141:563.
30. Bosso, J.V., Schwartz, L.B., and Stevenson, D.D. 1991. Tryptase and histamine release during aspirin-induced respiratory reactions. J. Allergy Clin. Immunol. 88:830.
31. Calhoun, W.J., Swensen, C.A., Dick, E.C., Schwartz, L.B., Lemanske, Jr., R.F., and Busse, W.W. 1991. Experimental rhinovirus 16

tern of prostanoids distinct from the acute response but including PGD_2 at levels a few percent of those seen in the acute response (7). The origin of this prostanoid in the lower airways is not clear. In the conjunctivae only the acute response has been characterized with histamine, kinins and PGD_2 identified.

Studies with Pharmacologic Antagonists

Antihistamines: These agents have been in use for several decades and, while clearly useful in allergic inflammation of the upper airways and skin, their utility in the lower airways has not been demonstrated. It has never been clear whether this clinical efficacy is due to H1 antagonism, since local concentrations of histamine released at the reaction site should exceed their ability to block the receptor. With some antihistamines, particularly the new generation of non-sedating agents, other, putatively non-H1 effects have been noted which include inhibition of mediator release and effects on inflammatory cell infiltration (10–11). We have demonstrated that with topical nasal application certain antihistamines are potent inhibitors of mediator release (9); it is our opinion that these studies should be pursued in both the upper and lower airways. Moreover, at least one study has shown that antihistamines in combination with an anti-leukotriene agent, have a definite, additive effect in the treatment of lower airways disease (12).

Anti-sulfidopeptide leukotrienes: These antagonists represent a major breakthrough by the pharmaceutical industry. Several compounds have been developed and clinical trials have been ongoing for the last few years. Thus far, it is evident that these antagonists can have an effect on the acute and late phase response to antigen and can positively influence airways function in asthmatics (13–15). This is a rapidly growing area.

Antagonists of platelet-activating factor: The profound biological activities of platelet-activating factors led many of us to hypothesize that antagonists of this mediator would have dramatic clinical effects. However, preliminary studies with the first generation of inhibitors have been disappointing. To our knowledge, no efficacy in model systems or in disease states has been observed. The recent cloning of the PAF receptor may well lead us to the next generation of drugs.

Antagonists of kinins: A first generation of kinin antagonists has been produced by modifying the amino acid sequence of the nonapeptide, bradykinin. While these antagonists have *in vitro* activity and some efficacy in animal models, they have not been successful in human challenge models. A second generation of peptide kinin antagonists has been developed and will soon enter clinical trials.

Studies with Enzyme Blockers.

Aspirin and other non-steroidal anti-inflammatory drugs are potent inhibitors of the cyclooxygenase pathways which generate prostaglandins. These drugs have been tried in human disease and in antigen challenge models. The results have been equivocal, probably because the synthesis of all prostanoids is inhibited, blocking both pro- and anti-inflammatory effects. Prostaglandin D_2 and its metabolites are proinflammatory while prostaglandin E_2 is probably anti-inflammatory, but both are inhibited equally. There is a clear subset of asthmatic individuals who are dramatically worsened by aspirin whereas a few others are helped. We will need more selective agents in order to assess the role of prostanoids in the disease. On the other hand, inhibitors of the other branch of arachidonic acid metabolism, the 5 lipoxygenase pathways, have been shown to be useful in animal models and in the first trial they were found to inhibit the generation of both leukotriene B_4 and the sulfidopeptide leukotrienes and to have clinical efficacy, at least in one human antigen challenge model (16). The same inhibitor was also effective in attenuating the cold, dry air-induced bronchospastic reaction in asthmatic patients (17).

Cells

Cellular Influx After Antigen Administration.

In the upper airways eosinophils begin to appear in as little as 3 hours after antigen administration and continue to accumulate for several hours (18). Basophils increase in the same time frame, as do the neutrophils, but to a lesser degree. There is a clear correlation between eosinophil numbers and the eosinophil-derived toxic proteins and between histamine levels and basophil infiltration (19). Corticosteroids block both the basophil and eosinophil infiltrate and the clinical response (19). In the skin, the cellular infiltration appears somewhat later, beginning when late phase mediator levels increase at 6 or 7 hours and peaking at 12 hours. Eosinophils and basophils are increased 20 to 30 fold over a saline challenged site, whereas neutrophils are only slightly increased (6,11). Biopsy studies show that the same dramatic increase in eosinophils and basophils occurs in the tissue. As in the nose, corticosteroids decrease the late phase reaction and ablate eosinophil and basophil infiltration, without having a significant effect on neutrophil accumulation (20). An antihistamine, Cetirizine, on the other hand, blocks eosinophil and basophil infiltration only partially and has the same partial effect on the clinical expression of disease (11). In our most recent work we have shown that the same pattern of cellular infiltration occurs in the lower airways 24 hours after antigen challenge through a wedged bronchoscope (7). Eosinophils may represent 20 to 80% of the infiltrating cells, and basophils represent up to several percent of the total. There is no difference in the neutrophil accumulation at the antigen challenged as opposed to the saline challenged site. Work by several European investigators suggests that Cetirizine decreases the eosinophil infiltration after antigen challenge of the lungs and decreases the severity of the late airways response to antigen. Thus, studies in all three human models show that antigen challenge leads to the selective accumulation of eosinophils and basophils; it appears that the neutrophils are not selectively drawn to the site of an IgE-antigen interaction.

The Role of Inflammatory Cells in Allergic Disease

Mast cells: These cells are responsible for the acute release of mediators after antigen exposure and are also felt to be a causal force in recruiting inflammatory cells to the late response. While this may result from the release of chemotactic mediators, it is more likely to be due to the recently reported ability of these cells to generate proinflammatory cytokines (e.g., IL 3, 4, 5) (21). Galli et al. have provided clear evidence for the role of mast cells in allergic inflammation in studies utilizing mast cell deficient animals.

Basophils: There is little question that the mediator release observed in the late phase reaction is derived from the basophil. The question of what secretogogue is operative has been referred to in other reviews (22): We believe that histamine releasing factor(s) are causal. Mediator release may well be important in the pathogenesis of late phase inflammation by increasing vascular permeability to allow both serum enzyme systems and cells into the tissues. A lessening of the late phase response with leukotriene antagonists, and particularly with a combination of antihistamines and leukotriene antagonists, suggests that mediator release plays such a role. In murine species the basophil can also generate proinflammatory cytokines (23).

Eosinophils: Work, predominately by Gleich et al., has characterized a variety of cytotoxic eosinophil proteins (24). *In vitro* experiments show that these proteins are capable of destroying epithelial cell surfaces at concentrations which apparently occur *in vivo* in disease states. Since epithelial tissue damage clearly occurs in allergic inflammation, it seems likely that the eosinophil plays a significant role. Epithelial damage may contribute to the induction or worsening of lower airway nonspecific reactivity by exposing sensory nerve endings (25).

Lymphocytes: Studies of lymphocyte infiltration in human allergic reactions are in an early state. Quantified as "mononuclear cells", there is a modest increase in the skin. Characterized as CD4 or CD8 positive cells, there is a similar increase. Preliminary biopsy studies of tissue from asthmatics examined by in situ hybridization reveal that these cells have mRNA for proinflammatory cytokines (26). Clearly, then, lymphocytes have a potential role in the pathogenesis of allergic inflammation.

The Cytokine-Inflammatory Cell Interaction.

Recruitment: Given the failure of chemotactic factors to play a demonstrable *in vivo* role in the recruitment of eosinophils and basophils, we currently favor the hypothesis that recruitment is the result of a cytokine-inflammatory cell/cytokine-endothelial cell interaction which leads to the development of enhanced function and/or expression of complementary adhesion molecules. It is now clear that cytokines such as IL-1, TNF, and IL-4 can induce or enhance the expression of adhesion molecules on vascular endothelium. To date, adhesion molecules which have been identified as potential contributors to the margination and transendothelial migration of circulating leukocytes include intercellular adhesion molecule-1 (ICAM-1, CD54), vascular cell adhesion molecule-1 (VCAM-1), and endothelial-leukocyte adhesion molecule-1 (ELAM-1) (27). Evidence for the potential importance of cytokines and adhesion molecules in allergic inflammation is rapidly accumulating. For example, it is known that IL-1 is released during human cutaneous allergic reactions (28), and treatment of asthmatic primates with anti-ICAM-1 antibody reduces antigen-induced airways hyperreactivity and bronchoalveolar eosinophilia (29). Endothelial cell activation and adhesion molecule expression occurs in the skin within hours of allergen challenge, and can be prevented in antigen-challenged skin explants using a combination of anti-IL-1 and anti-TNF antisera (30,31). Of particular relevance to the present discussion are the recent observations that while eosinophils and basophils can bind to each of the three endothelial adhesion molecules mentioned above, the neutrophil cannot bind to VCAM-1 (32). This may partly explain the enrichment of eosinophils and basophils (compared to neutrophils) observed at sites of allergic inflammation. Since IL-4 has now been shown to selectively induce expression of VCAM-1, while having little effect on ELAM-1 or ICAM-1 expression, local production of IL-4 may play an important role in promoting eosinophil and basophil recruitment *in vivo* (33).

Up-regulation/activation: Another area of cytokine-inflammatory cell interaction concerns the "activation" of inflammatory cells. In a sense this phenomenon has been appreciated since we introduced the term *releasability* at the 9th International Congress, to account for the characteristic of basophils from different patients releasing more or less effectively to different stimuli (34). Interleukin 3 treatment of basophils renders these cells far more responsive to antigen or to anti-IgE (35). Moreover, such treatment makes an incomplete secretogogue such as C5a (which normally causes only histamine release) complete (i.e., also causing leukotriene release) (36). Basophils derived from both the upper and the lower airways 24 hours after antigen challenge remain viable and express a pattern of surface markers consistent with cell activation (37). With respect to the eosinophil, the situation is more defined. A larger proportion of eosinophils from bronchial lavage 24 hours after antigen challenge have the so called "hypodense" phenotype than is seen in peripheral blood (38). Culture of eosinophils *in vitro* with IL-3, IL-5 or GM-CSF leads to a similar phenotype (39). In these *in vitro* experiments, cytokine treatment of eosinophils results in a priming response in which the cells are rendered more responsive to secretogogue-induced mediator production. *In vivo* the situation is more complex. The hypodense eosinophils obtained after lavage may be either up or down regulated with respect to their response to secretogogues, suggesting that the hypodense phenotype can be associated with multiple functional states.

In the future it may well be that the cytokines made by lymphocytes, macrophages and mast cells and which modulate the function of the inflammatory cells will be considered the "mediators" of most critical importance. Moreover, we will be able to test this hypothesis with novel antagonists: naturally occurring cytokine antagonists and soluble receptors.

References

1. Naclerio, R.M., Meier, H.C., Kagey-Sobotka, A., Adkinson, N.F. Jr., Meyers, D.A., Norman, P.S., and Lichtenstein, L.M. 1983. Mediator release after nasal airway challenge with allergen. Am. Rev. Respir. Dis. 128:597.
2. Creticos, P.S., Peters, S.P., Adkinson, N.F., Jr., Naclerio, R.M., Hayes, E.C., Norman, P.S., and Lichtenstein, L.M. 1984. Peptide leukotriene release after antigen challenge in patients sensitive to ragweed. N. Eng. J. Med. 310:1626.
3. Proud, D., Togias, A., Naclerio, R.M., Crush, S.A., Norman, P.S., and Lichtenstein, L.M. 1983. Kinins are generated *in vivo* following nasal airway challenge of allergic individuals with allergen. J. Clin. Invest. 72:1678.
4. Castells, M., and Schwartz, L.B. 1988. Tryptase levels in nasal-lavage fluid as an indicator of

the immediate allergic response. J. Allergy Clin. Immunol. 82:348.

5. Naclerio, R.M., Proud, D., Togias, A.G., Adkinson, N.F., Jr., Meyers, D.A., Kagey-Sobotka, A,. Plaut, M., Norman, P.S., and Lichtenstein, L.M. 1985. Inflammatory mediators in late antigen-induced rhinitis. N. Eng. J. Med. 313:65.
6. Charlesworth, E.N., Hood, A.F., Soter, N.A., Kagey-Sobotka, A., Norman, P.S., and Lichtenstein, L.M. 1989. Cutaneous late-phase response to allergen. Mediator release and inflammatory cell infiltration. J. Clin. Invest. 83:1519.
7. Liu, M.C., Hubbard, W.C., Proud, D., Stealey, B., Galli, S., Kagey-Sobotka, A., Bleecker, E.R., and Lichtenstein, L.M. 1991. Immediate and late inflammatory responses to ragweed antigen challenge of the peripheral airways in asthmatics: cellular, mediator, and permeability changes. Am. Rev. Respir. Dis. 144:51.
8. Wenzel, S.E., Irani, A.A., Sanders, J.M., Bradford, T.R., and Schwartz, L.B. 1986. Immunoassay of tryptase from human mast cells. J. Immunol. Methods 86:139.
9. Togias, A.G., Naclerio, R.M., Warner, J., Proud, D., Kagey-Sobotka, A., Nimmagadda, I., Norman, P.S., and Lichtenstein, L.M. 1986. Demonstration of inhibition of mediator release from human mast cells by azatadine base: *In vivo* and *in vitro* evaluation. JAMA 255:225.
10. Naclerio, R.M., Kagey-Sobotka, A., Lichtenstein, L.M., Freidhoff, L., and Proud, D. 1990. Terfenadine, an H-1 antihistamine, inhibits histamine release *in vivo* in the human. Am. Rev. Respir. Dis. 142:167.
11. Charlesworth, E.N., Kagey-Sobotka, A., Norman, P.S., and Lichtenstein, L.M. 1988. Effects of cetirizine on mast cell mediator release and cellular traffic during the cutaneous late phase response. J. Allergy Clin. Immunol. 83:905.
12. Eiser, N., Hayhurst, M., and Denman, W. 1989. The contribution of histamine and leukotriene release to the production of early and late asthmatic responses to antigen. Am. Rev. Respir. Dis. 139:A462.
13. Taylor, I.K., O'Shaughnessy, K.M., Fuller, R.W., and Dollery. C.T. 1991. Effect of cysteinyl-leukotriene receptor antagonist ICI 204.219 on allergen-induced broncho-constriction and airway hyperreactivity in atopic subjects. Lancet 337:690.
14. Findlay, S.R., Easley, C.B., Glass, M., and Barden, J.M. 1990. Effect of the oral leukotriene antagonist ICI 204.219 on antigen-induced bronchoconstriction in patients with bronchial asthma. J Allergy Clin. Immunol. 85:197.
15. Hendeles, L., Davison, D., Blake, K., Harman, E., Cooper, R., and Margolskee, D. 1990. Leukotriene D_4 is an important mediator of antigen-induced bronchoconstriction attenuation of dual response with MK-571, a specific LTD_4 receptor antagonist. J. Allergy Clin. Immunol. 85:197.
16. Knapp, H.R. 1990. Reduced allergen-induced nasal congestion and leukotriene synthesis with an orally active 5-lipoxygenase inhibitor. N. Eng. J. Med. 323:1745.
17. Israel, E., Demarkarian, R., Rosenberg, M., Sperling, R., Taylor, G., Rubin, P., and Drazen, J.M. 1990. The effects of 5-lipoxygenase inhibition on asthma induced by cold, dry air. N. Eng. J. Med. 323:1740.
18. Bascom, R., Pipkorn, U., Lichtenstein, L.M., and Naclerio, R.M. 1988. The influx of inflammatory cells into nasal washings during the late response to antigen challenge. Am. Rev. Respir. Dis. 138:406.
19. Bascom, R., Wachs, M., Naclerio, R.M., Pipkorn, U., Galli, S.J., and Lichtenstein, L.M. 1988. Basophil influx occurs after nasal antigen challenge: effects of topical corticosteroid pretreatment. J. Allergy Clin. Immunol. 81:580.
20. Charlesworth, E.N., Kagey-Sobotka, A., Schleimer, R.P., Norman, P.S., and Lichtenstein, L.M. 1991. Prednisone inhibits the appearance of inflammatory mediators and the influx of eosinophils and basophils associated with the cutaneous late-phase response to allergen. J. Immunol. 146:671.
21. Plaut, M., Pierce, J.H., Watson, C.J., Hanley-Hyde, J., Nordan, R.P., and Paul, W.E. 1989. Mast cell lines produce lymphokines in response to cross-linkage of $FC_{\epsilon}RI$ or to calcium ionophores. Nature 339:64.
22. Lichtenstein, L.M., and Bochner, B.S. 1991. The role of basophils in asthma. Ann. N. Y. Acad. Sci. 629:48.
23. Seder, R.A., Paul, W.E., Dvorak, A.M., Sharkis, S.J,. Kagey-Sobotka, A., Niv, Y., Finkelman, F.D., Barbieri, S.A., Galli, S.J., and Plaut, M. 1991. Mouse splenic and bone marrow cell populations that express high-affinity Fc epsilon receptors and produce interleukin-4 are highly enriched in basophils. Proc. Natl. Acad. Sci. USA 88:2835.
24. Gleich, G.J., Frigas, E., Filley, W.V., and Loegering, D.A. 1984. Eosinophils and bronchial inflammation. In: Asthma: Physiology, immunopharmacology and treatment. A.B.

Kay, K.F. Austen, L.M. Lichtenstein, eds. London: Academic Press, p. 195.
25. Barnes, P.J. 1986. Neural control of human airways in health and disease. Am. Rev. Respir. Dis. 134:1289.
26. Hamid, Q., Azzawi, M., Ying, S., Moqbel, R., Wardlaw, A.J,. Corrigan, C.J., Bradley, B., Durham, S.R., Collins, J.V., Jeffery, P.K., Quint, D.J., and Kay, A.B. 1991. Expression of mRNA for interleukin-5 in mucosal bronchial biopsies from asthma. J. Clin. Invest. 87:1541.
27. Springer, T.A. 1990. Adhesion receptors of the immune system. Nature 346:425.
28. Bochner, B.S., Charlesworth, E.N., Lichtenstein, L.M., Gillis, S., Dinarello, C.A,. Derse, C.P., and Schleimer, R.P. 1990. Interleukin-1 is released at sites of human cutaneous allergic reactions. J. Allergy Clin. Immunol. 86:830.
29. Wegner, C.D., Gundel, R.H., Reilly, P., Haynes, N., Letts, L.G., and Rothlein, R. 1990. Intercellular adhesion molecule-1 (ICAM-1) in the pathogenesis of asthma. Science 247:456.
30. Kyan-Aung, U., Haskard, D.O., Poston, R.N., Thornhill, M.H., and Lee, T.H. 1991. Endothelial leukocyte adhesion molecule-1 and intercellular adhesion molecule-1 mediate the adhesion of eosinophils to endothelial cells *in vitro* and are expressed by endothelium in allergic cutaneous inflammation *in vivo*. J. Immunol. 146:521.
31. Leung, D.Y.M., Pober, J.S., and Cotran, R.S. 1991. Expression of endothelial-leukocyte adhesion molecule-1 in elicited late phase allergic reactions. J. Clin. Invest. 87:1805.
32. Bochner, B.S., Luscinskas, F.W., Gimbrone, M.A., Newman, W., Sterbinsky, S.A., Derse-Anthony, C., Klunk, D., and Schleimer, R.P. 1991. Adhesion of human basophils, eosinophils, and neutrophils to IL-1-activated human vascular endothelial cells: Contributions of endothelial cell adhesion molecules. J Exp Med 173:1553.
33. Schleimer, R.P., Sterbinsky, S.A., Kaiser, J., Klunk, D.A., Tomioka, K., Newman, W., Luscinskas, F.W., Gimbrone, M.A., Jr., McIntyre, B.W., and Bochner, B.S. 1991. Interleukin-4 induces adherence of human eosinophils and basophils but not neutrophils to endothelium: Association with expression of VCAM-1. J. Immunol., in press.
34. Lichtenstein, L.M., and Conroy, M.C. 1977. The "releasability" of mediators from human basophils and granulocytes. In: Allergy and clinical immunology. E. Mathov, T. Sindo, and P. Naranjo, eds. Amsterdam: Excerpta Medica, p. 109.
35. Schleimer, R.P., Derse, C.P., Friedman, B., Gillis, S., Plaut, M., Lichtenstein, L.M, and MacGlashan, D.W. Jr. 1989. Regulation of human basophil mediator release by cytokines. I. Interaction with antiinflammatory steroids. J. Immunol. 143:1310.
36. Kurimoto, Y., deWeck, A.L., and Dahinden, C.A. 1989. Interleukin 3-dependent mediator release in basophils triggered by C5a. J. Exp. Med. 170:467.
37. Georas, S.N., Liu, M.C., and Bochner, B.S. 1991. Altered CD11b and Leu-8 expression on bronchoalveolar lavage granulocytes following local antigen challenge in allergic subjects. Am. Rev. Respir. Dis. 143:A45.
38. Kroegel, C., Liu, M.C., Hubbard, W.C., Lichtenstein, L.M., and Bochner, B.S. 1991. Segmental lung antigen challenge of allergic subjects induces the local activation and recruitment of eosinophilic leukocytes. Am. Rev. Respir. Dis. 143:A45.
39. Silberstein, D.S., Austen, K.F., and Owen, W.F. Jr. 1989. Hemopoietins for eosinophils. Hematology/Oncology Clinics of North America 3:511.

A New Cellular Assay for the Diagnosis of Allergy (SLT-ELISA)

A. L. de Weck, K. Furukawa, C. Dahinden, F. E. Maly*

When triggered *in vitro* by allergen or other basophil agonists, sensitized blood basophils not only release histamine but also produce various sulfidoleukotrienes (LTC4, LTD4, LTE4). These sulfidoleukotrienes (sLT) may now be detected by a unique monoclonal antibody detecting all three sLT moieties in a single very sensitive ELISA assay. Accordingly, an assay could be developed in which the reaction of basophils to various allergens, either when isolated as mononuclear cell suspensions or in diluted whole blood, can be easily assessed, especially when the reactive cells have been preincubated for a short period with a priming cytokine (e.g. IL3, IL5). Such an assay may advantageously replace histamine release and may also be applicable to the diagnosis of some pseudo-allergies.

Inflammatory Mediators

The release of inflammatory mediators by various types of blood or tissue cells upon interaction with different stimulants is a common feature of inflammatory processes occurring in a number of acute or chronic diseases, such as rheumatic or kidney diseases. In allergic reactions, the release of histamine by blood basophils and/or tissue mast cells has long been considered a major feature. The determination of histamine in supernatants from suspensions of isolated blood leukocytes from allergic patients *in vitro*, following interaction with allergens to which they are sensitive, is a procedure which has been extensively used in allergy research (1). However, a widespread and routine diagnosis of allergies based on blood cellular assays has up to now been prevented by the facts that (a) such determinations require numerous manipulations and (b) cannot be effected easily in whole blood with most techniques but only on isolated cells, and that (c) histamine determination requires cumbersome and expensive fluorometric or radioimmunoasssays. However, investigations in several laboratories have indicated that, when applied on a routine basis, the histamine release assay provides interesting diagnostic possibilities and correlates well with the patient's clinical history and with skin tests (2,3,4). At present, the only diagnostic method widely used *in vitro* is the serologic determination of allergen-specific IgE antibodies by various types of radio-immunological or immunoenzymatic assays (e.g. RAST assay). Such assays, however, only detect the occurrence of antibodies but do not reflect the most relevant pathophysiological feature of the allergic reaction, namely the production of inflammatory mediators by the reactive cells upon interaction with the responsible allergen(s). It has been shown that mediator release may vary considerably among individuals possessing similar levels of allergen-specific IgE and that histamine release correlates with the intensity of allergic symptoms. For that reason, practical and reliable cellular assays would be most desirable for the routine diagnosis of allergic and other inflammatory diseases. The object of the present paper is to describe a novel cellular assay for that purpose.

The sulfidoleukotrienes (sLT) LTC4, LTD4 and LTE4 are inflammatory mediators which were previously collectively called Slow Reactive Subtance of Anaphylaxis (SRS-A). They are synthesized in many cell types, such as tissue mast cells, blood basophils, macrophages, eosinophils and kidney mesangial cells. They play an important role in pathological events of inflammation and allergic reactions, particularly in IgE-mediated allergic reactions (5). It is of particular interest that blood basophils generate sLT in response to allergens in an IgE-dependent manner (6), particularly when pretreated with the cytokines IL-3, IL-5 and GM-CSF (7). Theoretically, therefore, on the basis of current knowledge, determination

* Institute of Clinical Immunology, Inselspital, Bern, Switzerland.

of basophil sLT production in response to suspected allergens could be of interest in the diagnosis of allergies. In practice, however, this goal has not yet been achieved, essentially because of multiple technical difficulties. The object of the present paper is the combination of various procedures by which a routine can be established for *in vitro* cellular diagnostic assay for allergies and other inflammatory diseases. Such an assay involves the following steps (Fig.1): (I) optimal enhancement of the reactive capacity of blood leukocytes, in particular of basophils, by pretreatment with priming agents; (II) stimulation of blood leukocytes to production of sLT by specific allergens in the detection of allergies; and (III) detection of SLT.

Diagnostic Assay for Allergies

Optimal enhancement of the reactive capacity of blood leukocytes, in particular of basophils, by pretreatment with priming agents

Our group has described (7) the fact that preincubating blood leukocytes for a relatively short time (5–10 minutes) with a special group of cytokines, namely IL-3 (interleukin 3), IL-5 (interleukin 5), GM-CSF (granulocyte/monocyte colony stimulating factor) or NGF (nerve growth factor) has the effect of considerably enhancing the capacity of these cells to produce and release mediators when challenged with appropriate stimulants, such as allergens (for leukocytes of sensitized allergic patients) or

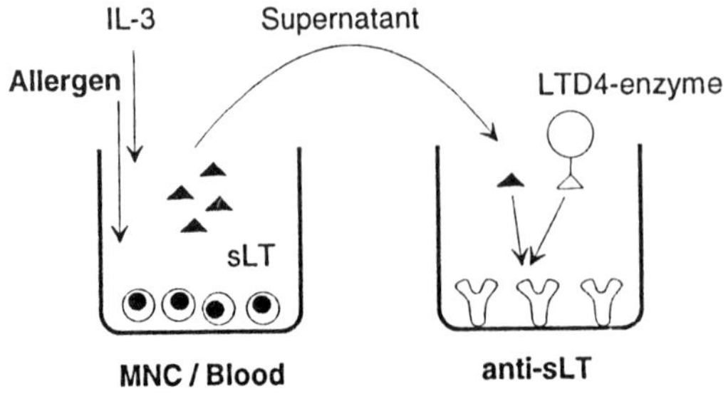

Figure 1. Schematic representation of the SLT-ELISA assay for allergy diagnosis.

non specific mediator releasing factors such as complement components C5a and C3a, various basic peptides, or bacterial-derived structures, such as formyl-methyl-peptide (fMLP). This phenomenon has been described as "priming". However, all experiments performed up to now have been performed on isolated leukocytes obtained by gradient centrifugation, a procedure which is cumbersome and possibly eliminates some of the cellular reaction partners also involved, such as monocytes and platelets, as well as some of the blood plasma factors which may influence the outcome of the reaction. We have now achieved similar results by pretreatment of diluted whole blood with purified human recombinant cytokines or with appropriately prepared supernatants of cultures from activated lymphoid cells. Maximal priming is required for obtaining high sensitivity and release of SLT from the smallest possible number of blood cells and volume of blood.

Stimulation of Blood Leukocytes to Production of sLT by Specific Allergens in the Detection of Allergies.

Following appropriate pretreatment and "priming", as described above, the blood leukocytes, isolated by gradient centrifugation, or as a suspension in whole diluted blood, are set up in the presence of specific allergens (such as pollen extracts, house dust mite extracts, etc.) in a suitable medium for a period of several minutes to one hour. In a classical experimental set up, as shown in Fig. 2, the blood leukocytes of putative allergic patients are set up with various doses of allergen extract in fluid form. After the required period of incubation, the cells are centrifuged and the supernatants harvested and analyzed separately for the amount of SLT produced in the SLT ELISA assay described below. For preparation of basophil-containing peripheral blood mononuclear cell suspensions (MNC) blood anticoagulated with 10 mM EDTA is mixed with 0.25 volumes of 6% dextran and the erythrocytes are allowed to sediment for 90 minutes at room temperature. Leukocytes are pelleted from the supernatant by centrifugation (150 g, 20 min at room temperature) and resuspended in HA buffer (20 mM Hepes, 125 mM NaCl, 5 mM KCl, 0.5 mM glucose and 0.025% BSA). The cells are then further fractionated by Ficoll-Hy-

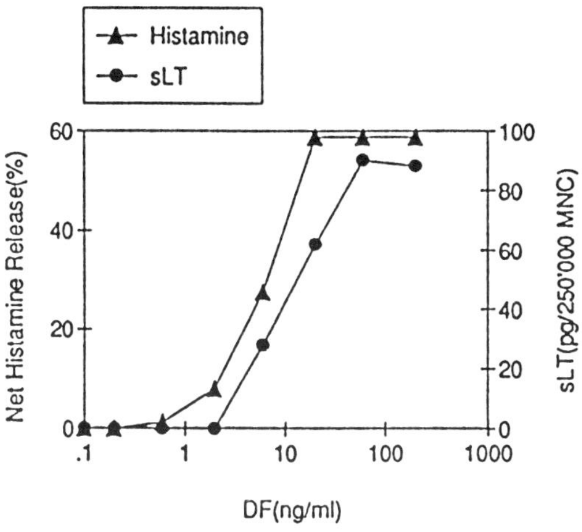

Figure 2. Allergen-triggered sLT generation and histamine release of isolated human mononuclear cells (MNC): MNC (250,000/ well) from a mite allergic donor were stimulated in microtiter wells with increasing amounts of Dermatophagoides farinae (DF) allergen. Supernatants were harvested after 40 minutes and generation of sLT and release of histamine were determined by ELISA and RIA respectively. Spontaneous histamine release was 1.2%. Data are duplicate means (range < 15%).

paque density gradient (specific gravity 1.077) centrifugation (600 g, 40 min at room temperature). MNC are harvested from the interphase, washed 3 times (150 g, 10 min at 4C) in HA buffer and are finally resuspended in HACM buffer (HA buffer supplemented with 1 mM CaCl2 and 1 mM MgCl2 at a cell density of 10^7 or 5 x 10^6 cells/ml. For generation of sLT by mononuclear cells, 100 microliters/well of MNC suspension in HACM buffer are heated at 37C for 10 min in flat-bottomed microtiter plates. IL 3 or GM-CSF (50 microliters, final concentration 10 ng/ml) or HACM buffer are added for 10 min before adding the stimulant (50 microliters, allergen extract or non specific stimulant such as C5a or fMLP). The reaction is stopped 40 min after the addition of stimulants by cooling the microtiterplate on ice. After centrifugation (600 g, 5 min at 4C), 100 microliters of supernatant are transferred into the ELISA assay microtiter plate and assayed for sLT as decribed below.

As shown in Fig. 2, the isolated MNC (250,000/microwell) of an individual allergic to the house dust mite Dermatophagoides pteronyssinus generate sLT in response to increasing doses of the relevant allergen. These sLT were easily detected by sLT-ELISA and their release was accompanied by a correlated release of histamine. Since MNC contain about 1% basophils, and as only 100 microliters of the total incubate (250 microliters) are used for sLT measurements, the sLT-ELISA detects generation of sLT from about 1,000 basophils. Changing incubation volume and supernatant volume used for sLT-ELISA may allow working with even fewer mononuclear cells. For clinical routine applications, the practicability of the sLT assay would be much improved if isolation of mononuclear cells could be by-passed and the test performed directly in whole blood. Indeed, the inclusion of blood plasma proteins in the SLT-ELISA assay does not markedly affect SLT recovery in the SLT-ELISA assay which varies from 70–90% depending upon the plasma concentration. Therefore, detection of sLT generated in diluted whole blood upon stimulation by allergen has become feasible. For this assay, venous whole blood is drawn into suitable closed containers with heparin (final concentration 12 U/ml). 100 microliters per well of heparinized blood diluted 1:4 with HACM buffer are pipetted into microtiterplates, after which the procedure is identical with that described above for isolated mononuclear cells. As shown in Fig. 3, the allergen Dermatophagoides pteronyssinus stimulates release of sLT in diluted whole blood from a mite allergic individual. In contrast, an irrelevant allergen, Phleum pratense, to which this individual is not allergic, does not cause significant release of sLT even in cells preincubated with IL3. The specificity of the mite allergen-induced sLT generation is further demonstated by the fact that non allergic individuals show no sLT generation when challenged with either allergen, with or without IL 3 "priming". For this test, only 25 microliters of whole blood are required, which is eminently suitable for multiple routine assays in the same individual. The results shown in Fig. 3 reflect sLT generation by approximately 100–300 basophils and are in the range expected from experiments with isolated MNC. As shown in Fig. 4, there is an excellent correlation between the results obtained with diluted whole blood and with isolated MNC. This is in contrast to the experience made with histamine release performed in parallel on the same supernatants. There, the correlation is

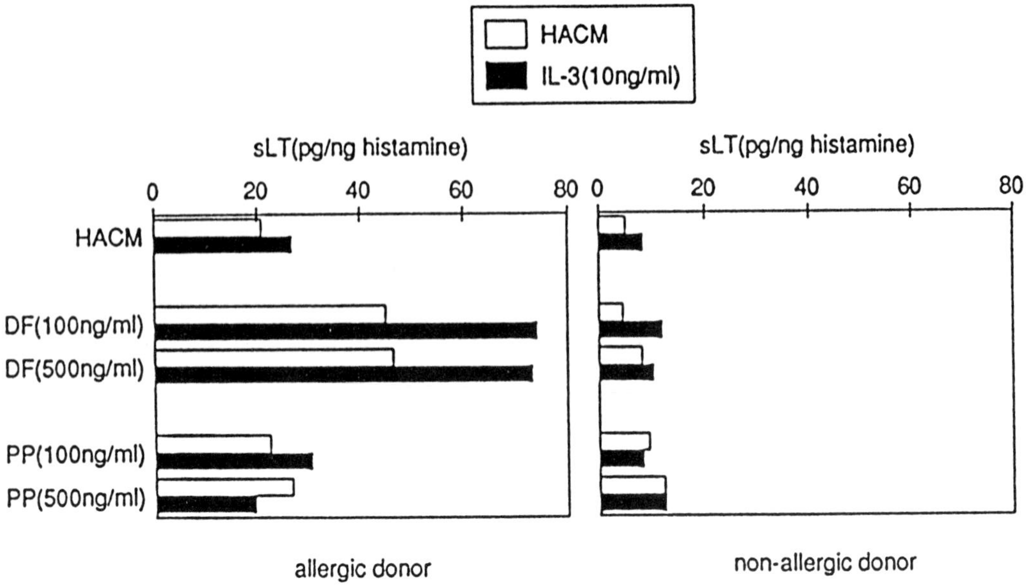

Figure 3. ELISA detection of allergen-triggered sLT generation in diluted whole blood.
Heparinized blood (25 µl/well) from a mite-allergic donor (left panel) and a non allergic donor (right panel) was stimulated with Dermatophagoides farinae (DF) or Phleum pratense (PP) extract, with (solid columns) or without (open columns) prior addition of IL 3 (10 ng/ml). Supernatants were harvested after 40 min. at 37C and sLT content was measured by ELISA. Data are means of duplicates with ranges < 15%. For easy comparison, sLT are given with reference to total histamine present in the sample, a measure of blood basophil content, i. e. as pg sLT per total amount of hitamine (ng).

much less impressive, obviously due to interference of some cells and/or plasma proteins with histamine determination.

The correlation between the SLT-ELISA test and skin tests in allergic patients has been tested up to now in a limited number of patients and with a limited number of allergens. The results, shown in Table 1, are quite encouraging.

Theoretically. a similar procedure could be used for detecting the production of sLT in other circumstances and for the diagnosis of other diseases than IgE specific allergy. For example, the capacity of blood leukocytes to produce sLT when challenged with a number of non specific stimulants, such as components C5a or C3a, as well as with bacterial structures like fMLP (results not shown) may be used for evaluating the reactive capacity of the blood cells in various types of immunodeficiencies and of inflammatory diseases, like rheumatic diseases. The spontaneous production of sLT by blood or tissue cells, including biological fluid (e. g. synovial fluid), may be used for assessment of inflammatory disease activity. In a similar way, the new tests could also be used for the diagnosis of so-called pseudo-allergies, in which inflammatory cells produce the same mediators as in IgE- mediated allergies but where the triggering mechanism is different. A classical example is seen in the intolerance reactions to aspirin and other non steroidal anti-inflammatory drugs (NSAIDs). In that case, the drugs induce the production and release of histamine and sLT in intolerant patients by some other mechanism than Ig-E mediated basophil activation. The precise mechanism is, however, not yet known. The whole blood, encompassing all possible reactive cells, offers a medium mimicking the *in vivo* situation. The new sLT test could possibly offer the possibility to explore for diagnostic purposes a number of other allergies and pseudo-allergies, hitherto difficult or impossible to detect *in vitro*, such as intolerance reactions to foods and food additives, drugs and other chemical agents, air pollutants, etc. Such investigations are currently under way.

Detection of SLT

A key element in the new assay is the method developed for assessing all sLTs quantitatively in a single, easy to perform, immunoenzymatic assay. Up to now, the preferred analytical methods for the determination of leukotriene (LT) concentrations in biological material have been High Pressure Liquid Chromatography (HPLC) and Radioimmunoassay (RIA). The advantage of the HPLC method is that several LTs may be determined in one assay. This is, however, outweighed by the disadvantage that detection is limited to the nanogram range and that every sample has to be purified extensively before being applied to HPLC. This precludes HPLC as a routine diagnostic method. In contrast, the RIA is a very sensitive analytical method and may be used without any purification of samples, such as serum, plasma or cell culture supernatants. The RIA, however, has the disadvantages of using radioactive reagents, an increasingly objectionable procedure, and encompassing high production costs. Furthermore, up to recently, only polyclonal antibodies of sufficient affinity and avidity for LT have been available for such assays. In particular, only a few polyclonal antibodies of high specificity for LTC 4 have been described (8,9). Decisive progress was made possible by the availability of monoclonal antibodies strictly specific for LTC4, the primary sLT produced by activated cells, and LTD4 and LTE4, which are the main metabolites of LTC 4. In this way, it

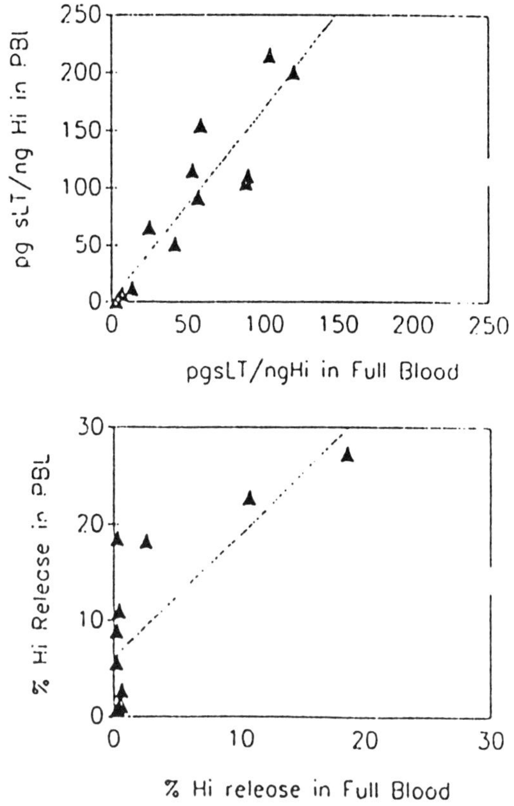

Figure 4. Correlation between sLT formation and histamine release in whole diluted blood or in isolated MNC. Cells triggered by anti-IgE Le27 monoclonal antibody (10 ng/ml).

Table 1. Correlation of Skin Test with SLT-ELISA Assay

Patient		6-Grasses	Birch	D.Pteron.	Mugwort	Plantain
1.	ST	...+++	Neg	+++	Neg	Neg
	ELISA	110*	0	75	0	0
2.	ST	Neg.	Neg	+++	Neg	Neg
	ELISA	0	0	120	0	0
3.	ST	+++	+++	Neg	Neg	Neg.
	ELISA	220	90	0	0	0
4.	ST	+++	Neg.	+++	Neg.	++
	ELISA	90	0	100	0	40
5.	ST	Neg	Neg.	Neg.	Neg.	Neg.
	ELISA	0	0	0	0	0

n = 25 r = 1.0

* Results expressed in pg sLT / 100.000 cells

has become possible to assess all relevant sLT products of activated cells in a single radioimmuno- or immunoenzymatic assay. With such a monoclonal antibody, an ELISA assay has recently been described (10). In this assay , LTE4 is conjugated to bovine serum albumin and coated to the wells of a microtiter plate. Biotinylated anti-sLT monoclonal antibody is reacted with the analytical sample containing sLT, followed by incubation in the microtiter plate coated with LTCE4-BSA and revelation with avidin-coupled peroxidase. This procedure has several disadvantages for a routine assay: (a) its sensitivity is not optimal (about 100 picograms), requiring thereby larger quantities of cells; (b) the preparation of the reagents is cumbersome and their stability suboptimal; (c) the amount of expensive synthetic LTE4 required is quite large; and (d) accuracy is not satisfactory when using samples with high protein loads, such as biological and tissue fluids. This led us to search for alternative ELISA procedures aimed at increasing sensitivity, reducing manipulation steps, improving preparation and quality of the reagents as well as making it possible to perform sLT assays in biological fluids. In our current procedure, the monoclonal anti-SLT antibody is coated onto microtiterplates without any modification, either directly, or indirectly with the help of an anti-mouse IgG antibody. Upon incubation of the analytical sample with such a coated microwell (Fig. 1), sLTs produced by the cells are directly bound. The revealing step of the assay is provided by mere addition of an LTD4-alkaline phosphatase conjugate, the binding of which is inhibited in direct corelation to the amount of sample sLT bound. Such a simplified sLT inhibition ELISA assay requires substantially less synthetic leukotriene for conjugate production, shows improved sensitivity and reagent stability, and allows simple and effective determination of sLT generated by small numbers of basophils in whole blood. (Precise description of the assays and of their application for diagnostic purposes will be given elsewhere, e.g., Furukawa, S., Tengler, R., de Weck, A.L., and Maly, F.E. 1991 (submitted): Simplified sulfidoleukotriene ELISA using LTD4-conjugated phosphatase for study of allergen-induced leukotriene generation by isolated mononuclear cells and diluted whole blood.)

References

1. Lichtenstein, L.M., Norman, P.S., Winkenwerder, W.L., and Osler, A.G. 1966. *In vitro* studies of human ragweed allergy: Changes in cellular and humoral activity associated with specific desensitization. J. Clin. Invest. 45:1126.
2. Lichtenstein, L.M. 1973. IgE antibody measurement in ragweed hay fever. Relationship to clinical severity and the results of immunotherapy. J. Clin. Invest. 52:472.
3. Siraganian, R. 1977. Automated histamine analysis for *in vitro* allergy testing. J. Allergy Clin. Immunol. 59:214.
4. Gamboa, P.M., Castillo, J.G., Oehling, A., Wong, E., and de la Cuesta, C.G. 1989. Variations of histamine release in an atopic population. I. Clinical situation and seasons. Allergol. et Immunopathol. 17:73.
5. Schleimer, R.P., MacGlashan, D.W., Peters, S.P., Naclerio, R., Proud, D., Adkinson, N.F., and Lichtenstein, L.M. 1984. Inflammatory mediators and mechanisms of release from purified human basophils and mast cells. J. Allergy Clin. Immun. 74:473.
6. Mita, H., Yui, Y., Yasueda, H., Kajita, T., Saito, H., and Shida, T. 1986. Allergen-induced histamine release and immunoreactive leukotriene C4 generation from leukocytes in mite sensitive asthmatic patients. Prostaglandins 31: 869.
7. Bischoff, S.C., Brunner, T., de Weck, A.L., and Dahinden, C.A. 1990. Interleukin 5 modifies histamine release and leukotriene generation by human basophils in response to diverse agonists. J. Exp. Med. 172:1577.
8. Reinke, M., Hoppe, U., Röder, T., Bestmann, H.J., Mollenhauer, J., and Brune, K. A monoclonal antibody against the sulfidoleukotrienes LTC4, LTD4 and LTE4. 1991. Biochim. Biophys. Acta 1081:274.

Monitoring of Inflammatory Cells in Asthma

Jean Bousquet, Pascal Chanez, Alison M. Campbell, Ingrid Enander, Philippe Godard, François-B. Michel*

Inflammation plays a key role in asthma, and the management of asthma is based upon anti-inflammatory treatments. The characterization of inflammation of the airways may be attempted clinically and on the basis of pulmonary function measurements. However, these methods are only approximative, and markers of inflammation are favored. These markers may be measured for research purposes in bronchial biopsies and bronchoalveolar lavage fluid, but in routine they should be meaured in peripheral blood or urine. Eosinophil markers include granule proteins such as ECP, EPX and MBP. Their levels in BAL fluid are significantly correlated with the severity of asthma but serum levels of these proteins do not clearly differentiate asthmatics and normal subjects. They may, however, be helpful for following the efficacy of anti-inflammatory treatments in an individual patient. Markers of lymphocyte activation such as serum sIL-2 receptor were found to correlate with the severity of asthma. Histamine and tryptase are released by mast cells but their levels in plasma or urine are only inconstantly correlated with acute asthma. Hyaluronic acid derived from fibroblasts is another interesting marker but more studies are needed. In urine, metabolites of leukotrienes are elevated in acute asthma but their titration requires highly sophisticated techniques. Markers of macrophages and epithelial cells are still lacking.

Although the first pathologic observations on patients who died from an asthma attack made just after the turn of the century described eosinophil inflammation and shedding of the epithelium, for many years the major basic mechanism of asthma remained bronchial obstruction whereby bronchospasm, mucosal edema and mucous hypersecretion played a major role. However, since the early 1980's the concept of asthma has evolved to an inflammatory disease in which epithelial shedding, eosinophils, mast cells, macrophages and lymphocytes appear to play a significant role (1,2). Other features of inflammation are likely to be observed in asthma since the histologic hallmarks of any chronic inflammation also include proliferation of fibroblasts and blood vessels, and increased connective tissue and reparation. Cells participating in the airway inflammation may be deleterious, and may also regulate the inflammation and participate in the reparation of the tissues. However, in 1991, our knowledge is mostly targeted to the deleterious effects of inflammatory cells, and very little is known about their contributory role in the processes of healing following inflammation. The monitoring of airway inflammation in asthma is critical in the management of asthma in which anti-inflammatory drugs take a major part. However, it is still very difficult to find accurate markers that can be serially measured in blood.

Methods Assessing Bronchial Inflammation in Asthma

The severity of asthma is of course monitored clinically by symptoms, pulmonary function studies, serial records of peak flow rates and/or the study of nonspecific bronchial hyperreactivity. However, attempts are made to obtain biologic markers that may be useful to monitor asthma. These markers, however, can also be used for the diagnosis of asthma, usually by the examination of eosinophils or their secretory products. Although bronchoscopy is favored to better understand the pathophysiological mechanisms of asthma, this technique cannot be applied to all patients, nor can it be used serially except for research purposes.

---

* Clinique des Maladies Respiratoires, Hopital l'Aiguelongue, 34059-Montpellier-Cedex, France and Pharmacia Diagnostics AB, Uppsala, Sweden.
Acknowledgements: The authors thank Dr. G. Barnéon, J.Y. Lacoste, T.H. Lee, R. Poston, J. Simony-Lafontaine, C. Peterson, P. Venge and P. Vic for their help in performing the studies and for fruitful discussions.

Sampling: Bronchial Biopsies

The first pathological observations on patients who died from an asthma attack were made in the nineteenth century, but until 1980 few pathological studies had been done in living asthmatics, and it was uncertain whether post-mortem findings represented a common feature in all asthmatic patients since: (a) in the vast majority of cases they had been made on only the most severe asthmatic patients who died from an asthma attack; (b) it was not known if the asthma attack leading to death was precipitated by a viral infection capable of altering the bronchial epithelium; (c) the smoking status was usually unknown and some patients may have been suffering from asthma and chronic bronchitis; and (d) the classification of COPD has changed over the years. In the 1980's, fiberoptic bronchoscopy made access to the bronchi easier, and techniques such as electron microscopy, immunohistochemistry or in situ hybridization have significantly improved our knowledge. However specimens from biopsies may not be adequate to quantify the inflammation of asthma since: (a) they examine only pathological abnormalities of large airways; (b) their size is very small; (c) they do not take into account the possible heterogeneity of the lesions; (d) submucosal edema (due to asthma or to the biopsic procedure) is often present and makes quantitation difficult and uncertain; and (e) the specimens (particularly epithelium) may be altered by the biopsic procedure and by the fixation.

Sampling: Bronchoalveolar Lavage (BAL)

BAL was initiated in asthmatics in the early 1980's in asthmatics (3) and greatly improved our understanding of asthma. It examines an ill-defined segment of the lung including small and large airways as well as alveoli so that although the heterogeneity of the lesions is taken into account, cells and mediators which have recovered originate from ill-defined sites of the lung. Quantitative measures are easy but BAL fluid (BALF) analysis only represents an indirect measure of bronchial inflammation as: (a) mediators may be degraded or only released in situ and therefore may be undetectable in BALF (most cytokines, except IL-1 and TNF, are usually undetectable in BALF by enzyme or radioimmunoassay); and (b) the dilution of the fluid is unknown, and the use of markers such as albumin and/or urea is still under evaluation. It has been proposed that BALF should be separated into several aliquots, and that the first wash is more related to bronchi, but this observation needs confirmation. It is also possible to have a true bronchial wash by means of balloons and catheters, but this technique is difficult, only applicable to large airways, and the volume of fluid recovered is relatively small. However, combining results of BALF and biopsies for similar markers appears to improve examinations of the inflammation of the bronchi better than either technique alone.

Sampling: Bronchial Brushing

This technique allows the examination of epithelial cells but contamination by other cell types should always be examined by immunocytochemistry with anti-cytokeratin antibodies. Cells recovered may be used for functional *in vitro* studies (4).

Samling: Sputum

Sputum is easy to study but its examination requires a perfect specimen that is seldom obtained except with precise techniques such as sputum induced by distilled water (5). Mouth contamination is frequent and quantitative studies cannot be made. When possible BALF should be used instead of sputum.

Sampling: Peripheral Blood

Many studies have been performed in peripheral blood (venous or arterial). Venous blood is easily accessible on a large scale from patients, and markers may be measured serially, but many studies were inconclusive since: (a) inflammatory markers or cells do not only derive from the lung; and (b) they may be completely altered.

Sampling: Urine

The titration of metabolites of leukotrienes (LTE_4) (6), thromboxanes or histamine (methyl-histamine or N-τ-methylimidazole acetic acid) has been used in asthmatics. Levels were found to be often increased after allergen or exercise challenge but only inconstantly increased in chronic and/or acute asthma. For metabolites of eicosanoids the technique of titration is extremely sophisticated (e.g., gas chromatography with mass spectrometry), and cannot be used in routine.

Characteristics of Markers Tested

The characteristics of the markers tested vary with their use: research or routine use for monitoring of asthma. For both research and routine use markers should fulfill the following criteria: (a) They should be released by cells that are pertinent to airways inflammation (and reparation) in asthma, and, if possible, they should be specific of a single cell type; and (b) the titration of the marker or its metabolites should be specific and sensitive. For routine use blood or urine markers must fulfill other criteria: (a) the titration of the marker or of its metabolites must not require very expensive and/or sophisticated techniques and should be performed in many laboratories; (b) if possible, the titration should not be modified by the sampling procedure; (c) pilot studies should have demonstrated that the marker is released during challenge in asthmatic subjects; and (d) studies in a large number of patients should have demonstrated: (i) that the levels of the marker are increased in chronic asthmatics; and (ii) that these levels are correlated with the severity of the disease and (iii) are decreased during effective anti-inflammatory treatment.

Epithelium Damage in Asthma

For many years epithelial cells were considered to have the simple role of a barrier participating in mucous secretion and removal of noxious agents by their cilia. More recently these cells were found to have a much broader activity including the release of eicosanoids, endopeptidases degrading neuropeptides, fibronectin participating in the regeneration of the normal epithelium, as well as possibly a role in immune function by way of their capacity for antigen presentation.

Epithelial Abnormalities in Asthma: Epithelial Shedding

In patients who died from an asthma attack, bronchial epithelium usually presents as having been shed, with separation of the mucosal cells leaving an intact basal cell layer. Changes in the epithelium have almost been found constantly in living asthmatic patients, but more often in moderately severe to severe patients than in mild asthmatic subjects. When the epithelial cells are present, the epithelium has a "fragile" appearance, the ciliated cells appearing swollen, vacuolized and often showing loss of cilia. Separated columnar cells may appear normal and are still attached to each other at their luminal surface, but they often undergo a necrosis. Epithelial cells recovered by brushing are significantly less viable in asthmatics than in normal subjects. However both partial epithelial shedding and increase of goblet cells can be observed in normal non-smoking subjects due to artifacts of the biopsic procedure. The shedding of ciliated epithelial cells from basal cells may be due to eosinophil granule proteins, the release of TNF by macrophages or oxygen free radicals released by several cell types. The loss of the bronchial epithelium layer causes a denudation of nerve endings as shown by electron microscopy.

Epithelial Abnormalities in Asthma: Inflammatory Infiltrate

Patients with an intact epithelium have an increased number of inflammatory cells among epithelial cells. These consist of granulated and degranulated eosinophils, lymphocytes, forms of lymphocytes transitional to plasma cells, activated macrophages and partly degranulated mast cells. In some severe asthmatic patients with a long course of the disease, neutrophils have also been found. These cells are target cells easily accessible to allergens or non-specific irritants.

Epithelial Abnormalities in Asthma: Metabolic Activity

In asthma, epithelial cells obtained by bronchial brushing were shown to release a greater amount of 15-HETE, PGE_2, fibronectin and endothelin spontaneously or after stimulation (4). Epithelial cells from asthmatic patients have an increased expression of Class II antigens and ICAM-1 and often express *c-fos* proto-oncogen suggesting their activation. 15-HETE is a biological mediator with the potential for influencing the inflammatory response through its chemotactic activity and by inducing the release of mucus glycoprotein from human airways in culture. It was also shown to enhance the early bronchoconstrictor response to inhaled allergen in atopic asthmatic subjects. Fibronectin is a large glycoprotein present in the extracellular matrix involved in epithelial cell adhesion and regeneration, suggesting an important role in the repair mechanisms of epithelial cell injury. Endothelin is one of the most potent bronchoconstrictor agents and a growth factor.

Markers of Epithelium in Monitoring of Asthma

There is no single blood or urinary marker of epithelium. In research, epithelium of asthmatics can be easily studied by recovering cells by brushing. A significant correlation has been found between nonspecific airway hyperreactivity and epithelial shedding studied in bronchial biopsies. In the sputum, epithelial cells can be recovered but the value of this finding remains to be understood.

Inflammation of the Submucosa

The bronchial submucosa often shows edema, blood vessel dilatation and a mixed cell infiltrate. These inflammatory cells include eosinophils, mast cells and mononuclear cells but in some patients the infiltrate cannot be found using hematoxylin-eosin staining since cells may be completely degranulated and only visible under conditions of immunohistochemistry or electron microscopy.

Involvement of Eosinophils in Asthma

For many years eosinophils were considered as cells offering protection against allergic inflammation since they release histaminase or arylsulfatase that can counteract the effects of mediators. However, after 1979, studies in parasitic inflammation led to more adequate investigations of the deleterious role of eosinophils. Eosinophils have been found in increased numbers in bronchial biopsies, especially when specimens were examined by immunohistochemistry using monoclonal antibodies against ECP and/or MBP. These cells are usually located beneath the basement membrane and are in an activated stage. They release large amounts of cationic proteins as shown by titration of ECP in the BALF. Most asthmatics, including those with mild asthma, have eosinophils in their bronchi, and there is a significant correlation between activated eosinophils and the severity of asthma. Both allergic and non-allergic asthmatics have a bronchial eosinophilia (1). Eosinophils appear to play a major deleterious role in asthma by the release of highly toxic products (MBP, ECP, EDN or EPX, oxygen free radicals) and it has been suggested that eosinophils play a role in the shedding of the epithelium, therefore confirming the hypotheses of eosinophil-induced damage of the bronchi.

Markers of Eosinophils in Monitoring of Asthma

Markers of eosinophils have been largely studied in asthma. In the BALF, ECP is increased during the late phase reaction following an allergen challenge (7). Significant correlations were observed between BALF markers (ECP and EPX in particular) and asthma severity assessed by the clinical score of Aas of the pulmonary function (1,8). MBP levels were significantly correlated with nonspecific bronchial hyperreactivity (9). There is a significant correlation between ECP and EPX levels in BAL fluid (Figure 1). ECP levels in the BALF significantly decrease during high-dose inhaled corticosteroid treatment (10).

In serum the data are not yet completely clear. Plasma values of ECP are significantly influenced by the sampling technique (11). Mean levels of ECP, EPX or MBP are not largely different between asthmatics and controls (12–15) and there is no indication that ECP levels are correlated with the severity of asthma. On the other hand, ECP and EPX may be useful markers in the serum of follow-up patients under anti-inflammatory treatments (10,13,14) but more data are needed before a definite conclusion can be made. Eosinophil

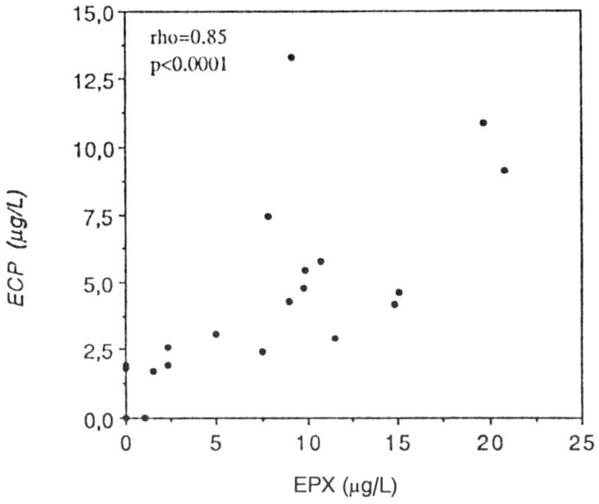

Figure 1. Correlation between BALF levels of ECP and EPX in asthmatics.

counts in peripheral blood and BAL have been correlated with the severity of asthma (clinical score and/or pulmonary function or nonspecific bronchial hyperreactivity) (1) and decreased levels have been found after anti-inflammatory treatment. Increased eosinophil counts and MBP levels have been found in sputum of asthmatics but most studies were designed to improve the diagnosis of asthma rather than monitor its severity. Eosinophil chemotactic activities can be measured in plasma and were found to increase during a pollen season or after allergen challenge (16). When the titration of these putative markers becomes available, they may prove useful in the monitoring of asthma.

Involvement of Metachromatic Cells in Asthma

Mast cells have been found in the bronchi of normal subjects and asthmatic patients. They are degranulated in asthmatics as suggested by the titration of tryptase, histamine and PGD_2 in the BAL fluid and shown by electron microscopy. There was no difference in mast cells in allergic and non-allergic asthma. Mast cells are often found adjacent to blood vessels and appear to be intimately related to bronchial smooth muscle. These cells were shown to release cytokines that may amplify the vaso-active phase of the allergic inflammation as well as attract inflammatory cells. Basophils are probably important cells of the nasal late phase reaction, but at the present their role in asthma is far from being confirmed.

Markers of Metachromatic Cells in Monitoring of Asthma

Histamine was found inconstantly increased in BALF but significant correlations were observed between its levels and nonspecific bronchial hyperreactivity (17) or the severity of asthma assessed by pulmonary function tests (18). In plasma and urine, histamine or methylhistamine can be titrated accurately using sensitive techniques. However, histamine levels in the urine are affected by bacterial contamination, and plasma values vary rapidly and are influenced by the sampling technique. Methylhistamine levels in urine are affected by food intake so that for optimal results subjects should fast for at least 3 hr prior to challenge test. These reasons may explain, at least partly, why plasmatic histamine or urinary methyl-histamine levels were inconstantly found to be increased in asthma (19). In acute asthma plasma histamine was found to be increased (20) but there is no definite data correlating the chronic severity of the disease with the levels of the marker in plasma or urine. After allergen challenge urinary methyl-histamine levels have been found to be increased (21). The presence of tryptase indicates a specific mast cell involved reaction, and its levels are increased in the BALF of pollen-allergic asthmatics after allergen challenge and in chronic asthmatics, but they were not correlated with severity in two studies (8,21). Tryptase levels are also elevated in the BALF of smokers. Data are lacking for blood levels of tryptase in chronic asthma.

Involvement of Lymphocytes in Asthma

T-lymphocytes are another major cell type of the mixed cell infiltrate. They often bear CD4+ receptors. In asthma, it has been observed that some cells express IL-2 receptors indicating that they are in an activated stage. T-cells are likely to play an important role in asthma (22). They may be involved in the formation of IL-4 and γ-IFN known to regulate the IgE synthesis in humans. In addition, T-lymphocyte products have the capacity to orchestrate directly the accumulation and activation of specific granulocyte effector cells at mucosal surfaces. Activated T-cells are a major source of hematopoietic cytokines (23) such as IL-3, GM-CSF and IL-5 involved in the differentiation, attraction and maturation of eosinophils. IL-5 can prolong the survival of eosinophils and activate them to the "hypodense" phenotype. IL-3 and GM-CSF have a role on basophil and mast cell differentiation, and GM-CSF and other T-cell dependent cytokines act on monocyte-macrophage differentiation. T-cells can also generate HRFs enhancing the releasability of basophils and lung mast cells. It therefore seems likely that T-cells may be responsible for initiating and possibly maintaining chronic inflammation from allergic and non-allergic origin.

Markers of Lymphocytes in Monitoring of Asthma

T-cell subsets and markers of activated lymphocytes have been studied in peripheral blood and BALF of asthmatic patients (24). Soluble IL-2-receptor in blood was found in one study (25) to correlate with the severity of asthma, although this could not be confirmed later (26).

Involvement of Macrophages in Asthma

Mononuclear phagocytes are the scavenger cells of the body but they have a much wider function in biology and pathology. They have a fundamental role in specific immunity by their accessory cell function. They are also metabolic cells playing a major role in chronic inflammation. The spectrum of their biologic activity is phenomenal and many of the products released are involved in inflammation, healing and repair. Although broncho-alveolar macrophages recovered by BAL have been extensively studied and are found to be hyperactive in asthma, little information was available on monocytes and macrophages in bronchial biopsies until recently. Using immunohistochemistry with different monoclonal antibodies it was shown in asthma that: (a) macrophages are increased in numbers (pan-macrophage marker); (b) many of these cells bear monocyte markers suggesting that they only recently developed from blood monocytes; and (c) class II antigen positive macrophages are increased, suggesting that they are in an activated stage (27). These cells were mainly found beneath the basement membrane and among epithelial cells. Thus, this study confirmed the role of airways macrophages in the pathogenesis of asthma. In asthmatics recovering from a recent exacerbation, BAL macrophages are often necrotic or apoptotic, whereas in stable asthmatics these patterns of cell death were not detected so often. These data combined with those of bronchial biopsies suggest that there is an increased turnover of macrophages in asthma. Finally, Cluzel et al. showed that the activation of BAL macrophages is significantly correlated with the severity of asthma (28). Airway macrophages appear to be in an activated stage and may release enzymes, eicosanoids, PAF, oxygen free radicals and TNF that might be deleterious for the bronchi. They can also synthesize and secrete a group of metalloproteinases having the capacity to degrade various extracellular matrix macromolecules including elastin. Macrophages may also be involved in the regulation of the airway inflammation through the secretion of cytokines and growth factors such as PDGF and in the priming of mast cell or eosinophil secretory processes as shown recently. These effects were found to enhance the release of vaso-active mediators involved in bronchoconstriction and mucous secretion. Finally, macrophages are likely to be involved in fibrosis. Thus the macrophage might well be the key cell of the bronchial inflammation and repair in asthma.

Markers of Macrophages in Monitoring of Asthma

To date there is no specific marker of macrophage activation that can be titrated in peripheral blood to monitor asthma inflammation. In the BALF, metabolic studies of macrophages may be used to assess their stage of activation and chemical mediators, and cytokines can be titrated. It has also been shown that the density of Percoll-fractionated macrophages was correlated with acute asthma (29).

Other Cell Types and Markers Released by Several Cell Types

Polymorphonuclear neutrophils may be involved in asthma but there is no solid information on these cells. In bronchial biopsies of asthmatic patients they are not often seen except in those with a severe and/or a long course of disease, or in smokers (27). Moreover, neutrophil-

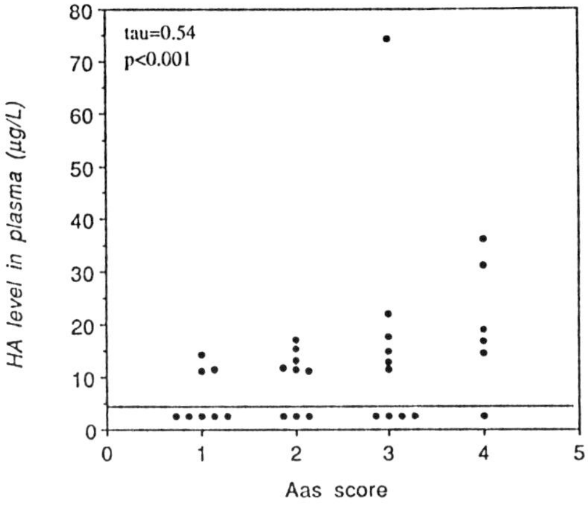

Figure 2. Correlation between the severity of asthma and hyaluronic acid levels.

specific myeloperoxidase is not increased in the BALF of non-smoking asthmatics (8). The importance of platelets in asthma still remains to be confirmed although it has been shown that they are activated in aspirin-induced asthma. Increased platelet factor 4 in blood was found in asthmatics but the relevance of this marker needs to be determined. Fibroblasts are structural cells of importance in inflammatory processes. In the asthmatic airways many fibroblasts have the form of myofibroblasts, characteristic of ongoing inflammation. Hyaluronic acid, a marker of fibroblast activation, is increased in the BALF of asthmatics, and its levels are significantly correlated with the levels of ECP and the severity of asthma (8). HA levels are also increased in peripheral blood of asthmatics (Figure 2). Sulfidopeptide leukotrienes can be released by eosinophils and metachromatic cells. LTC_4/D_4 levels were found increased in BALF (30) and arterial blood of chronic asthmatic patients. The urinary level of their end-product (LTE_4) was found to be increased in urine (by using highly sophisticated techniques not applicable to routine examinations) after allergen or exercise-challenge (6). PGD_2 is released by mast cells and macrophages and its levels are increased in BALF (31). The titration of cytokines in BALF, with techniques that did not use molecular biology, has usually proven inconclusive. A recent study showed that GM-CSF levels in plasma were significantly increased in patients with acute asthma by comparison to control subjects (26).

Reparation

Very little is known on the repair mechanisms in asthma. Collagen deposition was observed as well as elastolysis but there is no data on markers of reparation that can be used to monitor asthma.

References

1. Bousquet, J., Chanez, P., Lacoste, J.Y., et al. 1990. Eosinophilic inflammation in asthma. N. Engl. J. Med. 323:1033.
2. Djukanovic, R., Roche, W.R., Wilson, C.R.W., et al. 1990. Mucosal inflammation in asthma. Am. Rev. Respir. Dis. 142:434.
3. Godard, P., Chaintreuil, J., Damon, M., et al. 1982. Functional assessment of alveolar macrophages: Comparison of cells from asthmatic and normal subjects. J. Allergy Clin. Immunol. 170:88.
4. Campbell, A.M., Chanez, P., Lacoste, J.Y., Godard, P., Michel, F.B., and Bousquet, J. 1991. Epithelial cells obtained by brushing in normal subjects and asthmatics. Chest, in press.
5. Gibson, P.G., Girgis-Gabardo, A., Morris, M.M., et al. 1989. Cellular characteristics of sputum from patients with asthma and chronic bronchitis. Thorax 44:693.
6. Taylor, G.W., Taylor, I., Black, P., et al. 1989. Urinary leukotriene E4 after antigen challenge and in acute asthma and allergic rhinitis. Lancet I:584.
7. De Monchy, J.G.R., Kaufman, H.F., Venge, P., et al. 1985. Bronchoalveolar eosinophils during allergen-induced late reactions. Am. Rev. Respir. Dis. 131:373.
8. Bousquet, J., Chanez, P., Lacoste, J.Y., et al. 1991. Indirect assessment of bronchial inflammation in asthma by titration of mediators in bronchoalveolar lavage fluid. J. Allergy Clin. Immunol. 88:649.
9. Wardlaw, A.J., Dunnette, S., Gleich, G.J., Collins, J.V., and Kay, A.B. 1988. Eosinophils and mast cells in bronchoalveolar lavage in subjects with mild asthma. Am. Rev. Respir. Dis. 137:62.
10. Ådelroth, E., Rosenhall, L., Johansson, S-Å., Linden, M., and Venge, P. 1990. Inflammatory cells and eosinophilic activity in asthmatics investigated by bronchoalveolar lavage. The ef-

fects of antiasthmatic treatment with budesonide or terbutaline. Am. Rev. Respir. Dis. 142:91.
11. Venge, P., Dahl, R., Fredens, K., et al. 1983. Eosinophil cationic proteins (ECP and EPX) in health and disease. In: Immunobiology of the eosinophil. T. Yoshida and M. Torius, eds. New York: Elsevier, p. 163.
12. Durham, S.R., Loegering, D.A., Dunnette, S., Gleich, G.J, Kay. A.B. 1988. Blood eosinophils and eosinophil-derived proteins in allergic asthma. J. Allergy Clin. Immunol. 81:711.
13. Griffin, E., Hakansson, L., Formgren, H., Jôrgensen, P., Peterson, C., and Venge, P. 1991. Blood eosinophil number and activity in relation to lung function in patients with asthma and eosinophilia. J. Allergy Clin. Immunol. 87:548.
14. Venge, P., Dahl, R., and Peterson, G.B. 1988. Eosinophil granule protein in serum after allergen challenge of asthmatic patients and the effects of anti-asthmatic medication. Int. Arch. Allergy Appl. Immunol. 87:306.
15. Venge, P., Zetterström, O., Dahl, R., Roxin, R., and Olsson, I. 1977. Low levels of eosinophil cationic proteins in patients with asthma. Lancet II:373.
16. Hakannson, L., Rak, S., Dahl, R., and Venge, P. 1989. The formation of eosinophil and neutrophil chemotactic activity during a pollen season and after allergen challenge. J. Allergy Clin. Immunol. 83:933.
17. Casale, T.B., Wood, D., Richerson, H.B., et al. 1987. Elevated bronchoalveolar lavage fluid histamine levels in allergic asthmatics are associated with methacholine hyperreactivity. J. Clin. Invest. 79:1197.
18. Jarjour, N.N., Calhoun, W.J., Schwartz, L.B., and Busse, W.W. 1991. Elevated bronchoalveolar lavage fluid histamine levels in allergic asthmatics are associated with increased airway obstruction. Am. Rev. Respir. Dis. 144:83.
19. Löwhagen, O., Granerus, G., and Wetterqvist, H. 1979. Studies on histamine metabolism in intrinsic bronchial asthma. Allergy 34:395.
20. Simon, R.A., Stevenson, D.D., Arroyave, C.M., and Tan, E.M. 1977. The relationship of plasma histamine to the activity of bronchial asthma. J. Allergy Clin. Immunol. 60:312.
21. Keyzer, J.J., Kauffman, H.F., De Monchy, J.G.R., Keyzer-Udding, J.J., and De Vries, K. 1984. Urinary N^{τ}-methylhistamine during early and late allergn-induced bronchial-obstructive reactions. J. Allergy Clin. Immunol. 74:240.
22. Kay, A.B. 1991. Lymphocytes in asthma. Resp. Med. 85:87.
23. Hamid, G., Azzawi, M., Ying, S., et al. 1991. Expression of mRNA for interleukin-5 in mucosal bronchial biopsies from asthma. J. Clin. Invest 87:1541.
24. Kelly, C.A., Stenton, S.C., Ward, C., et al. 1989. Lymphocyte subsets in bronchoalveolar lavage fluid obtained from stable asthmatics and their correlations with bronchial responsiveness. Clin. Exp. Allergy 19:169.
25. Corrigan, C.J., and Kay, A.B. 1990. CD4 T-lymphocyte activation in acute severe asthma. The relationship to disease severity and atopic status. Am. Rev. Respir. Dis. 140:970.
26. Brown, P.H., Crompton, G.K., and Greening, A.P. 1991. Proinflammatory cytokines in acute asthma. Lancet 338:590.
27. Poston, R., Litchfield, P., Chanez, P., Lacoste, J.Y., Lee, T.K., and Bousquet, J. 1991. Immunohistochemical characterization of the cellular infiltration of asthmatic bronchi. Am. Rev. Respir. Dis., in press.
28. Cluzel, M., Damon, M., Chanez, P., et al. 1987. Enhanced alveolar cell luminol-dependent chemiluminescence in asthma. J. Allergy Clin. Immunol. 80:195.
29. Chanez, P., Bousquet, J., Couret, I., et al. 1991. Increased numbers of hypodense alveolar macrophages in patients with bronchial asthma. Am. Rev. Respir. Dis. 144:923.
30. Lam, S., Chan, H., LeRiche, J.C., Chan-Yeung, M., and Salari, H. 1989. Release of leukotrienes in patients with bronchial asthma. J. Allergy Clin. Immunol. 84:931.
31. Liu, M.C., Bleecker, E., Lichtenstein, L.M., et al. 1990. Evidence for elevated levels of histamine, prostaglandin D2 and other bronchoconstricting prostaglandins in the airways of subjects with mild asthma. Am. Rev. Respir. Dis. 142:126.

Progress in Diagnosis and Management of Atopic Dermatitis

Hugh A. Sampson*

Atopic dermatitis is a chronic form of eczema which has become more prevalent in the past several decades. Recent advances in the identification of cytokines and their effect on immune regulation have provided new insights into the immunopathogenesis of atopic dermatitis. Although there have been no recent "breakthroughs" in the diagnosis and management of atopic dermatitis, this new knowledge provides fertile ground for major advances in the near future.

Atopic dermatitis (AD) is one form of eczema which generally begins in infancy and is characterized by extreme pruritus, a chronically relapsing course, characteristic distribution, and an association with allergic rhinitis and asthma. Approximately 90% of children with AD will develop skin lesions by 2 years of age, while about 90% of all cases of AD will present by 5 years of age. The cumulative prevalence of AD has been increasing in the past 2 decades and is now believed to affect 10% to 15% of the population (1). A variety of factors are known to exacerbate flares of AD including irritants, heat, allergens, stress, and infection, but the underlying pathogenic mechanism (or mechanisms) remains unknown.

Phenotypic expression of AD is dependent upon both hereditary and environmental factors. The importance of genetics is underscored by the high (86%) concordance rate among monozygotic twin pairs compared to a 21% concordance rate in dizygotic twin pairs and siblings (2). The development or resolution of AD in bone marrow transplantation recipients indicate that bone marrow-derived cells are central to the immunopathogenesis of eczema. AD has developed in patients receiving bone marrow from donors with AD (3), and eczematous lesions have resolved in patients with Wiskott-Aldrich Syndrome following successful bone marrow engraftment (4). Environmental factors also may play a strategic role in the development of AD. Several studies have evaluated the effect of strict dietary elimination of major food allergens from infants at high risk for atopy. When infants and their lactating mothers were placed on strict allergen avoidance diets, they had significantly less AD compared to high risk infants on no dietary restrictions (5).

Atopic dermatitis is an erythematous papulovesicular eruption that evolves into scaly, lichenified plaques over time. Histological features of AD lesions are non-specific and depend on the stage of the lesion (6). *Acute* lesions are characterized by epidermal hyperplasia with focal intercellular edema, vesiculation, and infiltration of lymphocytes and monocytes. Perivenular infiltrations of lymphocytes, monocytes, and occasional neutrophils and eosinophils are prominent in the dermis. *Chronic* lesions show marked epidermal hyperplasia and dyskeratosis with marked fibrosis at all levels of the dermis, increased numbers of mast cells and Langerhans cells (LC's), and demyelination of cutaneous nerves. Immunohistochemical studies have revealed the following features: Infiltrating lymphocytes are predominantly $CD4^+$ T cells, LC's bear IgE on their surface (7), and a significant proportion of mast cells in lesional skin are lymphocyte-dependent M_T type (instead of M_{TC} type) (8), and eosinophil major basic protein (MBP) and cationic protein (ECP) are deposited in the dermis of eczematous lesions in most patients (9).

A number of abnormal physiologic and immunologic phenomena have been delineated in patients with AD, most of which vary in direct proportion to the extent of cutaneous lesions. Physiologic abnormalities include a decreased

* Division of Allergy/Immunology, The Johns Hopkins University School of Medicine, Baltimore, Maryland, USA.
Acknowledgements: Supported in part by AI-24439 from the National Institute of Allergy and Infectious Diseases and RR-00052 from the General Clinical Research Centers Program.

itch threshold, decreased and/or structurally altered ceremides from keratinocytes leading to increased transepidermal water loss, increased plasma linoleic acid levels and abnormal red cell phospholipids, increased cyclic-AMP phosphodiesterase activity in mononuclear cells, and paradoxical cutaneous vascular responses including white dermographism. *Immunological abnormalities* are characterized by overproduction of IgE and diminished T cell functions including decreased anamnestic antibody levels of recall antigens (e.g., tetanus, polio, etc.), decreased $CD8^+$ cells and increased CD4/CD8 ratio in the peripheral blood, depressed lymphocyte proliferation to antigens *in vitro*, cutaneous anergy with increased viral infections of the skin and decreased ability to develop sensitivity to contact allergens such as DNCB, and depressed chemotaxis of leukocytes and monocytes.

Recent advances in our understanding of cytokine production and interaction are providing new insight into the pathogenesis of AD. Studies in the mouse indicated that $CD4^+$ cells could be divided into TH_1 and TH_2 subpopulations (10). Activated TH_1 cells secrete predominantly IL-2 and interferon gamma (IFN) and to a lesser extent IL-3 and GM-CSF, and preferentially induce macrophage activation and delayed-type hypersensitivity. TH_2 cells produce primarily IL-4 and to a lesser extent IL-5, IL-6, IL-10, IL-3 and GM-CSF, and provide superior help for B cell responses. These subtypes have counter-regulatory roles in that IFN inhibits TH_2 cell proliferation and IL-10 inhibits TH_1 cells (11). Recent studies in man suggest that similar CD4 subtypes exist in man (12), and that allergen-specific T cell clones from patients with AD produced substantial amounts of IL-4 and minimal levels of IFN whereas non-allergen-specific T cell clones from AD patients or allergen-specific clones from non-atopic donors produced primarily IFN and minimal IL-4 (13). The presence of significant numbers of IL-4 secreting $CD4^+$ cells in AD patients may be of pathogenic significance since IgE production has been shown to be reciprocally regulated by IL-4 and IFN (14). In further studies it was found that virtually all $CD4^+$ cloned from eczematous lesions of AD patients were allergen-specific TH_2 cells, and that the IL-4 secreted was capable of inducing CD23 expression on antigen presenting cells (15). The local production of IL-4 by these infiltrating lymphocytes would promote CD23 expression on LC's, enabling them to present allergen more effectively. Recently it was shown that IgE^+-LC's were necessary to promote T cell responses to dust mite antigen *in vitro* (16). IgE^--LC's from AD patients or IgE^+-LC's preincubated with anti-IgE antibodies could not promote a T cell response to dust mite antigen, but the response to *Candida albicans* was no different when presented by IgE^+- or IgE^--LC's. These *in vitro* results correlated well with results of *in vivo* patch tests to these same antigens.

The role of IgE in the pathogenesis of AD has been suspected for many years. Food and airborne allergens may reach cutaneous mast cells, LC's, and lymphocytes by entering at mucosal surfaces and by being transported through the blood stream or infiltrating through minor breaks in the epidermis (17). As depicted in Figure 1, activation of mast cells leads to release of histamine, PGD_2 platelet-activating factor, and cytokines which may attract other cells (e.g., eosinophils, lymphocytes, and monocytes) in a late-phase response. Release of IL-4 and IL-10 by infiltrating lymphocytes would inhibit local TH_1 proliferation and cell-mediated responses and promote CD23 expression on LC's and monocytes leading to allergen-induced IL-1 release and the efficient presentation of allergens to T cells. IL-5 released by activated T cells (and possibly mast cells) would foster the infiltration and activation of eosinophils, which have been shown to play a central role in the pathogenesis of AD lesions, and IL-3 would promote local mast cell proliferation (M_T type). Repeated exposure to food and/or airborne allergens would result in chronic inflammation secondary to IgE-mediated Type-I and Type-IV hypersensitivity responses. In food allergic children, chronic food allergen ingestion has been shown to provoke "spontaneous" production of histamine-releasing factor from peripheral blood mononuclear cells (18), and to increase the number of "activated" eosinophils and basophils in the peripheral blood. While the underlying defect which results in the predominant TH_2 cell response to allergens remains to be elucidated, our understanding of the immunopathogenic mechanisms responsible for eczematous lesions in AD patients has progressed significantly in the last several years.

Despite the many exciting advances in our knowledge of immunopathogenic mechanisms, the diagnosis of AD remains dependent upon clinical criteria (19). Although the deposition

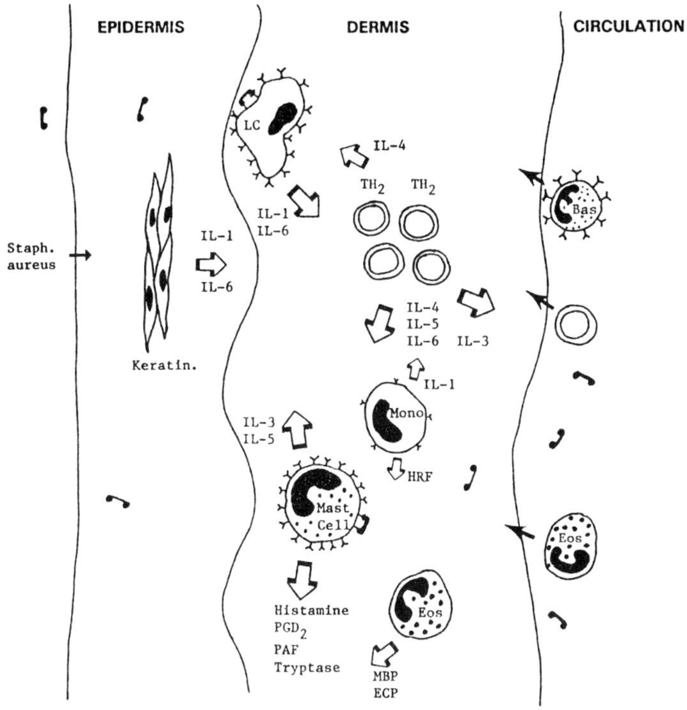

Figure 1. Allergen-induced activation of cutaneous mast cells and IgE±Langerhans cells results in the release of a number of mediators and cytokines which attract leukocytes, lymphocytes, and monocytes to the area promoting achronic cell-mediated inflammatory response. LC: Langerhans cell; Eos: eosinophil; Bas: basophil; Mono: monocyte; Keratin: keratinocyte.

of eosinophil MBP and ECP in the epidermis and dermis, and IgE^{+}-LC's are seen almost exclusively in lesional skin biopsies of AD patients, neither finding is pathognomonic. To determine the specificity of allergens suspected of provoking exacerbations of AD, the use of patch tests with airborne allergens appears promising (20). Dust mite sensitive patients with AD develop eczematous lesions with patch testing to dust mite, but a controlled trial demonstrating clinical improvement when patients are placed in mite-free environments has not yet been published (21). The double-blind placebo-controlled oral food challenge has proven to be the gold standard for diagnosing food hypersensitivity in AD patients. Whether a patch test technique might be useful in diagnosing food hypersensitivity remains to be established. Several scoring systems have been proposed to monitor disease activity in AD patients (1), but all are cumbersome and no unanimity on criteria has been reached. Two recent reports suggested that serum ECP concentration may provide a useful marker of disease activity. Serum ECP levels were found to be elevated in patients with AD compared to patients with psoriasis, inhalant allergy, or controls (22,23). In one study, the ECP concentrations were shown to correlate directly with the extent of skin involvement (23).

Although no major breakthrough in the treatment of AD has yet occurred, our advances in understanding basic mechanisms have provided insight into the better use of therapies currently at hand, and prospects for developing several new strategies. Pruritus and dry skin with secondary damage due to scratching remain the hallmark of AD. Use of *hydration and emollients* to circumvent the patient's deficient epidermal water barrier can significantly reduce itching. A number of studies investigating the anti-pruritic effect of *antihistamines* have concluded that histamine plays a minor role in the itchy skin of AD patients and that other mediators (e.g., neuropeptides, cytokines) are primarily responsible for the pruritus. However, two antihistamines (hydroxyzine and cetirizine) appear to reduce itching and have several unique properties which may favor their use in AD. Not only are these drugs effective H_1-receptor antagonists, but they also block IgE-mediated late-phase mast cell release of PAF (24) and the recruitment of neutrophils, eosinophils, and basophils into allergen-challenged skin blisters (25). Several uncontrolled trials of topical or oral *sodium cromoglycate* or the newer *nedocromil sodium* suggested some beneficial results. However, most recent controlled trials have failed to show any beneficial effects in the treatment of AD patients (26). *Phosphodiesterase inhibitors* have also been promoted for their antipruritic effect, but in a recent double-blind controlled trial of papaverine (the most promising agent), no beneficial effect was detected (27). *Corticosteroids* (primarily topical), with their broad immunomodulatory effects on LC's, lymphocytes, and the late-phase of the IgE-mediated response, continue as the mainstay of therapy in AD. Ultraviolet light therapy and psoralen photochemotherapy (*PUVA*) have been shown to induce remission in many patients with AD (28), probably due to their suppressive effect on LC's and possibly on cutaneous mast cells. However, the almost inevitable relapse following treatment, and the skin aging and increased risk of skin cancer with prolonged therapy discourage their use in children and limit their use in adults.

Several immunomodulatory approaches to the treatment of AD appear somewhat promising and may lead to more effective forms of therapy. A recent double-blind, placebo-controlled cross-over trial of *cyclosporin* (5 mg/kg/day)in adults with refractory AD demonstrated significant benefit when compared to placebo (29). Interestingly, pruritus was noted to decrease dramatically within 2 to 4 days, suggesting the inhibition of a "pruritogenic cytokine"(30). Unfortunately the hepatotoxic and immunosuppressive effects of this drug will preclude its use except in the most refractory cases of adults with AD. Early reports on the beneficial effects of topical cyclosporin were not borne out in a larger controlled trial. *Thymopentin* (TP5) is a synthetic pentapeptide corresponding to amino acid residues 32 through 36 of human thymopoietin, and which has been shown to promote differentiation of thymocytes and enhance T cell function. In a 6 week double-blind, controlled trial, 48 AD patients received daily subcutaneous TP5 injections and 52 received placebo (31). Subjects treated with TP5 experienced a significant decrease in their total severity scores compared to the placebo-treated group. Significant differences were not seen until the 6 week exam suggesting that the onset of action of TP5 may be delayed. No significant adverse effects were seen. IFN inhibits TH_2 cell functions including IgE synthesis and upregulation of CD23 receptors on a variety of cells (e.g. LC's, monocytes, lymphocytes, etc.). In a double-blind, controlled trial of recombinant IFN in the treatment of moderate to severe AD, 40 patients received daily subcutaneous injections of IFN, and 43 received placebo for 12 weeks (32). Physician and patient severity scores were significantly improved in subjects treated with IFN compared to placebo. In addition, blood eosinophil counts and spontaneous *in vitro* IgE synthesis by peripheral blood lymphocytes were decreased in the treated group. *Injection therapy* with mite allergen-antibody complexes appeared to have some beneficial effect in an uncontrolled study of 10 adults with AD and dust mite sensitivity (32). Significant improvement was noted in all patients after 3 to 4 months of therapy, and 6/10 were in complete or near-complete remission at 1 year. The lack of placebo control and the complexity of preparing specific antibody-antigen complexes for each patient temper the enthusiasm for this approach.

Significant advances in our understanding of the immunopathogenesis of AD have not yet translated into major advances in the diagnosis and treatment of this disorder. However, promising "first generation" immunomodulatory therapies provide hope for major advances in the coming years.

References

1. Rajka, G. 1989. Atopic dermatitis: Clinical aspects. In: Essential aspects of atopic dermatitis. G. Rajka, ed. Berlin: Springer-Verlig, p 4.
2. Schultz-Larsen, F., Holm, N.V., and Henningsen, K. 1986. Atopic dermatitis. Agenetic-epidemiologic study in a population based twin sample. J. Am. Acad. Dermatol. 15: 487.
3. Agosti, J.M., Sprenger, J.K., Lum, L.G., et al. 1988. Transfer of allergen-specific IgE-mediated hypersensitivity with allogeneic bone marrow transplantation. N. Engl. J. Med. 319:1623.
4. Saurat, J.-H. 1985. Eczema in primary immune deficiencies. Acta Derm. Venerol. (Stockholm) 114:125.
5. Zeiger, R.S., Heller, S., Mellon, M.H., et al.

1989. Effect of combined maternal and infant food allergen avoidance on development of atopy in early infancy: A randomized study. J. Allergy Clin. Immunol. 84:72.
6. Soter, N.A. 1989. Morphology of atopic dermatitis. Allergy 44 (Supp. l9):16.
7. Bruynzeel-Koomen, C., Wichen, D.F., Toonstra, J., et al. 1986. The presence of IgE molecules on epidermal Langerhans cells in patients with atopic dermatitis. Arch. Dermatol. Res. 278:199.
8. Irani, A.M., Sampson, H.A., Schwartz, L.B. 1989. Mast cells in atopic dermatis. Allergy 44 (Suppl. 9):31.
9. Leiferman, K.M. 1991. A current perspective on the role of eosinophils in dermatologic diseases. J. Am. Acad. Dermatol. 24:1101.
10. Mosmann, T.R., Cherwinski, H., Bond, M.W., et al. 1986. Two types of murine helper T cell clone. I. Definition according to profiles of lymphokine activities and secreted proteins. J. Immunol. 136:2348.
11. Fiorentino, D.F., Zlotnik, A., Vieira, P., et al. 1991. IL-10 acts on the antigen-presenting cell to inhibit cytokine production by TH1 cells. J. Immunol. 146:3444.
12. Romagnani, S. 1991. Human TH1 and Th2 cells. Doubt no more. Immunol. Today 12:256.
13. Wierenga, E.A., Snoek, M., de Groot, C., et al. 1990. Evidence for compartmentalization of functional subsets of CD4+ T lymphocytes in atopic patients. J. Immunol. 144:4651.
14. Pene, J., Rousset, F., Briere, F., et al. 1988. IgE production by normal human B cells induced by alloreactive T cell clones is mediated by IL-4 and suppressed by IFN. J. Immunol. 141:1218.
15. van der Heifden, F L., Wierenga, E.A., Bos, J.D., et al. 1991. High frequency of IL-4-producing CD4+ allergen-specific T lymphocytes in atopic dermatitis lesional skin. J. Invest. Deramtol. 97:389.
16. Mudde, G.C., van Reijsen, .FC., Boland, G.J., et al. 1990. Allergen presentation by epidermal Langerhans' cells from patients with atopic dermatitis is mediated by IgE. Immunol. 69:335.
17. Sampson, H.A. 1990. Pathogenesis of eczema. Clin. Exper. Allergy 20:459.
18. Sampson, H.A., Broadbent, K.R., Bernhisel-Broadbent, J. 1989. Spontaneous release of histamine from basophils and histamine-releasing factor in patients with atopic dermatitis and food hypersensitivity. N. Engl. J. Med. 321:228.
19. Hanifin, J.M., Rajka, G. 1980. Diagnostic features of atopic dermatitis. Acta Dermatol. Venereol. 92 (Suppl.):44.
20. Adinoff, A.D., Tellez, P., Clark, R.A.F. 1988. Atopic dermatitis and aeroallergen contact sensitivity. J. Allergy Clin. Immunol. 81:736.
21. Beck, H.-I., Bjerring, .P, Harving, H. 1989. Atopic dermatitis and the indoor climate. The effect from preventive measures. Acta Derm. Venereol. (Stockholm) 1989:162.
22. Kapp, A., Czech, W., Krutman, J., et al. 1991. Eosinophil cationic protein in sera of patients with atopic dermatitis. J. Am. Acad. Dermatol. 24:555.
23. Jakob, T., Hermann, K., Ring, J. 1991. Eosinophil cationic protein in atopic eczema. Arch. Dermatol. Res. 283:5.
24. Michel, L., De Vos, C., Rihowx, J.-P., et al. 1988. Inhibitory effect of oral cetirizine on *in vivo* antigen-induced histamine and PAF-acether release and eosinophil recruitment in human skin. J. Allergy Clin. Immunol. 82:101.
25. Charlesworth, E.N., Kagey-Sabotka, A., Norman, P.S., et al. 1989. Effect of cetirizine on mast cell-mediator release and cellular traffic during the cutaneous late-phase reaction. J. Allergy Clin. Immunol. 83:905.
26. David, T.J. 1991. New approaches to the treatment of atopic dermatitis in childhood. Pediatr. Rev. Commun. 5:145.
27. Berth-Jones, J., Graham-Brown, R.A.C. 1990. Failure of papaverine to reduce pruritus in atopic dermatitis: a double-blind, placebo-controlled cross-over study. Br. J. Dermatol. 122:553.
28. Atherton, D.J., Cababott, F., Glover, M.T., et al. 1988. The role of psoralen chemotherapy (PUVA) in the treatment of severe atopic eczema in adolescence. Br. J. Dermatol. 118:791.
29. Sowden, J.M., Berth-Jones, J., Ross, J.S., et al. 1991. Double-blind, controlled, crossover study of cyclosporin in adults with severe refractory atopic dermatitis. Lancet 338:137.
30. Ross, J.S., Camp, R.D.R. 1990. Cyclosporin A in atopic dermatitis. Br. J. Dermatol. 122 (Suppl. 36):41.
31. Leung, D.Y.M., Hirsch, R.L., Schneider, L., et al. 1990. Thymopent in therapy reduces the clinical severity of atopic dermatitis. J. Allergy Clin. Immunol. 85:927.
32. Schneider, L.C., Hanifin, J., Cooper, K., et al. 1991. Recombinant interferon-gamma therapy reduces the clinical severity of atopic dermatitis. J. Allergy Clin. Immunol. 87:235.
33. Leroy, B.P., Lachapelle, J.M., Somville, M. M, et al. 1991. Injection of allergen-antibody complexes is an effective treatment of atopic dermatitis. Dermatologica 182:98.

Progress in Early Detection of Atopic Disease

Stefan Croner*

The prevalence of atopic diseases is increasing in northwestern Europe and probably also in the rest of the westernized world. Cord blood IgE in combination with the family history of atopic disease seems at the present to be the most valuable tool for the prediction of early, multiple and more severe forms of atopic disease, but still only identifies a small proportion of all children who subsequently do develop atopic disease. Cord blood IgE cannot, without modifications, be recommended as a single test for identifying infants for allergy preventive programs. Other methods, such as genetic markers of atopic constitution, may develop in the near future to improve early identification of infants "at risk" of atopic disease.

Incidence and Prevalence of Atopic Disease

The prevalence of atopic diseases in childhood and adolescence, i.e. bronchial asthma (AB), allergic rhinoconjunctivitis (ARC) and atopic dermatitis (AD) is increasing in the industrialized (1,2,3,4) as well as in developing countries (5). The increased morbidity is claimed to be valid and not simply due to changes in diagnostic fashions (3). The prevalence of AB in children 6–18 years of age varies between 1.6 and 10%. In the Nordic countries the prevalence of AB was around 1–1.4% in the 1950's (6). In the 1980's corresponding figures in Sweden were 2.4–4% (4,7). The prevalence of ARC in Swedish schoolchildren in 1960 was 2.4% (8) while in the 80's it was 7.4% (7). The prevalence of AD was 7.8% (7). A remarkable increase has been noticed in northern parts of Sweden both in school children and in conscripts aged 18 (9). Possible explanations for this regional increase may be a deterioration in indoor environment with increased exposure to particles, evaporation from building materials, mites and animal proteins. Due to this increase in atopic diseases the search for reliable methods for prediction of these diseases has been intense during the last decades.

Laboratory Parameters for Prediction and Early Detection of Atopic Disease in Infancy and Childhood

Hyperproduction of IgE and of specific IgE antibodies are hallmarks of atopic diseases. Elevated total IgE (10,11,12), IgE antibodies in serum (13) and in skin (14,15) in healthy infants, children and adolescents have been found to precede the development of clinical disease.

IgE in Amniotic Fluid

Two studies have shown that determination of IgE in amniotic fluid (AF) might be useful in predicting atopic disease in infancy (16,17). In a different study, on the other hand, in 83 children followed for 1 year, AF-IgE was of no predictive value (18). Amniocentesis for the purpose of AF-IgE determination is too risky and the possibility of contamination with maternal blood is obvious.

IgE in Cord Blood

When using a sensitive assay such as Phadebas IgE PRIST® (10,19) or the even more sensitive IgE RIA Ultra® assay (Pharmacia Diagnostics AB, Uppsala Sweden, 1985) low levels of IgE can be detected in the blood of newborns. During the last 20 years, quite a number of investigations have been performed in several countries establishing the value of CB-IgE as a predictor of atopic disease in childhood (11,12,20,21,22,23). The Phadezym IgE PRIST®, an enzyme immunoassay, correlated

* Deptartment of Pediatrics, Faculty of Health Sciences, University Hospital, S-58185 Linköping, Sweden.

well with Phadebas IgE PRIST® (r=0.97) in 300 German newborns (24). Using a cut-off level of 0.9 kU/l, 15 of 23 children (65%) with an elevated CB-IgE developed atopic disease by 18 months of age. CB-IgE assayed by PACIA, a particle counting immunoassay, in an unselected series of 190 Belgian newborns had a sensitivity of 70% in children with a CB-IgE level ≥1.2 kU/l (25). In a Danish cohort of 1,189 infants, CB-IgE concentration 0.3 kU/l assayed by IgE RIA Ultra was the best cut-off level for prediction of atopic disease up to 5 years of age (26). In our cohort of 1,654 children followed up to 11 years of age, children having a high CB-IgE (≥0.9 kU/l) had a 5-fold risk for developing bronchial asthma (4).

Other studies have failed to show a good predictive capacity of CB-IgE. Among 115 Swedish high-risk infants followed-up to 18 months of age, the sensitivity was only 10% and the specificity 82% of CB-IgE concentration ≥0.9 kU/l (27). Similar results were found in other groups of Swedish high risk infants (28,29). Among 788 British infants followed to 1 year of age the sensitivity of CB-IgE was 9% but the specificity reached 78%, using 0.6 kU/l as cut-off level (30). In a cohort of 546 Danish children, no correlation was found between a CB-IgE ≥1.0 kU/l and subsequent disease up to 7 years of age (31). The discrepancies may partly be due to differences in the populations under study. Studies including selected groups of high-risk infants cannot be compared with whole population-based studies. It is probable that nowadays mothers-to-be are more conscious about the allergy risk with lower allergenic exposure of the fetus as a result. Health education may have led to lower cigarette smoking during pregnancy. Allergy preventive programs including manipulation of maternal food intake, prolonged breast feeding, later introduction of allergenic foods to the babies, avoidance of pets during the first years of life in combination with changes in the indoor and outdoor environment since 1975 have all changed the allergen load on the fetus and infant. These facts have made comparisons of studies during the last decades on the value of CB-IgE screening difficult. Several investigations in other countries and populations have shown that CB-IgE levels among neonates seem to have only minor variations: e.g. Chinese (32), and in black Americans (33). But significant differences in the median CB-IgE concentrations were, however, demonstrated between black and white ethnic groups in South Africa (34).

CB-IgE may be influenced by the month of birth and the child's sex, but gestational age does not seem to have considerable influence on the concentration (35). Among 1,074 umbilical cord sera probes from newborns in a healthy population in Tucson, Arizona, CB-IgE was higher in boys and in infants who developed AD before 9 months of age (36). CB-IgE varied according to the month of birth with a trough in September. A significant correlation between IgE levels at birth and 9 months of age was observed. Maternal cigarette smoking (37) as well as medication during pregnancy with progesterone (12) or metoprolol (38), a beta-adrenergic receptor blocking agent, increase CB-IgE significantly. CB-IgE levels, however, were unaffected by maternal smoking in the recent Arizona study (36).

IgE During the First Week of Life

Transfer of minimal amounts of blood from a mother to her fetus or admixture of maternal blood when collecting cord blood may occur and can be revealed by the presence in cord blood of IgA and/or specific IgE antibodies also present in maternal blood (39,40). In order to avoid the problems of contamination, blood sampling during the first week of life has been advocated. Among 83 Swedish infants with a family history (FH), 22 had CB-IgE ≥0.9 kU/l while a lower value on days 4–5 was found in half of these children (40). But cord blood may be difficult to obtain on a routine basis for mass screening. In order to avoid this problem, a Japanese group recently presented a high positive predictive value of IgE assayed by DELFIA®, measured on filter paper blood, collected from the heels of neonates on day 4–5. 90% of 389 infants with an FH and high IgE levels in filter paper blood developed atopic disease by 18 months of age (41).

IgE-Binding Factors in Cord Blood

Two classes of receptors for IgE have been identified, i. e. the high-affinity receptor Fc epsilon RI on basophils and mast cells and the low-affinity Fc epsilon RII (CD23) present on lymphocytes, platelets, eosinophils and macrophages (42). CB-CD23 levels, measured by

Table 1. Prevalence (%) of childhood bronchial asthma by age and sex in Taipei city in 1974, 1985 and 1991

Age (yr)	Boy 1974	Boy 1985	Boy 1991	Girl 1974	Girl 1985	Girl 1991	Average 1974	Average 1985	Average 1991
7	2.41	7.46	8.32	1.85	5.01	6.18	2.10	6.24	7.25
8	1.59	7.01	8.99	1.92	4.97	5.60	1.76	6.00	7.30
9	1.41	7.41	8.14	1.34	5.16	5.01	1.41	6.28	6.58
10	1.97	6.18	8.89	1.31	4.03	5.05	1.65	5.12	7.02
11	1.81	5.61	7.14	1.36	4.08	4.50	1.22	4.83	5.99
12	1.45	5.93	7.10	0.74	3.99	3.94	1.09	4.96	5.52
13	0.92	5.01	6.91	0.81	3.22	4.02	0.86	4.10	5.47
14	1.37	5.08	6.73	0.82	3.44	3.48	1.08	4.21	5.11
15	1.30	4.11	4.94	0.86	3.61	3.27	1.03	3.85	4.11
Mean	1.45	5.99	7.32	1.15	4.17	4.34	1.30	5.07	5.80
Total number studied	11,481	72,466	45,458	12,197	74,9079	47,013	23,678	147,373	92,471

sidered thoroughly answered and could be used for analysis. The recovered rate of 82% was comparable to 78% in the 1974 study and 85% in 1985. There were 45,458 boys and 47,013 girls. The prevalence of bronchial asthma for each age group is listed in Table 1. In the three surveys, the prevalence of asthma decreased, regardless of sex, as the children grew up, and for each age group boys were affected more often than girls (1.26:1 in 1974, 1.44:1 in 1985 and 1.69:1 in 1991). The average prevalence of childhood asthma (in 7–15-year-olds) in 1974 was 1.45% for boys and 1.15% for girls; the figures for 1985 were 5.99% and 4.17%, respectively, and 7.32% and 4.34%, respectively, in 1991. Thus, in the past 17 years in Taipei, the prevalence of childhood asthma in school children increased 5-fold in boys and 3.8-fold in girls, with a mean of 4.5-fold. In addition to the increase in prevalence, the severity of bronchial asthma also increased. The percentage of asthmatic children with a frequency of attack of greater than 12 times per year was 9.2% in 1974 and 19.4% in 1991 (data not shown). As shown in Table 2,the prevalence of allergic rhinitis for boys was 9.91% in 1985 and 25.33% in 1991 (a 2.6-fold increase), and the figures for girls were 6.14% and 15.78%, respectively, which also showed a 2.6-fold increase.

It is interesting to note that the prevalence of atopic eczema and urticaria did not change during the period of 1974 to 1985; however, there was a sharp increase of both diseases in the 1991 survey (Table 2). The increase in atopic eczema was 2.9-fold and the figure for urticaria was nearly the same (2.94-fold). In contrast to bronchial asthma and allergic rhinitis, no sex difference was found for dermatologic allergy.

Neither sex nor the age of onset influenced the prognosis of allergic diseases. In general, 35–40% of atopic children outgrew their diseases before 15 years of age (data not shown).

Table 2. Prevalence (%) of childhood allergic diseases in Taipei city in 1974, 1985 and 1991

Allergic disease	Boy 1974	Boy 1985	Boy 1991	Girl 1974	Girl 1985	Girl 1991	Average 1974	Average 1985	Average 1991
Bronchial asthma	1.45	5.99	7.32	1.15	4.17	4.34	1.30	5.06	5.80
Allergic rhinitis		9.91	25.33		6.14	15.78		7.84	20.67
Atopic eczema	1.53	1.20	4.05	1.33	1.27	3.63	1.43	1.23	3.84
Urticaria	2.84	2.15	7.38	2.00	2.46	6.22	2.32	2.30	6.79
Total		19.25	44.05		14.04	29.97		16.43	37.10

Discussion

A number of recent studies strongly indicate that bronchial asthma is an increasing worldwide problem. There is an upward trend for hospitalization rates (2,4–6), mortality rate (7,8) and prevalence (3,10,11) of bronchial asthma. The increase is the more surprising as mortality has been falling in most conditions for which there is effective prevention or treatment (12) and thus there are still arguments for regarding the increasing prevalence of bronchial asthma from the methodological point of view (1).

During the period of 17 years from 1974–1991, we conducted three studies of the prevalence of childhood allergic diseases in Taipei city, the capital of the Republic of China. The methods used in these studies have been the same throughout the period. The same questionnaire and school, school children of the same age (7–15 years), and the same season (early spring) were studied in these three surveys, thus eliminating several important variables which may otherwise influence the results.

The prevalence of bronchial asthma continued to rise in the past 6 years in Taipei, i. e. from 5.07% in 1985 to 5.80% in 1991. Allergic rhinitis also increased from 7.84% in 1985 to 20.67% in 1991, with a 2.6-fold increase in both boys and girls. These data indicate that both bronchial asthma and allergic rhinitis increase at the same time. Fleming et al. (13) also reported a similar tendency.

It is interesting to note that the prevalence of atopic eczema and urticaria remained unchanged during the period from 1974 to 1985; however, it increased 2.9-fold in 1991. Taylor et al. also found a definite increase in eczema since the 1939–45 war (14).

Finally, the age of onset of allergic disease in those born in 1984 was much younger than those born in 1976 (data not shown). This fact, in conjunction with the general increase in the prevalence of atopy, highly suggests that environmental factors must play an important role in the occurrence of allergic disease.

References

1. Cookson, J.B. 1987. Prevalence rates of asthma in developing countries and their comparison with those in Europe and North America. Chest 91:97S
2. Evans, R. III, Mullally, D.I., and Wilson, R.W. 1987. National trends in the morbility and mortality of asthma in the US. Prevalence, hospitalization and death from asthma over two decades. Chest 91:65S
3. Hsieh, K.H., and Shen, J.J. 1988. Prevalence of childhood asthma in Taipei, Taiwan, and other Asian Pacific countries. J. Asthma 25:73.
4. Mitchell, E.A. 1985. International trends in hospital admission rates for asthma. Arch. Dis. Child 60:376
5. Halfon, N., and Newacheck, P.W. 1986. Trends in the hospitalization for acute childhood asthma, 1970-84. Am. J. Public Health 76:1308.
6. Gergen, P.J., and Weiss, K.B. 1990. Changing patterns of asthma hospitalization among children: 1979–1987. JAMA 264:1688.
7. Sly, R.M. 1988. Mortality from asthma in children 1978–1984. Ann. Allergy 60:433.
8. Burney, P.G.J. 1986. Asthma mortality in England and Wales: Evidence for a further increase. Lancet 2:323.
9. Weiss, K.B.,and Wagener, D.K. 1990. Changing patterns of asthma mortality: Identifying target populations at high risk. JAMA 264:1683.
10. Gergen, P.J., Mullally, D.I., and Evans, R. III. 1988. National survey of prevalence of asthma among children in the United States. Pediatrics 81:1.
11. Burney, P.G.J., Chinn, S., and Rona, R.J. 1990. Has the prevalence of asthma increased in children? Evidence for the national study of health and growth 1973–86. Br. Med. J. 300:1306.
12. Charlton, J.R.H., and Velez, R. 1986. Some international comparisons of mortality amenable to medical intervention. Br. Med. J. 281:1191.
13. Fleming, D.M., and Crombie, D.L. 1987. Prevalence of asthma and hay fever in England and Wales. Br. Med. J. 294:279.
14. Taylor, B., Wadsworth, J., Wadsworth, M., and Peckham, C. 1984. Changes in the reported prevalence of childhood eczema since the 1939–45 war. Lancet 2:1255.

Epidemiology of Asthma in Australia

Ann J. Woolcock*

In order to understand the causes of asthma, studies are needed of its prevalence and associated risk factors in populations in which the prevalence and severity of the disease vary. This paper describes the prevalence of asthmatic symptoms, bronchial hyperresponsiveness (BHR), atopy and risk factors for asthma in populations of children living in different parts of Australia, New Zealand (NZ), Indonesia and Papua New Guinea (PNG). In NZ and Australian Caucasians, the prevalence of wheezing, of BHR and of asthma is higher than in children in Indonesia, PNG and Australian Aborigines. Furthermore, the death rates for asthma in the 5–34 age group are higher in Australia and NZ than in other countries, particularly the USA. The most important risk factor for asthma in Australian children is atopy followed by a family history of asthma, respiratory illness before the age of 2 years and being born in Australia. Of all the allergens, the house dust mite presents the most important risk for both BHR and for persistent asthma. House dust mite numbers are very high in houses in Australia and NZ and this may account for the high prevalence of the disease. However, it seems likely that factors other than exposure to HDM allergen are operating to cause the differences between populations. Genetic factors and the protective role of exposure to bacteria at an early age in PNG and Indonesian children must be considered. The possibility needs to be explored that widespread use of beta agonists in early childhood in Australasia increases disease severity.

Asthma is a disease of the airways that makes them prone to excessive narrowing. This paper deals with some aspects of the prevalence and mortality of asthma in populations of children in Australia and its neighbouring countries. All the data reported have been published or submitted for publication. Similar methods were used to collect the prevalence data in all the studies reported here and included measurements of symptoms, bronchial responsiveness, atopic status and other risk factors for asthma. Death rates are also an important source of epidemiological data and are shown for the 5 to 34 year old age group. The prevalence of acute attacks of asthma is not discussed.

Classification of Asthma for Epidemiology

Wheezing is very common in Australian children. Between 29 and 40% of children aged 7 to 10 years wheeze at some time in their lives (1,2,3). However, not all children who have wheezed have asthma and it is important to distinguish those children in whom wheezing may be associated with an adverse outcome. The outcomes of asthma are not known and it is unlikely that important progress will be made in understanding and treating the disease until long-term studies of the likely causal factors and the natural history of different forms of the disease are undertaken. A classification of the disease is needed in order to undertake long-term studies. It is proposed that the classification shown in Table 1 can be used in order to: (a) determine differences in prevalence between populations (in Australia and its neigh-

Table I: Symptoms: wheeze, chest tightness or cough lasting for more than 3 weeks. BD: bronchodilator therapy; DRC: dose response curve to histamine or methacholine; PD_{20}: dose of histamine or methacholine in micromols causing a 20% fall in FEV1. Plateau is the maximal fall in FEV_1.

	SYMPTOMS			BD THERAPY		DRC	
	PREVIOUS	LAST YEAR	EVERY MONTH	PAST	EVERY MONTH	PD_{20} µMOL	PLATEAU % Δ FEV_1
CURRENT							
PERSISTENT	+	+	+	+	+	< 8	> 60
EPISODIC	±	+	-	±	-	2 - 52	30 - 50
REMISSION	+	-	-	+	-	1 - 10	30 - 50
POTENTIAL	-	-	-	-	-	4 - 10	?
TRIVIAL WHEEZE	+	+	-	-	-	> 8	< 40

* Institute of Respiratory Medicine, Royal Prince Alfred Hospital, Camperdown, NSW 2050, Australia.

bours); (b) follow the natural history and thus to determine prognosis and outcomes; (c) determine the risk factors for each form; and (d) target appropriate interventions to reduce morbidity.

Persistent Asthma

This is defined as the presence of symptoms of wheezing, chest tightness or persistent cough in the last 12 months. This form of the disease may be mild, moderate or severe. It is always accompanied by BHR with values for $PD_{20} < 4.0$ µmols.

Episodic Asthma

This is defined as intermittent symptoms of asthma, at intervals of 2 or more months, in the last 12 months, severe enough to require treatment. PD_{20} is usually > 8.0 µmols.

Asthma in Remission

This is defined as a previous diagnosis of asthma but no symptoms or treatment for 12 months. PD_{20} varies between 1 and 10 µmols.

Trivial Wheeze

This is defined as symptoms of asthma not sufficiently severe to require treatment or to interfere with life style. The PD_{20} is usually > 8.0 µmols.

Potential Asthma

Defined as the absence of symptoms with BHR. The PD_{20} is < 8.0 µmols.

The usefulness of this classification in terms of outcome still has to be assessed.

Methods

In all studies, questionnaire data from parents have been collected, together with data on spirometric function, a histamine inhalation test (4) or a methacholine challenge test (5) and skin prick tests using common aeroallergens. The details of the methods used are given in the references (1,4,5,6). In some communities dust has been collected from houses and bedding for measurement of numbers of house dust mites (7).

Populations Studied

Figure 1 and Table 2 show the numbers of children in Australia and its neighbouring countries who have been studied to obtain data about allergic and asthmatic status. Populations of Caucasian children have been studied in New South Wales in Sydney (Villawood), Newcastle (Belmont) and Wagga Wagga, and in Western Australia in Busselton. Other populations studied include Indonesian children in Bali (8), PNG adults in the Asaro valley (9) and children in Goroka (10), New Zealand children in Auckland (11) and Dunedin (5) and Aboriginal children in Australia (12) studied in Northern Queensland. In all studies random or entire population samples of children were obtained and studied at school.

Results

The prevalence of persistent asthma is shown in Figure 1 and Table 2. In Australia the prevalence of persistent asthma is about 7% in Caucasian children. On the basis of PD_{20} values as described by Yan et al. (4), this is severe in 1%, moderate in 2% and mild in 4%. Not shown on the Figure are the prevalence of other forms of asthma, which are less easy to define in cross-sectional studies. In Australian children about 4% have episodic asthma or asthma in remission and 15% have trivial wheezing without asthma. Overall, about 26% of the Australian children studied by our group were said, by their parents, to have wheezed at some time in their lives. Table 2 shows the prevalence of symptoms (ever and within the previous year), BHR and atopy in groups of Caucasian children in Australia. The results for Aboriginal children have not yet been published. Little variation exists between Caucasian children in Australia. The lowest values were found in the coastal towns of Belmont, and Busselton and the highest in the inland town of Wagga Wagga. Children in NZ have slightly higher prevalences of BHR and symptoms than those in

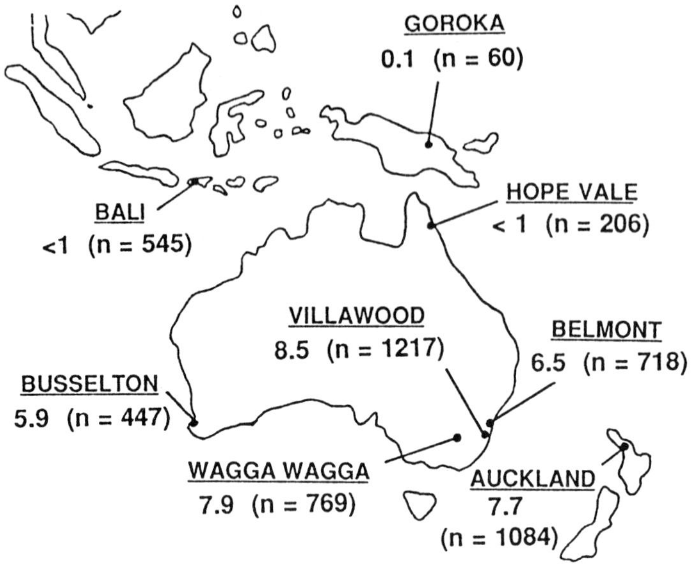

Figure 1. A map showing the numbers of children (%) studied in various parts of Australia and neighbouring countries together with the prevalence of persistent asthma as defined in the text.

Australia while in PNG and Indonesia the prevalence of BHR is very much lower.

Figure 2 shows the prevalence of atopy (one or more skin test wheals greater than 2 mm) and of BHR ($PD_{20} < 8.0$ µmols) in the same populations as shown in Figure 1. Figure 3 shows the relationship between the prevalence of these two findings. The data for the "Asaro" population (9) in the PNG highlands are for adults living in an area close to Goroka. In general there was a close correlation, but Balinese children had a low prevalence of BHR. Figure 4 shows the percentage of children with atopy in Belmont, Australia and in Bali in Indonesia, divided into 4 groups: normals, those with symptoms of wheeze without BHR (trivial wheeze as defined above), those who have BHR without wheeze (? potential asthma) and those with both (persistent asthma). In Australia the overall prevalence of atopy in Belmont was 29% and atopy was significantly increased in the group with BHR ($p > 0.01$) and those with persistent asthma ($p < .001$). In Indonesia there was no relationship between atopy and the group of children with BHR. In fact, those with asthma were not atopic.

Australian children with persistent asthma almost always have other markers of the dis-

Table 2. Prevalence (%) of wheeze, BHR and atopy in populations of children

	WW	B'MONT	VILL	B'TON	BALI	DUNEDIN	AUCKLAND
N.	1371	993	1217	885	545	815	1084
AGE	8–10	8–10	8–11	7–15	7–17	9	8–10
WH	26.3	21.5	26.6	21.4	5.3	26.9	26.0
R WH	15.2	11.7	17.7	11.0	5.3	19.6	15.1
Total BHR	19.6	15.5	15.3	11.6	2.2	22.0	20.1
BHR +R WH*	7.9	6.5	8.5	5.9	0.4	13.5	7.7
TOTAL ATOPY	30.6	29.3	31.9	34.5	26.2	–	–
HDM ATOPY	7.8	12.2	11.5	16.6	16.2	–	–

BHR = Bronchial Hyperresponsiveness; B'MONT: Belmont; B'TON: Busselton; R WH: Recent Wheeze; VILL: Villawood; WH: Wheeze; WW: Wagga Wagga; *: Persistent asthma.

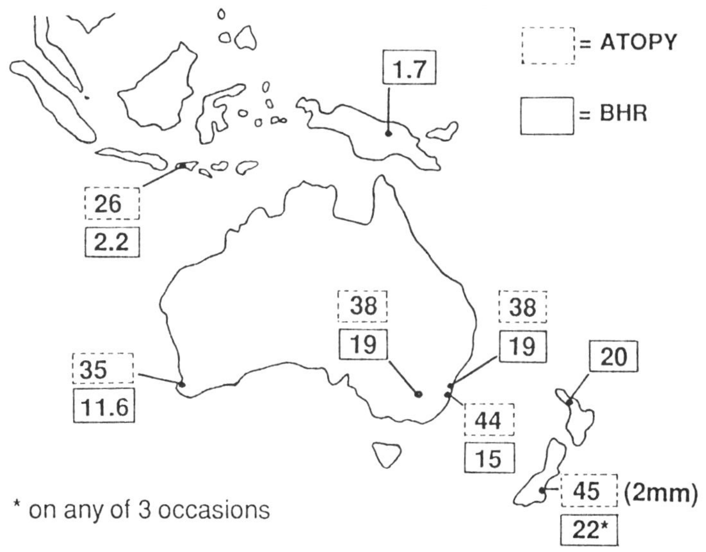

Figure 2. The prevalence of atopy (%), (based on skin prick tests) and of BHR found in the populations shown in Figure 1.

ease including atopy, family history of asthma and a history of respiratory illness before the age of 2 years. The most common allergen associated with asthma is the house dust mite. High numbers of house dust mites have been reported from houses in Australia (7) and NZ (13). In most populations in Australia pollens are not a risk factor for asthma in the absence of house dust mite allergy (14).

Figure 5 shows the adjusted odds ratios for the risk factors for a group of children living in Villawood near Sydney. Being born in Australia was a risk factor, but sex and race were not. In addition, eating fish meals on a regular basis was protective when the data were adjusted for the other factors.

Figure 6 shows the death rates per 100,000 for 5–34 year olds (the age group for which the death certificates are most reliable) in Australia, New Zealand and the USA. It shows that, overall, there has been little change in death rates in Australia apart from a small epidemic of deaths in the mid-1960s and little change in the USA, with two epidemics in NZ. Overall Australia and NZ have higher death rates than the USA. No data are available for PNG and Indonesia.

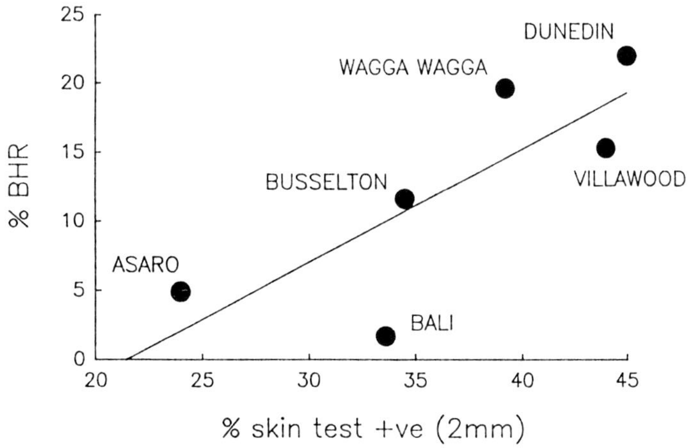

Figure 3. The relationship between the prevalence of BHR and of atopy in the populations shown in Figure 2 with the addition of some adult data from the Asaro valley in the Highlands of PNG.

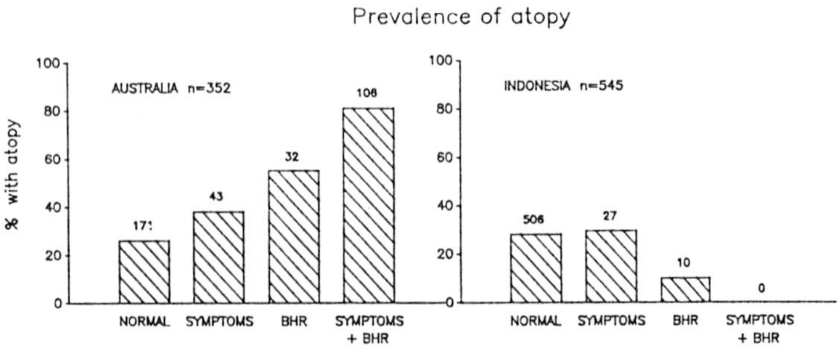

Figure 4. Percentage of children in Australia (Belmont) and Indonesia (Bali) who were atopic. Normal: no symptoms and no BHR; Symptoms: wheeze or cough in the last year without BHR; BHR: $PD_{20} < 8.0$ micromols without symptoms; and Symptoms plus BHR: persistent asthma.

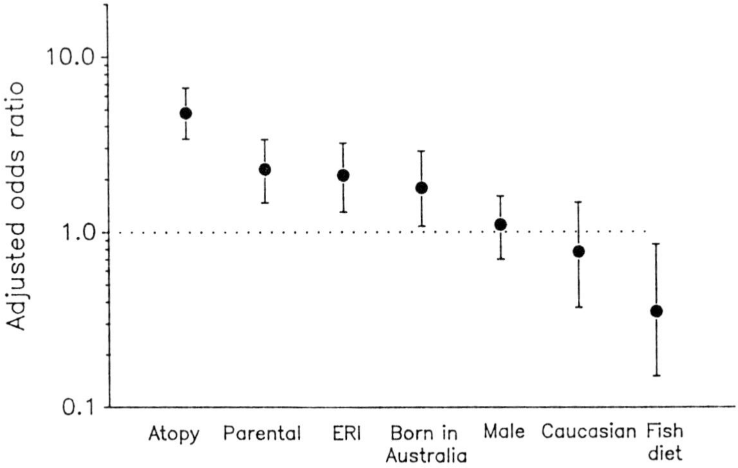

Figure 5. Adjusted odds ratios for risk factors for the presence of BHR in 1,217 children in Villawoos, NSW. Atopy = any positive skin test > 2 mm; Parental: asthma present in one or both parents; ERI: early respiratory illness.

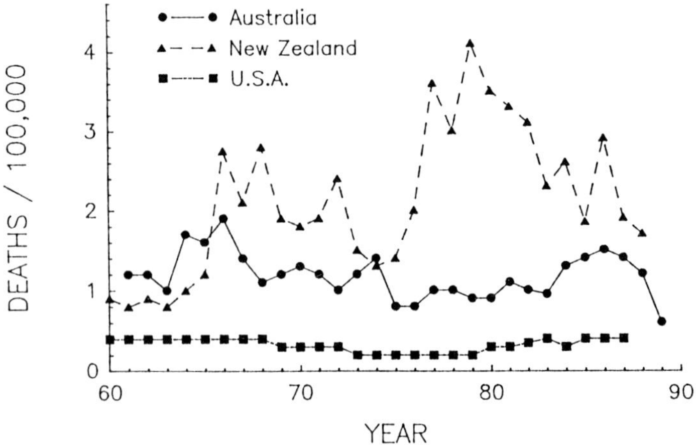

Figure 6. Mortality per 100,000 due to asthma between 1960 and 1990, in Australia, New Zealand and USA for 5 to 34 year olds.

Discussion

These studies, all using similar methods, allow us to make some firm conclusions about the epidemiology of asthma in the Australasian area. Firstly it is clear that allergy, BHR, symptoms and asthma are more common in Australia and NZ than in the two other countries. There appears to be a strong relationship in these countries between atopy and BHR, and the asthma appears to be severe with higher mortality than in other countries such as the USA. The reasons are not known for these differences in prevalence of persistent asthma, BHR, atopy and asthma deaths between Australia and NZ on the one hand and Indonesia, PNG and Aboriginal children on the other. They probably result from a combination of factors including differences in exposure to allergen as infants, differences in immunological responses to allergens, continuing exposure to high concentrations of indoor allergens during childhood and perhaps to differences in methods of treatment. There is now reason to believe that the epidemics of death may have been due, at least in part, to the long-term regular use of high doses of potent beta agonists which can increase the severity of asthma (15). If this is true, it could mean that drug therapy plays a role not only in the epidemics of deaths but in the overall severity and prevalence of persistent asthma in Australia and NZ. However, drug treatment is probably not the only factor causing deaths in these countries and the cause seems to involve a number of factors (16). The role of allergen pollution is still to be defined. It is known that death may occur during episodes of environmental pollution that cause severe attacks (17).

An opportunity now exists (a) to examine more closely the likely risk factors for asthma in the different populations, (b) to confirm the proposed classification, (c) to define the associated risk factors within each classification and (d) to make hypotheses about the causes and natural history of asthma. In general, the possibilities for the increased prevalence of the disease in children in Australia and NZ include higher exposure to house dust mite and other allergens in the first year of life, perhaps lack of protection afforded by early colonisation with bacteria and perhaps to the greater use of beta agonist drugs.

References

1. Britton, W.J., Woolcock, A.J., Peat, J.K., Sedgwick, C.J., Lloyd, D.M., and Leeder, S.R. 1986. Prevalence of bronchial hyperresponsiveness in children: The relationship between asthma and skin reactivity to allergens in two communities. Int. J. Epidemiol. 15:202.
2. Bauman, A.E. 1991. Public health approaches to asthma. PhD Thesis, University of Sydney, New South Wales, Australia.
3. Robertson, C.F., Heycock, E., Bishop, J., Nolan, T., Olinsky, A., and Phelan, P.D. 1991. Prevalence of asthma in Melbourne school children: Changes over 26 years. B. M. J. 302:1116.
4. Yan, K., Salome, C., and Woolcock, A.J. 1983. Rapid method for measurement of bronchial responsiveness. Thorax 38:760.
5. Sears, M.R., Jones, D.T., Holdaway, M.D., Hewitt, C.J., Flannery, E.M., Herbison, G.P., and Silva, P.A. 1986. Prevalence of bronchial reactivity to inhaled methacholine in New Zealand children. Thorax 41:283.
6. Peat, J.K., Salome, C.M., Sedgewick, C.J., Kerrebijn, J., and Woolcock, A.J. 1989. A prospective study of bronchial hyperresponsiveness and respiratory symptoms in a population of Australian school children. Clin. Exp. Allergy 19:299.
7. Green, W.F., Woolcock, A.J., Stuckey, M., Sedgewick, C., and Leeder, S.R. 1986. House dust mites and skin tests in different Australian localities. Aust. N. Z. J. Med. 16:639.
8. Woolcock, A.J., and Konthen, P.G. 1990. Lung function and asthma in Balinese and Australian children. Joint International Congress, 2nd Asian Pacific Society of Respirology and 5th Indonesian Association of Pulmonologists, Bali, Indonesia.
9. Woolcock, A.J., Peat, J.K., Keena, V.A., Smith, D., Molloy, C., Simpson, A., Middleton, P., Vallance, P., Alpers, M., and Green, W. 1989. Asthma and chronic airflow limitation in the highlands of Papua New Guinea: Low prevalence of asthma in the Asaro Valley. Eur. Respir. J. 2:822.
10. Turner, K.J., Dowse, G.K., Stewart, G.A., and Alpers, M.P. 1986. Studies on bronchial hyperreactivity, allergic responsiveness and asthma in rural and urban children of the Highlands of Papua New Guinea. J. Allergy Clin. Immunol. 77:558.
11. Asher, M.I., Pattemore, P.K., Harrison, A.C., Mitchell, E.A., Rea, H.H., Stewart, A.W., and

Woolcock, A. J. 1988. International comparison of the prevalence and severity of asthma symptoms and bronchial hyperresponsiveness. Am. Rev. Respir. Dis. 138:524.
12. Veale, A., Salome, C., Thompson, J., and Woolcock, A.J. 1991. Asthma and atopy on two remote Aboriginal communities. The Thoracic Society of Australia and New Zealand, 1991 Annual Scientific Meeting. Victoria, Australia.
13. Abbott, J., Cameron, J., and Taylor, B. 1981. House dust mite counts in different types of mattresses, sheepskins and carpets, and a comparison of brushing and vacuuming collection methods. Clin. Allergy 11:589.
14. Peat, J.K., and Woolcock, A.J. 1991. Sensitivity to common allergens: Relation to respiratory symptoms and bronchial hyperresponsiveness in children from three different climatic areas of Australia. Clin. Exp. Allergy, in press.
15. Sears, M.R., Taylor, D.R., Print, C.G., Lake, D.C., Li, Q., Flannery, E.M., et al. 1990. Regular inhaled beta-agonist treatment in bronchial asthma. Lancet 336:1391.
16. Sears, M.R., Rea, H.H., Beaglehole, R., Gillies, A.J., Holst, P.E., O'Donnell, T.V., Rothwell, R.P., and Sutherland, D.C. 1985. Asthma mortality in New Zealand: A two year national study. N.Z. Med. J. 98:271.
17. O'Hollaren, M.T., Yunginger, J.W., Offord, K.P., Somers, M.J., O'Connell, E.J., Ballard, D.J., and Sachs, M.I. 1991. Exposure to an aeroallergen as a possible precipitating factor in respiratory arrest in young patients with asthma. N. Engl. J. Med. 324:359.

Epidemiology of Allergic Diseases in Children

Bengt Björkstén, N.-I. Max Kjellman*

The epidemiology of childhood allergy has changed over the past decades and there seems to be a documentable increased incidence of allergic diseases, particularly in industrialized countries. Various environmental influences, particularly air pollution and exposure to tobacco smoke, have been suggested as explanations for the apparent increase. Even when all of the suggested environmental influences are taken together, however, they cannot adequately explain the increase. The symptoms of allergic disease and the dominating allergens vary with age. During the first years of life symptoms from the skin and gastrointestinal tract dominate and the offending allergens are mainly introduced with the food. Wheezy bronchitis occurs in up to 20% of all young children before 18 months of age. As the incidence of childhood asthma is about 5–8%, most cases of infant wheezing are not an indication of asthma. Allergic rhinoconjunctivitis is unusual before 5 years of age and then increases to a peak prevalence in adolescence. The increased susceptibility for environmental factors in early infancy seems to be limited to infants with a genetic propensity for allergy. Infants at risk should be identified early and preventive measures, particularly avoidance of exposure to tobacco smoke, should be encouraged. For efficient primary, secondary and tertiary prevention, large epidemiological studies on well-defined populations are needed to increase our knowledge about the relative importance of the various environmental factors that influence the sensitization and development of allergy, trigger symptoms and increase severity of disease.

Reasons for the apparent increase in childhood IgE mediated allergy are poorly understood. The allergic diseases include bronchial asthma, allergic rhinitis, conjunctivitis and urticaria, atopic dermatitis and gastrointestinal allergy. Although the risk of developing allergic disease is largely determined by genetic factors, they obviously cannot explain the observed increase in the prevalence, as the genetic determinants in man have not changed appreciably over only a few generations. Therefore, environmental factors must be responsible for this development. Their impact is particularly strong on infants with a genetic predisposition for allergy (Fig. 1). Several recent studies have focussed on the epidemiology of sensitization and on how to predict and possibly prevent the development of allergic disease (primary prevention). Modification of various environmental factors also plays a major role in secondary and tertiary prevention, i. e. the prevention of symptoms of allergic disease and the prevention of progression of inflammation as a consequence of disease. In this review the epidemiology of environmental influences will be summarized, with emphasis on primary prevention.

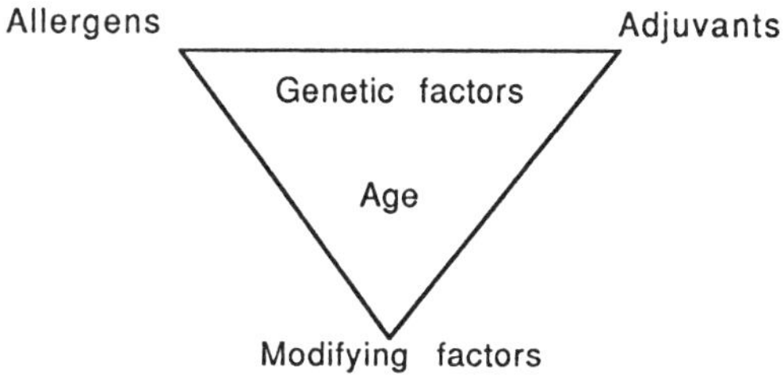

Figure 1: The development of allergic disease in a genetically predisposed individual is influenced by allergen exposure (e. g. potency and concentration of allergen and the duration of exposure) and by the simultaneous presence of adjuvant factors, e. g. air pollution. The responsiveness in the individual also varies with age and with the presence of individual modifying factors like concurrent infections and, possibly, psychological stress.

* Department of Pediatrics, Faculty of Health Sciences, University of Linköping, S-581 85 Linköping, Sweden.

Natural History

The highest incidence (new cases appearing during a given year) of allergy appears in infants and adolescents. The prevalence of a disease, i.e. presence of symptoms at any time during the past 12 months, depends on the incidence, the age of the subjects and the natural history of the disease, including healing and change to a latent phase. The accumulated incidence (sick presently or previously) of a disease in a particular region should therefore increase with age, unless there has been a dramatic reduction in the prevalence, as a consequence of efficient prevention, reduced exposure to allergens or adjuvant factors or improved treatment.

Recent Scandinavian studies show a total accumulated incidence of one or more of the allergic diseases in over 30% of adolescents and young adults (1,2). In prospective studies the prevalence of asthma in childhood is 3–5%, while the accumulated incidence is around 8% (1,3). Similar and higher figures have been reported from other industrialized countries (4).

The incidence of allergic disease has been repeatedly studied over 10–20 years with a similar methodology (2,5). These studies indicate that there is an observable increased incidence over time, although none of them conclusively proves this. The clinical symptoms of allergic disease vary with age. Symptoms from the skin, i.e. dermatitis and urticaria, and gastrointestinal tract dominate in infants, and the offending allergens are mainly introduced with the food. Thus, the dominating allergens in infants include cow's milk, egg and soy. From the second year of life wheezing becomes increasingly common and inhaled allergens become important as triggers of symptoms. Wheezy bronchitis occurs before 18 months of age in up to 20% of all young children (6). Wheezing in older children is however often associated with asthma (6). The wheezing is diagnosed as asthma either when the episodes of wheezing recur three times, or when at the first time there is a relation to exposure to a particular allergen. Allergic rhinoconjunctivitis is not commonly seen before 5–6 years of age and then increases to a peak prevalence in adolescence. The incidence of allergic disease is higher in boys than in girls, at least in infants and young children (1). In adolescents, however, there seem to be no sex differences. Children with biparental family history of allergic disease begin to have symptoms at an earlier age than children with less pronounced or no family history of allergy (7).

Immunological Aspects

Many epidemiological studies clearly indicate that various environmental influences play a particularly important role in individuals with a genetically determined propensity to allergic disease (4,8). The genes for atopy appear to be widely distributed, since over 30% of newborn babies have at least one family member, i.e. a parent, brother or sister, with a history of allergic disease (7). Many babies with a predisposition for allergic disease can be identified already at birth by various methods (9,10). They include the presence of certain clinical signs as dry skin, which may be observed already in the Maternity Ward, and various laboratory tests. Only a carefully obtained family history and determination of serum IgE antibodies are presently useful in clinical practice. Increased levels of IgE in umbilical cord blood, i.e. over 0.6 to 1.3 kU/l are strongly associated with an increased risk for allergy during childhood (1,10). The clinical value of IgE determinations in allergy prediction is, however, unfortunately limited by the low sensitivity of the test and by technical problems. As the maternal IgE levels, even in healthy non-atopic mothers, are usually more than 100 times higher than in a healthy newborn baby, even a minor contamination with maternal blood may cause falsely elevated IgE levels in the cord blood. After birth IgE antibody determinations may also be of value for prediction of allergy, and demonstration of high levels of IgE antibodies in an apparently healthy child with no present or previous history of allergy is associated with subsequent development of atopic disease, usually appearing within the next few years (11). Several observations indicate that atopic disease is associated with a defective suppression of the normal IgE antibody formation (9). As a consequence, the atopic individual responds with a prolonged IgE antibody formation against commonly encountered antigens, while the normal non-atopic individual under similar cirumstances may only respond with a brief low-grade response. Clinical observations and experimental studies (12) indicate that the conditions under which the first encounter with an allergen occur in early infancy may influence the immune response to it later in life.

Geographical Variations

Genetic factors may explain why the prevalence of, e. g., asthma is extremely high in certain isolated islands. Variations in allergens cannot, however, explain the pronounced differences in the prevalence of atopic disease in various countries, as potential allergens are present in most parts of the world. The apparently higher rate of allergic disease in affluent industrialized societies has been ascribed to an increased awareness, as other, more severe, diseases become less common. According to this notion, asthma and rhinoconjunctivitis would not be as readily observed in a poor Third World country, where severe intestinal and respiratory infections are common and would mask less life threatening allergic symptoms. Further, very few properly performed epidemiological studies have been reported from poor countries, as there is an obvious lack of adequate statistical records on the prevalence of various diseases. There are, however, a few studies indicating a de facto lower prevalence of allergic disease in less developed societies. A longitudinal study of asthma in a previously isolated population in Papua New Guinea is of particular interest in this respect (13). Asthma was previously unknown in the population. As they became increasingly exposed to Western life-style, blankets and new food items including more proteins were introduced, and their way of life changed in other ways. House dust mites could now be isolated in extremely high numbers from the blankets. Parallel to the changes in life style there has been a pronounced increase in the prevalence of asthma among adults. The studies clearly indicate that environmental factors can profoundly affect the incidence of allergic disease. The reasons for this increase, however, remain poorly understood. The varying prevalence of allergy in different parts of the world is probably not due to racial differences. In a study of 21,000 school children in Birmingham a similar prevalence of asthma was observed in native British children and in Black and Asian children, provided that they were born in England (14). In contrast, children born in the West Indies or in Asia and then moving with their parents to Britain had a significantly lower prevalence of asthma and wheezing. Similarily, a much higher prevalence of asthma, rhinitis and/or eczema was recorded in Tokelauan children living in New Zealand than in Tokelau (15). Similar differences have been observed in Black urban and rural children in South Africa (16) and in Somali infants born in Rome and in Somalia (17). In conclusion, living conditions, rather than genetic background appears to account for the pronounced regional differences in allergy prevalence.

Environmental Influences

Many nonspecific environmental factors appear to facilitate sensitization to allergens (see Table 1). They include air pollutants like ozone, sulfur dioxide and nitrogen dioxide. In a recent Japanese study it was found that the closer people lived to a motorway, the more likely they were to suffer from allergic rhinoconjuctivitis and sensitivity to red cedar tree pollen (18). It seems that exhaust particles from cars could increase the risk for sensitization to pollen. Possibly, pollutants covering pollen and other allergens influence their potency. Increased air pollution has also been offered as an explanation for an increased prevalence of hay fever and skin prick test positivity to allergens (3) in Europe. In the latter study, sensitivity to inhaled allergens like pollen and animal dander was much more common in urban than rural areas, even though the allergen exposure was more pronounced in the latter. Tobacco smoke

Table 1. Environmental factors influencing the development of allergic disease:— Foetal exposure to pharmaceutical drugs

- Intensity and type of early exposure to allergens, e. g. season of birth, exposure to furred pets, type of infant feeding
- Infections
- Exposure to tobacco smoke
- Air pollution indoors and outdoors
- Living conditions, e. g. quality of house and ventilation
- Psychological factors?

Asthma Morbidity and Mortality in the U.S.

Robert A. Goldstein*, Kevin B. Weiss**

It appears that asthma morbidity and mortality in the U.S have been increasing. Estimates from the National Health Interview survey, conducted by the U.S. National Center for Health Statistics, suggest an almost 35 percent increase in asthma prevalence for persons of all ages between 1979 and 1987. The trend may be higher for children. Data from the U.S. vital records system and hospitalization surveys suggest morbidity and mortality are increasing as well. From 1979 to 1987 U.S. hospitalizations in children and adolescents under 17 years old increased 4.5 percent per annum (see Figure 1) (1). The largest increase was found in children under 5 years of age. Among children this age, blacks had nearly 1.8 times the increase of whites. This increase in asthma hospitalization occurred during a period of decrease for hospitalization for respiratory diseases and does not appear to be directly related to a concurrent shift in diagnostic coding of bronchitis/bronchiolitis to asthma (2).

U.S. asthma mortality rates during this period also rose. From 1980 to 1987 mortality rates for persons of all ages increased from 2,891 to 4,360. For children and young adults, 5 to 34 years of age, asthma mortality rates increased by 6.2 percent per annum during this same time period (see Figure 2) (3). The rate of increase was faster for those children aged 5 to 14 years than for asthmatics 15 to 34 years old. Asthma mortality is known to exhibit regional variation (4). However, small-area geographic analyses of mortality trends in the U.S. revealed four areas with persistenly high asthma mortality. Two of these four areas, Cook County Illinois, and New York City, have been driving much of the national mortality trend for children and younger adults. Neither changes in ICD coding nor improved recognition of asthma seem to explain this recent increase in mortality (3).

A number of studies have demonstrated that asthma hospitalization rates exhibit unexplained small area geographic variation (see Figure 3) (5,6,7). A recent study of asthma hospitalizations between New York City neighborhoods has demonstrated large variations in rates: 16-fold differences in hospitalization, 25-fold differences in mortality. Geographic variation in asthma hospitalization and mortality rates were found to be highly correlated (r=0.67) with the highest rates concentrated in the city's poorest neighborhoods (6).

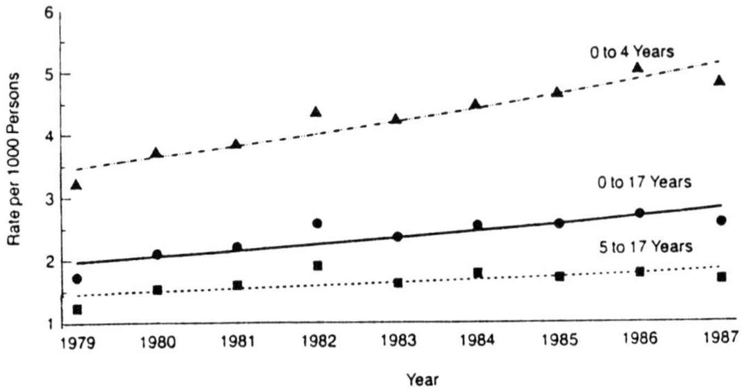

Figure 1. Asthma hospitalization rates per 1000 persons for US children and youths aged 0 to 17 years. Symbols represent observed rates; lines, predicted trends based on log-linear regression. From the National Center for Health Statistics, National Hospital Discharge Survey.

---

* Division of Allergy, Immunology, and Transplantation, National Institute of Allergy and Infectious Diseases, National Institutes of Health, Washington, D.C.

** Departments of Health Care Sciences and Medicine, George Washington University Medical Center and Center for Health Policy Research, George Washington University, Washington, D.C.

Figure 2. Trends in US asthma mortality among persons aged 5 to 34 years under *International Classification of Diseases-Eighth Revision* (left) and *International Classification of Diseases-Ninth Revision* (right). From the National Center for Health Statistics, US Vital Records.

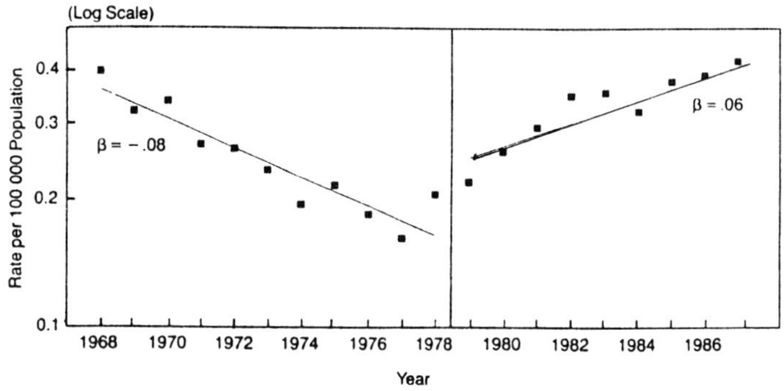

These recent studies suggest poverty to be an important independent risk factor for asthma hospitalizations and mortality. Data will soon be published that suggest poverty is an important risk factor in the prevalence of this condition as well. Although there is considerable speculation on the actual mechanisms by which poverty contributes to asthma morbidity and mortality, there is little science to enlighten our understanding in this area.

The reason for the increasing trends are not known. A number of determinant factors have been implicated, including: health care delivery, clinical management, and changes in indoor/outdoor environment, and changes in diagnostic classification. There have been a number of studies which identified how each of these factors can independently contribute to excessive asthma morbidity. Yet to date, there have been no studies to determine how these factors may dynamically be contributing to the increasing trends.

Although the main focus of this presentation is the changing epidemiology of asthma in the U.S., any changes must be viewed in the context of international epidemiologic patterns. In this regard, there is evidence that asthma mortality rates in other countries may have either ceased to decline or have increased during recent years (e.g., New Zealand, Denmark, France, Germany, and England and Wales). There is also evidence that asthma prevalence is increasing in Finland, Sweden, and South Wales. Collectively, this information would suggest that the prevalence of asthma may be increasing and the recent increasing trends are to some degree occurring independently of issues of health care delivery. This evidence would suggest that these recent increases could be related to new changes in clinical management, such as enhanced or earlier clinical diagnostic trends or related to changes in treatment and symptom control. However, the multi-national aspects of these increasing trends do not implicate issues such as health care access or many of the issues of clinical management. This multi-national trend may suggest changes in diagnostic classification, pharmacotherapy, or perhaps environmental factors.

Perhaps one of the more important epidemi-

Figure 3. Age-adjusted asthma hospitalization rates Children ages 1–19 years, 1979–82, Maryland Counties and Baltimore City Districts.

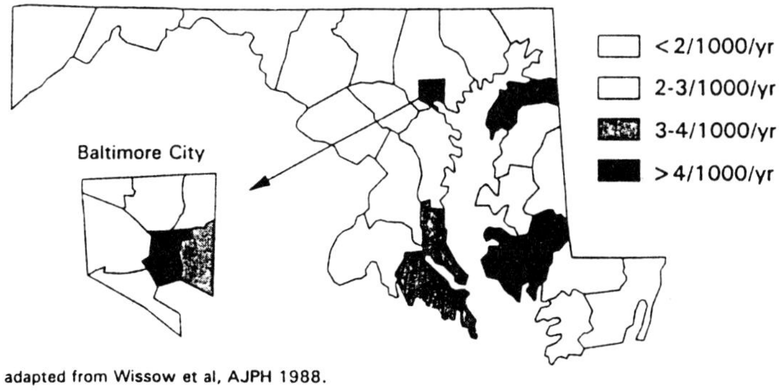

ologic findings to emerge in the past few years is the possible relationship between asthma prevalence, morbidity (specifically hospitalizations) and mortality in relationship to urbanization (see The National Health Interview Study). The U.S. studies of asthma mortality have pointed to higher prevalence in urban versus rural areas (8). Recent studies of mortality have identified the inner city as having extremely high asthma mortality rates (3,7). Some of this effect is related to poverty. However, poverty does not appear to explain all of the effect of urbanization. So, it appears that a better understanding of the effects of the environment, both indoor and outdoor, associated with a modern urban environment might bring us a long way in our understanding in the causation and clinical expression of this disease.

The National Institute of Allergy and Infectious Diseases has recently undertaken a 5 year, multi-site study to further our understanding of the factors that are associated with the disproportionate morbidity from asthma that is affecting minority populations in U.S. inner cities. This study is being conducted in two phases. First a one year epidemiologic study will be conducted to further elucidate factors associated with poor clinical outcomes. The second phase of this study will attempt a multi-disciplinary clinical intervention to reduce morbidity.

In summary, it becomes near certain that the patterns of asthma epidemiology are changing. The reasons for these changes in the epidemiologic expression of this condition are not clear. During the past few years, poverty and urbanization have emerged as clear risk factors in the expression of this disease. There is mounting evidence that to some degree, the increasing morbidity from asthma is a multi-national problem as well. Much new epidemiologic work is needed to help us understand these changing trends.

References

1. Weiss, K.B., and Wagener, D.K. 1990. Asthma surveillance in the United States: A review of current trends and knowledge gaps. Chest 90:179.
2. Gergen, P.J., and Weiss, K.B. 1990. Changing patterns of asthma hospitalization among U.S. children 0–17 years of age: 1979-1987. JAMA 264:1688.
3. Weiss, K.B., and Wagener, D.K. 1990. Changing patterns of asthma mortality: Identifying target populations at high risk. JAMA 264:1683.
4. Sly, R.M. 1988. Mortality from asthma 1979–84. J. Allergy Clin. Immunol. 82:705.
5. Wissow, L.S., Gittlesohn, A.M., Szklo, M., et al. 1988. Poverty, race, and hospitalization for childhood asthma. Am. J Public Health 78:777.
6. Perrin, J.M., Homer, C.J., Berwick, D.M., et al. 1989. Variations in rates of hospitalizations of children in three urban communities. N. Engl. J. Med. 320:1183.
7. Carr, W., Zeitel, L., and Weiss, K.B. 1992. Variations in asthma hospitalizations and mortality in New York City. Am. J. Public Health 82:59.
8. Evans, R. III, Mulally, D.I., Wilson, R.W., et al. 1987. National trends in the morbidity and mortality of asthma in the U.S. Chest 91 (suppl 6):65S.

Epidemiology of Bronchial Asthma in Japan

Terumi Takahashi, Mitsuru Adachi*

In the past 30 years, the prevalence rate of asthma has been increasing about three-fold, and in the past ten years, two-fold in Japan. The reason for this increase can be attributed to the increase in environmental air pollution such as auto exhaust and also to the increase in allergens, especially Dermatophagoides (pyroglyphidae), due to changes in housing environment and life style. Rate of death from asthma seems to be on a plateau at present. However, it is alarming that deaths in mild and moderate cases are slightly increasing. Classification of adult asthma based on the onset age showed that 77.3% of total asthmatics experienced the onset at the age of 20 or older, and this type of asthma was found to be severer and more intractable than childhood onset asthma. Thus, adult onset asthma needs some special attention.

Prevalence Rate of Asthma: Are Asthmatic Patients Increasing?

In the past, the prevalence rate of bronchial asthma in Japan was considered to be about 1% of the population. However, since the nineteen sixties, industrial type air pollution due to exhaust from petrochemical complexes in several factory districts, including Kawasaki City and Yokkaichi City, and so on, and environmental pollution due to industrial wastes, has become serious, and the increase in prevalence rate of asthma in these areas has been observed. The recent prevalence rate has increased two-fold in the past 10 years, according to the Health and Welfare Ministry's survey, as shown in Figure 1 (1). What factors are allowing the increase in prevalence rate of asthma?

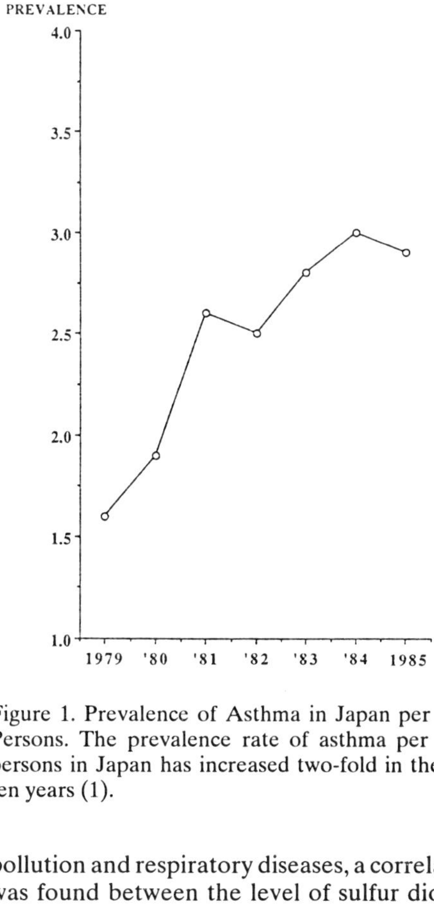

Figure 1. Prevalence of Asthma in Japan per 1,000 Persons. The prevalence rate of asthma per 1,000 persons in Japan has increased two-fold in the past ten years (1).

Air Pollution

According to Yoshida et al.'s survey in Yokkaichi city (2), which divided the city into 13 sections and analyzed the relationship between air pollution and respiratory diseases, a correlation was found between the level of sulfur dioxide (SO_2) and the prevalence rate in asthmatic patients older than 50 years (Figure 2). As to younger patients, Odashima reported that, in their survey which classified 70 asthmatic children into a younger juvenile group (3–7 years old) and an older juvenile group (8–19 years old), they found a significant correlation between the levels of suspended particulate matter (SPM) and episodes of asthma in every ten-day period in 1985 and 1986 in the younger juvenile group (Figure 3) with gamma = 0.429,

* First Department of Internal Medicine, School of Medicine, Showa University, 1-5-8 Hatanodai, Sinagawa-ku, Tokyo 142, Japan.

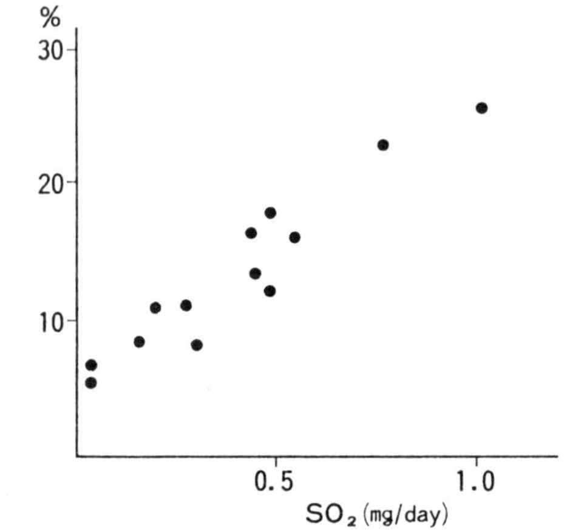

Figure 2. Relationship between SO_2 Concentration and Prevalence of Asthma. In Yokkaichi City, one of the heavily polluted factory areas in Japan, a correlation between the level of sulfur dioxide (SO_2) and the prevalence rate was found in asthmatic patients older than 50 years (2).

and p, while no apparent correlation was found in the older juvenile group (3).

In order to study the effects of air pollution by auto exhaust on respiratory systems of people living in areas with heavy traffic, Ono et al. conducted investigations on respiratory conditions of residents along one specific road with heavy traffic in Tokyo using the ATS-DLD questionnaire and examined the level of pollutants (NO_2 and SPM) in their houses (4). After excluding cases which had the origin of pollutants (cigarettes, open fuel heaters, etc.) wihin the house, both NO_2 and SPM levels tended to be high in the air, and the prevalence rate of respiratory symptoms was highest both in children and adults living in the area nearest to the main road (within 20 m), and these people showed "asthmatic symptoms" in a significantly higher rate than the residents in other areas (Figure 4). These effects on their health can be considered to result from auto exhausts. Since regulations on industrial exhaust have been tightened, the type of air pollution has changed from the industrial type (main pollutants: SO_2 and falling soot particles), a typical example of which was the Yokkaichi type of asthma in the past, to the life style related type (main pollutants: NO_2 and SPM).

However, there is a report showing that, in Izu-Ohshima, an island more than 100 km away from Tokyo and where air pollution cannot be considered serious, the prevalence rate in children is 6.8% (5). Taking these facts into consideration, we cannot attribute the cause for increasing prevalence of asthma to air pollution alone. What, then, is the largest factor contributing to the increase in asthma?

Increase in House Dust and Mites due to Changes in Housing Environment and Life Style

There is a good possibility that the increase in house dust and mites due to changes in housing conditions can explain the observed increase in the prevalence rate of asthma. The positivity ratio of skin reaction in asthmatic patients to

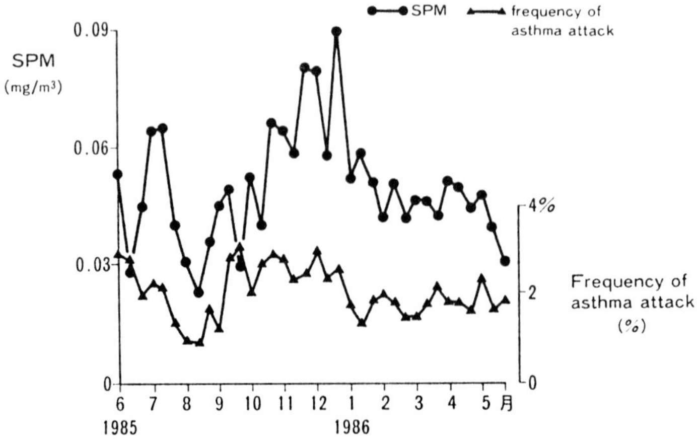

Figure 3. Relationship between Frequency of Asthma Attacks and Suspended Particulate Matter (SPM) Concentration in Childhood Asthma. 70 asthmatic children were classified into a younger juvenile group (3–7 years old) and an older juvenile group (8–19 years old); in the former group, a significant correlation was found between the levels of suspended particulate matter (SPM) and the frequency of asthma attacks within each ten day period examined (3).

Figure 4. Relationship between Asthmatic Symptoms and Concentration of Air Pollutants (NO_2 and SO_2). Effects of auto exhaust on respiratory conditions were examined along a main road. Both NO_2 and SPM levels tended to be high, and people living in the area nearest to the main road showed the highest prevalence rate of respiratory symptoms, and they had "asthmatic symptoms" in a significantly higher rate than the residents in other areas (4).

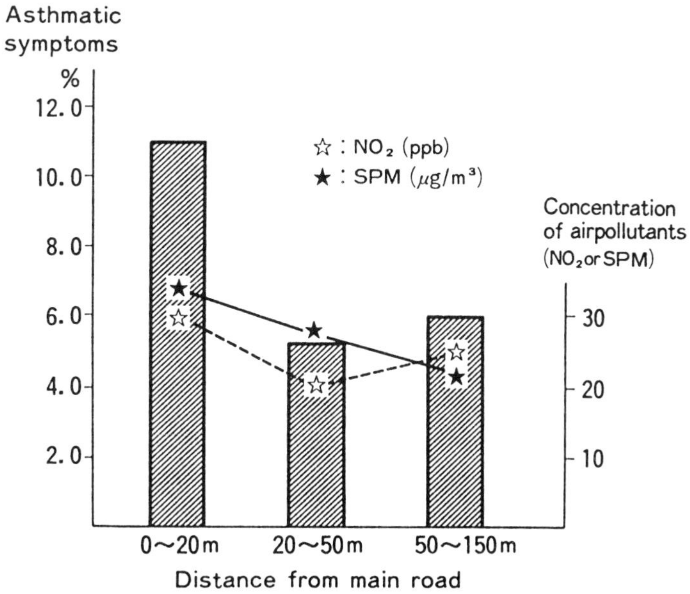

Figure 5. The Change in Number of Mites in House Dust (Tokyo). The total number of mites increased in the years studied, from 1965 to 1975, and then further to 1985, especially in the summer period rather than in winter. Besides, the proportion of pyroglyphidae in the total mites is increasng (7).

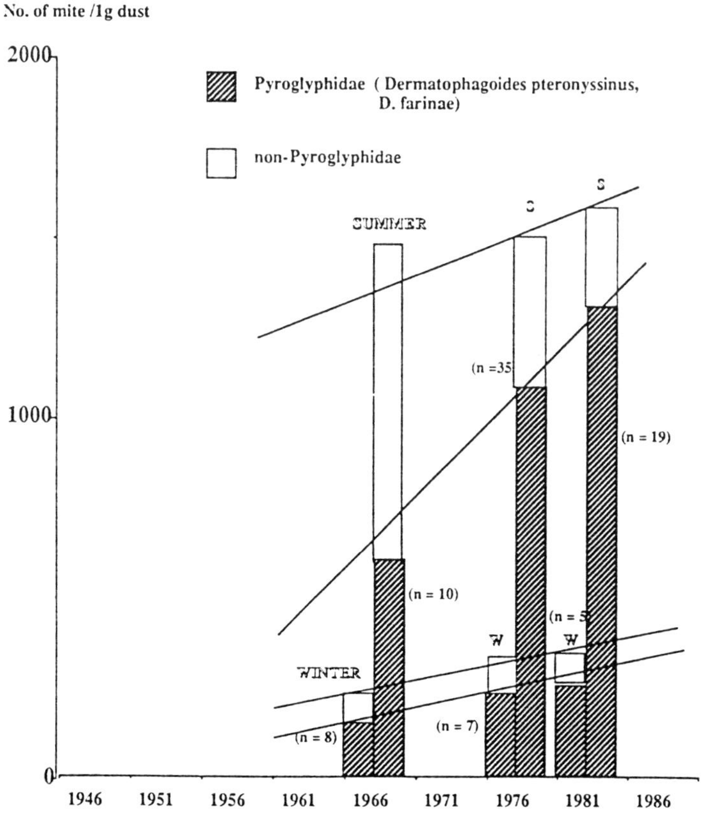

various allergens was examined (6). The highest positivity was recorded for house dust and mites. It was shown that the total number of mites increased throughout the years, from 1965 to 1975, and then further to 1985, and it increased stronger in summer periods rather than in the winter (7) (Figure 5). Besides, not only the total number of mites but also the proportion of pyroglyphidae in the total mites is increasing. The number was not more than 500 per 1 g of fine house dust in 1970, but it increased about 2.5-fold on the average in the nineteen eighties. This tendency is also obvious in Western countries, as reported by Bronswijk et al. in 1971. It is conceivable that the changes in housing environment are closely related to the increase in the number of mites in houses. These changes can largely be attributed to housing environment and life style changes.

Japan can be considered as belonging to a subtropical climate when the high humidity and temperature during summer are considered, and traditional Japanese houses consisted of wood and paper with elevated floors which provided good ventilation for adapting to the hot and humid summer time and rainy season. However, the modern trend towards Westernization introduced a new style of house structure, life style and interior decoration. For example, air-tight and highly insulated materials such as concrete or new synthetic building materials are now used for Japanese houses which are substantially smaller than American or European ones. Besides, residential areas are densely built-up. All of these changes contribute to making ventilation less sufficient and to increasing the humidity of the rooms. Traditional habits such as general house cleaning in the whole community at the end of the year tend to be lost, and the increase in the number of working women makes it difficult to sun-dry bed-quilts or tatami mats frequently. The changes in housing environment and life style described above are plausible reasons for the increase in mite-induced allergic asthma.

Death From Asthma

According to the statistical survey conducted by the Health and Welfare Ministry of Japan, the asthma mortality in Japan reached a maximum in the nineteen fifties, when nearly 20 persons per 100,000 in the population died of asthma; subsequently the rate decreased and can be regarded as having reached a plateau for the last 10 years, being about 5 deaths per 100,000 at the present (8). The asthma mortality in Japan is not much different from the rate observed in Europe and North America, and has been almost constant for the last several years with but a slightly increasing tendency. On the other hand, as shown in Figure 6, there is an alarming tendency towards an increase in the mortality of mild or moderate cases (8). The reasons for this mortality have not been fully clarified yet, but may involve patients who did not adequately understand the seriousness of their condition, or, possibly, physicians in charge who did not have sufficient understanding of the conditions of their patients.

Adult Onset Asthma: Special Attention Needed

The classification of bronchial asthma generally employed at present includes those proposed by Swineford, Rackeman, Scadding, and so on. However, a simple classification is not always applicable to adult bronchial asthma clinically, and it is frequently observed that the classification of asthma for one and the same patient differs with physicians.

A joint survey conducted by two groups revealed that in about 80% of asthma cases, the

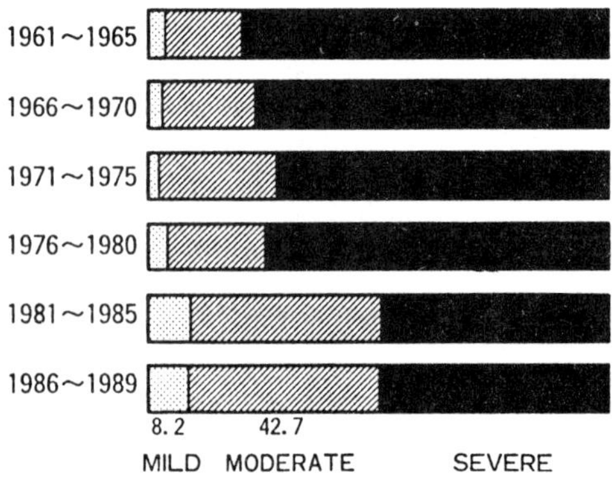

Figure 6. Deaths from Asthma and Clinical Severity. There is an alarming tendency for an increase in the mortality of mild or moderate cases (8).

Figure 7. Clinical Classification of Adult Asthma. Patients were classified into these three types. In about 80% of the asthma cases, onset was after the patient became 20 years old (9).

(N=2585)

	Childhood asthma	Age of onset	No. of patient (%)
Childhood onset asthma	Yes	0~15 y.o.	311 (11.1)
Adult onset asthma	No	20 y.o.~	2157 (77.3)
Adult recurrent asthma	Yes	16~19 y.o.	15 (0.5)
	Yes	20 y.o.~	102 (7.7)

onset occurred after the patients had become 20 years old, and therefore it became apparent that adult asthma is not a simple extension of childhood asthma (9). The study was done in a total of 37 institutions throughout Japan, and questionnaires were given to asthma patients who were hospitalized or visited the relevant hospital during the study period of 5 days from 18 through 22 September, 1989. In the questionnaire form, patients were asked to enter such items as sex, age, age at which the first episode of asthma was experienced, complications and so on, and the corresponding physician in charge was asked to enter the status of steroid use. Based on the content of nearly 2,800 questionnaire cards recovered and considered eligible, the patients were classified into three types as shown in Figure 7: Childhood onset asthma in which the onset occurred at 15 years or younger, adult onset asthma in which onset occurred at 20 years or later, and adult recurrent asthma. Patients who answered that they once had a history of childhood asthma and yet experienced the re-onset of asthma at the age of 20 years or later were classified into adult recurrent asthma.

As shown in Figure 8 (9), incidences of aspirin hypersensitivity, systemic steroid regular use, severe cases, regular use of anti-asthma drugs and the infectious type as classified by the Swineford method were significantly higher in adult onset asthma cases. This suggests that adult onset asthma needs special attention.

The classification method employed here was based on the age of the onset of asthma, and this simple classification allowed patients to answer questionnaire cards from their own disease history easily, and therefore has advantages in the actual clinical setting where standardized classification by cause, mechanisms and so on is not established yet. We thus propose the use of such a practical classification by the age of onset internationally in the future.

ADULT ONSET ≫ CHILDHOOD ONSET

* REGULAR USE OF SYSTEMIC CORTICOSTEROIDS (P<0.001, 7,23)
* REGULAR USE OF ANTI ASTHMA DRUGS (P<0.001, 1.68)
* SEVERE ASTHMA (P<0.05, 1.86)
* ASPIRIN SENSITIVE (P<0.05, 2.31)
* INFECTIOUS TYPE (NON ATOPIC) (P<0.001, 7.23)

Figure 8. Clinical Features of Adult Onset Asthma (p-value, odds). The incidences of aspirin hypersensitivity, systemic steroid regular use, severe cases, regular use of anti-asthma drugs and infectious type as classified by the Swineford method were significantly higher in adult onset asthma cases (9).

References

1. Nakamura, S. 1991. Epidimiology of asthma. Journal of Therapy 73:4.
2. Yoshida, K. 1966. Air pollution and asthma in Yokkaichi. Arch. Environ. Health 13:763.
3. Odashima, H. 1989. Air pollution and asthma. In: Are atopic deseases increasing ? T. Miyamoto, ed. Tokyo: International Medical Publication, p. 46.
4. Ono, M. 1991. Air pollution and asthma. Health Sciences 7:127.
5. Inoue, K. 1983. Epidemiology of childhood asthma in Oshima (non polluted area). Jap. J. Allergology 32:138.
6. Miyamoto, T. 1989. The positive ratio of skin test to various allergens in patients with bronchial asthma. In: Bronchial asthma and chronic brochites. T. Takahashi, ed. Tokyo: Medical View Publication, p. 14.
7. Takaoka, M. 1989. The changes of environmental situations of Japanese houses – relationship with increasing of house dust mite. In: Are atopic deseases increasing? T. Miyamoto, ed. Tokyo: International Medical Publication, p. 54.
8. Matsui, S., and Nakazawa T. 1991. Mortality of asthma. The Journal of Therapy 73:123.
9. Akiyama, K. 1991. Adult brochial asthma in Japan. Jpn. J. of Thoracic Diseases.

International Variations of Asthma Therapy

Timothy J. H. Clark*

Asthma questionnaires and analysis of prescriptions for asthma between countries show substantial variations in the way asthma is managed throughout the world. Epidemiological studies also show great variations in prevalence and asthma mortality between countries, and the relation between these measures of asthma and its treatment requires further analysis. In many countries asthma mortality seems to be on the increase, but this may represent greater awareness of asthma and hence better diagnosis. The increase is also only related to the population at large and not to those at risk. Thus increased prevalence and/or severity of asthma might explain the apparent increase in fatalities. These considerations make it difficult to assess the impact that treatment has on asthma deaths, but a number of studies have suggested that treatment is related to fatalities. Whether this is solely a function of asthma severity or an unexpected adverse effect of treatment remains to be clarified. Fortunately, there is now growing agreement between countries as to guidelines for treatment which may reduce the scale of global differences in management and enable a better understanding of the link between treatment for morbidity and asthma outcome.

There is growing interest in comparisons of care of asthma between different countries. In part this is stimulated by innate curiosity, but the differences in asthma fatalities between the countries have prompted a more scientific examination of differences in care and in particular medication. The differences in asthma medication between nations are likely to have many explanations and the link between asthma treatment and outcome measures such as fatalities and absenteeism from work or school is likely to be complex. Despite these problems an inspection of variations of asthma therapy between countries does provide useful information.

Observed Differences

There have been relatively few studies of differences in medication and asthma management between countries, and no study so far has been entirely satisfactory. Enquiries have fallen into two main categories; the first asks clinicians in different countries how they manage asthma and the second looks at information about prescriptions.

Clinician Questionnaires

A substantial enquiry into the treatment preferences of clinicians was carried out in Europe in the mid 1990s by Vermiere and Colleagues (1). The members of the European Society of Pneumology (SEP) were surveyed with a questionnaire which included questions about diagnosis and general management in addition to medication for acute and chronic asthma. This survey was clearly biased by its limitation to those members of the European Society who chose to respond and by the fact that the respondents included different specialities which made the analysis of responses even more difficult to interpret. An attempt was made to extend the survey to include pediatricians and general practitioners but the results can only be seen as a preliminary attempt to see if major variations were likely to exist between the European countries. The results confirmed that major differences in asthma medication were likely to occur and these applied particularly to the management of chronic asthma. There were very wide differences of opinion about the role of immunotherapy, and substantial differences arose with preferences for treatment of chronic asthma. In general bronchodilators were the preferred choice for this treatment but inhaled anti-inflammatory treatment was favored by physicians in some countries. Inhaled steroids were employed far more frequently than oral steroids, which suggested that the indications

* National Heart & Lung Institute, Dovehouse Street, London SW3 6LY, United Kingdom.

Table 1. % Value of Major Drug categories in selected countries for 1985.

	UK	USA	JAPAN	GLOBAL
Beta agonist inhaled	35	28	5	22
Beta agonist oral	5	16	32	15
Xanthines	14	36	13	27
Inhaled steroids	22	7	1	8
Inhaled anti allergic	14	3	6	7
Oral anti allergic	1	0	40	10
Others	9	9	3	10

Global % bronchodilator 64+% (22+% inhaled)
% anti-inflammatory 25+%

for inhaled steroids were no longer confined to substitution for oral medication.

Drug Prescriptions

Differences in physician preference between countries have also come from an analysis of prescriptions. The most secure data are those based upon prescriptions by value, which unfortunately weight the results in favor of expensive medications. What is required is a detailed breakdown of actual prescriptions, but in the absence of this the percentage value of the asthma market in each country is the best information available to date. Such information as shown in Table 1 demonstrates once again that there are very wide differences in prescribing habits between countries. The share of the market is likely to be dominated by treatment for chronic asthma, and on that assumption one can discern a number of patterns of prescriptions. The first consists of those countries which mainly prescribe bronchodilators. This is by far the largest group of countries, but within this group there are variations with some countries having a preference for oral theophylline e.g. the USA, with others more likely to prescribe inhaled beta agonists. As this group very much dominates the rest of the world it may account for the observation that nearly three quarters of all prescriptions by value are for bronchodilators taking the world as a whole. The other group of countries, e.g. the UK, also has a preponderance of bronchodilator prescriptions but a much larger proportion of the asthma market is devoted to inhaled anti-inflammatory medication of which inhaled steroids predominate. In these countries the use of inhaled therapy is likely to be greater than in the major category where oral medication still predominates. Japan is in a category of its own with a very much greater use of oral anti allergic treatment; and inhaled therapy is infrequent.

Trends

The information from surveys and analysis of prescriptions can only yield broad generalizations, but some further information can be obtained from trends revealed by further surveys and analysis of prescriptions (see Table 2). Vermiere carried out further surveys within

Table 2. % value of Major Drug categories in selected countries for 1989 (1985 in brackets).

	UK	USA	JAPAN	GLOBAL
Beta agonist inhaled	32 (35)	33 (28)	7 (5)	27 (22)
Beta agonist oral	4 (5)	13 (16)	25 (32)	12 (15)
Xanthines	8 (14)	31 (36)	17 (13)	23 (27)
Inhaled steroids	39 (22)	9 (7)	2 (1)	15 (8)
Inhaled anti allergic	9 (14)	4 (3)	5 (6)	6 (7)
Oral anti allergic	0 (1)	0 (0)	44 (40)	10 (10)
Others	7 (9)	11 (9)	1 (3)	9 (10)

Global % bronchodilator 62+% (64% 1985)
% bronchodilator inhaled 27% (22% 1985)
% anti inflammatory 31% (25+% 1985)

Belgium and proposed a new international survey 1991 and 1992. His preliminary results are in keeping with those from a review of prescription data, as they show a trend towards inhaled therapy in general and inhaled anti-inflammatory medication in particular. Despite these trends, if allowance is made for the costs of prescriptions it is likely that over 80% of asthma medication throughout the world continues to be bronchodilator therapy.

Causes for International Variations

The reasons for the observed differences in variation of asthma therapy cannot be analysed with any precision at this stage. There are likely to be a number of explanations all of which require closer examination. Setting the scene for most differences are likely to be such general factors as the wealth of the nation and the type of health service it can afford. The traditional use of bronchodilators is in part related to their availability and their cheapness, and for some countries very expensive treatments cannot be widely available and this will distort any analysis.

In addition to these general factors must be included the health service provision in general and access to care in particular. Even within the most affluent societies there are variations in patient access to care and this may account for some of the observed differences in fatalities which have initiated the examination of variations in therapy. There is growing concern in the USA about the differences in asthma mortality between the urban black population and the more affluent white members of society, and one explanation for this might be access to skilled care (2). Access to care and the provisions of the health service might produce a substantial variation within a country but also affect the prescribing habits between countries.

Another general factor that requires more detailed examination is the nature and scale of medical education particularly with respect to asthma treatment. The results of the European Survey suggested differences between North and South Europe which might be based upon teaching traditions, and this was suggested by the analysis of results from Belgium by Vermiere which showed differences between French speaking and Dutch speaking physician preferences. Prescribing preferences start at medical school and are known to be difficult to dislodge, so international variations are likely to be deep seated and are unlikely to be amenable to rapid convergence even if the best therapy for patients could achieve international agreement.

Epidemiology

The importance of the general background factors mentioned above needs be remembered when explanations are sought in terms of epidemiological information. Thus differences in asthma treatment might result from differences in prevalence and severity as well as types of asthma between the countries so it will be necessary to link the epidemiology of asthma with national variations in treatment with measures of outcome such as absenteeism and fatalities. Such linkage is in a very early and primitive stage but must remain the end result of any such enquiry (3).

Asthma Fatalities and Treatment

The starting point for the growing interest in international variations of asthma treatment was the asthma epidemic of deaths in the mid 1960s. This epidemic affected different countries in an inconsistent manner, with some countries such as England and Wales showing the epidemic very clearly and others such as the USA appearing to avoid it. As the epidemic of deaths was thought to be related to the excessive use of high dose Isoprenaline inhalers, the link with asthma therapy and fatalities between different countries became of interest to epidemiologists and others. The relationship between high dose Isoprenaline inhalers and asthma fatalities was never proved and remains only circumstantial. In the 1970s Isoprenaline was largely replaced with selective beta agonists such as Salbutamol, and the use of inhaled beta agonist therapy rose substantially without any return of asthma deaths. This gave comfort to those who felt that other explanations were required than high doses of inhaled beta agonists for the asthma fatality epidemic.

This complacency was challenged in New Zealand in the mid to late 1970s when another epidemic of deaths occurred which appeared to be related to excessive use of bronchodilators. This was initially thought to be associated with the introduction of long acting oral Theophyllines (4) but subsequent studies have more clearly implicated beta agonists (5,6) and in particular Fenoterol (7). An examination of variations in asthma prescribing and asthma fatalities might further help unravel the causes for the asthma epidemics, and this has led to comparisons of asthma prevalence between the countries as well as further more detailed examinations of asthma fatality rates in the various countries (8).

Morbidity and Mortality

The alleged relations between therapy and asthma fatalities are a paradox as modern therapy can clearly reduce morbidity, but of course this short term beneficial action does not exclude the possibility of a longer term risk. Theophylline medication is known to be associated with toxicity and some fatalities but other treatments are not; of these, only beta agonists are implicated as a possible cause for some asthma fatalities. This possibility has been further developed by the recent observations from New Zealand by Sears et al. that chronic Fenoterol therapy may in fact not improve morbidity in comparison with intermittent treatment, and may even make it worse (9). These observations require confirmation and further clarification but reinforce those who are concerned about the risks of beta agonist therapy taken on a regular basis. The relationship between beta agonist prescriptions and fatalities has been observed again in the more recent New Zealand outbreak of deaths but this relationship applies to all forms of asthma therapy, and follows the increase in fatalities with a time lag of up to two years (see Figure 1). This suggests that asthma fatalities stimulated patients and clinicians to recognize the need for an increased scale of treatment with the changes in therapy following and being led by the changes in fatalities. This observation and the failure to see a correlation between beta agonist prescriptions and fatalities in other countries where beta agonist usage has grown markedly over the past decade mean we cannot come to any definite conclusion about the relationship between therapy and asthma fatalities but we clearly need to resolve this issue as soon as possible.

Analysis of trends in asthma fatalities is further obscured by our failure to relate deaths to the at risk population, i. e. those with asthma. Instead fatalities are related to the general population and ignore the possibility that the variations may be based on differences in prevalence and severity of asthma. In the meantime the urgency surrounding this issue is lessened by a general agreement that therapy for chronic asthma should be based on anti-inflammatory medication rather than bronchodilators which

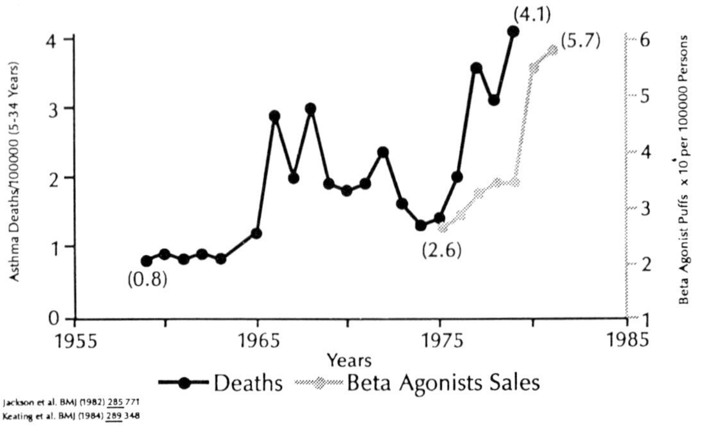

Figure 1. Relation between asthma mortality in New Zealand and sales of beta agonists. Data from references 5 and 6.

may lead to a substantial change in prescribing habits and reduce the risks of chronic bronchodilator therapy if they exist.

Asthma Guidelines

In the past few years there has been a convergence of views about asthma treatment which may lead to a reduction in the marked variations that presently exist between countries. As observed in the trends of prescriptions there is greater use of inhaled therapy and more frequent use of anti-inflammatory medication (10). There has also been a major change in attitude towards symptoms with the emphasis now on preventing symptoms rather than symptomatic treatment which reacted to them. The goals of therapy are to keep the patient well and free from asthmatic episodes with as near normal lung function as possible, and the avoidance of side effect liability (11). If these guidelines can achieve the goals of therapy set for them patient care will improve and international variations in asthma therapy will be reduced. This is clearly a worthwhile goal.

References

1. Vermeire, P.A., Wittesaele, W.M., Janssens, E., and DeBacker, W.A. 1986. European audit of asthma therapy. Chest 90:58.
2. Sly, R.M. 1988. Mortality from asthma 1979–1984. J. All. and Clin. Immunol. 82:705.
3. Holland, W.W. (Ed.) 1988. European Community atlas of avoidable death. Oxford: Oxford University Press.
4. Wilson, J.D., Sutherland, D.C., and Thomas, A.C. 1981. Has the change to beta agonists combined with oral theophylline increased cases of fatal asthma? Lancet 1:1235.
5. Jackson, R.T., Beaglehole, R., Rea, H.H., and Sutherland, D.C. 1982. Mortality from asthma: A new epidemic in New Zealand. Brit. Med. J. 285:731.
6. Keating, G., Mitchell, E.A., Jackson, R., Beaglehole, R., and Rea, H.H. 1984. Trends in sales of drugs for asthma in New Zealand, Australia and the United Kingdom 1975–1981. Brit. Med. J. 289:348.
7. Grainger, J., Woodman, K., Pearce, N., Grant, J., Burgess, C., Keane, A., and Beasley, R. 1991. Prescribed fenoterol and death from asthma in New Zealand 1981–7: A further case-control study. Thorax 46:105.
8. Mitchell, E.A., Anderson, H.R., Freeling, P., and White, P.T. 1990. Why are hospital admissions and mortality rates for childhood asthma higher in New Zealand than in the United Kingdom? Thorax 45:176.
9. Sears, M.R., Taylor, D.R., Punt, C.G., Lake, D.C., Li, Q., Flannery, E.M., Lucas, M.K., and Herbison, G.P. 1990. Regular inhaled beta agonist treatment in bronchial asthma. Lancet 336:1391.
10. Barnes, P.J. 1989. A new approach to the treatment of asthma. New Eng. J. Med. 321:1517.
11. Hargreave, F.E., Dolovich, J., and Newhouse, M.T.(Eds.) 1990. The assessment and treatment of asthma: A conference report. J. All. and Clin. Immunol. 85:1098.

Genetics of Chi t I Hypersensitivity

X. Baur, H. P. Rihs, C. Tautz*

189 individuals exposed to *Chi t I* have been HLA-D typed for DQB and DRB. The IgE-specific immune response to *Chi t I* is associated with sequences specific to DQB1*1 and DRB1*1. Individuals not sensitized to any other common allergen show the strongest association. Preliminary studies in 154 individuals indicate that DQA type 0501 is reduced in *Chi t I* responders. And finally, there is evidence for different mechanisms in the immune response to *Chi t I* of atopic and non-atopic people.

We have studied the IgE-specific immune response to the allergen *Chi t I* which represents the 12 hemoglobin molecules of the insect species Chironomus thummi. This non-biting midge of the Diptera family lives in water-rich areas. Chironomidae swarms, as well as their debris, were found to cause bronchial asthma and allergic rhinitis after environmental exposure. In addition, approximately 18% of aquarists using freeze-dried larvae ("red mosquito larvae") of the species Chironomus thummi as fish food become sensitized. Our previous studies demonstrated that immunologically cross-reacting hemoglobin molecules (*Chi t I*) are major allergens of Chironomidae. The primary and tertiary structures of *Chi t I* component III are known, and several of its B- and T-cell epitopes have been identified. Therefore, it is an adequate model to study the genetic bases of exposed individuals' immune response. Since associations between the IgE specific immune response to certain purified allergens and the HLA-system had been reported, especially by David Marsh and coworkers, our interest focussed on a potential association between the HLA class II system and the immune response to *Chi t I*.

The presentation of antigenic fragments to the T-cell-receptor is known to depend on the structure of HLA class II molecules forming a groove that binds the immunogenic peptides. In the region of chromosome 6 coding for the HLA-class II genes we find one pair of A- and B-genes coding for DP- and one pair coding for DQ molecules. In case of DR, there is one essentially non-polymorphic A gene and 4 coding polymorphic B genes, namely DRB1, 3, 4 and 5. The DRB2 gene is a pseudogene. Within the first domains of the HLA-DQB molecules considerable variability exists. HLA-DQA, on the other hand, is less variable. In the case of HLA-DR, only the B-chain is variable. The hypervariable regions in the first domain of DQB, DQA and the DRB chains can be detected on the DNA level by hybridization with sequence-specific oligonucleotides (SSOs). The DRB 1 gene (as well as the other class II genes) consists of 6 exons. The second exon codes for the variable first domain of the DRB 1 polypeptide. There are four hypervariable regions, namely amino acid sequences 9–13, 25–38, 57–60 and 67–74.

During the last 2 years, a panel of 189 persons exposed to *Chi t I* was HLA-D typed in our laboratory using PCR amplification with subsequent dot-blotting. The second exons of the class II genes were specifically amplified in the polymerase chain reaction with thermostable Taq polymerase and specific primers, e. g. for DQB, DQA or DRB in the presence of dNTPs. After the denaturation step, the primers anneal to the target DNA, and the polymerase elongates the complementary strands with the help of the deoxynucleotides in the sample. This cycle is repeated 30 times. Thus the target DNA is amplified up to 1 million times. We amplified the second exons of DQB1, of DQA1 and of DRB1, 3, 4, 5 respectively by using specific primers from the labs of David Marsh and Sasazuki. Equal amounts (10 to 50 ng) of the alkali denaturated amplified DNA were then spotted onto a nylon membrane and fixed by baking at 80°C. Figure 1 shows an example of the DRB-typing with radioactive labelled oligonucleotides. You can see four different hybridizations of the same filter. After hybridization, the

* Professional Associations' Research Institute for Occupational Medicine (BGFA), Ruhr University of Bochum, Germany.

Figure 1: Hybridizations of the target DNA sequence with a sequence specific oligonucleotide (SSO).

SSO			C	GAC	CCC	GGC	GGA	CGG	CG		
target sequence	...	ACG	CCG	CTG	GGG	CCG	CCT	GCC	GCC	...	+
not detected	...	ACG	CTG	CTG	GGG	*CTG*	CCT	GCC	GCC	...	–
sequences	...	ACG	CCG	CTG	GGG	*CGG*	*CTT*	*GAC*	GCC	...	–

Table 1: Association of the sensitization to *Chi t I* with SSOs specific for DQB1, DRB or DQA genes

SSO	Specificity	HVR	group A + B Pat. (n=61)	Contr. (n=128)	group A (non-atopic) Pat. (n=27)	Contr. (n=95)
Q4	3.1, 3.3	3	38%	44%	22%	42%
Q5	1.1, 1.19	3	39%	27%	52%	28%*
Q6	DQB1*2	3	36%	33%	37%	28%
R1	DRB1*1	1	33%	21%	44%	22%*
R3	DRB1*4	1	18%	28%	22%	26%
R7	1, 4.14	4	41%	29%	52%	30%
R10	DRB3*52a	4	18%	32%	1%	35%*

Contr.: control group; Pat.: patient group.

Table 2: HLA-DRB and -DQB types in a panel exposed to *Chi t I.*

Type	group A + B Pat. (n=61)	Contr. (n=128)	p	group A (non-atopic) Pat. (n=27)	Contr. (n=95)	p
DQw1	77%	68%	0.26	85%	71%	0.2
DQw1.1	33%	21%	0.11	44%	23%	0.05*
DQw3	46%	61%	0.07	37%	61%	0.04++
DQW3.1	31%	40%	0.31	19%	37%	0.12
DR1	33%	20%	0.09	44%	22%	0.04*
DR4	18%	28%	0.18	22%	26%	0.85
DRw11	18%	25%	0.37	19%	23%	0.8
DRw52	51%	61%	0.24	44%	62%	0.15
DRw52a	8%	18%	0.12	11%	35%	0.03++

filters were washed under stringent conditions and exposed to an X-ray film. So far, we investigated 16 SSOs for DQB1, 14 for DQA and 26 for DRB1, 3, 4, 5.

The filter was hybridized at first with a framework oligonucleotide probe which recognizes all DQB, DQA or DRB sequences to check the concentration of the applied DNA. Afterwards, hybridizations with SSOs followed resulting in the recognition of DQB, DQA or DRB sequences. A difference of only one nucleotide in the sequence can be detected by specific washing after hybridization (see Fig. 1).

We studied 189 *Chi t I*-exposed people devided into two subgroups: (a) group A (non-atopics): 95 controls and 27 *Chi t I*-sensitized subjects not sensitized to any other allergen; and (b) group B (atopics): 67 individuals sensitized to one or more common allergens; 34 of them had an additional IgE specific immune response to *Chi t* I. The IgE level was measured by RAST. Rast values > 0.35 U/ml were considered as positive.

Results

Sequences specific to DQB1 subtype 1.1 are more common in *Chi t I* responders than in non-responders. Sequences determining DRB1*1 are more frequently found in sensitized individuals. The associations of SSOs Q5 and R1 are significant in group A (non-atopics not sensitized to any common allergen). Furthermore, SSO R10 is distinctly less present in non-atopic responders. No significant correlation was found in group B, i.e. the atopics (Table 1).

When the results of hybridizations with different SSOs are combined to determine specific HLA-DQ or -DR subtypes, DQw1.1 and DR1 are more frequent in responders to *Chi t I* (Table 2). DQw1.1 is in linkage disequilibrium with DR1 and DR10. Which of the two HLA molecules is responsible for the presentation of specific *Chi t I* fragments still has to be determined. These associations are again significant in group A. In contrast, DQw3 and DRw52a are more frequent in non-responders (significant for group A).

Conclusions

Preliminary results obtained in DQA typing of 154 individuals exposed to *Chi t I* using 14 non-radioactively labelled SSOs indicate a reduction of 0501 in *Chi t I* responders.

The Atopic IgE Response and Chromosome 11

William O. C. M. Cookson*

Atopy is recognised as familial and many studies have conceded a major genetic effect controlling IgE levels. A gene for atopy, defined in a number of ways, is shown to be linked to the long arm of chromosome 11. Some genetic heterogeneity may be present. The finding allows new approaches to characterising the defects underlying atopy. The first benefit may be the recognition of at risk infants before sensitisation takes place.

It has long been recognised that there is a familial component to atopy, implying the presence of an underlying genetic predisposition. Early workers felt that the syndrome best fitted an autosomal dominant pattern of inheritance, without complete penetrance (1,2). These authors studied the inheritance of the whole syndrome, without defining its component parts. Later studies concentrated on the inheritance of specific illnesses such as asthma or hay fever. In these circumstances a pattern of inheritance was much harder to define (3,4).

After reaginic activity was shown to be mediated by Immunoglobulin E, an elevated total serum IgE was recognised as a concomitant of allergic disease. Workers then concentrated on the genetics of this parameter, presumably because it was quantifiable in a way not possible with symptoms alone. Bazaral et al. (5) studied IgE levels in infants and mothers, concluding that there was a presumptive fit to the Hardy-Weinberg distribution, and that this was consistent with simple Mendelian heredity of basal IgE levels. A subsequent study by the same investigators (6) showed identical twins to be highly concordant for total serum IgE, and that this effect was not linked to HLA haplotypes.

Marsh and his colleagues (7) studied many families for the inheritance of total IgE. They found that there was no simple pattern of Mendelian inheritance of the high IgE trait, but that a model in which high IgE was recessive best fitted the data. Gerrard et al. (8) studied families with complex segregation analysis, also concluding that a major locus controlled IgE levels, with a recessive allele determining high IgE levels, but that also other genes, even many, influenced the trait. Blumenthal et al. (9), however, considered that a dominant allele coded for high IgE levels.

Boreki et al. studied a Canadian population for the inheritance of atopy, and looked at the problem in a number of ways. They found that if the total serum IgE was the only measure of atopy, then an autosomal recessive pattern of inheritance best fitted the data. When they included symptoms in their definition, they then found that a dominant pattern of inheritance best explained their findings (10).

Cookson and Hopkin considered that elevated specific IgE, detectable either in the serum or by prick skin tests, was also a marker for the atopic state. They found that when atopy was defined in this way there was an apparent dominant pattern of inheritance, which correlated closely, although not completely, with the symptoms of atopic disease (11). Eighty-five per cent of subjects with IgE elevations had either wheeze or rhinitis, compared to 15% of controls. However, only 35% considered themselves to have hay-fever, and 30% to have asthma. The penetrance of this trait was high, about 90%, but was not complete, so that some atopic children did not have demonstrably atopic parents.

All of these studies of atopy and IgE responsiveness have been made more difficult by confounding factors. The most notable of these are age and smoking. The prevalence of atopy and the total serum IgE rise steeply through childhood to a peak in the teens, and then decline steadily thereafter (12). The skin tests and specific IgE titres follow a similar pattern, although they diminish at a rate slower than the total serum IgE. Smoking elevates the total IgE to an uncertain degree (13), so that studies of the

* Nuffield Department of Clinical Medicine, John Radcliffe Hospital, Headington, Oxford OX3 9DU, Great Britain.
Acknowledgement: Grant support from The Wellcome Trust.

genetics of atopy need to avoid smokers and individuals older than 45 to define the phenotype with clarity. A further confounding factor is the extreme commonness of the atopic syndrome, as more than 40% of the population may carry the atopic trait. This high prevalence means that many families will contain homozygous individuals, obscuring patterns of inheritance.

Despite these difficulties in understanding the clinical genetics, which are not completely resolved, there is agreement that a major locus controls the level of IgE responses in the population, and almost certainly the same locus affects the prevalence of atopic illnesses.

Cookson et al. followed their investigations of the clinical genetics of IgE responsiveness (IgER) by a linkage study to try and determine a chromosomal localisation for the gene (or genes). They found linkage between IgER and a marker (λms51) on the long arm of chromosome 11 (14). The lod score was about 5 (or odds of 10^5:1 in favor of linkage). A subsequent study of 64 small families by the same group (15) reproduced the initial findings. A feature of this study was the greatly increased male/female recombination ratio. A third investigation, carried out in Japan (16) has also found positive evidence for linkage.

The linkage study has been criticized because of the definition of atopy used, and the lod score method of analysis of results. Lod scores are sensitive to assumptions about penetrance and gene frequency, and the model of inheritance used. Sib-pair analysis, although less sensitive, is much more robust in finding linkage associations. Table 1 shows that linkage with chromosome 11 may be detected by using skin tests or total IgE as markers of atopy.

The presence of linkage implies a gene on chromosome 11 which controls the presence or absence of atopy in an individual. An eventual aim of genetic research is to characterise the gene, and if possible to devise pharmacologic control of its action. It will also be possible to assess genetic risk of atopy early in life, with subsequent potential for avoidance of sensitising factors at critical stages of development.

A final consideration in the genetic control of IgE synthesis is the restriction of the IgE response to specific allergens by class II molecules of the HLA complex. Much of this work has been carried out by Marsh (18), who has shown significant associations between HLA type and some allergen components. This finding may also permit risk assessment, particularly when allergy is to small antigens, such as industrial compounds.

Table 1. Allele sharing, identity by descent, parent of origin not taken into account. 743 subjects, 144 two-generation families.

	Alleles Shared			
Phenotype	2 or 1	0	X^2	(p:1df)
Atopy	144	31	6.48	0.011
Skin Test 3mm	87	13	7.68	0.006
ELISA	90	14	7.38	0.007
Total IgE	36	4	4.80	0.028
Symptoms	134	26	6.53	0.001

References

1. Cooke, R.A., & van der Veer, A. 1916. Human sensitisation. J. Immunol. 1:201.
2. Schwartz, M. 1952. Heredity in bronchial asthma. Acta Allergol. 5:suppl. 2.
3. Edfors-Lubs, M.L. 1971. Allergy in 7,000 twin pairs. Acta Allergol. 26:249.
4. Sibbald, B., and Turner-Warwick, M. 1979. Factors influencing the prevalence of asthma in first degree relatives of extrinsic and intrinsic asthmatics. Thorax 34:332.
5. Bazaral, M., Orgel, H.A., and Hamburger, R.N. 1971. IgE levels in normal infants and mothers and an inheritance hypothesis. J. Immunol.107:794.
6. Bazaral, M., Orgel, H.A., and Hamburger, R.N. 1974. Genetics of IgE and allergy: Serum IgE levels in twins. J. Allergy Clin. Immunol. 54:288.
7. Marsh, D.G. 1976. Allergy: A model for studying the genetics of human immune response. In: Molecular and biologic aspects of the acute allergic reaction (Nobel Symposium No. 33). S.G.O. Johansson, K. Strandberg, and B. Unvas, eds. London: Plenum, p. 23.
8. Gerrard, J.W., Horne, S., Vickers, P., et al. 1974. Serum IgE levels in parents and children. J. Pediatr. 85:660.
9. Blumenthal, et al. 1981. Genetic transmission of serum IgE levels. Am. J. Med. Genet. 10:219.
10. Boreki, I., et al. 1985. Demonstration of a common major gene with pleiotrophic effects on Immunoglobulin E and allergy. Genet. Epidemiol. 2:327-8.

11. Cookson, W.O.C.M., and Hopkin, J.M. 1988. Dominant inheritance of atopic IgE responsiveness. Lancet i:86.
12. Cline, M.G., and Burrows, B. 1989. Distribution of allergy in a population sample residing in Tuscon, Arizona. Thorax 44:425.
13. Barbee, R.A., et al. 1987. A longitudinal study of serum IgE in a community cohort: Correlations with age, sex, smoking, and atopic status. J. Allergy Clin. Immunol. 79:919.
14. Cookson, W.O.C.M., et al. 1989. Linkage between IgE responses underlying asthma and rhinitis and chromosome 11q. Lancet i:1292.
15. Young, R.P., et al. 1991. Confirmation of linkage between atopic IgE responsiveness and chromosome 11q in 64 nuclear families. Cytogen. and Cell Genet. 58:1974.
16. Shirakawa, T., et al. 1991. Linkage between IgE responses underlying asthma and rhinitis (atopy) and chromosome 11q in Japanese families. Cytogen. and Cell Genet. 58:1970.
17. Vercelli, D., and Geha, R.S. 1989. The IgE system. Ann. Allergy 63:4.
18. Marsh, D.G., Meyers,D.A., and Bias, W.B. 1981. The epidemiology and genetics of atopic allergy. New Eng. J. Med. 305:1551.

Molecular Genetic Studies of Human Immune Responsiveness to Ragweed Pollen Allergens

David G. Marsh, Balaram Ghosh, Thorunn Rafnar, Shau-Ku Huang*

Immunogenetic factors of atopic allergy can best be analyzed by considering two classes of genetic controls, of *overall* and of *specific* IgE response, which, together with non-genetic factors, determine the patterns of specific IgE antibodies seen in different individuals. HLA-D genes are important determinants of specific responsiveness to small allergens like the *Amb* V homologues (M_r = 4400–5000), where the association is with DR2/Dw2 (DR2.2). For certain allergens of 'intermediate complexity' (M_r = 10,000–15,000), we have observed an apparent interaction between genetic regulation of IgE, and of HLA-D genes. We have cloned and sequenced three *Amb* V cDNAs and/or genomic DNAs and have expressed the proteins in *E. coli* as 50–100% active molecules in Ab-binding assays and 100% active in T-cell assays. In collaborative studies, we have obtained the 3D structures of two *Amb* V molecules by NMR spectroscopy, which will facilitate analysis of the epitopes. We have analyzed the polymorphic second exons of HLA-DRB, DQA and DQB genes of 69 atopic Caucasians and found no sequence that is unique to *Amb a* V responders; however, virtually all IgE Ab responders to *Amb a* V possess DNA sequences normally associated with the DR2.2 phenotype. From sequence and Ab data from individuals having unusual combinations of HLA-DR and DQ specificities, we infer that probably a DR, but not a DQ, MHC Class II molecule is involved in the presentation of a major *Amb a* V epitope. This was confirmed using human T-cell clones and lines and HLA-specific MAbs; we found that the DRab1 heterodimers of DR2.2 (and of DR2.12, predominant in Orientals) are the principal Class II molecules that present a major *Amb a* V epitope. Analysis of the b1 polypeptide sequences of DR2 molecules was completely compatible with this hypothesis.

We believe that the old notion of a single gene determining atopic allergy, reviewed in (1,2) and recently revived (3), is too simplistic, considering the complexity of the disease. In order to analyze the genetic basis of allergy, we need to appreciate the *multifactorial* (multiple genetic and environmental) determinants which lead to the heightened IgE responsiveness characteristic of severely atopic subjects, the different antibody (Ab) specificities exhibited by different patients, and the different clinical manifestations: allergic rhinitis, asthma, atopic dermatitis, etc. We propose that immunogenetic factors in allergy can best be analyzed by breaking down the problem into *overall* IgE response and *specific* immune response aspects. On the one hand, gene(s) that are *not* linked to the human major histocompatibility complex (MHC) play an important role in overall IgE production (4); on the other hand, MHC Class II, T-cell receptor (TcR) and immunoglobulin (Ig) genes are all determinants of specific immune responsiveness (5). The pattern of specific IgE Ab responsiveness seen in any given individual is dependent on the complex interaction between these genetic and a array of non-genetic factors. The expression of allergic disease in its various manifestations no doubt requires the involvement of further genetic and non-genetic factors determining, for example, the inflammatory response seen in asthma. However, the focus here will be on the immunogenetics of overall and, more particularly, of antigen- (Ag-) specific IgE responsiveness.

Family Studies

We have extensively studied the genetics of allergic responsiveness in families and unrelated atopic subjects (4–10). Our family studies suggest that one major factor determining the inheritance of high total serum IgE level (nor-

* Johns Hopkins Asthma and Allergy Center, Baltimore, MD 21224, USA.
Acknowledgements: This work was supported by the NIH Grants Nos. AI19727 and AI20059, by an Irvington Fellowship (to S.-K.H.) and a Jack Center Award (to T.R.).

mally associated with high IgE-Ab responsiveness) is recessive (6,9,10), although the cutpoints between low and high IgE vary in the different studies. Several of our study families illustrate that it is possible for two completely non-atopic individuals with low total serum IgE levels to have highly atopic offspring with high serum IgEs (cf. Fig. 1). However, some families exhibit a dominant or codominant pattern of inheritance; therefore, recessive inheritance is by no means the complete picture. In our early research (6), we found that the overall concordance in the levels of specific skin-test sensitivity to an array of highly purified allergens in pairs of siblings who had inherited the identical HLA haplotypes from their parents were essentially the same as sib pairs who had inherited the completely opposite haplotypes; however, pairs of siblings having similar *high* total serum IgE levels were significantly more alike ($p = 0.001$) in their patterns of skin-test sensitivities than sib pairs having high and low IgE levels. From this finding, we postulated that IgE-regulating gene(s) are more important in determining overall IgE Ab responsiveness to an array of inhalant allergens than are specific, HLA-linked *Ir* genes.

HLA-D Association Studies in Unrelated Subjects

The above findings seem to present a dilemma. It is apparent from animal and human studies that the initiation of an IgE Ab response requires 'Ag processing' by an Ag-presenting cell (APC), and subsequent presentation of a fragment of the Ag by an MHC Class II molecule (HLA-DR, DQ or DP) to a TcR on a $CD4^+$, T_{H2}-like cell. We initially investigated Ag-specific responsiveness toward the simplest allergen we could find, namely *Amb a* V ($M_r = 5000$; 45 aas; ref. 11), which we felt confident would represent a truly limiting immunogenic stimulation: We found a striking association with the HLA-DR2, Dw2 (DR2.2) phenotype (12,13). (DR2 is defined by serology and Dw2 by MLR typing.) Subsequently, we found an HLA-DR5 association with responsiveness to a different, small ragweed allergen, *Amb a* VI (14) and weaker DR3 associations with responsiveness to three different rye grass allergens, *Lol p* I, II and III (15,16). Using DNA typing of HLA-D-region genes (discussed below), we continued

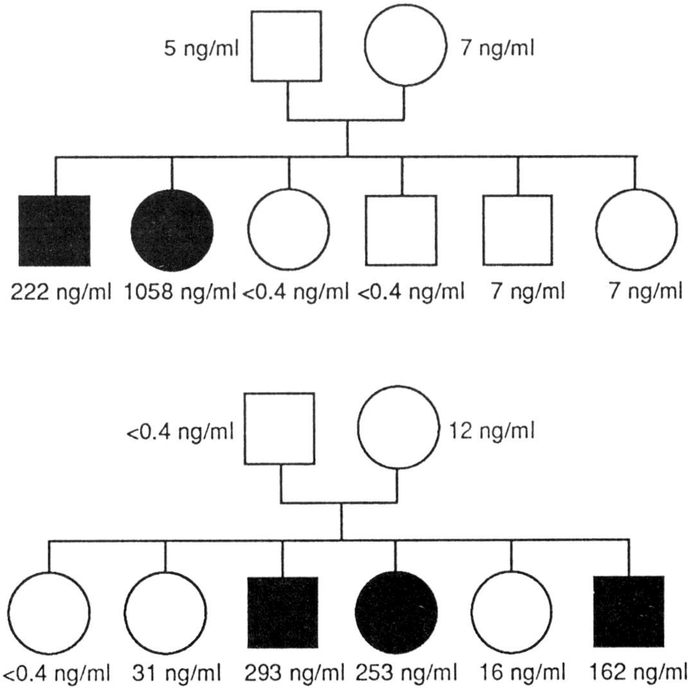

Figure 1. Examples of two families (#50 and #798) that show distribution patterns of total serum IgE levels (and associated atopic disease) that are compatible with recessive inheritance of high IgE responsiveness. Total IgE levels are given beside the symbols of the family members. The subjects shown in closed symbols exhibit symptoms of atopic allergy and have positive skin tests to common inhalant allergens; all other subjects are negative by both criteria. These families form part of the cohort studied by Meyers et al. (8–10).

to search for further associations (and confirm previous associations) in population studies, both of our local patients (17–21) and as part of the large international collaborative study on *HLA and Allergy*, for the *Eleventh International Histocompatibility Testing Workshop*, Yokohama, Japan, November, 1991 (22).

The finding of weaker HLA associations for certain allergens of 'intermediate complexity,' like *Lol p* II and *Lol p* III (M_r = 11,000), led us to investigate a possible interaction between the IgE-regulating gene(s) and HLA-linked *Ir* genes. For example, we examined the frequency of DR3 versus total IgE in atopic individuals who are positive or negative to *Lol p* III (16). In the positive group, we found that the frequency of DR3 varied according to the total serum IgE level of the individual; there is a striking association between DR3 and immune responsiveness to *Lol p* III at low total IgE level, but this association disappears in individuals having high total serum IgE levels. *Lol p* III$^+$ individuals with high total IgE, like *Lol p* III$^-$ individuals, possess a frequency of DR3 indistinguishable from the normal Caucasian population frequency of DR3. This finding suggests an interrelationship between genetic regulation of IgE on the one hand and HLA-linked *Ir* genes on the other. Our interpretation is that people who cannot make IgE very well may have a limiting population of T_{H2}-like cells and, as a result, may need to express a Class II molecule that is optimal for the recognition of a major *Lol p* III epitope in order to be able to produce IgE Ab to this Ag.

Molecular and Cellular Studies of the *Amb* V Allergens and Their Epitopes

We have focused on the *Amb* V homologues because of their relatively simple antigenic structures and the striking HLA-D associations observed. Interestingly, we found essentially no cross-reactivity between *Amb a* V and *Amb t* V (from short and giant ragweeds) at the B-cell (Ab) level (23), although they share 45–50% aa sequence identity; *Amb p* V (from western ragweed) is partially crossreactive with *Amb a* V and is non-crossreactive with *Amb t* V (24). Our studies using *Amb a* V-specific human T-cell clones and lines from DR2.2$^+$ subjects showed no cross-stimulation by *Amb t* V and *Amb p* V (25), although both of these *Amb* V homologues were able to inhibit stimulation of the T cells by *Amb a* V, with DR2.2$^+$ APCs (Fig. 2). These results show that

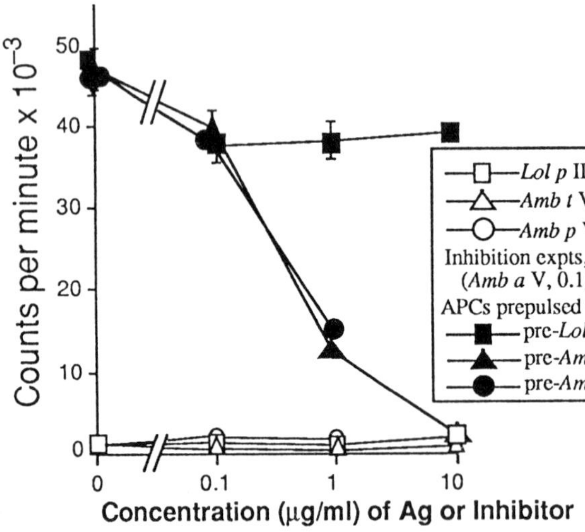

Figure 2. Blocking of *Amb a* V stimulation of the proliferative response of a DR2.2-restricted human T-cell clone by *Amb t* V or *Amb p* V. *Open symbols*, direct T-cell stimulation with *Lol p* III (control Ag), *Amb t* V and *Amb p* V. *Closed symbols*, inhibition of presentation of *Amb a* V (0.1 μg/ml) by prepulsing APCs with *Lol p* III (control), *Amb t* V or *Amb p* V. T cells (5 x 10^4/ml) and irradiated autologous PBMCs (5 x 10^5/ml) were used in all experiments. Proliferation of the T-cells was monitored by the incorporation of ^{3}H-thymidine (expressed in cpm). This experiment shows no direct T-cell stimulation by *Amb t* V or *Amb p* V, although both Ags show inhibition of *Amb a* V stimulation. (Adapted from ref. 25.)

Figure 3. Nucleotide sequence of *Amb t* V cDNA and its encoded amino acids. Numbers above the sequences indicate nucleotides and below the sequences amino acid residues. The translation-termination codon is marked by an asterisk. The two possible translation-initiation codons and the polyadenylation signal are shown in bold type. In some 3'-end clones, additional sequences, CAAATGCTT (25%) or AAATGCT (25%) are present immediately before the poly-A sequence. (From ref. 26.)

```
          1                          27
          ACATTTCATAGTTTAAAGAAATTATC ATG AAG AAC
                                     Met Lys Asn
                                     -33
36
ATA TTT ATG CTT ACA CTT TTT ATT CTT ATT ATT ACT TCG ACC ATT
Ile Phe Met Leu Thr Leu Phe Ile Leu Ile Ile Thr Ser Thr Ile
-30                 -25                 -20
81
AAG GCT ATA GGA TCC ACA AAT GAA GTC GAT GAA ATA AAA CAA GAA
Lys Ala Ile Gly Ser Thr Asn Glu Val Asp Glu Ile Lys Gln Glu
-15                 -10                  -5
126
GAC GAT GGA CTT TGT TAT GAG GGG ACC AAT TGT GGT AAA GTG GGC
Asp Asp Gly Leu Cys Tyr Glu Gly Thr Asn Cys Gly Lys Val Gly
  1               5                  10                  15
171
AAA TAC TGT TGT AGC CCC ATT GGG AAG TAC TGT GTC TGT TAT GAT
Lys Tyr Cys Cys Ser Pro Ile Gly Lys Tyr Cys Val Cys Tyr Asp
                 20                  25                  30
216                                          *
TCC AAG GCA ATA TGC AAC AAA AAT TGT ACT TAA TGAATGTCACTA
Ser Lys Ala Ile Cys Asn Lys Asn Cys Thr
                 35                  40
261                         289
AGCACACAATATAAAAATAATTACAGTTT(A)n
```

the allergens are not crossreactive at the T-cell level in this system; however, they suggest that peptides from all three Ags (generated within the APCs) can compete with one another in binding to the Ag-presenting Class II molecule. The latter result is compatible with our findings that responsiveness to all three *Amb* V molecules is associated with DR2.2 (12, 13, 23, 24). In further studies, we obtained evidence suggesting that a peptide close to the C-terminus of *Amb a* V (residues 31–44) may contain the major Class II-binding (Ia) epitope (25).

We have recently cloned and sequenced all three *Amb* V cDNAs and/or genomic DNAs using polymerase chain reaction (PCR) and anchored-PCR technologies (26,27; cf. Fig. 3, and ref. 30). The clones can all be expressed in the pGEX vector in *E. coli* as 50–100% active molecules in terms of Ab-binding, and 100% active in T-cell assays (28,31). Furthermore, we have recently collaborated with Drs. Luciano Mueller and William Metzler (Bristol-Meyers-Squibb Labs, New Jersey) to obtain the complete, refined three-dimensional structures of the *Amb a* V and *Amb t* V molecules by NMR spectroscopy (32). These data will facilitate the analysis of the epitopes on these rather unique, highly disulfide-bonded, small allergen molecules. We are, therefore, now in a position to prepare site-directed mutants of known structure for further analysis of Ia/T-cell, as well as B-cell, epitopes in this model allergen system.

Analysis of HLA-D-Region Genes

We have examined the molecular basis of specific immune responsiveness to the *Amb* V allergens using both molecular biologic and cellular immunologic approaches. We focussed on the polymorphic second exons of HLA-DRB and DQB genes that encode the Ag-binding portions of Class II molecules. In 17 selected individuals (*Amb a* V responders and non-responders), we amplified the respective gene segments using the PCR and sequenced the products (17,19). We also analyzed the polymorphic regions of the DRB, DQA and DQB genes of these 17 and a further 52 individuals using dot-blot analyses with sequence-specific oligonucleotides (SSOs) (17, 33). We found no sequence that was *unique* to *Amb a* V responders; however, virtually all people producing IgE Ab to *Amb a* V possessed the DRB1*1501 and DRB5*0101 sequences normally associated with the DR2.2 phenotype. We also examined some people having unusual *combinations* of DRB and DQB alleles, which are not normally found together on the same chomosome (in linkage disequilibrium) in Caucasians. Two such individuals, CSz and #218, who were *Amb a* V responders, had the DRB sequences normally associated with DR2.2, but had DQB specificities not usually found with

DR2.2. Conversely, we found one *non*-responder individual, JMc, who had the DQB1*0602 (DQw1) allele usually associated with DR2.2, but did not have the DRB1*1501 and DRB5*0101 sequences. From these data we infer that probably a DR, but not a DQ, MHC Class II molecule is involved in the presentation of a major *Amb a* V epitope.

T-Cell Studies

We tested this hypothesis using *Amb a* V T-cell clones derived from a DR2.2⁺, *Amb a* V responder subject (29). Cells from different patients or B-cell lines were used as APCs to present *Amb a* V epitopes to the TcRs on the cloned T cells. The autologous APCs presented the Ag very well, as did the APCs of all the individuals having DR2.2 (including CSz and #218, but not JMc), or the closely related DR2.12 specificity that is common in Orientals. APCs of individuals (or B-cell lines) having *any other* DR2 variant did not present *Amb a* V to the T-cell clones. In blocking experiments, we found that anti-DR monoclonal Abs (MAbs) inhibited Ag presentation, but anti-DQ and anti-DP MAbs had no effect (Figs. 4a and b). These data strongly support a role for a DR molecule in *Amb a* V presentation, but do not address the question: "which DR molecule, αβ1 or αβ?" To resolve this issue we used MAb Hu30, which is specific for the αβ1 Class II molecules of DR2 haplotypes. This MAb inhibited *Amb a* V presentation both by DR2.2

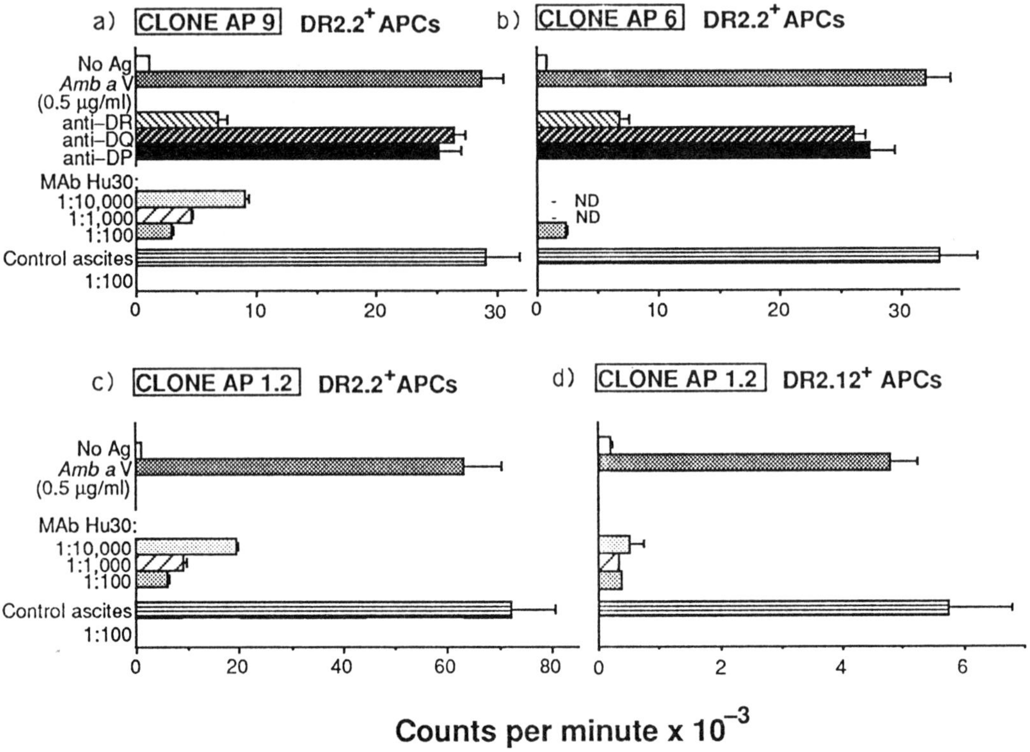

Figure 4. Inhibition of *Amb a* V-induced proliferation of three human T-cell clones by anti-HLA-D MAbs. Proliferation of the T-cells was monitored by the incorporation of ^{3}H-thymidine (expressed in cpm). Purified anti-DR, anti-DQ and anti-DP MAbs (Figs. a and b) were used at 1 µg/ml; ascites fluid containing Hu30 MAb (anti-ab1 of DR2), shown in all figures, was used at dilutions of 1:100–1:10,000. APCs from the autologous donor (DR2.2⁺) were used in Figs. a–c and APCs from a DR2.12⁺ subject were used in Fig. d. Inhibition of T-cell proliferation was found using anti-DR and anti-ab1 MAbs, but not with anti-DQ, anti-DP, or a control ascites fluid (1:100) containing a MAb of an irrelevant specificity. (Adapted from ref. 29.)

and DR2.12 APCs (Fig. 4), showing that the respective $\alpha\beta1$ heterodimers, DR(α, $\beta1$*1501 and DR(α, $\beta1$*1502), are the principal Class II molecules that present a major *Amb a* V epitope.

We compared the polypeptide sequences of DR$\beta1$*1501 and 1502 which are involved in presentation of *Amb a* V, versus those of DR$\beta1$*1601 (DR2.21) and DR$\beta1$*1602 (DR2.22) which are not. We found that these two groups differ from each other at aa residues 67, 70 and 71 that are postulated to point into the Ag-binding groove. Notably, *uncharged* residues, 70 (Gln) and 71 (Ala) are present in *Amb a* V responders, but *charged* residues 70 (Asp) and 71 (Arg) are present in non-responders to *Amb a* V.

Conclusions

The HLA-D-association studies, together with molecular and cellular studies of model systems like *Amb a* V, help us to understand the genetic and molecular basis of human immune responsiveness to allergens. This approach is directly relevant to studies of atopic allergy and asthma and is of more general relevance in understanding the molecular basis of human immune responsiveness and susceptibility to immunologic diseases.

References

1. Weiner, A., Zieve, I., and Fries, J. 1936. The inheritance of allergic disease. J. Ann. Eugen. 7:141.
2. Marsh, D.G. 1975. Allergens and the genetics of allergy. In: The antigens, Vol. III. M. Sela, ed. New York: Academic Press, p. 271.
3. Cookson, W.O.C.M., Sharp, P.A., Faux, J.A., and Hopkin, J.M. 1989. Linkage between immunoglobulin E responses underlying asthma and rhinitis and chromosome 11q. Lancet i:1292.
4. Meyers, D.A., Hasstedt, S.J., Marsh, D.G., Skolnick, M., King, M.C., Bias, W.B., and Amos, D.B. 1983. The inheritance of immunoglobulin E: Linkage analysis. Amer. J. Med. Genet. 16:575.
5. Marsh, D.G. and Blumenthal, eds. 1990. Genetic and environmental factors in clinical allergy. Minneapolis: University of Minnesota Press.
6. Marsh, D.G., Bias, W.B., and Ishizaka, K. 1974. Genetic control of basal serum immunoglobulin E level and its effect on specific reaginic sensitivity. Proc. Nat. Acad. Sci. 71:3588.
7. Marsh, D.G., Meyers, D.A., and Bias, W.B. 1981. The epidemiology and genetics of atopic allergy. New Engl. J. Med. (Medical Progress Series) 305:1551.
8. Meyers, D.A., Freidhoff, L.R. and Marsh, D.G. 1986. Predicting skin-test sensitivity and total serum IgE levels in family members. J. Allergy Clin. Immunol. 77:608.
9. Meyers, D.A., Beaty, T.H., Freidhoff, L.R., and Marsh, D.G. 1987. Inheritance of total serum IgE (basal levels) in man. Amer. J. Hum. Genet. 41:51.
10. Meyers, D.A., Beaty, T.H., Colyer, C.R., and Marsh, D.G. 1992. Genetics of total serum IgE levels: A regressive model approach to segregation analysis. Genet. Epidemiol., in press.
11. Mole, L.E., Goodfriend, L., Lapkoff, C.B., Kehoe, J.M., and Capra, J.D. 1975. The amino acid sequence of allergen Ra5. Biochemistry 14:1216.
12. Marsh, D.G., Hsu, S.H., Roebber, M., Ehrlich-Kautzky, E., Freidhoff, L.R., Meyers, D.A., Pollard, M.K., and Bias, W.B. 1982. HLA-Dw2: A genetic marker for human immune response to short ragweed pollen allergen Ra5. I. Response resulting primarily from natural antigenic exposure. J. Exp. Med. 155:1439.
13. Marsh, D.G., Meyers, D.A., Freidhoff, L.R., Ehrlich-Kautzky, E., Roebber, M., Norman, P.S., Hsu, S.H., and Bias, W.B. 1982. HLA-Dw2: A genetic marker for human immune response to short ragweed pollen allergen Ra5. II. Response after ragweed immunotherapy. J. Exp. Med. 155:1452.
14. Marsh, D.G., Freidhoff, L.R., Kautzky, E.E., Bias, W.B., and Roebber, M. 1987. Immune responsiveness to *Ambrosia artemisiifolia* (short ragweed) pollen allergen *Amb a* VI (Ra6) is associated with HLA-DR5 in allergic humans. Immunogenetics 26:230.
15. Freidhoff, L.R., Ehrlich-Kautzky, E., Meyers, D.A., Ansari, A.A., Bias, W.B., and Marsh, D.G. 1988. Association of HLA-DR3 with human immune response to *Lol p* I and *Lol p* II allergens in allergic subjects. Tissue Antigens 31:211.
16. Ansari, A.A., Freidhoff, L.R., Meyers, D.A., Bias, W.B., and Marsh, D.G. 1989. Human

immune responsiveness to *Lolium perenne* grass pollen allergen *Lol p* III (Rye III) is associated with HLA-DR3 and DR5. Hum. Immunol. 25:59.
17. Marsh, D.G., Zwollo, P., Huang, S.K., Ghosh, B., and Ansari, A.A. 1990. Molecular studies of human response to allergens. Cold Spring Harbor Symp. Quan. Biol. 54:459.
18. Ansari, A.A., Shinomiya, N., Zwollo, P. and Marsh, D.G. 1991. HLA-D gene studies in relation to immune responsiveness to a grass allergen, *Lol p* III. Immunogenetics 33:24.
19. Zwollo, P., Ehrlich-Kautzky, E., Ansari, A.A., Scharf, S.J., Erlich, H.A., and Marsh, D.G. 1991. Molecular studies of human immune response genes for the short ragweed allergen, *Amb a* V. Sequencing of HLA-D second exons in responders and non-responders. Immunogenetics 33:141.
20. Marsh, D.G., Shinomiya, N., Shinomiya, M., and Kautzky, E.E. 1991. Molecular analysis of the HLA-D association with immune responsiveness to *Amb a* VI. J. Allergy Clin. Immunol. 87:204.
21. Eura, M., Freidhoff, L.R., Ehrlich-Kautzky, E., Heymann, P., Platts-Mills, T.A.E., Roebber, M., Matthiesen, F., Løwenstein, H., and Marsh, D.G. 1991. HLA-DPB polymorphism and IgE responsiveness to specific allergens. 11th International Histocompatibility Testing Workshop and Conference, Yokohama, Japan, Abs. No. PS-I12-6, p. 235.
22. Marsh, D.G., Blumenthal, M.N., Ishikawa, T., Ruffilli, A., Sparholt, S. and Freidhoff, L.R. 1992. HLA and allergy. Histocompatibility testing, 1991. Oxford Univ. Press, in press.
23. Roebber, M., Klapper, D.G., Goodfriend, L., Bias, W.B., Hsu, S.H., and Marsh, D.G. 1985. Immunochemical and genetic studies of *Amb t* V (Ra5G), an Ra5 homologue from giant ragweed pollen. J. Immunol. 134:3062.
24. Marsh, D.G., Zwollo, P., Freidhoff, L., Golden, D.B.K., Ansari, A.A., Kautzky, E.E., Meyers, D.A., and Holland, C.L. 1990. Studies of human immune response to the *Amb* V (Ra5) homologues. J. Allergy Clin. Immunol. 85:201.
25. Huang, S. K., and Marsh, D.G. 1991. Human T-cell responses to ragweed allergens: *Amb* V homologues. Immunol. 73:363.
26. Ghosh, B., Perry, M.P., and Marsh, D.G. 1991. Cloning the cDNA encoding the *Amb t* V allergen from giant ragweed (*Ambrosia trifida*) pollen. Gene 101:231.
27. Ghosh, B., and Marsh, D.G. 1991. cDNA cloning of *Amb* V allergens from ragweed *(Ambrosia)* pollens. FASEB J. 5:A1662. (Abs.)
28. Rafnar T., Ghosh, B., Huang, S.-K., Metzler, W.J., Mueller, L., and Marsh, D.G. 1992. Expression and analysis of the highly disulfide-bonded *Amb* V allergens from ragweed. Internat. Symp.-Workshop on Molecular Biology and Immunology of Allergens, Vienna, Austria, Feb., 1992, in press. (Abs.)
29. Huang, S. K., Zwollo, P., and Marsh, D.G. 1991. Class II MHC restriction of human T-cell responses to short ragweed allergen, *Amb a* V. Europ. J. Immunol. 21:1469.
30. Ghosh, B., Perry, M.P., and Marsh, D.G. Molecular cloning and sequence analysis of the gene encoding the *Amb a* V allergen from short ragweed (*Ambrosia artemisiifolia*) pollen. Submitted for publication.
31. Rafnar T., Ghosh, B., Huang, S.-K., Metzler, W.J., Mueller, L., and Marsh, D.G. Expression of cystine-rich ragweed allergens in *E. coli*: Confirmation of the structural and immunological identity of recombinant and native *Amb t* V for epitope studies. In preparation.
32. Metzler, W.J., Valentine, K., Roebber, M., Friedrichs, M., Marsh, D.G., and Mueller, L. Solution structures of ragweed allergen *Amb t* V. Submitted for publication.
33. Marsh et al. Unpublished observations.

Section VIII

Nasal Allergy: Pathophysiology and Management of Nasal Congestion

Nasal Congestion as a Symptom of Nasal Allergy

Minoru Okuda, Hideji Tanimoto, Takao Watase, Masaki Ohnishi, Ruby Pawankar, Shuifang Xiao*

By questionnaire or interrogation, we examined the most troublesome nasal symptoms, the severity and duration of nasal blockage, the relation of nasal blockage to other nasal symptoms, the severity and duration of nasal blockage to other nasal symptoms, and to the quality of life, and subsequent symptoms in patients with house dust allergy or pollen allergy. As a result, nasal blockage was found to be the most troublesome nasal symptom, was moderate to severe in half of the patients with perennial allergy, persisted for a long time after an allergen attack, and its severity could not be correlated well with other nasal symptoms like sneezing and discharge but correlated very well with the impairment of quality of life, also leading to various subsequent symptoms. Furthermore, measurement of nasal airway resistance (NAR) and blood flow in the inferior turbinate revealed that nasal obstruction persisted for almost a whole day after and without nasal allergen provocation in many patients with nasal allergy; an increase in nasal airway resistance similar to the late phase response was noted in some patients; and an increase in nasal blood flow was observed after nasal provocation. Administration of a vasoconstrictor nasal spray reduced the increase in nasal blood flow and nasal airway resistance but did not bring it down to normal values, suggesting that organic changes in the mucosal tissues as well as congestion contribute to nasal blockage. It can be concluded that nasal blockage is the most troublesome symptom, especially for the quality of life in patients with nasal allergy because of the subsequent symptoms and its persistence over a long period, which may be due to both organic changes in the mucosal tissues as well as congestion.

Nasal blockage is caused by different pathological conditions of the nose and epipharynx, and often hampers the quality of life by impairment of sleep, normal breathing, sense of smell and psychological status. In patients with allergic rhinitis, nasal blockage is also the most troublesome symptom.

Many books on rhinology and nasal allergy cover the mechanisms of nasal obstruction, methods of assessment and clinical characteristics such as incidence, circadian change, aggravating factors and response to H_1 blocker (1, 2). However, as far as we know, the clinical significance of nasal blockage in allergic rhinitis has rarely been documented in detail. Thus, we will now present the clinical aspects of nasal blockage in correlation with the quality of life in patients with nasal allergy, based on the study of patients with house dust allergy and Japanese cedar pollen allergy in our clinic.

The Severity of Nasal Blockage

The severity of the symptoms of nasal allergy was classified into four grades as follows. The degree of sneezing was graded by the average number of attacks per day. Even if a patient sneezed many times during the period of a single attack, it was counted as one. The degree of discharge was expressed as the number of times the patient had to blow his nose, also being counted as one, if it was during the period of a single attack. The degree of nasal blockage was evaluated by a combination of duration and severity (mouth-breathing). Disturbances in the quality of life were graded by the extent to which the patient's daily routine work was hampered. At first we examined the patients' symptoms by interrogation. 94.1% of 212 patients with house dust allergy complained and 57.3% of 131 patients with Japanese cedar pollen allergy complained during the season. The total percentage of patients with moderate or severe nasal blockage was 51.8% and 21.2% respectively, which shows that many patients are troubled with nasal blockage.

* Dept. of Otolaryngology, Nippon Medical School, Japan.

Relationship Among the Degree of Different Nasal Symptoms in Allergy

We also examined the relationship between the severity of each nasal symptom in 220 patients with house dust allergy and found that Spearman's correlation coefficient was 0.474 ($p<0.001$) between sneezing and discharge, 0.147 (NS) between sneezing and blockage, and 0.081 (NS) between discharge and blockage. This result suggested that the mechanisms of sneezing and discharge correlate well with each other but differ from the mechanism of nasal blockage. Previously, we (3) proposed that both sneezing and discharge are reflex mediated symptoms due to stimulation of irritant receptors of sensory nerve endings with chemical mediators which are released from sensitized mast cells, since (a) unilateral allergen challenge induces nasal secretion on the contralateral side as well as the challenged side; (b) unilateral vidian neurectomy inhibited production of nasal secretion completely on the neurectomized side, but did not affect the contralateral side on allergen challenge to the neurectomized side; and (c) administration of topical anesthesia to the inferior turbinate on the provoked side inhibited nasal secretion on both the provoked and unprovoked sides. Contrary to nasal secretion, nasal obstruction did not change concomitantly on the contralateral side, in unilateral nasal stimulation. Nasal obstruction was measured in 23 patients as increased nasal airway resistance (NAR) by the anterior method of rhinonanometry (MRR-1100 Nihon-koden, Japan) and was expressed as the resistance (cn H_2O/L/sec) to natural expiratory airflow of the combined nasal cavities. In unilateral challenge with allergen, NAR increased on the challenged side in most cases but was inconsistent on the contralateral side.

Effect of Nasal Blockage on the Quality of Life of the Patients

We examined the relationship between the extent to which the quality of life was hampered and nasal or ocular symptoms in 220 patients with house dust allergy and 131 patients of Japanese cedar pollen allergy. The extent to which the quality of life was hampered correlated well with sneezing (0.303 for house dust allergy, 0.456 for pollinosis in Spearman's correlation coefficient), discharge (0.271, 0.529, for house dust and pollinosis, again), blockage (0.489, 0.669) and ocular symptoms (not examined, 0.479). The coefficient was largest in nasal blockage suggesting that blockage is the most important factor responsible for hampering the quality of life in both perennial rhinitis and pollen allergy.

The Reason Why Nasal Blockage Strongly Hampers the Quality of Life in Nasal Allergy

In our questionnaire assessment, 31 patients with house dust allergy having nasal blockage as the most troublesome nasal symptom, had mouth-breathing (21 patients), sore throat (15), disturbed sleep (10), nervous irritation (6), snoring (7) and headache (5), all of which impaired the quality of life. Another factor which contributes to the impairment of quality of life may be the persistence of nasal blockage over a longer period in allergy, when compared with other nasal symptoms. Patients with perennial allergic rhinitis had nasal blockage intermittently as well as during the period of an attack of allergy. We found that a moderate to severe degree of nasal blockage persisted in 25.4% of patients even after the other symptoms, i.e., sneezing and discharge, almost disappeared. The severity of nasal blockage correlated well during the period of attack and in the intermittent period too ($r=0.747$).

To confirm the above results, we measured the NAR every two hours from 8:00 A.M. to 8:00 P.M. for 12 hours in 17 patients with house dust allergy and 24 normal controls without nasal allergen challenge. In the allergy group the NAR increased significantly at 2:00 P.M. and 6:00 P.M., while in the control group NAR was almost stable. Furthermore, we examined the changes in NAR in 14 patients with Japanese cedar pollen allergy after nasal challenge, out of season. Immediately after challenge the NAR increased and persisted for 12 hours with a small peak at the 9th hour after challenge which seems to be the late phase allergic reaction. On the other hand, sneezing induced by allergen challenge subsided within a few minutes, and nasal secretion reached a peak within 5 min and returned to baseline within 20 min after provocation. These experimental results clearly show that nasal blockage lasts for a longer period after allergen challenge than sneezing and discharge.

The Reason Why Nasal Blockage Persists for a Longer Period

There is general agreement that nasal blockage, objectively nasal obstruction, is caused as a result of local vasodilatation, i.e., congestion, by direct effect of chemical mediators on the capacity vessels. We measured the blood flow of the nasal mucosa of the inferior turbinate by the hydrogen clearance method (4) in patients with varied nasal diseases and normal controls. Blood flow increased in rhinosinusitis and allergic rhinitis (1.19 ± 0.40 ml/min/g) when compared with normal (0.93 ± 0.08 ml/min/g) and vasomotor rhinitis.

We also measured the blood flow before and after nasal challenge with an allergen containing paper disc on the inferior turbinate, and found that the flow decreased in the mucosa close to the area of contact of the allergen disc, whereas it decreased in the area 10 mm away from the disc (from 1.12 ± 0.27 to 1.30 ± 0.24 ml/min/g) suggesting the co-existence of contraction of the resistance vessels with dilatation of the capacity vessels. The increased blood flow in 32 patients with allergic rhinitis reduced (from 1.19 ± 0.04 to 0.91 ± 0.29 ml/min/g) within 5 minutes on administration of a nasal spray containing a vasoconstrictor, tetrahydrozoline nitrate, in a concentration of 1 mg/ml. The above results show that congestion of the inferior turbinate increases after allergen challenge and responds to treatment with a vasoconstrictor.

We also measured NAR before and 5 min. after administration of a vasoconstrictor spray, epirenamine (1:5,000 solution), in 45 patients with allergic rhinitis, and found that in 22 out of 45 patients examined NAR was greater than the normal value (2.0 cm/H_2O/L/sec (P: 100Pa) or less). In 11 patients with NAR less than 4 but more than 2.1 the NAR became normal after the spray; but also in 11 patient with NAR more than 4.1 the NAR was reduced but did not come down to normal values, suggesting that nasal blockage is not always reversible.

The above results suggested that we should consider some factors as well as congestion as the reason why nasal blockage persists for a longer period. We (5) examined histopathological sections from 106 patients with perennial allergic rhinitis and noted definitive edema in 60.3%, and marked proliferation of connective tissue fibers in 37.3%. The former may be caused by the stimulation of chemical mediators of allergy to the subepithelial small vessels, and the latter may be produced after repeated allergic attacks. The edema in acute allergic attack may not return to the baseline for a short time.

Conclusion

Nasal blockage is the most troublesome nasal symptom in allergy, and differs from sneezing and discharge in its mechanism of onset (direct and indirect stimulation to the vessels in blockage, versus indirect reflex-mediated phenomenon in sneezing and discharge). Nasal blockage is the most important cause in the impairment of the quality of life in patients with nasal allergy, because of the subsequent symptoms and its tendency to persist over a longer period. Nasal blockage persists for a long period due to irreversible organic changes in the mucosal tissues together with reversible congestion of the mucosal vessels.

References

1. Goldman, J.L. 1987. Rhinology. New York: John Wiley & Sons.
2. Settipane, G.A. 1991. Rhinitis. Providence: Oceanside Pub.
3. Okuda, M., and Mygind, N. 1980. Pathophysiological basis for topical steroid treatment in the nose. Asthma and rhinitis. N. Mygind and T.J.H. Clark (eds.). London: Bailliere Tindal.
4. Tanimoto, H., Okuda, M., Yagi, T., and Ohtsuka, H. 1983. Measurement of the blood flow of the nasal mucosa by the hydrogen clearance method. Rhinology 21:59.
5. Okuda, M. 1991. Nasal allergy. Tokyo: Kanehara Pub.

Mediators and Nasal Blockage in Allergic Rhinitis

P. H. Howarth, S. Walsh, A. Napper, K. Harrison, C. Robinson, K. Rajakulasingam*

Nasal blockage is a troublesome and common manifestation of rhinitis. While with chronic disease, mucosal hypertrophy will give rise to persistent limitation of nasal airflow on account of collagen deposition, it is the intention of this review to concentrate not on these mechanisms but on those relevant to reversible changes in nasal airflow. The reversible changes in nasal airflow that occur in rhinitis are related to nasal obstruction arising due to a combination of three potential mechanisms: engorgement of the venous sinusoids within the turbinates and septum, plasma protein leakage from fenestrated mucosal capillaries leading to mucosal oedema, and physical obliteration of the nasal lumen by secretions. The favorable response to topical vasoconstrictors suggests that the prominent mechanisms are vascular. The basis for these vascular changes is an alteration in the neurohumeral regulatory balance.

To allow for rapid changes in nasal airflow and to permit conditioning of inspired air, the nasal vasculature represents a complex network of subepithelial fenestrated capillaries and a deeper plexus of cavernous venous sinusoids. The superficial vessels are regulated by arteriolar tone, such that increased flow produces vasodilation and extravascation of fluid through the fenestrated endothelial wall, which are co-responses for warming and humidifying cool dry air. The residual volume of blood within the venous sinusoids reflects a balance between the tone of arteriovenous anastomoses and venous drainage. Engorgement of venous sinusoids within the turbinates and septum will obstruct the nasal cavity increasing nasal airways resistance and limiting airflow. These sinusoids are under sympathetic regulation, with a constant input limiting sinusoidal engorgement such that a reduction in sympathetic activity, either endogenously or as a consequence of therapeutic intervention, results in engorgement and nasal blockage. Conversely alpha-adrenoceptor agonists reduce nasal resistance by both constricting the venous plexi and diminishing superficial nasal blood flow. Para-sympathetic stimulation induces superficial vasodilation and a degree of nasal obstruction. This response may, in part, be related to the co-release of vasoactive intestinal peptide (VIP) as Ipratropium bromide, a potent antimuscarinic agent, while modulating cholinergic glandular secretion has no influence on the associated nasal blockage. In addition to the autonomic control, the local antidromic release of neuropeptides following sensory neural stimulation may contribute to changes in nasal vascular tone, as in rodents substance P (SP) and calcitonin gene related peptide (CGRP) exhibit both vasodilator and vasopermeable actions. While substance P receptors and these neuropeptides have been localized to nasal tissue, their exact contribution to vascular homeostasis in health and disease within the nasal airways still requires further evaluation.

In addition to these neural regulatory mechanisms, humoral factors will have local effects on nasal blood flow, either through a direct vascular action or through modification of neural tone. It is the local release of mediators from activated inflammatory cells that is responsible for the reversible nasal blockage associated with allergic rhinitis (1). From an understanding of the cellular and mediator changes in association with disease expression and from a knowledge of the nasal actions of those individual mediators along with an assessment of how either specific receptor antagonism or synthesis inhibition modifies the development or expression of nasal blockage in naturally occurring rhinitis, it is possible to build up a profile of mediators relevant to nasal blockage and their respective contributions to allergic rhinitis.

* Medicine I, Level D, Centre Block, Southampton General Hospital, Tremona Road, Southampton, UK.

Cellular and Mediator Changes in Allergic Rhinitis

Both the cytological examination of nasal smears and immunohistochemical and transmission electronmicroscopic evaluations of nasal biopsies have been undertaken in naturally occurring seasonal and perennial allergic rhinitis and also in laboratory provoked allergic exacerbations of rhinitis. In the normal nose, nasal mucosal cytology identifies the presence of epithelial cells (ciliated and non-ciliated columnar cells), goblet cells, lymphocytes and basal cells. There are few neutrophils and rarely any eosinophils or metachromatic cells. Nasal biopsy findings are similar; other than beneath the epithelial basement membrane, mast cells are present, largely in a non-degranulated state. In allergic rhinitis there is an increase in nasal mucosal eosinophils in both smears and biopsy, although this is not an invariable finding, with 69% of a population of school children with allergic rhinitis (n=60) having nasal eosinophilia compared to only 7% of children (n=70) who had no seasonal nasal symptoms (2). In adults similar findings exist with a significant correlation being reported between the seasonal increase in eosinophils, pollen count and symptom expression (3).

In addition to these changes in eosinophils, studies in seasonal rhinitis have identified elevations in metachromatic cells in nasal smears, histamine-containing cells in nasal lavage and mast cells in the nasal mucosa (3–6). These changes appear predominantly epithelial with only one study finding submucosal increments in seasonal mast cell numbers (7). With allergen challenge, the changes in metachromatic cells recovered from the nasal airway lumen in the late response have characteristics of basophils rather than mast cells (8). This cellular identification is based on electronmicroscopic appearances, in that basophils are smaller than mast cells, have a segmented nucleus, contain fewer and larger granules, possess fewer cytoplasmic filaments and are characterised by the presence of glycogen particles and aggregates within the cytoplasm. In addition, the basophil differs from the mast cell in not generating prostaglandin D_2 on immunological degranulation while releasing histamine and producing comparable quantities of leukotriene C_4. Consistent with these late changes in lumenal "basophil-like"cells, nasal lavage during the late response recovers increased quantities of histamine but not prostaglandin D_2. While giving insight into the cellular responses to high dose allergen exposure, there is, however, uncertainty as to the relevance of these late findings to clinical disease, in which symptoms often are a reflection of repeated lower concentration allergen exposure within the environment. Consistent with this, electronmicroscopic evaluation of nasal biopsies usually identifies mast cells and mast cell degranulation (4,6) with only the occasional cell having basophil-like appearances. Despite these reservations about the relationship between the late response to allergen challenge within the nose and clinical disease, nasal allergen challenge has, however, been used in conjunction with nasal lavage to investigate mediator changes in association with symptom development following allergen nasal insufflation in rhinitis.

Following nasal allergen challenge in allergic rhinitis, sequential nasal lavage identifies, during the immediate response, the local release of histamine, tryptase, prostaglandin (PG)D_2, leukotriene (LT) B_4 and LTC_4 in association with the development of nasal pruritus, sneezing, rhinorrhoea and nasal blockage (9–10). While histamine, LTC_4 and LTB_4 are not specific for mast cells, the parallel identification of PGD_2 and tryptase release is strongly suggestive of a mast cell origin for these mediators of immediate hypersensitivity (12). In addition increased recovery of the kinins, bradykinin and kallidin (lysyl-bradykinin), has also been described (13). Both bradykinin and kallidin are potent vasoactive peptides derived respectively by their cleavage from high and low molecular weight kininogens by kallikrein and like enzymes. As tryptase possesses kallikrein-like activity, it is likely that this will, in part, contribute to the kinin generation identified in allergic rhinitis during the immediate nasal response. Nasal lavage in the late response identifies elevated levels of histamine and kinins but not PGD_2. Under clinical situations the identification of distinct disease related mediator changes has been less successful, due to variability in baseline levels, especially with histamine. Nasal lavage identifies high levels of histamine in the absence of disease expression, although nasal challenge produces immediate symptoms which are antagonised by the H_1-receptor blockade, suggesting both that tachyphylaxis may occur with continued histaminergic stimulation and that rate of change of histamine exposure may also be relevant to the initiation of symptoms. Despite these limitations, increased levels of LTC_4 and kinins have both been described in naturally occurring rhinitis (14–15).

Mediator Relevance to Nasal Blockage

To investigate the relevance of these mediators identified in relationship with disease expression, to the generation of nasal blockage, studies have been undertaken with nasal insufflation in which the nasal response to stimulation has been objectively monitored by measurement of nasal airflow and the pressures required to achieve the flow. From these recordings measurements can be derived of nasal airways resistance. In addition nasal lavage measurements of albumin or the albumin/protein ratio in association with challenge can be used as an index of plasma protein and fluid leak from the fenestrated superficial capillaries.

Histamine

Nasal insufflation with histamine induces a transient nasal blockage that is dose dependent and an increase in nasal vascular permeability. While the effects of histamine on nasal vascular permeability are readily inhibited by H_1-receptor antagonism, those on nasal obstruction are only partially reduced. Furthermore the combination of an H_1 and H_2 receptor antagonism provides little additional protection raising the possibility that H_3-receptor stimulation by histamine may contribute to nasal blockage. In rodents, H_3-receptors have been localized to pre-synaptic, perivascular nerve terminals, where they regulate sympathetic tone, the stimulation thus reducing post ganglionic neurotransmission (16). Thus, H_3-receptor stimulation would promote nasal blockage. Consistent with these findings H_1-receptor blockade has no influence on naturally occurring nasal blockage in seasonal allergic rhinitis (17). As the effect of histamine on nasal blockage with challenge is small and requires supraphysiological doses, it is, however, more likely that alternative mediators have greater relevance to clinical disease expression.

Kinins

Kinin nasal challenge produces a dose-dependent increase in nasal airways resistance and an increase in nasal vascular permeability (6,18,19). These effects are mediated by bradykinin β2-receptor stimulation (20). A comparative investigation of the nasal effects of bradykinin and histamine has identified that bradykinin is more potent on a molar basis, with the relative doses required to produce a 100% increase in NAR being 57 mM and 141 mM respectively. There are, however, as yet no clinical trials of either bradykinin β2 receptor antagonists or kinin synthesis inhibitors to permit a positioning of the relative importance of kinins in the genesis of nasal blockage.

Leukotrienes

Nasal insufflation with LTC_4 and LTD_4 has been shown to induce nasal blockage and to increase nasal mucosal blood flow (21–22). In addition these leukotrienes are known to promote microvascular permeability. The effects of LTC_4 on nasal blockage are more pronounced both in magnitude and duration of effect than histamine, when comparable doses are used in nasal challenge (21). A recent report, investigating the effect of a new 5-lipoxygenase inhibitor, A-64077, on allergen-provoked nasal blockage, identified significant protection in comparison to placebo (23). The further evaluation of this compound or receptor specific antagonists in clinical disease will provide further evidence to assess the relevance of these eicosanoids to nasal allergy and nasal blockage.

Prostaglandins

We have investigated the nasal effects of PGD_2 and have found the nose to be extremely sensitive to nasal PGD_2 insufflation, with a 100% increase in nasal airways resistance being induced by 7 μM PGD_2 (24). Thus on a molar basis PGD_2 is approximately 200× more potent than histamine in inducing nasal blockage. Consistent with this, oral acetyl-salicylic acid pretreatment reduces the nasal obstructive response to nasal allergen challenge by approximately 60% (25). The poor response to cyclooxygenase inhibition in seasonal allergic rhinitis has questioned the relative contribution of prostanoids to allergic rhinitis. This may be related to the production of leukotrienes limiting the clinical efficacy or to the production of prostanoids by non-cyclooxygenase pathways involving free radical formation (26). It will only be with the development of specific prostaglandin D_2 receptor antagonists that the contribution of this prostanoid to nasal blockage will be clarified.

Neuropeptides

Substance P containing nerves are present in the nasal mucosa in a perivascular, periglandular and an epithelial distribution and substance P nasal insufflation has been shown to produce a dose-dependent nasal blockage (27). Furthermore, it has recently been reported that the nasal response to substance P is exaggerated during natural exposure to allergen in seasonal rhinitics (28). In both instances, however, the dose producing nasal blockage also produced facial flushing and in some instances hypotension, suggesting that this induced effect on nasal airflow was only occurring at supraphysiological levels of stimulation. Thus again until specific pharmacological intervention can be investigated it is difficult to place the potential role of neuropeptides in nasal blockage in perspective with chemical mediators.

Conclusion

The difficulty in treating nasal blockage, other than by physiological antagonism with vasoconstrictors or by eradication of the inflammatory cell populations within the nasal mucosa and epithelium by corticosteroids, is likely to relate to the identification that a number of chemical mediators and peptides may all contribute to the genesis of this symptom. Nasal challenge studies suggest the importance of PGD_2 and leukotrienes in particular but until receptor specific antagonists are available for clinical investigation the further dissection of their relative contributions cannot adequately be achieved. In addition to considerations of potency, considerations to the relevant quantities of mediators present within the nasal mucosa are obviously of relevance. While PGD_2 is solely released by activated mast cells, LTC_4 will be released by activated mast cells, basophils and eosinophils. In addition to an understanding of the end organ effects of released mediators, an advanced understanding of the factors which regulate transendothelial migration, endothelial cell adhesion, cell chemotaxis and cell activation is likely to provide additional indirect mechanisms whereby the development of nasal obstruction may be prevented. While these approaches are attractive propositions, a detailed analysis of their relevance is beyond the scope of this review and interference with the end organ effects of released mediators provides a more immediate means of intervention.

References

1. Howarth, P.H. 1989. Allergic rhinitis: A rational approach to therapy. Respiratory Medicine 83:179.
2. Miller, R.E., Paradise, J,K., Friday, G.A., Fireman, P., and Voith, D. 1982. The nasal smear for eosinophils. Its value in children with seasonal allergic rhinitis. Am. J. Dis. Child. 136:1009.
3. Pipkorn, U., Karlsson, G., and Ennerback, L. 1988. The cellular response of the human allergic mucosal to natural allergen exposure. J. Allergy Clin. Immuno. 82:1046.
4. Enerback, L., Pipkorn, U., and Olaffsson, A. 1986. Intraepithelial migration of mucosal mastcells in hay fever: Ultrastructural observations. Int. Arch. Allergy Appl. Immunology 81:289.
5. Okuda, M., Ohtsuka, H., and Kawabori, S. 1985. Studies on nasal surface basophilic cells. Ann. Allergy 54:69.
6. Howarth, P.H., Wilson, S., Lau, L., and Rajakulasingam, K. 1991. The nasal mast cell and rhinitis. Clin. and Exp. Allergy 21 (Suppl 2):3.
7. Viegas, M., Gomez, E., Brooks, J., and Davies, R.J. 1987. The effect of the pollen season on nasal mast cell numbers. Br. Med. J. 294:414.
8. Bascom, R., Wachs, M., Naclerio, R. M., Pipkorn, U., Galli, S,J., and Lichtenstein, L.M. 1988. Basophil influx occurs after nasal challenge: Effects of topical corticosteroid pretreatment. J. Allergy Clin. Immunol. 81:580.
9. Naclerio, R. M., Meier, H. L., Kagey-Sabotka,

A., Adkinson, N.F., Meyers, D.A., Norman, P.S., and Lichtenstein, L.M. 1983. Mediator release after nasal airway challenge with allergen. Am. Rev. Resp. Dis. 128:597.
10. Creticos, P.S., Adkinson, N.F., Kagey-Sabotka, A., et al. 1985. Nasal challenge with ragweed pollen in hay fever patients. J. Clin. Invest. 76:2247.
11. Castells, M., and Schwartz, L.B. 1988. Tryptase levels in nasal-lavage fluid as an indicator of the immediate allergic response. J. Allergy Clin. Immunol.83:348.
12. Howarth, P.H., and Holgate, S.T. 1990. Basic aspects of allergic reactions. In: Childhood rhinitis and sinusitis pathophysiology and treatment. C.K. Naspitz, and D.G. Tinkelman, eds. New York: Marcel Dekker, p. 1.
13. Proud, D., Togias, A., Naclerio, R.M., Crush, S.A., Norman, P.S., and Lichtenstein, L.M. 1983. Kinins are generated in vivo following nasal airway challenge of allergic individuals with allergen. J. Clin. Invest. 72:1678.
14. Volovitz, B., Osur, S.L., Berstein, J.M., and Ogra, P.L. 1988. Leukotriene C4 release in the upper respiratory mucosa during natural exposure to ragweed in ragweed-sensitive children. J. Allergy Clin. Immunol. 82:414.
15. Svensson, C., Anderson, M., Persson, C.G.A., Venge, P., Alker, U., and Pipkorn, U. 1990. Albumin, bradykinin and eosinophilic cationic protein on the nasal mucosal surface in patients with hay fever during natural allergen exposure. J. Allergy Clin. Immunol. 85:823.
16. Ishikawa, S., and Sperelakis, N. 1987. A novel class (H3) of histamine receptors on perivascular nerve terminals. Nature 327:158.
17. Howarth, P.H., and Holgate, S.T. 1984. Comparative trials of two non-sedative H1-antihistamines, terfenadine and astemizole for hay fever. Thorax 39:668.
18. Proud, D., Reynolds, C.J., Lacorpa, S., Sabotka, A.K., Lichtenstein, L.M., and Naclerio, R.M. 1988. Nasal provocation with bradykinin induces symptoms of rhinitis and a sore throat. Am. Rev. Resp. Dis. 137:613.
19. Rajakulasingam, K., Polosa, R., Lau, L.C.K., Church, M., K., Holgate, S.T., and Howarth, P.H. Nasal effects of bradykinin and capsaicin: Influence on microvascular leakage and role of sensory neurones. J. Appl. Physiol., in press.
20. Rajakulasingam, K., Polosa, R., Holgate, S.T., and Howarth, P.H. 1991. Comparative nasal effects of bradykinin, kallidin and [des-arg]-bradykinin in atopic rhinitic and normal volunteers. J. Physiol. 437:557.
21. Miadonna, A., Tedeschi, A., Leggiere, E., Lorini, M., Colco, G., Sala, A., Qualizza, R., Froldi, M., and Zannussi, C. 1987. Behaviour and clinical relevance of histamine and leukotrienes C4 and B4 in grass pollen-induced rhinitis. Am. Rev. Resp. Dis. 136:357.
22. Olsson,. P., and Bende, M. 1984. Leukotriene D_4 increases mucosal blood flow in humans. Prostaglandins 27:599.
23. Knapp, H.R. 1990. Reduced allergen-induced nasal congestion and leukotriene synthesis with an orally active 5-lipoxygenase inhibitor. New Engl. J. Med. 323:1745.
24. Howarth, P.H., Walsh, S., and Robinson, C. 1991. The comparative nasal effects of prostaglandin D_2 in normal and rhinitic subjects. In: Advances in prostaglandin, thromboxane and leukotriene research. B. Sammuelsson, S.E. Dahlen, J. Fritsch, and P. Hedquist, eds. New York: Raven Press, 20:157.
25. Brooks, C.D., and Karl, K.J. 1988. Hay fever treatment with combined antihistamine and cyclooxygenase-inhibiting drugs. J. Allergy Clin. Immuno. 81:1110.
26. Morrow, J.D., Hill, K.E., Burk, R.F., Namour, T.M, Badr, K., and Roberts, L.J. 1990. Prostanoids can be generated in vivo by a non-cyclooxygenase pathway involving free radical formulation. In: Proc. of 7th International Conference on Prostaglandins and Related Compounds. Fondazione-Giovanni Lorenzini, Italy, p. 12.
27. Devillier, P., Dessanges, J.F., Rakotosihanaka-Ghaem, A., Boushey, H.A., Lockhart, A., Marsac, J. 1988. Nasal response to substance P and methacholine in subjects with and without allergic rhinitis. Eur. Resp. J. 1:356.
28. Frossand, N., Fajac, I, Burry, A., Braunstein, G., Lacronique, J., LeGall, G., Marsae, J., and Lockhart A. 1991. Nasal responses to substance P are potentiated during the pollen season in patients with allergic rhinitis. In: Proc. of XIV International Conference of Allergology and Clinical Immunology. Toronto: Hogrefe and Huber, p. 116.

The Role of Cytokines in the Pathogenesis of Allergic Rhinitis

Tommy C. Sim, Rafeul Alam, J. Andrew Grant*

Allergic rhinitis is characterized by an acute reaction with mediator release from mast cells followed by recruitment of leukocytes during the late-phase response. Cytokines have a fundamental role in the pathogenesis of this syndrome by regulation of IgE synthesis, expression of endothelial adhesion molecules, and by recruitment and activation of inflammatory leukocytes. Histamine releasing factors represent one group of cytokines that modulate the function of basophils and mast cells; the most important cytokine stimulating secretion of basophils is monocyte chemotactic and activating factor. Therapy directed towards blockade of vasoactive mediators, as well as against this intense inflammatory response induced by cytokines, is essential for management of allergic rhinitis.

The purpose of this review is to discuss the potential role of a series of soluble oligopeptides, known as cytokines, in the recruitment and activation of inflammatory cells in allergic reactions of the upper airways. Previous investigations of the pathobiologic features of allergic rhinitis have focussed on the measurement of biochemical mediators, peptides, and enzymes and the enumeration of recruited leukocytes (1). However, the past decade has seen a rapid growth in the list of cytokine polypeptides regulating the action of various immunocompetent cells. The study of these cell-derived polypeptides has led to a tremendous interest in their biologic activity and clinical use. There is increasing evidence that interactions between cytokines, vascular endothelium, and leukocytes are of major importance in the course of late allergic reactions and the chronic inflammation seen in naturally occurring allergic rhinitis and other atopic disorders (2).

The Late-Phase Response

In his initial description of allergic rhinitis, Blackley (3) described both an immediate as well as a persistent clinical response following grass pollen exposure. The late-phase reaction (LPR) to experimental nasal antigen challenge is characterized by the influx (or perhaps the differentiation from precursor cells) of basophils, eosinophils, neutrophils, and mononuclear cells (4). The LPR has been observed in the nose, lungs, and skin with antigen challenge. The LPR most closely resembles the chronic allergic disease state in many clinical settings (5). The recrudescence of symptoms in the LPR is associated with influx of inflammatory cells and release of mediators, and cytokines may be significantly involved.

The Role of Cytokines

The regulatory function of many immunocompetent cells is mediated by the secretion of cytokines. The availability of recombinant cytokines has been foremost in establishing their individual activities; in addition, monoclonal antibodies directed against individual cytokines have facilitated purification and improved the specificity of bioassays for individual cytokines. Now that specific characteristics have been assigned to each cytokine, it has become clear that some have crucial roles in the evolution of allergic inflammatory processes. The isotype switching of B cells is carefully regulated by cytokines. Interleukin (IL)-4, synthesized by T cells, is most important for this differentiation, and potent antibodies to IL-4

* Division of Allergy and Immunology, Department of Internal Medicine, The University of Texas Medical Branch at Galveston, Galveston, Texas, USA.
Acknowledgements: Supported in part by grants AI27864 and AI22940 from the US National Institutes of Health, the Sealy and Smith Foundation, and the Norwich Eaton Research Award of the American College of Allergy and Immunology.

can block expression of IgE after primary sensitization (6). Interferon (IFN)-gamma, another T cell product, antagonizes the effects of IL-4 (7). However, in a controlled trial of IFN-gamma in seasonal allergic rhinitis, neither was the synthesis oflgE suppressed nor were clinical symptoms ameliorated (8).

A number of observations support the theory that the coordinated expression of cytokines is paramount to the successful initiation and maintenance of inflammation (2). To support this concept, many cytokines have been found to have significant proallergic actions. These include IL-3, IL-4, IL-5 and granulocyte-macrophage colony-stimulating factor (GM-CSF), cytokines released by Th2 cells. The expression of messenger RNA for these cytokines has been observed in the LPR to cutaneous allergen challenge (9) and in mucosal biopsies from asthmatic subjects (10). IL-1, IL-3, and GM-CSF can activate basophils of highly allergic subjects and cause histamine release (11). On the other hand, we have previously described a distinct group of cytokines called histamine releasing factors (HRF) (12,13). HRF represent a heterogeneous group of cytokines produced by a variety of cells including lymphocytes, monocytes, macrophages, platelets, and neutrophils. Recently we have shown that the predominant species of HRF synthesized by blood mononuclear cells is monocyte chemotactic and activating factor (14). HRF have been recovered from cutaneous LPR (15), bronchoalveolar lavage fluid (16), and nasal washings (17). Although the clinical significance of HRF is unknown, it has been suggested that HRF might have a seminal role in the pathogenesis of allergic and other inflammatory disorders such as asthma (18), allergic rhinitis (17), atopic dermatitis (19), chronic idiopathic urticaria (20), and idiopathic pulmonary fibrosis (21).

Other regulatory functions of cytokines include activation of inflammatory cells, stimulation of further cellular production of cytokines, and synthesis and release of other proinflammatory mediators such as arachidonic acid metabolites and platelet activating factor (22). Recent exciting findings have implicated the mast cell as a source of cytokines that may be important in allergic reactions. These cytokines include both endothelial-activating cytokines such as IL-1 and TNF, and cytokines that can prime and aid in the recruitment of leukocytes such as IL-3, IL-5, and GM-CSF (23). Secretion of these cytokines is stimulated by antigen after a lag period of approximately 2 to 4 hours. Thus, mast cells may participate in immediate hypersensitivity reactions by releasing vasoactive mediators, as well as in the LPR by recruitment of cells to sites of inflammation via production of proallergic cytokines.

Cytokines and Endothelial Cell Adhesion Molecules

Endothelial cells express a series of adhesion molecules such as intercellular adhesion molecule-1 (ICAM-1), endothelial-leukocyte adhesion molecule-1 (ELAM-1), and vascular cell adhesion molecule-1 (VCAM-1). These molecules are instrumental in directing the traffic of the inflammatory cell to the target tissue (24). The role of endothelial adherence proteins in inflammation *in vivo* has recently been studied. They have been observed in various forms of dermatitis, at sites of delayed type hypersensitivity reactions in human skin, and in biopsy tissues taken from allergic subjects after intradermal antigen challenge (25,26). In an animal model of asthma, infusion of anti-ICAM antibody reduced antigen-induced bronchoalveolar eosinophilia and airways hyperreactivity (27). Thus, production of endothelial-activating cytokines, together with expression of adhesion molecules, may be an important mechanism by which leukocytes are recruited to sites of allergic inflammation. Several studies have provided evidence that cytokines regulate the recruitment of leukocytes, a hallmark of chronic allergic reactions. Cytokines can act as communication signals between endothelial cells and leukocytes. IL-1, tumor necrosis factor (TNF), IL-4, IL-8, GM-CSF, and IFN-gamma induce de novo synthesis and expression of specific adhesion molecules which promote the interaction of cells in the circulation with vascular endothelium (28,29). Bochner et al. (30) showed that IL-1 stimulates the expression of endothelial adhesion molecules essential for binding of basophils, eosinophils and neutrophils, and suggested that this is a critical event in leukocyte recruitment in allergic inflammation.

Nasal Cytokines

Review of the published data, many of which were obtained from the investigations made by Denburg and Dolovich, demonstrates that levels of cytokines such as IL-6, IL-8 and GM-CSF can be detected from culture supernatants (31,32). They have used human nasal polyp-derived fibroblasts and endothelial cells as well as epithelial cells from human upper airway scrapings. In a series of experiments, the same investigators successfully used conditioned media from these structural cells in inducing differentiation of human hematopoietic progenitor cells to histamine-containing, basophilic cells and eosinophils (33). Using monoclonal antibodies to human hemopoietic cytokines, as well as oligonucleotide probes for messenger RNA derived from transcription of genes encoding these cytokines, they established that nasal epithelial cells and fibroblasts derived from patients with allergic rhinitis express and secrete GM-CSF, IL-6, and IL-8. The principal active cytokine responsible for precursor cell growth and differentiation was GM-CSF derived from culture supernatants. Furthermore, they also showed that GM-CSF from conditioned media was the factor supportive of eosinophil activation and survival (34). In summary, the results of these *in vitro* studies suggest that cytokines may have a role in the process whereby leukocytes proliferate or are locally recruited, primed, or activated in inflamed tissues during responses initiated by antigen or other stimuli. However, further *in vivo* studies are required to clearly establish whether cytokines are produced *in vivo* in allergic diseases, and if they are responsible for initiation or exacerbation of the inflammatory processes underlying these diseases.

To test the hypothesis stated above, we recently recovered HRF activity from nasal lavage fluids, and observed significant modulation by topical corticosteroids of HRF activity in the nasal lavages of symptomatic ragweed-allergic patients. Briefly, we evaluated the possible role of cytokines in allergic rhinitis, and found that one of the proinflammatory cytokines, HRF, could be measured reproducibly in nasal lavage fluid from large numbers of subjects, both atopic and normal subjects (17). We also evaluated the effects of the state-of-the-art therapy, intranasal steroids, in a group of 30 individuals suffering with seasonal allergic rhinitis (36). We demonstrated that the concentration of HRF dramatically decreased in the steroid-treated patients when compared with the placebo group (Table I). Moreover, there was a statistically significant correlation in the net decrease of HRF activity and clinical improvement. This study is the first description of corticosteroid-induced inhibition of cytokine recovery in nasal lavages from allergic patients.

These studies suggest that corticosteroids may possibly act at the level of cytokine synthesis or release. Short-term treatment with corticosteroids does not affect mediator release from mast cells, nor do these drugs inhibit immediate allergic responses. However, these agents strongly inhibit LPR. We speculate that cytokines, such as HRF, have a significant role in the pathogenesis of LPR and that the blockade of cytokine synthesis is one mechanism of action of corticosteroids in allergic rhinitis. Because measurement of HRF requires a tedious bioassay, we attempted to extend these studies to evaluate highly characterized recombinant cytokines. The first cytokine we have investigated in allergic rhinitis is IL-1 which typically rises during the immediate as well as the LPR to antigen challenges in the skin (35). Initially we were unsuccessful in measuring IL-1 in nasal lavages. In an effort to improve the sensitivity, we developed a novel recovery technique and subsequently found that IL-1 could be easily detected immediately after antigen challenge as well as during the late allergic re-

Table I. Effect of beclomethasone on clinical symptom scores and recovery of HRF activity from nasal lavages of patients with seasonal allergic rhinitis. Fifteen patients were studied in each group.

	SYMPTOM SCORES		HRF ACTIVITY (%)	
	Placebo	Beclomethasone*	Placebo	Beclomethasone*
Before	4.8 ± 1.8	5.0 ± 1.3	33 ± 22	37 ± 25
After	5.5 ± 1.9	1.7 ± 1.6	35 ± 26	24 ± 20

* $p < 0.05$

Table II. Changes in symptom scores and recovery of IL-1 in nasal secretions after allergen challenge in eight subjects with allergic rhinitis.

TIME AFTER CHALLENGE (hr)	SYMPTOM SCORES	IL-1 (pg/ml)
Nasal lavage	0.0 ± 0.0	0.0 ± 0.0
Diluent	0.0 ± 0.0	0.0 ± 0.0
Decongestant	0.2 ± 0.7	0.0 ± 0.0
5 AU allergen dose	5.7 ± 2.5*	11.9 ± 33.6
50 AU allergen dose	6.9 ± 1.6*	6.2 ± 17.7
500 AU allergen dose	6.8 ± 2.4*	51.0 ± 27.2*
Post 1 hr	4.0 ± 1.4*	35.8 ± 12.4*
2 hr	2.4 ± 1.5	11.4 ± 1.3
3 hr	1.8 ± 1.6	35.1 ± 15.0*
4 hr	2.5 ± 2.3	55.2 ± 27.4*
5 hr	3.8 ± 2.8*	78.5 ± 24.3**
6 hr	5.1 ± 2.9*	38.0 ± 9.7*
7 hr	3.4 ± 3.2*	10.6 ± 3.0
8 hr	2.4 ± 3.2	4.6 ± 1.3
9 hr	1.4 ± 1.8	0.0 ± 0.0
10 hr	1.0 ± 1.2	0.0 ± 0.0

* $p < 0.01$ **$p < 0.001$

action (Table II)(37). Again, there has been a correlation between nasal symptoms and recovery of the cytokine. Very recently, we also successfully measured another proallergic cytokine, GM-CSF, in nasal secretions during the LPR (37). Our findings that these cytokines are secreted after nasal antigen challenge in allergic subjects but not after diluent challenge, support the suggestion that these proinflammatory cytokines may contribute to the pathogenesis of nasal allergic response.

Conclusions

It is becoming increasingly apparent that the field of immunology has only begun to appreciate the impact of cytokines on the inflammatory process. Attempts to clarify the exact role of these local mediators during inflammation should be addressed at various levels of investigations. The implication is that by manipulating the activity of the cytokines, in the future one may be able to modulate the inflammatory response. Although the contribution of molecular biologists to the cytokine field has been immeasurable, continued advances should be done to elucidate the nature of agonistic as well as antagonistic cytokines, define the structure of cytokine receptors, develop specific antagonists by site-directed mutagenesis, and understand the regulatory mechanisms of transcriptions of cytokine genes. This information will be necessary to truly understand the role of cytokines in health and disease as well as provide new therapeutic approaches.

References

1. Iliopoulos, O., Proud, D., Adkinson, N.F., et al. 1990. Relationship between the early, late and rechallenge reaction to nasal challenge with antigen: Observations on the role of inflammatory mediators and cells. J. Allergy Clin. Immunol. 86:851.
2. Schleimer, R.P., Benenati, S.V., Friedman, B., and Bochner, B.S. 1991. Do cytokines play a role in leukocyte recruitment and activation in the lung? Am. Rev. Respir. Dis. 143:1169.
3. Blackley, C.H. 1973. Experimental researches on the causes and nature of catarrhous aestivus. London: Balliere, Tindal, Cox.
4. Bascom, R., Pipkorn, U., Lichtenstein, L.M., and Naclerio, R.M. 1988. The influx of inflammatory cells into nasal washings during the late response to antigen challenge: Effect of systemic steroid pretreatment. Am. Rev. Respir. Dis. 138:406.
5. Gleich, G.J. 1982. The late phase of the immunoglobulin E-mediated reactions: A link between anaphylaxis and common allergic diseases? J. Allergy Clin. Immunol. 70:160.

6. Ohara, J. 1989. Interleukin-4: Molecular structure and biochemical characteristics, biological function, and receptor expression. In: Cytokines and cell growth. J.M. Cruse, and R.E. Lewis, eds. Basel, Switzerland: Karger.
7. Snapper, C.M., and Paul, W.E. 1987. Interferon-gamma and B cell stimulatory factor-1 reciprocally regulate Ig isotype production. Science 236:944.
8. Li, J.T., Yunginger, J.W., Reed, C.E., et al. 1990. Lack of suppression of IgE production by recombinant interferon-gamma: A controlled trial in patients with allergic rhinitis. J. Allergy Clin. Immunol. 85:934.
9. Kay, A.B., Ying, S., Varney, V., et al. 1991. Messenger RNA expression of the cytokine gene cluster, interleukin 3(IL-3), IL-4, IL-5 and granulocyte/macrophage colony-stimulating factor, in allergen-induced late phase cutaneous reactions in atopic subjects. J. Exp. Med. 173:775.
10. Hamid, Q., Azzawi, M., Ying, S., et al. 1991. Expression of mRNA for interleukin-5 in mucosal bronchial biopsies from asthma. J. Clin. Invest. 87:1541.
11. Alam, R., Welter, J.B., Forsythe, P.A., et al. 1989. Comparative effect of recombinant IL-1, -2, -3, -4, and -6, IFN-gamma, granulocyte-macrophage colony stimulating factor, tumor necrosis factor-alpha, and histamine releasing factors on the secretion of histamine release from basophils. J. Immunol. 142:3431.
12. Thueson, D.O., Speck, L.S., Lett-Brown, M.A., and Grant, J.A. 1979. Histamine releasing activity (HRA). I. Production by mitogen- or antigen-stimulated human mononuclear cells. J. Immunol. 123:626.
13. Grant, J.A., Alam, R., and Lett-Brown, M.A. 1991. Histamine-releasing factors and inhibitors: Historical perspectives and possible implications in human illness. J. Allergy Clin. Immunol. 88:683.
14. Alam, R., Lett-Brown, M.A., Forsythe, P.A., Anderson-Walters, D.J., Kenamore, C., Kormos, C., and Grant, J.A. Monocyte chemotactic and activating factor (MCAF) is a potent histamine releasing factor for basophils. J. Clin. Invest. 89:723.
15. Warner, J., Pienkowski, M., Plaut, M., Norman, P.S., and Lichtenstein, L.M. 1986. Identification of histamine releasing factor(s) in the late phase of cutaneous IgE-mediated reactions. J. Immunol. 136:2583.
16. Alam, R., Welter, J., Forsythe, P.A., Lett-Brown, M.A., Rankin, J., Boyars, M., and Grant, J.A. 1990. Detection of histamine release inhibitory factor- and histamine releasing factor-like activities in bronchoalveolar lavage fluids. Am. Rev. Respir. Dis. 141:666.
17. Sim, T.C., Forsythe, P.A., Alam, R., Welter, J.B., Lett-Brown, M.A., and Grant, J.A. 1990. Evaluation of histamine releasing factor in nasal washings from individual subjects [Abstract] J. Allergy Clin. Immunol. 85:156.
18. Alam, R., Kuna, P., Rozniecki, J., and Kuzminska, B. 1987. The magnitude of spontaneous production of histamine releasing factor by lymphocytes *in vitro* highly correlates with state of bronchial hyperreactivity in patients with asthma. J. Allergy Clin. Immunol. 79:103.
19. Sampson, H.A., Broadbent, K.R., and Bernhisel-Broadbent, J. 1989. Spontaneous basophil histamine release and histamine releasing factor in patients with atopic dermatitis and food hypersensitivity. N. Engl. J. Med. 321:228.
20. Claveau, J., Lavoie, A., Brunet, C., Bedard, P.M., and Hebert, J. 1991. Idiopathic chronic urticaria: Contribution of histamine-releasing factor (HRF) to pathogenesis [Abstract]. J. Allergy Clin. Immunol. 87:223.
21. Broide, D.H., Smith, C.M., and Wasserman, S.I. 1990. Mast cells releasing factor in bronchoalveolar lavage fluid. J. Immunol. 145:1838.
22. Alam R. 1991. Novel concepts in allergy and asthma: Interleukins and other cytokines as mediators. Insights Allergy 6:1.
23. Plaut, M., Pierce, J.H., Watson, C.J., et al. 1989. Mast cell lines produce lymphokines in response to cross-linkage of FcE RI or to calcium ionophores. Nature 339:64.
24. Pober, J.S., and Cotran, R.S. 1990. The role of endothelial cells in inflammation. Transplantation 50:537.
25. Kyan-Aung, U., Haskard, D.O., Poston, R.N., Thornhill, M.H., and Lee, T.H. 1991. Endothelial leukocyte adhesion molecule-1 and intercellular adhesion molecule-1 mediate the adhesion of eosinophils to endothelial cells *in vitro* and are expressed by endothelium in allergic cutaneous inflammation *in vivo*. J. Immunol. 146:521.
26. Leung, D.Y.M., Pober, J.S., and Cotran, R.S. 1991. Expression of endothelial-leukocyte adhesion molecule-1 in elicited late phase allergic reactions. J. Clin. Invest. 87:1805.
27. Wegner, C.D., Gundel, R.H., Reilly, P., Haynes, N., Letts, L.G., and Rothlein, R. 1990. Intercellular adhesion molecule-1 (ICAM-1) in the pathogenesis of asthma. Science 247:456.

28. Pober, J.S., Gimbrone, M.A., Lapierre, L.A., et al. 1986. Overlapping patterns of activation of human endothelial cells by interleukin-1, tumor necrosis factor, and immune interferon. J. Immunol. 137:1893.
29. Schleimer, R.P., and Rutledge, B.K. 1986. Cultured human vascular endothelial cells acquire adhesiveness for neutrophils after stimulation with interleukin-1, endotoxin, and tumor-promoting phorbol diesters. J. Immunol. 136:649.
30. Bochner, B.S., Luscinskas, F.W., Gimbrone, M.A., et al. 1991. Adhesion of human basophils, eosinophils, and neutrophils to interleukin-1-activated human vascular endothelial cells: Contributions of endothelial cell adhesion molecules. J. Exp. Med. 173:1553.
31. Keith, P., Wong, D., Liehl, E., Ceska, M., Denburg, J., and Dolovich, J. 1991. *In vivo* assessment of airway inflammation in nasal polyposis. Presence of IL-8 and albumin in nasal lavage fluid [Abstract]. J. Allergy Clin. Immunol. 87:139.
32. Ohtoshi, T., Zhou, X., Gauldie, J., et al. 1991. Human upper airway epithelial cell and fibroblast IL-8 production and its modulation by steroids [Abstract]. J. Allergy Clin. Immunol. 87:174.
33. Ohtoshi, T., Vancheri, C., Cox, G., et al. 1991. Monocyte-macrophage differentiation induced by human upper airway epithelial cells. Am. J. Respir. Cell Mol. Biol. 4:255.
34. Denburg, J.A. 1991. Basophils, mast cells and eosinophils and their precursors in allergic rhinitis. Clin. Exp. Allergy. 21:253.
35. Bochner, B.S., Charlesworth, E.N., Lichtenstein, L.M., et al. 1990. Interleukin-1 is released at sites of human cutaneous allergic reactions. J. Allergy Clin. Immunol. 86:830.
36. Sim, T.C., Hilsmeier, K.A., Alam, R., and Grant, J.A. 1992. Effect of topical corticosteroids on the recovery of histamine releasing factors in nasal washings of patients with allergic rhinitis. Am. Respir. Dis., in press.
37. Sim, T.C., Hilsmeier, K.A., Alam, R., and Grant, J.A. 1992. Measurement of interleukin-1 and granulocyte-macrophage colony-stimulating factor in nasal secretions after antigen challenge (abstract). J. Allergy Clin. Immunol 89:287.

Section IX

The Role of PAF and the Importance of PAF Antagonists in Respiratory Diseases

Platelet Activating Factor and Airway Inflammation

Peter J. Barnes*

PAF is a potent mediator of airway inflammation and closely mimics many of the pathophysiological features of asthma. It induces airway narrowing which is indirect, and is partly mediated by release of leukotriene D_4. It may be partly due to airway oedema, and is a potent inducer of microvascular leak in the airways. PAF also causes mucus hypersecretion and impairs mucociliary clearance. PAF is a potent activator of airway inflammatory cells, and this effect may underlie its ability to induce increased airway responsiveness in several species, including normal human subjects. PAF is a potent activator of eosinophils, and causes eosinophil accumulation and degranulation. Potent PAF receptor antagonists have now been developed, which may be useful in the management of chronic asthma, although preliminary reports suggest that they have little effect in acute airway challenge. Inhibitors of PAF synthesis may be more valuable in the future.

Platelet activating factor (PAF) has many inflammatory effects on the airways and closely mimics the pathophysiological features of asthma (1,2). It is released by many of the inflammatory cells which have been implicated in asthmatic inflammation, including macrophages, eosinophils, endothelial cells, platelets, neutrophils and possibly mast cells.

PAF Receptors

The effects of PAF are mediated by surface receptors, which may be detected on several cell types by radioligand binding (3). Using the labelled antagonist [^{3}H]WEB 2086, specific binding sites have been characterised in human and guinea pig lung (4) and leukocytes (5,6). The recent cloning of a PAF receptor from guinea pig lung (7) may now make it possible to determine whether distinct subtypes of receptor exist, as suggested by some of the functional studies (8).

PAF Effects on Airways

Airway Calibre

PAF causes bronchoconstriction *in vivo* in several species, including humans, which is usually indirect, since PAF has no constrictor effect on airway smooth muscle *in vitro*. The airway narrowing which occurs acutely in normal human subjects may be markedly reduced by prior treatment with a potent leukotriene D4-antagonist such as ICI 204,219, indicating that PAF must release LTD_4 from cells resident in the airways (9).

Microvascular Leak

PAF is potent at inducing microvascular leakage and plasma exudation in animal airways, and this effect appears to be mediated directly on postcapillary venules (10). The rapid induction of plasma exudation is likely to contribute to the airway narrowing induced by PAF, as demonstrated in guinea pigs *in vivo* after inhalation of PAF (11). While it is not possible to measure plasma exudation directly in human airways, indirect evidence that inhaled PAF causes airway oedema is provided by the demonstration that the airway narrowing after PAF inhalation is only partially inhibited by a β-agonist, which completely blocks the constrictor response to a cholinergic agonist (12).

Airway Secretions

PAF also has potent effects on the airway epithelium; in guinea pig trachea it stimulates ion transport and increases intercellular spaces so that the epithelium becomes more permeable (13). PAF also increases mucus secretion in human airways (14), and therefore may contribute to the formation of mucus plugs in asthma, which are composed of mucus glycoproteins and plasma proteins.

* Department of Thoracic Medicine, National Heart and Lung Institute, London SW3 6LY, UK.

Airway Hyperresponsiveness

The property of PAF which has attracted most interest is its ability to cause increased airway responsiveness in every animal species in which it has been tested, including humans (15,16). The degree of increased responsiveness is small and only demonstrable when airway reactivity can be measured precisely. Airway hyperresponsiveness in asthma has been linked to eosinophilic inflammation in the airways (17), and the increased responsiveness seen after PAF may reflect the ability of PAF to induce eosinophil infiltration and activation. PAF antagonists inhibit the eosinophil infiltration into guinea pig airways induced by PAF and allergen, and also inhibit the increased airway responsiveness after allergen (18).

Effects on Eosinophils

PAF has potent effects on eosinophils. *In vitro* PAF is a potent chemoattractant of human eosinophils (19) and promotes adherence of eosinophils to vascular endothelium (20). PAF inhalation stimulates eosinophil infiltration into guinea pig lungs, and this effect is markedly enhanced by cytokines such as GM-CSF and IL-5 (21). PAF directly activates human and guinea pig eosinophils *in vitro*. PAF-receptors have been demonstrated in high density on eosinophils using [^{3}H]WEB 2086 as a radioligand (22), and PAF causes degranulation and release of cyclooxygenase and superoxide anions from eosinophils (23–25). PAF also induces the formation of hypodense eosinophils (26), presumably by degranulating them. The molecular mechanisms by which PAF leads to degranulation appear to involve entry of Ca^{2+} via receptor-operated channels and stimulation of phosphoinositide hydrolysis to release Ca^{2+} from intracellular stores (27). Eosinophils from asthmatic patients appear to show an exaggerated response to PAF; this may indicate that these eosinophils have been "primed", possibly by exposure to cytokines (28). Activated eosinophils appear to cause shedding of ciliated epithelium *in vitro* presumably via the release of basic proteins and oxygen free radicals (29). This may be relevant to the development of airway hyperresponsiveness since epithelial damage may cause loss of a barrier, exposure of sensory nerves, loss of a relaxant substance and the loss of enzymes such as neutral endopeptidase which degrades bronchoconstrictor peptides.

Therapeutic Implications

Whether PAF plays an important role in human asthma will only be answered when the effects of potent and specific PAF antagonists have been given in clinical trials. Several potent antagonists have now been developed, and some are currently being tested in asthmatic patients. Potent antagonists such as WEB 2086 inhibit ex vivo platelet activation by PAF and the skin response to intradermal PAF after oral administration (30), but preliminary studies with orally administered WEB 2086 show no effect on allergen challenge including the increase in airway responsiveness (31). More potent PAF antagonists may be necessary and a potent antagonist UK 74,505 is capable of completely blocking the airway and neutropaenic response to PAF for up to 24 hours (32). Since PAF may be produced locally in the airways in high concentrations, it may prove difficult to antagonize its effects by oral antagonists, however. PAF may function as a "paracrine" mediator which is only active on cells in the immediate vicinity of the cell producing PAF. PAF then activates neighboring cells to produce PAF and the inflammatory effect spreads locally. It may therefore be necessary to give the antagonists by inhalation, in order to achieve high enough local concentrations. Alternatively it may be preferable to develop drugs which inhibit the synthesis of PAF, and either phospholipase A_2 antagonists or PAF acetyltransferase inhibitors may be needed, particularly if intracellular PAF (which may be inaccessible to the effects of PAF antagonists) has effects on cell function. There is some evidence that subtypes of PAF receptor exist, so that in the future it may prove possible to develop antagonists which are more selective for certain subtypes of PAF-receptor (e.g., on eosinophils).

References

1. Barnes, P.J., Chung, K.F., and Page, C.P. 1988. Platelet-activating factor as a mediator of allergic disease. J. Allergy Clin. Immunol. 81:919.

2. Barnes P.J., and Henson P.M. 1990. Platelet activating factor. In: The lung. R. Crystal, J.B. West, P.J. Barnes, N. Chernick, and E. Weibel, eds. New York: Raven Press, p.49.
3. Dent G., Ukena D., and Barnes P.J. 1989. PAF Receptors. In PAF and human disease. P.J. Barnes, C.P. Page, P.M. Henson, eds. Oxford: Blackwell, p.58.
4. Dent, G., Ukena, D., Sybrecht, G.W., and Barnes, P.J. 1989. [^{3}H]WEB 2086 labels platelet activating factor receptors in guinea pig and human lung. Eur. J. Pharmacol. 169:313.
5. Dent, G., Ukena, D., Chanez, P., Sybrecht, G.W., and Barnes, P.J. 1989. Characterization of PAF receptors on human neutrophils using the specific antagonist, WEB 2086: correlation between receptor binding and function. FEBS Lett. 244:365.
6. Ukena, D., Dent, G., Birke, F.W., Robaut, C., Sybrecht, G.W., and Barnes, P.J. 1988. Radioligand binding of antagonists of platelet-activating factor to intact human platelets. FEBS Lett. 228:285.
7. Honda, Z., Nakamura, M., Miki, I., Minami, M., Liatanase,T., Seyama, Y., Okado, H., Toh, H., Ito, K., Miyamoto, T., and Shimizu, T. 1991. Cloning by functional expression of guinea pig lung platelet activating factor (PAF) receptor. Nature 349:342.
8. Kroegel, C., Yukawa, T., Westwick, J., and Barnes, P.J. 1989. Evidence for two platelet activating receptors on eosinophils: dissociation between PAF induced intracellular calcium mobilization, degranulation and superoxide anion generation. Biochem. Biophys. Res. Commun. 162:511.
9. Kidney, J.C., Ridge, S., Chung, K.F., and Barnes, P.J. 1991. Inhibition of PAF-induced bronchoconstriction by the oral leukotriene antagonist ICI 204,219 in normal subjects. Am. Rev. Respir. Dis. 142:A811.
10. Evans, T.W., Chung, K.F., Rogers, D.F., and Barnes, P.J. 1987. Effect of platelet activating factor on airway vascular permeability: Possible mechanisms. J. Appl. Physiol. 63:479.
11. Tokuyama, K., Lotvall, J.O., Barnes, P.J., and Chung, K.F. 1991. Mechanism of airway narrowing caused by platelet activating factor: role of airway microvascular leakage. Am. Rev. Respir. Dis. 143:1345.
12. Chung, K.F., Dent, G., and Barnes, P.J. 1989. Effects of salbutamol on bronchoconstriction, bronchial hyper-responsiveness and leukocyte responses induced by platelet activating factor in man. Thorax 44:102.
13. Rogers, D.F., Alton, E.F.W., Aursudkij, B., Boschetto, P., Dewar, A., and Barnes, P.J. 1991. Effect of platelet activating factor on formation and composition of airway fluid in the guinea pig trachea. J. Physiol. 431:643.
14. Goswami, S.K., Omashi, M., Stathas, P., and Marom, Z.A.M. 1989. Platelet-activating factor stimulates secretion of respiratory glycoconjugate from human airways in culture. J. Allergy Clin. Immunol. 84:726.
15. Cuss, F.M., Dixon, C.M.S., and Barnes, P.J. 1986. Effects of inhaled platelet activating factor on pulmonary function and bronchial responsiveness in man. Lancet 2:189.
16. Kaye, M.G., and Smith, L.J. 1990. Effects of inhaled leukotriene D4 and platelet activating factor on airway reactivity in normal subjects. Am. Rev. Respir. Dis. 141:993.
17. Gleich, G.J., Flavahan, N.A., Fujisawa, T., and Vanhoutte, P.M. 1988. The eosinophil as a mediator of damage to respiratory epithelium: A model for bronchial hyperreactivity. J. Allergy Clin. Immunol. 81:776.
18. Lellouch-Tubiana, A., Lefort, J., Simon, M-T., Pfister, A., and Vargaftig, B.B. 1988. Eosinophil recruitement into guinea pig lungs after PAF-acether and allergen administration. Modulation by prostacyclin, platelet depletion and selective antagonists. Am. Rev. Respir. Dis. 137:948.
19. Wardlaw, A.J., Moqbel, R., Cromwell, O., and Kay, A.B. 1986. Platelet activating factor. A potent chemotactic and chemokinetic factor from human eosinophils. J. Clin. Invest. 78:1701.
20. Kimani, G., Tonnesen, M.G., and Henson, P.G. 1988. Stimulation of eosinophil adherence to human vascular endothelial cells *in vitro* by platelet activating factor. J. Immunol. 140:3161.
21. Sanjar, S., Smith, D., Kings, M.A., and Morley, J. 1990. Pretreatment with rh-GMCSF, but not rh-IL3, enhances PAF-induced eosinophil accumulation in guinea-pig airways. Br. J. Pharmacol. 100:399.
22. Ukena, D., Kroegel, C., Yukawa, T., Sybrecht, G., and Barnes, P.J. 1989. PAF-receptors on eosinophils: identification with a novel ligand [^{3}H)WEB 2086. Biochem. Pharmacol. 38:1702.
23. Kroegel, C., Yukawa, T., Dent, G., Chanez, P., Chung, K.F., and Barnes, P.J. 1988. Platelet activating factor induces eosinophil peroxidase release from human eosinophils. Immunology 64:559.
24. Kroegel, C., Yukawa, T., Dent, G., Venge, P., Chung, K.F., and Barnes, P.J. 1989. Stimula-

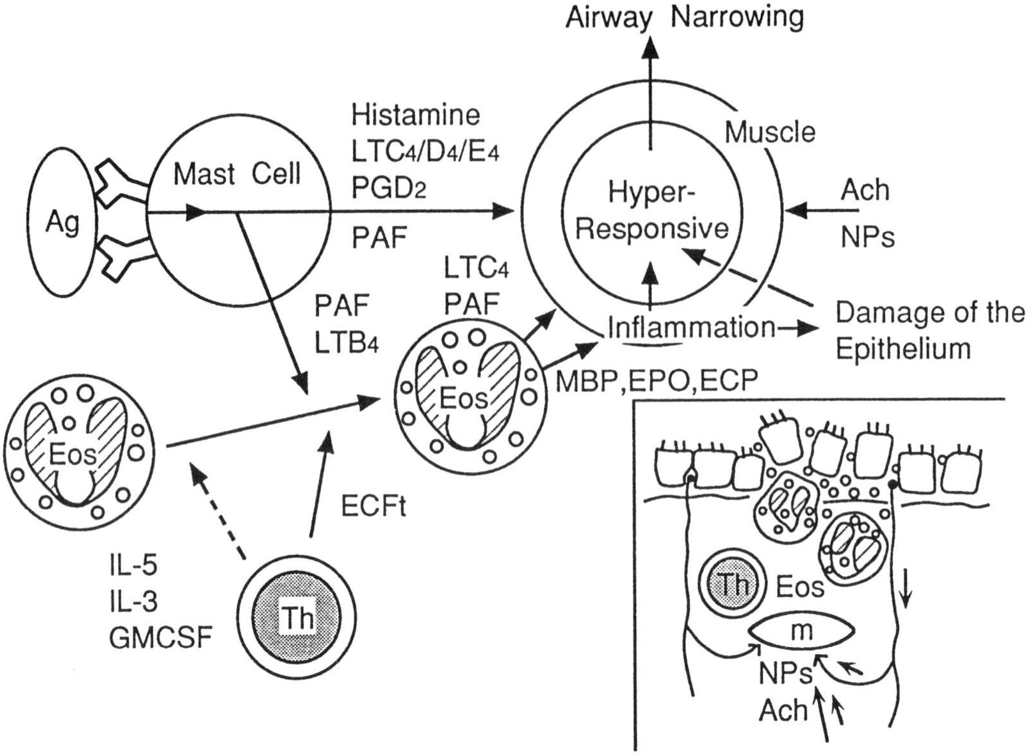

Figure 1: Possible roles of PAf and eosinophiles in antigen-induce airway responses in Allergic Asthma (Makno, S. Pharma Medica, (Medikaru-byu, Tokyo), 9, 12, 1991, partially modified).

cells in the bronchial mucosa, and the density of CD25(+) cells shows positive correlation with that of eosinophils, again confirming the working hypothesis (3).

Effects of PAF Antagonist on Antigen-Induced Airway Responses and Eosinophil Infiltration in the Airway in a Model of Actively Sensitized Guinea Pigs (1st Experiments) (4)

Based on these clinical observations, and in order to examine the roles of PAF on antigen-induced airway responses and eosinophil migration in the airway, the suppressive effect of a PAF antagonist, WEB 2086, was examined on these responses in actively sensitized guinea pigs. For active sensitization, Hartley male guinea pigs were exposed to aerosols of 10 mg/ml solution of ovalbumin (OA) for 10 minutes daily for 10 days and received 2 booster sensitization inhalations every 7 days. One week after the last inhalation the animals were challenged by the inhalation of 20 mg/ml OA solution for 5 minutes. Sixty mg of diphenhydramine was given intraperitoneally 30 minutes before the antigen challenge. This model of experimental asthma showed immediate and late-phase airway narrowing followed by airway hyperresponsiveness 24 hours and 5 days after the antigen challenge, being similar to allergen-induced airway responses of human allergic asthma. Eosinophil infiltration shows 2 peaks at 6 hours and 24 hours after the challenge and remains for at least 5 days. A PAF antagonist, WEB 2086, 3 mg/kg, which was given intravenously 15 minutes before and 3 hours after the antigen challenge, did not suppress immediate airway narrowing, but it did suppress late-phase airway narrowing and post-late-phase airway hyperresponsiveness, and also eosinophil migration 6 and 24 hours after the challenge, significantly. These observations suggest that PAF has important roles in antigen-induced eosinophil migration in the airway and possibly resultant late-phase airway narrowing and post-late-phase airway hyperresponsiveness.

Possible Contribution of T-Cell Factors to PAF-Induced Eosinophil Migration in the Skin of Mice (2nd Experiment) (5)

Since eosinophil infiltration showed a significant correlation with lymphocyte infiltration in the airway of asthmatic patients, and T-cell-derived IL-5 enhances PAF-induced migration in Boyden's chamber, it is suggested that T-cells in the human airway release IL-5 and enhance eosinophil chemotaxis induced by PAF *in vivo*. In order to examine this possibility, PAF-induced eosinophil infiltration was measured in normal and actively sensitized BALB/C mice, since in the actively sensitized model, T-cells are considered to be sensitized and release T-cell factors which stimulate eosinophils. Male BALB/C mice were sensitized by intraperitoneal injection of 1 µg of OA with 5 mg of aluminum hydroxide twice with the interval of 2 weeks, and 1 week after the last immunization of 10 µg of PAF was injected intradermally. Eosinophil infiltration, which was measured 6 hours after the injection, was significantly higher in sensitized mice as compared to normal non-sensitized mice, confirming the hypothesis. In order to examine whether T-cell-derived factors enhance PAF-induced eosinophil migration at the site of PAF injection, IL-5 was injected 60 minutes before PAF injection in the skin of BALB/C mice, and eosinophil infiltration in the skin was examined 6 hours after the PAF injection. Locally injected IL-5, from 250 to 1000 units/site, enhanced PAF-induced eosinophil migration dose-dependently. These observations suggest that T-cell sensitization enhances PAF-induced eosinophil migration at least in part by the release of IL-5.

Effects of Active Sensitization on PAF-Induced Airway Responses and Eosinophil Infiltration in Guinea Pigs (3rd Experiment) (6)

We observed that PAF played an important role in immediate and late-phase airway narrowings and post-late-phase airway hyperresponsiveness in antigen-induced airway responses and eosinophil infiltration in sensitized guinea pigs, and, in the second experiment, sensitization enhanced eosinophil infiltration. Based on these observations, we examined the effects of sensitization on exogenous PAF-induced airway responses. Guinea pigs were actively sensitized in the same method as in the first experiment by inhalation sensitization of OA. One week after the last OA inhalation, animals inhaled the aerosols of PAF solution until respiratory resistance increased by 100% of the baseline value. The dose-response curve shifted to the right significantly by sensitization. Late-phase airway narrowing, which was defined as more than 50% increase of respiratory resistance 3 to 8 hours after PAF inhalation, was not observed in non-sensitized control animals, but narrowing was observed in most of the sensitized animals. Eosinophil infiltration, which occurred 6 and 24 hours after the PAF inhalation, was significantly higher in sensitized animals as compared to non-sensitized animals, though sensitized animals exposed approximately half the amount of PAF as compared to non-sensitized animals. The observations of this experiment show that sensitization enhances PAF-induced immediate and late-phase airway narrowings and eosinophil infiltration in the late-phase, and suggest that eosinophils may participate in late-phase airway narrowing.

Conclusion

In bronchial asthma PAF attracts eosinophils to the airway. Attracted eosinophils are activated by T-cell factors including IL-5, and contribute to late-phase airway narrowing by releasing PAF and LTC_4, and to post-late-phase airway hyperresponsiveness by releasing toxic granule proteins and resultant damage of the bronchial epithelium. Inhibition of the production of PAF or blocking the effects of PAF would be one of the major approaches in the treatment of bronchial asthma.

References

1. Makino, S. 1990. Eosinophils and airway hyperresponsiveness. In: Inflammation and mediators in bronchial asthma, D.K. Agrawal and R.G. Townley, eds. CRC, p. 115.
2. Ohashi, Y., Motojima, S., Fukuda, T., and Makino, S. 1990. Relationship between bronchial reactivity to inhaled acetylcholine, eosinophil infiltration and a widening of the intercellular space in patients with asthma. Jpn. J. Allerg. 39:1541.
3. Fukuda, T. 1990. Eosinophils, neutrophils and lymphocytes. Jpn. J. Thor. Dis. 28 (suppl):82.
4. Arima, M., Yukawa, T., Terashi, Y., Sagara, H., and Makino, S. 1991. Involvement of platelet-activating factor (PAF) in ovalbumin antigen-induced late asthmatic response and increase of airway hyperresponsiveness in a guinea pig experimental model of asthma. Jpn. J. Allerg. 40:141 (with English abstract).
5. Arima, M., Yukawa, T., Terashi, Y., Sagara, H., and Makino, S. 1991. Platelet-activating factor (PAF)-induced late asthmatic response in sensitized but not in non-sensitized guinea pigs. Am. Rev. Respir. Dis. 143:A153.
6. Yukawa, T., Terashi, Y., Terashi, K., Arima, H., Sagara, S., Motojima, S., Fukuda, T., and Makino, S. Sensitization primes platelet-activating factor-induced accumulation of eosinophils in mice skin lesion, contribution of cytokines to the response. J. Lipid. Mediator, in press.

Experimental Models of Lung Hypersensitivity and Hyperresponsiveness : A Reappraisal of the Role of Inflammatory Cells and Mediators

Michel Bureau, Eliane Coëffier, Stéphanie Desquand, Jean Lefort, Marina Pretolani, B. Boris Vargaftig*

Few disease models are tailored for the human diseases in every detail. The guinea-pig model for asthma overestimates the role of histamine, and must be tailored in order to provide useful results for testing the different classes of potential anti-allergic drugs. With these reservations in mind, it provides important information for mediator inhibition and antagonism and for the different correlations between immediate hypersensitivity, cell migration/activation and nonspecific bronchopulmunary hyperreactivity. In particular, eosinophil participation can be readily controlled and the consequences of stimulation with antigen or with specific mediators can be studied in many details. When studied with the reservations in mind, the guinea-pig is a very useful tool in studies on pathology and pharmacology of allergic diseases, asthma in particular.

Anti-allergic drugs addressed to the bronchopulmonary system reduce acute bronchoconstriction and the increased vascular permeability and/or affect the inflammatory component which accounts for bronchopulmonary hyperresponsiveness.

Intervention of Mediators and Pharmacological Control Using the Guinea-Pig Model

The present concepts concerning the role of mediators in allergic and intrinsic asthma originate paradoxically from studies on the mode of action of non-steroidal anti-inflammatory drugs, which inhibit cyclooxygenase derivatives formation. However, this class of agents has no indication in allergy. In fact, other arachidonate derivatives from the lipoxygenase pathway, such as the peptido-leukotrienes (LTC_4, LTD_4, LTE_4) and LTB_4 are more important than prostanoids for allergy in general, and for asthma in particular. Peptido-LT induce bronchoconstriction in guinea-pigs and many of their accepted antagonists or the inhibitors of 5-lipoxygenase reduce allergen-induced bronchoconstriction, but preferentially when cyclooxygenase is inhibited and the effects of histamine are antagonized. LTC_4 and LTD_4 also provoke bronchoconstriction in guinea-pigs which involves the endogenous formation of thromboxane (Tx)A_2 (1,2). Since the mechanism by which cyclooxygenase inhibition uncovers the lipoxygenase-dependent bronchoconstriction is undefined, the guinea-pig model applied for this purpose is in fact tailored to demonstrate the participation of lipoxygenase and peptido-leukotrienes in lung anaphylaxis. This does not mean that the antagonists of peptido-LT or the inhibitors of 5-lipoxygenase will not exhibit anti-allergic properties, but indicates that caution is needed to interpret the results when acute guinea-pig anaphylaxis is used as a model.

Platelet-activating factor (PAF), which was discovered within the frame of immunology (3), activates inflammatory cells and induces hypotension, pulmonary hypertension, bronchoconstriction, leucopenia, thrombocytopenia and increased vascular permeability (reviews in 4,5). All these properties are compatible with a role of this lipid mediator in allergic reactions in guinea-pigs (6,7) and rabbits (8). The effects of PAF are not inhibited by cyclooxygenase inhibitors or by histamine antagonists, supporting its potential involvement in allergic situations. Two PAF antagonists, compounds BN 52021 and WEB 2086, blocked *in vitro* and *in vivo* antigen-induced bronchoconstriction and the release of mediators from perfused

* Unité de Pharmacologie cellulaire, Unité Associée Institut Pasteur-INSERM n 285, 25, rue du Dr. Roux, 75015, Paris, France.

lungs in the case of passively sensitized guinea-pigs (9–11). By contrast, both antagonists were shown to be inactive when tested on actively sensitized animals (10,12,13). Other investigators demonstrated the effectiveness of PAF antagonists against anaphylactic shock, but only under protection by anti-histamine drugs (14). In fact, the variable effects of PAF antagonists in guinea-pig allergy appear to be less dependent on the difference between active and passive anaphylaxis or on the presence of anti-histamine drugs than on the essential role of the booster injection of antigen which is administered during active sensitization of guinea-pigs (12,13). The booster injection is usually delivered in order to augment the formation of specific antibodies. However, we could demonstrate that, even if unperceived clinically because of the low amounts of antigen delivered, the booster injection behaves as a micro-antigen challenge leading to acute airway inflammation and subsequent lung hyper-responsiveness to various mediators, including PAF and LTD_4 (15). Indeed, the changes in lung reactivity develop within 2–4 days after the booster injection of the antigen, which is administered 14 days after the first sensitizing injection. Concomitantly with lung hyperresponsiveness, the number of eosinophils found in the bronchoalveolar lavage (BAL) fluid of boosted guinea-pigs more than doubles as compared to non-immunized or non-boosted animals (16). This airway inflammation may be traced by markers. In this model, prophylactic anti-asthma drugs, which do not interfere with the acute manifestations of experimental asthma, may prevent the development of hyperresponsiveness. This is the case of nedocromil sodium and cetirizine which, when administered to the guinea-pigs during the interval between the booster injection and the day of lung removal, reduced hyperresponsiveness and the increased numbers of eosinophils in the BAL (16 and unpublished results).

The Increased Vascular Permeability

The guinea-pig model of immediate hypersensitivity is also characterized by an increased lung vascular permeability. This phenomenon can be induced by the exogenous administration of inflammatory mediators originating from granulocytes (LTB_4 or C5a and the peptide secretagogue formyl-L-methionyl-L-leucyl-phenylalanine - fMLP) or from other cell types (PAF, histamine or bradykinin) (17). The increased vascular permeability and the accompanying leucocyte recruitment into the airways induced by fMLP in the guinea-pig are not affected by aspirin, even though bronchoconstriction is so. All *in vivo* effects of fMLP in the guinea-pig are inhibited by the systemic administration of pertussis toxin (18,19), but whether granulocytes are needed or not for the permeability effects has not been established. Since antigen-induced effects in the guinea-pig bronchial vascular permeability are suppressed by anti-histamines, it is likely that histamine is centrally involved. Indeed, histamine augments powerfully the bronchial and tracheal vascular permeability, a property shared with PAF.

The vascular effects of histamine and of the other mediators released by antigen interfere with the consequences of anaphylactic shock. Thus, the intra-tracheal administration of antigen to passively sensitized guinea-pigs is followed by a marked recruitment of leucocytes into the airways. Paradoxically, the extent of cell recruitment that follows anaphylactic shock is lowered in actively sensitized animals, even though they are more responsive to antigen (Bureau *et al.*, in preparation). In fact, the combination of antagonistic mepyramine (anti-H_1) and cimetidine (anti-H_2) uncovers a very consistent leucocyte recruitment by preventing the marked vascular effects of antigen.

Mechanisms of Bronchial Hyperreactivity

Bronchial hyperreactivity is expressed as a lowered threshold and an augmented response to standard bronchoconstrictor agents. Experimental models of airway hyperreactivity are usually based on the exposure of sensitized animals to the specific antigen. This is followed within a few hours by bronchial provocations with agonists such as acetylcholine or serotonin to show a shift in their dose-response curves. This *in vivo* approach allows modulating the establishment or the expression of hyperresponsiveness by treating the animals before the antigen exposure or later, just before the administration of the unspecific agonists. The *in vivo* approach lacks some correlations between hyperresponsiveness and *in situ* cell activation, characterized by mediator formation and release. This correlation can be achieved by using the *in vitro* approach on guinea-pig perfused lungs (see above), since the different dynamic processes (effects on intra-pulmonary resistance, lung weight as expression of water gain) can be linked to the release of mediators (15,20–23). According to the quantity and nature of the mediators involved, conclusions can be drawn regarding the kinetics of the release, the cell sources and the specificity of the different interferences. Furthermore, lungs can be collected after whatever required *in vivo* maneuvers (cell depletion, drug administration), and antigenic or other challenges by the intravascular (intra-arterial) or intratracheal routes. Finally, the effect of potential inhibitors can be investigated by performing the experiments in the presence or absence of drugs in the perfusing medium.

The Place of Eosinophils

The involvement of inflammatory cells during the late phase reaction and bronchial hyperreactivity is usually determined by the evaluation of the cell composition of the BAL from challenged animals or, more precisely, by light and/or electron microscopy. Nevertheless, the determination of the mediator content of the BAL is hindered by metabolism and by intrinsic difficulties of BAL collection during bronchoconstriction and enhanced vascular permeability. For this reason, experiments with isolated cells allow determining their state of activation by measuring specific markers and mediators following the application of appropriate stimuli. Among the various cells which play a central role in asthma, attention is focused mostly on eosinophils, particularly because their mechanism of recruitment is a potential target for drug modulation. Indeed, eosinophils are found in the bronchial sub-mucosa of asthmatic patients (24) and of guinea-pigs challenged with PAF or antigen (25). The rapid migration of mature eosinophils should account for the early enrichment of lungs with those cells, but other mechanisms are likely to explain the delayed phase. These mechanisms include local differentiation of circulating precursors and distal proliferation and differentiation, particularly at the bone-marrow compartment.

Cell recruitment into the lungs requires the up-regulation of adhesive proteins at the level of the endothelium and is expected to be followed by epithelial shedding which accounts for hyperresponsiveness. Once in the airways, eosinophils release cytotoxic proteins to the respiratory epithelium (26,27), thus exposing sub-mucosal structures, essentially nerve terminals, which are otherwise protected from the environment. Nevertheless, it is important to recognize that the presence of eosinophils by itself explains neither epithelial shedding nor hyperresponsiveness. Indeed, cationic proteins other than those originating from eosinophils also induce bronchial hyperreactivity in the rat (Coyle *et al.*, submitted). In addition, the intense hypereosinophilia which follows human or animal infection by parasites is not accompanied by asthma symptoms in general, or by epithelium damage in particular. It is thus likely that, in addition to recruitment, other mechanisms are required for the full expression of the capacity of eosinophils to intensify and perpetuate asthma. This suggests that a partial stimulus, such as sensitization, leads to cell migration, but that an additional component, such as antigen provocation, is needed to fully induce eosinophil-dependent damage.

The importance of antigen provocation for increased cell activation has been underlined by experiments showing an *ex vivo* priming of eosinophils collected from BAL of sensitized and challenged guinea-pigs. Indeed, these cells respond *in vitro* with an enhanced migration to LTB_4, PAF and C5a. These results indicate that, under those conditions, eosinophils have been activated *in vivo* by the antigen challenge. These results support the concept that atopy is essential for the expression of the activity of the different mediators of inflammation.

It has been demonstrated that the intradermal injection of PAF to allergic humans induces a marked eosinophilic infiltration, whereas non-allergic controls show only non-specific neutrophil recruitment (28,29). These results

ness to histamine: relationship to diurnal variation of peak flow rates and improvement after bronchodilators. Thorax 37:423.

4. Juniper, E.F,. Frith, P.A., and Hargreave, F.E. 1981. Airway responsiveness to histamine and methacholine: relationship to minimum treatment to control symptoms of asthma. Thorax 36:575.
5. Beasley, R., Roche, W.R., Roberts, J.A., and Holgate, S.T. 1989. Cellular events in the bronchi in mild asthma and after bronchial provocation. Am. Rev. Respir. Dis. 139:806.
6. Kirby, J.G., Hargreave, F.E., Gleich, G.J., and O'Byrne, P.M. 1987. Bronchoalveolar cell profiles of asthmatic and nonasthmatic subjects. Am. Rev. Respir. Dis. 136:379.
7. Juniper, E.F., Frith, P.A., Dunnett, C., Cockcroft, D.W., and Hargreave, F.E. 1978. Reproducibility and comparison of responses to inhaled histamine and methacholine. Thorax 33:705.
8. Cockcroft, D.W., Killian, D.N., Mellon, J.J.A., and Hargreave, F.E. 1977. Bronchial reactivity of inhaled histamine: A method and clinical survey. Clin. Allergy 7:235.
9. Holgate, S.T,. Mann, J.S., and Cushley, M.J. 1984. Adenosine as a bronchoconstrictor mediator in asthma and its antagonism by methylxanthines. J. Allergy Clin. Immunol. 74:302.
10. Anderson, S.D. 1985. Exercise-induced asthma. The state of the art. Chest 87:191.
11. O'Byrne, P.M., Ryan, G., Morris, M., McCormack, D., Jones, N.L., Morse, J.L.C., and Hargreave, F.E. 1982. Asthma induced by cold air and its relation to nonspecific bronchial responsiveness to methacholine. Am. Rev. Respir. Dis. 125:281.
12. Cockcroft, D.W., Ruffin, R.E., Dolovich, J., and Hargreave, F.E. 1977. Allergen-induced increase in non-allergic bronchial reactivity. Clin. Allergy 7:503.
13. Hargreave, F.E., Ryan, G., Thomson, N.C., O'Byrne, P.M., Latimer, K., Juniper, E.F., and Dolovich, J. 1981. Bronchial responsiveness to histamine or methacholine in asthma: Measurement and clinical significance. J. Allergy Clin. Immunol. 68:347.
14. Adelroth, E., Morris, M.M., Hargreave, F.E., and O'Byrne, P.M. 1986. Airway responsiveness to leukotrienes C4 and D4 and to methacholine in patients with asthma and normal controls. N. Engl. J. Med. 315:480.
15. Cushley, M.J., and Holgate, S.T. 1985. Adenosine induced bronchconstriction in asthma. Role of mast cell mediator release. J. Allergy Clin. Immunol. 75:272.
16. Fuller, R.W., Dixon, C.M., Cuss, F.M., and Barnes, P.J. 1987. Bradykinin-induced bronchoconstriction in humans: Mode of action. Am. Rev. Respir. Dis. 135:176.
17. Ramsdale, E.H., Otis, J., Klein, P., Hargreave, F.E., and O'Byrne, P.M. 1991. The effect of a long acting B_2-adrenoceptor agonist, Formoterol, on methacholine airway responsiveness in asthmatic subjects. Am. Rev. Respir. Dis. 143:998.
18. Ryan, G., Latimer, K.M., Juniper, E.F., Roberts, R.S., and Hargreave, F.E. 1985. Effect of beclomethasone dipropionate on bronchial responsiveness to histamine in controlled non-steroid-dependent asthma. J. Allergy Clin. Immunol. 75:25.
19. Juniper, E.F., Kline, P.A., Vanzieleghem, M.A., Ramsdale, E.H., O'Byrne, P.M., and Hargreave, F.E. 1990. Effect of long-term treatment with inhaled corticosteroids on airway hyperresponsiveness and clinical asthma in nonsteroid dependent asthmatics. Am. Rev. Respir. Dis. 142:832.
20. Dutiot, J.I., Salome, C.M., and Woolcock, A.J. 1987. Inhaled corticosteroids reduce the severity of bronchial hyperresponsiveness in asthma but oral theophylline does not. Am. Rev. Respir. Dis. 136:1174.
21. Juniper, E., Kline, P., Vanzieleghem, M., and Hargreave, F. 1991. Reduction of Budesonide after a year of increased use: A randomized controlled trial to evaluate whether improvements in airway responsiveness and clinical asthma are maintained. J. Allergy Clin. Immunol. 87:483.
22. Bel, E.H., Timmers, M.C., Hermans, J., Dijkman, J.H., and Sterk, P.J. 1990. The long-term effect of nedocromil sodium and beclomethasone dipropionate on bronchial responsiveness to methacholine in nonatopic asthmatic subjects. Am. Rev. Respir. Dis. 141:21.
23. Anderson, S., Seale, J.P., Ferris, L., Schoeffel, R., and Lindsay, D.A. 1979. An evaluation of pharmacotherapy for exercise-induced asthma. J. Allergy Clin. Immunol. 64:612.
24. Manning, P.J., Watson, R.M., Margolskee, D.J., Williams, V., Schartz, J.I, and O'Byrne, P.M. 1990. Inhibition of exercise-induced bronchoconstriction by MK-571, a potent leukotriene D4 receptor antagonist. N. Engl. J. Med. 323:1736.
25. Latimer, K.M., O'Byrne, P.M., Morris, M.M., Roberts, R., and Hargreave, F.E. 1983. Bronchoconstriction stimulated by airway cooling: Better protection with combined inhalation of terbutaline sulphate and cromolyn sodium

than with either alone. Am. Rev. Respir. Dis. 128:440.

26. Israel, E., Juniper, E.F. Callaghan, J.T, Mathur, P.N., Morris, M.M., Dowell, A.R., Enas, G.G., Hargreave, F.E. Drazen, J.M. 1989. Effect of a leukotriene antagonist, LY171883, on cold air-induced bronchoconstriction in asthmatics. Am. Rev. Respir. Dis. 140:1348.
27. Anderson, S., Schoeffel, R., and Finney, M. 1983. Evaluation of ultrasonically nebulized solutions for provocative testing in patients with asthma. Thorax 38:284.
28. O'Byrne, P.M., Dolovich, J., and Hargreave, F.E. 1987. State of the art: Late asthmatic responses. Am. Rev. Respir. Dis. 136:740.
29. Cartier, A., Thomson, N.C., Frith, P.A., Roberts, R., and Hargreave, F.E. 1982. Allergen-induced increase in bronchial responsiveness to histamine: Relationship to the late asthmatic response and change in airway caliber. J. Allergy Clin. Immunol. 70:170.
30. Cockcroft, D.W., and Murdock, K.Y. 1987. Protective effect of inhaled albuterol, cromolyn, beclomethasone and placebo on allergen-induced early asthmatic responses, late asthmatic responses and allergen-induced increases in bronchial responsiveness to inhaled histamine. J. Allergy Clin. Immunol. 79:734.
31. Freitag, A., Watson, R.M., Matsos, G., Eastwood, C., and O'Byrne, P.M. 1991. The effect of treatment with an oral platelet activating factor anatgonist (WEB 2086) on allergen-induced asthmatic responses. Am. Rev. Respir. Dis. 143:A15.
32. Gibson, P.G., Girgis-Gabardo, A., Hargreave, F.E., Morris, M.M., Matoli, S., Kay, J.M , Dolovich, J., and Denberg, J. 1989. Cellular characteristics of sputum from patients with asthma and chronic bronchitis. Thorax 44:693.
33. Pin, I., Freitag, A.P., O'Byrne, P.M., Girgis-Gabardo, A., Denberg, J.A., Dolovich, J., and Hargreave, F.E. (1991). Changes in cellular profile of induced sputum after allergen-induced asthmatic responses. J. Allergy Clin. Immunol. 87: A249.

Effect of Paf-Antagonists in Animal Models

Hubert O. Heuer*

From different preclinical models of asthma there is evidence that paf-antagonists (as represented by the hetrazepines apafant, WEB 2086, and bepafant, WEB 2170) inhibit some pathological features of asthma. These are inhibition of allergen-induced bronchoconstriction, antigen-associated infiltration of eosinophils, lung-edema formation by antigen, late phase reaction and bronchial hyperresponsiveness to antigen. In addition the formation and release of inflammatory mediators (such as leukotrienes, prostaglandins, thromboxanes, and histamine) are inhibited *in vivo*, although a direct interaction of selective paf-antagonists with these mediators has been excluded. The involvement of paf in a sequence of pathophysiological events including other mediators, and the possibility of interactive synergism, strengthen the view that antagonists of paf may have effects extending beyond those assumed for a single mediator.

Platelet-Activating Factor (Paf) Mimicking the Pathophysiology of Bronchial Asthma

Platelet activating factor (paf, paf-acether) was originally described as being released from basophils sensitized to IgE and stimulated by antigen (1). Paf is released into the systemic circulation (2) and from sensitized lungs (3) upon antigen challenge. In relation to asthma both increased levels of paf-like activity in the bronchoalveolar lavage fluid (4) and in sputum as well as increased level of lyso-paf after allergen provocation (5) in plasma in patients with late phase response, have been reported. The evidence that paf may be involved in the *pathophysiology of asthma* was initially derived from its ability to bronchoconstrict at low doses (6) as well as its properties as an inflammatory mediator (7). The bronchoconstrictive action as well as the edema-inducing action of paf is shared by other putative mediators of inflammation like histamine, thromboxane and leukotrienes; but in contrast to previous mediators paf is the hitherto sole mediator which in addition simultaneously increases the mucus secretion (8) and recruits platelets and eosinophils (9) from the extravascular space into the lungs. Since an important role in the pathogenesis of asthma is attributed to eosinophils, it is of interest that paf is among the most potent chemotactic factors for eosinophils (10). Furthermore paf can mimic the late-phase response at least in animals which also respond to antigen with a late phase reaction (11) and may induce bronchial hyperreactivity in different species including man (12). In addition there is support that paf may down-regulate the beta-receptors in human lung tissue (13).

Antagonism of Endogenous paf in Disease-Related "Animal Models of Asthma"

As outlined above paf can reproduce most of the symptoms and pathophysiological changes in asthma which can also be induced by antigen. In spite of this, it must be recognized that paf is not the sole mediator in asthma and other mechanisms may also be involved. This same complexity applies to *in vivo* animal models of asthma. Since we do not know the real cause of human bronchial asthma and the pathophysiological mechanisms involved therein, there is no perfect animal model of asthma which is satisfactory for prediction of the therapeutic value of new agents. Care has to be taken when drawing conclusions from a complex *in vivo* model, when the effect of a single therapeutic agent or antagonist is used to predict the causative contribution of a mediator or mechanism to this system. Conclusions can be misleading

* Department of Pharmacology, Boehringer Ingelheim Pharmaceuticals, Inc., 900 Ridgebury Rd., Ridgefield, CT 06877-0368, USA.

when a single agent fails to show any protective effect because the putative protection may be hidden by the deleterious effects of other preceding mediators or mechanisms. Thus failure of a selective agent should not necessarily exclude a contribution of the respective mediator or mechanism to the system. Therefore the compound should be reinvestigated in the presence of drugs which will remove these masking influences before definite conclusions can be drawn.

The results obtained with structurally different or even the same type of antagonists of paf in models of *in vivo anaphylaxis* are divergent, although most authors do report at least some protective action during passive anaphylaxis in the guinea pig (14,15). The divergent results may be due to differing experimental conditions (e. g., testing in the absence of a small dose of an antihistamine, antigen load during challenge, booster sensitization, etc.) and the different potency and bioavailibility of paf antagonists *in vivo*. Paf seems to be more important in passive anaphylaxis and during challenge with the antigen by the inhaled route (16). In active anaphylaxis paf-antagonists seem to be more effective when animals are once sensitized compared to a booster sensitization regimen (17,18) but paf-antagonists can still block anaphylaxis in boosted animals (18).

The contribution of paf to airway inflammation and recruitment of inflammatory cells (particularly eosinophils) and associated late phase reaction and bronchial hyperreactivity may be more prominent than its putative contribution to acute bronchoconstriction. With respect to airway microvascular leakage there are contradictory results as to whether paf-antagonists inhibit antigen-induced microvascular leakage. In one set of experiments a paf-antagonist failed to block leakage at a dose which inhibited paf-induced leakage (19). Other results are in favor of a paf-antagonist blocking antigen-induced microvascular leak (20).

Concerning *infiltration of eosinophils into the lungs*, selective paf-antagonists blocked eosinophil and leukocyte infiltration in the bronchial walls or the appearance of the cells in bronchoalveolar fluid of sensitized guinea pigs (9), rabbits (21) or monkeys (22). A few studies have, however, failed to show this effect. Therefore further work is needed to identify the conditions under which paf-antagonists block antigen-induced eosinophil-infiltration.

The *late phase response* to antigen and its inhibition by selective paf-antagonists has been shown in models for investigating the late phase reaction produced by antigen inhalation to diferent species including allergic guinea pigs (23), rabbits (21) and monkeys (22). This result is in accordance with the reported effect of a paf-antagonist in another model of late phase response in allergic sheep (11). Inhibition of antigen-increased bronchial responsiveness by selective paf-antgonists has been reported by several authors in guinea pigs (24), rabbits (21) and other species (25).

Since other mediator antagonists like antihistamines, and agents directed against the action or biosynthesis of leukotrienes or thromboxanes also provide more or less significant protection against the above mentioned changes, the question arises why these selective paf-antagonists share the inhibitory action with these agents. This occurs although these selective paf-antagonists have been shown not to have direct antihistaminic activities or to interfere with the biosynthesis of leukotrienes or thromboxanes. Furthermore this raises the question of synergistic interaction between paf and other mediators like histamine, thromboxanes and leukotrienes and the positive feedback loops between these mediators (20,26,27). For example paf has been described as releasing histamine from sensitized lung tissue (26) and vice versa histamine releases paf (27). These positive feed-back enhancement mechanisms between paf and different mediators and the sequence of mediator release may also be particularly involved in interaction between paf and eicosanoids (28). This paf-induced release of other mediators like thromboxanes, histamine, and leukotrienes during antigen-induced alterations is inhibited by selective paf-antagonists (20,26,28). Furthermore this inhibition by structurally unrelated but selective paf-antagonists occurs although these paf-antagonists are neither antagonists of histamine nor direct inhibitors of thromboxane or leukotriene biosynthesis. Therefore, e. g., the necessity for a small dose of an antihistamine in models of anaphylaxis *in vivo* may reflect that amount of histamine which is not released by or does not synergize with paf. This indicates that a small dose of antihistamine discloses the following paf-predominated phase. Furthermore this suggests that the selective paf-antagonists may even indirectly antagonize not only paf but also the synergism under *in vivo* conditions, as a consequence of the known synergism between paf and histamine, thromboxane, leukotrienes and other mediators. Due to this synergism of paf with other mediators and the amplifier role of paf, the antagonism of paf by selective paf-antagonists may go beyond the antagonism of just this particular mediator under *in vivo* conditions. On the other hand the interference with this synergism and interaction with other mediators may require higher doses of a particular paf-antagonist than required compared to just antagonizing paf (18). Although there is no conclusive rationale, ongoing priming towards paf (as can occur during booster-sensitization: 18) may also require a higher dose of a paf-antagonist to block this increased sensitivity to paf. The synergism, interaction with other mediators and priming towards paf may have to be considered for the real role of paf in its micro-environmental network and disease.

Concluding Remarks

In summary, the results derived from animal models which focus on diverse aspects of the complex pathophysiology of asthma, provide increasing support that selective paf-antagonists antagonize different symptoms of bronchial asthma. Clinical studies in human bronchial asthma will clarify the real pathophysiological significance of paf in relation to and in interaction with other mediators involved in bronchial asthma.

References

1. Benveniste, J., Henson, P.M., and Cochrane, C.G. 1972. Leukocyte-dependent histamine release from rabbit platelets; the role of IgE, basophils, and a platelet-activating-factor. J. Exp. Med. 136:1356.
2. Pinckard, R.N., Farr, R.S., and Hanahan, D.J. 1979. Physicochemical and functional identity of rabbit platelet-activating factor (Paf) released *in vivo* during IgE anaphylaxis with paf released *in vitro* from IgE sensitized basophils. J. Immunol. 123:1847.
3. Chignard, M., Le Couedic, J.P., Andersson, P., and Brange, C. 1986. Use of steroidal antiinflammatory drug provides further evidence for a potential role of PAF-acether in bronchial anaphylaxis. Int. Arch. Allergy Appl. Immunol. 81:184.
4. Court, E.N., Goadby, P., and Hendrick, D.J. 1987. Platelet-activating factor in bronchoalveolar lavage fluid from asthmatic subjects. Br. J. Clin. Pharmacol. 24:258.
5. Nakamura, T., Morita, Y., Kuriyama, M., Ishihara, K., Ito, K., and Miyamoto, T. 1987. Platelet-activating factor in late asthmatic response. Int. Arch. Allergy Appl. Immunol. 82:57.
6. Vargaftig, B.B., Lefort, J., Chignard, M., and Benveniste, J. 1980. Platelet-activating factor induces a platelet-dependent bronchoconstriction unrelated to the formation of prostaglandin derivatives. Eur. J. Pharmacol. 65:185.
7. Camussi, G., Pawlowski, J., and Tetta, C. 1983. Acute lung inflammation induced in the rabbit by local instillation of 1-O-octadecyl-2-acetyl-sn-glyceryl-3-phosphorylcholine or of native platelet activating factor. Am. J. Pathol. 112:78.
8. Hahn, H.-L., Purnama, I., Lang, M., and Sonnwald, U. 1986. Effects of platelet activating factor on tracheal mucus secretion, on airway mechanics and on circulating blood cells in live ferrets. Eur. J. Resp. Dis. 69, Suppl. 146:277.
9. Lellouch-Tubiana, A., Lefort, J., Simon, M.T., Pfister, A., and Vargaftig, B.B. 1988. Eosinophil recruitment into guinea-pig lungs after PAF-acether and allergen administration: Modulation by prostacyclin, platelet depletion and selective antagonists. Am. Rev. Resp. Dis. 137:948.
10. Wardlaw, A.J., Moqbel, R., Cromwell, O., and Kay, A.B. 1986. Platelet activating factor. A potent chemotactic and chemokinetic factor for human eosinophils. J. Clin. Invest 78:1701.
11. Stevenson, J.S., Tallent, M., Blinder, L., and Abraham, W.M. 1987. Modification of antigen-induced late responses with an antagonist of platelet activating factor (WEB 2086). Fed. Proc.46:1461.
12. Cuss, F.M., Dixon, C.M.S., and Barnes, P.S. 1986. Effects of inhaled platelet activating factor on pulmonary function and bronchial responsiveness in man. Lancet 2:189.
13. Agrawal, D.K., and Townley, R.G. 1987. Effect of platelet-activating factor on beta-adrenoceptors in human lung. Biochem. Biophys. Res. Commun. 143:1.
14. Casals-Stenzel, J. 1987. Effects of WEB 2086, a novel antagonist of platelet activating factor, in active and passive anaphylaxis. Immunopharmacology 13:117.
15. Lagente, V., Touvay, C., Randon, J., Des-

quand, S., Cirino, M., Vilain, B., Lefort, J., Braquet, P., and Vargaftig, B.B. 1987. Interference of the paf-acether antagonist BN 52021 with passive anaphylaxis in the guinea-pig. Prostaglandins 33:265.
16. Heuer, H., and Casals-Stenzel, J. 1988. Effect of the PAF-antagonist WEB 2086 on anaphylactic lung reaction: Comparison of inhalative and intravenous challenge. Agents and Actions, Suppl. 23:207.
17. Desquand, S., Lefort, J., Dumarey, C., and Vargaftig, B.B. 1990. The booster injection of antigen during active sensitization of guinea pigs modifies the anti-anaphylactic activity of the paf-antagonist WEB 2086. Br. J. Pharmacol. 100:217.
18. Heuer, H.O. 1991. WE 2347: Pharmacology of a novel very potent and long acting hetrazepinoic paf-antagonist and its action in repeatedly sensitized guinea pigs. J. Lipid Mediators 4:39.
19. T.W. Evans, G. Dent, D.F. Rogers, B. Aursudkij, K.F. Chung, and P.J. Barnes 1988. Effect of a PAF antagonist, WEB 2086, on microvascular leakage in the guinea-pig and platelet aggregation in man, Br. J. Pharmacol. 94:164.
20. Christy, L.J., Stewart, A.G., and Dusting, G.J. 1988. Platelet-activating factor and leukotrienes in rat pulmonary anaphylaxis, Proc. Australian Physiol. Pharmacol. Society, 19:94.
21. Metzger, W.J., Ogden-Ogle, C., and Atkinson, L.B. 1988. Chronic platelet activating factor (paf) aerosol challenge induces *in vivo* and *in vitro* bronchial hyperresponsiveness. FASEB J. 2:1252.
22. Gundel, R.H., Letts, L.G., and Wegner , C.D. 1991. The role of platelet activating factor in airway inflammation, airway responsiveness, and pulmonary function in monkeys. Ann. N.Y. Acad. Sci. 629:205.
23. Hutson, P.A., Holgate, S.T., and Church, M.K. 1988. Effect of WEB 2086 on early and late airway responses to ovalbumin challenge in conscious guinea-pigs. Br. J. Pharmacol. 95 (Proc. Suppl.):770P.
24. Coyle, A.J., Urwin, S.C., Page, C.P., Touvay, C., Villain, B., and Braquet, P. 1988. The effect of the selective PAF-antgonist BN 52021 on PAF and antigen induced bronchial hyperreactivity and eosinophil accumulation. Eur. J. Pharmacol. 148:51.
25. Soler, M., Sielczak, M.W., and Abraham, W.M. 1989. Platelet-activating factor (PAF) contributes to antigen-induced airway hyperresponsiveness and inflammation in allergic sheep: modulation by a selective PAF-antagonist. J. Appl. Physiol. 67:406.
26. Pretolani, M., Lefort, J., Malanchere, E., and Vargaftig, B.B. 1987. Interference by the novel PAF-acether antagonist WEB 2086 with the bronchopulmonary responses to PAF-acether and to active and passive anaphylactic shock in guinea pigs. Eur. J. Pharmacol. 140:311.
27. McIntyre, T.M., Zimmerman, G.A., Satoh, K., and Prescott, S.M. 1985. Cultered endothelial cells synthetize both platelet-activating factor and prostacyclin in response to histamine, bradykinin and adenosine triphosphate. J. Clin. Invest. 76:271.
28. Jancar, S., and Sirois P. 1988. Effects of paf and antigen on guinea pig lungs: inhibition by ginkgolides. In: Ginkgolides: Chemistry, biology, pharmacology and clinical perspectives. P.Braquet ed., vol. 1. Barcelona: J.R. Prous Science Publishers, p. 283.

Section X

Current Perspectives in Food Allergy

vents an immune response on subsequent parenteral administration of the same antigen (3). This immune tolerance pertains to delayed hypersensitivity reactions, and therefore to the T lymphocytes, but also to the production of IgM, IgG and IgE antibodies, and therefore constitutes a physiological means of preventing occurrence of an allergy.

Abnormal Response to Food Allergens: Food Allergy

Epidemiology has difficulty in identifying the frequency with which food allergy occurs, undoubtedly because the clinical signs are very varied and range from anaphylactic shock and Quincke's oedema, to urticaria and atopic dermatitis, to rhinitis and asthma, to diarrhoea, aphthous stomatitis and abdominal pain, even to some types of migraine and nephrotic syndromes. IgE antibodies are produced locally. In rodents synthesis is effected exclusively by plasma cells situated in the mesenteric ganglia; immunoglobulin then binds with the mast cells of the intestinal membrane (4). In humans, however, the two cell types (IgE plasma cells and mast cells activated by the antibody) are both evident in the intestinal membrane. The situation is exactly the same in patients infected with giardia intestinalis (5) and in those presenting with a food allergy (6) as shown below. Biopsies were obtained during endoscopic examination from the jejunum in 120 control subjects and in 220 patients with food allergy. None of them was infested by gut parasites. Jejunal biopsies were also taken in 10 patients with giardiasis before and after efficient treatment with metronidazole. Immunofluorescence staining was used to identify mucosal plasma cells. Immunoglobulin-containing cells were counted according to the tissue unit method. In control subjects, the mean number of IgA, IgM, IgG, IgD and IgE cells in three adjacent tissue units were 97, 17, 8, 1 and 1. In food-allergic patients, the mean numbers were 90, 17, 5, 1 and 16 respectively. Sensitization was admitted if the number of IgE cells for 3 tissue units was 6 or more. This was found in all of the intestinal samples from the 220 allergic patients and in none of the control subjects. Before treatment with metronidazole, the mean numbers of IgA, IgM, IgG, IgD and IgE cells in patients with giardiasis were 81, 26, 15, 7 and 24. After treatment, the numbers were 124, 20, 15, 5 and 6 respectively. A less invasive method will produce the same result. IgE was determined by the Phadebas paper disc double antibody radioimmunoassay technique (PRIST, Pharmacia) in the faecal extracts of 75 control subjects and of 177 patients with food allergy diagnosed by the radio-allergo-sorbent-test (RAST, Pharmacia) positivity. None of them was infested by gut parasites. IgE was also determined in the faecal extracts of 16 patients with intestinal parasite infestation. Blood was not detected in any of the faecal samples. IgE was found in faeces from no healthy subjects, in 12 of 16 patients (75%) with parasite infestation and in 142 of 177 patients (80%) with food allergy (7).

Gut Response to Allergen Challenge

After challenge with an allergen, histamine and other mediators are released by intestinal mast cells. Histamine induces a disruption of the intercellular junctions between the epithelial cells as shown by electron microscopy in the small gut of rabbits. As a consequence, intestinal permeability is increased (8). Intestinal permeability was measured in 100 fasting healthy subjects and in 136 patients with food allergy by oral administration to both groups of 5 g of mannitol, a marker of absorption of small molecules and of 5 g of lactulose, a marker of abnormal absorption of large molecules and subsequent measurement of urinary excretion of mannitol and lactulose. In healthy subjects, mean 5 hour urinary excretion of mannitol was 14.20% (SD 3.60) and of lactulose it was 0.30% (SD 0.15). The mean mannitol lactulose/mannitol ratio was 0.20.

In the fasting state, the 136 patients with food allergy (presenting mainly with atopic dermatitis and urticaria) exhibited a main urinary recovery of mannitol of 13.88% (SD 4.18), not statistically different from that in healthy subjects; mean recovery of lactulose in the patients was 0.46% (SD 0.33), significantly greater than in healthy subjects ($p < 0.001$). After ingestion of food allergen by the patients, mean mannitol recovery fell to 12.69% (SD 4.93) and mean recovery of lactulose rose to 1.10% (SD 0.84), this value being significantly different ($p < 0.0005$) from that observed in the fasting patients. On challenging the patients after they had taken 300 mg sodium cromoglycate, mean mannitol and lactulose recoveries were 13.39 (SD 4.72) and 0.61 (SD 0.40) respectively. The lactulose clearance was significantly different ($p < 0.0005$) from that measured on challenging patients unprotected by sodium cromoglycate. Histamine released by intestinal mast cells also influences the intestinal muscular layers. Oro-caecal transit time as measured by the lactulose hydrogen breath test has been studied in 15 healthy subjects and in 10 patients with food allergy. In fasting conditions oro-caecal transit time was no different in controls than in patients. Oral allergen challenge did not modify oro-caecal transit time in controls, but in allergic patients, it dropped from 117 (range 50–240) to 75 (range 30–180) minutes. Abnormalities of small bowel motility induced by allergen challenge were also prevented by pretreatment with sodium cromoglycate. Under sodium cromoglycate cover the mean oro-caecal transit time was 99 minutes (range 40–240).

Effect of Long-Term Treatment with Sodium Cromoglycate on Local IgE Synthesis

At the time of diagnosis, patients were advised to take daily 800 mg sodium cromoglycate and to reduce the consumption of recognised allergens. Some patients were compliant and some reported being non-compliant. They were studied again 6 or 12 months later. Three separate studies were carried out: on the levels of plasma food-specific IgE, on the levels of faecal IgE and on the density of jejunal IgE plasma cells respectively. In 32 patients who adhered to treatment the numbers of food sensitizations and inhalant sensitizations identified at the time of diagnosis were 117 and 40 respectively. One year later the RAST classes were equal or increased for 56 foods and reduced for 121; the RAST of inhalant sensitizations was equal or higher for 36 allergens and lower for 4 allergens. In 32 patients not complying to sodium cromoglycate treatment, there were initially 96 food allergies and 41 respiratory allergies. One year later, the classes of RAST for foods were equal or higher for 76 foods and lower for 20; for inhalant sensitizations, 35 results remained the same or became higher, and 6 reductions were observed.

A comparable study, but one which focussed on the jejunal plasma cell count, was carried out using four compliant and five non-compliant patients without parasitic infestation. After one year, the mean number of plasma cells counted in three tissue units in the compliant subjects went from 74 to 82 for IgA, from 19 to 14 for IgM, from 5 to 6 for IgG, from 0 to 1 for IgD and from 24 to 9 for IgE. In the non-compliant subjects, under the same conditions, the mean number of cells changed from 85 to 87 for IgA, from 16 to 27 for IgM, from 6 to 6 for IgG, from 1 to 1 for IgD and from 19 to 20 for IgE. Finally, the levels of faecal IgE expressed in IU/g dry weight were measured at the time of diagnosis and 6 months later in two groups of subjects. In 25 patients compliant with sodium cromoglycate treatment, the faecal IgE level changed from 84 (SEM 29) to 21 (SEM 21) IU/g dry weight ($p < 0.005$). In 15 non-compliant patients the level of faecal IgE changed from 46 (SEM 17) to 99 (SEM 64) IU/g dry weight (insignificant variation). In 16 patients interruption of effective treatment with cromoglycate resulted in a corresponding change in faecal IgE level from 10 (SEM 5) to 39 (SEM 13) IU/g dry weight ($p < 0.005$).

Conclusions

Any doubt as to the existence of food allergy could now be dispelled in view of the cumulative evidence showing local production of IgE and in view of intestinal functional abnomalies induced by contact with an allergen. It would seem that oral desensitization is a possible therapy (9), benefiting from long-term treatment with sodium cromoglycate which acts not only as an anti-allergic treatment, but also as an immunoregulator, as has already been demonstrated *in vitro* (10).

References

1. André, C., André, F., Druguet, M., and Fargier, M.C., 1978. Response of anamnestic IgA-producing cells in the mouse gut after repeated intragastric immunization. Advances in Experimental Medicine and Biology 107:583.
2. André, C., Lambert, R., Bazin, H., and Heremans, J.F. 1974. Interference of oral immunization with the intestinal absorption of heterologous albumin. Eur J. Immunol. 4:701.
3. André, C., Heremans, J.F., Vaerman, J.P., and Cambiaso, C.L. 1975. A mechanism for the induction of immunological tolerance by antigen feeding: Antigen antibody complexes. J. Exp. Med. 142:1509.
4. Mayrhofer, G., Bazin, H., and Gowans, J.L. 1976. Nature of cells binding anti-IgE in rats immunized with Nippostrongylus brasiliensis: IgE synthesis in regional nodes and concentration in mucosal mast cells. Eur. J. Immunol. 6:537.
5. Gillon, J., André, C., Descos, L., Minaire, Y., and Fargier, M.C. 1982. Changes in mucosal immunoglobulin-containing cells in patients with giardiasis before and after treatment. The Journal of Infection 5:67.
6. André, C., André, F., Descos, L., and Cavagna, S. 1989. Diagnosis of food allergy by enumerating IgE-containing duodenal cells. Gut 30:751.
7. André, F., André, C., Colin, L., and Descos, L. 1990. Diagnosis of food allergy by dosage of IgE in faecal extracts. Gut 31:611
8. André, C., André, F., and Colin, L. 1989. Effects of allergen ingestion challenge with and without cromoglycate cover on intestinal permeability in atopic dermatitis, urticaria and other symptoms of food allergy. Allergy 44:47.
9. Lafont, S., André, C., André, F., Gillon, J., and Fargier, M.C., 1982. Abrogation by subsequent feeding of antibody response, including IgE, in parenterally immunized mice. J. Exp. Med. 155:1573.
10. Kimata, H., Yoshida, A., Ishioka, C., and Mikawa, H. 1991. Disodium cromoglycate (DSCG) selectively inhibits IgE production and enhances IgG4 production by human B cells *in vitro*. Clin. Exp. Immunol. 84:395.

The Immunology of Allergic Gastroenteritis

Dean D. Metcalfe*

Eosinophilic gastroenteritis is a disease characterized by peripheral eosinophilia, gastrointestinal symptoms, and an eosinophilic infiltration of the bowel wall. This disease occurs in all age groups and in any segment of the gastrointestinal tract. The etiology is largely unknown, although food allergy has been demonstrated to play a major role in many cases. Cytokine imbalance with an increase in interleukin 5 (IL-5) and decrease in gamma interferon is noted in involved tissues. The course is usually benign, and responds to diet and/or steroid administration.

Eosinophilic gastroenteritis is an unusual disease characterized by peripheral eosinophilia, gastrointestinal symptoms, and eosinophilic infiltration of the gastrointestinal wall. The esophagus, stomach, small intestine, colon, and rarely extraintestinal organs may be involved. In approximately one half of the cases, allergic features suggest the etiology may be related to food hypersensitivity. The incidence of eosinophilic gastroenteritis is not known, although more than 150 cases have been reported. Males are affected slightly more than females, and the disease may occur at any age, although the peak age of onset is in the third decade of life. Most patients with food-dependent forms are under the age of 20 years (1,2). The disease is sporadic in distribution, although familial eosinophilic gastroenteritis has been reported (3).

The etiology of eosinophilic gastroenteritis is largely speculative, although an IgE-dependent mast cell-mediated mechanism has been suggested as the basis of this disorder in patients with an immunologic reaction to food antigens (4). Allergic diseases, including childhood food allergies, eczema, urticaria, allergic rhinitis, bronchial asthma, and a family background for allergy are common in patients with eosinophilic gastroenteritis (5). Many patients have peripheral eosinophilia, an elevated serum IgE level and radioallergosorbent tests (RASTs) positive for specific IgE to food antigens (2,6). Results of RASTs or skin tests may be accompanied by a symptomatic response to food challenge (7,8). In addition, mononuclear cells containing IgE have been identified in the lamina propria of the intestine, and the number of IgE containing cells and eosinophils has been reported to decrease after an appropriate elimination diet, which was accompanied by clinical improvement (9). Finally, a therapeutic response to corticosteroid, cromolyn sodium, or ketotifen, each of which may inhibit the release of chemical mediators from mast cells and/or the resulting inflammatory reaction, suggests the allergic nature of this disease in some individuals.

Not all patients with eosinophilic gastroenteritis, however, are atopic, and not all cases can be explained by food allergy (10). Only approximately one half of patients with eosinophilic gastroenteritis have findings consistent with atopy. The other patients do not report a personal or family history of allergy, and do not have positive skin tests for food allergens, an elevation in serum IgE, or adverse reactions to foods. Even in patients with suspected food hypersensitivity, however, withdrawal of suspected foods may fail to relieve symptoms, and there may be a poor correlation between the results of skin tests to specific food antigens and the results of an elimination diet.

Other etiologies including viral infections, parasitic infestations, and malignancies, have been considered as an explanation for eosinophilic gastroenteritis in patients without obvious food allergies. Viral infections have been proposed because of the observation that eosinophilic gastroenteritis may follow viral gastroenteritis. A history of flu-like symptoms, laboratory data including viral cultures and serologies, gastric histology showing inclusion

* Mast Cell Physiology Section, Laboratory of Clinical Investigation, National Institute of Allergy and Infectious Diseases, National Institutes of Health, Bethesda, Maryland, 20892, USA.
Acknowledgement: The author thanks Mrs. Belinda Richardson for her assistance in the preparation of this manuscript.

bodies, and spontaneous remissions in a few weeks are consistent with this hypothesis. Several patients have had evidence of infection with cytomegalovirus or parainfluenza virus (11). Interestingly, it has been reported that certain viral infections may also provoke allergic reactions by preferentially depressing T-suppressor cells, thereby allowing T-helper cells to stimulate IgE production (12). Moreover, the increased absorption of antigen through mucosa damaged by a viral infection may stimulate immune responses.

Parasite infestation is often suggested by peripheral eosinophilia and eosinophilic infiltrations of tissues. Eosinophilic gastroenteritis associated with Schistosoma, the herring parasite Eustoma rotundatum and Angiostrongylus costaricensis has been reported (13,14,15). However, this possibility can usually be eliminated. Eosinophilia with nonhematopoietic malignancy has been described in patients with carcinoma of the lung, stomach, kidney, thyroid, uterus, and ovary (16,17,18,19,20). Mature eosinophils infiltrate uninvolved tissues as well as the tumor (20). The peripheral eosinophilia and the abdominal symptoms may resolve after resection or chemotherapy of the tumor (18). Eosinophil (chemotactic and/or proliferating) factor(s) were advocated to explain these findings (20). Other diseases occurring with eosinophilic gastroenteritis include scleroderma, polymyositis, dermatomyositis, polyarteritis nodosa, dermatitis herpetiformis and gluten-sensitive enteropathy, agammaglobulinemia, chronic interstitial pulmonary fibrosis, and hypothyroidism. The significance behind such associations is not understood but the gastrointestinal disease may proceed the development of these disorders by years.

The biologic function of the eosinophil has long been debated. It is, however, generally accepted that eosinophils are part of host defense mechanisms against parasitic infestations. Eosinophils are heterogeneous in terms of their density and activity. The hypodense cells are more cytotoxic, have increased numbers of receptors, and are metabolically more active. The regulation of eosinophil production and maturation is complex, and incompletely understood. T lymphocyte-derived IL-5, which is also known as eosinophil differentiation factor, is critical for the development of eosinophils, and acts on blast cells induced by IL-3 or G-CSF (21). Moreover, IL-5 has a marked chemokinetic effect on eosinophils as well as a chemotactic effect (22).

Recently, we reported that gastric biopsies from patients with eosinophilic gastroenteritis associated with severe allergies to foods have normal to increased levels of IL-5 message when compared to normal biopsies (23). Peripheral blood lymphocytes secreted increased amounts of IL-5, similar to lymphocytes from patients with active parasitic infections. Perhaps more interesting was the observation that gamma-interferon levels were below normal in affected tissues.

Lacking a precise knowledge of the etiology and pathogenesis in eosinophilic gastroenteritis, any proposed classification may change with time. The first classification of eosinophilic gastroenteritis was proposed by Ureles et al. based on the histopathologic findings (24). They defined two major classes of disease. Class I disease was considered to be diffuse eosinophilic gastroenteritis, in which the gastrointestinal wall was infiltrated by mature eosinophils accompanied by prominent peripheral blood eosinophilia. Class II disease was a circumscribed eosinophil-infiltrated granuloma, in which there was a circumscribed granuloma, taking the form of either a pseudotumor or a polyp, massively infiltrated by eosinophils but unassociated with peripheral eosinophilia. The diffuse infiltrative form (class I) has now been further divided into three types by linking the most-affected layer of tissue with presenting symptoms and signs (25). In this classification scheme as shown in Table 1, type I disease is predominantly mucosal and characterized by symptoms of diffuse mucosal damage (26). Type II disease is predominantly a muscle layer disease with symptoms of gastrointestinal obstruction due to thickening and rigidity of the gut. Type III disease is predominantly a subserosal disease with eosinophilic ascites. More than one site may be involved in a given patient. There is a tendency for the mucosal type to have more allergic features than the other two types, and an exclusion diet produces a better therapeutic effect in the mucosal type. The subserosal type, which accounts for approximately 10% of the reported cases, is the least frequent of the three types of eosinophilic gastroenteritis and develops either subsequent to or concomitant with the development of other forms. Colonic or esophageal involvement, isolated or combined, is also be-

Table 1. Clinical manifestations of eosinophilic gastroenteritis related to the depth of the maximal disease process.

Type	Predominant involvement	Manifestations
I	Mucosal	Abdominal pain Nausea Vomiting Diarrhea Weight loss Growth retardation Fecal blood loss Iron deficiency anemia
II	Muscular	Abdominal pain Nausea Vomiting Pyloric or intestinal obstruction Weight loss Early satiety
III	Subserosal	Ascites Abdominal pain Nausea Vomiting Diarrhea

ing recognized more frequently, suggesting that the designation of this disease as gastroenteritis is too limiting.

The term allergic gastroenteropathy has also been used for a childhood disease characterized by anemia, edema, hypoalbuminemia, hypogammaglobulinemia, peripheral blood eosinophilia, marked eosinophilic infiltration in the gastrointestinal mucosa, excessive gastrointestinal protein loss, growth retardation, and manifestations of allergy (27). There is considerable clinical and histological overlap between reported cases of allergic gastroenteropathy and the mucosal type of eosinophilic gastroenteritis, perhaps justifying their inclusion into a single disease category.

Eosinophilic gastroenteritis most commonly affects the stomach and the small bowel. Esophageal, colonic or rectal involvement is infrequent. Typically, the gastric antrum is included. The duodenum, and to a lesser extent the jejunum, tend to be affected in association with the stomach rather than alone. The infiltrated bowel is thickened and swollen with induration, edema, hyperemia and nodularity, sometimes obstructing the lumen. The rugal folds of the stomach or intestinal valves of the small intestine are enlarged. There may be multiple small, discrete mucosal ulcerations. The serosa appears reddened with yellow or grayish patches. In colonic involvement, the mucosa is erythematous, granular and friable. In children, the appendix may be involved in which case eosinophilic gastroenteritis may present as acute appendicitis. Regional lymphadenopathy is sometimes quite marked, and ascites may be present. Eosinophilic infiltrations of other organs such as the liver, spleen, gallbladder, and pancreas have been described (24). Involvement of the prostate, peritoneum, biliary tracts or urinary bladder is very rare.

A pronounced eosinophilic infiltration and associated edema are the most characteristic histologic features of eosinophilic gastroenteritis (1). The lamina propria or submucosa is usually heavily infiltrated by eosinophils. Eosinophilic infiltration is extremely focal and variable. There is a tendency to perivascular aggregation of the eosinophils. In some instances, large numbers of eosinophils are observed in the subserosal layer or in the muscle coat with separation of the muscle bundles. The degree of tissue eosinophilia bears no relationship either to the number of eosinophils in the peripheral blood or to the extent of the gut involvement (1). The sinusoids of enlarged regional lymph nodes are engorged with mature eosinophils, but the nodes are otherwise normal.

Clinical manifestations depend on the area of maximal gastrointestinal involvement and more particularly the depth of the maximal disease process (Table 1). In patients with mucosal involvement, cramping periumbilical pain, postprandial nausea, vomiting, and loose watery diarrhea are common. Weight loss due to malabsorption may progress to cachexia. Generalized edema secondary to protein-losing enteropathy is seen in patients with widespread mucosal involvement. In patients with predominantly muscle layer involvement, manifestations of intermittent gastric or small bowel obstruction are seen. Epigastric pain, nausea, vomiting, and weight loss are frequent. Nocturnal regurgitation, heartburn, hematemesis, or melena may be encountered. Duodenal involvement may result in biliary obstruction. The chief manifestation of subserosal involvement is ascites. Abdominal distension, pain, and diarrhea are the usual symptoms. Nausea and vomiting may occur. Eosinophilic pleural effusions may also be noted. The patients with colonic or rectal involvement experience recurrent cramping lower abdominal pain, weight loss, and frequent liquid, blood-streaked stools. Esophageal involvement presents with intermittent dysphagia, epigastric pain, or vomiting. When the appendix is infiltrated with eosinophils, the clinical signs and symptoms may be indistinguishable from acute suppurative appendicitis.

The most characteristic laboratory finding in eosinophilic gastroenteritis is a prominent eosinophilia (up to 80%) in the peripheral blood. The eosinophils are mature and show no abnormality in morphology. The bone marrow may be infiltrated with eosinophils but reveals no evidence of a blood dyscrasia. The total white blood count is frequently elevated. The erythrocyte sedimentation rate is usually normal. There may be varying degrees of iron-deficiency anemia. Stools are usually positive for occult blood, and may contain gross blood. Charcot-Leyden crystals, presumably from extruded mucosal eosinophils, may be found on microscopic examination of the stool. The ascites when present is invariably an exudate and contains many eosinophils. Abnormal D-xylose absorption tests may be indicative of mucosal disease. Hypoalbuminemia secondary to protein-losing enteropathy or malabsorption is occasionally seen. Elevated serum IgE levels are associated with forms of disease associated with atopy. Specific IgE and positive skin reactions to food antigens may be detected.

Radiological findings, while not diagnostic, are helpful in the differential diagnosis. In mucosal disease, gastric lesions are most prominent in the antrum with a cobblestone appearance of the mucosa, prominent folds, luminal narrowing and large polypoid filling defects (28). The changes in the small bowel include spasm, with patchy thickening and distortion of the folds, more prominent in the jejunum. In the muscular pattern, changes in the stomach are usually limited to the antrum, producing a radiological appearance of hypertrophic pyloric stenosis or focal irregular narrowing of the distal antrum. When muscular thickening is diffuse, an appearance simulating scirrhous carcinoma may be produced. Segments of small intestine may show irregular narrowing or a pipestem appearance with no mucosal folds. If eosinophilic gastroenteritis involves only the subserosa, radiological findings will be those of ascites. In addition, mucosal or muscular bowel involvement frequently accompanies the subserosal type. When esophageal involvement is present, the radiological findings may include mucosal irregularities or narrowing of the lumen.

The diagnosis of eosinophilic gastroenteritis depends upon a biopsy specimen of the bowel wall which reveals a marked eosinophilic infiltration in a patient with peripheral eosinophilia and characteristic gastrointestinal symptoms. Endoscopic or peroral biopsy may show characteristic abnormalities in patients with mucosal disease, but patients with infiltration of deeper layers may require full thickness biopsies. Abnormalities in the gastric antrum are more constant and profound, suggesting biopsy of this site is the most sensitive and discriminating for diagnosis, even when gastric involvement is not suspected (29). The intestinal lesions are often patchy and multiple biopsies may be required. Assessment of eosinophil infiltration in the rectum is only satisfactory if the biopsy includes submucosal tissue.

A personal and family history of atopy are common. An increased IgE level, iron deficiency anemia, and hypoproteinemia may be present. The patient may show positive skin tests to food antigens, and food specific IgE antibodies may be detected in the serum. Symptoms may be related to exposure to specific foods (7,30). Challenge with a suspected food may provoke a severe exacerbation of symptoms and should not routinely be performed, although food challenge may aid in diagnosis under carefully controlled conditions.

The differential diagnosis of eosinophilic gastroenteritis includes a variety of diseases with gastrointestinal manifestations and peripheral eosinophilia. Eosinophilic gastroenteritis and cow's milk allergy in children have similar features. Both disorders have peripheral eosinophilia, iron deficiency anemia secondary to blood loss in the stools, protein-losing enteropathy, and eosinophilic infiltration of the stomach and small intestine. In cow's milk allergy the disease is transient, presents in the first year of life, remits on withdrawal of milk from the diet, and is not always associated with IgE-mediated reactions, even though children with this disease have peripheral and tissue eosinophilia. The term milk-sensitive enteropathy has been proposed as more appropriate than cow's milk allergy. In contrast, eosinophilic gastroenteritis is a chronic disease that generally has its onset later in childhood, does not respond to simple dietary changes, is associated with atopy and immediate hypersensitivity reactions to multiple foods, and usually requires corticosteroid therapy to establish remission. The relationship between these groups remains undefined (30). Other disorders to consider include lymphoma, gastrointestinal carcinoma, peptic ulcer disease, inflammatory fibroid polyp, intestinal parasite infestation, polyarteritis nodosa, and the hypereosinophilic syndrome. Hypereosinophilic syndrome is characterized by widespread parenchymal infiltration and damage of extraintestinal organs, as well as the bowel, in contrast to the limited involvement of the gastrointestinal tract with eosinophilic gastroenteritis. Eosinophilic gastroenteritis thus has a more benign course than hypereosinophilic syndrome. In infants with small bowel involvement, intestinal lymphangiectasia, immune deficiency, and celiac disease should be considered. Findings in the large bowel are those of a colitis. Such features may simulate Crohn's disease or ulcerative colitis.

The ideal treatment of eosinophilic gastroenteritis is to identify and remove the causative antigens if they exist. In pediatric cases, milk, egg, and wheat flour are most commonly incriminated. Administration of an elemental, hypoallergenic diet should result in a rapid clinical recovery. Replacement of cow's milk with soy formula is successful in the treatment of children with cow's milk protein allergy, but there is a tendency to develop sensitivity to soy protein when it is fed during an active disease process. It may be necessary to rest the inflamed bowel, using an elemental diet or total parenteral nutrition for a short period before attempting to broaden the diet.

In adults, the causative agents are usually not as evident. Withdrawal of various foods may fail to provide predictable amelioration of symptoms. There may be a poor correlation between results of skin tests to specific foods and the results of elimination diets. Patients may experience exacerbations and remissions seemingly independent of dietary management. A trial of an elimination diet is justified, however, in those patients with an atopic diathesis. In the absence of a clinically suspected food sensitivity, trial elimination diets should be based upon results of skin tests and RASTs. Some patients with food hypersensitivity have anaphylactic episodes following exposure to certain foods. Such patients must be identified and instructed to avoid the incriminated foods. These patients must be prepared to self-administer epinephrine if a systemic reaction should occur following inadvertent exposure.

In most patients with eosinophilic gastroenteritis who fail to respond to elimination diets, steroids have been successful. The response is usually rapid. Steroid therapy is sometimes required for months or even years. An alternate day schedule is preferred to reduce steroid-induced side effects for those who require long-term steroids. Cromolyn sodium and ketotifen, inhibitors of mediator release from mast cells, have been used in some patients. Childhood cases show better results than adult cases (31,32). Trials with such drugs are reasonable as these drugs have negligible side effects. Classic antihistamines are of little benefit. Surgery is reserved for those who present with severe obstructive symptoms not responsive to conservative therapy, or those who present with bowel perforation. It is possible that bowel obstruction can be managed with steroids if detected early. A few patients have shown a persistent remission after surgical excision of the involved bowel segment.

The long-term prognosis of patients with eosinophilic gastroenteritis is generally good. Pediatric patients with this disease usually respond to an elimination diet when the disease is related to food sensitivity. Frequently the sensitivity to foods resolves by the age of two or three. However, some patients have recurrent symptoms after a short period of improvement on an elimination diet. Adult patients may experience chronic recurrent disease. The recurrent symptoms can be managed by dietary manipulation and steroid therapy. Fatal cases are very rare, and have been due to bowel perforation, paralytic ileus, or other complications.

References

1. Johnstone, J.M., and Morson, B.S. 1978. Eosinophilic gastroenteritis. Histopathology 2:335.
2. Thounce, J.Q., and Tanner, M.S. 1985. Eosinophilic gastroenteritis. Arch. Dis. Child 60:1186.
3. Keshavarzian, A., Saverymuttu, S.H., Tai, P.C., Thompson, M., Barter, S., Spry, C.J.F., and Chadwick, V.S. 1985. Activated eosinophils in familial eosinophilic gastroenteritis. Gastroenterology 88:1041.
4. Caldwell, J.H., Mekhjian, H.S., Hurtubise, P.E., and Beman, F.M. 1978. Eosinophilic gastroenteritis with obstruction: Immunological studies of seven patients. Gastroenterology 74:825.
5. Lucak, B.G., Sansaricq, C., Snyderman, S.E., Greco, A., Fazzini, E.P., and Bazaz, G.R. 1982. Disseminated ulcerations in allergic eosinophilic gastroenterocolitis. Am. J. Gastroenterol. 77:248.
6. Elkon, K.B., Sher, R., and Seftel, H.C. 1977. Immunological studies of eosinophilic gastroenteritis and treatment with disodium cromoglycate and beclomethasone dipropionate. S. Aff. Med. J. 52:838.
7. Caldwell, J.H., Sharma, H.M., Hurtubise, P.E., and Colwell, D.L. 1979. Eosinophilic gastroenteritis in extreme allergy: Immunopathological comparison with nonallergic gastrointestinal disease. Gastroenterology 77:560.
8. Caldwell, J.H., Tennenbaum, J.I., and Bronsterin, H.A. 1975. Serum IgE in eosinophilic gastroenteritis: Response to intestinal challenge in two cases. N. Engl. J. Med. 292:1388.
9. Jenkins, H.R., Pincott, J.R., Soothill, J.F., Milla, P.J., and Harries, J.T. 1984. Food allergy: The major cause of infantile colitis. Arch. Dis. Child 59:326.
10. Leinbach, G.E., and Rubin, C.E. 1970. Eosinophilic gastroenteritis: A simple reaction to food allergens? Gastroenterology 59:874.
11. Edelman, M.J., and March, T.L. 1964. Eosinophilic gastroenteritis. Amer. J. Roentgen. 91:773.
12. Frick, O.L., German, D.F., and Mills, J. 1979. Development of allergy in children: 1. Association with virus infections. J. Allergy Clin. Immunol. 63:228.
13. Ashby, B.S., Appleton, P.J., and Dawson, I. 1964. Eosinophilic granuloma of gastrointestinal tract caused by herring parasite Eustoma rotundatum. Br. Med. J. 1:1141.
14. Hesdorffer, C.S., and Ziady, F. 1982. Eosinophilic gastroenteritis: A complication of schistosomiasis and peripheral eosinophilia? A case report and review of the pathogenesis. S. Aft. Med. J. 61:591.
15. Silvera, C.T., Ghali, V.S., Roven, S., Heimann, J., and Gelb, A. 1989. Angiostrongyliasis: A rare cause of gastrointestinal hemorrhage. Am. J. Gastroenterol. 84:329.
16. Goetzl, E.J., Tashjian, A.H., Rubin, R.H., and Frank, K. 1978. Production of a low molecular weight eosinophil polymorphonuclear leukocyte chemotactic factor by anaplastic squamous cell carcinomas of human lung. J. Clin. Invest. 61:770.
17. Miller, W.M., Adcook, K.J., Moniot, A.L., Raymond, L.W., Hutcheson, J., and Elliott, R.C. 1977. Progressive hypereosinophilia with lung nodules due to thyroid carcinoma. Chest 71:789.
18. Reshef, R., Manaster, J., Ezekiel, E., Suprun, H., and Manor, E. 1987. Malignant tumor masquerading as eosinophilic gastroenteritis. Isr. J. Med. Sci. 23:281.
19. Sala, A.M., and Stein, R.J. 1937. A case of carcinoma of cervix with a blood picture simulating chronic aleukemic eosinophilic leukemia. Am. J. Cancer 29:125.
20. Tsutsumi, Y., Ohshita, T., and Yokoyama, T. 1984. A case of gastric carcinoma with massive eosinophilia. Acta Pathol. Jpn. 31:117.
21. Yamaguchi, Y., Suda, T., Suda, J., Eguchi, M., Miura, Y., Harada, N., Tominaga, A., and Takatsu, K. 1988. Purified interleukin 5 supports the terminal differentiation and proliferation of murine eosinophilic precursors. J. Exp. Med. 167:43.
22. Yamaguchi, Y., Hayashi, Y., Sugama, Y.,

Miura, Y., Kasahara, T., Kitamura,S., Torisu, M., Mita, S., Tominaga, A., Takatsu, K., and Suda, T. 1988. Highly purified murine interleukin 5 (IL-5) stimulates eosinophili function and prolongs *in vitro* survival. IL-5 as an eosinophil chemotactic factor. J. Exp. Med. 167:1737.
23. Jaffe, J.S., Mullin, G.E., Braun-Elwert, L., Metcalfe, D.D., and James, S.P. 1991. IL-5 RNA production in gastric mucosa in eosinophilic gastroenteritis. J. Allergy Clin. Immunol. 87:349 (839A).
24. Ureles, A.L., Alschibaja, T., Lodico, D., and Stabins, S.J. 1961. Idiopathic eosinophilic infiltration of the gastrointestinal tract, diffuse and circumscribed: A proposed classification and review of the literature with two additional cases. Am. J. Med. 30:899.
25. Klein, N.C., Hargrove, R.L., Sleisenger, M.H., and Jeffries, G.H. 1970. Eosinophilic gastroenteritis. Medicine (Baltimore). 49:299.
26. Metcalfe, D.D. Eosinophilic gastroenteritis. In: Food allergy: Immunology and allergy clinics of North America. J.A. Anderson, ed. Philadelphia: W.B. Saunders, in press.
27. Waldmann, T.A., Wochner, R.D., Laster, L., and Gordan, R.S. 1967. Allergic gastroenteropathy: A cause of excessive gastrointestinal protein loss. N. Engl. J. Med. 276:761.
28. Marshak, R.H., Lindner, A., Maklansky, D., and Gelb, A. 1981. Eosinophilic gastroenteritis. JAMA 245:1677.
29. Katz, A.J., Goldman, H., and Grand, R.J. 1977. Gastric mucosal biopsy in eosinophilic (allergic) gastroenteritis. Gastroenterology 73:705.
30. Katz, A.J., Twarog, F.J., Zeiger, R.S., and Falchuk, Z.M. 1984. Milk-sensitive and eosinophilic gastroenteropathy: Similar clinical features with contrasting mechanisms and clinical course. J. Allergy Clin. Immunol. 74:72.
31. Heatley, R.V,. Harris, A., and Atkinson, M. 1980. Treatment of a patient with clinical features of both eosinophilic gastroenteritis and polyarteritis nodosa with oral sodium cromoglycate. Dig. Dis. Sci. 25:470.
32. Kravis, L.P., South, M.A., and Rosenlund, M.L. 1982. Eosinophilic gastroenteritis in the pediatric patient. Clin. Pediatr. 21:713.

Diagnosis of Food Allergy

Luisa Businco, Barbara Bellioni, Vanda Ragno*

The initial diagnostic approach of food allergy (FA) is to take a detailed history and to perform a careful physical examination in the gastrointestinal, cutaneous and respiratory systems. Subsequently, verification of the relationship between the symptom(s) and the ingestion of the offending food(s) is mandatory, and finally a determination of the immunologic mechanism involved should be performed with *in vivo* and *in vitro* tests. However the underlying immunologic mechanisms may be difficult to document, and the only immunologic mechanism easily proven in current practice is the IgE-mediated one. The double-blind-placebo-control-food-challenge (DBPCFC) is the gold standard for the diagnosis of FA. In children not able to swallow capsules, the food can be masked in other items. Patients with a history of anaphylactic life threatening reactions and strongly positive prick test and/or Rast to the offending food should not be challeged. Concerning the *in vivo* tests: Prick tests have low sensitivity and specificity; however, when strongly positive, they are indicative of allergy. The methods used for specific IgE detection (Rast, Fast, CLA) show the same limitations as the prick tests.

Definition

The diagnosis of FA in infancy and in childhood is a challenge both for the pediatrician and allergist because it can be easily accomplished only when there is a relation between the ingestion of the offending food(s) and the onset of the symptoms, and when it can be demonstrated that these symptoms are the consequence of an immunological reaction. However, the underlying immunologic mechanisms may be difficult to document, and the only immunologic mechanism easily proven in current practice is the IgE-mediated one. When an immunological reaction cannot be proven, the symptoms should be defined as food intolerance. Since the term "allergy" comprises symptoms and sensitization, these two components should be carefully investigated when dealing with a child suffering from FA. The term "symptomatic sensitization" indicates that a patient has objectively reproducible symptoms after the ingestion of the offending food, and the symptoms are associated with positive *in vivo* and/or *in vitro* response to the immunologic tests. On the contrary "asymptomatic sensitization" indicates positive response to the immunologic test, despite negative response to the challenge test.

Clinical History and Manifestations

The first step in achieving the diagnosis of FA is a thorough history which should provide precise information to support or to rule out FA. If parents refer typical symptoms such as angioedema, urticaria or anaphylaxis, which immediately occur after the ingestion of the offending food, the clinical history may be so obvious that no other diagnostic tests are necessary. Unfortunately the clinical history is only occasionally useful, and more frequent and especially in atopic dermatitis (AD) it does not provide valuable information (1). A large spectrum of manifestations involving different organs may be associated with FA (2). Some manifestations are immediate and severe (anaphylaxis, angioedema, laryngospasm) while others have a more insidious and chronic clinical course (diarrhea, urticaria, AD). There is a unanimous consensus in the literature that several manifestations are due to FA (anaphylaxis, angioedema, urticaria, AD, contact urticaria, vomiting, diarrhea, respiratory symptoms), while for others (headache, altered behavior, irritable bowel syndrome) the consensus is not unanimous.

* Allergy and Clinical Immunology Division, Department of Pediatrics, University " La Sapienza", Medical School of Rome, Viale Regina Elena 324, OO161, Rome, Italy.

Diagnosis

The manifestations due to FA are not pathognomonic and no reliable laboratory tests are available; therefore the diagnosis should be done with the challenge test. If this test is positive, and if in addition the immunological tests are positive, FA is a likely diagnosis. Occasionally, however, if the symptoms resolve during the diagnostic elimination diet and the offending food can be identified, then an open challenge will generally still be useful to confirm the diagnosis and there will be no need for the DBPCFC. On the contrary, if the symptoms do not improve during an appropriate diagnostic elimination diet, then the diagnosis of FA should be reconsidered. Finally we would like to point out that many parents of very young children frequently have incorrect concepts about foods triggering symptoms in their children. However, in the majority of these cases the association between the ingestion of the food under suspicion and the appearence of the symptoms is a coincidence. In such cases there is no need for a DBPCFC; that is, a reintroduction of the incriminated food into the diet when the symptoms disappear, will convince the parents that the food can be well tolerated.

Diagnostic Elimination Diet

Since there are as yet no laboratory tests for the diagnosis of FA which obviate the need for careful clinical assessment, a "diagnostic" foods elimination diet should be given for no more than 4 weeks (3). With good results (and infants' compliance) we have been using a home-made meat diet prepared as suggested by Rezza: lamb meat 100 g, rice flour 70 g, olive oil 40 g, Calcium 500 mg, Vitamin D 400 IU, water up to 1 liter (4). This diet provides 750 calories per liter. One of the major advantages of this diet is that it can be adapted to the individual patient; vegetables, other types of fruit and meat, wheat flour and other nutrients can be added to the diet according to the age and weight of the child, and the doctor's judgement.

Food Challenge Test

The DBPCFC is the gold standard for the diagnosis of FA, therefore capsules should be filled by someone else who is not involved in the diagnostic procedure (5,6). The most common offending foods are available in dry state at the grocery. In children not able to swallow capsules, the food can be masked in other forms. An appropriate elimination diet should be given up to 4 weeks before the challenge in order to obtain the disappearence of the symptoms. Before the DBPCFC is given, the patient must be symptom free or, if AD is present, the severity score of the skin lesions must be significantly improved. In infants with chronic diarrhea and severe malnutrition, the challenge test should not be performed until a period of improvement of the clinical condition with weight gain. Patients with a history of anaphylactic life-threatening reactions and a strongly positive prick test and/or Rast test to the offending food should not be challeged. Although over the last decade DBPCFC has been considered the gold standard for the diagnosis of FA, up to now there is no general agreement on some details regarding the procedure of how to perfom the challenge test; nonetheless, we suggest the following points: First, the test should always be performed under medical supervision in an office or in the hospital setting and the child should be carefully supervised for 4 hours. Medical equipment for the managment of anaphylaxis should be at hand. Second, if the response to the challenge test is unequivocal, then the diagnosis is definitive and no further tests, as suggested in the past, should be necessary. Third, symptoms may appear after a few minutes or hours; nevertheless in many cases they may not appear until after a few days (colitis, AD). Fourth, although there is no general agreement on the amount of the offending food to be administered in the challenge test, it would be advisable to begin with small quantities, gradually increasing the doses. It has been recommended to increase the dose up to 8 g of the food in dry form. If this amount is tolerated, the challenge is negative, and then the food can be given openly in its natural form, and according to various authors no reaction will occur (1,5,6). Fifth, there is no general agreement on how to mask the taste and the color of the offending food and the vehicle to use for this purpose, if the child cannot swallow the capsules. Usually we mask cow's milk in soy milk (if the child is not soy-sensitive), and other foods can be masked in different fruit juices such as orange, apple, pineapple, etc. Sixth, there is no general agreement on how to increment the dose and how long challenges with other foods should be separated. We generally double the dose every 30 minutes until symptoms occur or 8 g of the food is ingested in a single challenge without reaction. We separate challenges with different foods by one week. Seventh, and finally, placebo controls are necessary when symptoms are equivocal or when the clinical course of the disease is fluctuating as in AD. There is no general agreement on the substance to be used as placebo. We usually employ soy milk, if the child is not allergic to it.

Prick Tests and Specific IgE Detection

Prick tests have low sensitivity and specificity; however when strongly positive, they are indicative of allergy (6,7). Many factors may affect the skin reactivity (age, drugs, potency and quality of the extract, etc). In many circumstances it may be useful to directly use fresh food. The methods used for specific IgE detection (Rast, Fast, CLA) show the same limitations as the prick tests (6–9).

Other Diagnostic Tests

Other tests to detect type III immunoreactions (antibodies belonging to class IgG, IgA, and IgM to foods, or circulating immunocomplexes) or to type IV (such as the lymphocyte response *in vitro* to foods or the production of lymphokines) or the basophil degranulation test are not recommended in current clinical practice due to lack of standardization. The eosinophil count in peripheral blood, nasal secretions and faecal mucous may be useful when significant variations are observed in relation to the ingestion of a given food. Other useful data after the challenge test may be the appearance of (hidden) blood in the faeces or a 50% reduction of xilosemia (colitis, etc.).

Diagnosis of FA in Children with AD

The diagnosis of FA in children with AD confronts allergists with one of their most demanding challenges (10). The fluctuating clinical course of the diseases and the large variety of the environmental triggering factors make the identification of the offending food(s) rather difficult. The identification of the offending food(s) is difficult since Skin Test and RAST yield varying results in terms of sensitivity, specificity, and predicted positive and negative values (11,12). Since foods are common triggering factors of AD in infancy and in childhood, it would seem obvious that elimination diets should be useful in the identification of the offending food(s) in these patients. However as stressed by Sampson, "historical information and elimination diets were rarely helpful" and only DBPCFC's were useful for the diagnosis (1). In the studies by Sampson (1,5), eggs, peanuts and CM elicited 70% of the positive DBPCFCs. Less than 15% of the children reacted to more than two foods. Employing two foods for challenges, we have obtained a similar percentage of positive reactions (75%) (11,12). Children with AD are frequently reported to be allergic to a broad spectrum of foods. This assumption is usually endorsed by the high number of positive skin and RAST tests to foods found in AD children. Even though a wide variety of different foods is consumed by children, CM, egg and wheat, which are the foods most common in the Italian diet, accounted for more than 93% of the positive responses (11,12). These data should be taken into account to eliminate the nutritional problems of too restrictive a diet. Foods commonly described to induce hypersensitivity such as citrus fruit, chocolate and strawberries, failed to trigger positive responses in the children studied by us (11,12).

Conclusion

In conclusion the diagnosis of FA has been considered for many years as a dilemma. However, in the last decade a number of studies has shown that this diagnosis can be correctly achieved with a rational procedure which includes: a detailed history, verification of the symptoms with objective methods and, finally, demonstration of specific immunological reaction.

References

1. Sampson, H.A. 1988. The role of food allergy and mediator release in atopic dermatitis. J. Allergy Clin.Immunol. 81: 635.
2. Businco, L., Benincori, N., and Cantani, A. 1984. Epidemiology,incidence and clinical aspects of food allergy. Ann. Allergy 53:615.
3. Benincori, N., Cantani, A., Picarazzi, A., Osmelli, S., and Businco, L. 1986. Management of atopic dermatitis by elimination diet: A useful but difficult approach. In: Proceedings of the First Latin Food Allergy Workshop. L. Businco and F. Ruggeri, eds. Rome: Fison Spa Publisher, p.95.
4. Businco, L., Benincori, N., Cantani, A., Tacconi, L., and Picarazzi, A. 1985. Chronic diarrhea due to cow's milk allergy. A 4 to 10 year follow-up study. Ann. Allergy. 55:844.
5. Sampson, H.A. 1989. Role of immediate hypersensitivity in the pathogenesis of atopic dermatitis. Allergy 44, Suppl 9:52.
6. Cummings, N., and Bock, A. 1988. Clinical methods for diagnosis in food allergy. In: Series clinical pediatrics, Vol V. L.T. Chiaramonte, A.T. Scheider, and F. Lifshitz, eds. New York: M. Dekker Inc, p. 289.
7. Bahana, S.L. 1987. The dilemma of pathogenesis and diagnosis of food allergy. Immunol. Allergy Clin. North Am. 7:48.
8. Aas, K. 1978. The diagnosis of hypersensitivity to ingested foods. Reliability of skin prick tests and the radioallergosorbent tests with different materials. Clin. Allergy 8:39.
9. Benincori, N., Novarino, D., Cantani, A., Di Cicco, C., Messina, E., Perlini, R., and Businco, L. 1983. On the reliability of RAST in childhood food allergy. Allergol. Immunopathol. 11:255.
10. Businco, L., and Cantani, A. 1989. Food allergy and atopic dermatitis. Allergy Today 3:9.
11. Businco, L., Ziruolo, M.G, Ferrara, M., Benincori, N., Muraraoro, A., and Giampietro, P.G. 1989. Natural history of atopic dermatitis: An updated review and personal experience of a five year follow-up. Allergy 44, Suppl. 9:70.
12. Meglio, P., Giampietro, P., Farinella, F., Cantani, A., and Businco, L. 1989. Personal experience in the diagnostic procedures in children with atopic dermatitis and food allergy. Allergy 44, Supl 9, 165.

Management of Food Allergy

Minoru Baba*

Interest in food allergy has been increasing in clinical practice, due to its high incidence, especially in infancy and early childhood. The management of food allergy includes: (a) elimination of causative foods, (b) symptomatic treatment, and (c) natural growing out of the phase. Elimination of causative food allergen is effective when single foods alone are causative agents. In our sample for egg and milk allergy cases, 66.7% and 82.8% were successful respectively. When oral DSCG was given to food allergy patients for 6 months or much longer, the results were as follows: Of 47 cases, 12 cases (25.5%) were not effective, 16 cases (34.0%) were moderately effective, and 10 cases (21.3%) were markedly so. It is thus concluded that oral DSCG is one of the highly preferable drugs to be used for the treatment of food allergy. Applying heat to foods was observed here to change the allergenicity: When boiled egg was given to raw egg-sensitive bronchial asthma patients, 10 of 18 cases (55.6%) could take egg without any complications and roasted egg was taken in 12 cases of 18 cases (66.7%). In many food allergy cases, natural growing out can be expected. In patients with cow's milk and egg allergy, rates for growing out were checked at 3, 6, and 9 years of age: 62.5% of the milk allergy patients had outgrown the allergy at 3 years of age, 78.6% at 6 years, and 87.5% at 9 years. 51.2% of egg allergy patients outgrew the allergy at 3 years of age and 82.4% at 9 years. As for the reason why food allergy can be outgrown during child development, the role of secretory IgA in the intestine is confirmed here.

In the past decade, interest in food allergy has been increasing in clinical practice, due to its high incidence, especially in infancy and early childhood. Foods play an important role as causative allergens in some cases of atopic dermatitis, which is consequently sensitized with age to inhalants and develops further allergic symptoms, such as asthma. We have called such a developing process in a number of allergic diseases the "Allergy March" (1).

In Japan, the incidence of atopic dermatitis is estimated at 10 to 20% of all children, and that of bronchial asthma is estimated at about 4 to 5%. It is not yet clear what percentage of such allergic diseases is related to foods as causative allergens. But, from our clinical experience, in about 20 to 30% of infantile atopic dermatitis and to a lesser extent in bronchial asthma, some kind of foods play an important role.

Over the past 15 years we have been studying the significance of foods as a direct causative allergens of atopic diseases, and we have tried to understand its importance in two key dimensions. One is the role of various foods as direct allergens that cause symptoms, which we call the "promoter" effect. In some allergic diseases there is no doubt as to this connection. The other possible role of food is to set the "Allergy March" in motion, which we label the "initiator" effect.

The topic of my paper concerns only food as direct allergens, with special emphasis on treatment. In Table 1, the difficulty of the diagnosis of food allergy is shown. In a sample of 108 atopic children who visited our clinic, the patients kept to an elimination diet, avoiding some particular kind of foods for 6 months to 1 year and 6 months. Their symptoms, however, did not improve. All cases were checked and elimination and provocation tests and immunological studies were performed. Subsequently, we found 16 of 108 cases were definitely allergic to some kind of foods but 77.8 % were not allergic to any kind of foods. What does this result mean? I think the diagnosis of food allergy is very difficult and it gives us the warning that we should be careful in applying this diagnosis.

Table 1. Diagosis of Food Allergy: Its Pitfalls

Food Elimination 108 Cases → No Improvement 92 / Worsening 16 Cases → Recheck →

→ Food Allergy
- No. 84 Cases (77.8%) → Misdiagnosed
- Yes 16 Cases (14.8%)
- ? 8 Cases (7.4%)

* Department of Pediatrics, Doai Memorial Hospital, 2-1-11, Yokoami, Sumida-ku, Tokyo 130, Japan.

Table 2. Clinical Symptoms and Causative Food Allergens (1985–1989)

Food	Case		Clinical Symptom			
			G.I.	Resp.	Skin	Others
Egg	118	(34.6%)	68	32	42	3
Egg White	42	(12.3%)	28	16	25	
Milk	62	(18.2%)	29	11	42	2
Beef	13	(3.8%)	9	4	3	
Chicken	24	(7.0%)	19	3	11	
Pork	11	(3.2%)	8	4	2	
Deer	2	(0.6%)		1	2	
Ice Cream	16	(4.7%)	3	9	9	
Rice	3			1	2	
Wheat	4			2	2	
Soy Bean	9	(7.3%)	3	1	6	
Buckwheat	6		3	2		3
Peanut	3			2	1	
Bonito	5		2		3	
Crab	5			1	4	
Mackerel	4	(6.0%)			4	
Tuna	3				3	
Shrimp	3				3	
Kiwi Fruit	2				2	
Papaya	1				1	
Pimento	2	(2.3%)			2	
Orange	2				2	
Spinach	1			1	1	
	341		172 (50.4%)	90 (26.4%)	172 (50.4%)	8 (2.3%)

Table 2 shows a profile of clinical symptoms and causative allergens in allergic diseases which we confirmed and treated in the past 4 years. The most frequent allergen is egg (egg white). About half of the cases are caused by egg; the next most frequent agent is cow's milk. Recently, cases caused by some kind of cereals, such as rice, wheat, or buckwheat, have been reported in Japan. As clinical symptoms, gastrointestinal and skin symptoms are frequent; relatively rare, on the other hand, are cases of anaphylactic shock after consumption of egg, milk or buckwheat.

The management of food allergy is shown in Table 3. The first level denotes the elimination of causative food allergen: When causative allergen is confirmed, complete food elimination should be attempted. As to the question of how long an elimination diet should be continued, we recommend a check-up every 6 months to ascertain whether the eliminated food is still causative. The second level is symptomatic treatment: For each symptom, the most effective treatment should be tried. Thus we should not adhere only to attempts at finding the causative allergen. Prompt and suitable treatment should be started as early as possible. The third level is not a medical treatment; rather, in many food allergy cases, especially in children, natural outgrowth can be expected. I will show the data later.

Table 3. Management of Food Allergy

1. Elimination of Causative Allergen

2. Symptomatic Treatment
   Topical
   Anti-Allergic Drug—Prevention

3. Expect Natural Outgrowing

Table 4 shows the clinical results of eliminating causative foods. In these cases, eliminations were continued for at least one year. All cases were allergic to single foods. In egg and milk allergy cases, 66.7% and 82.8% were successfully treated respectively. In rice and buckwheat allergic children, eliminations were effective as well.

Table 4. Elimination of Causative Food Allergen

	Cases	Successful	?
Egg	48	32 (66.7%)	16 (33.3%)
Milk	29	24 (82.8%)	5 (17.2%)
Soy Bean	3	2 (66.7%)	1 (33.3%)
Rice	2	2 (100.0%)	0 (0 %)
Buckwheat	5	5 (100.0%)	0 (0 %)

All Cases : Allergic to Single Food

Table 5 also exemplifies the clinical results of elimination of causative foods. All cases were allergic to two food allergens. When children, for example, were allergic to both egg and milk, 75.5% were successful in treatment, whereas children allergic to egg and soybean had a 66.7% rate of success.

Table 5. Elimination of Causative Food Allergens

	Cases	Successful	?
Egg + Milk	8	6 (75.5%)	2 (25.5%)
Egg + Soy Bean	3	2 (66.7%)	1 (33.3%)
Milk + Soy Bean	2	1 (50.0%)	1 (50.0%)
Egg + Rice	2	0 (0 %)	2 (100.0%)

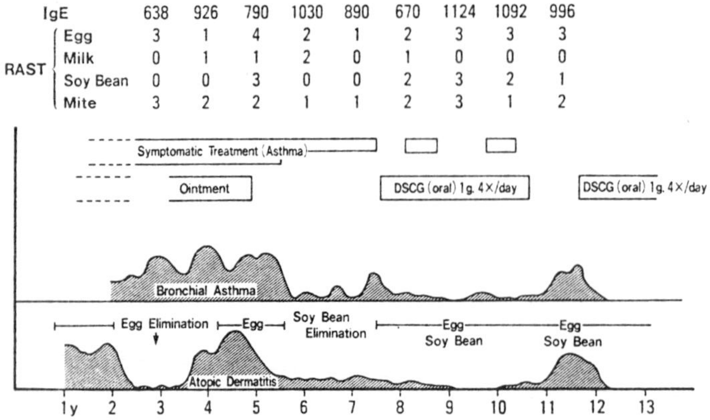

Figure 1. Effect of Oral DSCG in Egg and Soy Bean Allergy (Atopic Dermatix, Bronchial Asthma) T. T. boy

Figure 1 shows a case of food allergy treated by oral DSCG. The boy presented with skin exanthema in early infancy and subsequently developed bronchial asthma. For both diseases, only symptomatic treatments were tried. When he visited our clinic, he was found to be allergic to egg, and so egg elimination was initiated. At 4 years of age, he was found to be allergic to soy bean as well. Elimination of soy bean has proved effective in the treatment of both atopic dermatitis and bronchial asthma. At 7 years of age, we started oral DSCG. Since then, egg and soy bean were not eliminated but clinical symptoms have nonetheless subsided.

Figure 2 exemplifies the case of a child who was also allergic to egg, and was treated by oral DSCG: The patient, a 1 year old girl at admission to our hospital, was almost unconscious and her lips were cyanotic. She was in shock. We treated symptomatically and after 30 minutes she became fairly well. After this event, she was followed up in our hospital. We performed several tests trying to find causative allergens. We talked with her parents and found that her shock had been caused by egg intake. Complete egg elimination was initiated but at around one and half years of age, she started to take egg and egg products. Soon after that, she developed the symptoms of atopic dermatitis. Her skin symptoms subsided after egg elimination. At 3 years and 9 months oral DSCG was started. Since then, her skin symptoms have almost disappeared, even when she eats eggs again. In these two cases, oral DSCG was effective and the children could carry on daily life without elimination of causative food allergen.

Table 6 shows the results of the treatment of food allergy by oral DSCG. 47 cases (including 8 respiratory, 16 gastrointestinal and 23 dermatological diseases) were treated by oral

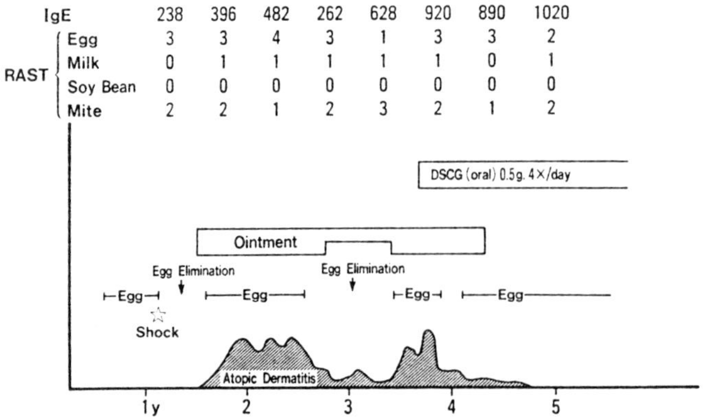

Figure 2. Effect of Oral DSCG in Egg Allergy (Shock, Atopic Dermatis) S. Y. girl

Table 6. Results of Treatment of Food Allergy DSCG (oral)

Symptom	Cases	Treatment Period	Slightly Effective	Moderately Effective	Markedly Effective	Not Effective
Resp.	8	6m-1y8m	2	4	1	1
GI	16	8m-2y6m	3	6	3	4
Skin	23	4m-2y6m	4	6	6	7
	47		9 (19.2%)	16 (34.0%)	10 (21.3%)	12 (25.5%)

Table 8. Outgrow Rate at 3, 6, 9 years of Age Milk and Egg Allergy (6m. of Age)

	3y.	6y.	9y.
Milk Allergy	62.5% (20/32)	78.6% (22/28)	87.5% (14/16)
Egg Allergy	51.2% (22/43)	72.2% (26/36)	82.4% (14/17)

DSCG for 6 months or much longer. In most cases, weak corticosteroid ointment and symptomatic medicine were applied. Effectiveness of oral DSCG was evaluated by the severity of attack in bronchial asthma, by objective skin symptoms and subjective complaints in atopic dermatitis and by gastrointestinal symptoms in GI allergy. Out of 47 cases, 12 cases (25.5%) were not effective. 9 cases (19.2%) were slightly effective, while 16 cases (34.0%) were moderately so, and 10 cases (21.3%) were markedly effective. From these results, it is concluded that oral DSCG is one of the highly preferable drugs to be used for the treatment of food allergy.

It has been observed that allergic causative foods are sometimes eaten without any complications after they have been subjected to heating. The change in allergenicity by heating is shown in Table 7. 10 out of 18 cases of bronchial asthma patients whose symptoms were caused by raw egg were given boiled egg without subsequently developing any complications, and 12 cases could take roasted egg without any reactions. The reason why heated food loses or decreases its allergenicity has not yet been elucidated. But it is clinically very important that food allergic patients can eat boiled or roasted food without any symptomatic complications.

Finally I would like to present the data of outgrowing food allergy (Table 8). All patients were demonstrably allergic to cow's milk or egg at 6 months of age. They were followed up if they were still allergic to cow's milk or egg more than several times. At 3, 6 and 9 years of age, they were checked by provocation tests. 62.5% of milk allergy patients had outgrown their symptomatic reaction at 3 years of age, 78.6% at 6 years of age, and 87.5% at 9 years of age. 51.2% of egg allergy patients outgrew their reactions by 3 years of age, and 82.4% by 9 years.

As for the reason why food allergies can be outgrown during development, several reasons are conceivable. At present, I think the most

Table 7. Effect of Egg Allergy by Heating

Symptom	Raw Egg +	Boiled 15 min. +	Boiled 15 min. −	Roasted Egg +	Roasted Egg −
Asthma	18	8	10 (55.6%)	6	12 (66.7%)
Atopic Dermatitis	24	17	7 (29.1%)	6	18 (75.0%)
Urticaria	6	4	2 (33.3%)	1	5 (83.3%)

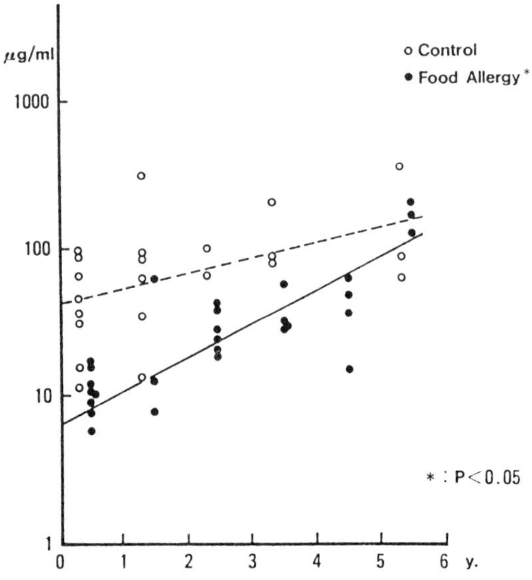

Figure 3. Secretary IgA and Its Development

important is the role of secretory IgA in the intestine. We studied secretory IgA (2,3,4) in saliva in food allergy patients and in a control group (Figure 3). Secretary IgA is considered to play a role in defense and to prevent the penetration of food allergens through the intestinal mucosa. Consequently, atopic children are easily sensitized by food allergens when their diet includes strong allergenic foods, for example, egg in early infancy. Fortunately, the amount of secretory IgA in saliva gradually increases as children grow up, and it reaches normal levels at around 7 or 8 years of age. This explains why food allergy manifestations in early infancy often disappear by the time children reach elementary school.

References

1. Baba, M., and Yamaguchi, K. 1989. "The Allergy March": Can it be prevented? Allergy Clin. Immunol. News 1:71.
2. Baba, M. 1989. Establishment and development of allergic diseases in childhood. Possibilities of prediction and prevention. Jap. J. Allergol. 38:1061.
3. Noma, T., Yoshizawa, I., Kawano, Y., Ito, M., Baba, M., and Yata, J. 1987. Allergen-induced IL2 responsiveness in lymphocytes from patients with atopic dermatitis and/or bronchial asthma. Jap. J. Allergol. 36:1075.
4. Yamaguchi, K., Mukoyama, T., and Baba, M. 1985. Secretory IgA in saliva of asthmatic children. Jap. J. Allergol. 34:234.

Additives in Allergic or Pseudo-Allergic Reactions

Mario Sánchez-Borges*/**, Raúl Suárez-Chacón*

98 patients with chronic idiopathic urticaria, angioedema or anaphylactoid reactions were studied in order to determine the prevalence of sensitivity to tartrazine, sodium benzoate and sodium metabisulfite in those diseases. By means of double-blind placebo-controlled challenges, sensitivity to any of the studied food additives in the whole group was observed in 29.6%, and in patients with chronic urticaria/angioedema it was found in 26.9%. Sensitivity to tartrazine was observed in 22.4% of the chronic urticaria/angioedema patients and correlated with benzoate and metabisulfite sensitivity. Benzoate sensitivity in chronic urticaria/angioedema was found in 32.4%, and also occurred more often in patients with simultaneous tartrazine or metabisulfite sensitivity. Metabisulfite sensitivity in chronic urticaria/angioedema presented in 18.1% of the cases, while aspirin sensitivity was found in 42.1% of those patients. Non-steroidal anti-inflammatory drugs (NSAIDs) intolerance, but not food additive intolerance, was more prevalent in atopic individuals. We conclude that food additive intolerance in patients with chronic urticaria/angioedema is more prevalent than previously recognized. In addition, we suggest that patients suitable for additive challenge be selected according to their medical history of previous adverse reactions to NSAIDs or to processed foods.

The process of industrialization has introduced a number of changes in the way of living which have progressively expanded from developed countries to the rest of the world. One of those changes which has more directly influenced humans is the exposure to a number of chemicals through industrial foods and drugs. Therefore, it is not surprising that some deleterious effects induced by such products, which are foreign to the normal constituents of the human body, are becoming apparent.

Adverse effects of dyes, preservatives, antioxidants, and other chemical compounds present in foods and drugs have been described by a number of investigators (1–8). However, the prevalence of reactions to food additives in the general population is largely unknown. There are also reports of additive reactions in selected patient subsets, such as patients with urticaria, asthma or anaphylactoid reactions. For example, it is suspected that less than 10% of patients with chronic urticaria and angioedema are sensitive to tartrazine and other food additives. Stevenson et al. found only one out of 24 subjects (4%) with chronic idiopathic urticaria/angioedema who was sensitive to tartrazine (1). Other authors have published rates of sensitivity to tartrazine in patients with chronic urticaria between 8 and 36%, but none of those studies were adequately controlled (5,9–10).

In the case of sodium benzoate, it has been observed that it exacerbates symptoms in less than 10% of the chronic urticaria patients challenged (7), but again sensitivity rates vary widely between 3 and 44% according to the different authors (10–12). There have also been isolated case reports of urticaria/angioedema due to sulfites. Simon observed no positive metabisulfite challenges in 25 patients with chronic urticaria/angioedema (7). Two cases of anaphylaxis related to sulfite ingestion have been described. One out of 130 patients with idiopathic anaphylaxis had positive challenges to sodium metabisulfite in three studies reviewed by Simon (7). One systemic reaction (IgE mediated?) to a sulfite skin test has also been reported. On the other hand, sulfites may induce severe attacks of asthma (4).

The purpose of the present study was to investigate the prevalence of reactions to three food additives (tartrazine, sodium benzoate and sodium metabisulfite) in patients with unexplained urticaria, angioedema or anaphylaxis.

---

* National Center for Oncology and Hematology, Health Ministry of Venezuela.
** Centro Médico-Docente "La Trinidad".

Materials and Methods

Patients: 98 consecutive patients suffering unexplained urticaria, angioedema or generalized anaphylactoid reactions were studied. Inclusion criteria were acute or chronic urticaria or angioedema, or symptoms of anaphylactoid reaction plus previous repeated adverse reactions to NSAIDs (mainly aspirin) or a history suggestive of reactions to foods containing additives (colored, canned, preserved, industrially produced). 68 patients were female, 30 male, aged 3 to 60 years (average age 27.9 ± 15.3 years). 49 (50%) were atopic, as demonstrated by personal and family history of atopic diseases (asthma, rhinitis, atopic eczema, food allergy) plus at least one positive immediate type skin test to inhalant allergens, which were done by the prick method. A history of symptoms triggered by NSAIDs was found in 57 patients (58.1%) (Table I). Clinical diagnosis for this group of patients is presented in Table II, and consisted of chronic urticaria in 46 patients, chronic angioedema in 19, acute urticaria and angioedema in 13, chronic urticaria and angioedema in 13, and idiopathic anaphylactoid reactions in 7.

Challenge procedures: 161 oral challenges were carried out in the 98 study patients. Double-blind placebo controlled challenges were done with Tartrazine (T) (FDC Yellow #5) 50 mg, Sodium Benzoate (B) 100 mg, Sodium Metabisulfite (SMB) 100 mg, and Aspirin 250 mg in adults, 125 mg in children. Each challenge was done on a separate day, and if positive the interval between challenges was 7 days. All anti-histamines, sympathomimetics, corticosteroids and sodium cromolin were discontinued 72 hours before the procedure. Astemizole was witheld for 1 month before the challenge. Test reagents, as well as lactose placebo, were given in identical opaque capsules and patients were observed for 3 hours in the office. The patient was seen again after 24 hours in order to confirm any delayed reaction. To assess the response to the challenge, we followed the procedure described by Stevenson et al. which utilizes the "rule of nines" (1). Pulse rate and blood pressure were measured every 30 minutes during the observation period.

Table 1. Demographics of Study Population (n = 98).

			%
AGE	RANGE 3-60 YEARS (27.9+/-15.3)		
SEX	FEMALE	68	69.3
	MALE	30	39.6
NSAID SENSITIVITY		57	58.1
ATOPY		49	50.0

Table 2. Clinical Diagnosis in 98 Patients Challenged with Food Additives.

CLINICAL DIAGNOSIS	NUMBER OF PATIENTS
CHRONIC URTICARIA	46
CHRONIC ANGIOEDEMA	19
ACUTE URTICARIA / ANGIOEDEMA	13
CHRONIC URTICARIA / ANGIOEDEMA	13
IDIOPATHIC ANAPHYLAXIS	7
TOTAL	98

Statistical Analysis: The Chi-square test was used to compare differences between proportions. Significance level was $p < 0.05$.

Results

The results of double-blind placebo-controlled challenges are presented separately for each additive and aspirin. There were no major modifications of vital signs, and no asthma attacks were observed during the challenges.

Tartrazine Challenges

74 patients were submitted to challenge with tartrazine. 16 reacted positive (21.6%). In Table III it can be observed that positive responses were not associated to the patient's sex, atopy, or previous adverse reactions to NSAIDs. However, patients who reacted to tartrazine also reacted more frequently to benzoate and metabisulfite ($p < 0.05$). Positive responses occurred in 4 out of 9 patients with chronic urticaria/angioedema (44.4%), in 9 out of 34 of those with chronic urticaria (27.2%), and in 2 out of 11 with acute urticaria/angioedema (18.1%), in 1 out of 5 with anaphylactoid reactions (20%) and in 0 out of 15 patients with chronic angioedema (0%).

Table 3. Results of tartrazine Challenges (n = 74).

	+/n	%	P value*
Number of positive challenges	16/74	21.6	–
Female	13/54	24.0	–
Male	3/20	15.0	n.s.
Atopic	7/16	43.7	–
Non Atopic	9/16	56.2	n.s.
NSAID (+), T Ch (+)	10/16	62.5	–
NSAID (+), T Ch (-)	38/58	65.5	n.s.
B Ch (+), T Ch (+)	5/ 7	71.4	–
B Ch (+), T Ch (-)	7/32	21.8	<0.05
SMB Ch(+), T Ch(+)	1/ 1	100.0	–
SMB Ch(+), T Ch(-)	1/10	10.0	<0.05
Asa Ch(+), T Ch(+)	1/ 4	25.0	–
Asa Ch(+), T Ch(-)	3/ 4	75.0	n.s.

*Chi-square test. NSAID: Non steroidal anti-inflammatory drugs. T Ch: Tartrazine challenge. B Ch: Benzoate challenge. SMB Ch: Metabisulfite challenge. Asa Ch: Aspirin challenge. n.s.: not significant

Table 4. Results of Benzoate Challengs (n = 74).

	+/n	%	P value *
Number of positive challenges	15/46	32.6	–
Female	10/29	34.4	–
Male	3/20	15.0	n.s.
Atopic	4/15	26.6	–
Non Atopic	11/15	73.3	n.s.
NSAID (+) B Ch(+)	9/15	60.0	–
NSAID (+) B Ch(-)	21/31	67.7	n.s.
T Ch (+) B Ch(+)	5/12	41.6	–
T Ch (+), B Ch(-)	2/27	7.4	<0.05
SMB Ch(+), B Ch(+)	2/ 2	100.0	–
SMB Ch(+), B Ch(-)	0/ 5	0	<0.05
Asa Ch (+), B Ch(+)	2/ 3	66.6	–
Asa Ch (+), B Ch(-)	1/ 3	33.3	<0.05

* Chi-square test. NSAID: Non steroidal anti-inflammatory drugs. T Ch: Tartrazine challenge. B Ch: Benzoate challenge. SMB: Metabisulfite challenge. Asa Ch: Aspirin challenge. n.s.: not significant.

Benzoate Challenges

Challenges with sodium benzoate were performed in 46 patients. Positive responses occurred in 15 (32.6%). There were no associations with whether the patient was male or female, atopic, or had previous reactions to NSAIDs. Again, an increased reaction rate to benzoate was observed in patients who also reacted to tartrazine and metabisulfite (P < 0.05) (Table IV). Responses to benzoate were observed in 60% of patients with chronic urticaria/angioedema (3/5), in 38% of those with chronic urticaria (8/21), in 40% of patients with acute urticaria/angioedema (2/5), in 25% of patients with anaphylactoid reactions (1/4), and in 9% of patients with chronic angioedema (1/11).

Metabisulfite Challenges

16 patients were challenged with sodium metabisulfite. Only two patients (12.5%) presented urticarial manifestations, as shown in Table V. There was no clear relationship to sex, atopy, or history of NSAID intolerance. As already mentioned, a positive reaction to metabisulfite challenge occurred more often in patients with tartrazine and benzoate sensitivity. The 2 patients who reacted to metabisulfite had chronic urticaria, which gives a reaction rate of 33.3% (2/6), whereas metabisulfite challenges were negative in 3 patients with chronic angioedema, in 3 with acute urticaria/angioedema, in 2 with chronic urticaria/angioedema, and in 2 with idiopathic anaphylaxis.

Aspirin Challenges

25 patients were challenged with aspirin. 10 of them experienced adverse skin reactions after challenge (40%). These patients were not significantly different in regard to sex, presence of atopic diseases, nor did they evidence increased rates of reactions to tartrazine or benzoate, when compared to the subjects with negative aspirin challenges (Table VI). Positive challenges were seen in 3 out of 3 patients with chronic urticaria/angioedema (100%), in 3 out of 11 patients with chronic urticaria (27.2%), in 2 out of 5 patients with chronic angioedema (40%), in 1 out of 4 patients with acute urticaria (25%), and in 1 out of 2 patients with idiopathic anaphylaxis (50%).

Correlation Between Atopy and NSAID Sensitivity

We investigated the prevalence of NSAID sensitivity in atopic and non atopic patients in our study group. 36 out of 49 atopic patients were

Table 5. Results of Metabisulfite Challenges (n = 16).

	+/n	%	P value*
Number of positive challenges	2/16	12.5	–
Female	1/11	9.0	–
Male	1/ 5	20.0	n.s.
Atopic	0/ 2	0	–
Non Atopic	2/ 2	100.0	n.s.
NSAID(+), SMB Ch(+)	1/ 2	50.0	–
NSAID(+), SMB Ch(-)	6/14	42.8	n.s.
T Ch(+), SMB Ch(+)	1/ 2	50.0	–
T Ch(+), SMB Ch(-)	1/11	9.0	<0.05
B Ch(+), SMB Ch(+)	2/ 2	100.0	–
B Ch(+), SMB Ch(-)	0/ 5	0	<0.05

*Chi-square test. NSAID: Non steroidal anti-inflammatory drugs. T Ch: Tartrazine challenge. B Ch: Benzoate challenge. SMB Ch: Metabisulfite challenge. n.s.: not significant

Table 6. Results of Aspirin Challenges (n = 25).

	+/n	%	p value*
Number of positive challenges	10 / 25	40.0	–
Female	8 / 17	47.0	–
Male	2 / 8	25.0	n.s.
Atopic	7 / 10	70.0	–
Non atopic	6 / 15	40.0	n.s.
T Ch(+), Asa Ch(+)	1 / 4	25.0	–
T Ch(+), Asa Ch(–)	1 / 8	12.5	n.s.
B Ch(+), Asa Ch(+)	2 / 2	100.0	–
B Ch(+), Asa Ch(–)	0 / 2	0	<0.05

*Chi-square test. T Ch: Tartrazine challenge. Asa Ch: Aspirin challenge. B Ch: Benzoate challenge. n.s.: not significant.

sensitive to NSAID (73.4%), whereas 22 out of 49 non atopic individuals were NSAID sensitive (44.8%). As shown in Figure 1, this difference was statistically significant, which means that NSAID sensitivity was more prevalent in atopic subjects.

Results of Additive Challenges in Young Patients

We analyzed separately the results of food additive and aspirin challenges in our group of patients 3 to 18 years old, in order to find out if there were any differences with older ages. This young subject group included 27 patients, 20 female and 7 male. Average age was 9.44 ± 4.5 years. 17 of them (62.9%) were atopic. Clinical diagnosis was chronic urticaria in 11 patients, chronic angioedema in 6, chronic urticaria/angioedema in 5, acute urticaria in 3, and acute urticaria/angioedema in 2. Sensitivity to NSAID was present in 14 out of the 27 children

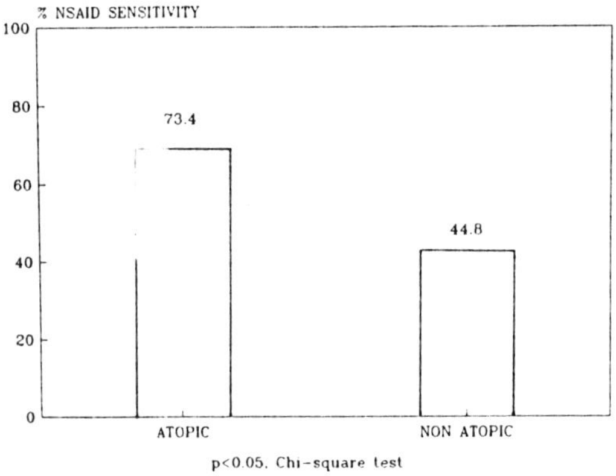

Figur 1. Correlation between atopy and NSAID sensitivity. ($p < 0.05$. Chi-square test)

and adolescents (51.8%). Challenge results for this group are presented in Figure 2, and were as follows: 8 of the 27 challenges were positive to any one of the additives (29.6%). Out of 17 tartrazine challenges, 4 were positive (23.5%); of 9 benzoate challenges, 4 were positive (44.4%); out of 2 metabisulfite challenges, none resulted positive (0%); and of 6 aspirin challenges, 4 resulted positive (66.6%). As depicted in Figure 2, there were no statistically significant differences between children and adults in regard to prevalence of atopy or NSAID sensitivity, but the overall rate of positive challenges to any of the additives, to tartrazine, benzoate or aspirin, were significantly higher in children than in adults, whereas the reaction rate to metabisulfite was significantly lower in children.

Discussion

The prevalence of pseudoallergic reactions to food and drug additives in the general population has not been determined, since there are very few reports on the subject. Young et al. found a rate of 0.026% in a survey of 18,582 persons (13). A Danish study reported 0.1% and a paper from the European Economic Community gave a rate of 0.03 to 0.5% (14). In the present study, which included 98 patients, 136 food additive challenges and 25 aspirin

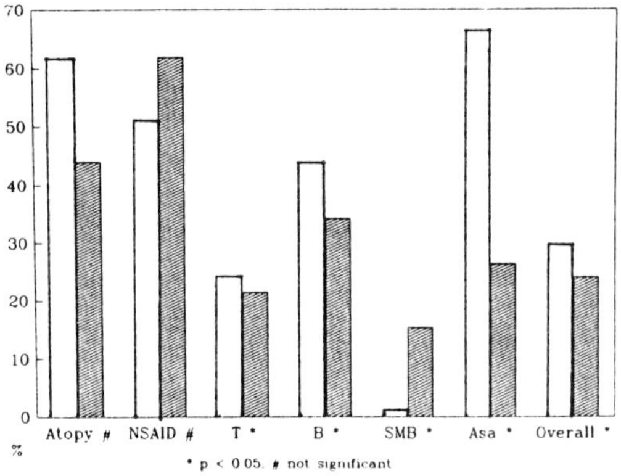

Figur 2. Comparison of challegende patients according to age □ Children ▨ Adults Tartrazine B Benzoate SMB Metabisulfite Asa Aspirin
(* $p < 0.005$. # not significant).

challenges, the number of individuals who reacted at least to one of the additives was 29, which gives a reaction rate of 29.6% in this selected group.

A few studies on the prevalence of tartrazine sensitivity in different patient subsets have been published. The general population prevalence is unknown, although rates of 1:1,000 to 1:100,000 have been mentioned. In aspirin sensitive patients, percentages between 15 to 100% of tartrazine sensitivity were initially proposed, but more recent studies from Stevenson and coworkers found only one tartrazine-sensitive patient out of 24 aspirin-sensitive patients (1). In the present study we found that 1/4 (25%) of patients with positive aspirin challenges also had positive tartrazine challenges, and in patients with NSAID sensitivity (as derived from medical history of past reactions to NSAIDs) the tartrazine reaction rate was 62.5% (Table III), although tartrazine positive challenges were not statistically more frequent in patients with positive or negative history. These results are much higher than the ones reported by Stevenson.

The prevalence of reactions to food or drug additives in patients with chronic urticaria and angioedema is also unknown (7). Stevenson et al. reported a 4% reaction rate to tartrazine in chronic idiopathic urticaria/angioedema (1), since only one out of 24 patients had positive challenges. In 9 studies reviewed by Stevenson, 8 to 100% of patients with chronic urticaria/angioedema reacted to tartrazine, but most of these studies were not controlled (1). In our group of patients, selected according to the presence of previous reactions to NSAIDs or a history suggestive of additive sensitivity, we observed an overall reaction rate of 22.4% (13/58) to tartrazine in patients with chronic urticaria, chronic angioedema, or both.

Sodium benzoate has been mentioned as an exacerbating factor in less than 10% of patients with chronic urticaria (7). There is another report, from Sweden, which found that 11% of the cases of chronic urticaria were related to benzoate ingestion (15). We challenged 46 patients and obtained 15 positive responses (32.6%) (Table IV). 12 of those positive challenges were present in 37 patients suffering chronic urticaria/angioedema (32.4%). There was no correlation between benzoate sensitivity and sex, atopy or previous adverse reaction to NSAIDs.

In the case of sulfites, there have been isolated case reports of urticaria and angioedema attributed to sulfites contained in foods. However, the investigators from Scripps Clinics could not find any positive reaction in 25 patients challenged with sulfites. We observed only 2 patients out of 16 challenges (12.5%), who reacted to blind challenges with sodium metabisulfite. Both patients were not atopic, had chronic urticaria, and one of them had previous history of NSAID sensitivity (Table V).

Only 25 of our patients were challenged with aspirin, and 10 positive responses were obtained (40%). Aspirin sensitivity was not associated with sex, presence of atopic diseases, reactivity to tartrazine, benzoate or metabisulfite (Table VI). However, when we compared the overall NSAID sensitivity, including patients with positive NSAID adverse reaction history and those with positive aspirin challenges, there was an increased rate of NSAID reactions in atopic patients (Figure 1).

Another issue which is worthy of further discussion is the correlation found between reactions to challenges with the three different additives. We observed a correlation between positive reactions to tartrazine with positive reactions to benzoate and metabisulfite. Benzoate positive challenges also correlated with positive reactions to metabisulfite (Tables III, IV, and V). There was no correlation between aspirin positive challenges and sensitivity to tartrazine, and in the case of benzoate the number of patients challenged is too low to draw any conclusions (Table VI). Ros et al. found a significant association between sensitivity to benzoate, azo dyes and aspirin (16).

In regard to the young patient population, some authors have suggested that tartrazine intolerance is rare in children (17). There are very few published studies about food additive sensitivity in children. One by Supramaniam and Warner, who selected for challenge children who improved their chronic urticaria symptoms through an additive-free diet, found 25.5% positive tartrazine challenges, 14.8% benzoate challenges, 8.3% metabisulfite challenges, 2,3% aspirin challenges, and overall additive reactivity of 55.8% (3). These results differ from ours, with the exception of tartrazine sensitivity rate, which is quite similar. Interestingly, although these authors mentioned that atopy was not frequent in their patients (only 11.6% of patients had positive immediate-type skin tests), all of their atopic patients gave positive additive challenges mainly to tartrazine. In fact, all positive challenges to tartrazine occurred in atopic patients.

From our results we conclude: (A) Overall additive sensitivity (to tartrazine, benzoate, and metabisulfite) in patients with chronic urticaria/angioedema was found in 26.9%. (B) Tartrazine sensitivity in patients with chronic urticaria/angioedema was found in 22.4%; benzoate sensitivity in those patients was observed in 32.4%; metabisulfite sensitivity presented in 18.1% and aspirin sensitivity in 42.1%. (C) There is an increased rate of NSAID intolerance, but not of additive intolerance, in atopic patients. (D) Patients sensitive to tartrazine have an increased risk of reactions to benzoate and metabisulfite, and patients sensitive to benzoate also have increased risk for metabisulfite sensitivity. (E) Tartrazine, benzoate and aspirin sensitivity was more prevalent in children than in adults, but metabisulfite sensitivity occurred more frequently in adults. Thus: Food additive intolerance in patients with chronic urticaria/angioedema may be more prevalent than previously recognized.

References

1. Stevenson, D.D., Simon, R.A., Lumry, W.R., and Mathison, D.A. 1986. Adverse reactions to tartrazine. J. Allergy Clin. Immunol. 78:182.
2. Simon, R.A. 1984. Adverse reactions to drug additives. J. Allergy Clin. Immunol. 74:623.
3. Supramaniam, G., and Warner, J.O. 1986. Artificial food additive intolerance in patients with angio-oedema and urticaria. Lancet 2:907.
4. Stevenson, D.D., and Simon, R.A. 1981. Sensitivity to ingested metabisulfites in asthmatic subjects. J. Allergy Clin. Immunol. 68:26.
5. Settipane, G.A., Chafee, H., Postman, M., and Levine, M.I. 1976. Significance of tartrazine sensitivity in chronic urticaria of unknown etiology. J. Allergy Clin. Immunol. 57:541.
6. Simon, R.A. 1986. Adverse reactions to food additives. N. Engl. Reg. Allergy Proc. 7:533.
7. Simon, R.A. 1989. Adverse reactions to food and drug additives. In: Progress in allergy and clinical immunology. W.J. Pichler, B.M. Stadler, C.A. Dahinden, A.R. Pecoud, P. Frei, C.H. Schneider, A.L. de Weck, eds. Toronto: Hogrefe & Huber Publishers, p. 467.
8. Lessof, M.H., Murdoch, R.D., Pollock, I., and Young, E. 1989. Intolerance to food and food additives. In: Progress in allergy and clinical immunology. W.J. Pichler, B.M. Stadler, C.A. Dahinden, A.R. Pecoud, P. Frei, C.H. Schneider, A.L. de Weck, eds. Toronto: Hogrefe & Huber Publishers, p. 353.
9. Thune, P., and Granholt, A. 1975. Provocation tests with antiphlogistic and food additives in recurrent urticaria. Dermatologica 151: 360.
10. Michaelsson, G., and Juhlin, L. 1973. Urticaria induced by preservatives and dye additives in food and drugs. Br. J. Dermatol. 88:525.
11: Schneider, A.T., and Codispoti, A.J. 1988. Allergic reactions to food additives. In: Food allergy. A practical approach to diagnosis and management. L.T. Chiaramonte, A.T. Schneider, F. Lifshitz, eds. New York: Marcel Dekker, p. 117.
12. Doeglas, H.M.G. 1975. Reactions to aspirin and food additives in patients with chronic urticaria, including the physical urticarias. Br. J. Dermatol. 93:135.
13. Young, E., Patel, S., Stoneham, M., Rona, R., and Wilkinson, J.D. 1987. The prevalence of reaction to food additives in a survey population. J. Roy. Coll. Phys. 21:241.
14. Moneret-Vautrin, D.A. 1986. Food antigens and additives. J. Allergy Clin. Immunol. 78:1039.
15. Juhlin, L. 1981. Recurrent urticaria: Clinical investigation of 330 patients. Br. J. Dermatol. 104:369.
16. Ros, A.M., Juhlin, L., and Michaelsson, G. 1976. A follow-up study of patients with recurrent urticaria and hypersensitivity to aspirin, benzoates and azo dyes. Br. J. Dermatol. 95:19.
17. Mathews, K.P. 1980. Management of urticaria and angioedema. J. Allergy Clin. Immunol. 66:347.

Sulfite Additives Causing Allergic or Pseudoallergic Reactions

Brunello Wüthrich*

Sulfiting agents are widely used in the food and beverage industry as well as in many pharmaceutical preparations as preservatives and antioxidants. It is well recognized that sulfites can induce a wide range of anaphylactoid reactions, including urticaria, asthmatic attacks and anaphylaxis in sensitive individuals, mainly in an asthmatic population. No one single pathogenetic mechanism is responsible for sulfite-induced reactions. An IgE-mediated hypersensitivity reaction may occur in a few patients. A reflex bronchoconstriction to sulfur dioxide by stimulating irritant receptors in asthmatics with bronchial hyperreactivity is well known. A third possible mechanism involves sulfite oxidase deficiency. The diagnosis of sulfite-sensitivity is based on placebo-controlled oral provocation tests with either capsules, neutral solutions or acid solutions of metabisulfite. Besides the avoidance of sulfited foods and drugs, prophylaxis with cromolyn sodium may be useful in asthmatics.

Sulfur dioxide and a variety of sulfiting agents such as sodium or potassium sulfite, bisulfite or metabisulfite (Table I) are widely used in the food and beverage industry as sanitizers for containers and fermentation equipment, and in many foods and beverages as preservatives to prevent spoilage by controlling bacterial growth, and as antioxidants for the prevention of browning of fruits, vegetables and seafoods (Table II). In addition, sulfites are used in the pharmaceutical industry in many preparations acting parenterally, orally, by inhalation or by topical application (1,2,3).

Table I. Classification of sulfites

Sulfur dioxide	SO_2	E 220
Sulfites (SO_3^-)	Na_2SO_3	E 221
	Ca SO_3	E 226
Bisulfites (HSO_3^-)	Na HSO_3	E 222
Metabisulfites or	Na S_2 O_5	E 223
Disulfites (S_2O_5)	K_2 S_2 O_5	E 224

E: European code

Table II. Foods and beverages commonly preserved with sulfur dioxide and/or sulfites

Wines, beers and other fermented beverages.
Cider and wine vinegars, pickled vegetables.
Salads, mushrooms, avocado.
Shrimps and other seafoods.
Dried and packaged fruits and vegetables.
Potatoes: frozed, peeled, dried, baked, fried, chips.
Processed, preserved food and beverages.

Since the first descriptions in 1973–1977 (4,5,6), it is well recognized that sulfites can induce a wide range of anaphylactoid reactions, including itching, flush, urticaria, angioedema, nasal congestion, laryngeal oedema, diarrhea, abdominal pain, headache and more often life-threatening asthmatic attacks (7,8,9,10). Several cases of anaphylaxis have been described in patients who were eating restaurant meals with extremely high levels of sulfites such as at salad bars (11,12). The FDA has received reports of at least 12 deaths that may be associated with sulfited restaurant foods up to 1986 (13). There are case reports of adverse reactions to sulfites in foods from several investigators in several different countries (14–21), and a number of studies conducted with double-blind controlled challenge tests (22). Food handlers may react to sulfites with a contact eczematous reaction, usually of the hands (23), while asthmatics can experience anything from mild wheezing to severe asthmatic episodes following ingestion of sulfite-containing foods. The exact prevalence of sulfite sensitivity in the normal population is not known. Reports from different groups indicate that 2–5% of asthmatics in the United States may be sulfite sensitive (24,25,26,27). The following case history of a patient seen recently at our allergy unit is a typical example of such a sensitivity reaction to sulfites.

* Allergy Unit, Department of Dermatology, University Hospital, Zurich, Switzerland.

Case History

A 36-year old dental hygienist with a 5 year history of bronchial asthma and rhinitis of the intrinsic type, but without aspirin intolerance, experienced a generalized itching, the feeling of heat, redness in the face, swelling of the lips, tachycardia and chest tightness while she was eating a salad in the canteen of the dental institute of the university. This meal consisted of cottage cheese, tomatoes, cucumbers, carrots, beans and pineapples with an Italian dressing and tea. She reported that she had had three similar episodes in the past and that she noted the appearance of asthma and rhinitis after alcoholic beverages. Skin and RAST tests were negative for inhalants, foodstuffs and additives as well as an oral provocation test with benzoic acid (total 400 mg). A placebo-controlled oral challenge test with sodium metabisulfite in capsules was performed in a single-blind fashion, beginning with the dose of 1 mg. The challenge was positive after 25 mg with a decrease in FEV1 of 24% (Fig. 1). In addition the patient complained of blockage of the nose, feeling of heat, redness in the palms and shortness of breath. The final diagnosis was: "Restaurant syndrome with an anaphylactoid reaction due to sulfite sensitivity; intrinsic asthma and rhinitis without aspirin and benzoic acid intolerance."

Pathogenesis of Reactions to Sulfites

Whatever the chemical structure or route of administration, sulfites come in contact with acidic salivary, bronchial or gastric secretions, promoting the generation of sulfur dioxide (27) (Fig. 2). In addition, sulfite radicals may be absorbed through the sublingual or bronchial mucosa and act as haptens. It is well established that sulfur dioxide, even inhaled or taken orally in solution, is a powerful irritant to the bronchial tree, probably by stimulating irritant receptors. The reactivity to inhaled sulfur dioxide in asthmatic patients likely correlates with the degree of underlying bronchial hyperreactivity. Sulfur dioxide is believed to produce bronchoconstriction through cholinergic reflex mechanisms. Effectively, it has been shown that atropine can block the airway response to challenge with sulfiting agents (28). However, this mechanism, which is likely to explain the asthmatic attacks, cannot be the cause of anaphylactoid reactions, including urticaria, angioedema and shock, so a mechanism associated with mast cells or basophil activation is likely to be involved. Few sensitive individuals, not necessarily atopics, exhibited positive scratch, prick or intracutaneous tests to sulfite solutions at 10 mg/ml or at 0.1 mg/ml, suggesting an IgE-mediated mechanism (10,21,29,

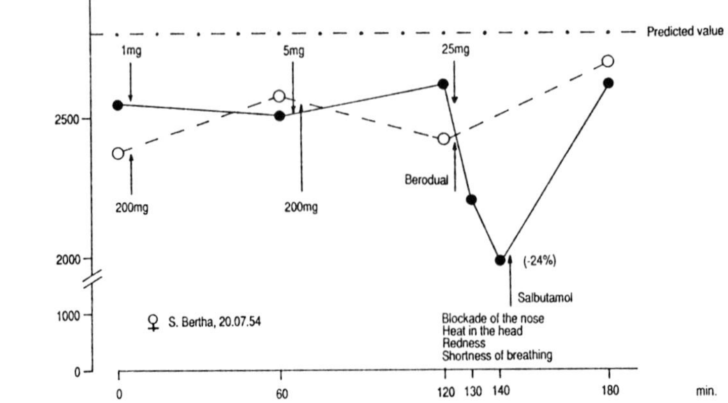

Fig. 1. Positive challenge test with natrium disulfite (natrium metabisulfite) capsules at a dosage of 25 mg. Negative challenge with benzoic acid.

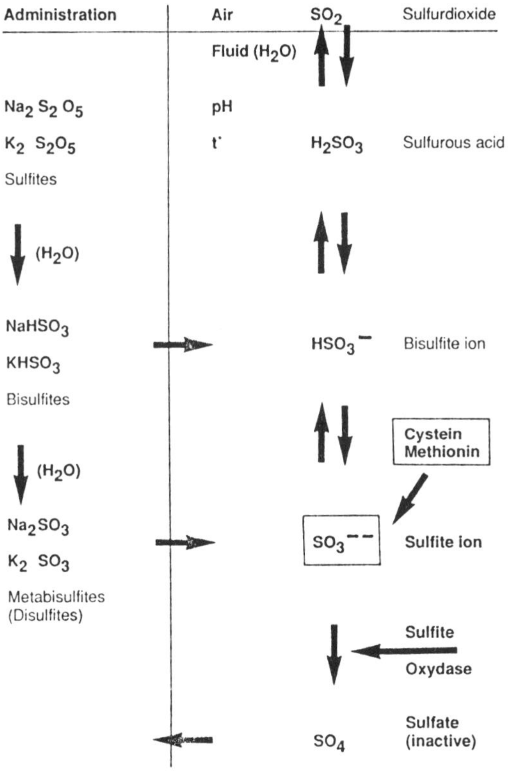

Fig. 2. Metabolism of sulfites.

30,31). A nonspecific histamine release can be excluded, as normal persons and the majority of sulfite-sensitive patients failed to react to skin testing. With the sera from sulfite-sensitive individuals a passive transfer of skin reactivity has been successful (30,31). Moreover, the effect was abolished by heating the sera to 56°C for 30 minutes, which suggested the presence of thermolabile reaginic antibodies. However, to date, specific IgE to sulfites itself or in conjugated form have not been demonstrated with the RAST technique. Recently, a dose-response curve of metabisulfite-induced basophil histamine release could be demonstrated in a non-asthmatic patient with urticaria and angioedema following provocative challenge with sodium metabisulfite (10). It seems accurate to state that, although probably rare, IgE-mediated sulfite sensitivity does exist (10).

Finally, a deficiency in the enzyme sulfite oxidase, which metabolizes sulfates to inactive sulfaces, has been proposed as a possible mechanism for the adverse reactions (32) (Fig. 2). During the metabolism of sulfur containing amino-acids, such as methionine and cysteine, significant amounts of sulfite (up to 1000 mg/day) are produced but are rapidly and completely oxidized by the sulfite oxidase. Jacobsen and Simon (33) found six subjects who had decreased sulfite oxidase activity in skin fibroblasts compared to normal controls. After considerable exogenous exposure to sulfites in polluted air, foods and drugs, the levels of the enzyme would be insufficient, so that some sulfite radicals are available to provoke asthma via tracheobronchial reflexes or via activation of mast cells or basophils. Further investigations must be conducted to confirm this hypothesis.

Diagnosis of Sulfite-Sensitivity

The diagnosis of sulfite sensitivity can be suspected after a history of adverse reactions to foods which are likely to be preserved by sulfites, i.e., wine or prepacked meals. Skin prick, scratch or intracutaneous tests can identifiy some individuals with a probable IgE-mediated mechanism, particularly if an anaphylactic reaction with urticaria and angioedema is reported. Provocative challenge tests under standardized conditions with measurement of pulmonary function in properly prepared patients with stable asthma and under intensive-care are the only effective methods to establish diagnosis. Patients can be challenged with either capsules, neutral solutions, or acid solutions of metabisulfite, according to published protocols (Tables III and IV) (34,35). A single-

Table III. Capsule and neutral-solution metabisulfite challenge

- Administer placebo (powdered sucrose) in capsule form. Measure FEV1.
- Administer capsules containing 1, 5, 25, 50, 100 and 200 mg of potassium metabisulfite at 30-minute intervals. Measure FEV1 30 minutes after administering each dose and if the patient becomes symptomatic.
- If no response, administer 1, 10 and 25 mg of potassium metabisulfite in water-sucrose solution at 30-minute intervals. Measure FEV1 30 minutes after each dose and if symptoms occur. Positive response is indicated by a decrease in FEV1 of 20% or more.

(after Bush et al. [34]).

Table IV. Acid-solution metabisulfite challenge

– Dissolve 0,1 mg of potassium metabisulfite in 20 ml of a sulfite-free lemonade crystal solution. Have the patient swish the solution around for 10 to 15 seconds, then swallow.
– Measure FEV1 10 minutes after the first dose. Then, administer 0.5, 1, 5, 10, 15, 25, 50, 75, 100, 150 and 200 mg per 20 ml of the solution at ten minute intervals. Measure FEV1 10 minutes after each incremental increase in dose. Positive response is signified by a decrease in FEV1 of 20% or more.

(after Bush et al. [34])

blind provocation test with placebo and sulfite additives is enough for diagnosis in daily allergological practice. It was shown that these provocation tests with sulfites are highly reproducible regarding results (positive or negative), although the threshold provocative dose can vary with the passage of time (10). The double-blind procedure as a golden standard is only needed for scientific purposes, as repeated challenges pose significant risks for the patient.

In our unit 245 placebo-controlled oral single-blind challenges with sodium disulfite in capsules (1,5,20,50–100–200 mg) have been performed in patients with a suspected history of sulfite-sensitivity. Fifty-seven challenges were positive (15%) with a great variety of objective and subjective symptoms (Table V). The cumulative dose which elicited reactions varied from 5 mg up to 350 mg. Two of the 15 positive asthmatics reacted with a life-threatening status asthmaticus after doses of 12.5 and 50 mg (Fig. 3). Only one of the disulfite-positive patients had an aspirin intolerance.

Management of Sulfite-Sensitive Patients

Avoidance of sulfiting agents in food and drugs is the objective therapy, but because of the ubiquitous nature of this food additive such avoidance is often difficult, especially when eating in a restaurant and also when travelling. In Europe sulfite additives are coded, in conformance with the European list, from E 220 to E 226 (Table I), but in each country the legislation concerning the declaration of additives contained in foods and drugs is quite variable. In Switzerland sulfite containing foods must be labeled if they contain more than 20 mg $S0_2$ per kg or per liter. Wines are excluded from declaration, although one liter of wine may contain up to 250 mg sulfite. It has been estimated that eating foods prepared at home without drinking beer or wine would lead to ingestion of only 2 to 3 mg/day of sulfites (normal people tolerate a dose of 400 mg sulfites/day during 3 weeks without side-effects), but a restaurant meal with seafoods, potatoes and preserved salads can contain 25 to 250 mg, not including the amount in alcoholic beverages. In the USA in August 1986, the FDA banned the use of sulfites in any foods served as fresh in restaurants (13,36). Currently, the highest levels can be found in dry fruits (such as apricots), potatoes, wine, and some seafoods. Processed foods with more than trace amounts of sulfites (10 ppm $S0_2$) must have sulfite-containing labels on package materials. Wine bottled after January, 1988, must also bear a label with a sulfite inscription. FDA regulations concerning sulfite use in potatoes remains pending (36).

All patients with a diagnosis of sulfite-sensitivity who have experienced a severe reaction should carry with them emergency medication, including a metered-dose Epinephrin-Inhaler and an Epinephrin-Injection (Adrenaline), despite its sulfite preservative (9,27,34). In case of mild bronchospastic reactions to inhaled sulfur dioxide a prophylactic treatment with a vagolytic agent (28), e.g. Atrovent (Ipratropium bromide), may be useful. Recently, in a pilot study conducted at the National Jewish Center in Denver it was shown that the administration of cromolyn sodium (20 mg) prior to metabisulfite challenge markedly attenuated

Table V. Oral challenges with metabisulfate in capsules, 5 to 200 mg Dosis

Diagnosis	N=245	Positive n = 57	15.00%
Asthma	87	15	17.25%
Extrinsic	36	7	19.40%
Intrinsic	51	8	15.70%
Urticaria/ Angioedema	99	17	17.20%
Rhinitis	38	7	18.40%
Local anesthetic reactions	21	5	24.00%

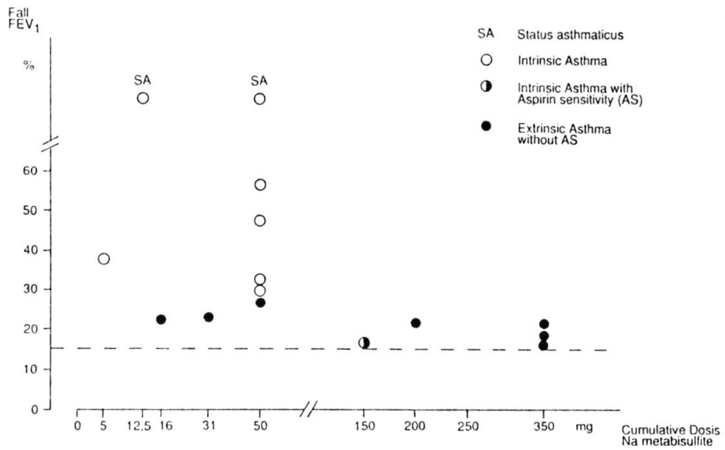

Fig. 3. Fall of the FEV1 in % of the initial value and thresold cumulative dose of natrium metabisulfites in 15 asthmatics with positive challenge test.

the bronchoconstrictive response in nine of ten patients (37). In one patient the initial positive challenge with metabisulfite was followed on different days by placebo challenge, without reaction, then by metabisulfite after treatment with cromolyn, but no significant bronchoconstriction occurred, and finally by another challenge with metabisulfite which was again positive. So in this patient a desensitization effect of repeated tests does not explain the protective effect of cromolyn, a mast cell stabilizing agent. Other studies have suggested that the protective effect of cromolyn in sulfite-sensitive asthmatics may be dose-related (38,39). In a case of sulfite-induced urticaria the oral administration of cromolyn (400 mg) 30 minutes before the challenge with 25 mg potassium metabisulfite failed, however, to give protection (40). Other studies will be necessary to confirm cromolyn's effect on metabisulfite-induced adverse reactions.

References

1. Koepke, J.W., Selner, J.C., and Dunhill, A.L. 1983. Presence of sulfur dioxide in commonly used bronchodilator solutions. J. Allergy Clin. Immunol. 72:504.
2. Kolly, M., Pécoud, A., and Frei, P.C. 1989. Additives contained in drug formulations most frequently prescribed in Switzerland. Ann. Allergy 62:21.
3. Fisher, A.A. 1989. Urticaria, asthma, and anaphylaxis due to sodium sulfite in an antifungal cream complicated by treatment with aminophylline in an ethylenediamine-senstive person. Cutis 44:19.
4. Kochen, J. 1973. Sulfur dioxide, a respiratory tract irritant even if ingested. Pediatrics 52:145.
5. Prenner, B.M., and Stevens, J.J. 1976. Anaphylaxis after ingestion of sodium bisulfite. Ann. Allergy 37:180.
6. Freedman, B.J. 1977. Asthma induced by sulphur dioxide, benzoate and tartrazine contained in orange drinks. Clin. Allergy 7: 407.
7. Stevenson, D.D., and Simon, R.A. 1981. Sensitivity to ingested metabisulfites in asthmatic subjects. J. Allergy Clin. Immunol. 68:26.
8. Jamieson, D.M., Guill, M.F., Wray, B.B., and May, R.J. 1985. Metabisulfite sensitivity: Case report and literature review. Ann. Allergy 54:115.
9. Simon, R.A. 1986. Sulfite sensitivity. Ann. Allergy 56:281.
10. Sokol, W.N., and Hydick, I.B. 1990. Nasal congestion, urticaria, and angioedema caused by an IgE-mediated reaction to sodium metabisulfite. Ann. Allergy 65:233.
11. Settipane, G.A. 1987. The restaurant syndrome. N. Engl. Reg. Allergy Proc. 8:39.
12. Howland, W.C., and Simon, R.A. 1989. Sulfite-treated lettuce challenges in sulfite-sensitive subjects with asthma. J. Allergy Clin. Immunol. 83:1079.
13. Food and drug administration. Sulfiting agents: Revocation of GRAS status for use on fruits and vegetables intended to be served or sold raw to consumers. Final rule. Fed. Reg. 1986. 51:25012.
14. Carmona, J.G.B., and Picon, S.J. 1987. Asma por sensibilizacion a sulfitos. Rev. Esp. Alergol. Inmunol. Clin. 2:23.

15. Boner, A.L., Guarise, A., Vallone, G., et al. 1990. Metabisulfite orale challenge: Incidence of adverse responses in chronic childhood asthma and its relationship with bronchial hyperreactivity. J. Allergy Clin. Immunol. 85:479.
16. Drouet, M., Sabbah, A., Le Sellin, J., et al. 1990. Syndrome de Fernand Widal et intolérance aux sulfites. Problèmes thérapeutiques en général et ORL en particulier. Allergie et Immunologie 22:91.
17. Hong, S.P., Park, H.S., Lee, M.K., and Hong, C.S. 1989. Oral provocation tests with aspirin and food additives in asthmatic patients. Yonsei Med. J. 30:339.
18. Kleinhans, D., and Galinsky, T. 1982. Zur möglichen Provokation eines Bronchialasthmas und einer Urtikaria durch Natriumdisulfit. Zwei Fallbeobachtungen. Allergologie 5:120.
19. Nichol, G.M., Nix, A., Chung, K.F., and Barnes, P.J. 1989. Characterisation of bronchoconstrictor response to sodium metabisulphite aerosol in atopic subjects with and without asthma. Thorax 44:1009.
20. Van Bever, H.P., Docx, M., and Stevens, W.J. 1989. Food and food additives in severe atopic dermatitis. Allergy 44:588.
21. Wüthrich, B., and Huwyler, T. 1989. Das Disulfit-Asthma. Schweiz. med. Wschr. 119:1177.
22. Simon, R.A. 1989. Sulfite challenge for the diagnosis of sensitivity. Allergy Proc. 10:357.
23. Fisher, A.A. 1989. Reactions to sulfites in foods: Delayed eczematous and immediate urticarial, anaphylactoid, and asthmatic reactions. Cutis 44:187.
24. Simon, R.A., Green, L., and Stevenson, D.D. 1982. The incidence of metabisulfite sensitivity in an asthmatic population. J. Allergy Clin. Immunol. 69:118 (Abstract).
25. Buckley, C.E., Saltzmann, H.A., and Sicker, H.O. 1985. The prevalence and degree of sensitivity to ingested sulfites. J. Allergy Clin. Immunol. 77:144 (Abstract).
26. Bush, R.K., Taylor, S.L., Holden, K., et al. 1986. Prevalence of sensitivity to sulfiting agents in asthmatic patients. Am. J. Med. 81:816.
27. Nicklas, R.A. 1989. Sulfites: A review with emphasis on biochemistry and clinical application. Allergy Proc. 10:349.
28. Simon, R.A., Goldgar, G., and Jacobsen, D. 1984. Blocking studies in sulfite sensitive asthmatics. J. Allergy Clin. Immunol. 73:136.
29. Twarog, F.J., and Leung, D.Y.M. 1982. Anaphylaxis to a component of isoetharine (sodium bisulfite). J. Am. med. Ass. 248:2030.
30. Yang, W.H., Purchase, E.C.R., and Rivington, R.N. 1986. Positive skin tests and Prausnitz-Küstner reactions in metabisulfite-senstive subjects. J. Allergy Clin. Immunol. 78:443.
31. Boxer, M.B., Bush, R.K., and Harris, K.E. 1988. The laboratory evaluation of IgE antibody to metabisulfites in patients skin test positive to metabisulfites. J. Allergy Clin. Immunol. 78:443.
32. Stevenson, D.D., and Simon, R.A. 1984. Sulfites and asthma (Editorial). J. Allergy Clin. Immunol. 74:469.
33. Jacobsen, D.W., Simon, R.A., and Singh, M. 1984. Sulfite-oxidase deficiency and cobalamine protection in sulfite-sensitive asthmatics. J. Allergy Clin. Immunol. 73:135.
34. Bush, R.K., Zoratti, E., and Taylor, S.L. 1990. Diagnosis of sulfite and aspirin sensitivity. Clin. Reviews in Allergy 8:159.
35. Simon, R.A. 1989. Sulfite challenge for the diagnosis of sensitivity. Allergy Proc. 10:357.
36. Simon, R.A. 1989. Adverse reaction to food and drug additives. In: Progress in allergy and clinical immunology. W.J. Pichler, B.M. Stadler, C.A. Dahinden, A.R. Pécoud, P. Frei, C.H. Schneider, eds. Hans Lewiston, NY: Huber Publishers, p. 467.
37. McClellan, M.D., Wanger, J.S., and Cherniack, R.M. 1990. Attenuation of the metabisulfite-induced bronchoconstrictive response by pretreatment with cromolyn. Chest 97:826.
38. Koenig, J.Q., Marshall, S.G., van Belle, G., et al. 1988. Therapeutic range cromolyn dose-response inhibition and complete obliteration of SO_2-induced bronchoconstriction in atopic adolescents. J. Allergy Clin. Immunol. 81:897.
39. Myers, D.J., Bigby, B.G., and Boushey, H.A. 1986. The inhibition of sulfur dioxide-induced bronchoconstriction in asthmatic subjects by cromolyn is dose dependent. Am. Rev. Respir. Dis. 133:1150.
40. Belchi, J., Florido, J.F., and Estrada, J.L., et al. 1991. Sulfite-induced urticaria. Schweiz. med. Wschr. 121, Suppl. 40/II:93.

Section XI

Mediator Release and its Modulation

Structural Characterization of Secretory Granule Neutral Proteases in Mouse and Human Mast Cells

H. Patrick McNeil, K. Frank Austen*

In similarity to other hematopoietic cells such as lymphocytes and tissue macrophages, mast cells of human and rodent origin are heterogeneous, with at least two distinct subclasses definable based upon tissue distribution, histochemical staining properties, and biochemical characteristics of protein and lipid components (1). In rodents, mast cells found in association with blood vessels in loose connective tissue, such as in skin and skeletal muscle, and in the peritoneal fluid (serosal mast cells: SMC) are termed connective tissue mast cells (CTMC), whereas those situated in the intestinal lamina propria are termed mucosal mast cells (MMC). MMC characteristically increase dramatically during helminth infection of mice or rats, in response to $CD4^+$ T-lymphocyte derived cytokines (2). In contrast, CTMC are considered to be at a stage independent of T-cell products. Two types of human mast cells have also been described immunochemically by the presence in the secretory granules of either tryptase alone (MC^T) or both tryptase and chymase (MC^{TC}). Although MC^T and MC^{TC} may not be exactly analogous to the rodent MMC and CTMC respectively, there are a number of common features including a similar tissue distribution of the two subclasses (1,3). Of the many biologically active compounds produced by mast cells, the secretory granule proteases appear to be cell specific products, although cytotoxic T-lymphocytes contain a related but distinct set of enzymes. Human tryptase has been used as an immunohistological mast cell specific marker (4), and as a measure of mast cell activation in allergic diseases (5). While the function of mast cell proteases remains uncertain, their abundance (50% of total cellular protein) and cellular specificity argue for an important biological role.

Neutral Proteases in Mouse Mast Cells

Of all species examined thus far, the proteases in mouse mast cells have been characterized most extensively. Mast cell proteases can be divided into three categories: serine proteases of either (i) chymotryptic- or (ii) tryptic-like substrate specificities (chymases and tryptases respectively), and (iii) a carboxypeptidase-A which cleaves C-terminal aromatic or aliphatic amino acids. At least six serine proteases, termed mouse mast cell protease (MMCP) -1 to -6 have been identified by complete or N-terminal amino acid sequencing of purified proteins (6). Based on a comparison to the pancreatic proteases, MMCP-1 to -5 are chymases, whereas MMCP-6 is a tryptase. MMCP-1 was the first chymase purified biochemically from MMC enriched intestines of Trichinella spiralis infected mice (7). The complete amino acid sequence of the mature enzyme was determined (8), and recently the gene encoding this enzyme has been cloned (9). The N-terminal amino acid sequences of MMCP-2 to -6 were determined by analysis of the respective proteins purified from secretory granules of Kirsten sarcoma virus-transformed mast cells (KiSV-MC) and SMC (6). The N-terminal sequence in MMCP-2 was very similar to the rat MMC protease, rat mast cell protease (RMCP)-2 (10), and cDNAs encoding MMCP-2 were isolated from a KiSV-MC cDNA library using the rat basophilic leukemia cell-derived RMCP-2 cDNA as a probe (11). In addition, cDNAs encoding MMCP-4 (12), MMCP-5 (13), MMCP-6 (14), and mast cell carboxypeptidase-A (MC-CPA) (15), have been isolated using degenerate oligonucleotides designed from knowledge of the N-terminal amino acid

* Department of Medicine, Harvard Medical School, and Department of Rheumatology and Immunology, Brigham and Women's Hospital, Boston, MA 02115, USA.
Acknowledgements: This work was supported in part by Grants AI-22531, HL-36110 and RR-05950 from the National Institutes of Health, and in part by a grant from the Hyde and Watson Foundation.

sequences of the respective enzymes. In each case, the complete structure of the proteases has been deduced from the nucleotide sequence of the consensus cDNAs. The genes encoding MMCP-1 (9), MMCP-2 (43), MMCP-4 (12), MMCP-5 (13), and MMCP-6 (14), have also been isolated and characterized. Two other related genes (an MMCP-4 like gene designated MMCP-L (12), and a MMCP-5 pseudogene [44]), have been identified in the mouse genome, indicating the diversity of this gene family. Apart from variations in intron length, the genomic organization of the chymase genes is identical to that of other members of the hematopoietic cell granule protease superfamily which includes neutrophil cathepsin G (16), and the cytolytic T-lymphocyte chymases (17). However, the MMCP-6 gene displays a distinct genomic structure, possessing an additional intron between the transcription initiation and translation initiation codons (14).

The cloning of these mouse mast cell protease genes has enabled studies to determine the expression of each protease mRNA in the different mast cell subsets with a sensitivity that has not been possible with immunochemical techniques used in the rat and human systems (Table I). Despite significant homologies between the protease genes, it has been possible to prepare gene-specific cDNA fragments of each protease cDNA. Using these probes, it has been found that CTMC (as represented by SMC) express mRNA for MC-CPA, the chymases MMCP-4 and MMCP-5, and the tryptase MMCP-6. SMC also contain MMCP-3 protein. In contrast, MMC contain MMCP-1, and express mRNA for the chymase, MMCP-2. By RNA blot analysis, MMC also contain a transcript(s) reacting with probes for MMCP-4 and MMCP-L (12). However, it has recently been found that these probes exhibit 85% and 80% homology respectively with the analogous nucleotide sequence in MMCP-1 (9), and it is possible that the hybridization seen with the MMCP-4 and MMCP-L probes in parasitic infected intestinal RNA may be due to the MMCP-1 transcript. Thus, no protease identified to date is definitively present in both subclasses of mature mast cells. MMC do not express MC-CPA, or the tryptase MMCP-6, although the possibility of MMC expressing an additional uncharacterized mouse tryptase should be considered.

The protease probes have also proved useful in examining the differentiation of mast cell subtypes from bone marrow progenitors. The differentiation/maturation of mast cells is thought to occur as a result of exposure of progenitor cells to combinations of cytokines, initially in the bone marrow, and subsequently in various tissue microenvironments. At least six cytokines, active in mast cell differentiation and

Table I. Expression of secretory granule proteases in mouse and human mast cells.

	MOUSE MAST CELLS			HUMAN MAST CELLS	
PROTEASE	BMMC	MMC	SMC	MC^{T}	MC^{TC}
(A) Mouse Proteases					
MMCP-1	–	+	–		
MMCP-2	–	+	–		
MMCP-3	?	?	+		
MMCP-4	–	–	+		
MMCP-5	+	–	+		
MMCP-6	+	–	+		
MC-CPA	+	–	+		
(B) Human Proteases*					
Skin Chymase				–	+
Skin Tryptase				–	+
Lung Tryptase				+	–
MC-CPA				–	+

* Data for expression of human proteases in each subclass is tentative.

growth, have been defined, including the $CD4^+$ T-cell derived factors IL-3 (18), IL-4 (19), IL-9 (20), and IL-10 (21), and the fibroblast products c-kit ligand (22), and nerve growth factor (23). Mast cells also produce many of these cytokines (24), suggesting possible autocrine stimulation of mast cell growth. When mouse bone marrow cells are cultured *in vitro* in the presence of IL-3, or stimulated T-lymphocyte conditioned media, an apparently homogeneous population of bone marrow-derived mast cells (BMMC) is obtained (25). BMMC are immature cells, possessing small granules which contain low amounts of histamine and neutral protease activities. However, BMMC are able to differentiate into either MMC or CTMC when injected into mast cell deficient $WBB6F_1$-W/W^v mice (26). By RNA blot analysis, BMMC express abundant quantities of mRNAs encoding MC-CPA, the chymase, MMCP-5, and the tryptase, MMCP-6 (13). Thus, although similar by histochemical and biochemical characteristics, BMMC are not *in vitro* equivalents of MMC. Furthermore, when BMMC differentiate into MMC, the genes encoding MC-CPA, MMCP-5, and MMCP-6 must be suppressed, and those for MMCP-1 and MMCP-2 induced. Preliminary evidence suggests that cytokine IL-10 may be at least partially instrumental in this gene regulation (27). Since BMMC acquire CTMC characteristics when cocultured with mouse 3T3 fibroblasts, the fibroblast derived cytokines c-kit ligand (28), and nerve growth factor are likely to operate to induce expression of MMCP-3 and MMCP-4. These studies also indicate that the MC-CPA, MMCP-5 and MMCP-6 genes are expressed early in mast cell development, whereas the MMCP-1, MMCP-2, and MMCP-4 chymase genes are expressed later, possibly in the tissue microenvironment. This cytokine-induced regulation of protease gene expression is likely to occur through the control of DNA-binding proteins present in the nucleus of mouse mast cells. Recently, BMMC, KiSV-MC, and SMC have been shown to express all three members of the GATA DNA-binding protein family (29). Furthermore, activation of a proximal promoter in the mouse MC-CPA gene was found to be regulated by GATA binding proteins (29). The GATA binding motif is also present in the 5′-flanking regions of many of the mast cell protease genes identified so far, suggesting a possible role in transcriptional regulation of these genes. Additionally, a DNA sequence identified as an enhancer region in pancreatic proteases (30), and in RMCP-2 (31), is present in the 5′-flanking of the MMCP-1, MMCP-4 and MMCP-5 (45) genes. This motif is not present in the tryptase gene, but a 44 base pair sequence present in the MMCP-6 gene 5′-flanking is highly conserved in an equivalent region of the human skin tryptase gene, indicating the possibility of this representing a tryptase specific regulatory region (14).

In addition to exploring questions of gene expression and regulation, the cloning of the mouse mast cell proteases has provided detailed information about the structure of these enzymes without the need to purify the proteins biochemically. All the neutral proteases are synthesized as preproenzymes, with hydrophobic signal peptides of between 15 to 19 amino acids which are predicted to be cleaved in the endoplasmic reticulum, and activation peptides of 94 amino acids in MC-CPA, 10 amino acids in MMCP-6 and acidic dipeptides in the chymases MMCP-1, -2, -4, and -5. Activation of pro-MMCP-6 to the mature enzyme requires cleavage of a Gly-Ile bond in similarity to the dog and human tryptases, whereas the chymases and MC-CPA are activated by cleavage of a Glu-Ile bond. The prepro-peptides in MMCP-1, MMCP-2, and MMCP-4 are identical, but distinctly different from that in MMCP-5 which more closely resembles the sequence in dog mastocytoma chymase. In addition, the activation dipeptide in MMCP-5 consists of a Gly-Glu sequence compared to a Glu-Glu which is found in all other rodent mast cell chymases. This, and a number of other novel structural features (see below) indicate that MMCP-5 represents a distinct subset from the other mouse mast cell chymases. Examination of the predicted amino acids forming the substrate binding domains of the mast cell chymases indicates that most containa Ser^{176} residue (analogous to the Ser^{189} in chymotrypsin which confers specificity for cleavage of amino acids with aromatic side chains), although MMCP-1 and MMCP-5 possess a Thr and Asn respectively at this site. MMCP-5 also contains a novel Val^{199} in an otherwise highly conserved region of the substrate binding region (Table II). MMCP-6 possesses an Asp^{188} analogous to Asp^{189} in trypsin which is the critical substrate binding residue for cleavage of peptide bonds at basic amino acid residues. Analysis of the amino acid

Table II. Activation peptides and amino acid residues forming the substrate binding cleft of mast cell chymases

Chymase	Activation Peptide	Amino Acid Residues Forming the Substrate Binding Cleft (176)	(197–199)	(207)
MMCP-1	Glu-Glu	Thr	Ser-Tyr-Gly	Ala
MMCP-2	Glu-Glu	Ser	Ser-Tyr-Glu	Ala
MMCP-4	Glu-Glu	Ser	Ser-Tyr-Gly	Ala
MMCP-5	Gly-Glu	Asn	Ser-Tyr-Val	Ala
RMCP-1	ND	Ser	Ser-Tyr-Gly	Ala
RMCP-2	Glu-Glu	Ala	Ser-Tyr-Gly	Ala
Dog Chymase	Glu-Glu	Ser	Ser-Tyr-Gly	Ala
Hum Skin Chymase	Gly-Glu	Ser	Ser-Tyr-Gly	Alaq

ND: not determined

content of each protease indicates the chymases MMCP-1 and MMCP-2 are weakly basic at neutral pH whereas MMCP-4, MMCP-5 and MC-CPA are strongly basic with net charges of +12 to +17. This is consistent with the association of the latter proteases with heparin proteoglycans forming a macromolecular complex in the secretory granules of CTMC, whereas MMCP-1 and MMCP-2 appear to be less tightly bound to the chondroitin sulfate proteoglycans present in MMC. The tryptase MMCP-6 is on the other hand weakly acidic at neutral pH.

Neutral Proteases in Human Mast Cells

Human mast cells contain the same three classes of proteases in their secretory granules as described above in the mouse. A human MC-CPA has been purified from skin and the N-terminal amino acid sequence was found to be nearly identical to mouse MC-CPA (32). Because of this homology, cDNAs were isolated encoding human MC-CPA by screening a human lung cDNA library with the mouse cDNA (33). The human gene has also been isolated and extensively characterized (34).

A cDNA encoding human lung tryptase was isolated using anti-tryptase antibodies to screen a cDNA expression library (35), and more recently cDNAs distinct from lung tryptase were cloned from human skin using a dog tryptase cDNA as a probe (36). These skin tryptase cDNAs exhibited some variability which most likely is due to allelic variations, although there is some evidence that they represent the products of separate genes. The gene encoding one of these cDNAs has also been isolated, and exhibits an identical intron/exon organization to the mouse and dog tryptase genes (36). Although anti-tryptase antibodies are reactive with both MC^{T} and MC^{TC} cells, it is not clear which of the two tryptases identified above is contained in each cell subtype. The use of in situ hybridization with probes specific for each cDNA would allow this question to be addressed.

There is evidence for at least two chymases in human mast cells. Human skin chymase has been purified, the N-terminal amino acid sequence determined (37), and the enzyme has been localized to skin MC^{TC} cells by immunohistology (3). In addition to skin chymase, it appears that human skin mast cells contain a 'cathepsin G-like' enzyme which has not been further characterized (37). Since the N-terminal amino acid sequence of skin chymase exhibited considerable homology with the corresponding sequence of dog mastocytoma chymase, the dog cDNA was used as a probe to isolate the gene encoding human skin chymase from a genomic library (38). The deduced amino acid sequence of human skin chymase exhibits considerable homology with dog chymase (83%) and with MMCP-5 (75%) but much less similarity to the other rodent chymases (54–61%), suggesting MMCP-5 is the mouse analogue of human skin chymase. Interestingly, both human skin chymase and MMCP-5 possess the unusual Gly-Glu activation peptide, compared to a Glu-Glu dipeptide present in other rodent and dog chymases. The presence of skin chymase in MC^{TC} adds further support to the idea that these are the human equivalent of mouse CTMC which express MMCP-5. MC^{TC} cells also contain human MC-CPA (39), analogous to the distribution of mouse MC-CPA in murine CTMC. The isolation and N-terminal amino acid sequencing of a chymase from human heart which exhibited striking amino acid homology with human skin chymase (40), raised the possibility that this enzyme represented an additional mast cell chymase. However, the recent cloning of this enzyme indicates it to be identical to human skin mast cell chymase (41), although cellular localization has yet to be determined.

Genomic DNA blot analysis using a human skin chymase probe indicates the presence in the human genome of at least one additional homologous gene (38). As noted above, although mast cell heterogeneity in human mast cells has been defined using antibodies raised against human tryptase, skin chymase, and human MC-CPA, the degree of heterogeneity may have been underestimated by analogy with the diversity present in mouse mast cells. Further cloning of human mast cell chymases should enable this question to be addressed, by the use of in situ hybridization, protease specific anti-peptide antibodies, and further developments in the *in vitro* culture of human mast cells (42).

Conclusions and Future Considerations

Recent advances using molecular biology and *in vitro* cell culture systems, have expanded our understanding of the diversity and structural characteristics of secretory granule neutral proteases in mast cells of both mouse and human origin. The cloning of these protease genes will allow studies aimed at delineating the cellular mechanisms which regulate transcriptional control of expression of the respective mRNAs. The availability of cDNA probes to investigate cytokine induced gene regulation represents a major advance in achieving this aim. The greatest gap in our knowledge of mast cell proteases is their physiologic role, and the protein substrates which they act upon. The use of the protease cDNAs in prokaryotic and eukaryotic expression systems to produce recombinant enzymes, will facilitate these studies and also provide the capability to specifically mutate the proteins at critical sites. Elucidation of the function of the mast cell neutral proteases will no doubt unravel further the role of these cells in various inflammatory disease states.

References

1. Irani, A.M., and Schwartz, L.B. 1989. Mast cell heterogeneity. Clin. Exp. Allergy. 19:143.
2. Enerback, L. 1986. Mast cell heterogeneity: The evolution of the concept of a specific mucosal mast cell. In: Mast cell differentiation and heterogeneity. A.D. Befus, J. Bienenstock, and D.A. Denburg, eds. New York: Raven Press, p. 1.
3. Irani, A.A., Schechter, N.M., Craig, S.S., DeBlois, G., and Schwartz, L.B. 1986. Two types of human mast cells that have distinct neutral protease compositions. Proc. Natl. Acad. Sci. USA. 83:4464.
4. Schwartz, L.B. 1985. Monoclonal antibodies against human mast cell tryptase demonstrate shared antigenic sites on subunits of tryptase and selective localization of the enzyme to mast cells. J. Immunol. 134:526.
5. Schwartz, L.B., Metcalfe, D.D., Miller, J., Earl, H., and Sullivan, T. 1987. Tryptase levels as an indicator of mast cell activation in systemic anaphylaxis and mastocytosis. N. Engl. J. Med. 316:1622.
6. Reynolds, D.S., Stevens, R.L., Lane, W.S., Carr, M.H., Austen, K.F., and Serafin, W.E. 1990. Different mouse mast cell populations express various combinations of at least six distinct mast cell serine proteases. Proc. Natl. Acad. Sci. USA 87:3230.
7. Newlands, G.F.J., Gibson, S., Knox, D.P., Grencis, R., Wakelin, D., and Miller, H.R.P. 1987. Characterization and mast cell origin of a chymotrypsin-like proteinase isolated from intestines of mice infected with Trichinella spiralis. Immunology 62:629..
8. LeTrong, H., Newlands, G.F.J., Miller, H.R.P., Charbonneau, H., Neurath, H., and Woodbury, R.G. 1989. Amino acid sequence of a mouse mucosal mast cell protease. Biochemistry 28:391.
9. Huang, R., Blom, T., and Hellman, L. 1991. Cloning and structural analysis of MMCP-1, MMCP-4 and MMCP-5, three mouse mast cell

specific serine proteases. Eur. J. Immunol. 21:1611.
10. Benfey, P.N., Yin, F.H., and Leder, P. 1987. Cloning of the mast cell protease, RMCP II. J. Biol. Chem. 262:5377.
11. Serafin, W.E., Reynolds, D.S., Rogelj, S., Lane, W.S., Conder, G.A., Johnson, S.S., Austen, K.F., and Stevens, R.L. 1990. Identification and molecular cloning of a novel mouse mucosal mast cell serine protease. J. Biol. Chem. 265:423.
12. Serafin, W.E., Sullivan, T.P., Conder, G.A., Ebrahimi, A., Marcham, P., Johnson, S.S., Austen, K.F., and Reynolds, D.S. 1991. Cloning of the cDNA and gene for mouse mast cell protease 4. J. Biol. Chem. 266:1934.
13. McNeil, H.P., Austen, K.F., Somerville, L.L., Gurish, M.F., and Stevens, R.L. 1991. Molecular cloning of the mouse mast cell protease 5 gene. J. Biol. Chem. 266:20316.
14. Reynolds, D.S., Gurley, D.S., Austen, K.F., and Serafin, W.E. 1991. Cloning of the cDNA and gene of mouse mast cell protease 6. J. Biol. Chem. 266:3847.
15. Reynolds, D.S., Stevens, R.L., Gurley, D.S., Lane, W.S., Austen, K.F., and Serafin, W.E. 1989. Isolation and molecular cloning of mast cell carboxypeptidase A. J. Biol. Chem. 264:20094.
16. Hohn, P.A., Popescu, N.C., Hanson, R.D., Salvesen, G., and Ley, T.J. 1989. Genomic organization and chromosomal localization of the human cathepsin G gene. J. Biol. Chem. 264:13412.
17. Lobe, C.G., Upton, C., Duggan, B., Ehrman, N., Letellier, M., Bell, J., McFadden, G., and Bleackley, R.C. 1988. Organization of two genes encoding cytotoxic T lymphocyte specific serine proteases CCPI and CCPII. Biochemistry 27:6941.
18. Rennick, D., Lee, F., Yokota, T., Arai, K., Cantor, H., and Nabel, G. 1985. A cloned MCGF cDNA encodes a multilineage hematopoietic growth factor: Multiple activities of interleukin 3. J. Immunol. 134:910.
19. Smith, C., and Rennick, D. 1986. Characterization of a murine lymphokine distinct from interleukin 2 and interleukin 3 (IL-3) possessing a T-cell growth factor activity and a mast cell growth factor activity that synergizes with IL-3. Proc. Natl. Acad. Sci. USA. 83:1857
20. Hultner, L., Druez, C., Moeller, J., Uyttenhove, C., Schmitt, E., Rude, E., Dormer, P., and Van Snick, J. 1990. Mast cell growth enhancing activity (MEA) is structurally related and functionally identical to the novel mouse T cell growth factor P40/TCGFIII (interleukin 9). Eur. J. Immunol. 20:1413.
21. Thompson-Snipes, L., Dhar, V., Bond, M.W., Mosmann, T.R., Moore, K.W., and Rennick, D.M. 1991. Interleukin 10: A novel stimulatory factor for mast cells and their progenitors. J. Exp. Med. 173:507.
22. Nocka, K., Buck, J., Levi, E., and Besmer, P. 1990. Candidate ligand for the c-kit transmembrane kinase receptor: KL, a fibroblast derived growth factor stimulates mast cells and erythroid progenitors. EMBO J. 9:3287.
23. Matsuda, H., Kannan, Y., Ushio, H., Kiso, Y., Kanemoto, T., Suzuki, H., and Kitamura, Y. 1991. Nerve growth factor induces development of connective tissue type mast cells in *vitro* from murine bone marrow cells. J. Exp. Med. 174:7.
24. Gordon, J.R., Burd, P.R., and Galli, S.J. 1990. Mast cells as a source of multifunctional cytokines. Immunology Today 11:458.
25. Razin, E., Stevens, R.L., Akiyama, F., Schmid, K., and Austen, K.F. 1982. Culture from mouse bone marrow of a subclass of mast cells possessing a distinct chondroitin sulfate proteoglycan with glycosaminoglycans rich in N-acetylgalactosamine-4-6-disulfate. J. Biol. Chem. 257:7229.
26. Nakano, T., Sonoda, T., Hayashi, C., Yamatodani, A., Kanayama, Y., Yanamura, T., Asai, H., Yonezawa, T., Kitamura, Y., and Galli, S.J. 1985. Fate of bone marrow derived cultured mast cells after intracutaneous, intraperitoneal, and intravenous transfer into genetically mast cell deficient W/Wv mice. J. Exp. Med. 162:1025.
27. Ghildyal, N., McNeil, H.P., Gurish, M.F., Austen, K.F., and Stevens, R.L. 1992. Transcriptional regulation of the mucosal mast cell protease, MMCP-2 by interleukin 10 and interleukin 3. J. Biol. Chem., in press.
28. Gurish, M.F., Ghildyal, N., McNeil, H.P., Austen, K.F., Gillis, S., and Stevens, R.L. 1992. Differential expression of secretory granule proteases in mouse mast cells exposed to interleukin 3 and c-kit ligand. J. Exp. Med., in press.
29. Zon, L.I., Gurish, M.F., Stevens, R.L., Mather, C., Reynolds, D., Austen, K.F., and Orkin, S.H. 1991. GATA binding transcription factors present in mast cells regulate the promoter of the mast cell carboxypeptidase A gene. J. Biol. Chem. 266:22948..
30. Boulet, A.M., Erwin, C.R., and Rutter, W.J. 1986. Cell specific enhancers in the rat ex-

ocrine pancreas. Proc. Natl. Acad. Sci. USA 83:3599.
31. Sarid, J., Benfey, P.N., and Leder, P. 1989. The mast cell specific expression of a protease gene, RMCP II, is regulated by an enhancer element that binds specifically to mast cell transacting factors. J. Biol. Chem. 264:1022.
32. Goldstein, S.M., Kaempfer, C.E., Kealey, J.T., and Wintroub, B.U. 1989. Human mast cell carboxypeptidase. purification and characterization. J. Clin. Invest. 83:1630.
33. Reynolds, D.S., Gurley, D.S. Stevens, R.L., Sugarbaker, D.J., Austen, K.F., and Serafin, W.E. 1989. Cloning of cDNAs that encode human mast cell carboxypeptidase A, and comparison of the protein with mouse mast cell carboxypeptidase A and rat pancreatic carboxypeptidases. Proc. Natl. Acad. Sci. USA 86:9480.
34. Reynolds, D.S., Gurley, D.S., and Austen, K.F. 1992. Cloning and characterization of the novel gene for mast cell carboxypeptidase A. J. Clin. Invest. 89:273.
35. Miller, J.S., Westin, E.H., and Schwartz, L.B. 1989. Cloning and characterization of complementary DNA for human tryptase. J. Clin. Invest.84:1188.
36. Vanderslice, P., Ballinger, S.M., Tam, E.K., Goldstein, S.M., Craik, C.S., and Caughey, G.H. 1990. Human mast cell tryptase: Multiple cDNAs and genes reveal a multigene serine protease family. Proc. Natl. Acad. Sci. USA 87:3811.
37. Schechter, N.M., Irani, A.M., Sprows, J.L., Abernethy, J., Wintroub, B., and Schwartz, L.B. 1990. Identification of a cathepsin G-like proteinase in the MC^{TC} type of human mast cell. J. Immunol. 45:2652.
38. Caughey, G.H., Zerweck, E.H., and Vanderslice, P. 1991. Structure, chromosomal assignment, and deduced amino acid sequence of a human gene for mast cell chymase. J. Biol. Chem. 266:12956.
39. Irani, AM.A., Goldstein, S.M., Wintroub, B.U., Bradford, T., and Schwartz, L.B. 1991. Human mast cell carboxypeptidase. Selective localization to MC^{TC} cells. J.Immunol. 147:247
40. Urata, H., Kinoshita, A., Misono, K.S., Bumpus, F.M., and Husain, A. 1990. Identification of a highly specific chymase as the major angiotensin II forming enzyme in the human heart. J. Biol. Chem. 265:22348.
41. Urata, H., Kinoshita, A., Perez, D.M., Misono, K.S., Bumpus, F.M., Graham, R.M., and Husain, A. 1991. Cloning of the gene and cDNA for human heart chymase. J. Biol. Chem. 266:17173.
42. Furitsu, T., Saito, H., Dvorak, A.M., Schwartz, L.B., Irani, A.M.A., Burdick, J.F., Ishizaka, K., and Ishizaka, T. 1989. Development of human mast cells *in vitro*. Proc. Natl. Acad. Sci. USA 86:10039.
43. Gurish, M.F., Austen K.F., and Stevens R.L. Unpublished results.
44. McNeil, H.P., Austen, K.F., and Stevens, R.L. Unpublished results.
45. McNeil, H.P., Austen, K.F., and Stevens, R.L. Unpublished results.

Tyrosine Phosphorylation Coupled to IgE Receptor-Mediated Signal Transduction and Histamine Release

Reuben P. Siraganian*, Marc Benhamou*, Volker Stephan*, Jorge S. Gutkind**, Keith C. Robbins**

Cross-linking of FcεRI (for all abbreviations, see below) in rat basophilic leukemia (RBL-2H3) cells resulted in tyrosine phosphorylation of several proteins, the most prominent having an M_r of 72 kDa (pp72). Tyrosine phosphorylation was rapid, detectable 15 sec after stimulation and correlated with both the time-course and antigen dose for histamine release. Reversal of FcεRI crosslinking stopped histamine release and caused a rapid loss of pp72 tyrosine phosphorylation. The receptor-mediated pp72 tyrosine phosphorylation was still induced in the absence of calcium in the medium. There was no pp72 tyrosine phosphorylation by protein kinase C activation with phorbol 12-myristate 13-acetate. Similarly, the calcium-ionophore A23187 induced histamine release in the absence of pp72 tyrosine phosphorylation. The activation of G proteins by 3 different methods resulted in phosphatidylinositol hydrolysis and histamine release but not in pp72 tyrosine phosphorylation. Therefore, pp72 tyrosine phosphorylation was not induced by G protein activation or as a consequence of phosphatidylinositol hydrolysis. The tyrosine kinase inhibitor genistein decreased in parallel antigen-induced tyrosine phosphorylation of pp72 and histamine release but did not inhibit phosphatidylinositol hydrolysis. Therefore tyrosine phosphorylation of pp72 is functionally linked to FcεRI-mediated signal transduction leading to histamine release. Furthermore, pp72 tyrosine phosphorylation represents a distinct, independent signalling pathway induced specifically by aggregation of the FcεRI.

Aggregation of the high affinity IgE receptor (FcεRI) on mast cells, basophils, and related cultured cell lines such as rat basophilic leukemia cells (RBL-2H3 cells), initiates a number of biochemical events leading to cell degranulation (1–4). These include increased phospholipase C (PI-PLC) activity resulting in phosphatydylinositol (PtdIns) hydrolysis, stimulation of phospholipase A2 and D, a rise in intracellular free calcium concentration ($[Ca^{2+}]i$), increased calcium influx into the cell and membrane depolarization. Activation of PI-PLC results in generation of inositol-1,4,5-trisphosphate and 1,2-diacylglycerol, that induce, respectively, the release of intracellular calcium and the activation of protein kinase C (PKC) (5,6). These secondary messengers are thought to initiate a cascade of biochemical events leading to the release of histamine and other mediators from RBL-2H3 cells. FcεRI activation may regulate intracellular second messengers through intermediate guanine nucleotide-binding (G) proteins (7,8). The stimulation of G proteins by guanosine 5′-[γ-thio]triphosphate (GTPγS) or aluminum fluoride complexes results in PtdIns hydrolysis and histamine release. However, none of these events can totally account for the degranulation signal (9).

Protein-tyrosine kinases of the receptor class mediate cell growth responses to environmental signals such as epidermal growth factor and platelet-derived growth factor (10,11). However, tyrosine phosphorylation by non-receptor class of tyrosine kinase may play a role in other biological events in the cell; for example, de-

* Laboratory of Immunology
** Laboratory of Cellular Development and Oncology, National Institute of Dental Research, National Institutes of Health, Bethesda, MD 20892, USA.

The abbreviations used are: RBL-2H3, rat basophilic leukemia 2H3 cell line; FcεRI, the high-affinity receptor for immunoglobulin E; m3-mAchR, human subtype-3 muscarinic acetylcholine receptor; GTPγ, guanosine 5′-(3-O-thio) triphosphate; $[Ca^{2+}]_i$, concentration of intracellular free calcium; PKC, protein kinase C; PMA, phorbolmyristate acetate; PI-PLC, phosphatydylinositol-specific phospholipase C; PtdIns, phosphatidylinositol., granulation by fully differentiated cells such as platelets (12), neutrophils (13) and chromaffin cells (14,15). We therefore initiated a series of studies to explore the role of tyrosine phosphorylation in the process of histamine release from basophils.

In the present experiments RBL-2H3 cells cultured as previously described, were sensitized with mouse hybridoma IgE and stimulated to secrete by specific antigen or anti-FcεRI specific antibodies (16,17). Histamine released was measured and the corresponding cell pellets were analyzed for protein-tyrosine phosphorylations. In some experiments, cells were stimulated in the absence of external calcium. The cell pellets were lysed, proteins were fractionated by SDS-PAGE and electrotransferred to nitrocellulose sheets. Phosphorylated proteins were detected using anti-phosphotyrosine antibodies (18, 35,36).

FcεRI-Aggregation and Protein Tyrosine Phosphorylations

There was tyrosine phosphorylation of several proteins in lysates from IgE-sensitized cells stimulated with antigen. The most prominent phosphoprotein had a relative molecular mass of 72 kDa (pp72). Additional but fainter bands were observed at 38, 57, 62,77, 110 and 130 kDa. In contrast, IgE or antigen alone failed to induce tyrosine phosphorylation. As an independent means of activating the FcεRI, RBL-2H3 cells were incubated with the anti-FcεRI monoclonal antibody BC4 in the absence of IgE or antigen. This also resulted in histamine release and a pattern of tyrosine phosphorylations similar to that observed in sensitized cells stimulated with antigen. These findings demonstrated that tyrosine phosphorylation was coupled to FcεRI activation and suggested that phosphorylation on tyrosine residues was involved in signal transduction leading to histamine release.

The relationship of FcεRI aggregation and tyrosine phosphorylation to histamine release was examined further in antigen dose-response and time-course experiments. The degree of tyrosine phosphorylation correlated with the extent of histamine release over a wide dose range of antigen. In time-course studies, FcεRI-aggregation induced tyrosine phosphorylation of pp72 was detectable as early as 15 sec after the addition of antigen. Band intensity peaked by 10-15 min and remained unchanged for another 30 min. The extent of histamine release correlated with the degree of tyrosine phosphorylation. Experiments demonstrated that protein tyrosine phosphorylation required continued receptor cross-linking. When the antigen-dependent bridging of FcεRI was disrupted by the addition of excess hapten, further histamine release ceased and tyrosine phosphorylation of pp72 was rapidly lost. Therefore tyrosine phosphorylation was an early event following FcεRI stimulation and was functionally linked to signal transduction leading to degranulation.

Relationship of pp72 Tyrosine Phosphorylation to PKC Activation

Activation of FcεRI in RBL-2H3 cells results in the hydrolysis of phosphatidylinositols with the release of inositol triphosphates, an increase in intracellular calcium and activation of protein kinase C (PKC). Direct activation of PKC by the addition of phorbol myristate acetate (PMA) to RBL-2H3 cultures does not induce exocytosis but potentiates the release of histamine induced by calcium ionophores (19,20). PMA treatment of RBL-2H3 cells did not induce histamine release or pp 72 tyrosine phosphorylation. Therefore, PKC does not directly activate tyrosine phosphorylation of this protein. In cells depleted of PKC by the overnight incubation with PMA, tyrosine phosphorylation of pp72 was still observed following FcεRI-mediated stimulation, although both tyrosine phosphorylation and histamine release were reduced approximately 50%. Therefore, the FcεRI-induced tyrosine phosphorylation of pp72 was not dependent on PKC, although PKC may play a role in modulating protein tyrosine phosphorylation and histamine release.

Effect of Calcium on FcεRI-Induced Tyrosine Phosphorylation

The calcium-ionophore A23187 induces degranulation in RBL-2H3 cells by a mechanism that circumvents the IgE receptor complex and results in an increase in intracellular calcium ([Ca2+]i). There was no pp72 tyrosine phosphorylation when cells were stimulated with ionophore to release histamine. Furthermore, stimulation with A23187 together with activation of PKC with PMA also failed to induce pp72 tyrosine phosphorylation. Therefore, FcεRI-mediated tyrosine phosphorylation of pp72 is not induced by a major rise in free cytosolic calcium in the presence or absence of PKC activation. Moreover, tyrosine phosphorylation of pp72 is coupled to functional FcεRI signaling but is independent of the exocytotic-process itself.

In the absence of extracellular calcium, no degranulation occurs from RBL-2H3 cells in response to FcεRI-mediated triggering, but minimal increases in [Ca2+]i have been observed (21,22). The kinetics and the extent of tyrosine phosphorylation were similar in the presence or absence of extracellular calcium. Therefore, increased intracellular calcium is neither sufficient nor required for the FcεRI dependent tyrosine phosphorylation of pp72.

Relationship of G Proteins and pp72 Phosphorylation

The next series of studies (35) investigated the relationships among FcεRI-mediated protein-tyrosine phosphorylation of pp72, activation of G proteins and PtdIns hydrolysis. Three different approaches were used to stimulate G proteins in RBL-2H3 cells. In the first strategy, RBL-2H3 cells were stimulated with AlF_4-complexes to activate phospholipase C and release histamine. Although there was 15-63% histamine release there was no detectable phosphorylation of pp72. In the second approach, RBL-2H3 cells were permeabilized with streptolysin O and stimulated to secrete with GTPγS. TheGTPγS is thought to stimulate G proteins, to increase PtdIns hydrolysis and release histamine (7,23,24). In permeabilized cells, both antigen-IgE and GTPγS caused PtdIns hydrolysis and histamine secretion. However, there was pp72 phosphorylation only following FcεRI-mediated cell activation. In a third type of experiment, G protein activation and protein tyrosine phosphorylation were studied in RBL-2H3 cells expressing the human m3-muscarinic receptor (m3-mAchR). Activation of the m3-mAchR in many cells results in PtdIns hydrolysis by coupling to a stimulatory G protein (25). RBL-2H3 cells do not have muscarinic receptors and do not secrete on the addition of carbachol. Using a retrovirus vector, two different cloned RBL-2H3 cell lines were isolated each expressing the m3-AchR. In both of these cell lines, crosslinking of FcεRI with antigen or activation of the m3-mAchR by carbachol induced dose-dependent PtdIns breakdown and histamine release. FcεRI but not muscarinic receptor stimulation caused strong tyrosine phosphorylation of pp72. Thus, activation of G proteins by a variety of different means resulted in increased PtdIns hydrolysis and the release of histamine without inducing tyrosine phosphorylation of pp72. Therefore G proteins activation and G protein mediated PtdIns hydrolysis alone are not sufficient to induce pp72 tyrosine phosphorylation.

Relationship of pp72 Tyrosine Phosphorylation and PtdIns Hydrolysis

To determine whether PtdIns hydrolysis was secondary to tyrosine phosphorylation of pp72, we investigated the effect of the tyrosine kinase inhibitor genistein on pp72 phosphorylation, hydrolysis of PtdIns and histamine release. This compound specifically inhibits tyrosine kinase activity but has only minimal effects on serine and threonine kinases (26). Genistein caused a dose-dependent inhibition of all tyrosine phosphorylated proteins including pp72 (IC_{50} = 34 μg genistein/ml) and in parallel inhibited histamine release up to 88% at a concentration of 100 μg/ml (IC_{50} = 31 μg genistein/ml).

Experiments also investigated the effect of genestein on both histamine release and PtdIns hydrolysis. Although there was dose dependent inhibition of histamine release, total PtdIns hydrolysis was minimally affected by genistein.

Only at the highest concentration of genistein (100 µg/ml) was there a moderate decrease ofPtdIns breakdown (18%), probably due to nonspecific effects. Similar results were obtained with genistein in antigen dose response experiments.

Activation of PI-PLC results in the generation of inositol 1,4,5-trisphosphate, which acts both as a secondary messenger to release intracellular calcium and plays a role in the influx of extracellular calcium. The pattern of inositol phosphates generated in RBL-2H3 cells, when analyzed by HPLC anion exchange chromatography, was very similar in the absence or presence of genistein. Although there were some minor changes in some of the other inositol phosphates, there was no inhibition in the generation of inositol-1,4,5-trisphosphate in the presence of genistein. In RBL-2H3 cells, phospholipase C activation can be detected as early as 5-10 s after antigen stimulation (27). However, there were no significant differences in the amount of inositol-1,4,5-trisphosphate generated in the absence or presence of 60 µg/ml genistein at any time-points studied. These findings demonstrate that pp72 tyrosine phosphorylation is unlikely to be the signal for antigen induced activation of PI-PLC since inhibition of tyrosine phosphorylation by genistein did not affect total PtdIns hydrolysis, nor did it inhibit the generation of the secondary messenger inositol 1,4,5-trisphosphate. Therefore, unlike a number of other receptor systems (e.g., T-cell receptor), the generation of inositol phosphates is not secondary to the activation of PI-PLC by tyrosine phosphorylation (28–30).

Tyrosine Phosphorylation of Other Proteins During Degranulation

Stimulation of cells by antigen or the calcium-ionophore A23187 led to tyrosine phosphorylation of a 110-kDa protein (pp110) whereas pp72 tyrosine phosphorylation was induced only by antigen triggering. The tyrosine phosphorylation of pp110 was also observed by carbachol activation of the cells expressing the G protein-coupled m3 muscarinic receptor. In contrast to the tyrosine phosphorylation of pp72, the antigen-induced pp110 tyrosine phosphorylation required extracellular calcium, was absent in cells depleted of protein kinase C and was detected between 1 and 5 min after stimulation. The protein-tyrosine kinase inhibitor genistein blocked both histamine release and tyrosine phosphorylations induced by A23187. Furthermore, protein kinase C activation induced pp110 tyrosine phosphorylation but not histamine release demonstrating that pp110 tyrosine phosphorylation alone is not sufficient for degranulation. Therefore, tyrosine phosphorylation of pp72 is associated with the early steps of IgE receptor-generated signalling, whereas pp110 tyrosine phosphorylation occurs secondary to calcium influx and to protein kinase C activation (36).

Discussion

Protein-tyrosine kinases or phosphatases could account for the increased phosphorylation of proteins following RBL-2H3 cell activation. Several protein-tyrosine kinases belonging to the SRC family are expressed in RBL-2H3 cells (18,35). It has recently been suggested that $p56^{lyn}$ is associated withthe FcεRI in RBL-2H3 cells and is activated following antigen stimulation (31). In addition, the protein-tyrosine phosphatase, CD45, is detectable at low levels in these cells (unpublished observations). The level of protein phosphorylation is due to the balance between protein tyrosine kinase and phosphatase activities within the cell (32,33). Therefore, changes in protein tyrosine phosphorylation could be due to an alteration in protein tyrosine phosphatase activity. We have recently observed that monoclonal antibodies against the protein tyrosine phosphatase CD45 specifically inhibit the FcεRI-mediated triggering of human basophils (34).

Model for Protein Tyrosine Phosphorylation Events

The present study provides a model for the events that are initiated by the crosslinking of the FcεRI. Aggregation of the receptor results in the increased tyrosine phosphorylation of pp72 as an early signal; in parallel there is activation of a PI-PLC pathway that results in the release of inositol phosphates, a rise in $[Ca^{2+}]i$, the influx of extracellular calcium and the activation of PKC. Tyrosine phosphorylation of pp72 is a FcεRI specific, distinct pathway, that is independent of previously described metabolic events. This event is important for histamine secretion as demonstrated by the parallel inhibition by genistein of protein tyrosine phosphorylation and cell degranulation. However, cell stimulation in the absence of extracellular calcium established that activation of the tyrosine phosphorylation pathway alone is not sufficient to induce degranulation. Therefore, tyrosine phosphorylation of pp72 is another component of the complex network of biochemical events initiated by aggregation of FcεRI that contribute to intracellular signalling. There is a second specific protein-tyrosine phosphorylation event in RBL-2H3 cells. The pp110 tyrosine phosphorylation was induced following stimulation by either FcεRI aggregation or A23187 and appears to be downstream of PKC activation. Tyrosine phosphorylation of pp110 required extracellular calcium and was induced by ionophore or PKC activation. Thus, pp110 phosphorylation was secondary to calcium influx, and PKC activation and may be required for secretion regardless of the pathway of cell activation.

References

1. Metzger, H., Alcaraz, G., Hohman, R., Kinet, J.P., Pribluda, V., and Quarto, R. 1986. The receptor with high affinity for immunoglobulin E. Annu. Rev. Immunol. 4:419.
2. Siraganian, R. P. 1988. Mast cells and basophils. In: Inflammation: Basic principles and clinical correlates. J.I. Gallin, I.M. Goldstein, and R. Snyderman, eds. New York: Raven, p. 513.
3. Beaven, M.A. and Cunha-Melo, J.R. 1988. Membrane phosphoinositide-activated signals in mast cells and basophils. Prog. Allergy 42:123.
4. Cunha-Melo, J.R., Dean, N.M., Moyer, J.D., Maeyama, K., and Beaven, M.A. 1987. The kinetics of phosphoinositide hydrolysis in rat basophilic leukemia (RBL-2H3) cells varies with the type of IgE receptor cross-linking agent used. J. Biol. Chem. 262:11455.
5. Oliver, J.M., Seagrave, J., Stump, R.F., Pfeiffer, J.R., and Deanin, G.G. 1988. Signal transduction and cellular response in RBL-2H3 mast cells. Prog. Allergy 42:185.
6. Nishizuka, Y. 1988. The molecular heterogeneity of protein kinase C and its implications for cellular regulation. Nature 334:661.
7. Ali, H., Collado-Escobar, D.M., and Beaven, M.A. 1989. The rise in concentration of free Ca^{2+} and of pH provides sequential, synergistic signals for secretion in antigen-stimulated rat basophilic leukemia (RBL-2H3) cells. J. Immunol. 143:2626.
8. Wilson, B.S., Deanin, G.G., Standefer, J.C., Vanderjagt, D., and Oliver, J.M. 1989. Depletion of guanine nucleotides with mycophenolic acid suppresses IgE receptor-mediated degranulation in rat basophilic leukemia cells. J. Immunol. 143:259.
9. Cunha-Melo, J.R., Gonzaga, H.M., Ali, H., Huang, F.L., Huang, K.P., and Beaven, M.A. 1989. Studies of protein kinase C in the rat basophilic leukemia (RBL-2H3) cell reveal that antigen-induced signals are not mimicked by the actions of phorbol myristate acetate and Ca^{2+} ionophore. J. Immunol. 143:2617.
10. Hunter, T., and Cooper, J.A. 1985. Protein-tyrosine kinases. Annu. Rev. Biochem. 54:897.
11. Ullrich, A., and Schlessinger, J. 1990. Signal transduction by receptors with tyrosine kinase activity. Cell 61:203.
12. Golden, A., and Brugge, J.S. 1989. Thrombin treatment induces rapid changes in tyrosine phosphorylation in platelets. Proc. Natl.Acad. Sci. U.S.A. 86:901.
13. Gutkind, J.S., and Robbins, K.C. 1989. Translocation of the FGR protein-tyrosine kinase as a consequence of neutrophil activation. Proc. Natl. Acad. Sci. U.S.A. 86:8783.
14. Parsons, S.J., and Creutz, C.E. 1986. p60c-src activity detected in the chromaffin granule membrane. Biochem. Biophys. Res. Commun. 134:736.
15. Grandori, C., and Hanafusa, H. 1988. p60c-src is complexed with a cellular protein in subcellular compartments involved in exocytosis. J. Cell Biol. 107:2125.
16. Barsumian, E.L., Isersky, C., Petrino, M.G., and Siraganian, R.P. 1981. IgE-induced histamine release from rat basophilic leukemia cell lines: Isolation of releasing and nonreleasing clones. Eur. J. Immunol. 11:317.
17. Basciano, L.K., Berenstein, E.H., Kmak, L., and Siraganian, R.P. 1986. Monoclonal antibodies that inhibit IgE binding.J. Biol. Chem. 261:11823.
18. Benhamou, M., Gutkind, J.S., Robbins, K.C., and Siraganian, R.P. 1990. Tyrosine phospho-

rylation coupled to IgE receptor-mediated signal transduction and histamine release. Proc. Natl. Acad. Sci. U.S.A. 87:5327.

19. Sagi-Eisenberg, R., Lieman, H., and Pecht, I. 1985. Protein kinase C regulation of the receptor-coupled calcium signal in histamine-secreting rat basophilic leukaemia cells. Nature 313:59.
20. White, K.N., and Metzger, H. 1988. Translocation of protein kinase C in rat basophilic leukemic cells induced by phorbol ester or by aggregation of IgE receptors. J. Immunol. 141:942.
21. Stump, R.F., Oliver, J.M., Jr., Cragoe, E.J., and Deanin, G.G. 1987. The control of mediator release from RBL-2H3 cells: Roles for Ca^{2+}, Na+, and protein kinase C1. J. Immunol. 139:881.
22. Mohr, F.C., and Fewtrell, C. 1987. The relative contributions of extracellular and intracellular calcium to secretion from tumor mast cells. Multiple effects of the proton ionophore carbonylcyanide m-chlorophenylhydrazone. J. Biol. Chem. 262:10638.
23. Cockcroft, S., and Gomperts, B.D. 1985. Role of guanine nucleotide binding protein in the activation of polyphosphoinositide phosphodiesterase. Nature 314:534.
24. Ishizaka, T. 1989. Role of GTP-binding protein in histamine release from mast cells. Clin. Immunol. Immunopathol. 50:20.
25. Peralta, E.G., Winslow, J.W., Ashkenazi, A., Smith, D.H., Ramachandran J., and Capon, D.J.. 1988. Structural basis of muscarinic acetylcholine receptor subtype diversity. Trends Pharmacol. Sci. Suppl:6.
26. Akiyama, T., Ishida, J., Nakagawa, S., Ogawara, H., Watanabe, S., Itoh, N., Shibuya, M., and Fukami, Y. 1987. Genistein, a specific inhibitor of tyrosine-specific protein kinases. J. Biol. Chem. 262:5592.
27. Pribluda, V.S., and Metzger, H. 1987. Calcium-independent phosphoinositide breakdown in rat leukemia cells. Evidence for an early rise in inositol 1,4,5-trisphosphate which precedes the rise in other inositol phosphates and in cytoplasmic calcium. J. Biol.Chem. 262:11449.
28. Klausner, R.D., and Samelson, L.E. 1991. T cell antigen receptor activation pathways: The tyrosine kinase connection. Cell 64:875.
29. Mustelin, T., Coggeshall, K.M., Isakov, N., and Altman, A. 1990. T cell antigen receptor-mediated activation of phospholipase C requires tyrosine phosphorylation. Science 247:1584.
30. June, C.H., Fletcher, M.C., Ledbetter, J.A., Schieven, G.L.,Siegel, J.N., Phillips, A.F., and Samelson, L.E. 1990. Inhibition of tyrosine phosphorylation prevents T-cell receptor-mediated signal transduction. Proc. Natl. Acad. Sci. U.S.A. 87:7722.
31. Eiseman, E., and Bolen, J.B. 1990. src-related tyrosine protein kinases as signaling components in hematopoietic cells. Cancer Cells 2:303.
32. Hunter, T. 1989. Protein-tyrosine phosphatases: The other side of the coin. Cell 58:1013.
33. Fischer, E.H., Charbonneau, H., and Tonks, N.K. 1991. Protein tyrosine phosphatases: A diverse family of intracellular and transmembrane enzymes. Science 253:401.
34. Hook, W.A., Berenstein, E.H., Zinsser, F.U., Fischler, C., and Siraganian, R.P. 1991. Monoclonal antibodies to the leukocyte common antigen (CD45) inhibit IgE-mediated histamine release from human basophils. J. Immunol., in press.
35. Stephan, V., Benhamou, M., Gutkind, J.S., Robbins, K.C., and Siraganian, R.P. 1991. FcεRI-induced protein tyrosine phosphorylation of pp72 in rat basophilic leukemia cells (RBL-2H3): Evidencefor a novel signal transduction pathway unrelated to G protein activation and phosphatidylinositol hydrolysis. Submitted for publication.
36. Benhamou, M., Stephan, V., Gutkind, J.S., Robbins, K.C., and Siraganian, R.P. 1991. IgE Receptor-mediated stimulation of rat basophilic leukemia (RBL-2H3) cells induces early and late proteintyrosine phosphorylations. Submitted for publication.

Role of Phospholipases in Mast Cell Activation

Donald A. Kennerly*

The emerging importance of lipid second messengers, such as 1,2-diacylglycerol (DAG), motivates a review of the pathways by which DAG is formed. Increasing evidence points to the importance of receptor dependent activation of phospholipase D (PLD) in the accumulation of DAG by a two step "Indirect Pathway" involving: PLD-mediated conversion of phosphatidylcholine (PC) to phosphatidic acid (PA) followed by the formation of DAG from PA by phosphatidic acid phosphohydrolase (PA-PHase). Activation of PC-PLD may be important not only in the indirect formation of DAG, but also because increasing evidence suggests that the direct product of PC-PLD (PA) or a metabolic derivative of PA (lyso-PA) may act as second messengers. In addition to PC-PLD, receptor-dependent activation of phospholipase A2 (PLA_2) occurs in the mast cell and may be important in the formation of inflammatory lipids such as eicosanoids and platelet activating factor (PAF) as well as in a regulatory capacity. Some of these phospholipases are active in the secretory granule of mast cells and, coupled with data bearing on the regulation of PLD, suggest the hypothesis that receptor dependent activation of a granule associated PC-PLD may be important in the lipid changes necessary to facilitate the fusion of the granule membrane with the plasma membrane.

This brief review will focus on the biochemical processes associated with exocytosis of secretory granules caused by aggregation of high affinity IgE receptor (Fcε-RI) on mast cells. It will not seriously address important differences between different mast cell models, but rather will stress important common findings. Further, what follows will principally explore a single class of second messengers, effectors and mediators: those that are themselves lipids or derived from membrane lipids.

Structural and Effector Functions of Membrane Lipids

Biologically relevant membranes are formed from phospholipids, cholesterol, glycolipids and proteins and have a characteristic bilayer structure as a consequence of the amphipathic nature of phospholipids. Membranes are important biochemical barriers in the cell that allow functional compartmentalization within and between cells, but obstruct the flow of information from the extracellular environment to the interior of the cell. Mast cells and basophils share with all secretory cells the regulated ability to undergo exocytosis despite the fact that this process is energetically highly unfavorable. During exocytosis, granules not only must become physically approximated with the plasma membrane (perhaps facilitated by cytoskeletal elements), but also must overcome a very significant thermodynamic barrier to membrane fusion. To overcome this energy hurdle, cells must locally synthesize either specialized proteins or lipids that can form non-bilayer membrane structures capable of facilitating membrane fusion, but that do not result in loss of integrity of either the plasma membrane or granule membrane, a feat of some consequence. The fusion of adjacent membranes illustrated in Figure 1 can be promoted by endogenous lipids such as 1,2-diacylglycerol termed "fusogens" that act by facilitating the formation of lipid intermediates (IMI and ILA) necessary for exocytosis (1).

Elements of Intracellular Signaling

Structural and functional diversity demand that each cell have the ability to recognize a large subset of extracellular molecules, and to translate an extracellular binding event into an

* University of Texas Southwestern Medical Center, Department of Internal Medicine, Dallas, TX, USA.
Acknowledgements: The author was supported by the NIH (R01-AI22277) and by the Burroughs Wellcome Fund (Developing Investigator in Immunopharmacology of Allergic Diseases).

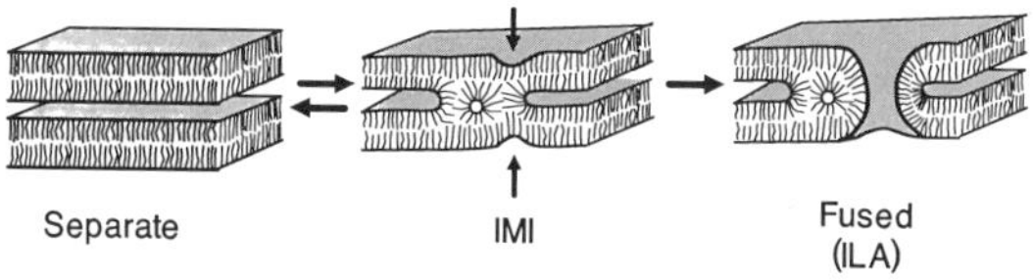

Figure 1. Mechanism of membrane fusion. The formation of lipids having small hydrophilic head groups results in the reversible formation of inverted micellar intermediates (IMIs) that facilitate the formation of fusion pores termed interlaminar attachments (ILAs) (1).

amplified intracellular biochemical signal that causes an appropriate cellular response, a task requiring a variety of structures and/or mechanisms. First, recognition by the target cells requires an appropriate cell surface or intracellular receptor. Most cells distinguish between receptors that are occupied by a ligand versus those that are not; presumably the result of a conformational change in an intracellular signal transducing domain. The capacity of each mast cell to respond vigorously to a variety of different antigens, however, requires the existence of Fcε-RI and the subsequent generation of antigen specificity by tightly associated antigen specific IgE. Exocytosis occurs not as the result of ligand binding, but in response to physical approximation (often referred to as "crosslinking") of IgE bearing Fcε-RI by multivalent antigens (2). By one or more of several mechanisms (beyond the scope of the current review), plasma membrane receptor activation causes rapid changes in the intracellular levels of regulatory molecules termed second messengers that function both to amplify receptor-mediated signals and to rapidly alter the activity of one or more enzymes or nonenzymatic proteins critical to a relevant regulated function of the cell. In contrast to the wide variety of extracellular bioinformation molecules and their respective receptors, the repertoire of intracellular second messenger molecules is somewhat restricted, although more new second messengers will undoubtedly be described in the future. The most extensively studied second messengers include: cyclic-AMP (cAMP), cyclic-GMP (cGMP), inositol 1,4,5-trisphosphate (IP_3), 1,2-diacylglycerol (DAG), Ca^{2+} and arachidonic acid (AA)-derived eicosanoids. Most commonly, second messengers function by changing the activity of an increasing number of second messenger responsive protein kinases that each alter the activity of a different subset of target proteins by phosphorylating them and that collectively cause the specific receptor dependent cellular response.

Early Mast Cell Studies of Lipid Metabolism: The "PI Cycle" and Protein Kinase C (PKC)

Subsequent to the initial description of receptor enhanced labeling of phosphoinositides (PI) and phosphatidic acid (PA) by ^{32}Pi in pancreas (3), virtually all cells have been shown to have this capacity in response to stimulation by one or more appropriate receptors (Figure 2; reviewed by Hokin, 4). Fcε-RI enhanced activity of this pathway, initiated by PI specific phospholipase C (PI-PLC) in mast cells, was shown by ourselves and others (5–7). Extensive studies in the RBL-2H3 mast cell line by Beaven and his colleagues (reviewed in 8) have characterized Fcε-RI dependent hydrolysis of phosphoinositides by PI-PLC. The mechanisms by which phospholipases act are shown in Figure 3. Protein kinase C (PKC) was initially described by Nishizuka and ultimately found to represent a family of molecules that are responsive to two different second messengers: DAG and Ca^{2+} (reviewed in 9). Given an appropriate membrane surface containing the phospholipid phosphatidylserine (PS), membrane associated DAG causes PKC to translocate from the cytosol to the membrane,

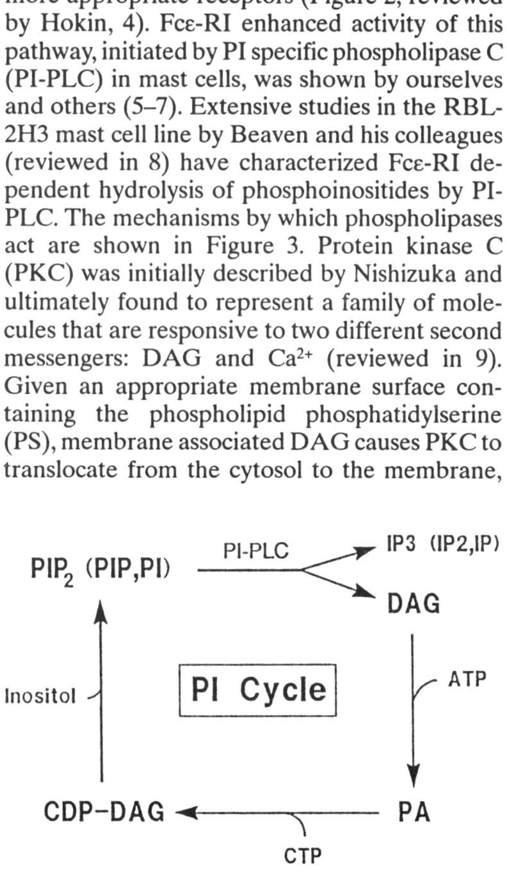

Figure 2. Phosphoinositide metabolism. Abbreviations: PIP_2: phosphatidylinositol 4,5-bisphosphate; PIP: phosphatidylinositol 4-phosphate; PI: phosphatidylinositol; DAG: 1,2-diacylglycerol; PA: phosphatidic acid; CDP-DAG: cytidyl-DAG.

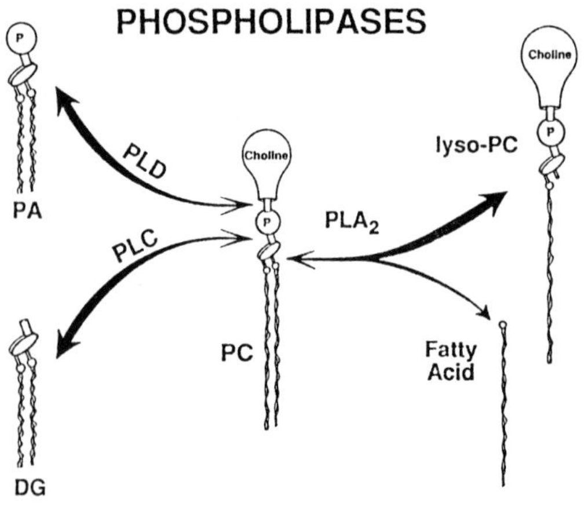

Figure 3. Mechanisms of phospholipases. Abbreviations: PLD: phospholipase D; PLC: phospholipase C; PLA_2: phospholipase A_2 P: phosphate.

and to increase its affinity for Ca^{2+}, so that at permissive and physiologically relevant $[Ca^{+2}]_{cytosol}$ PKC will become active. Because DAG is an intermediate in the PI cycle, its ability to activate PKC led to the attractive hypothesis during the early 1980s that the importance of the PI cycle was to generate DAG that regulates PKC. The potential importance of the minor phosphoinositide PI 4,5-bisphosphate (PIP_2) was brought to the fore by the description in 1983 (10) of the ability of PI-PLC hydrolysis of (PIP_2) not only to form DAG, but also to form the water soluble product, inositol 1,4,5-trisphosphate (IP_3), a compound able to act as a second messenger as the result of its capacity to control $[Ca^{+2}]_{cytosol}$ by interacting with an intracellular IP_3 receptor (11). Because PIP_2 hydrolysis results in the formation of two second messengers that synergistically activated PKC [DAG and Ca^{2+} (via IP_3)], receptor dependent PI-PLC activity was felt by many to be both necessary and sufficient for activation of mast cells. PKC activation was shown to increase as the result of Fcε-RI stimulation of mast cells (12).

Role of Phosphatidylcholine Metabolism in Mast Cells

As to the role of PC in DAG accumulation: Recent studies have called into question the singular importance of phosphoinositide hydrolysis in signal transduction that involves

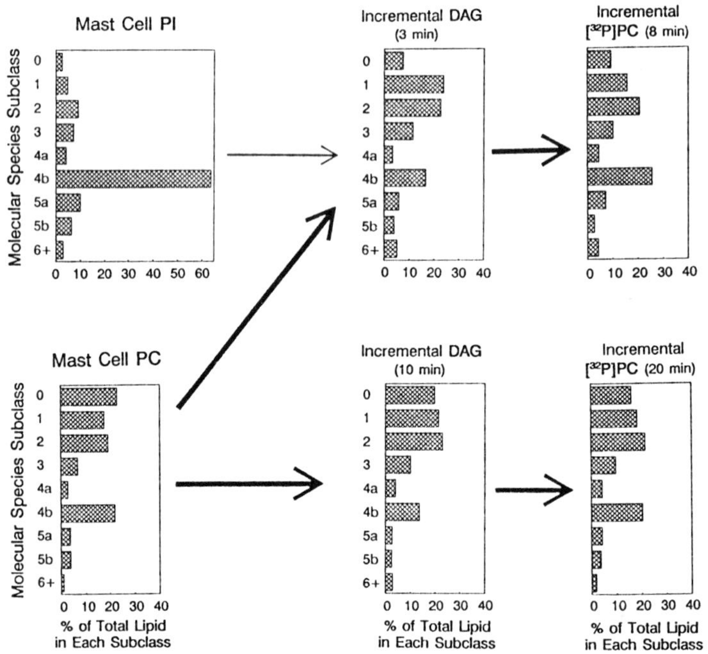

Figure 4. Molecular species analysis of the metabolic origin of DAG in Fcε-RI stimulated mast cells. Cellular phospholipids and DAG were isolated and separated into different molecular species subclasses based on degree of unsaturation of fatty acids (13). DAG mass in Fcε-RI stimulated cells doubled at 3 min and was increased 3 fold at 10 min. The similar patterns of DAG and PC (vs. PI compared to DAG) indicate that DAG accumulating in Fcε-RI stimulated mast cells is primarily derived from PC. The similarity of patterns of $[^{32}P]PC$ and DAG (in ^{32}Pi prelabeled mast cells) indicates the existence of Fcε-RI dependent PC resynthesis.

cellular lipid metabolism. First, the quantitative presence of PIP_2 and PIP in many tissues is not sufficient to explain the increases in DAG that were observed as the result of receptor stimulation. Second, molecular species analysis, a method used to evaluate the precursor-product relationship of glycerol based lipids, showed that most of the DAG accumulating after Fcε-RI stimulation in mast cells could not be derived from PI (13). Figure 4 demonstrates that the DAG accumulating as the result of Fcε-RI stimulation bears striking resemblance to PC, an observation suggesting that Fcε-RI dependent PC hydrolysis is more important than is PI hydrolysis in Fcε-RI dependent DAG accumulation. These findings have been extended to other cells (14) and it is now evident that many of the hormones that induce PI turnover also cause PC hydrolysis (reviewed in 15).

Potential Mechanisms of PC Conversion to DAG in Mast Cells: Phospholipase C (PLC) vs. Phospholipase D (PLD)

Figure 5 illustrates that two mechanisms might be involved in the formation of DAG from PC: a "Direct Pathway" involving PC-PLC and/or an "Indirect Pathway" initiated by PC-PLD. Several lines of evidence support the primary importance of PC-PLD and the Indirect Pathway over

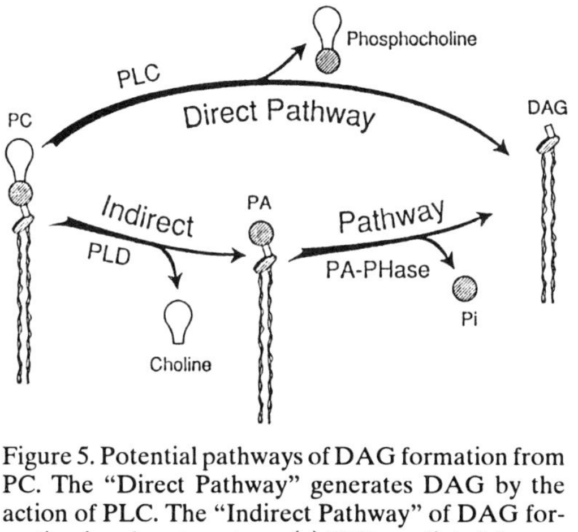

Figure 5. Potential pathways of DAG formation from PC. The "Direct Pathway" generates DAG by the action of PLC. The "Indirect Pathway" of DAG formation involves two steps: (a) PLD mediated formation of choline and PA and (b) subsequent conversion of PA to DAG by phosphatidic acid phosphohydrolase PA-PHase.

PC-PLC and the Direct Pathway in mast cells. First, accumulation of ([^{3}H]palmitoyl)PA increased in Fcε-RI stimulated cells slightly before labeled DAG did, an observation most consistent with the PA acting as a substrate for DAG formation (by PA phosphohydrolase [PA-PHase]) rather than a product of the phosphorylation of DAG (16). Second, Fcε-RI stimulation of [^{3}H]palmitate prelabeled mast cells in the presence of low concentrations of ethanol was accompanied by receptor dependent formation of the phosphatidylethanol (PEt), the transphosphatidylation product catalyzed exclusively by PLD (17). Third and most recently, we developed methods to assess the relative importance of PC-PLD vs. PC-PLC during mast cell activation by examining the water soluble products of these reactions (18). Figure 6 demonstrates that Fcε-RI stimulation is associated with a rapid and dramatic increase in the levels of intracellular choline (16), the product of PC-PLD activation (Figure 5). Recent unpublished observations by ourselves demonstrate in the mast cell that PC-PLD activity appears to be regulated by both Ca^{+2} and PKC. Although the intracellular levels of choline increase in Fcε-RI stimulated cells, phosphocholine mass (a measure of PC-PLC activity) declined with stimulation (Figure 6), an observation undermining the importance of PC-PLC in the genesis of receptor dependent DAG generation. Control experiments have ruled out direct conversion of phosphocholine to choline as an explanation for these findings (16). Consistent with the proposed importance of PC-PLD in receptor dependent DAG accumulation is our observation of significant PA-PHase activity. This enzyme is the second and a necessary element in the formation of DAG from PC via the Indirect Pathway by converting PA to DAG (Figure 5; Duffy & Kennerly, 1991, manuscript in review). Our experiments demonstrate that mast cell PA-PHase activity is not associated with the isoform responsible for structural lipid biosynthesis, but rather is richly represented in the secretory granule membrane, the regulatory implications of which are discussed in detail in a subsequent section. PC-PLD may be important not only from the perspective of generating DAG via the Indirect Pathway, but also as the result of the potential importance of PA as a second messenger and/or effector. Proposed mechanisms by which PA may exert important effects include: Ca^{+2} dependent membrane phase changes (19), increased membrane permeability

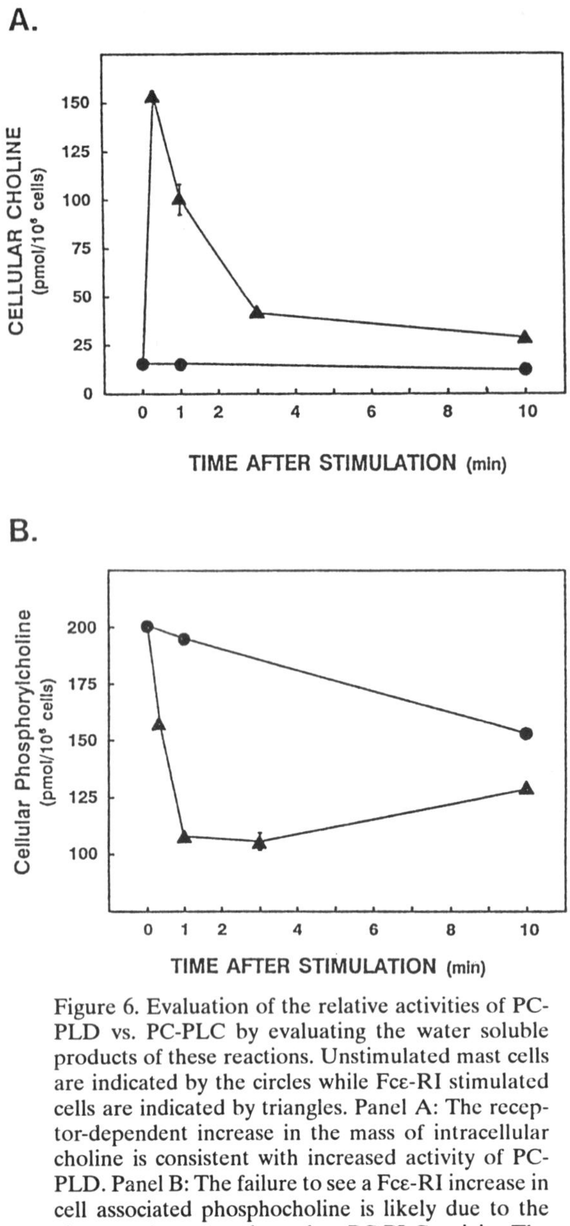

Figure 6. Evaluation of the relative activities of PC-PLD vs. PC-PLC by evaluating the water soluble products of these reactions. Unstimulated mast cells are indicated by the circles while Fcε-RI stimulated cells are indicated by triangles. Panel A: The receptor-dependent increase in the mass of intracellular choline is consistent with increased activity of PC-PLD. Panel B: The failure to see a Fcε-RI increase in cell associated phosphocholine is likely due to the absence of receptor dependent PC-PLC activity. The transience of the increase in choline and the decrease in phosphocholine mass in stimulated cells are likely the result of consumption of these compounds during Fcε-RI dependent PC resynthesis (data not shown).

to Ca^{+2} in membranes containing PA (20), substitution of PA for PS for PKC binding to membranes (21), regulation of the activity of the GAP protein (important in the activation of cellular ras) (22) and, in provocative studies, activation of a distinct protein kinase (23). In recent experiments lyso-PA (the product of phospholipase A_2 [PLA_2]–catalyzed hydrolysis of PA and a frequent contaminant of commercial preparations of PA) has been shown to act as a second messenger by liberating Ca^{+2} from intracellular sites at concentrations well below those causing cytotoxicity (24). In the mast cell, Fcε-RI stimulation causes an increase in [^{32}P]lyso-PA in ^{32}Pi prelabeled cells (Fagan, Kennerly & Sullivan, unpublished observations).

Phospholipase A_2 (PLA_2) Activation: a role in both lipid mediator biosynthesis and signal transduction

In addition to a role for PLA_2 hydrolysis of PC in the genesis of arachidonic acid and lyso-PAF for receptor dependent biosynthesis of lipid mediators (eicosanoids and PAF, respectively), data from several groups suggest that PLA_2 mediated hydrolysis of phospholipids may play an important role in regulating exocytosis. Stimulation of mast cells is associated with increased PLA_2 activity in mast cells that is both Ca^{2+} and GTP[S] augmented (25). Also, preliminary data from Ishizaka's group (American Academy of Allergy and Immunology presentation, 1990) demonstrate (a) that Fcε-RI stimulation of glycerol prelabeled cells results in accumulation of labeled lyso-PI and lyso-PE in addition to lyso-PC and (b) that pharmacologic inhibition of PLA_2 by an agent devoid of PI-PLC antagonist properties is accompanied by a dose related inhibition of granule secretion. Several mechanisms may contribute to a regulatory role for PLA_2 activation in mast cell exocytosis. First, lyso-phospholipid products of PLA_2 have surface active properties (detergent-like) and have been proposed to be important in the fusion of granule membranes with each other and with the plasma membrane. Recent models of membrane fusion suggest, however, that the ability of lipids to enhance non-cytolytic membrane fusion is principally associated with the genesis of lipids with biophysical parameters typical of DAG, not lyso-phospholipids (26). Second, lyso-PC has been shown to weakly substitute for PS in the association of PKC with membranes (21), but because no deficiency of PS has thus far been demonstrated in mast cells, the importance of this property of lyso-PC is speculative. Third, fatty acid products of PLA_2 activation might exert a variety of regulatory activities: (a) arachidonic acid derived eicosanoids may modify processes important to mast cell activation including PI hydrolysis (27); (b) arachidonic acid has been shown to activate some isoforms of PKC (9); and (c) both oleic acid and arachidonic acid have been shown to rather selectively activate PLD in several models (28) suggesting that PLA_2 activation may result in increased PLD activity. Finally, PLA_2 mediated lyso-PA synthesis may have the Ca^{2+} regulatory effects described previously.

A Working Hypothesis: Different Subcellular Roles for DAG

The model illustrated in Figure 7 grew out of our unpublished observation that pharmacologic activation of mast cell PKC using PMA dramatically enhanced PLD activity. This finding was initially concerning because of the implication that a positive feedback loop might exist (DAG → ↑ PKC → ↑ PLD → ↑ PA → ↑ DAG, etc.). Moreover, a number of other observations were also difficult to integrate into a satisfactory model: (a) that mast cells can undergo exocytosis in the absence of PI hydrolysis (29); (b) that acute phorbol ester mediated PKC activation has only modest effects on receptor mediated mast cell exocytosis when added alone (30); (c) that antagonists of PKC successfully block Fcε-RI mediated secretion (31); and (d) that depletion of mast cell PKC (by prolonged exposure to PMA) has only modest effects on Fcε-RI mediated exocytosis (32). A second important concept that helped form our model is that DAG and other lipid second messengers differ from water soluble second messengers in that its hydrophobicity prevents it from rapidly entering the cytosol and moving from the membrane where it is generated to other organelles. Thus, generating DAG in different locations may well result in *site specific* activation of PKC, a process potentially resulting in fundamentally different effects on cell function by a single lipid second messenger depending on where it is generated.

The model (Figure 7) integrates these concepts into the working hypothesis that a positive feedback loop involving PKC mediated activation of PLD may be limited to the secretory granule where it might help to drive (either directly or indirectly) the membrane fusion associated with exocytosis. We propose that granules possess DAG removal pathways that antagonize increases in local DAG levels, probably by converting DAG to PC (the right hand portion of Figure 4 demonstrates Fcε-RI augmented [^{32}P]PC synthesis from DAG in ^{32}Pi prelabeled mast cells). But because DAG removal is limited, exceeding a certain rate of DAG formation in any given granule (as the result of an Fcε-RI mediated increase in the PLD initiated Indirect Pathway) will initiate an accelerative cycle (DAG → ↑ PKC → ↑ PLD → ↑ PA → ↑ DAG, etc.). We suggest that perhaps this explosive local production of

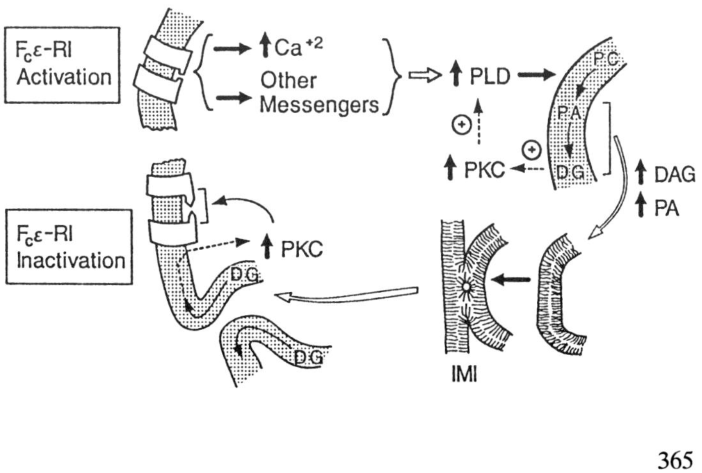

Figure 7. Working hypothesis regarding the role of PLD in exocytosis of mast cell granules.

DAG may represent a "biochemical commitment" of the granule to undergo fusion/exocytosis as the result of rapid accumulation of fusogenic lipids such as DAG (1,26). This hypothesis could explain the morphologic observation that granules display an "all or none" swelling response in Fcε-RI stimulated mast cells (33). This concept is consistent with Chock's data and proposals relating to the assembly of lipids stored in the granule matrix into membrane that is integrated into the perigranule membrane during mast cell activation (34).

Two attractive corollaries of this model emerge. First, exocytosis of secretory granules might usefully be viewed in probabilistic terms. In an unstimulated cell, the frequency of granules exceeding the concentration of DAG required for self sustaining DAG formation (by the PKC augmented PLD initiated Indirect Pathway) is low, though not zero, consistent with the observed existence of a low rate of spontaneous exocytosis. Receptor dependent enhancement of granule-associated DAG formation by the PLD-initiated Indirect Pathway could increase the probability that any given granule will exceed its threshold for irreversible "commitment" and thus drives secretion. Second, delivery of DAG to the plasma membrane by exocytosis of DAG rich granules might provide appropriate negative feedback by reducing pro-exocytotic signals generated in the plasma membrane, perhaps as the result of PKC-mediated down regulation of Fcε-RI responsiveness and/or by facilitating the generation of second messengers that more directly down regulate PLD.

References

1. Siegel, D.P., Burns, J.L., Chestnut, M.H., and Talmon, Y. 1989. Intermediates in membrane fusion and bilayer/nonbilayer phase transitions imaged by time-resolved cryo-transmission electron microscopy. Biophys. J. 56:161.
2. Ishizaka, T., and Ishizaka, K. 1978. Triggering of histamine release from rat mast cells by divalent antibodies against IgE receptors. J. Immunol. 120:800.
3. Hokin, R.R., and Hokin, L.E. 1953. Enzyme secretion and the incorporation of ^{32}P into the phospholipids of pancreas slices. J. Biol. Chem. 203:967.
4. Rana, R.S., and Hokin, L.E. 1991. Role of phosphoinositides in transmembrane signaling. Physiol. Rev. 70:115.
5. Kennerly, D.A., Sullivan, T.J., and Parker, C.W. 1979. Activation of phospholipid metabolism during mediator release from stimulated rat mast cells. J. Immunol. 122:152.
6. Cockcroft, S., and Gomperts, B.D. 1979. Evidence for a role of phosphatidylinositol turnover in stimulus-secretion coupling: studies with rat peritoneal mast cells. BiochemJ. 178:681.
7. Ishizuka, Y., Imai, A., and Nozawa, Y. 1984. Polyphosphoinositide turnover in rat mast cells stimulated by antigen. Biochem. Biophys. Res. Comm. 123:875.
8. Beaven, M.A., and Cunha-Melo, J.R. 1988. Membrane phosphoinositide-activated signals in mast cells and basophils. In: Progress in allergy. E.L. Becker edition. 42:123.
9. Bell, R.M., and Burns, D.J. 1991. Lipid activation of protein kinase C. J. Biol. Chem. 266:4661.
10. Fein, A., Payne, R. Corson, D.W., Berridge, M.J., and Irvine, R.F. 1984. Photoreceptor excitation and adaptation by inositol 1,4,5-trisphosphate. Nature 311:157.
11. Mignery, G.A., Newton, C.L., Archer, 3d, B.T., and Sudhof, T.C. 1990. Structure and expression of the rat inositol 1,4,5-trisphosphate receptor. J. Biol. Chem. 265:12679.
12. White, J.R., Pluznik, D.H., Ishizaka, K., and Ishizaka, T. 1985. Antigen induced increase in protein kinase C activity in plasma membranes of mast cells. Proc. Nat. Acad. Sci. (USA) 82:8193.
13. Kennerly, D.A. 1987. Diacylglycerol metabolism in mast cells: Analysis of lipid metabolic pathways using molecular species analysis of intermediates. J. Biol. Chem. 262:16305.
14. Pessin, M.S., Baldassare, J.J., and Raben, D.M. 1990. Molecular species analysis of mitogen-stimulated 1,2-diglycerides in fibroblasts. J. Biol. Chem. 265:7959.
15. Exton, J.H. 1990. Signaling through phosphatidylcholine breakdown. J. Biol. Chem. 265:1.
16. Dinh, T.T., and Kennerly, D.A. 1991. Assessment of receptor dependent activation of phosphatidylcholine hydrolysis by both phospholipase D and C. Cell Regulation 2:229.
17. Gruchalla, R.S., Dinh, T.T., and Kennerly, D.A. 1990. An indirect pathway of receptor-mediated 1,2-diacylglycerol formation in mast cells I: IgE receptor-mediated activation of phospholipase D. J. Immunol. 144:2336.
18. Gruchalla, R.S., Dinh, T.T., Truett, A.P., and

Kennerly, D.A. 1990. Isolation and enzymatic assay of choline and phosphocholine present in cellular extracts with picomole sensitivity. Biochem. J. 270:63.
19. Boughriet, A., Ladjadj, M., and Bicknell-Brown, E. 1988. Calcium-induced condensation-reorganization phenomena in multilamellar vesicles of phosphatidic acid. Biochem.Biophys. Acta 939:523.
20. Blau, L., and Weissmann, G. 1988. Transmembrane calcium movements mediated by ionomycin and phosphatidic acid in liposomes with Fura-2 entrapped. Biochemistry 27:5661.
21. Oishi, K., Raynor, R.L., Charp, P.A., and Kuo, J.F. 1988. Regulation of protein kinase C by lysophospholipids, potential role in signal transduction. J. Biol. Chem. 263:6865.
22. Tsai, M.H., Yu, C.L., Wei, F.S., and Stacey, D.W. 1989. The effect of GTPase activating protein upon ras is initiated by mitogenically responsive lipids. Science 243:522.
23. Bocckino, S.B., Wilson, P.B., and Exton, J.H. 1991. Phosphatidate-dependent protein phosphorylation. Proc. Nat. Acad. Sci. USA 88:6210.
24. Jalionk, K., van Corven, E.J., and Moolenaar, W.H. 1990. Lysophosphatidic acid, but not phosphatidic acid, is a potent Ca^{2+} mobilizing stimulus for fibroblasts. J. Biol. Chem. 265:12232.
25. Narasimhan, V., Holowka, D., and Baird, B. 1990. A guanine nucleotide-binding protein participates in IgE receptor-mediated activation of endogenous and reconstituted phospholipase A2 in a permeabilized cell system.
26. Siegel, D.P., Banschbach, J., Alford, D., Ellens, H., Lis,L.J., Quinn, P.J., Yeagle, P.L., and Bentz, J. 1989. Physiological levels of diacylglycerols in phospholipid membranes induce membrane fusion and stabilize inverted phases. Biochemistry 28:3703.
27. Gladari, S.H., Morris, H.R., and Di Marzo, V. 1990. Novel interactions between second messengers in rat basophilic leukemia (RBL-1) cells. Biochemistry International 22:379.
28. Chalifour, R., and Kanfer J.N. 1982. Fatty acid activation and temperature perturbation of rat brain microsomal phospholipase D. J. Neurochem. 39:299.
29. Saito, H., Ishizaka, K., and Ishizaka, T. 1989. Effects of nonhydrolyzable guanosine phosphate on IgE-mediated activation of phospholipase C and histamine release from rodent mast cells. J. Immunol. 143:250.
30. Heiman, A.S., and Crews, F.T. 1985. Characterization of the effects of phorbol esters on rat mast cell secretion. J.Immunol. 134:548.
31. Gilfillan, A.M., Wiggan, G.A., and Welton, A.F. 1990. The effects of protein kinase C inhibitors staurosporine and H7 on the IgE dependent mediator release from RBL-2H3 cells. Agents Actions 30:418.
32. Marquardt, D.L., and Walker L.L. 1989. Pretreatment with phorbol esters abrogates adenosine responsiveness. J.Immunol. 142:1268.
33. Schmauder-Chock, E.A., and Chock, S.P. 1990. Mechanism of secretory granule exocytosis: Can granule enlargement precede pore formation? Histochemical J. 19:413.
34. Chock, S.P., and Schmauder-Chock, E.A. 1990. A new model for the mechanism of stimulus-secretion coupling. BioFactors 2:133.

Regulation of Leukotriene Generation

Shigekatsu Kohno*, Hideki Yamamura*, Takeshi Nabe*, Michiaki Horiba**, Katsuya Ohata*

A highly potent and selective peptide leukotriene (p-LT) antagonist, MCI-826 was found to inhibit the antigen-specific anaphylactic immunoreactive (i-) LTC_4 release without effect on the histamine release from the isolated human lung fragments and purified mast cells. When the human lung mast cells were incubated with radiolabeled [^{3}H]arachidonic acid (AA) and then challenged with antigen, only minute but obvious amounts of [^{3}H]AA incorporated into the cells were found to be transformed into prostaglandin (PG)D_2 and LTC_4. The treatment of the cells with LTB_4 and p-LTs, especially LTC_4 and LTE_4 induced marked enhancement of anaphylactic PGD_2 and LTC_4 formation. The enhanced anaphylactic release of arachidonate metabolites including PGD_2 and LTC_4 by LTC_4 and LTE_4 were greatly reduced by the pretreatment of islet activating protein (IAP), which inhibits some cellular signal transduction by interfering a kind of G-proteins. In addition, IAP considerably inhibited the anaphylactic release of the metabolites. On the other hand, from the mouse bone marrow-derived mast cells (BMMC), which are known to form large amounts of p-LTs, either MCI-826 or LTC_4 hardly affected the anaphylactic i-LTC_4 or p-LT release, although obvious specific binding in the crude cell membrane to LTC_4 was found. The binding to LTD_4 or LTE_4 was hardly detected in the membrane. These results indicate that LTs specifically stimulate the arachidonate formation of the human lung mast cells,in contrast to BMMC, during anaphylaxis, probably through their receptors.

We have reported that a highly potent, selective and competitive inhibitor of 5-lipoxygenase, which is the first enzyme to form LTs, a benzoquinone derivative, AA-861 dose-dependently inhibits the p-LT, or slow reacting substance of anaphylaxis (SRS-A) release from human, guinea pig and monkey (*Macaca irus*) lung fragments or rat peritoneal cells over species (1). On the other hand, the compound does not influence the histamine release at least from human and guinea pig lung fragments, indicating that histamine release from these species is not modulated by the arachidonate 5-lipoxygenase metabolites at all.

In 1973, it was reported that one of the chromone derivatives, FPL55712 is a selective SRS-A antagonist (2). Since then, many p-LT antagonists with chromone and other structures have been presented. *(E)*-2,2-diethyl-3′-[2-[2-(4-isopropyl) thiazoyl]ethenyl]succinanilic acid (MCI-826), which was synthesized from modification of LTD_4 structure using computer analysis, is one of the most potent and highly specific p-LT antagonists. The antagonistic activity of this compound to LTD_4 and LTE_4 is more than 100 times as potent as that of FPL 55712, when assessed by the specific binding experiments in the guinea pig crude lung membrane and the contraction of isolated guinea pig tracheal muscle preparation. The compound also greatly reduced the antigen-induced contractions of not only isolated human bronchi but also lung parenchymas, suggesting that p-LTs largely contribute to the antigen-induced pulmonary contractions. In this paper, we describe the effect of p-LT antagonists on the release of LTs as well as histamine and the effect of LTs on the anaphylactic mediator release *in vitro*.

Materials and Methods

Preparation of the Passively Sensitized Human Lung Fragments and Purified Mast Cells

Macroscopically normal human lung parenchymas were cut into pieces of 0.5 × 1 × 1 mm in size with the McIlwain tissue chopper. After washing with Tyrode's solution, one part of the lung fragments was passively sensitized with 5-fold dilution of mite sensitive human atopic serum (RAST score = 4) for 2 hrs at 37°C for

* Department of Pharmacology, Kyoto Pharmaceutical University, Misasagi-Nakauchi, Yamashina, Kyoto 607, Japan;

** Department of Pneumology, Ogaki Municipal Hospital, Minaminokawa, Ogaki, Gifu 503, Japan.

Scheme 1. Principal procedure for isolation, purification and passive sensitization of human lung mast cells.

Human lung fragments

- Digestion by deoxyribonuclease(10μg/ml) and collagenase(145μ/ml) in Ca^{++}-free and 0.1% BSA-containing Tyrode's solution at 37°C for 20min
- Filtration on nylon mesh(100μm)

Residual tissue

2nd to 6th filtrate

- Centrifugation(4°C, 200xg, 7min)

Pellet / Supernatant

- Purification by centrifugation(4°C, 400xg, 15min) on discontinuous layer of 70% and 55% Percoll solution

Partially purified human lung mast cells

- Culture at $2x10^6$ cells/ml as total cells in 10% FCS-containing GIT medium at 37 °C for 24hr
- Addition of human atopic serum(RAST score =4, 0.5ml/15ml cell suspension)
- Culture at 37°C for 24hr
- Harvest of nonadherent cells and loosely adhered cells on the culture flask

Cultured and passively sensitized mast cells

- Purification by centrifugation(4°C, 400xg, 12min) on discontinuous layer of 80, 70, 60, 55, 50 and 40% Percoll solution

Passively sensitized, purified mast cells

experiments of mediator release. The other part was subjected to the procedure as shown in Scheme 1 for obtaining the isolated, passively sensitized mast cells. After the final purification by Percoll discontinuous gradient, the purity of mast cells was 40–80%.

Conditions of Culture of BMMC

The conditions of proliferation and culture (3), and passive sensitization of mouse (BALB/c) bone marrow-derived mast cells (BMMC) are described in Scheme 2. BMMC (purity > 98%) cultured for 5 weeks were used for mediator release and binding assay of p-LTs. In the binding assay, the mast cells were not passively sensitized.

Incorporation of Radiolabeled [^{3}H]AA into the Purified Human Lung Mast Cells

The purified, passively sensitized human lung mast cells were incubated with radiolabeled [^{3}H]AA as following conditions : $7 \times 10^5 - 4.0 \times 10^6$ mast cells/experiment in 8–20 ml of 0.1% BSA-containing and Ca^{++}-free Tyrode's solution were incubated with 250 – 750μCi of [5,6,8,9,11,12,14,15-^{3}H(N)]AA at 37°C for 2 hrs. The cells were washed twice and resuspended at 2×10^4 mast cells/ml with the same Tyrode's solution. The amount of [^{3}H]AA incorporated into the cells was 16 to 30%.

Anaphylactic LT and Histamine Release

The passively sensitized human lung fragments (100 mg wet tissue/ml), human lung mast cells (2×10^4 mast cells/ml) or BMMC (10^5 BMMC/ml) suspended in 0.1% BSA- and/or gelatin-containing and Ca^{++}-free Tyrode's solution were incubated with $CaCl_2$ at final concentrations of 1.8×10^{-3} M at 37°C for 5 min, treated with drugs, LTs or vehicle for 5 min and challenged with 5×10^{-6} g/ml mite extracts (from *Dermatophagoides farinae*) for 15 min in human lung fragments, 30 min in human lung mast cells, and with 10^{-5} g/ml dinitrophenylated Ascaris suum extracts (DNP-As) for 20 min in BMMC experiments, respectively. After completion of the reaction, the anaphylactic filtrate on gauze in the fragment experiment or the cell suspension was centrifuged at 1,700 × g for 20 min at 4°C. Resultant supernatants were stored at -80C until assay or purification of mediators.

Assay of Histamine and LTs

Histamine was assayed by fluorometrical method after purification by ion exchange column of high performance liquid chromatography (HPLC) (4). LTs in the non-radioactive experiments were radioimmunoassayed after purification by Amprep C-18 reversed phase column chromatography [estimated as immunoreactive (i-) LTB_4 or i-LTC_4] or further by HPLC using C-18 reversed phase column (5). In the radioactive experiments, all of the specimens were subjected to the Amprep column chromatography and HPLC. The radioactivity of the fractions from the HPLC was counted.

Scheme 2 Principal procedure for culture and passive sensitization of mouse bone marrow-derived mast cells (BMMC).
*: α-medium supplemented 20% heat-inactivated horse serum, 60 μg/ml kanamycin, 10^{-4} M nonessential amino acid and 10^{-4} M 2-mercaptoethanol.
**: Male 8 week-old BDF_1 mouse spleen cells (2×10^6 cells/ml) were cultured for 5 days at 37°C in α-medium supplemented 300 fold dilution of pokeweed mitogen, 10% fetal calf serum, 60 μg/ml kanamycin, 10^{-4} M nonessential amino acid and 10^{-4} M 2-mercaptoethanol.

Bone marrow cell from BALB/c mice (♂)

- ← Suspension at 10^6 cells/ml with α-medium* containing 10% conditioned medium(CM)[3]**
- ← Culture at 37°C in 5% CO2 and 95% air
- ← Exchange of the half culture medium with fresh α-medium containing 10% CM weekly to 3 weeks after starting of culture
- ← Culture at 10^5 cells/ml in fresh α-medium containing 20% CM weekly from 3 to 5 weeks after starting of culture
- ← Addition of rat anti-dinitrophenylated Ascaris suum serum (48hr PCA titer: 256x, 1ml/10ml cell suspension)
- ← Sensitization at 37°C for 24hr under culture

↓

Passively sensitized bone marrow-derived mast cells (BMMC)

Binding Assay of p-LTs Using BMMC Crude Membrane Fraction

The crude membrane fraction from 10^9 BMMC was obtained by sedimentation technique following cell disruption by sonication as usual method. The crude membranes (95 μg protein/tube) were incubated with radiolabeled $[^3H]LTC_4$ (16 nCi, Sp. activity 40 Ci/mmol), $[^3H]LTD_4$ (200 nCi, 168 Ci/mmol) and $[^3H]LTE_4$ (200 nCi, 183 Ci/mmol), respectively, with or without respective 1 μM cold p-LTs in 400 μl of the medium containing 10 mM serine-borate complex, 10 mM cysteine, 10 mM $CaCl_2$, 10 mM $MgCl_2$, 10 mM glycine and 50 mM HEPES (pH 7.4) at 0°C for 1 hr.

Results

Effect of p-LT Antagonists on the LT and Histamine Release from Human Lung Fragments and Mast Cells, and BMMC

Figure 1 shows the results of the influence of MCI-826 and FPL 55712 on the anaphylactic release of i-LTs and histamine from human lung fragments. MCI-826 did not inhibit the histamine release at all. On the other hand, the compound inhibited i-LTC_4 as well as i-LTB_4 release. The inhibition, which was not seen over 20%, appeared to be almost constant, irrespective of concentrations of the drug used. In the same manner as the results of the lung fragment experiments, no inhibition and almost constant inhibition by MCI-826 of anaphylactic histamine and i-LTC_4 release, respectively, from purified human lung mast cells was observed. FPL 55712 showed, however, a concentration dependent inhibition of not only i-LTB_4 and i-LTC_4, but also histamine release from the lung fragments.

Effect of LTs on the Histamine Release from Human Lung Mast Cells and BMMC

LTB_4, LTC_4, LTD_4 and LTE_4 at concentrations of 10^{-8} and 10^{-7} M did not affect the anaphylactic histamine release from the purified human lung mast cells.

Effect of p-LTs on the Release of $[^3H]PGD_2$ and $[^3H]LTC_4$ from the Purified Human Lung Mast Cells

The influence of LTB_4, LTC_4, LTD_4 and LTE_4 at 10^{-9} - 10^{-7} M on the release of $[^3H]PGD_2$ and $[^3H]LTC_4$ from the purified human lung mast cells, into which $[^3H]$AA had been incorporated, was assessed. In the incubation conditions of 2×10^4 mast cells/ml with antigen at 37°C for 30 min, either $[^3H]LTD_4$, $[^3H]LTE_4$ or $[^3H]LTB_4$ was released less than 1/10 of LTC_4 into the medium. Therefore, as for LTs in some experiments, only

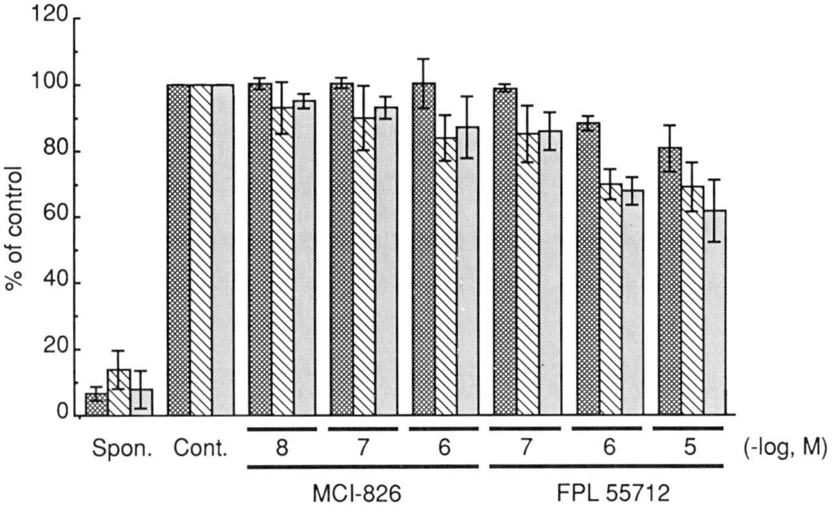

Figure 1. Effect of MCI-826 and FPL 55712 on the anaphylactic histamine, immunoreactive (i-) LTB_4 and i-LTC_4 release from passively sensitized human lung fragments. Drugs were added 5 min before antigen (5×10^{-5} g/ml mite extracts from Dermatophagoides farinae). Respective mediators (/g wet tissue) released were: histamine (spontaneous 0.29–0.47 μg, control 3.04–5.43 μg, content in the tissue 15.2–23.6 μg), i-LTB_4 (spontaneous 1.37–4.49 ng, control 13.2–26.1 ng) and i-LTC_4 (spontaneous 2.10–32.3 ng, control 75.1–168 ng). Each column represents mean ± S.E. of 3 experiments.

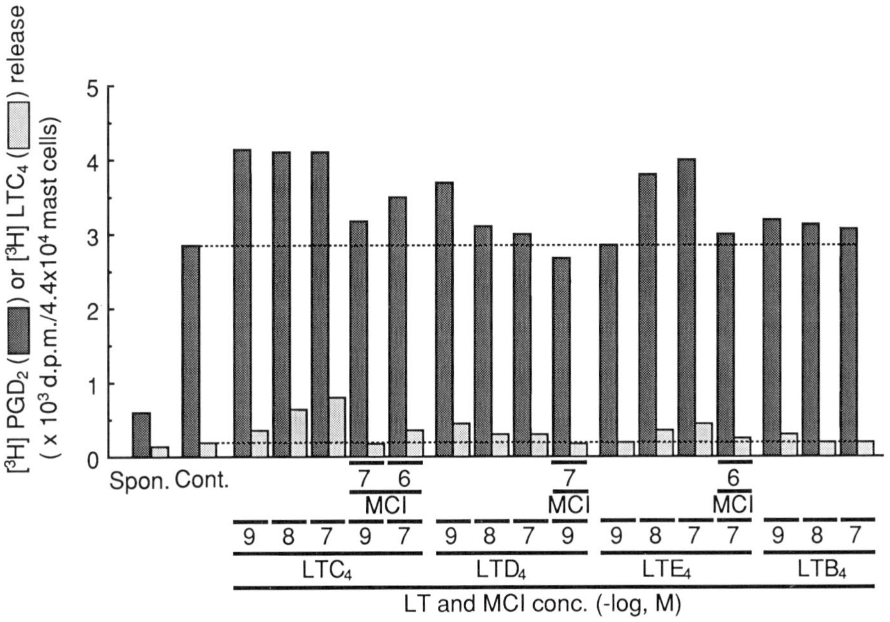

Figure 2. Effect of LTs (10^{-9}–10^{-7} M) and their combination with MCI-826 (MCI, 10^{-7} or 10^{-6} M) on anaphylactic $[^3H]PGD_2$ and $[^3H]LTC_4$ release from the passively sensitized, purified human lung mast cells. Purified human lung mast cells (3.3×10^6 mast cells, purity 46%), which had been incubated with $[^3H]$arachidonic acid (350 μCi, incorporation into cells 23%), were suspended at 2×10^4 mast cells/ml with 0.1% BSA-containing and Ca^{++}-free Tyrode's solution. After preincubation at 37°C for 5 min, and treatment with 1.8×10^{-3} M $CaCl_2$ for 5 min and then LTs for 5 min, the mast cells were challenged with antigen (5×10^{-6}/ml mite extracts) for 30 min. Each column represents mean of triplicate determinations.

radioactivity of LTC_4 fraction from HPLC of the sample was measured. Figure 2 shows the results. Either LT, especially LTC_4 and LTE_4, surprisingly enhanced anaphylactic release of $[^3H]PGD_2$ and $[^3H]LTC_4$. Respective enhancements by p-LTs were partially or completely inhibited by MCI-826. In addition to the results, by the treatment of indomethacin (1 μg/ml), increased amounts of $[^3H]LTC_4$ released anaphylactically was clearly found and this was further enhanced by the coexistence of either LT (Fig. 3).

Effect of Islet Activating Protein (IAP) on the Anaphylactic Release of Enhanced $[^3H]$arachidonate Metabolites by LTC_4 and LTE_4

Figure 4 represents the effect of pretreatment of IAP on the anaphylactic release of $[^3H]$arachidonate metabolites including $[^3H]PGD_2$ and $[^3H]$p-LTs in the presence or absence of LTC_4 and LTE_4. The markedly enhanced release by both of LTC_4 and LTE_4 was greatly reduced and still the anaphylactic release without these LTs was also fairly diminished by the protein.

Specific Binding of p-LTs to BMMC Crude Membrane

Substantial amounts of $[^3H]LTC_4$ specifically bound to the BMMC crude membrane were found (4,870 ± 2,074 dpm/mg protein, mean ± SD, N = 5), but those of $[^3H]LTD_4$ and $[^3H]LTE_4$ were negligible (LTD_4 : 543 ± 1,600 dpm, LTE_4 : 822 ± 1,808 dpm/mg protein).

The Effect of p-LTs on the Anaphylactic Release of $[^{14}C]$ or LTs from BMMC

When challenged with antigen, about 1.3% of $[^{14}C]$AA incorporated into BMMC were released as $[^{14}C]$LTs, among which $[^{14}C]LTC_4$ was the major component, and $[^{14}C]LTB_4$ and $[^{14}C]LTD_4$ were 1/3 and 1/10, respectively. $[^{14}C]LTE_4$ was not detected as significant amounts. The treatment of 10^{-8} – 10^{-6}M LTC_4

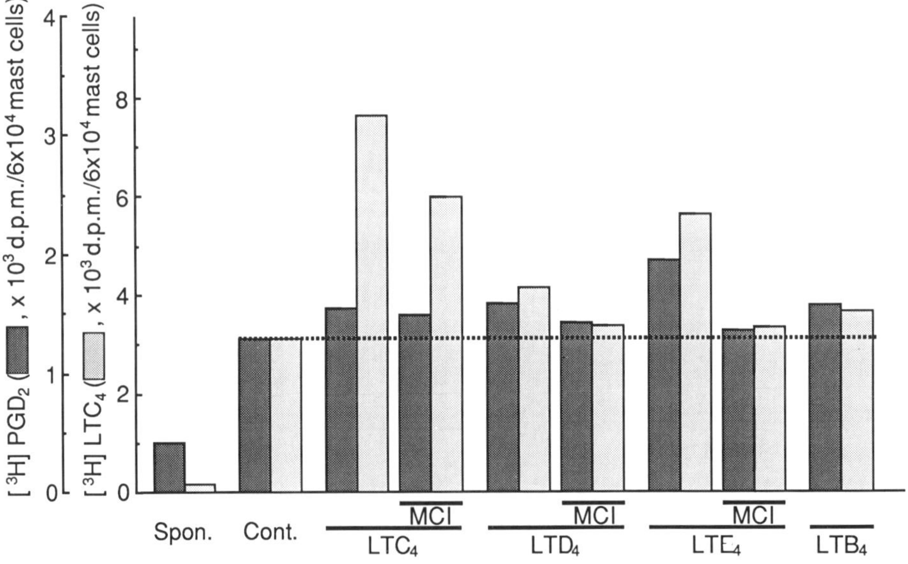

Figure 3. Effect of LTs (10^{-7} M) and their combination with MCI-826 (MCI, 10^{-6} M) on anaphylactic $[^3H]PGD_2$ and $[^3H]LTC_4$ release from the passively sensitized, purified human lung mast cells in the presence of indomethacin (10^{-6} g/ml). Purified human lung mast cells (2.3×10^6 mast cells, purity 55%), which had been incubated with $[^3H]$arachidonic acid (500 μCi, incorporation into cells 27%), were suspended at 2×10^4 mast cells/ml with 0.1% BSA-containing and Ca^{++}-free Tyrode's solution. After preincubation at 37°C for 5 min, and the treatment with indomethacin and 1.8×10^{-3} M $CaCl_2$ for 5 min, and respective LTs for 5 min, the mast cells were challenged with antigen (5×10^{-6} g/ml mite extracts) for 30 min. Each column represents mean of triplicate determinations.

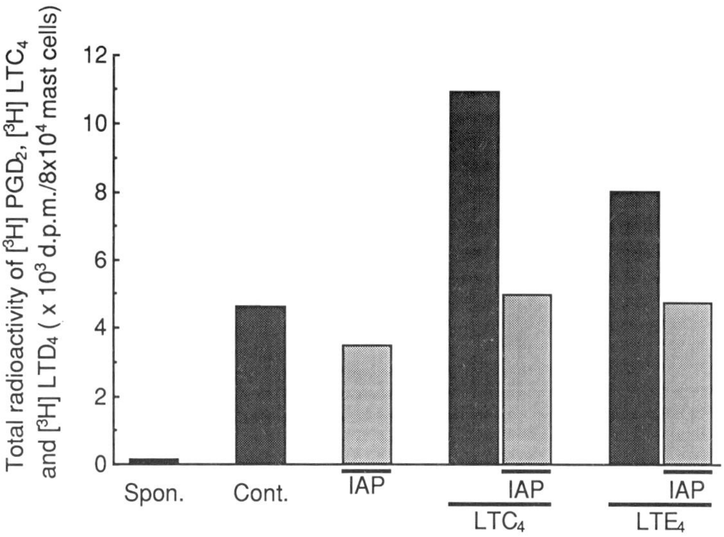

Figure 4. Effect of islet activating protein (IAP), LTC_4 and LTE_4, and the combination of IAP + LTC_4 and IAP + LTE_4 on anaphylactic [^{3}H]arachidonate metabolite release from passively sensitized, purified human lung mast cells. Purified human lung mast cells (7×10^5 mast cells, purity 62%), which had been incubated with [^{3}H]arachidonic acid (250 μCi, incorporation into cells 16%) at 37°C for 2 hrs, were resuspended at 2×10^4 mast cells/ml, treated with or without 3×10^{-8} g/ml IAP at 37°C for 3 hrs, washed 3 times with BSA-containing Tyrode's solution, treated with or without 10^{-7} M LTC_4 or LTE_4 at 37°C for 5 min and challenged with antigen (5×10^{-6} g/ml mite extracts) for 30 min. Radioactivities of [^{3}H]PGD_2, [^{3}H]LTC_4 and [^{3}H]LTD_4 of the sample from HPLC following partial purification by Amprep C-18 reversed column were summed as arachidonate metabolites. Each column represents mean of triplicate determinations.

slightly enhanced the anaphylactic release of [^{14}C]LTC_4 but suppressed that of [^{14}C]LTD_4 (Fig. 5). When [^{14}C]LTC_4 and [^{14}C]LTD_4 were summed as amount of [^{14}C]p-LTs, the treatment of LTC_4 did not consequently influence the total [^{14}C]p-LT release (Fig. 6). Similar to the results, $2 \times 10^{-9} - 2 \times 10^{-7}$ M LTD_4 did not show any significant effect on the anaphylactic release of [^{14}C]LTC_4 from the cells.

Discussion

In the current study, we demonstrated that the purified human lung mast cells and BMMC were different in behaviors to p-LT antagonists and p-LTs on the LT release. That is, first, a highly potent and selective p-LT antagonist, MCI-826, irrespective of concentrations almost constantly inhibited anaphylactic i-LTC_4 release from the human lung mast cells without effect on the histamine release. In contrast, either anaphylactic LT or histamine release from BMMC was not affected by the compound. Second, p-LTs, especially LTC_4 and LTE_4 markedly enhanced the anaphylactic release of not only LTC_4 or p-LTs but also PGD_2 from the human lung mast cells.

On the other hand, LTC_4 and LTD_4 did not substantially influence the anaphylactic release of LTC_4 from the BMMC. These results clearly indicate that p-LTs specifically and potently stimulate the release of arachidonic acid from phospholipid(s) from the human lung mast cells during anaphylaxis. Furthermore, the result of IAP experiments strongly suggests that the enhanced release is activated through IAP-sensitive G-protein. The present results are very different from the report about monkey lung fragment experiment, in which LTC_4 and LTD_4 induce negative feedback regulation (6).

The stimulation of arachidonate formation by LTs can be induced through LT receptors because MCI-826 and IAP potently inhibited the formation. However, it was not specified

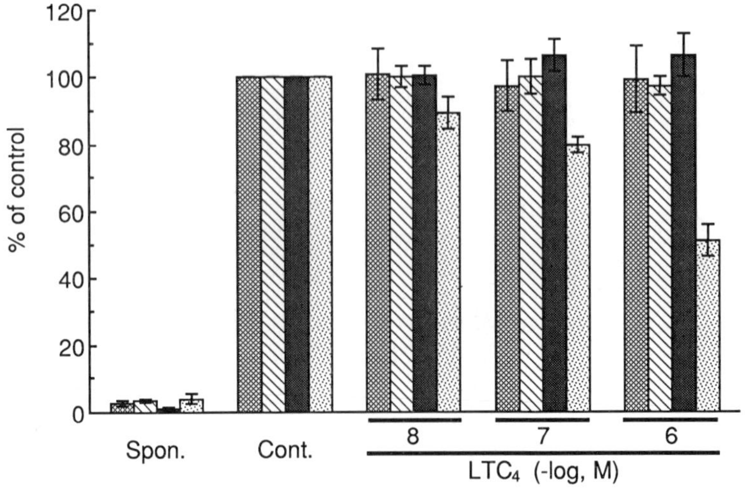

Figure 5. Effect of LTC_4 on anaphylactic histamine and [^{14}C]LT release from mouse bone marrow-derived mast cells (BMMC). BMMC, which had been incubated with [^{14}C]arachidonic acid (0.18 μCi/10^6 BMMC/ml) in the conditioned medium- and BSA-containing Tyrode's solution at 37°C for 3 hr (incorporation of [^{14}C]AA into BMMC 15.6 ± 1.48%, N = 3), were resuspended at 10^5 BMMC/ml, treated with LTC_4 at indicated concentrations for 5 min and challenged with antigen (10^{-5} g/ml dinitrophenylated Ascaris suum extracts) for 20 min. Each column represents mean ± S.E. of 3 experiments. Anaphylactic release of histamine, [^{14}C]LTB_4, [^{14}C]LTC_4 and [^{14}C]LTD_4 were 0.43 ± 0.09, 5.8 ± 1.50, 13.0 ± 4.34 and 1.70 ± 0.16 pmole/10^6 BMMC, respectively.

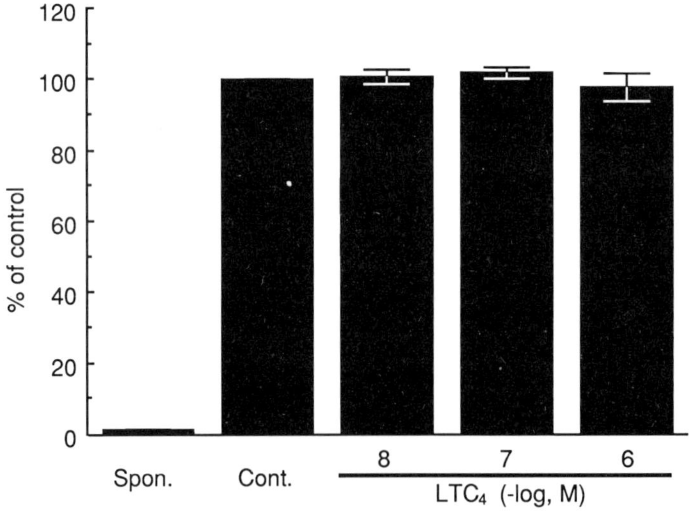

Figure 6. Effect of LTC_4 on anaphylactic [^{14}C]p-LT release from mouse bone marrow-derived mast cells (BMMC). [^{14}C]p-LTs released from BMMC were calculated as the sum of [^{14}C]LTC_4 and [^{14}C]LTD_4 shown in Fig.5.

which LT receptor is responsible for that because serine-borate complex and cysteine which inhibit the enzymes to transform LTC_4 to LTD_4 and LTD_4 to LTE_4, respectively, showed almost complete or great inhibition of not only anaphylactic LT but also histamine release. At least LTE_4 receptor may be involved since LTE_4 does not convert to LTD_4 or to further metabolites in the present condition.

Finally, arachidonic acid formation and resultant release of its metabolites including PGD_2 and LTs by (positive feedback regulation of) LTs may aggravate atopic diseases, especially asthma because some of these metabolites have potent biological activities.

References

1. Kohno, S.W., Ohata, K., Maki, Y., Horie, T., Yoshimoto, T., and Yamamoto, S. 1985. Potent and selective 5-lipoxygenase inhibitors : Cirsiliol and AA-861. In: Advances in prostaglandin, thromboxane, and leukotriene research. O. Hayaishi and S. Yamamoto eds. New York: Raven Press, 217.
2. Augstein, J., Farmer, J.B., Lee, T.B., Sheard, P., and Tattersall, M.L. 1973. Selective inhibitor of slow reacting substance of anaphylaxis. Nature (New Biol.) 245:215.
3. Nakahata, T., Speicer, S.S., Contey, J.R. and Ogawa, M. 1982. Clonal assay of mouse mast cell colonies in methylcellulose culture. Blood 60:352.
4. Yamatodani, A., Fukuda, H., Wada, H., and Watanabe, T. 1985. High performance liquid chromatographic determination of plasma and brain histamine without previous purification of biological samples: Cation-exchange chromatography coupled with post column derivatization fluorometry. J. Chromatogr. 344:115
5. Watanabe-Kohno, S., Shimizu, T., Mizuta, J., Ogino, K., Yamamura, H., and Ohata, K. 1990. Effect of procaterol on the isolated airway smooth muscle and release of anaphylactic chemical mediators from the isolated lung fragments. Arzneim.-Forsch./Drug Res. 40:669.
6. Weichman, B.M., Hostelley, L.S., Bostick, S.P., Muccitelli, R.M., Krell, R.D., and Greason, J. G. 1982. Regulation of the synthesis and release of slow-reacting substance of anaphylaxis from sensitized monkey lung. J. Pharmacol. Exp. Ther. 221:295

Human Histamine Releasing Factors

Allen P. Kaplan, Piotr Kuna, Sesha Reddigari, Joost Oppenheim, Doreen Rucinski*

Histamine Releasing Factors (HRF) are a group of molecules derived from mononuclear cells (T or B lymphocytes, monocytes) (1–4), platelets (5), and neutrophils (6,7) which induce histamine release from basophils or mast cells. Such factors may have importance in cell-cell communication that is seen during late phase allergic reactions (8) in which protracted histamine release is found (9), chronic urticaria (10), or rheumatic diseases such as scleroderma (11). In each of these disorders there is activation of basophils and/or mast cells in relation to surrounding mononuclear cells without any evident IgE-dependent mechanism or activation of complement to release anaphylatoxins (12). We have previously described the fractionation of supernatants from activated mononuclear cells and platelets and isolated three separate proteins possessing HRF activity. These had molecular weights of 8–10 Kd, 15–17 Kd, and 35–41 Kd (13) and an extensive review of the subject has been recently published (14). In this review, I will focus on the 8–10 Kd fraction which contains three molecules relevant to HRF activity. One of these, termed MCAF (macrophage chemotactic and activating factor), is the most potent cytokine with HRF activity thus far identified (15). The second is a mixture of CTAP III and its degradation product NAP-2 (16). These are primarily platelet-derived proteins with HRF activity that are of lesser potency but are plentiful in amount (17). Finally, interleukin 8 (17) is contained in this fraction and it is a potent inhibitor of cytokine-induced histamine release (HRIF) (18,19).

Results

Table I is a partial listing of the molecules containing those that are relevant to the "HRF phenomenon". These have been called the "intecrine" group of molecules. All are 8–10 Kd, bind heparin although with varying affinities, and have similar structural features and significant amino acid sequence homology. Two subgroups, termed a and b, are shown. The factors listed within a particular subgroup are more closely related structurally. The molecules thus far identified to have HRF or HRIF activity are highlighted.

Table 1.

The "Intercrine" Cytokine Family

Subfamily A	Subfamily B
Platelet Factor 4	**MCAF**
CTAP III / β-Thromboglobulin / **NAP 2**	RANTES
Interleukin 8 (NAP 1)	LD 78 (MIP 1α)
Melanoma Growth Factor (GRO)	ACT 2 (MIP 1β)
Macrophage Inflammatory Peptide (MIP-2)	I-309
Chromosome 4 8-10 kD Bind Heparin 4 Cysteines Cys-X-Cys Free N-terminus	Chromosome 17 8-10 kD Bind Heparin 4 Cysteines Cys-Cys Blocked N-terminus

When HRF supernatants were sequentially fractionated by gel filtration, accell QMA ion exchange chromatography and preparative elution from SDS gels, a major form of HRF was identified which had a single broad band at 8–12 Kd upon SDS gel electrophoresis (13). When a comparable gel was transferred to nitrocellulatose, the band divided into an upper and lower half, and each half had been sequenced, the result shown in Figure 1 was obtained. The upper half of the band had a sequence virtually identical to that of Connective Tissue Activating Peptide III or CTAP III (20), a platelet-derived protein shown to activate fibroblasts to produce collagen and proteoglycan. The lower half of the band aligned with the CTAP III sequence if it began with residue 16, i.e., it lacked the N-terminal 15

* Division of Allergy, Rheumatology, and Clinical Immunology, SUNY - Stony Brook, Health Sciences Center, Stony Brook, NY 11794, USA.

Figure 1. Amino acid sequence of the 8–10 Kd form of HRF as eluted from SDS gels. The upper half of the band (HRF-1) corresponds to CTAP III while the lower half of the band (HRF-2) represents NAP-2.

N-terminal sequence comparison of CTAP III and HRF

	1---2---3--4---5---6---7---8---9--10--11-12--13-
CTAP III:	ASN-LEU-ALA-LYS-GLY-LYS-GLU-GLU-SER-LEU-ASP-SER-ASP
HRF 1:	ASN-LEU-ALA-LYS-GLY-LYS-GLU-GLU-SER-LEU-ASP-SER-ASP
HRF 2:	

	14--15--16-17--18--19--20--21--22--23-24--25--26
CTAP III:	-LEU-TYR-ALA-GLU-LEU-ARG-CYS-MET-CYS-ILE-LYS-THR-THR
HRF 1:	-LEU-TYR-ALA-GLU-LEU---------------MET
HRF 2:	ALA-GLU-LEU-ARG--------MET-CYS-ILE-LYS-THR-THR

	-27-28--29-30--31-32--33-34--35--36--37--38-39--40
CTAP III:	-SER-GLY-ILE-HIS-PRO-LYS-ASN-ILE-GLN-SER-LEU-GLU-VAL-ILE
HRF I:	
HRF 2:	-SER-GLY-ILE-HIS-PRO-LYS-ASN-ILE-GLN-SER-LEU-GLU-VAL-ILE

amino acids. This corresponds to Neutrophil Activating Peptide-2 (NAP-2) (16) which can be derived from CTAP III by cleavage with elastase (20). We prepared a monoclonal antibody to CTAP III and isolated CTAP III from platelet-derived supernatants by affinity chromatography and demonstrated that it lacked NAP-2. We then cleaved the material with elastase and isolated the NAP-2 product by rechromatography using the same affinity column. Figure 2 shows the difference in mobility of CTAP III and NAP-2 as assessed by SDS gel electrophoresis. When tested separately, they gave an identical dose response of histamine release between 1–20_µg/ml (~10^{-6}M) (21). This material is a relatively weak form of HRF on a molar basis, but it is plentiful. One ml of platelets release about 35 µg of protein.

If crude HRF supernatants are subjected to Accell QMA anion exchange chromatography, the effluent contains the 8–10 Kd form(s) of HRF while the 15–17 Kd and 35–41 Kd moieties bind to the column. If we remove CTAP III/NAP-2 from this fraction by affinity chromatography, residual HRF activity at the same molecular weight is found. The proportion is highly variable depending in large part upon the percentage of platelet contamination of

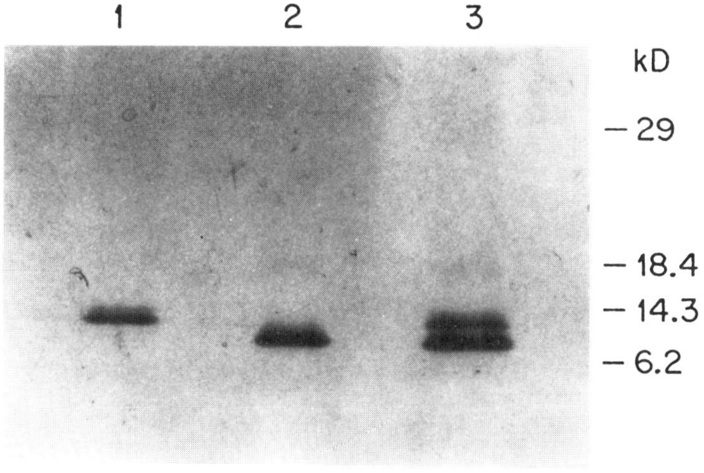

Figure 2. SDS gel electrophoresis of purified CTAP III, NAP-2, and a mixture of the two proteins.

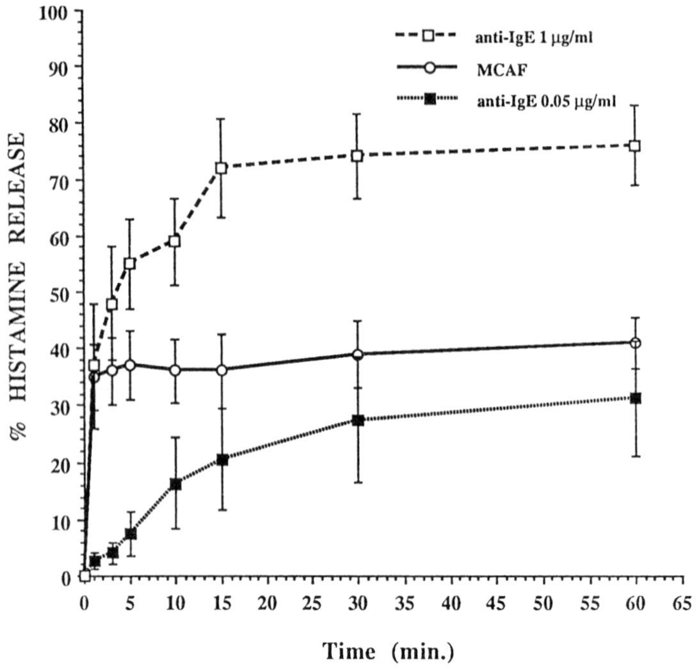

Figure 3. Time course of histamine release by 10^{-7}M MCAF (800 ng/ml) compared to anti-IgE tested at concentrations of 50 ng/ml and 1 µg/ml.

mononuclear cell preparations (removal of 99% of platelets leaves a platelet monoclonal cell ratio of 1:1). We thus considered the possibility that two other related cytokines that are contained in this fraction and possess the same molecular weight possess HRF activity. These are MCAF (22) and interleukin 8 (23). Both are monocyte/macrophage products, the first a monocyte activator (autocoid) and chemotactic factor and the second a neutrophil activator and chemotactic factor. Synonyms for these in the literature are MCP-1 for MCAF and NAP-1 for interleukin 8 (24,25).

MCAF was found to give a dose response release of histamine from human basophils starting at concentrations as low as 10-11M with peak activity reached at 10^{-7}M. Basophils of approximately 90% of subjects tested respond to it regardless whether the donors are atopic or not. The rate of histamine release is extremely rapid; a peak dose of 800 ng/ml yields maximal histamine release within a minute which is even faster than that seen with an optimal concentration (1 µg/ml) of anti-IgE (Figure 3). Although the percent histamine release seen with MCAF was comparable to that obtained with anti-IgE, basophil release of leucotriene C_4/D_4 was far less with MCAF. Thus, MCAF appeared to cause rapid release of basophil granules, but did not activate the pathway for release of lipid mediators. When the basophil population was purified to 85% basophils, the release with MCAF was augmented compared to that seen with mixed leucocytes. Thus, the very rapid effect plus an augmentation of histamine release when basophils are purified suggests a direct effect on the basophil surface rather than an indirect effect mediated by some other cell type. Priming of basophils with interleukins 3 or 5 led to augmented release of histamine by MCAF, but a low dose of MCAF did not augment other secretagogues.

Interleukin 8 was first reported to cause histamine release from basophils, but the concentration required was 10^{-6}M or greater (26). Cells primed with IL3, however, appeared to release histamine at lower IL8 concentrations (27). We reassessed the effect of IL8 upon basophils and found little or no histamine release in most subjects tested with only an occasional positive at 10^{-6}M or more. When we preincubated basophils with IL8, there was inhibition of histamine release induced by various HRF containing fractions, CTAP III/NAP-2, or interleukin 3 (19). Inhibition was detectable at concentrations as low as 10^{-11}M and peak inhibition was

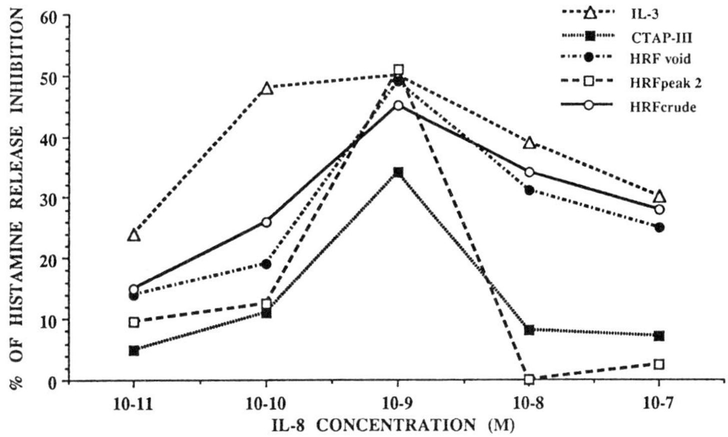

Figure 4. Dose response inhibition of IL8 upon a variety of forms of HRF, CTAP III/NAP-2, and IL3. In each instance, preincubation with IL8 inhibits histamine release and peak inhibition is seen at 10^{-9}M.

found at 10^{-9}M (Figure 4). There was less inhibition at higher concentrations perhaps due to a partial agonist effect. There was no inhibition by IL8 upon anti-IgE or FMLP induced histamine release. These preparations of HRF correspond to the initial description of HRIF (18).

Discussion

The aforementioned data deal solely with the HRF's and related factors present in the 8–10 Kd fraction obtained from mononuclear cell/platelet supernatants. The 15–17 Kd and 35–41 Kd forms of HRF appear thus far to be separate gene products and lack the properties of the "intecrine" factors listed in Table I. It is clear that the concept of HRF is over-simplified in that there are multiple factors which possess histamine-releasing capability and these may be made by different cell types. It is clear that CTAP III/NAP-2 is primarily a platelet product although production by mononuclear cells has not been ruled out. MCAF and IL8 were discussed as monocyte-derived factors although it is already clear that a variety of other cell types can produce them. HRF's have been shown to be released from T lymphocytes, B lymphocytes, monocytes, platelets, and neutrophils and further work will be needed to distinguish which form(s) is made by which cell. The potency of different histamine releasing factors is also important to consider. CTAP III/NAP-2 are not potent on a molar basis, but the concentrations released are high and therefore may contribute to inflammatory conditions. IL3 and GM-CSF are likewise of low to intermediate potency, but only a small percentage of subject basophils is responsive to them, and those are primarily atopic subjects. On the other hand, MCAF is routinely positive in at least 90% of basophils tested, whether from atopic subjects or not, and it is very potent. Priming of basophils by cytokines is a mechanism by which basophil responsiveness is heightened. Thus, augmented responses seen with basophils of atopic subjects may, in part, be due to *in vivo* priming. Interleukins 1,3,5, and GM-CSF have been shown to be capable of priming basophils (16,28,29,30) and we have shown that IL3 and IL5 can each prime responses to MCAF.

Our data thus far suggest that the aforementioned HRF's react directly with basophils and do not require a cellular intermediate. MCAF as agonist and IL8 as antagonist have an effect within seconds and MCAF is more reactive with highly purified basophils than mixed leucocytes, thus the likelihood of an MCAF receptor or IL8 receptor on basophils appear likely. There are no data regarding the kinetics of histamine release by CTAP/NAP-2, although IL3 and GM-CSF are very slowly acting agonists for histamine release (31,32). IL3 receptors on basophils have been demonstrated (33). There are also data to suggest that HRF, or at least some forms of HRF, require cell surface IgE for basophils to be responsive (34,35). An interaction with IgE is therefore suggested rather than a separate receptor. It was further shown that IgE of some patients is required [IgE(+)] while IgE of non-responders is different [IgE(-)], perhaps a function of the carbohydrate attached (36). Non-allergic subjects possess IgE(-) and are HRF non-responsive while atopics are 50% IgE(+) and 50% IgE(-) (37). We have no evidence to suggest that either CTAP III/NAP-2 or MCAF require cell surface IgE and it is clear that responsiveness to each is not strictly dependent on atopic vs. non-atopic studies. However, the other molecular species of HRF need to be assessed for a requirement for cell surface IgE.

HRF activity (without definition of particular type) has been identified in bronchial secretions (38), late phase reactions (8), and may have a role in atopic dermatitis (39), or rheumatoid arthritis (40). In addition, immunotherapy for asthma appears to result in diminished HRF activity in activated mononuclear cell supernatants which may reflect diminished HRF production and/or increased HRIF production (41,42). Thus, the ratio of HRF to HRIF may have a critical role in the pathogenesis of allergic diseases, and therapeutic alteration of that ratio may affect the course of allergic diseases.

References

1. Thueson, D.O., Speck, L.S., Lett-Brown, M.A., and Grant, J.A. 1979. Histamine-releasing activity (HRA). II. Interaction with basophils and physicochemical characterization. J. Immunol. 123:633.
2. Thueson, D.O., Speck, L.S., Lett-Brown, M.A., and Grant, J.A. 1979. Histamine-releasing activity (HRA). I. Production by mitogen or antigen stimulated human mononuclear cells. J. Immunol. 123:623.
3. Kaplan, A.P., Haak-Frendscho, M., Fauci, A., Dinarello, C., and Halbert, E. 1985. A histamine-releasing factor from activated human mononuclear cells. J. Immunol. 135:2027.
4. Alam, R., Forsythe, P.A., Lett-Brown, M.A., and Grant, A.J. 1989. Cellular origin of histamine-releasing factor produced by peripheral blood mononuclear cells. J. Immunol. 142:3951.
5. Orchard, M.A., Kagey-Sobotka, A., Proud, D., and Lichtenstein, L.M. 1986. Basophil histamine release induced by a substance from stimulated platelets. J. Immunol. 136:2240.
6. White, M.V., and Kaliner, M.A. 1987. Neutrophils and mast cells. I. Human neutrophil-derived histamine releasing activity (HRA-N). J. Immunol. 139:1624.
7. White, M.V., Kaplan, A.P., Haak-Frendscho, M., and Kaliner, M. 1989. Neutrophils and mast cells. Comparison of neutrophil-derived histamine-releasing activity with other histamine-releasing factors. J. Immunol. 1412:3575.
8. Warner, J.A., Pienkowski, M.M., Plaut, M., Norman, P.S., and Lichtenstein, L.M. 1986. Identification of histamine releasing factor(s) in the late phase of cutaneous IgE-mediated reactions. J. Immunol. 136:2583.
9. Charlesworth, C.N., Hood, A.F., Soter, N.A., Kagey-Sobotka, A., Norman, P.S., and Lichtenstein, L.M. 1989. Cutaneous late-phase response to allergen. Mediator release and inflammatory cell infiltration. J. Clin. Invest. 83:1519.
10. Kaplan, A.P. 1985. Urticaria and angioedema. In: Allergy. A.P. Kaplan, ed. New York: Churchill Livingstone, p. 439.
11. Clamen, H. 1989. On scleroderma. Mast cells, endothelial cells, and fibroblasts. JAMA 262:1206.
12. Cochrane, C.G., and Muller-Eberhard, H.J. 1968. The deviation of two distinct anaphylatoxin activities from the third and fifth component of human complement. J. Exp. Med. 127:371.
13. Baeza, M.L., Reddigari, S.R., Haak-Frendscho, M., and Kaplan, A.P. 1989. Purification and further characterization of human mononuclear cell histamine-releasing factor. J. Clin. Invest. 83:1204.
14. White, M.V., Baer, H., Kubota, Y., and Kaliner, M.D. 1989. Neutrophils and mast cells. Characterization of cells responsive to neutrophil derived histamine releasing activity. J. Allergy Clin. Immunol. 84:773.
15. Kuna, P., Reddigari, S.R., Rucinski, D., Oppenheim, J.J., and Kaplan, A.P. 1991. Monocyte chemotactic and activating factor is a potent histamine releasing factor for human basophils. J. Exp. Med. 175:489.
16. Baeza, M.L., Reddigari, S.R., Kornfeld, D., Ramani, N., Smith, E.M., Hossler, P.A., Fischer, T., Castor, C.W., Gorevic, P.G., and Kaplan, A.P. 1990. Relationship of one form of human histamine releasing factor to connective tissue activating peptide-III. J. Clin. Invest. 85:1516.
17. Castor, C.W., Miller, J.W., and Walz, D.A. 1983. Structural and biological characteristics of connective tissue activating peptides (CTAP-III), a major human platelet derived

growth factor. Proc. Natl. Acad. Sci., USA 80:765.
18. Alam, R., Welter, J., Forsythe, P.A., Lett-Brown, M.A., Rankin, J.A., Boyars, M., and Grant, A. 1990. Detection of histamine release inhibitory factor- and histamine releasing factor-like activities in bronchoalveolar lavage fluids. Am. Rev. Respir. Dis. 141:666.
19. Kuna, P., Reddigari, S.R., Kornfeld, D., and Kaplan, A.P. 1991. Interleukin 8 inhibits histamine release from human basophils induced by histamine releasing factors, connective tissue activating peptide III, and interleukin 3. J. Immunol. 147:1920.
20. Walz, A., and Baggiolini, M. 1990. Generation of the neutrophil activating peptide NAP-2 from platelet basic protein or connective tissue-activating peptide III through monocyte proteases. J. Exp. Med. 171:449.
21. Reddigari, S.R., Miragliotta, G.F., Kuna, P., Kornfeld, D., Baeza, M.L., Castor, C.W., and Kaplan, A.P. Connective tissue activating peptide III and its derivative neutrophil activating peptide-2 release histamine from human basophils. J. Allergy Clin. Immunol. In press.
22. Matsushima, K., Morishita, K., Yoshimura, T., Lavu, S., Kobayashi, Y., Lew, W., Appella, E., Kung, H.F., Leonard, E.J., and Oppenheim, J.J. 1988. Molecular cloning of a human monocyte-derived neutrophil chemotactic factor (MDNCF) and the induction of MDNCF mRNA by interleukin 1 and tumor necrosis factor. J. Exp. Med. 167:1883.
23. Leonard, E.J., and Yoshimura, T. 1990. Human monocyte chemoattractant protein-1 (MCP-1). Immunology Today 11:97.
24. Yoshimura, T., Robinson, E.A., Tanaka, S., Appella, E., and Leonard, E.J. 1989. Purification and amino acid analysis of two human monocyte chemoattractants produced by phytohemagglutinin-stimulated human blood mononuclear leukocytes. J. Immunol. 142:1956.
25. Schrr, J.M., Mrowietz, U., Morita, E., and Christophers, E. 1987. Purification and partial biochemical characterization of a human monocyte-derived, neutrophil-activating peptide that lacks interleukin 1 activity. J. Immunol. 139:3474.
26. White, M.V., Yoshimura, T., Hook, W., Kaliner, M.A., and Leonard, E.J. 1989. Neutrophil attractant/activation protein-1 (NAP-1) causes human basophil histamine release. Immunol. Lett. 22:151.
27. Dahinden, C.A., Kurimoto, Y., De Weck, A.L., Lindley, I., Dewald, B., and Baggiolini, M. 1989. The neutrophil-activating peptide NAF/NAP-1 induces histamine release and leukotrine release by interleukin 3-primed basophils. J. Exp. Med. 170:1787.
28. Massey, W.A., Randall, T.C., Kagey-Sabotka, A., Warner, J.A., MacDonald, S.M., Gillis, S., Allison, A.C., and Lichtenstein, L.M. 1989. Recombinant human IL-1a and -1b potentiate IgE-mediated histamine release from human basophils. J. Immunol. 143:1875.
29. Bischoff, S.C., De Weck, A.L., and Dahinden, C.A. 1990. Interleukin 3 and granulocyte/macrophage-colony-stimulating factor render human basophil responsive to low concentration of complement component C3a. Proc. Natl. Acad. Sci., USA 87:6813.
30. Bischoff, S.C., Brunner, T., De Weck, A.L., and Dahinden, C.A. 1990. Interleukin 5 modifies histamine release and leukotriene generation by human basophils in response to diverse agonists. J. Exp. Med. 172:1577.
31. Haak-Frendscho, M., Arai, N., Arai, K.-I., Baeza, M.L., Finn, A., and Kaplan, A.P. 1988. Human recombinant granulocyte-macrophage colony-stimulating factor and interleukin 3 cause basophil histamine release. J. Clin. Invest. 82:17.
32. MacDonald, S.M., Schleimer, R.P., Kagey-Sobotka, A., Gillis, S., and Lichtenstein, L.M.»; . Recombinant IL-3 induces histamine release from human basophils. J. Immunol. 1989142:3527.
33. Lopez, A.M., Lyons, A.B., Eglinton, J.M., Park, L.S., To, L.B., Clark, S.C., and Vadas, M.A. 1990. Specific binding of human interleukin-3 and granulocyte-macrophage colony-stimulating factor to human basophils. J. Allergy Clin. Immunol. 85:99.
34. Schulman, E.S., Liu, P.C., Proud, D., McGlashan, J., D.W., Lichtenstein, L.M., and Plaut, M. 1985. Human lung macrophages induce histamine release from basophils and mast cells. Am. Rev. Resp. Dis. 131:230.
35. MacDonald, S.M., Lichtenstein, L.M., Proud, D., Plaut, M., Naclerio, R.M., MacGlashan, D.W., and Kagey-Sobotka, A. 1987. Studies of IgE-dependent histamine releasing factors: Heterogeneity of IgE. J. Immunol. 139:506.
36. MacDonald, S.M., White, J.M., Kagey-Sobotka, A., and Lichtenstein, L.M. 1988. Is glycosylation the basis of IgE heterogeneity? Clin. Res. 36:602 (Abst.).
37. Fisher, R.H., Kagey-Sobotka, A., Proud, D., Naclerio, R.M., and Lichtenstein, L.M. 1987. Histamine releasing factor: Release mecha-

nisms and responding population. J. Allergy Clin. Immunol. 79:248 (Abst.).
38. Broide, D.H., Smith, C.M., and Wasserman, S.I. 1990. Mast cells and pulmonary fibrosis. Identification of histamine releasing factor in bronchoalveolar lavage fluid. J.Immunol. 145:1838.
39. Sampson, H.A., Broadbent, K.R., and Bernhisel-Broadbent, J. 1989. Spontaneous release of histamine from basophils and histamine-releasing factor in patients with atopic dermatitis and food hypersensitivity. N. Engl. J. Med. 321:228.
40. Gruber, B., Poznansky, M., Boss, E., Partin, J., Gorevic, P., and Kaplan, A.P. 1986. Characterization and functional studies of rheumatoid synovial mast cells: Activation by secretagogues, anti-IgE, and a histamine-releasing lymphokine. Arth. Rheum. 29:944.
41. Kuna, P., Alam, R., Kuzminska, B., and Rozniecki, J. 1989. The effect of preseasonal immunotherapy on the production of histamine releasing factor (HRF) by mononuclear cells from patients with seasonal asthma: Results of a double blind placebo-controlled, randomized study. J. Allergy Clin. Immunol. 83:816.
42. Tung-Nan, L., and Kue-Hsiung, H. 1990. Altered production of histamine-releasing factor (HRF) activity and responsiveness to HRF after immunotherapy in children with asthma. J. Allergy Clin. Immunol. 86:894.

Characteristics of the Cytosolic Calcium Response During IgE-Mediated Stimulation of Human Basophils and Mast Cells

Donald MacGlashan*

In recent years, IgE-mediated stimulation of human mast cells and basophils has been shown to result in elevations of cytosolic free Ca^{++}, as long expected. However, single cell studies have shown that the response has several interesting properties. First, although the response is graded according to the magnitude of the stimulation, the single cell kinetics show properties of an all-or-nothing response. A typical response in the mast cell shows a variable quiescent period, following stimulation, followed by a rapid transition to a new elevated calcium level. In basophils, this new state is not stable. Instead, the response is characterized by oscillations or spiking of the cytosolic calcium. In an attempt to determine whether these oscillations are important to degranulation, we have studied the initial calcium response which is thought to be derived from the release of internal stores of calcium, the hypothesized source of oscillations. These recent studies in the human basophil indicate that the calcium response derived from internal stores is not responsible for degranulation.

Since the studies of Mongar and Schild in 1958, it has been known that the anaphylactic secretory response of mast cells required extracellular calcium. Later studies by Lichtenstein demonstrated a similar dependence in human basophils. In light of studies being done in other cell types at the time, these early studies suggested that an influx of calcium was obligatory for degranulation of mast cells and basophils. Over the intervening decades, studies have refined the initial observations so that today we know that cytosolic calcium concentrations do indeed increase following the crosslinking of cell surface IgE. However, little else is known concerning the role of the calcium elevation in degranulation or the mechanisms leading to increases in calcium. Although these fundamental pieces of knowledge are missing, there have been several important insights concerning the calcium response. For example, a generally accepted paradigm of the calcium response is that it is composed of two phases, the first of which is dependent on the release of intracellular stores of calcium and lasting from 10–200 seconds and the second which depends on the influx of calcium from the extracellular medium. Many details of the initial phase are well understood, but the mechanism by which extracellular calcium traverses the cell membrane and finds its way to the cytoplasm is still in hot debate. Another important insight into the calcium response is the recognition that the behavior of single cells is not reflected in the average population response and that the single cell calcium response might be frequency encoded rather than exerting its effects by the amplitude of the response. Elegant studies in the laboratories of Fewtrell and Webb (1,2) first made these observations in rat basophilic leukemia cells. This report will review our recent studies on single cell behavior of human mast cells and basophils and discuss recent evidence that the initial phase of the calcium response may have little to do with degranulation.

A perennial question in the study of mediator release for mast cells or basophils has been whether partial histamine release represents a fraction of the cells releasing all of their histamine, or all cells releasing a part of their histamine. Our interest in the role of calcium in the secretory response and the possibility of studying single cell calcium responses with new digital video microscope technology made it possible to address another form of this question. Instead of asking whether histamine release behaved in an all-or-nothing manner, we asked whether the calcium response behaved this way.

Two new technologies were required to an-

* Johns Hopkins University, Asthma and Allergy Center, 301 Bayview Blvd., Baltimore, Md. 21224, USA.

swer this question. The first depended on the development of a calcium sensitive fluorescent probe by Roger Tsien. This molecule has the special property that it changes its excitation spectrum when it binds a single calcium ion. This property means that calcium concentrations can be calculated without considering the cell thickness or change in dye intensity due to leakage from the cell cytoplasm. This property also means that single cells can be studied under the microscope. The second technology involved the creation of a microscope capable of quantitative measurements of light intensity for an entire field of cells. During the last 5 years, we have developed this technology in our laboratory and have begun studying the human mast cell and basophil calcium response following challenge with a number of stimuli. Initially, the response to IgE-dependent stimuli was examined.

The first studies noted that for histamine release of less than 50%, the calcium response occurred to varying extents in all cells in the microscopic field of view (histamine release was measured by removing some of the supernatant from the microscope chamber). In other words, we did not find only two populations of response, either non-response or response. The response was normally distributed about a mean (approximately a 300 nM change for cells showing 50% histamine release). We expected a wide distribution in the response since all biological responses are distributed about a mean behavior. We then verified that the response was a simple graded response, rather than all-or-nothing, by arranging the conditions to be suboptimal for release. This could be done by any of five methods. The simplest method involved comparing the two single cell calcium response distributions following stimulation with either an optimal concentration of anti-IgE antibody or sub-optimal (lower) concentrations of anti-IgE (3). We found that the distributions simply shifted to a lower mean net calcium response when the cells were challenged with a suboptimal concentration of anti-IgE. We have found the same behavior when suboptimal conditions were created by other methods. These include (a) comparing the response at two densities of cell surface IgE, (b) comparing desensitized cells to non-desensitized cells, (c) comparing two forms of the same antigen (one with weaker crosslinking properties), and (d) comparing normal cells to cells treated with a pharmacologic agent which inhibits or enhances the response. Therefore, in the context of the maximal or average calcium response, the behavior of single cells was graded in nature. We have seen that this is true of both human mast cells from various sources and human basophils. In addition, we have examined response distributions for several additional basophil behaviors. In all cases, including degranulation, the response is unimodal and graded according to the conditions of challenge. While there are situations where the response is definitely not Gaussian and somewhat skewed, the distributions have never been bimodal (non-response vs. response).

These results led to the conclusion that the single cell response was reflecting the population response, i. e., gradual changes in the magnitude of the response occurred at both levels. However, we were surprised to find that the kinetics of the response as determined by the population average was completely misleading. In mast cells, a close inspection of the early time-points following stimulation revealed that there was a quiescent period followed by an abrupt transition to a new steady state level or, following the initial abrupt transition, a slower gradual elevation to a somewhat higher calcium level (4). The remarkable fact was in the characteristics of the transition: Cells were asynchronously making this transition, although the nature of the transition was similar for nearly all cells. Lower levels of stimulation lead to longer quiescent periods but ultimately a similar abrupt transition would follow. The length of the quiescent period, the lagtime, increased with lower levels of stimulation, and the cells became more asynchronous. If the single cell kinetic curves were summed, the result was the slow gradual increase characteristic of the average population response. These results required a shift in our point of view: that is, the single cell response had characteristics that were a composite of all-or-nothing events and graded changes. At this time, we do not have an adequate model which would lead to these observations.

The kinetic response of human basophils differs from the mast cell. Following stimulation, there is a quiescent period, as in the mast cell, and an abrupt transition. However, the transition is not stable (4). Instead, a series of chaotic oscillations occurs, with calcium levels sometimes showing a sustained elevation upon which oscillations occur, or the oscillations occur during periods of resting calcium concentrations. Again, a summation of these single cell kinetics leads to the gradual response seen in the population average.

The occurrence of oscillations is not restricted to the basophil; a very small percentage of mast cells shows a few oscillations. Likewise, some basophils show mast cell characteristics. We believe this indicates that a similar underlying mechanism is operating in these two cell types. But the predominant behavior of these two cell types is distinguished by the presence of oscillations in basophils. A plot of the *average* net elevation in the cytosolic calcium concentration versus histamine release for mast cells and basophils shows that the EC50 for histamine release is 300 nM for mast cells and 100 nM for basophils. In other words, mast cells appear to require higher elevations in calcium to obtain the same histamine release. If, instead, the peaks of the oscillations are used to plot the basophil points in this relationship, the mast cell and basophil calcium-histamine release curves are similar. Thus, it becomes necessary to determine whether the basophil response is controlled by the oscillations and especially the peaks of the oscillations. We have begun a number of studies to address this question. One of these studies uses some of the knowledge gained from other cell systems.

As noted above, the general paradigm for the calcium response postulates that there are two phases. The first phase is dependent on the release of intracellular stores of calcium and the second phase is dependent on the entry of extracellular calcium. Despite the ultimate sources of calcium being different for these two phases of the response, it is generally believed (though still hotly debated) that extracellular calcium is routed to the cytoplasm through the same internal stores responsible for the first phase of the response. This implies that the same biochemical steps are involved in both the first phase and partially in the second phase, the sustained calcium response. The general belief is that by some mechanism, the second messenger, inositol 1,4,5 trisphosphate (IP3), is generated from cell membrane phospholipids, stimulates a specific receptor on endoplasmic reticulum-like (ER) organelles which in turn causes the ER to release calcium. Calcium in these ER stores is presumably maintained by the influx of extracellular calcium by means yet unknown. Thus, the sustained response should also depend on the sustained generation of inositol trisphosphate and its action on the specific receptor in the ER membrane. Studies of oscillations in other cell types suggest that they are also sustained by an IP3 driven mechanism. Therefore, a study of the initial phase of the response might indicate the importance of spiking or oscillatory events later in the reaction.

Suboptimal stimulation of basophils with anti-IgE antibody does not reveal a biphasic response; however, optimal and supraoptimal concentrations of anti-IgE do show a well-defined first and second phase. This is also true at the single cell level with the difference that the second phase is characterized by oscillations in cytosolic calcium. Our first clue that the initial phase might not affect degranulation was derived from studies where the calcium chelator, EGTA, was added to the reaction at the same time as the stimulus. Under these conditions, influx of extracellular calcium is blocked because the chelator effectively reduces the extracellular free calcium to very low levels (below cytosolic concentrations). The remaining cytosolic calcium response should be due to the release of internal stores of calcium. Under these conditions, the second phase is ablated for any stimulus. For a univalent stimulus like the bacterial peptide, fmet-leu-phe, the initial phase of the response is not effected and histamine release is inhibited by less than 10% (5). For supra-optimal anti-IgE antibody, the initial phase is also not effected but histamine release is inhibited 90–100%. Thus for these two stimuli, the initial phase of the response apparently leads to histamine release in one case (fmet peptide), while having no effect on release for IgE-mediated release. If the histamine release kinetics are compared for these two stimuli, we find that histamine release is complete within 1 minute following fmet peptide, and therefore occurs during the initial transient. However, following anti-IgE antibody, no histamine release occurs during the first phase; only during the second phase does release occur. The onset of the second phase can be determined with manganese. This metal ion only enters the cell when calcium channels are opened. However, it will quench the fura-2 fluorescence upon entering. This provides a way of determining the time of influx during the reaction. These studies indicate that influx does indeed occur only after the first 2 minutes of the reaction, at a time when the IgE-mediated histamine release occurs. Recent pharmacologic studies with cAMP active agents have found that they have no effect on the initial phase of the calcium response but do inhibit the second phase response to a degree which reflects their inhibition of histamine release. Not surprisingly, then, they have little effect on fmet peptide-induced release.

If the initial transient works for fmet peptide but not for anti-IgE, then maybe the source of the internal calcium may differ for these two stimuli, and it is the location of its release which is important to the degranulation apparatus. However, we have found that the source of the initial phase is probably the same for both stimuli. If basophils are first incubated with fmet peptide in the presence of EGTA to discharge the internal pool, then stimulation with supra-optimal anti-IgE leads to no initial phase. This experiment works in reverse as well. If the internal pool is discharged with the drug thapsagargin, both the initial phase following anti-IgE antibody and fmet peptide are inhibited. Therefore, the initial calcium response for both stimuli is probably coming from the same internal pool, and if it is responsible for degranulation, both stimuli should be unaffected by EGTA, and the kinetics of release should be similar.

We suggest that the initial transient during the fmet peptide response is coincidental and not responsible for histamine release. This belief is supported by single cell studies. Among different preparations of basophils, the peak of the initial transient following fmet peptide correlates with histamine release. This seems to indicate its involvement in degranulation. However, at the single cell level, there is no correlation. We have been able to measure the rough magnitude of the degranulation response in basophils by the appearance of fura-2 free regions that we believe are the large vacuoles that form during degranulation as observed by electron microscopy (6). When these morphologic changes are quantified and compared to the individual cell's calcium response, no correlation exists. There is another stimulus which can be used to probe the importance of these reactions. The anaphylatoxin, C5a, induces a response which is the natural analog to the fmet peptide and EGTA simultaneously. In other words, there is no second phase with this stimulus even in the presence of extracellular calcium. Yet cells also release histamine in response to C5a. However, unlike fmet peptide, among different basophil preparations, we have found no correlation between the height of the C5a-induced calcium response and subsequent histamine release.

These studies suggest to us that the initial phase of the response is a red-herring and unrelated to the degranulation response. If the oscillations in cytosolic calcium occur by a mechanism which depends on the continued release of calcium from the internal stores, as is usually suggested, then this conclusion about the initial transient suggests that oscillation peaks may have little to do with histamine release. However, these studies are continuing and we are currently beginning careful quantification of oscillations and the conditions which alter their appearance.

If calcium oscillations do not explain the difference in calcium sensitivity between mast cells and basophils, there must be another reaction taking place in basophils which may not be dominant in mast cells. The activation of protein kinase C may fulfill this role. One of the most obvious differences between mast cells and basophils is that the activation of PKC by phorbol esters causes degranulation in basophils (in the absence of a change in cytosolic calcium levels) but not mast cells. This review will not cover our studies on PKC, but only mention that we hypothesize that its involvement explains the mast cell/basophil difference.

References

1. Millard, P.J., Gross, D., Webb, W.W., and Fewtrell, C.. 1988. Imaging asynchronous changes in intracellular Ca2+ in individual stimulated tumor mast cells. Proc. Natl. Acad. Sci. U S A 85:1854.
2. Millard, P.J., Ryan, T.A., Webb, W.W., and Fewtrell, C. 1989. Immunoglobulin E receptor cross-linking induces oscillations in intracellular free ionized calcium in individual tumor mast cells. J. Biol. Chem. 264:19730.
3. MacGlashan, D.J. 1989. Single-cell analysis of Ca++ changes in human lung mast cells: graded vs. all-or-nothing elevations after IgE-mediated stimulation. J. Cell. Biol. 109:123.
4. MacGlashan, D.W., Jr., and Guo, C.B. 1991.

Oscillations in free cytosolic calcium during IgE-mediated stimulation distinguish human basophils from human mast cells. J. Immunol., in press.
5. MacGlashan, D.W., Jr., and Warner, J.A. 1991. Stimulus-dependent leukotriene release from human basophils: A comparative study of C5a and Fmet-leu-phe. J Leuk. Biology 49:29.
6. Warner, J.A., Bochner, B.S., and MacGlashan, D.W., Jr. 1990. Cytoskeletal rearrangement and shape change in human basophils. J. All. Clin. Immunol. 146:1a.

Antiinflammatory Effects of Cyclosporin A

Gianni Marone, Amato de Paulis, Anna Ciccarelli, Vincenzo Casolaro, Giuseppe Spadaro, Raffaele Cirillo*

Cyclosporin A (CsA) is a potent immunosuppressive agent widely used in the prevention/treatment of graft rejection. CsA is also effective in the treatment of some patients with several autoimmune diseases and preliminary evidence indicates that it may be useful in the management of severe allergic disorders. We investigated the effect of CsA and its analogs (CsC, CsD, CsG, and CsH) on the release of preformed (histamine) and *de novo* synthesized proinflammatory mediators (leukotriene C_4: LTC_4 and prostaglandin D_2: PGD_2) from human peripheral blood basophils and from mast cells isolated from lung parenchyma or skin tissues. Pharmacological concentrations (2.4–800 nM) of CsA rapidly inhibited the *in vitro* release of histamine, LTC_4 and/or PGD_2 from basophils and mast cells induced by immunologic (antigen and anti-IgE) and non-immunologic stimuli (A23187). The inhibitory effect of CsA and of its congeners was significantly correlated to their affinity for the cytosolic binding protein cyclophilin (CyP). *In vivo* administration of CsA (7 mg/kg) caused a significant reduction of *in vitro* basophil responsiveness to immunologic (anti-IgE) and non-immunologic stimuli (A23187 and f-Met-Leu-Phe) which peaked at 1–5 hrs after CsA administration and lasted for up to 18 hours. The inhibitory effect of CsA on the release of proinflammatory mediators from human basophils and mast cells may contribute to the therapeutic efficacy of CsA in several inflammatory diseases.

Cyclosporin A (CsA) is a lipophilic, cyclic undecapeptide (m.w. 1,203) extracted from *Tolypocladium inflatum Gams* (1). Several natural and synthetic structural congeners with substitutions or deletions on the ring structure have been identified or synthesized. Early studies by Borel and co-workers led to the theory that CsA is a selective immunosuppressive agent acting on defined subpopulations of immunocompetent cells (2). CsA significantly improved the initial and long-term survival of renal allografts (3), and has had an even greater effect on cardiac (4), hepatic (5), heart-lung (6), single-lung (7) and multiple-organ transplantation. For several years the immunosuppressive effect of CsA was commonly attributed to inhibition of lymphokine mRNA transcription (8). However, the drug is also proving effective in an increasing number of autoimmune (endogenous uveitis, rheumatoid arthritis, psoriasis, type I diabetes mellitus, Crohn's disease, primary biliary cirrhosis, etc.) (3,9–11) and inflammatory diseases (atopic dermatitis, severe chronic asthma, etc.) (12,13) suggesting that it may have multiple sites of action (3).

A number of proteins have been proposed as mediating the immunosuppressive activity of CsA. CsA binds to calmodulin (14), which is present in human immune cells (15,16). However, CsA does not specifically bind to calmodulin, and inactive (CsH) structural congeners of CsA bind to calmodulin equally well (17). Finally, intracellular concentrations of CsA do not correlate with calmodulin content. A second possible target of CsA effects are the CsA-binding proteins called cyclophilins (CyPs), discovered by Handschumacher et al. (18). This class of ubiquitous and abundant proteins is highly conserved among eukaryotic organisms, and is responsible for CsA uptake into the cell. CyPA refers to the originally discovered isoform (18), whereas CyPB refers to the isoform described by Price et al. (19) and CyPC refers to the isoform identified by Friedman and Weissman (20). Several observations indicate that CyP is involved in CsA's mechanism of action (21). When the specificity of CyP binding was examined with a series of CsA analogs, the

* Division of Clinical Immunology, Department of Medicine, University of Naples Federico II, Second School of Medicine, Via Sergio Pansini 5, 80131 Naples, Italy.
Acknowledgements: This work was supported in part by grants from the C.N.R. (Project F.A.T.M.A.: Subproject Prevention and Control of Disease Factors; Project No. 91.00081.PF41), the M.U.R.S.T. and "Ministero Sanità: Istituto Superiore di Sanità" AIDS Project 1990 (Rome, Italy).

immunosuppressive activity correlated with CyP binding (22). Second, CyP catalyzes the *cis-trans* isomerization of peptidyl-prolyl bonds, and CsA inhibits this enzymatic activity (23). It is still not clear whether the inhibition of peptidyl-prolyl-*cis,trans*-isomerase (PPIase) activity by CsA plays a critical role in lymphocyte signal transduction. However, there is now general agreement that CsA binding to CyPs is a first critical step in the drug's immunosuppressive activity. There are many unanswered questions regarding the ubiquitous nature of CyPs and the relative selectivity of CsA for only certain cell types. Perhaps binding to CyPs is necessary, but not sufficient, for immunosuppression and the complex CsA-CyPs inhibits some other component (24).

During recent years we investigated whether CsA inhibits biochemical events controlling the release of preformed (histamine) and *de novo* synthesized (leukotriene C_4: LTC_4 and prostaglandin D_2: PGD_2) mediators of inflammatory reactions from human basophils and mast cells by interacting with CyP. We selected this *in vitro* system for two reasons. First, the release of mediators from basophils and mast cells occurs in a few minutes and does not require protein synthesis (25). Second, this *in vitro* model is clinically relevant to a variety of inflammatory and autoimmune diseases such as uveoretinitis (26), rheumatoid arthritis (27), Crohn's disease (28), allergic diseases (29), scleroderma (30) and allergic encephalomyelitis (31).

Pharmacological concentrations of CsA (2.4–800 nM) caused a concentration-dependent inhibition of histamine and LTC_4 release from human basophils induced by anti-IgE, antigen or the Ca^{2+} ionophore A23187 (32). In contrast, phorbol myristate (TPA) and bryostatin 1, which directly activate different isoforms of protein kinase C (PKC) bypassing several biochemical steps of the release process, induced histamine release regardless of the presence of CsA. This suggests that the activation of PKC mediated by TPA and bryostatin 1 bypasses biochemical steps that are inhibited by CsA and that play a role in the release process in human basophils. Thus, CsA's inhibitory effect on the release process of basophils depends on the nature of the basophil stimulus, similar to the suppression of T cell function that also depends on the nature of the T cell stimulus (33).

Another interesting finding of this study was the extreme rapidity of the inhibitory effect of CsA. Inhibition of basophil histamine release was unaffected by different preincubation times (1 to 30 min) but, more important, CsA was effective in inhibiting mediator release throughout the release process (32). Thus, CsA is an extremely rapid inhibitor of mediator release from basophils and it probably interferes with biochemical events that occur during the release process. This finding agrees with the observation that CsA rapidly inhibits cytolytic T lymphocyte effector functions without affecting protein synthesis (34), presumably by binding to CyP.

CsA also inhibits the immunological release of preformed and *de novo* synthesized mediators from mast cells isolated from lung parenchyma and skin tissues. It concentration-dependently inhibited the *de novo* synthesis of LTC_4 and PGD_2 from lung mast cells (35,36) and of PGD_2 from skin mast cells (37). The inhibition of proinflammatory mediator release from basophils and mast cells is presumably mediated by the interaction with CyP. In fact, a series of CsA analogs (CsC, CsD, CsG, and CsH), which bind with decreasing affinity to CyP (18), showed a typical pattern of activity in these cells (32). CsH had no inhibitory effect and the rank order of potency CsA > CsG > CsC = CsD > > CsH is consistent with the different affinities of these analogs for CyP (18). Figure 1 shows the results obtained in a series of experiments in which CsA (2.4–800 nM) concentration-dependently inhibited histamine release from basophils, lung and skin mast cells, whereas CsH, which has low affinity for CyP (18), had no inhibitory effect. These observations are compatible with the theory that CsA inhibits the release of preformed and *de novo* synthesized chemical mediators from basophils and mast cells by interacting with CyP.

Recently, we extended these *in vitro* observations to a more complex *in vivo* system. In these experiments a single dose of CsA (7 mg/kg) or placebo was given orally to eight volunteers and the plasma level of CsA and basophil releasability were monitored up to 24 hrs. A single dose of CsA was sufficient to cause a rapid and significant (20–40%) inhibition of histamine release from basophils obtained *ex vivo* from these subjects and challenged *in vitro* with anti-IgE, f-Met-Leu-Phe (FMLP) and compound A23187. The inhibitory effect of

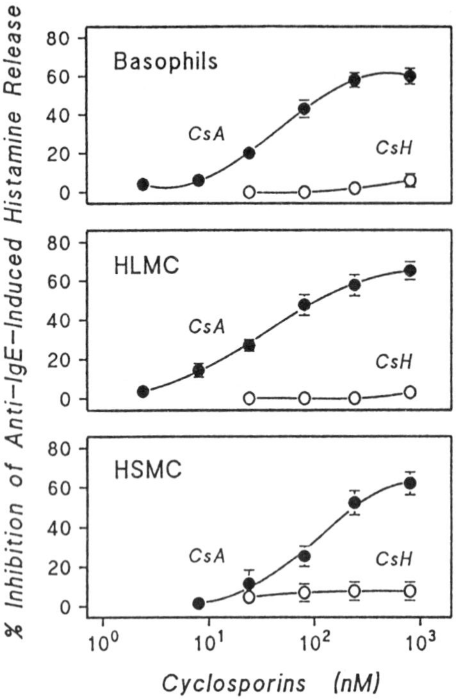

Figure 1. Effects of various concentrations of CsA and CsH on histamine release from human basophils, lung mast cells (HLMC), and skin mast cells (HSMC) induced by anti-IgE. Cells were preincubated 5 min with CsA or CsH and then incubated (30 min) with optimal concentrations of anti-IgE. Results are presented as mean ± S.E.M. of the percent inhibition caused by CsA and CsH in several experiments (basophils: n = 6; HLMC: n = 5; HSMC: n = 5).

CsA was extremely rapid, it peaked at 1–5 hrs and slowly decreased up to 18 hrs. This inhibitory effect was associated with a sharp increase in CsA blood level (max 500 ng/ml) and a rapid decrease within 5 hrs. Thus, it appears that the rapid inhibitory effect of CsA was correlated with a rapid absorption of the drug and persisted up to 18 hrs when CsA blood levels are almost undetectable. Presumably, CsA tightly bound to CyP in basophils exerts its antiinflammatory effect *in vivo* up to 18 hours. Another interesting finding of this study was the marked inhibitory effect of CsA administered *in vivo* on FMLP-induced histamine release from basophils. In fact, CsA had little or no effect on FMLP-induced histamine release from basophils *in vitro* (32). This indicates that *in vivo* CsA might have a more ample antiinflammatory activity than expected from *in vitro* observations.

These *in vitro* and *in vivo* findings are also important for two reasons. First, because they provide clear evidence that CsA exerts marked antiinflammatory effects, presumably mediated by the interaction with CyP and not dependent on protein synthesis and gene transcription. The second reason is the identification of human basophils and mast cells as the first inflammatory cells showing a high degree of sensitivity in the antiinflammatory effect of CsA. Basophils and mast cells play a major role in the pathogenesis of several inflammatory disorders through the release of chemical mediators. Besides allergic diseases (29), these cells are involved in the pathogenesis of autoimmune uveoretinitis (26), rheumatoid arthritis (27), Crohn's disease (28) and graft rejection (38). CsA treatment has proven effective in these conditions (3,9–11). In addition, there is growing evidence that CsA is effective in some patients with severe steroid-dependent asthma (12) and severe atopic dermatitis (13). Therefore, our *in vitro* and *in vivo* findings suggest that the antiinflammatory property of CsA may contribute to some of the drug's therapeutic effects.

Concluding Observations

Since CsA was discovered in 1970, information concerning its mechanism of action has grown enormously. CsA has been shown to be effective not only in the prevention/treatment of graft rejection, but also in a growing list of autoimmune and inflammatory diseases. Two major advances have been made during the last few years: the identification (18–20), purification and cloning (19,20,23) of human CyPA, CyPB, and CyPC as the cytoplasmic receptors for CsA and the discovery that, besides its well-known immunosuppressive effects, the drug also exerts marked antiinflammatory effects on human basophils and mast cells *in vitro* as well as *in vivo* (32,35–37). Both the immunosuppressive and the antiinflammatory activities of CsA appear to be mediated by binding to CyPs. Although binding of CsA to CyPs is necessary, but not sufficient, to exert its immunosuppressive and antiinflammatory effects, the inhibition of PPIase activity seems unrelated to these properties of CsA (24). The current hypothesis suggests that the CsA-CyP complex binds to and inhibits a component X (calcineurin) selectively in certain immune cells sensitive to the effects of CsA (24). This flood of new information has raised many interesting questions. The answer to these questions will lead to a better understanding of signal transduction mechanisms in human inflammatory cells, and presumably to a better tailoring of CsA treatment in various autoimmune and inflammatory diseases.

References

1. Borel, J.F. 1982. The history of cyclosporin A and its significance. In Cyclosporin A: Proceedings of an International Conference on Cyclosporin A. D.J.G. White, ed. New York: Elsevier Biomedical, p. 5.
2. Borel, J.F. 1976. Comparative study of *in vitro* and *in vivo* drug effects on cell-mediated cytotoxicity. Immunology 31:631.
3. Kahan, B.D. 1989. Cyclosporine. N. Engl. J. Med. 321:1725.
4. Oyer, P.E., Stinson, E.B., Jamieson, S.W., Hunt, S.A., Perlroth, M., Billingham, M., and Shumway, N.E. 1983. Cyclosporine in cardiac transplantation: A $2^1/_2$ year follow-up. Transplant. Proc. 15 (Suppl. 1):2546.
5. Starzl, T.E., Klintmalm, G.B.G., Porter, K.A., Iwatzuki, S., and Schröter, G.P.J. 1981. Liver transplantation with use of cyclosporin A and prednisone. N. Engl. J. Med. 305:266.
6. Reitz, B.A., Wallwork, J.L., Hunt, S.A., Pennock, J.L., Billingham, M.E., Oyer, P.E., Stinson, E.B., and Shumway, N.E. 1982. Heart-lung transplantation: Successful therapy for patients with pulmonary vascular disease. N. Engl. J. Med. 306:557.
7. The Toronto Lung Transplant Group. 1988. Experience with single-lung transplantation for pulmonary fibrosis. JAMA 259:2258.
8. Krönke, M., Leonard, W.J., Depper, J.M., Arya, S.K., Wong-Staal, F., Gallo, R.C., Waldmann, T.A., and Greene, W.C. 1984. Cyclosporin A inhibits T-cell growth factor gene expression at the level of mRNA transcription. Proc. Natl. Acad. Sci. USA 81:5214.
9. Nussenblatt, R.B., Rook, A.H., Wacker, W.B., Palestine, A.G., Scher, I., and Gery, I. 1983. Treatment of intraocular inflammatory diseases with cyclosporin A. Lancet 2:235.
10. Weinblatt, M.E., Coblyn, J.S., Fraser, P.A., Anderson, R.J., Spragg, J., Trentham, D.E., and Austen, K.F. 1987. Cyclosporin A treatment of refractory rheumatoid arthritis. Arthritis Rheum. 30:11.
11. Brynskov, J., Freund, L., Rasmussen, S.N., Lauritsen, K., Shaffalitzky de Muckadell, O., Williams, N., MacDonald, S., Tanton, R., Molina, F., Campanini, M.C., Bianchi, P., Ranzi, T., Quarto di Palo, F., Molchow-Moller, A., Thomsen. O., Tage-Jensen, U., Binder, V., and Riis, P. 1989. A placebo-controlled, double-blind, randomized trial of cyclosporine therapy in active chronic Crohn's disease. N. Engl. J. Med. 321:845.
12. Alexander, A., Barnes, N.C., and Kay, A.B. 1991. Cyclosporin A (CyA) in chronic severe asthma: A double-blind, placebo-controlled trial. Am. Rev. Respir. Dis. 143:A633.
13. Allen, B.R., Berth-Jones, J., Camp, R., Finlay, A., Graham-Brown, R., Marks, R., and Sowden, J.M. 1991. Ciclosporin in severe atopic dermatitis: A multicentre double-blind trial. In: 2nd Congress on Immunointervention in Autoimmune Diseases: The role of sandimmun (Ciclosporin). May 13-16, Paris, p. 84.
14. Colombani, P.M., Robb, A., and Hess, A.D. 1985. Cyclosporin A binding to calmodulin: A possible site of action on T lymphocytes. Science 228:337.
15. Marone, G., Columbo, M., Poto, S., and Condorelli, M. 1983. Inhibition of histamine release from human basophils *in vitro* by calmodulin antagonists. Clin. Immunol. Immunopathol. 28:334.
16. Marone, G., Poto, S., Columbo, M., Giugliano, R., Genovese, A., and Condorelli, M. 1984. Possible role of calmodulin in the control of lysosomal enzyme release from human polymorphonuclear leukocytes. J. Pharmacol. Exp. Ther. 231:678.
17. Hait, W.N., Harding, M.W., and Handschumacher, R.E. 1986. Calmodulin, cyclophilin and cyclosporin A. Science 233:987.
18. Handschumacher, R.E., Harding, M.W., Rice, J., Gruggs, R.J., and Speicher, D.W. 1984. Cyclophilin: A specific cytosolic binding protein for cyclosporin A. Science 226:544.
19. Price, E.R., Zydowsky, L.D., Jin, M., Baker, C.H., McKeon, F.D., and Walsh, C.T. 1991. Human cyclophilin B: A second cyclophilin gene encodes a peptidyl-prolyl isomerase with a signal sequence. Proc. Natl. Acad. Sci. USA 88:1903.
20. Friedman, J., and Weissman, I. 1991. Two cytoplasmic candidates for immunophilin action

similarity in the genetic regulation between anti-DNA, anti-histone and anti-retroviral gp70 antibodies in NZB/W F1 mice (23–25,32,33), provided that these antibodies share a common idiotope originated from immunoglobulin V region sequence homology. In any instance, once these critical antigens are identified, studies to define corresponding TCR repertoires and to develop specific immunotherapies by antibodies or vaccination protocols to prevent and treat the SLE will be facilitated.

References

1. Oksenberg, J.R., Stuart, S., Begovich, A.B., Bell, R.B., Erlich, H.A., Steinman, L., and Bernard, C.C.A. 1990. Limited heterogeneity of rearranged T cell receptor Vα transcripts in brains of multiple sclerosis patients. Nature 345:344.
2. Ben-Nun, A., Liblau, R.S., Cohen, L., Lehmann, D., Tournier-Lasserve,E., Rosenzweig, A., Jingwu, Z., Raus, J.C.M., and Bach, M.-A. 1991. Restricted T-cell receptor Vβ gene usage by myelin basic protein specific T-cell clones in multiple sclerosis: Predominant genes vary in individuals. Proc. Natl. Acad. Sci. USA 88:2466.
3. Wucherpfennig, K.W., Ota, K., Endo, N., Seidman, J.G., Rosenzweig, A., Weiner, H.L., and Hafler, D.A. 1990. Shared human T cell receptor Vβ usage to immunodominant regions of myelin basic protein. Science 248:1016.
4. Sottini, A., Imberti, L., Gorla, R., Cattaneo, R., and Primi, D. 1991. Restricted expression of T cell receptor Vβ but not Vα genes in rheumatoid arthritis. Eur. J. Immunol. 21:461.
5. Paliard, X., West, S.G., Lafferty, J.A., Clements, J.R., Kappler, J.W., Marrack, P., and Kotzin, B.L. 1991. Evidence for the effects of a superantigen in rheumatoid arthritis. Science 253:325.
6. Davies, T. F., Martin, A., Concepcion, E.S., Graves, P., Cohen, L., and Ben-Nun, A. 1991. Evidence of limited variability of antigen receptors on intrathyroidal T cells in autoimmune thyroid disease. New. Eng. J. Med. 325:238.
7. Posnett, D.N., Schmelkin, I., Burton, D.A., August, A., McGrath, H., and Mayer, L.F. 1990. T cell antigen receptor V gene usage. Increases in Vβ8$^+$ T cells in Crohn's disease. J. Clin. Invest. 85:1770.
8. Kontiainen, S., Toomath, R., and Feldmann, M. 1991. Selective activation of T cells in newly diagnosed insulin-dependent diabetic patients: Evidence for heterogeneity of T cell receptor usage. Clin . Exp.Immunol. 83:347.
9. Moebius, U., Manns, M., Hess, G., Kober, G., Büschenfelde, K-H. M., and Meuer, S.C. 1990. T cell receptor gene rearrangements of T lymphocytes infiltrating the liver in chronic active hepatitis B and primary biliary cirrhosis (PBC): oligoclonality of PBC-derived T cell clones. Eur. J. Immunol. 20:889.
10. Posnett, D.N., Gottlieb, A., Bussel, J.B., Friedman, S.M., Chiorazzi, N., Li,Y., Szabo, P., Farid, N.R., and Robinson, M.A. 1988. T cell antigen receptors in autoimmunity. J. Immunol. 141:1963.
11. Urban, J.L., Kumar, V., Kono, D.H., Gomez, C., Horvath, S.J., Clayton, J., Ando, D.G., Sercarz, E.E., and Hood, L. 1988. Restricted use of T cell receptor V genes in murine autoimmune encephalomyelitis raises possibilities for antibody therapy. Cell 54:577.
12. Sakai, K., Sinha, A.A., Mitchell, D.J., Zamvil, S.S., Rothbard, J.B., McDevitt, H.O., and Steinman, L. 1988. Involvement of distinct murine T-cell receptors in the autoimmune encephalitogenic response to nested epitopes of myelin basic protein. Proc. Natl. Acad. Sci. USA 85:8608.
13. Padula, S.J., Lingenheld, E.G., Stabach, P.R., Chou, C.J., Kono, D.H., and Clark, R.B. 1991. Identification of encephalitogenic Vβ-4-bearing T cells in SJL mice. Further evidence for the V region disease hypothesis? J. Immunol. 146:879.
14. Burns, F.R., Li, X., Shen, N., Offner, H., Chou, Y.K., Vandenbark, A.A., and Heber-Katz, E. 1989. Both rat and mouse T cell receptors specific for the encephalitogenic determinant of myelin basic protein use similar Vα and Vβ chain genes even though the major histocompatibility complex and encephalitogenic determinants being recognized are different. J. Exp. Med. 169:27.
15. Chluba, J., Steeg, C., Becker, A., Wekerle, H., and Epplen, J.T. 1989. T cell receptor β chain usage in myelin basic protein-specific rat T lymphocytes. Eur. J. Immunol. 19:279.
16. Banerjee, S., Behlke, M.A., Dungeon, G., Loh, D.Y., Stuart, J., Luthra, H.S., and David, C.S. 1988. Vβ6 gene of T cell receptor may be involved in type II collagen induced arthritis in mice. FASEB J. (Abstr.) 2:661.
17. Stamenkovic, I., Stegagno, M., Wright, K.A., Krane, S.M., Amento, E.P.,Colvin, R.B., Duquesnoy, R.J., and Kurnick, J.T. 1988. Clonal dominance among T-lymphocyte infil-

trates in arthritis. Proc. Natl. Acad. Sci. USA 85:1179.
18. Steinmetz, M., and Uematsu, Y. 1991. Heterogeneity of T cell repertoires in human autoimmune disease. Br. J. Rheumatol. (suppl. 2) 30:24.
19. Duby, A.D., Sinclair, A.K., Osborne-Lawrence, S.L., Zeldes, W., Kan, L.,and Fox, D.A. 1989. Clonal heterogeneity of synovial fluid T lymphocytes from patients with rheumatoid arthritis. Proc. Natl.Acad. Sci. USA 86:6206.
20. Wofsy, D., and Seaman, W.E. 1985. Successful treatment of autoimmunity in NZB/NZW F1 mice with monoclonal antibody to L3T4. J. Exp. Med. 161:378.
21. Sekigawa, I., Ishida, Y., Hirose, S., Sato, H., and Shirai, T. 1986. Cellular basis of *in vitro* anti-DNA antibody production. Evidence for T cell dependence of IgG-class anti-DNA antibody synthesis in the (NZB x NZW)F1 hybrid. J. Immunol. 136:1247.
22. Sekigawa, I., Okada, T., Noguchi, K., Ueda, G., Hirose, S., Sato, H., and Shirai, T. 1987. Class-specific regulation of anti-DNA antibody synthesis and the age-associated changes in (NZB x NZW)F1 hybrid mice. J. Immunol. 138:2890.
23. Yanagi, Y., Hirose, S., Nagasawa, R., Shirai, T., Mak, T.W., and Tada, T. 1986. Does the deletion within T cell receptor-β chain gene of NZW mice contribute to autoimmunity in (NZB x NZW)F1 mice? Eur. J.Immunol. 16:1179.
24. Hirose, S., Tokushige, K., Kinoshita, S., Nozawa, S., Nishimura, H., and Shirai, T. 1991. Contribution of the gene linked to T cell receptor β chain gene complex of NZW mice to the autoimmunity of (NZB x NZW)F1 mice. Eur. J. Immunol. 21:823.
25. Hirose, S., Ueda, G., Noguchi, K., Okada, T., Sekigawa, I., Sato, H., and, Shirai, T. 1986. Requirement of H-2 heterozygosity for autoimmunity in (NZB x NZW)F1 hybird mice. Eur. J. Immunol. 16:1613.
26. Hirose, S., Kinoshita, K., Nozawa, S., Nishimura, H., and Shirai, T. 1990. Effects of major histocompatibility complex on autoimmune disease of H-2-congenic New Zealand mice. Int. Immunol. 2:1091.
27. Acha-Orbea, H., and Palmer, E. 1991. Mls-a retrovirus exploits the immune system. Immunol. Today 12:356.
28. Kotzin, B.L., Kappler, J.W., Marrack, P.C., and Herron, L.R. 1989. T cell tolerance to self antigens in New Zealand hybrid mice with lupus-like disease. J. Immunol. 143:89.
29. Singer, P.A., and Theofilopoulos, A.N. 1990. T-cell receptor Vβ repertoire expression in murine model of SLE. Immunol. Rev. 118:103.
30. Ohgaki M., Ueda, G., Shiota, J., Nishimura, H., Hirose, S., Sato, H., and Shirai, T. 1989. Two distinct monoclonal natural thymocytotoxic autoantibodies (NTA) from New Zealand Black mouse. Clin. Immunol. Immunopathol. 53:475 .
31. Ueda, G., Hirose, S., and Shirai, T. 1991. An early activation antigen of murine T lymphocytes recognized by monoclonal autoantibody NTA204. Autoimmunity, in press.
32. Shirai, T., Ohta, K., Kohno, A., Furukawa, F., Yoshida, H., Maruyama, N., and Hirose, S. 1986. Naturally occurring antibody response to DNA is associated with the response to retroviral gp70 in autoimmune New Zealand mice. Arthritis Rheum. 29:242.
33. Shirai, T., Hirose, S., Okada, T., and Nishimura, H. 1991. Immunology and immunopathology of the autoimmune disease of NZB and related mouse strains. In: Immunological disorders in mice. B. Říhová, and V.Větvička, eds. Boca Ratton, Florida: CPC Press, p. 95.
34. Nishimura, H., Noguchi, K., Tokushige, K., Nozawa, S., Okamoto, H., Nagata, S., Tsurui, H., Hirose, S. and Shirai, T. T-cell receptor Vβ gene usage by spontaneously activated $CD4^+$ T cells in autoimmune disease-prone (NZB x NZW)F1 mice. Submitted for publication.

T Cell Subsets: Role of Cell Surface Structures

Chikao Morimoto, Stuart F. Schlossman*

A number of T-cell surface structures are now known to be involved in their activation. The primary pathway of clonal expansion of the T-cell occurs by means of antigen-recognition by the TCR/CD3 complex. However, several accessory interactions involving CD4:MHC Class II, CD8:Class I, CD2:LFA-3, LFA-1:ICAM-1 and CD28:B7 synergize with the TCR/CD3 complex in its response to foreign antigen. Cell adhesion and conjugate formation are now known to be important consequences of these binding events which contribute to the intracellular signals that may modify antigen-induced proliferation. Significantly, several additional structures (CD29 (4B4), CD26 (1F7, Ta1), CD31 (1F11) and CD45 (2H4)) define subsets of CD4 cells with distinct functional programs. Engagements of these structures by their respective ligands can also generate or modify intracellular signals leading to the expression of distinct functional programs of individual CD4 cells. It is our belief that a further understanding of the contribution of these surface structures to T cell regulation, migration, and localization should yield great insight into the pathogenetic mechanism of various autoimmune and immunodeficiency diseases.

A number of T-cell surface structures are now known to be involved in the activation of human T lymphocytes. The primary pathway of clonal expansion of the T-cell occurs by means of antigen-recognition by the TCR/CD3 complex. However, several accessory interactions involving CD4:MHC Class II, CD8:Class I, CD2:LFA-3, LFA-1:ICAM-1 and CD28:B7 synergize with the TCR/CD3 complex in this response to foreign antigen. Cell adhesion and conjugate formation are now known to be important consequences of these binding events. Moreover, these accessory interactions may also trigger intracellular signals that modify antigen-induced proliferation via the TCR/CD3 complex. The repertoire of cell surface structure expressed on antigen presenting cells will dictate a group of lymphocyte surface molecules that can be engaged in regions of cell-cell contact. We have examined several additional structures (CD29 [4B4], CD26 [1F7, Ta1], CD31 (1F11) and CD45 [2H4]) for their ability to further divide CD4 and CD8 populations into subsets of T-cells with distinct functional programs. For example, within the CD4+ subset, the CD4+CD45RA-CD29+ ($CD29^{high}$) CD26+ subset provides helper function for B cell Ig production, responds maximally to recall antigen and can induce CD8 cells to exert Class I-restricted cytotoxicity (1–4). The CD4+ CD45RA+ CD29- CD26-, CD31+ population, in contrast, can induce CD8 cells to suppress Ig synthesis, but provides poor helper function and responds poorly to recall antigens (1,2,4,5). Thus, the CD4+ subsets can be distinguished by the differential expression of isoforms of the CD45 family, CD29, CD26 and CD31. Not only do these subset defining molecules restrict the interactions between populations of cells but more importantly are integrally involved in the activation process. In this brief review, we will focus on the possible contribution of these structures in dictating helper functions.

The T200/leukocyte common antigen (LCA; CD45) is a family of lymphocyte cell surface glycoproteins ranging in molecular mass from 180 kDa to 220 kDa that is abundantly expressed on lymphocytes and other hematopoietic cells. The five different CD45 isoforms are generated by alternative splicing of three exons of a single gene, and distinct isoforms are expressed on T cell subsets (6–9). It was the differential expression of these isoforms on subsets of CD4 cells that attracted our laboratory to the characterization of the LCA family of antigens. The primary structures of five human CD45 isoforms have been predicted based on the nucleotide sequences of cloned CD45 cDNA (7,8). These isoforms have the same 707-amino acid cytoplasmic domain, 22-amino acid

* Division of Tumor Immunology, Dana Farber Cancer Institute, Harvard Medical School, 44 Binney Street, Boston, MA, 02115, USA.
Acknowledgements: This work is supported by NIH AI12069, AI29530, and AR33713.

transmembrane region, 23-amino acid signal peptide and 8-amino acid amino-proximal sequence, but differ from one another in that they contain extracellular domains of 552, 504, 486, or 391 amino acids depending on which combination of the alternatively spliced exons A, B and C are used. Although the functional role of CD45 is unclear, studies using anti-CD45 antibodies have implicated these molecules in several immunologic functions including the blocking of the induction of suppressor activity (10,11), and the inhibition of cytotoxic activity (12) and NK function (13). Additionally, anti-CD45 antibodies have been reported to augment T cell proliferation by PHA and autologous MLR (AMLR) (14,15). Ledbetter et al. suggested a regulatory role for CD45 based on their observation that heterologous antibody-mediated cross-linking of CD3 and CD45 on the surface of T cell prevents anti-CD3 from transducing an activation signal (16). It was shown that the two homologous domains of the intracytoplasmic region of CD45 share homology with a soluble protein tyrosine phosphatase (PTPase) and when isolated expressed the tyrosine phosphatase activity of CD45 (17,18). It is now known that CD45 is a member of a family of transmembrane receptors which functions in a specific signal transduction pathway via tyrosine dephosphorylation. This dephosphorylation pathway might be directly linked to the CD4/CD8 associated tyrosine kinase $p56^{lck}$, CD3/$p59^{fyn}$, $p72^{fyn}$ providing a possible mechanism for the regulatory role of CD45 in CD3-CD4 cross-linking and activation (19). As described above, although the cytoplasmic domain of CD45 has the PTPase activity, the precise role of the extracellular domain of each isoform or the identity of the natural ligand(s) of CD45 are still unknown. Nevertheless, engagement of individual isoforms of CD45 expressed on subsets of CD4 cells provides a model by which these structures play a potentially important role in T cell activation.

Synergistic signalling of the CD3/TCR also occurs through the VLA/integrin super gene family. These transmembrane glycoproteins are expressed on a variety of cell types including lymphocytes (20). The VLA protein family consists of a common β1 subunit CD29, non-covalently associated with different α chains to form different heterodimers (20). At least six VLA proteins have been identified based on their distinct α chains and many are known to function as cell surface receptors for the extracellular matrix components, fibronectin, collagen, and laminin. These structures have been implicated in a number of biological processes, including tissue organization, cell migration, embryogenesis, and tumor metastasis (20). While differentially expressed subsets of CD4 cells, their function in the immune system is largely unknown. Nevertheless, the observation that the fibronectin (FN) can synergize with the CD3/TCR pathway to promote $CD4^+$ T cell proliferation has provided an important insight into the mechanism by which extracellular matrix proteins modulate immune function (21). When plasma FN is crosslinked with anti-CD3 on culture plates, highly purified CD4 cells were maximally activated in a serum-free culture system. This anti-CD3/FN-dependent proliferation was specifically inhibited by anti-4B4 (CD29) (anti-VLA-β1) and anti-VLA-5 antibodies, suggesting that VLA-5 was the major functional FN receptor. Subsequently it was shown that VLA-4 also functions as a FN receptor but recognizes an alternatively spliced CS-1 domain of the FN which is distinct from the classical Arg-Gly-Asp-Ser (RGDS)-domain recognized by VLA-5 (22). As a cell receptor, VLA-4 has also been shown to bind to V-CAM, a molecule induced by inflammatory cytokines on endothelial cells (23). In contrast to other VLA proteins, which are distributed widely on a variety of cell types, the expression of VLA-4 is relatively restricted to myeloid and lymphoid cells (20). We showed that immobilized synthetic CS1 peptides, via their interaction with the VLA-4 receptor, can provide a signal which synergizes with anti-CD3 in promoting CD4 cell proliferation (24). Moreover, we demonstrated that CD4 cell proliferation induced by anti-CD3 plus native plasma FN is dependent on both VLA-4 and VLA-5, although the latter may be required for full function of the former. It is conceivable that VLA-4 might have a significant role in T cell function through its interaction with FN as one potential ligand and with endothelial cells as another. These structures may provide a mechanism for the binding, activation and migration of T cells through endothelial cells.

Another structure with unknown immunologic role that is involved in cellular adhesion to extracellular matrix proteins is a dipeptidyl peptidase IV (DPPIV) defined by the CD26 antibodies (25). Found on a number of tissue types in addition to T cells, DPPIV (CD26) is a membrane-associated intrinsic ectoenzyme that has a binding affinity for collagen (26). Anti-1F7 not only recognizes CD26 on the surface of a subset of CD4+ CD29+ T lymphocytes, but blocks both helper functions and the proliferative response of these cells to antigen (4). In addition, CD26 as a collagen receptor is of interest and may play a role in CD4 T cell activation. It is possible to activate human CD4 T cells by x-linking CD3 and collagen in a serum-free system (27). This activation can be inhibited by the addition of peptides containing either RGD sequences or Gly-Pro-X which is known to be a "substrate" for DPPIV activity. We have found that both the structure defined by 1F7 (CD26) and the VLA-3 complex synergize with CD3 in activating the CD4 cell. It is also important to note that both anti-VLA-3 and anti-CD-26 (1F7) can block collagen-induced CD4 cell activation.

Unexpectedly, we found that anti-CD26 not only modulated the surface expression of CD26, but also enhanced both the proliferative response and calcium mobilization of human T cells to either the TCR/CD3 or CD2 (28). In as much as the intracellular domain of CD26 consisted of only six amino acids, it is possible that the role of CD26 in T cell activation may be mediated in part by its linkage to an associated structure such as CD45, which is transducing an activation signal. We showed that CD26 is physically associated with CD45 as evidenced by the findings that CD26 comodulates CD45, and that the 180 kDa and 190 kDa isoforms of CD45 and coprecipitate with CD26 (29). These findings strongly suggest that CD26 may be closely associated with membrane linked CD45 protein tyrosine phosphatase on T cell surface, and further supports our findings that the modulation of CD26 results in enhanced tyrosine kinase activity, ζ chain phosphorylation, and T cell activation.

The preceding structures and others such as CD28 seem to play key roles in the helper pathway of T cell activation (30). CD31, in contrast, has focussed our attention to the much less well understood suppressor pathway. This molecule, also known as platelet-endothelial cell adhesion molecule-1; PECAM-1, gpIIa', has been shown to be a 120 kDa surface structure, having Ig-like extracellular domains and an overall structure similar to the cellular adhesion molecules (CAM) (31). CD31, though originally defined as a myelomonocytic differentiation antigen, is also found on platelets and a subset of lymphoid cells (32). We have recently investigated a novel anti-CD31 mAb, anti-1F11, which is reactive with both resting and activated human CD4 cells and can divide them into functionally distinct populations based upon their expression of CD31 (5). Resting CD4+ CD31+ cells, like their CD4+CD45RA+ counterpart, provided poor helper function for B cell IgG synthesis and responded maximally in auto-MLR and to ConA. CD4+CD31-cells, in contrast, responded maximally to recall antigens such as TT and provided excellent helper function. Of interest was the findings that CD31 is stably expressed on activated CD4+CD45RA+ cells. Thus, unlike CD45RA, CD45RO, or CD29, CD31 can differentiate subsets of CD4 cells having distinct functional and pattern of cytokine production even after activation. Perhaps of greater importance was the findings that anti-CD31 (1F11) mAb inhibited the generation of suppressor function in PWM-driven 1gG synthesis system, suggesting that CD31 may contribute to the function of resting and activated CD45RA+ T cells. Whether it contributes to the generation of suppression or in someway synergizes with CD45RA in enhancing this signal, is of great interest. In any event, CD31 appears to be the first adhesion molecule to be preferentially expressed by cells of the naive or CD45RA lineage.

A key feature of the molecules described above is that engagement by their respective ligands can generate or modify the functional programs of individual CD4 cells. Further understanding of the contribution of these surface structures to T cell activation, cell migration, and localization in tissues should provide new opportunities to alter the pathogenetic mechanisms involved in autoimmune and immunodeficiency diseases.

References

1. Morimoto, C., Letvin, N.L., Boyd, A.W., Hagen, M., Brown, H., Kornacki, M.M., and Schlossman, S.F. 1985. The isolation and characterization of the human helper inducer subset. J. Immunol. 134:3762.

2. Morimoto, C., Letvin, N.L., Distaso, J.A., Aldrich, W.R., and Schlossman, S.F. 1985. The isolation and characterization of the human suppressor inducer T cell subset. J. Immunol. 134:3762.
3. Kalish, R.S., Morimoto, C., and Schlossman, S.F., 1988. Generation of CD8(T8) cytotoxic cells has a preferential requirement of CD4+2H4-inducer cells. Cell Immunol. 111:379.
4. Morimoto, C., Torimoto, Y., Levinson ,G., Rudd, C.E., Schrieber, M., Dang, N.H., Letvin, N.L., and Schlossman, S.F. 1989. 1F7, a novel cell surface molecule, involved in helper function of CD4 cells. J. Immunol. 143:3430.
5. Torimoto, C., Rothstein, D.M., Dang, N.H., Schlossman, S.F., and Morimoto, C. 1992. CD31, a novel cell surface marker for CD4 cells of suppressor lineage, unaltered by state of activation. J. Immunol. 148:388.
6. Thomas, M.L. 1989. The leucocyte common antigen family. Ann. Rev. Immunol. 7:339.
7. Streuli, M., Hall, L.R., Saga, Y., Schlossman, S.F., and Saito, H. 1987. Differential usage of three exons generates at least five different mRNA's encoding human leukocyte common antigens. J. Exp. Med. 166:1548.
8. Ralph, S.J., Thomas, M.L., Morton, C., and Trowbridge, I.S. 1987. Structural variants of human T200 glycoproteins (leukocyte common antigen). EMBO J. 6:1251.
9. Rudd, C.E., Morimoto, C., Wang, L.L., and Schlossman, S.F. 1987. The subdivision of the T4 (CD4) subset is the basis of the differential expression of L-C/T200 antigens. J. Exp. Med. 166:1758.
10. Morimoto, C., Letvin, N.L., Rudd, C.E., Hagan, M., Takeuchi, T,, and Schlossman, S.F. 1986. The role of the 2H4 molecule in the generation of suppressor function in ConA activated T cells. J. Immunol. 137:3247.
11. Takeuchi, T., Rudd, C.E., Schlossman, S.F., and Morimoto, C. 1987. Induction of suppression following autologous mixed lymphocyte reaction: Role of 2H4 antigen. Eur. J. Immunol. 17:97.
12. Lefrancois, L., and Bevan, M.J. 1985. Functional modifications of cytotoxic T lymphocyte T200 glycoprotein recognized by monoclonal antibodies. Nature 314:449.
13. Newman, W., Fast, L.D., and Rose, L.M. 1983. Blockade of NK cell lysis is a property of monoclonal antibodies that bind to distinct region of T200. J. Immunol. 131:1742.
14. Ledbetter, J.A., Rose, L.M., Spooner, C.E, Beatty, P.G., Martin, P.J., and Clark, E.A. 1985. Antibodies to common leukocyte antigen p220 influences human T cell proliferation by modifying IL-2 receptor expression. J. Immunol. 135:1819.
15. Takeuchi, T., Rudd, C.E., Tedder, T.F., Schlossman, S.F., and Morimoto, C. 1989. amplification of suppressor inducer pathway with monoclonal antibody, anti-2H4 identifying a novel epitope of the common leukocyte antigen/T200 antigen. Cell Immunol. 118:68.
16. Ledbetter, J.A., Tonks, N.K., Fischer, E.H., and Clark, E.A. 1988. CD45 regulates signal transduction and lymphocyte activation by specific association with receptor molecules on T or B cells. Proc. Natl. Acad. Sci USA 85:8628.
17. Charboneau, H., Tonks, N.K., Walsh, K.A., and Fischer, E.H. 1988. The leukocyte common antigen (CD45): A putative receptor-linked protein tyrosine phosphatase. Proc. Natl. Acad. Sci USA 85:7812.
18. Streuli, M., Krueger, N.X., Tsai, A.Y., and Saito, H. 1989. A family of receptor-linked protein tyrosine phosphatase in human and drosophila. Proc. Natl. Acad. Sci USA 86:8698.
19. Rudd, C.E., Anderson,P., Morimoto, C., Streuli, M., and Schlossman, S.F. 1989. Molecular interactions, T-cell subsets and a role of the CD41CD8:p56^{lck} complex in human T cell activation. Immunol. Review 111:225.
20. Hemler, M.E. 1990. VLA proteins in the integrin family: Structures, functions, and their role on leukocytes. Ann. Rev. Immunol. 8:365.
21. Matsuyama, T., Yamada, A., Kay, J., Yamada, K.M., Akiyama, S.K., Schlossman, S.F., and Morimoto, C. 1989. Activation of CD4 cells by fibronectin and anti-CD3 antibody. A synergistic effect mediated by the VLA-5 fibronectin receptor complex. J. Exp. Med. 170:1133.
22. Wayner E.A., Garcia-Pardo, A., Humphries, M..J., MacDonald, J.A., and Carter, W.G. 1989. Identification and characterization of the T lymphocyte adhesion receptor for an alternative cell attachment domain (CS-1) in plasma fibronectin. J. Cell Biol. 109:1321.
23. Elices, M.J., Osborn, L., Takada, Y., Crouse, C., Luhowski, S., Memler, M.E., and Lobb, R.R. 1990. VCAM-1 on activated endothelium interacts with the Leukocyte integrin. VLA-4 at a site distinct from the VLA-4/fibronectin binding site. Cell 60:577.

24. Nojima, Y., Humphries, M.J., Mould, A.P., Komoriya, A., Yamada, K.M., Schlossman, S.F., and Morimoto, C. 1990. VLA-4 mediates CD3-dependent CD4+ T cell activation via the alternatively spliced domain of fibronectin. J. Exp. Med. 172:1185.
25. Hegen, M., Niedobitek, G., Klein, E., Stein, H., and Fleisher, B. 1990. The T cell triggering molecule Tp103 is associated with dipeptidyl aminopeptidase IV activity. J. Immunol. 74:431.
26. Hanski, C., Huhler, T., Gossran, R., and Reutter, W. 1988. Direct evidence for the binding of rat liver DPPIV to collagen in vitro. Exp. Cell Res. 178:64.
27. Dang, N.H., Torimoto, Y., Schlossman, S.F., and Morimoto, C. 1990. Human CD4 helper T cell activation: Functional involvement of two distinct collagen receptors, IF7 and VLA integrin family. J. Exp. Med. 172:649.
28. Dang, N.H., Torimoto, Y., Sugita, K., Daley, J.F., Schow, P., Prado, C., Schlossman, S.F., and Morimoto, C. 1990. Cell surface modulation of CD26 by anti-1F7 monoclonal antibody analysis of surface expression and human T cell activation. J. Immunol. 145:3963.
29. Torimoto, Y., Dang, N.H., Vivier, E., Tanaka, T., Schlossman, S.F., and Morimoto, C. 1991. Coassociation of CD26 (dipeptidyl peptidase IV) with CD45 on the surface of human T lymphocytes. J. Immunol., 147:2514.
30. Gimmi, C.D., Freeman, G.J., Gribben, J.G., Sugita, K., Freedman, A.S., Morimoto, C., and Nadler, L.M. 1991. B-cell surface antigen B7 provides a costimulatory signal that induces T cells to proliferate and secrete interleukin 2. Proc. Natl. Acad. Sci. USA 88:6575.
31. Newman, P,, Berndt, J.M., Gorski, J., White, G.C., Lyman, C., Paddock, C., and Muller, W.A. 1990. PECAM-1(CD31) cloning and relation to adhesion molecules of the immunoglobin gene superfamily. Science 247:1219.
32. Goyert, S.M., Fierro, E.M., Seremetis, S..V, Winchester, R.J., Silver, J., and Mattison, A.C. 1986. Biochemistry and expression of myelomonocytic antigens. J. Immunol. 137:3909.

Immune Abnormalities and Control of AIDS

John L. Fahey, Bo Hofmann, Pari Nishanian, Hong Bass*

HIV infection has three major effects on the immune system. *Immune deficiency* is manifested by reduced CD4 T cell levels and impaired immune functions. *Activation of immune system* cells is evident by increased production of soluble markers, such as serum neopterin, β2M, sIL-2R, sCD8, and IgA molecules. The surrogate markers that relate strongly to prognosis are the CD4 T cell numbers and serum neopterin and β2M levels (soluble activation markers). Activation contributes to several aspects of disease pathology, including development of neoplasia, immune dysfunction and increased virus production. *Specific immune response* to HIV includes antibodies that are essential for diagnosis. Specific cellular immunity also occurs. Anti-retroviral therapy such as zidovudine (AZT) results in a relatively short (4–12 week) period of maximum effect on the immune system. Serum activation markers respond more rapidly and are more sensitive to AZT than CD4 change. Immune-based therapies are directed at amplification of host-resistance to HIV, stimulation of T and B cell functions, transfer of specific antibody or cellular immunity, and vaccines for induction of protective humoral and cellular immunity.

The central importance of the damaged immune system was recognized when AIDS was first identified as a new disease 10 years ago. Immune deficiency was evident in reduced CD4 T lymphocyte levels and impaired functional tests. Opportunistic infections, due to impaired immune function were, and still are, the common cause of death. In addition, immune disregulation was evident in the occurrence of Kaposi's Sarcoma and B cell lymphoma. A major advance was identification of the HIV-1 virus as the etiologic agent of AIDS. This made possible the serologic tests essential for detection of HIV infection. Epidemiologic studies demonstrated the presence of a variable, but generally long, period of infection before clini-

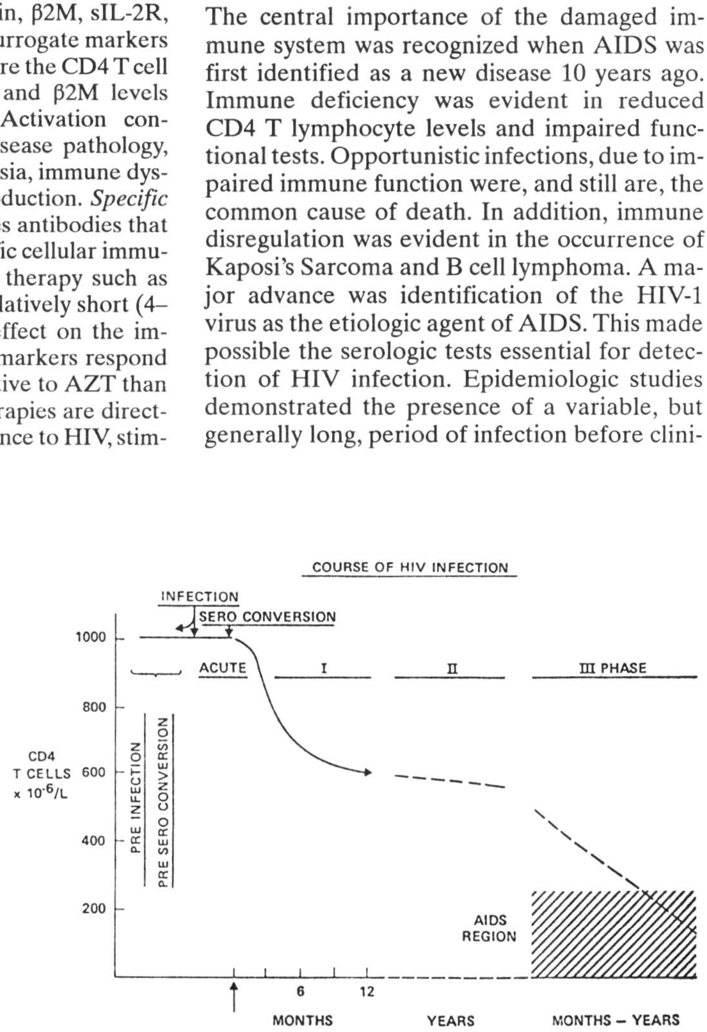

Figure 1. Schematic Representation of the Major Phases of CD4 T Cell Fall during HIV Infection. The first phase represents the changes occurring in the first year after seroconversion. The second phase depicts the period (or periods) of little or no progression in the CD4 fall. The third represents the period when CD4 levels are below 200/mm^3 and the patient is at risk for AIDS. The duration of phase II varies enormously between individuals in accord with the length of the asymptomatic period.

* Center for Interdisciplinary Research in Immunology and Disease (CIRID), Department of Microbiology and Immunology and the Jonsson Comprehensive Cancer Center, UCLA School of Medicine, Los Angeles, CA.
Acknowledements: Supported by NIH Grants AI23606, AI 27660, AI72631, CA09120.

cal symptoms became evident. The general pattern of CD4 T cell changes, illustrated in Figure 1, was established. Three phases are evident in the course of HIV infection. In the first phase a fall in CD4 T levels occurs. After several months, in most individuals, the CD4 T cell levels tend to plateau or fall at a very low rate (phase 2). Finally a stage (phase 3) is reached when the CD4 T cell depletion has advanced and opportunistic infections can occur (1). Clearly, HIV-infection causes reductions in CD4 T cell levels but the mechanisms are not well understood. The virus can be directly cytopathic or act via syncitial formation as well as by direct or indirect effects impairing CD4 T cell generation. Some infected persons continue to have aggressive disease with progressive fall in CD4 T cell levels and develop opportunistic infections relatively soon after the onset of HIV infection. Most individuals, however, have a prolonged course of infection. This appears to be due, at least in part, to specific immune responses to HIV that develop early in infection.

Specific Immune Response to HIV

Specific immune responses include specific antibodies against many different antigens on HIV proteins. Some antibodies are able to neutralize the HIV virus *in vitro*. Antibodies against the principle neutralizing domain (PND) of the V3 loop of the gp120 molecule may have neutralizing activity (2). Some antibodies elicit antibody dependent cellular cytotoxicity (ADCC), a potentially effective mechansism for controling HIV-infection. Unfortunately, however, none of the antibodies have been shown with certainty to relate strongly to prognosis. Further proof is needed of the significance of specific antibodies for modifying disease course. Cellular immunity to HIV has been demonstrated both in terms of proliferative response to specific HIV antigens and specific cell mediated cytotoxicity against gp120 antigens. Cell mediated immunity appears to increase after infection is established but subsides later in infection (3). Mechanisms of this failure later in infection are not certain. The implications are, however, that this loss of protective cellular immunity contributes to the progression of infection and disease.

Immunological Abnormalities in HIV Infection

Immune abnormalities induced by HIV infection include reduced CD4 T cell numbers, impaired immune function and inappropriate activation of immune cells (see Table I).

Reduced CD4 T Cell Numbers

Measurement of CD4 T lymphocyte numbers is essential for evaluation of HIV disease. Determinations of numbers or percentages of CD4 cells provide approximately the same information (4). The CD8 T cell number increase occurs promptly with infection and is accompanied by phenotypic changes indicative of activation such as HLA-DR and CD38 (5,6). CD8 T cell numbers, however, are not relevant to prognosis.

Impaired Immune Functions

Impairment of immune functions occurs early in disease, before CD4 T cells are below normal ranges (7,8). Furthermore, impaired proliferative responses have been shown to relate to prognosis (9) and to be independent of CD4 T cell level. Functional impairment appears to be caused by two separate mechanisms, one involving HIV proteins and the other via suppressor cytokines. The HIV proteins that have been identified as contributing to functional impairment include gp120 envelope proteins, p17gag protein and the tat protein. Suppressor cytokines that can impair proliferative capacity of T cells have been shown to be produced in excessive amounts during HIV infection and include TGF-beta (10) and, possibly, other factors as well. It seems probable that impaired immune functions contribute to lack of ability to contain HIV infection or to prevent opportunistic infections.

Table 1. Immune Abnormalities in HIV Infection

A. *CD4 Cell Deficiency*
B. *Impaired Functions*
C. *Immune Activation:*
  Increased levels of soluble products of activated immune cells
  Increased cytokines
  Increased Phenotypic Markers

Activation of Immune System

Generalized activation of the immune system occurs early in HIV infection but is not yet generally appreciated. Activation contributes to disease progression and relates (as well as CD4 T cell levels) to prognosis. Activation of the immune system in HIV infection involves the CD8 T cells, B cells and macrophages. Substantial increases of serum neopterin (from macrophages), β2M and soluble IL2 receptor (from T and B cells), soluble CD8 antigen (CD8 T cells) and serum IgA (B cells) occur. All of these markers relate to prognosis, especially serum neopterin and β2M (11–14). Furthermore, these serum immune activation markers are as good as CD4 T cell levels for indicating prognosis. Serum neopterin and β2M are independent of CD4 T cell levels. Thus, combinations of CD4 and neopterin or β2M measurements are superior to a single measure alone for determining prognosis (11,15,16). The significance of immune activation is summarized in Table II.

Table II. Immune Activation: Significance

A. Relates to Prognosis/Course of Disease,
 – Independent of CD4 Levels
B. Impairs Lymphocyte Function
C. Contributes to Neoplasia:
 – B cell lymphoma
 – Kaposi's Sarcoma
D. Increases HIV Production

Activation can be viewed as reflecting disease activity and as an index of the course of illness at least for several years. The CD4 T cells, on the other hand, can be viewed as measuring the stage that the disease has reached. This is an over-simplification but does permit some insight as to how the two measures can contribute together to assessing disease. Clearly combining these two measures adds substantially to the ability to assess prognosis (11,15,16). The mechanisms underlying increased production of the soluble immune activation markers involve increased production of cytokines including interferon-gamma, interferon alpha, IL-6, TNF-alpha and other cytokines and lymphokines (17–19). Mechanisms of immune activation have been investigated and one of the possibilities is the direct stimulation of many cells by HIV protein. Other hypotheses have involved the possible development of auto-immunity with antibodies and/or cell mediated immunity that stimulate lymphocytes. Development of neoplasia, especially Kaposi's Sarcoma and B cell lymphomas appears to relate to excessive production of cytokines. IL6 has been implicated with these neoplastic processes (20) and other cytokines may also play significant roles. Finally, activation contributes directly to disease progression. Increased production of the HIV virus requires activation of lymphoid cells (and presumably mononuclear cells) (18). Thus activation of the immune system via increased cytokine production plays a major role in pathogenesis.

Evaluation of Disease Course: Prognosis

Careful studies have indicated that both laboratory markers such as serum neopterin and β2M (11–16) and clinical (21,22) markers can contribute to evaluation of prognosis (Table III). The laboratory markers apply both to the occurrence of AIDS in asymptomatic or mildly symptomatic individuals with CD4 T cells over $200/mm^3$ (11–16). Laboratory markers such as serum neopterin and β2Mlevels as well as CD4 T cell levels are indicative of time to death in individuals with more advanced disease (AIDS: Kaposi's Sarcoma) and CD4 T cells under $200/mm^3$ (23,24). Clinical correlations have established that CD4 cell levels below 500/mm3 are an indication for zidovudine therapy, and CD4 levels under 200/mm3 are considered to be an indication for prophylactic administration of agents to control/prevent opportunistic infection.

Table III. Evaluation of Disease Course: Prognosis

A. CD4 T Cell Levels
B. Immune Activation Markers/Serum
C. Viral Load/p24 Antigen Serum
D. Fever
E. Candida Infection
F. Opportunistic Infections

Control of AIDS

A. Antiretroviral Treatment

Zidovudine (AZT) is a nucleoside analogue which is phosphorylated by cellular enzymes and incorporated into DNA by retroviral reverse transcriptase, thereby producing chain termination of viral DNA. Doses of about 1200 mg per day (given as divided doses) or 500–600 mg/day are most commonly employed. The improvement in the course of disease was documented in patients with AIDS and CD4 T cells under 200/mm^3 as well as in patients with mildly symptomatic disease and CD4 T cells between 200–500/mm^3. Improved performance status, weight gain and survival along with reduced frequency of life threatening illness were reported (25). Other nucleoside analogues, including dideoxycytidine (ddC) and dideoxyinosine (ddI) with potent antiretroviral activity are being used in conjunction with or as an alternative to AZT. AZT has effects on both the immune deficiency and on the immune activation of HIV infection. Mean CD4 T cell increases of about 50 CD4 T cells/mm^3 have been reported (26,27). Serum immune activation markers (which are increased by HIV infection) are reduced with a nadir at 2–8 weeks after onset of zidovudine treatment (28). A study was conducted with mildly symptomatic patients that were enrolled in ACTG protocol 016 and received either placebo or 1200 mg/d of AZT. In the AZT treated group substantial reductions were seen in the elevated serum neopterin and β2M levels. Less marked changes (increase) were noted in CD4. β2M showed return to the baseline levels by 6 months. Neopterin, however, showed more substantial mean reduction with a more prolonged and incomplete return of the mean level towards baseline. The changes in neopterin likely indicate continuing effects of AZT. Thus changes in both immune deficiency (CD4 lymphocytes) and in immune activation (serum neopterin and β2M) reflect the therapeutic effects of zidovudine. Changes in both CD4 and β2M have been shown to correlate with clinical outcome

B. Immune-Based Therapies

A variety of approaches to improving immune functions in HIV-infection (Table IV) have been explored (reviewed in 30).

Replacement Therapy

Antibody replacement has been undertaken with whole serum and concentrated IgG prepared from the serum of individuals with high titre antibodies to HIV. Whether these will be useful under circumstances such as in infants early in infection, in a prenatal period, or in adults with various stages of disease remains to

Table IV. Immune-Based Therapies in HIV Infection and AIDS

Replacement:	*Lymphokines and Cytokines*
Antibody Therapy	IL-2
Immune serum/Gamma Globulin	Interferon-alpha
Monoclonal Antibody to gp160	Interferon-beta
	Interferon-gamma
CD8 (Cytotoxic) T	*Hematopoetic Cytokines*
Cell enrichment	GM-CSF, G-CSF
Bone-Marrow Transplantation	Erythropoierin
Enrichment	
Vaccines for HIV-Infected Individuals	*Receptor Directed Therapy*
gp160 Vaccine Trials	Soluble CD4 Blocking
Killed HIV Vaccines	CD4-Ig Adhesins
	Immune Suppression
	General: Cyclosporine
	Specific Cytokine Reduction
	Block TNF-alpha

be determined. Specific monoclonal antibodies have been developed in two forms. Some are based on murine monoclonal or are partially murine monoclonal and the others are human IgG being grown in quantity from B cells immortalized by hybridization technics. Time is required to produce these in sufficient quantity and therapeutic trials lie ahead. Immune cell treatment trials have focussed on CD8 T cells taken from individuals with HIV infection which are partially purified and then amplified *in vitro* before return to the patient. Initial efforts indicate that these procedures can be carried out, but evaluation of their influence on the course of disease is incomplete. Bone marrow transplantation is again being explored in individuals with advanced disease. No therapeutic benefit was demonstrated without AZT co-treatment. The results of recent studies conducted with AZT are not yet available.

Vaccines in HIV-Seropositive Patients

Studies have been conducted with two types of vaccines: recombinant gp120 pepide (31) and killed HIV virus which is largely depleted of gp120 (32). The findings reported are similar: e. g., immune response better with CD4 (levels over 600/mm^3), humoral and cellular response to preparation-specific antigens, and (perhaps) stabilization of CD4 T cell levels.

Lymphokines and Cytokines

The approaches that were directed to improve immune functions were designed before the extent of HIV-induced immune activation was appreciated. However, recent studies have been conducted in conjunction with AZT. IL-2 administration was effective in causing some increases in CD4 cells when used in high dose and with better immune competence (CD4 T cells greater than 400/mm^3). Interferon alpha and beta had similar requirements. TNF alpha had no beneficial effect. Even at low dose levels, G-CSF and GM-CSF increased blood levels of polymorphonuclear leukocytes (32), but a reduced occurrence of OI is not certain.

Immune Suppression

Earlier hypotheses postulated that HIV infection resulted in autoimmune responses that accounted for CD4 destruction. Subsequent studies have failed to provide substantial evidence of causative antibodies or cell mediated immunity. Meanwhile, however, cyclosporine trials were initiated (34). Careful study indicates no benefit and, possibly, disadvantageous results from one schedule of cyclosporine administration (35).

Selectivly Blocking Cytokines

Because of the compelling evidence that activated immune cells produce substantial cytokines which in turn stimulate T cells and monocytes to produce HIV virus, several approaches are underway to inhibit production or to increase removal of specific cytokines. Several approaches to reduction of TNF-alpha are being explored using inhibitors of production and antibodies to TNF-alpha. Whether reductions in single cytokines will be effective is uncertain. Redundancy in the immune cytokines may require more complex approaches for effective therapy.

Clearly, immune cells are targets of immune destruction and dysregulation in HIV infection. Equally, immune cells are involved in disease pathogenesis. Thus immune-based therapies provide major opportunities for therapeutic interventions.

References

1. Phair, J., Munoz, A., Detels, R., et al. 1990. Risk of pneumocystis carinii pneumonia among men infected with HIV-1. NEJM. 322:161.
2. Javaherian, K., Langlois, A.J., LaRosa, G.J., et al. 1990. Broadly neutralizing antibodies elicited by the hypervariable neutralizing determinant in HIV-1. Science 250:1590.
3. Walker, B.D., and Plata, F. 1990. Cytotoxic T lymphocytes against HIV. AIDS 4:177.
4. Taylor, J.M.G., Fahey, J.L., Detels, R., and Giorgi, J.V. 1989. CD4 percentage, CD4 number and CD4:CD8 ratio in HIV infection: Which to choose and how to use. J. Acquir. Immune Defic. Syndrome 2:114.
5. Giorgi, J.V., and Detels, R. 1989. T cell subset alterations in HIV-infected homosexual men. Clin. Immunol. and Immunopath. 52:10.

6. Prince, H., Kleinman, S., Czaplicker, C., John, J., and Williams, A.E. 1990. Interrelationships between serologic markers of immune activation and T lymphocyte subsets in HIV infection. 3:525.
7. Lane, H.C., Depper, J.M., Green, W.C., et al. 1985. Quantitative analysis of immune function in patients with acquired immunodeficiency syndrome. NEJM. 313:79.
8. Hofmann, B., Jakobsen, K., Odum, N., et al. 1989. The HIV-induced immunodeficiency: Relatively preserved PHA as opposed to decreased PWM responses may be due to possibly preserved responses via CD2/PHA pathway. J. Immunol. 142:1874.
9. Hofmann, B., Lindhardt, B.O., Gerstoft, J., et al. 1987. The lymphocyte transformation response to pokeweed mitogen is a highly predictive parameter for the development of AIDS and AIDS-related symptoms in homosexual men with HIV antibodies. Brit. Med. J. 295:293.
10. Wahl, S.L., Hunt, D.A., Wong, H.L., et al. 1988. Tumor growth-factor-beta is a potent immunosuppressive agent that inhibits IL2 dependent lymphocyte proliferation. J. Immunol. 140:3026.
11. Fahey, J.L, Taylor, J.M.G., Detels, R., Hofmann, B., Melmed, R., Nishanian, P., and Giorgi, J.V. 1990. The prognostic value of cellular and serologic markers in infection with human immunodeficiency virus type 1. NEJM. 322:166.
12. Moss, A.R., Bacchetti, S., Osmond, D., et al. 1988. Seropositivity for HIV and development of AIDS or AIDS-related condition: three-year follow-up of the San Francisco General Hospital cohort. Br. Med. J. 296:745.
13. Fuchs, D., Jager, H., Popescu, M., et al. 1989. Immune activation markers to predict AIDS and survival in HIV-1 seropositives. Immunol. Letters 26:75.
14. Kramer, A., Wiktor, S.Z., Fuchs, et al. 1989. Neopterin: a predictive marker of acquired immune deficiency syndrome in human immunodeficiency virus infection. J. Acq. Immun. Def. Synd. 12:291.
15. Melmed, R.N., Taylor, J.M.G., Detels, R., Bozorgmehri, M., and Fahey, J.L. 1989. Serum neopterin changes in HIV-infected subjects: Indicator of significant pathology, CD4 T cell changes, and the development of AIDS. J. Acquir. Immune. Defic. Syndr. 2:70.
16. Osmond, D.H., Shiboski, S., Bacchetti, S., Winger, E.E., and Moss, A.E. 1991. Immune activation markers and AIDS prognosis. J. AIDS 5:505.
17. Huber, C., Batchelor, J.R., Fuchs, D., et al. 1984. Immune response associated production of neopterin. Release from macrophages is primarily under control of interferon-gamma. J. Exp. Med. 160:310.
18. Rosenberg, Z.F., and Fauci, A.S. 1990. Immunopathogenic mechanisms of HIV infection: Cytokine induction of HIV expression. Immunol. Today 11:162.
19. Breen, E.C., Rezai, A.R., Nakajima, K., Beall, G.N., Mitsuyasu, R.T., Hirano, T.,Kishimoto, T., and Martinez-Maza, O. 1990. Infection with HIV is associated with elevated IL-6 levels and production. J. Immunol. 144:480.
20. Miles, S.A., Rezai, A.R., Salazar-Gonzales, J. Martines-Maza, O., et al. 1990. AIDS Kaposi sarcoma-derived cells produce and respond to IL6. Proc. Natl. Acad. Sci. 87:4068.
21. Polk, B.E., Fox, R., Brookmeyer, R., et al. 1987. Predictors of AIDS developing in a cohort of seropositive men. NEJM. 315:61.
22. Munoz, A., Carey, V., Saah, A.J. Phair, J.P., Kingsley, L.A., Fahey, J.L, Ginzburg, H.M., and Polk, B.F. 1988. Predictors of decline in CD4 lymphocytes in a cohort of homosexual men infected with human immunodeficiency virus. J. Acquir. Immune. Defic. Syndr. 1:396.
23. Taylor, J., Afrashiabi, R., Fahey, J.L., Korn, E., Weaver, M., and Mitsuyasu, R. 1986. A prognostically significant classification of immune changes in AIDS with Kaposi's Sarcoma. Blood 67:666.
24. Krown, S.E., Niedzwiecki, D., Bhalla, R.B., Flomenberg, N., Bundow, D., and Chapman, D. 1991. Relationship and prognostic value of endogenous interferon alpha, β2M and neopterin serum levels in patients with Kaposi's Sarcoma and AIDS. J. AIDS 4:871.
25. Merrigan, T.C. 1991. Issues in the development of more effective antiviral therapies for HIV infection. In: Current issues in the management of patients with HIV infection (Therapeutic strategies in oncology). S. Krowon, ed. London: Mediscropt, p. 8.
26. Fischl, M.A., Richman, D.D., Hansen, N., et al. 1990. The safety and efficacy of zidovudine (AZT) in the treatment of mildly symptomatic human HIV-1 infection. Ann. Int. Med. 1121:727.
27. Volberding, P.A., Lagakos, S.W., Koch, M.A., et al. 1990. Zidovudine in asymptomatic human HIV infection. NEJM. 322:941.

28. Bass, H.Z., Hardy, W.D., Mitsuyasu, R.T., Taylor, J.M.G., Wang, Y.X., Fischl, M., Spector, A., Richman, D.D., and Fahey, J.L. 1991. Effects of zidovudine treatment on serum neopterin and β2M levels in mildly symptomatic HIV seropositive individuals. J. AIDS, in press.
29. Jacobson, M.A., Abrams, D.I., Volberding, P.A., et al. 1991. Surrogate markers for survival in patients with AIDS and AIDS related complex treated with zidovudine. Brit. Med. J. 302:73.
30. Fahey, J.L., and Schooley, R. 1991. Status of immune-based therapies in HIV infection and AIDS. Clin. Exper. Immunol. in press.
31. Redfield, P.R., Brix, D.L., Ketter, N., et al. 1991. A Phase I evaluation of the safety and immunogenicity of vaccination with recombinant gp160 in patients with early HIV infection. NEJM. 324:1678.
32. Levine, A.M., Henderson, B.E. Groshen S., et al. 1990. Immunization of HIV-infected individuals with inactivated HIV immunogen: Significance of HIV specific cell mediated immune response. VII Inter. Conf. on AIDS 337:204.
33. Mitsuaysu, R. 1991. The role of recombinant cytokines in patients with HIV disease. In: Current issues in the management of patients with HIV infection (Therapeutic strategies in oncology). S. Krowon, ed. London: Mediscript, p. 83.
34. Andrieu, J.M., Even, P., Venet, A., Tourani, J.M., et al. 1988. Effect of cyclosporin on T-cell subsets in HIV disease. Clin. Immunol. & Immunopath. 46:181.
35. Phillips, A., Wainberg, M.A., Coates, R., et al. 1989. Cyclosporin induced deterioration in patients with AIDS. Can. Med. Assoc. J. 140:1456.

The Factors Influencing Autoimmune Responses

Ivan M. Roitt*, Patricia R. Hutchings*, Kim I. Dawe*, Nazira Sumar*, Katherine B. Bodman*, Anne Cooke**

There are two classes of autoimmune disease, organ-specific and non-organ specific or systemic. That cells producing autoantibodies are selected by antigen is strongly suggested by the presence of mutations and high affinity antibody. T-cells are pivotal in all forms of autoimmunity as evidenced by the therapeutic benefit of anti-T-cell monoclonals such as anti-CD4, and the frequent development of high affinity IgG autoantibodies. The production of anergic T-cells by the use of non-depleting anti-CD4 in the presence of antigen is discussed with particular reference to its potential for immunological intervention in autoimmune disease. It is possible to identify T-cell epitopes in organ-specific autoimmunity by using pathogenic T-cell clones or hybridomas to identify the peptide sequences which are reactive. Antigen-specific therapy may ultimately be based on such peptide epitopes. The specificity of the T-cells in systemic autoimmunity is still obscure, but there is some evidence that reactivity with certain germ-line idiotypes can lead to the development of systemic autoimmunity. The possibility of stimulating B-cells specific for autoantigens such as DNA becomes feasible if a complex of antibody and DNA is taken up by these specific B-cells and processed idiotype is presented to T-helpers specific for those idiotype epitopes. Evidence is presented that there may be pre-existing defects in the target organ in certain organ-specific disorders, and the evidence for a glycosylation defect in the IgG in patients with Rheumatoid Arthritis is explored. It is noted that the spouses of probands with Rheumatoid Arthritis also tend to have this glycosylation defect and this raises the possibility of an effect due to an environmental factor, such as a microbial infection. Molecular mimicry of autoantigens by microbes can stimulate autoreactive cells by their cross-reactivity. It is emphasized that cross-reaction which gives rise to the priming of autoreactive T-cells could give rise to the establishment of a chronic autoimmune state. In animals with normal regulatory immune systems, such induced autoimmunity is ultimately corrected and it is only in animals where there are defects in regulation that autoimmunity persists. Thus, there are many factors giving rise to autoimmunity, and the diseases are rightly regarded as multifactorial in origin.

Two Classes of Autoimmune Disease

It is convenient to group autoimmune disease under two main headings, as first proposed by us many years ago (1). In the organ-specific diseases the immune process is directed to antigens within a specific organ and, as a result of aggressive action, lead to organ-specific lesions. Examples are Hashimoto's disease of the thyroid, pernicious anaemia affecting the stomach and myasthenia gravis involving autoimmunity to the acetylcholine receptors in the muscle endplate. By contrast, the non-organ specific diseases involving a systemic autoimmunity lead to the production of antibodies to autoantigens with a widespread organ and tissue distribution and correspondingly there is a more widespread location of the lesions, often considered to be representative of immune complex disease although this may be an over-simplified view. The rheumatological disorders, such as rheumatoid arthritis, SLE, scleroderma, dermatomyositis, Wegener's granulomatosis and so on, are the main contributors to this group of disorders. Fundamentally different underlying mechanistic processes may operate in the two groups of diseases as evident from the fact that there is frequent overlap of diseases within each group but far less between the groups.

Currently, there are cogent advocates of the view that a pre-existing autoimmune state is

* Department of Immunology, University College & Middlesex School of Medicine, London, W1P 9PG
** Dept. of Pathology, University of Cambridge, UK.
Reprinted with the kind permission of the *Journal of Autoimmunity 5, (2),* 1992, Supplement.

intrinsic to the immune system and that a regulated network of lymphocytes linked through autoantigen and idiotype anti-idiotype interactions forms a part of the normal physiology of the immune system (2). From this standpoint, failure to regulate this physiological autoimmune network leads to the emergence of pathogenic autoimmunity as evidenced by the appearance of destructive autoreactive T-cells and high affinity IgG autoantibodies.

B-Cells Producing Autoantibodies are Selected by Antigen

This is not an entirely self-evident proposition since B-cells can be stimulated by polyclonal activators and by idiotypic interactions. Perhaps the most convincing evidence that B-cells are selected by antigen is the existence of somatic mutations (3) and high affinity in the autoantibody response. T-cell driven somatic mutation of B-lymphocytes can only lead consistently to a high affinity antibody response if the appropriate B-cell mutants are selected by antigen itself in germinal centre structures. Additional support for the antigen-driven hypothesis comes from the occurrence of autoantibody responses to antigen clusters. The cluster may be represented by an intra-molecular linkage as for example in the occurrence of several epitopes on the same autoantigenic molecule (4). It is really difficult to envisage a mechanism which could account for the co-existence of antibody responses to different epitopes on the same molecule, except through a linkage dependent on the structure of the antigen molecule itself. The same considerations apply to autoimmunity directed to different molecular components of intracellular organelles such as nucleosomes or antigens linked within the same organ, such as thyroglobulin and thyroid peroxidase within the thyroid gland.

In a sense these arguments are circumstantial; and possibly the most direct evidence for the contention that autoimmunity is antigen driven, has been obtained by studies in the obese strain chicken which spontaneously develops thyroid autoimmunity with a chronic thyroiditis leading to complete atrophy of the gland and hypothyroidism. If the thyroid gland as a source of antigen is removed at birth, the chickens grow up without developing thyroid autoantibodies, i. e., in the absence of autoantigen thyroid autoimmunity does not arise. Furthermore, once the disease and the thyroid autoimmunity have been established, removal of the thyroid then leads to a gross decline of thyroid autoantibodies, usually to undetectable levels, again implying that maintenance of autoimmunity is antigen driven rather than depending upon some non-antigen source.

T-Cells

T-Cells: Pivotal in Organ-Specific Autoimmunity

The evidence for this is overwhelming, at least in experimental models of disease. For example, neonatal thymectomy inhibits the production of experimental allergic encephalomyelitis induced by myelin basic protein in Complete Freund's adjuvant. The spontaneous thyroiditis in the obese strain chicken is held in check by a combination of neonatal thymectomy plus Draconian injections of a turkey anti-chicken T-cell serum. Another spontaneous model of autoimmune disease, the diabetes in NOD mice, is crucially dependent upon the activity of T-cells since treatment with monoclonal anti-CD4 or anti-CD8, or preferably both, can completely inhibit the development of hypoglycaemia. Antigen-specific T-cell clones can themselves be shown to be capable of causing disease as has been demonstrated in experimental autoallergic encephalitis (5) and thyroiditis, and in NOD mice. Clearly it is far more difficult in the human to obtain direct evidence for pathogenic T-cell action and perhaps the nearest we can get at the moment is the demonstration that thyroid-specific T-cells are actually present in the thyroid of patients with thyrotoxicosis. T-cell clones were isolated which were driven by class II associated antigens present on the thyroid cells of the patients, and many but not all had specificity for peptides derived from the thyroid peroxidase molecule (6).

T-Cell Epitopes in Experimental Autoallergic Thyroiditis

With the knowledge that T-cell epitopes involve linear sequences of amino acids forming relatively small peptides, it is now feasible to seek to identify the T-cell epitopes responsible for autoimmune reactions with the view to developing possible immunotherapeutic intervention based upon such peptides which could be readily synthesized. Accordingly, with our interest in the thyroiditis produced by immunization with thyroglobulin in Complete Freund's adjuvant, we have attempted to identify the relevant T-cell epitopes and although the task is somewhat daunting in view of the fact that the molecule is made up of two chains each containing 2,760 amino acids, we were fortunate in having made the observation that thyroglobulin lacking iodine did not produce pathogenic autoimmunity (7). Since thyroglobulin has just four sites of thyroxine hormonogenesis, we concentrated our efforts on the peptides which covered these four regions and together with Mario Geysen and his colleagues, synthesized a series of 12-mer peptides overlapping by 11 residues, which systematically covered these sites. Thyroglobulin-specific T-cell hybridomas, derived from clones or lines which were themselves capable of inducing thyroiditis on transfer to a naive recipient, were used to identify the T-cell epitope. It is clear that the epitope is localised to the peptide sequence covering the thyroxine at residue 2553. The thyroxine side chain is extremely bulky and must protrude quite prominently from the MHC class II groove, but nonetheless its presence is mandatory for antigenic activity since replacement of this residue by any of the 20 natural amino acids leads to loss of recognition of the peptide by the T-cell hybridoma (8). The pathogenetic relevance of this thyroxine containing peptide is shown by the fact that cells taken from donors immunized with peptide in Complete Freund's adjuvant, and then cultured *in vitro* with the peptide, become highly activated and can transfer significant thyroiditis when injected into histocompatible recipients (unpublished observations).

Therapy with Non-Depleting Anti-CD4

Having identified an important T-cell epitope of thyroglobulin, it is clearly of interest to investigate possible strategies for exploiting the peptide in therapeutic strategies and we are particularly interested in the possibility of targetting the peptide to induce unresponsiveness in the antigen-specific T-cell population. We are encouraged by the observations of Waldmann and his colleagues (9) showing that treatment with a non-depleting monoclonal anti-CD4 in the presence of antigen induces a state of anergy in the T-cell population, which can be sustained by repeated exposure to antigen which, in the case of autoimmune diseases, might be adequately provided by natural presentation of autoantigenic moieties. The precise mechanisms underlying the production of anergy are perhaps still controversial, but there is no doubt that, given the right timing of the anti-CD4 and antigen injections, the treatment is effective and holds great promise.

We have found in our system that treatment with thyroid antigen in Complete Freund's together with a non-depleting anti-CD4 does in fact induce unresponsiveness with respect to the development of thyroiditis in response to subsequent challenge with a thyroiditogenic injection. Even more exciting are the observations by A. Cooke and her colleagues (unpublished) suggesting that T-cells from NOD mice which are already primed against pancreatic antigens can be held in check by treatment with non-depleting anti-CD4 monoclonals.

T-Cells are Critical in Systemic Autoimmunity

Non-depleting anti-CD4 treatment is also extremely effective when used in models of systemic autoimmunity such as the spontaneous SLE which develops in the New Zealand Black x White F1 cross (10). Beneficial effects of anti-CD4 therapy are also seen in patients with rheumatoid arthritis where there is a preponderance of activated T-cells in the diseased synovium. This emphasizes the point that T-cells are pivotal not only in organ-specific autoimmunity but also in the non-organ specific group of diseases. This is further supported by the finding that IgG autoantibodies in these disorders show somatic mutations and high affinity, properties which are very much dependent on the cooperative action of helper T-cells. Furthermore, knowing the role of MHC molecules in presentation of antigen to T-cells, associations such as those of rheumatoid arthritis with certain polymorphic sequences common to the HLA DR1 and DR4 molecules should be taken to imply a basic contribution by T-cell responses in the pathogenesis of disease.

What is painfully obvious is that in systemic autoimmunity we have very little idea of the identity of the antigens recognized by the T-cells. One possibility which has been seriously muted is that the T-cells do not see conventional antigen at all, clearly the case with DNA responses, but instead are devoted to the recognition of idiotype and in this view lupus, for example, would be an "idiotype disease". Some support for this view has been obtained in experiments in which a human monoclonal anti-DNA obtained from a patient with SLE, and bearing the germ-line idiotype labelled 16/6, was injected with Complete Freund's into BALB/c mice. The animals developed anti-DNA, immune complex glomerulonephritis, and produced their own 16/6 positive antibodies (11). Human 16/6 could only elicit mouse antibodies with the same idiotype, through the intermediary stage of an anti-16/6, either an antibody or a T-cell. In fact, T-cells with specificity for 16/6 idiotype were isolated by these authors and claimed to induce disease when transferred to new recipients. In another set of experiments, Schwartz and his colleagues (12) sequenced a monoclonal antibody from MRL/lpr mice which recognized the idiotype on an anti-ribonuclear protein and found that immunization with a peptide derived from the third complementarity determining region of the light chain elicited the production of anti-RNP. Since the immunogen was a peptide, it is highly likely that the first cells to respond were T-cells.

We thus have evidence that T-cells recognising appropriate idiotypes may provoke the formation of antibodies typical of lupus. Nonetheless, we earlier produced evidence showing that the B-cells were probably being selected by conventional autoantigen. The two ideas are not mutually exclusive since T-cell help for one component in an intermolecular complex can provide help for antibody formation to the second component. For example, DNA complexed with antibody bearing the 16/6 idiotype (present as a "natural antibody" ?) would be taken up by B-cells specific for anti-DNA through the surface receptor, and processed internally to yield idiotype related peptide which could be expressed on the surface in association with MHC class II. This could be recognized by T-helpers for 16/6 which, if they escape from normal regulation, would help the B-cell to become an antibody-forming cell secreting the immunoglobulin for which it was originally programmed, namely anti-DNA. Given a natural interlocking network of idiotypes and autoantigens as postulated much earlier in this article, such a mechanism would contribute to the formation of specific autoantibody clusters in systemic autoimmunity.

Is There a Pre-Existing Defect in the Target-Organ?

We should now turn our attention to evidence indicative of a pre-existing defect in the organs which become the target of autoimmune disease. Here, the evidence from spontaneous models of autoimmunity is likely to be more persuasive. Looking first at the obese strain chicken, studies by Sundick and colleagues (13) revealed that the uptake of iodine into the thyroid glands of animals in which endogenous TSH had been suppressed by thyroxine treatment, was far higher than that seen in a variety of normal strains. Furthermore, this was not due to any stimulating effect of the autoimmunity, since immunosuppressed animals showed even higher uptakes of radio-iodine. Interestingly, the Cornell strain, from which the obese strain was derived by breeding, showed yet higher uptakes of ^{131}I even though the animals do not develop spontaneous thyroiditis. This is indicative of abnormal thyroid behaviour which in itself is insufficient to induce autoimmune disease. That the Cornell strain thyroid possesses an abnormality which may predispose to the development of autoimmune thyroiditis, is seen by experiments in which lymphoid cells from older obese strain chickens with thyroid disease were transferred to other histocompatible recipients. Young obese strain chickens developed thyroiditis on receiving these lymphoid cells but normal strains did not. However, thyroiditis did develop in the Cornell strain of chickens suggesting that a combination of the autoaggressive lymphoid cells from the diseased OS chicken with the abnormally susceptible thyroid of the CS strain did provide the circumstances in which thyroiditis could develop (14).

Considerable excitement was generated by the findings of Bottazzo, Pujol-Borell and colleagues (15) that the thyroids of patients with autoimmune thyrotoxicosis expressed abundant MHC class II on their surface. As mentioned above, these surface class II molecules can present endogenous antigen to appropriate thyroid-specific T-cells, but a role of such antigen presentation in the initiation or perpetuation of autoimmunity is still debated. Although this issue is still unresolved, there remain certain pieces of evidence which indicate that a propensity to class II expression may be a feature of organs involved in certain spontaneous autoimmune diseases. For example, Wick and his colleagues (14) showed that thyroid cells from obese strain chickens in culture had a lower threshold for the induction of surface class II MHC by IFNγ than do cells from normal strains. A similar phenomenon was observed by Cooke et al. (16) regarding the induction of MHC class II by interferon-γ on the beta cells of the islets of Langerhans of diabetic-prone BB rats as compared with their diabetic-resistant cousins. What is striking about these results is that they parallel the events occurring in the human disease, since only the insulin-producing cells, but not the glucagon and somatostatin producing cells, in the diabetic pancreas express class II. Although normal human islets do not express class II when stimulated by IFNγ, a combination with tumour necrosis factor does upregulate the class II genes, but here the effect is seen on all three types of cells making up the islets of Langerhans. Conceivably, in spontaneous disease, there might be an agent such as an endogenous virus which turns on the cells' own TNF genes and this combined with an external source of IFNγ, possibly derived from infiltrating T-cells, could provide the trigger for expression of class II genes, thereby making the cells susceptible to the autoimmune disease processes.

IgG Glycosylation Defect in Rheumatoid Arthritis

Although there may be defects in the organisation of target organs in various autoimmune disorders, in only one instance has it been possible to discern an abnormality in the structure of the autoantigen itself, and that is in the case of immunoglobulin G in rheumatoid arthritis, where autoimmunity to this molecule is a dominant feature. It is now clear that the IgG molecules in both juvenile and adult forms of rheumatoid arthritis are significantly hypogalactosylated in that the percentage of biantennary sugars which lack galactose (G0%) is significantly higher than in IgG from normal individuals. These differences may endow the molecule with a greater propensity for self-association of IgG rheumatoid factor, thereby enhancing immune complex formation in the joint, or it may increase the propensity of IgG to be handled in a way which predisposes to the encouragement of autosensitization. Be that as it may, the occurrence of a high G0 percentage early in disease can be a valuable prognostic indicator (17). We know that it is a consequence of reduced galactosyltransferase (18), the enzyme which adds galactose to terminal N-acetyl glucosamine in the biantennary sugar molecule; and conceivably, other molecules of importance, including those released by T-cells, may show abnormal behaviour as a result of a lower galactose content. This is an obvious area for further study.

It is well known that the severity of rheumatoid arthritis is reduced late in pregnancy with an exacerbation post-partum. What was not expected, was that the degree of galactosylation of the patient's IgG should change pari passu with the disease state pre- and post-partum. In a series of cases, G0% levels fell markedly near to term in parallel with amelioration of disease, but soon after that the disease became more severe and was associated with a rise in the G0% (19). At the least, this suggests that the galactose content of the IgG is tracking the underlying pathological events with some fidelity. Another unexpected finding surfaced during a study on family members of probands with rheumatoid arthritis. It appeared that, unlike other family members without disease, the spouses actually had elevated percent G0 values. A further cohort of spouses of patients attending the clinic for RA confirmed this finding of decreased galactose content in IgG of the spouses. This indicates environmental elements, most likely infectious agents.

Molecular Mimicry of Autoantigens

There are many ways in which microorganisms could influence autoimmunity, but the mechanism which has attracted most interest is that of molecular mimicry between micro-organisms and autoantigens, including of course idiotypes. There are innumerable examples of cross-reactions at the B-cell level, or of sequence homology at the T-cell level, between microbial molecules and autoantigens (20). Ebringer has consistently championed cross-reactivity between HLA-B27 and certain strains of klebsiella in connection with ankylosing spondylitis, and more recently cross-reactivity between *Proteus mirabilis* and DR4 in relationship to rheumatoid arthritis (21). Homology between the highly conserved heat shock proteins in mycobateria and humans has also been highlighted as a potential contributory factor in the pathogenesis of the latter disease (2).

The scene was set many years ago independently by Weigle and Allison who envisaged a situation in which autoreactive B-cells which did not normally respond to autoantigens because of tolerance at the T-cell level, could be activated by cross-reacting microbial antigens which offered T-cell helper epitopes to which the individual was not tolerant. The problem with this system is that when the foreign microbe is eliminated by immune reactivity, there is no longer T-cell help and the autoreactive B-cell cannot be stimulated by endogenous autoantigen. Thus, a chronic autoimmune state cannot be established.

On the other hand, cross-reactivity at the T-cell level may lead to chronicity because of the nature of interactions with primed versus naive T-cells. We can illustrate the point by quoting the studies of Clayton, Sercarz and colleagues (22). They used the experimental allergic encephalomyelitis system, immunizing with myelin basic protein (MBP) in Complete Freund's. First they tolerized to the most immunogenic epitope, peptide no. I, and then showed that cross-reacting MBP could induce the brain lesions, whereas the mouse protein could not. In other words, mouse peptide no. II, which is the second encephalitogenic epitope, given as the whole protein, could not induce the brain lesions through production of autoreactive T-cells whereas heterologous guinea-pig MBP presented epitope II effectively and induced autoreactive T-cells capable of interacting with mouse MBP processed in the brain which acts as the target for these cells and leads to the production of brain lesions. In other words, the heterologous MPB epitope is presented more effectively to the naive T-cells than the homologous protein, but once it has stimulated the cells they are then able to react with processed homologous MBP because they have a higher avidity for the antigen processing cell. This is not a consequence of any change in the receptor because T-cell receptors do not mutate, but rather a consequence of increased expression of accessory molecules like CD2 and LFA-1 which give much stronger binding to the antigen presenting cells. Thus, when primed, the T-cells can react with peptides from endogenous protein which normally would remain cryptic (22), i.e. would not be presented in sufficient concentration to bind effectively and trigger the naive T-cell. Once triggered, the endogenous molecules can continue to stimulate the T-cells and so give rise to a chronic autoimmune state.

Regulatory Defects Contribute to the Development of Autoimmune Disease

It seems that the adventitious induction of autoimmunity by cross-reactivity through the mechanisms outlined above, may be regulated in normal animals. Let us look for example at the model in which rat red cells are used to break tolerance as a cross-reacting antigen with mouse erythrocytes in the mouse. The resulting antibodies give rise to positive Coomb's tests in which the presence of antibody on the red cells is revealed by a conventional antiglobulin reagent. If one continues to inject rat red cells at weekly intervals, the Coombs' test becomes positive and reaches a maximum at around 2 weeks, but thereafter declines in a normal mouse strain such as CBA. However, in other strains, where the tolerance mechanisms are less well ensconced, such as NZB (which eventually spontaneously develops an autoimmune haemolytic anaemia) and even more so in the SJL, the autoimmune state does not resolve and, in the case of the SJL, becomes so severe that the animals die shortly after the 4th injection, probably as the result of anaphylaxis. Thus, it appears that the normal mice had managed to regulate the induced autoimmune response, and further studies reveal that the mice at 4 weeks contain T-cells capable of transferring active suppression to a naive recipient which will then fail to make autoantibodies when challenged with rat red blood cells. At the T-cell level in experimental models such as allergic encephalomyelitis induced by MBP and the adjuvant arthritis produced by Freund's adjuvant alone, the diseases are also self-limiting apparently due to the operation of T-suppressor systems.

It is clear therefore that many different factors must operate together before a chronic autoimmune state becomes established; in a word, autoimmune diseases are multifactorial in origin.

References

1. Hijmans, W., Doniach, D., Roitt, I.M., and Holborow, E.J. 1961. Serological overlap between lupus erythematosus, rheumatoid arthritis, and thyroid autoimmune disease. B. M. J. ii:909.
2. Cohen, I.R., and Young, D.B. 1991. Autoimmunity, microbial immunity and the immunological homunculus. Imm. Today 12 (Apr):105.
3. Schlomchik, M., Mascelli, M., Shan, H., Radic, M.Z., Pisetsky, C., Marshak-Rothstein, A., and Weigert, M. 1990. Anti-DNA antibodies from autoimmune mice arise by clonal expansion and somatic mutation. J. Exp. Med. 171 (1):265.
4. Vincent, A., Whiting, P.J., Schluep, M., Heidenreich, F., Lang, B., Roberts, A., Willcox, N., and Newsom-Davis, J. 1987. Antibody heterogeneity and specificity in myasthenia gravis. Ann. N. Y. Acad. Sci. 505:106.
5. Ben-Nun, A., and Cohen, I.R. 1982. Experimental autoimmune encephalomyelitis (EAE) mediated by T cell lines: process of selection of lines and characterization of the cells. J. Immunol. 129:303.
6. Dayan, C.M., Londei, M., Corcoran, A.E., Grubeck-Loebenstein, B., James, R.S.L., Rappaport, B., and Feldmann, M. 1991. Autoantigen recognition by thyroid-infiltrating T-cells in Graves Disease. PNAS 88:7415.
7. Champion, B.R., Rayner, D.C., Byfield, P., Page, K., Chan, J., and Roitt, I.M. 1987. Critical role of iodination for T-cell recognition of thyroglobulin in experimental murine thyroid autoimmunity. J. Immunol. 139:3665.
8. Champion, B.R., Page, K.R., Parish, N., Rayner, D.C., Dawe, K., Biswas-Hughes, G., Cooke, A., Geysen, M., and Roitt, I.M. 1991. Identification of a thyroxine-containing self epitope of thyroglobulin which triggers thyroid autoreactive T cells. J. Exp. Med., 174:363.
9. Mathieson, P.W., Cobbold, S.P, Hale, G., Clark, M.R., Oliviera, D.B.G., Lockwood, C.M., and Waldmann, H. 1990. Monoclonal antibody treatment in systemic vasculitis. New Engl. J. Med. 323:250.
10. Carterton, N.L., Schimenti, C.L., and Wofsy, D. 1989. Treatment of murine lupus with F(ab')2 fragments of monoclonal antibody to L3T4. Suppression of autoimmunity does not depend on T helper cell depletion. J. Immunol. 142:1470.
11. Shoenfeld, M., and Mozes, E. 1990. Pathogenic idiotypes of autoantibodies in autoimmunity: Lessons from new experimental models of SLE. FASEB J. 4:2646.
12. Pucetti, A. Koizumi, T., Migliorini, P., Andre-Schwartz, J., Barrett, K.J., and Schwartz, R.S. 1990. An immunoglobulin light chain from a lupus-prone mouse induces autoantibodies in normal mice. J. Exp. Med. 171(6):1919.
13. Sundick, R.S. Bagchi, N., Livezey, M.D., Brown, T.R., and Mack, R.E. 1979. Abnormal thyroid regulation in chickens with autoimmune thyroiditis. Endocrinology (Baltimore) 105:493.
14. Wick, G., Kuhr, T., Kromer, G., and Hala, K. 1990. Genetic background, thyroid activity and autoimmune phenomena. In: The thyroid gland, environment and autoimmunity. H.A. Drexhage, J.J.M. de Vijlder and W.M. Wiersinga, eds. Amsterdam: Elsevier Science, p. 23.
15. Bottazzo, G.F., Pujol-Borrell, R., Hanafusa, T., and Feldmann, M. 1983. Hypothesis: Role of aberrant HLA-DR expression and antigen presentation in the induction of endocrine autoimmunity. Lancet ii:1115.
16. Walker, R., Cooke, A., Bone, A.J., Dean, B.M., van der Meide, P., and Baird, J.D. 1986. Induction of class II MHC antigens in vitro on pancreatic B cells isolated from BB/E rats. Diabetologia 29:749.
17. Young, A., Sumar, N., Bodman, K., Goyal S., Sinclair, H., Roitt, I., and Isenberg, D. 1991.

Agalactosyl IgG: an aid to differential diagnosis in early synovitis. Arthritis & Rheumatism, 34:1425.

18. Axford, J.S., Mackenzie, L., Lydyard, P.M., Hay, F.C., Isenberg, D., and Roitt, I.M. 1987. Reduced B-cell galactosyltransferase activity in rheumatoid arthritis. Lancet ii:1486.
19. Rook, G.A.W., Steele, J., Brealey, R., Whyte, A., Isenberg, D., Sumar, N., Nelson, L., Bodman, K.B., Young, A., Roitt, I.M., Williams, P., Scragg, I., Edge, C.J., Arkwright, P., Ashford, D., Wormald, M., Rudd, P., Redman, C., Dwek, R.A., and Rademacher, T.W. 1991. Changes in IgG glycoform levels may be relevant to remission of arthritis during pregnancy. J. Autoimmunity, 4:779.
20. Oldstone, M.B. 1989. Virus-induced autoimmunity: molecular mimicry as a route to autoimmune disease. J. Autoimmunity June: 2 Suppl:187.
21. Ebringer, A., Khalafpour, S., and Wilson, C. (1989). Rheumatoid arthritis and Proteus: a possible aetiological association. Rheumatol. Int. 9:223.
22. Clayton, J.P., Gammon, G.M., Ando, D.G., Kono, D.H., Hood, L., and Sercarz, E.E. 1989. Peptide-specific prevention of experimental allergic encephalomyelitis. J. Exp. Med. 169:1681.

Novel Immune Deficiencies: Defective Transcription of Lymphokine Genes

Emanuela Castigli, Raif S. Geha, Talal Chatila*

A 4-year-old female with severe combined immunodeficiency (SCID) had normal numbers of T cells in circulation and normal T cell subsets. However, her T cells proliferated poorly to mitogens and did not proliferate to antigens or to anti-CD3 mAb. Interleukin-2 (IL-2) receptor expression was normal but IL-2 synthesis was undetectable. The addition of recombinant IL-2 to a mitogen-stimulated culture resulted in normalization of the proliferative response. Northern blot analysis of total RNA derived from the patient's T cells revealed a weak or absent expression of mRNA coding for IL-2, IL-3, IL-4, and IL-5. In contrast, there were normal amounts of mRNA coding for granulocytic-macrophage colony-stimulating factor (GM-CSF). Tumor necrosis factor and IL-6 production were also normal. Nuclear run on transcriptional assays revealed markedly decreased levels of newly initiated nuclear transcripts coding for IL-2, IL-3, IL-4, and IL-5 and normal levels of GM-CSF transcripts in patient relative to control lymphocytes. Gel retardation assays suggest that the NFAT-1 nuclear transcription complex is abnormal in the patient. These results indicate that the patient's T cells suffered from a defect affecting the transcription of multiple T cell lymphokines and suggest that abnormalities affecting the production of T cell lymphokines may underlie some of the primary immunodeficiency diseases. Cellular and humoral immune responses to antigens are strictly dependent on the synthesis by activated T cells of a multitude of soluble factors. These factors include the interleukins (IL), interferon-γ, colony stimulating factors, tumor necrosis factor (TNF) α and β, transforming growth factor β, and other yet uncharacterized factors (1,2). We describe a case of primary severe combined immunodeficiency (SCID) with normal numbers and phenotypes of circulating lymphocytes which were deficient in their capacity to synthesize multiple lymphokines.

Case Report

The patient, who is a girl, is 3 years and 8 months old and was born at 37 weeks of gestation. The patient developed at 2 months of age a generalized vesicular eruption after exposure to a sibling with chicken pox. This was ultimately resolved following intravenous therapy with acyclovir. Investigation of her immune function at 6 months of age revealed normal lymphocyte count and phenotype, an absent delayed-type hypersensitivity response to a battery of seven antigens, impaired *in vitro* proliferation of T cells to mitogens, hypogammaglobulinemia (IgG 170 mg/ml; IgA < 1mg/ml; IgM 12 mg/ml), and low varicella zoster titiers (IgG titer, 1:16; IGM titer, < :8). Tests for HIV in the child and in the mother were negative. Tests for the activity of adenosine deaminase and purine nucleoside phosphorylase were normal. The patient was placed on intravenous γ-globulin, yet she suffered from progressive opportunistic infections including oral thrush and *Pneumocystis carinii* pneumonia, and failed to thrive. Two bone marrow transplants at 6 and 8 months of age were performed with a T cell-depleted haploidentical (paternal) bone marrow graft. Based on the observation that the patient's T cells failed to secrete detectable amounts of IL-2 upon stimulation with mitogens but proliferated well to the combination of mitogens and exogenous IL-2, the patient was started on intravenous IL-2 replacement therapy with a remarkable clinical response (3).

* Division of Immunology, Children's Hospital, Department of Pediatrics, Harvard Medical School, 300 Longwood Avenue, Boston, Massachusetts, 02115, U.S.A.
Acknowledgements: Grant support: NIH/1P01A128046, 1R29A130550-01, March of Dimes.

Results

Flow cytometric analysis of the patient's circulating lymphocytes at the age of 6 months revealed normal absolute numbers and percentages of T cells that expressed the T cell receptor/CD3 complex, CD4 and CD8. Despite their normal number and phenotype, the patient's lymphocytes failed to proliferate in response to the mitogenic anti-CD3 monoclonal antibody OKT3 to a mitogenic combination of anti-CD2 monoclonal antibodies, OKT11 + 9.6 or to phytohemaglutinin: see Table 1. The various mitogens tested induced the expression of the IL-2 receptor on the patient's T cells but to a lesser extent than that observed for control T cells. The secretion of IL-4 and of interferon-γ by the patient's T cells upon their activation by lectins or by agonistic antibodies was either severely defective or undetectable. In contrast, the monocyte-derived production of IL-6 and TNFα was normal. The impaired proliferation of the patient's T cells to mitogens was dramatically enhanced by IL-2 (Table 1).

Table 1. Immunologic Function of Patient and Control T Lymphocytes

Stimulus	{^{3}H} Thymidine incorporation (cpm) Patient	Control
A. Proliferative responses to mitogens		
Medium	538,336	1,911
Medium + IL-2	13,336	60,060
Anti-CD3 (OKT3)	720	22,680
Anti-CD3 + Il-2	67,785	198,090
Anti-CD2	673	183,487
Anti-CD2 + IL-2	298,610	268,160
PHA	25,583	365,690
PHA + IL-2	521,010	418,070

B. Lymphokine synthesis following PMA plus ionomycin stimulation.

	Patient	Control
Il-2 (Femtomoles/ml)	69	2,745
IFN-γ (U/ml)	75	782
IL-4 (pg/ml)	3	110
TNF-α (pg/ml)	400	370
IL-6 (ng/ml)	29	30

A) Recombinant IL-2 was used at 100 U/ml, all monoclonal antibodies were used at 1 μg/ml, and PHA-P was used at 10 μg/ml. Results are means of triplicate determinations. Similar results were found in five other experiments.

B) PMA was used in 20 mg/ml and ionomycin at 0.5 μM. Similar results were found in three other experiments.

The defective synthesis of multiple lymphokines by the patient's T cells could be the result of an abnormality affecting the transduction via cell surface receptors of signals necessary for the induction of lymphokine synthesis, e. g., elevation in free intracellular Ca^{2+} $[Ca^{2+}]i$, and activation of protein kinase C (PKC). (4). Alternatively the defective production of lymphokines by the patient's lymphocytes could have resulted from a more distal abnormality. Treatment of the patient's peripheral blood lymphocytes with the PKC activator PMA and the calcium ionophore ionomycin could induce only a modest synthesis of both IL-2 interferon-γ and IL-4. This suggested that the defective synthesis of lymphokines by the patient's peripheral blood T cells was related to an abnormality distal to the generation of second messengers which follows the engagement of the T cell receptor/CD3 complex (5).

T cell lines were generated from the patient's peripheral lymphocytes and were similar to the patient's peripheral blood T cells in their inability to secrete lymphokines upon stimulation with mitogens. Northern blot analysis of total cellular RNA isolated from these cell lines upon activation with PMA and ionomycin revealed profound decrease in the levels of mRNA coding for IL-2, IL-3, IL-4, IL-5, and interferon-γ with otherwise normal message size for each of these lymphokines (6). The time course for lymphokine mRNA accumulation in patient and in control lymphocytes was identical. The specificity of these abnormalities was suggested by normal mRNA levels found for two other genes transcribed by T cells, the cytokine GM-CSF and the T cell receptor-associated protein CD3γ.

The decreased lymphokine mRNA levels could result from a decreased rate of initiation of lymphokine gene transcription upon lymphocyte activation. Alternatively, it could result from enhanced degradation of lymphokine mRNA which is otherwise transcribed at a normal rate. To differentiate between these two possibilities, we used a nuclear run-off transcription assay. The results obtained showed that the rate of initiation of IL-2, IL-4 and IL-5 transcription upon cell activation was markedly decreased in the patient's T cells as compared to control lymphocytes (6). Thus the defect in the patient's lymphocytes involved a failure of initiation of lymphokine gene transcription. The defect in the patient's lymphocytes likely involves an abnormality affecting a regulatory factor that participates in the initiation of transcription of these lymphokines upon T cell activation.

Several DNA regulatory elements govern the transcription of IL-2. These include NFK-B, AP-1, Oct-1 and NFAT-1. In an attempt to further define the defect in this patient, we performed gel retardation assays using nuclear extracts from patient and control and labeled oligonucleotides corresponding to the consensus sequence of NFK-B,, AP-1, Oct-1 and NFAT-1. The migration of the NFAT-1 complex was faster in the patient than in controls. In contrast, migration patterns of the NFK-B, AP-1 and Oct-1 complexes were normal. The results suggest that the patient's defect involved a defective NFAT-1 binding complexes.

The causal relationship between defective IL-2 production by the patient's lymphocytes and her immunodeficiency state was highlighted by the complete correction of the poor *in vitro* proliferative responses of her lymphocytes to mitogens and the improvement in her clinical status upon initiation of IL-2 replacement therapy (3). Interestingly, despite the defective expression of multiple lymphokines, replacement therapy with IL-2 alone was sufficient to restore her immune function. IL-2 could upregulate the production of some lymphokines that are defectively expressed by the patient's lymphocytes, e. g., interferon-γ. Indeed IL-2 supplementation caused a modest increase in interferon-γ production by the patient's lymphocytes (data not shown). The function of other lymphokines such as IL-3 is to a large extent redundant with that of cytokines such as colony stimulating factors (e. g., GM-CSF), the production of which was apparently unaffected. This would account for the normal hematopoiesis observed in this patient.

References

1. Dinarello, C.A., and Mier, J.W. 1987. Lymphokines. N. Engl. J. Med. 317:940.
2. Kronke, M., Leonard, W.J., Depper, J.M., and Greene, W.C. 1985. Sequential expression of genes involved in human T lymphocyte growth and differentiation. J. Exp. Med. 161:1593.
3. Pahwa, R., Chatila, T., Pahwa, S., Paradise, C., Day, N.K., Geha, R.S, Schwartz, S.A., Slade, H., Oyaizu, N., and Good, R.A. 1989. Recombinant interleukin 2 therapy in severe combined immunodeficiency. Proc. Natl. Acad. Sci. USA 86:5069.
4. Chatila, T., Wong, R., Young, M., Miller R., Terhorst, C., and Geha, R.S. 1989. An immunodeficiency characterized by defective signal transduction in T lymphocytes. N. Engl. J. Med. 320:696.
5. Weiss, A., Imboden, J., Hardy, K., Manger, B., Terhorst, C., and Stobo, J. 1986. The role of the antigen receptor/T3 complex in T-cell activation. Annu. Rev. Immunol. 4:539.
6. Chatila, T.A., Castigli, E., Pahwa, R., Good, R., and Geha, R.S. 1990. Primary combined immunodeficiency resulting from defective transcription of multiple lymphokine genes. PNAS 87:10033.

Leukocyte Adhesion Molecules and Immunodeficiency

Kunihiko Kobayashi*, Shinya Matsuura**, Masato Tsukahara**, Kyoko Fujita**

A brief commentary is made here on leukocyte adhesion molecules, including the integrin family, immunoglobulin superfamily and selectin family. An immunodficiency disease called "Leukocyte adhesion deficiency" that is defective in expression of leukocyte adhesion molecules from the integrin family, LFA-1, Mac-1 and p150,95, is described with special reference to its clinical features and molecular defects. Some abnormal expression of a Fc-gamma receptor in neutrophils and new data concerning the molecular defects found in Japanese patients are also included.

All leukocytes, including granulocytes, monocytes/macrophages and lymphocytes, have the common feature of adhering to cell or tissue surfaces. This cell adherence is an essential step for the expression of a wide spectrum of cell-functions, such as migration, cell to cell interaction and cellular recognition. Investigations of molecular mechanisms in leukocyte adherence have disclosed several families of adhesion molecules: integrin family, immunoglobulin (Ig) superfamily and LEC-CAM (lectin-type cell adhesion molecule) family (1). Members of the integrin family consist of non-covalently associated alpha and beta subunits with one alpha and one beta stoichiometry. This family includes a number of cell-adhesion molecules, such as the leukocyte adhesion proteins of LFA-1, Mac-1 and p150,95, the platelet adhesion molecules of gpIIb/IIIa and gpIb/IIa, and the lymphocyte-surface antigens called VLA family proteins. Members of the Ig superfamily characteristically have the immunoglobulin domain structure in their molecules. They also include many membrane proteins. Among them, ICAM-1 and ICAM-2 are representative of the leukocyte adhesion molecules and are known as the counter receptors of a leukocyte integrin of LFA-1. Members of the LEC-CAM family, now alternatively called "selectins", characteristically contain a lectin-like domain in their amino terminus and bind with carbohydrate moieties. They are also expressed on a variety of cell surfaces, including leukocytes, platelets and endothelial cells. Deficiency of surface expression or dysfunction of these leukocyte adhesion molecules will lead to impairment of adhesion-related functions in leukocytes, and result in immunodeficient states. In fact, there is an immunodeficiency disease called "leukocyte adhesion deficiency", or LAD in short, which is characterized by the deficient expression of leukocyte integrins of LFA-1, Mac-1 and p150,95 on the cell surface of leukocytes (2). The disease is known to be inherited in an autosomal recessive fashion. There are more than 30 families with this disease in the world. In Japan, so far we have located three families with four patients still alive. One family with two patients, a sister and her brother, is in Yamaguchi prefecture (3,4), one in Miyagi prefecture (5) and one in Kumamoto prefecture (6).

Some Characteristics of Leukocyte Integrins of LFA-1, Mac-1 and p150,95

Figure 1 summarizes the molecular characteristics, cellular distributions, functions and ligands of LFA-1, Mac-1 and p150,95 (1). These three molecules share an identical beta subunit, now called CD18, and are distinguished by distinct alpha subunits designated as CD11a for LFA-1, CD11b for Mac-1 and CD11c for p150,95. The LFA-1 is expressed on all leukocytes, while the other two are expressed mainly on granulocyte lineages. The LFA-1 is mostly involved in the function of lymphocyte lineages, such as T cell

---

* Department of Laboratory Medicine, Hokkaido University School of Medicine, Sapporo 060 Japan;
** Department of Pediatrics Yamaguchi University School of Medicine, Ube 755 Japan.
Acknowledgments: This work was supported in part by a grant of the Ministry of Health and Welfare of Japan. Thanks are extended to Drs. Kishimoto and T.A. Springer for providing us with the CD18-probe.

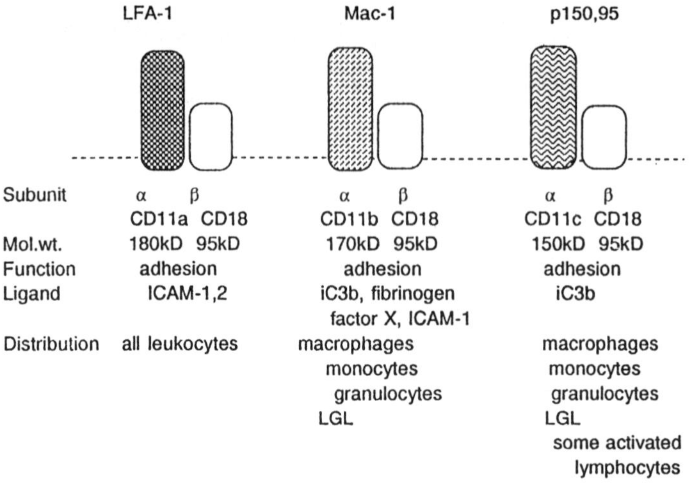

Figure. 1. Schematic representation of three leukocyte integrins of LFA-1, Mac-1 and p150,95, and their ligands, celluar distribution and functions.

cytotoxicity and natural killing. The Mac-1 and p150,95 bind with iC3b and promote the complement-dependent cellular functions.

Clinical Features of LAD

Recurrent non pustular bacterial skin infections are the most prominent feature of LAD, always progressing to ulcerative craters, or pyoderma gangrenosa, which are resistant to appropriate antibiotic therapies and heal very slowly with dysplastic eschars. Staphylococcal or gram-negative bacterial organisms are cultured from such lesions for up to several weeks, due to lack of neutrophil migration in the lesions. Separation of the umbilical cord delays many cases. Persistent gingivitis appears in all cases with eruption of primary dentition. Marked increase of peripheral leukocyte count with matured granulocytosis is a consistent laboratory finding (2). Most of these clinical features were seen in our Japanese LAD patients (3–6). It is interesting to note that the clinical symptoms seen in the LAD patients best fit the symptoms found in dysfunction of phagocytes but not those of lymphocytes, despite the fact that lymphocytes in LAD are defective in adhesion dependent functions, such as cytotoxicity, natural killing, T-T and T-B interactions.

Table 1. Some neutrophil function tests

Source of cells	Locomotion: Agarose plate (mm)	Boyden's chamber(mm): Random migation	Boyden's chamber(mm): Chemotaxis	Adhesion(%): Nylon fiber	Adhesion(%): Plastic dish (spreading)	Phagocytosis (Yeasts/100 neutrophils)	Nitroblue tetrazorium test(Δ OD)
Age-matched control	1.36	44.5	81.3	ND*	64.5	1004	0.50
Sister	0.17	21.1	37.5	12.5	4.6	302	0.77
Brother	0.12	24.7	42.6	23.5	9.6	195	0.60
Adult control	1.51	45.6	81.0	94.7	94.0	947	ND
Father	1.51	50.3	80.6	20.0	80.4	604	ND
Mother	0.91	49.6	98.1	43.8	76.2	917	ND

* not done

Leukocyte Function Tests

Table 1 summarizes neutrophil function tests determined for the brother and sister case of our LAD patients in Japan. Leukocyte locomotion is highly impaired especially when determined by the agarose plate method, a two dimensional migration test. However, by Boyden's chamber test, a three dimensional migration test, the impairment is no longer so obvious. Leukocyte adhesion on nylon fiber is highly affected. Leukocyte spreading (determined by examining cells adhered on plastic dishes by phase contrast microscopy) was highly impaired (Table 1 and Fig. 2). Scanning electron microscopic examination of patient's neutrophils adhered on a glass surface shows fragility and a decreased number of pseudopods (Fig. 2). Phagocytosis is also poor. However, a nitroblue-tetrazorium dye reduction test and intracellular bacterial killing are not affected at all. The neutrophil functions as determined for their parents show almost normality, with only the one exception of leukocyte adhesion on nylon fiber or leukocyte spreading, and the parents do not show any clinical symptoms of LAD at all.

Some Lymphocytic Functions

Table 2 represents some lymphocytic functions determined for the patients. Lymphocyte blastgenesis by PHA and PWM are normal. The number and proportion of CD4+ and CD8+ lymphocytes are within normal range. ADCC of lymphocytes determined by chicken red blood cell as target show normality in our patients, although other patients are reported to have a low ADCC (2). Natural killer activity is quite low. Other lymphocytic functions such as delayed cutaneous hypersensitivity and antibody synthesis are not affected in the patients.

Figure 2. Phase contrast microscopic (a,b) and scanning electron microscopic (c-f) finding of neutrophils from a control (right) and a patient (left).

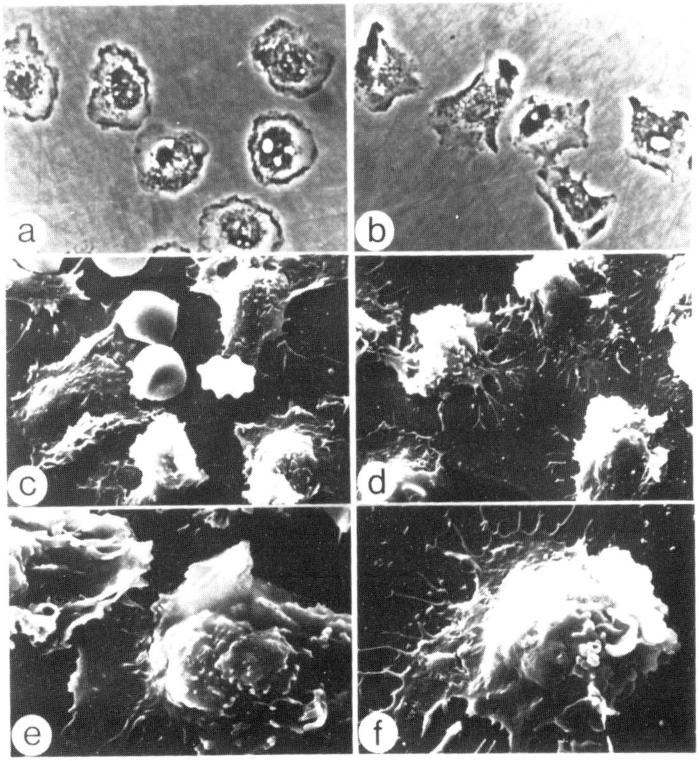

Table 2. Some lymphocytic function tests

	Blast formation (cpm) PHA	Con A	CD4+ (%)	CD8+ (%)	ADCC* (%)	NK** (%)
Sister	39946	25081	41	24	39	0.5
Brother	36696	33798	36	22	40	0.3
Control	37700–62400	24300–58200	38 ± 6.9	28.8 ± 6.5	41–72	35–45

* CRBC as target cells
** K562 as target cells

An Abnormal Expression of Fc-Gamma Receptor Type I(FcγRI) on Patient's Neutrophils

In the investigation of Fc-gamma receptor expression on patient's neutrophils and monocytes, we found that type I Fc-gamma receptor (FcγRI), which is normally expressed only on monocytes but not on neutrophils, was detected on patient's neutrophils by a flow cytometry with a mAb 32.3 specific for the FcγRI (not shown). This was an unexpected phenomenon. Thus we examined the phagocytosis of murine IgG2a-coated RBC by patient's neutrophils, since the murine IgG2a is known to be a ligand of the FcγRI. As shown in Table 3, the patient's neutrophils showed an enhanced phagocytosis of the IgG2a-coated RBC, whereas control neutrophils did not. This confirms the abnormal expression of FcγRI in the patient's neutrophils (7). Presumably, this is a compensatory reaction of the patient's neutrophils that lack the integrin adhesion molecules.

Examination of Molecular Defects in Japanese LAD

Molecular defects in LAD have been analyzed for a number of patients and several single base substitutions in the beta subunit (CD18) genes were defined as the pathogenetic events leading to the deficiency of three leukocyte integrins (8–10). Concerning the Japanese patients, we examined mRNA production by Northern blot analysis using a full-length cDNA of the CD18 as a probe (11). With poly(A)+RNA from the control, a band at 3.2 kb was hy-

Table 3. Phagocytosis of IgG2a-SRBC by neutrophils from an LAD patient

	TNP-SRBC	IgG2a-SRBC	IgG2b-SRBC
Controls	0.4 ± 0.5*	2.3 ± 2.2	0.6 ± 0.3
Patient	0.3 ± 0.3	11.4 ± 3.9	0.7 ± 0.2

* mean of triplicate determinations and SD

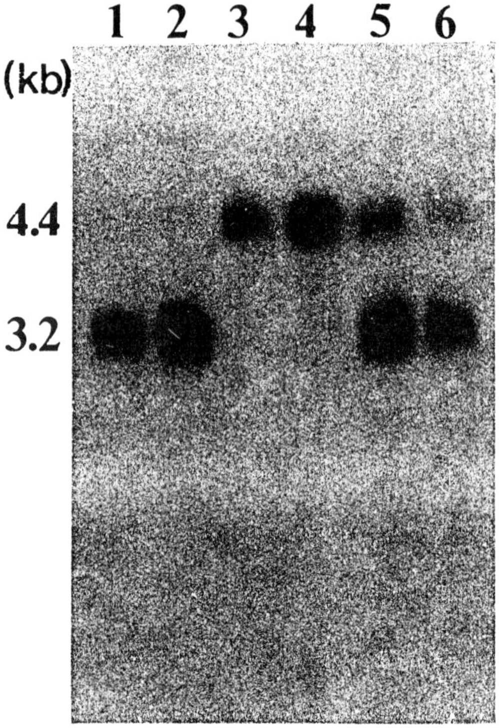

Figure 3. Northern blot analysis of poly(A)+mRNA from LAD patients and their family members using full-length cDNA of CD18 as a probe. 1, Kumamoto case; 2, Miyagi case; 3, Yamaguchi case (sister); 4, Yamaguchi case (brother); 5, Yamaguchi (father); 6, Yamaguchi (mother).

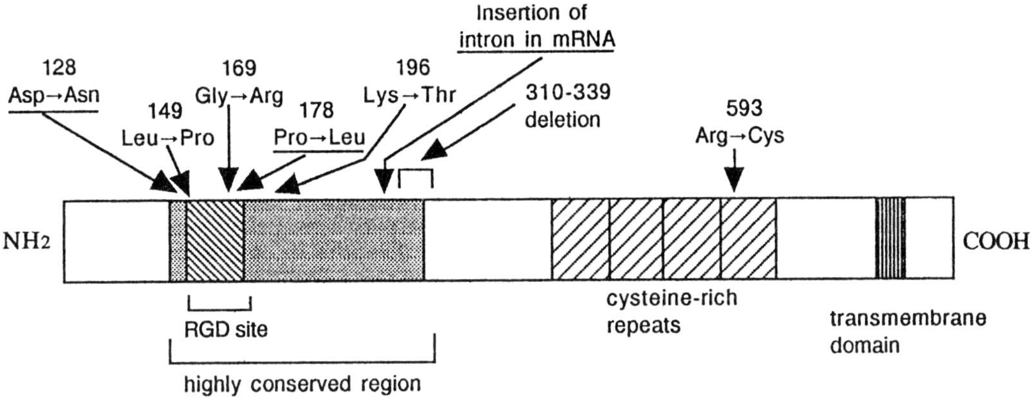

Figure 4. A schematic representation of amino acid mutations in CD18. Numbers on amino acids represent position of mutated amino acid. Amino acid mutations are from left to right. Mutations underlined are those identified in Japanese patients. A position where an intron was inserted in mRNA (Yamaguchi cases) is included in the figure.

bridized with the probe, consistent with the results described (12). The same 3.2 kb band was detected for the mRNA of patients from Kumamoto and Miyagi prefectures, while in the siblings from Yamaguchi prefecture a band of 4.4 kb instead of the normal 3.2 kb was detected. Parents of the Yamaguchi cases, both heterozygous carriers, showed two bands at 3.2 and 4.4 kb(Fig. 3). The aberrantly large mRNA found in our siblings was investigated by reverse transcription/polymerase chain reaction (RT/PCR) using a number of primers covering the whole CD18 cDNA. It was found that the aberrant mRNA represents abortive mRNA splicing of an entire intron of 1.2 kb. DNA sequence analysis of the putative exon-intron junction disclosed that the abortive mRNA splicing was due to a single base substitution of G for A at the consensus splice donor site of the intron. This insertion of intron introduces several termination codons in the aberrant mRNA, leading to a lack of translation of a complete CD18 polypeptide in our cases. The other two Japanese patients with normal sized CD18-mRNA were also analyzed by the RT/PCR, revealing that, in the Kumamoto patient, G at 454 was substituted for A, resulting in a substitution of aspartic acid at 128 into asparagine. In the Miyagi patient, C at 605 was substituted for T, leading to a change of proline at 178 into leucine. Fig. 4 summarizes our results together with those reported previously (8–10).

References

1. Springer, T.A. 1990. Adhesion receptors of the immune system. Nature 346:425.
2. Anderson, D.C. 1987. Leukocyte adhesion deficiency: An inherited defect in the Mac-1, LFA-1 and p150,95 glycoproteins. Ann. Rev. Med. 38:175.
3. Kobayashi, K., Fujita, K., Okino, F., and Kajii, T. 1984. An abnormality of neutrophil adhesion: Autosomal recessive inheritance associated with missing neutrophil glycoproteins. Pediatrics 73:606.
4. Fujita, K., Kobayashi, K., Uchida, M., and Kajii, T. 1986. Neutrophil adhesion abnormality with deficient surface membrane proteins (gp 110 and p98): The effect of their antibodies in the function of normal neutrophils. Pediatr. Res. 20:361.
5. Konno, T., Tsukamoto, J., Terasawa, M., Tsuchiya, S., and Tachibana, T. 1986. OKM-1(Mo1)/LFA-1 deficiency in a Japanese infant with recurrent infection. In: Primary immunodeficiency diseases. M.M. Eibl and F.S. Rosen, eds. Elsevier Science Publ. B.V., p. 315.
6. Nunoi, H., Yanase, Y., Higuchi, S., Tsuchiya, H., Yamamoto, J., Matsuda, I., Naito, M., Takahashi, K., Fujita, K., Uchida, M., Kobayashi, K., Jono, M., and Malech, H. 1988. Severe hypoplasia of lymphoid tissues in Mo1 deficiency. Human Pathol. 19:753.
7. Majima, T., Minegishi, N., Nagatomi, R., Ohashi, Y., Tsuchiya, S., Kobayashi, K., and

Konno, T. 1990. Unusual expression of IgG Fc receptors on peripheral granulocytes from patients with leukocyte adhesion deficiency (CD11/CD18 deficiency). J. Immunol. 145:1694.
8. Kishimoto, T.K., O'Conner, K., and Springer T.A. 1989. Leukocyte adhesion deficiency. Aberrant splicing of a conserved integrin sequence caused a moderate deficiency. J. Biol. Chem. 264:3588.
9. Arnaout, M.A, Danna, N., Gupta, S.K., Tonen, D.G., and Fathallah, D.M. 1990. Point mutation impairing cell surface expression of the common β subunit (CD18) in a patient with leukocyte adhesion molecule (Leu-CAM) deficiency. J. Clin. Invest. 85:972.
10. Wardlaw, J.A., Hibbs, M.L., Stacker, S.A., and Springer, T.A. 1990. Distinct mutation in two patients with leukocyte adhesion deficiency and their functional correlates. J. Exp. Med. 172:335.
11. Kishimoto, T.K., O'Conner, K., Lee, A., Roberts, T.M., and Springer, T.A. 1987. Cloning of the β subunit of the leukocyte adhesion proteins. Homology to an extracellular matrix receptor defines a novel supergene family. Cell 48:181.
12. Kishimoto, T.K., Hollander, N., Roberts, T.M., Anderson, D.C., and Springer, T.A. 1987. Heterogeneous mutations in the β subunit common to the LFA-1, Mac-1, and p150,95 glycoproteins cause leukocyte adhesion deficiency. Cell 50:193.

Section XIII

Inflammatory Cells and Cytokines in Allergy

T Lymphocytes in Allergic Disease

Christopher J. Corrigan, A. Barry Kay*

Activated T lymphocytes and eosinophils are features of the immunopathology of asthma and atopic allergic inflammation. Cells infiltrating these reactions have a Th2-type cytokine profile (i.e., express mRNA for the IL-3, IL-4, IL-5 and GM-CSF gene cluster). This preferential production of cytokines might explain, in part, local eosinophil accumulation, mast cell proliferation and enhanced IgE synthesis.

CD4 T ("helper") lymphocytes, after activation by antigen, have the capacity to elaborate a wide variety of protein mediators (cytokines or lymphokines). Cytokines have the capacity to regulate the differentiation, recruitment, accumulation and activation of specific granulocyte effector cells at mucosal surfaces. A full description of the properties of individual lymphokines is beyond the scope of this article, but the general properties of these mediators which are responsible for their pro-inflammatory actions may be summarised as follows: (A) They can increase the production of specific granulocytes from precursor cells both in the bone marrow and at sites of inflammation. (B) They can prolong the survival of specific granulocytes, thereby bringing about their accumulation in tissues. (C) Some lymphokines are directly chemotactic for specific granulocytes and can cause preferential adherence of specific granulocytes to vascular endothelium. (D) They can prime specific granulocytes for an enhanced response to physiological activating stimuli. And: (E) They influence the activation of B lymphocytes and the classes of antibodies which they produce in immune responses.

For example, CD4 T lymphocytes are a major source of IL-5. This has been shown to: (a) promote the differentiation of mature eosinophils from precursor cells (1,2); (b) prolong the survival of eosinophils *in vitro* from days to weeks, especially in the presence of fibroblasts or endothelial cells (3,4); (c) exhibit chemotactic activity for eosinophils but not neutrophils *in vivo*, although this effect was weak and requires further confirmation (5); (d) enhance the adhesion of eosinophils, but not neutrophils, to vascular endothelial cells; and (e) prime eosinophils for increased activity in a number of subsequent effector responses, including antibody-mediated killing of parasitic larvae, elaboration of lipid mediators and activation by platelet activating factor (4,6,7).

Similar effects on eosinophils were exhibited by interleukin (IL)-3 (8) and granulocyte/macrophage-colony stimulating factor (GM-CSF) (9,10). Interferon-gamma was shown to enhance eosinophil cytotoxicity (11). The fact that T lymphocyte clones from patients with the hypereosinophilic syndrome demonstrated IL-5-like activity (12) directly supports the hypothesis that eosinophil numbers and function may be regulated by T lymphocytes *in vivo*. Similarly, expansion and differentiation of mast cells in tissues was shown to be dependent on IL-3 and IL-4 (13). A deficiency of mucosal mast cells was demonstrated in the gastrointestinal tract of humans with defective T lymphocyte function (14). In nude mice, IL-3 restored the intestinal mucosal mast cell response to Strongyloides infection and facilitated worm expulsion (15).

These experiments emphasize the facts that activated CD4 T lymphocytes have the propensity to bring about selective accumulation and activation of specific granulocytes in tissues and that T lymphocyte-mediated granulocyte accumulation and activation need not be dependent on the presence of IgE, thus providing a unifying hypothesis for the pathogenesis of asthma in both atopic and non-atopic patients. CD4 T lymphocytes are therefore inflammatory cells in their own right and can no longer be regarded simply as "helper" cells for the production of antibody. T lymphocytes are not the

---

* Department of Allergy and Clinical Immunology, National Heart & Lung Institute, Dovehouse Street, London, SW3 6LY, UK.
Acknowledgements: Grant support from the Medical Research Council, UK.

only source of lymphokines. For example, GM-CSF was shown to be elaborated by macrophages, endothelial cells (16) and eosinophils (17).

Th1 and Th2 CD4 T Lymphocytes

The genes encoding IL-3, IL-4, IL-5 and GM-CSF are located relatively close together in the human genome, on the long arm of chromosome 5, raising the possibility that their expression may be at least in part coordinately regulated. There is now good evidence that this may be the case, at least in mouse T lymphocytes. Antigen-activated murine CD4 T lymphocyte clones can be divided into two broad types, called Th1 and Th2, according to the pattern of lymphokines they secrete (18). Th1 cells secrete IL-2, interferon-gamma, and TNF-beta, but not IL4, IL-5 and IL-6. Th2 cells secrete IL-4, IL-5 and IL-6 but not IL-2, interferon-gamma and TNF-beta. Other lymphokines, including IL-3 and GM-CSF are secreted by both cell types. The mechanisms which determine expression of Th1 or Th2 phenotypes are not completely understood. Interferon-gamma, when added to antigen-stimulated cultures of mouse CD4 T lymphocytes favored the expression of the Th1 phenotype (19), while another lymphokine secreted by Th2 cells, called "cytokine synthesis inhibitory factor" or IL-10, inhibited Th1 clone proliferation through an effect on antigen-presenting cells (20,21). Thus, products of Th1 clones have the capacity to inhibit the growth of Th2 clones, and vice versa.

The functional capacities of Th1 and Th2 CD4 T lymphocyte clones differ in a manner which reflects their respective patterns of lymphokine synthesis. Th2 clones, through their secretion of IL-4 and IL-5, serve as excellent helper cells for Ig synthesis by B lymphocytes *in vitro* (22), since both these lymphokines nonspecifically enhance B lymphocyte activation. In addition, by their secretion of IL-3, IL-4 and IL-5, Th2 clones favor the synthesis of IgE and the activation of mast cells and eosinophils, and are therefore strongly implicated in the pathogenesis of allergic and asthmatic inflammation.

In contrast to murine cells, human CD4 T lymphocyte clones stimulated at random using lectins do not fall cleanly into Th1 and Th2 patterns, and there are many examples of clones which secrete a mixture of lymphokines characteristic of both categories (23,24). Nevertheless, T lymphocytes with Th1 and Th2 type patterns of lymphokine secretion do appear to exist *in vivo*. These data can be reconciled with those from mice if it is assumed that precursors of Th1 and Th2 cells (Th0 cells) exist which secrete a mixture of Th1 and Th2 type lymphokines, and that these Th0 cells develop into Th1 or Th2 cells under the influence of extraneous factors such as their antigen specificity, the site of antigen presentation and the nature of the antigen presenting cells.

This discovery of a functional dichotomy of activated CD4 T lymphocytes, which have the propensity either to mediate delayed-type hypersensitivity reactions and suppress IgE synthesis (Th1) or to mediate allergic and asthmatic inflammation and promote IgE synthesis (Th2), is likely to have a profound impact on our understanding of allergic inflammation and inappropriate IgE synthesis.

Experimental Observations Implicating Activated CD4 T Lymphocytes in the Pathogenesis of Asthma and Allergic Inflammation

In two recent studies of bronchial biopsies obtained from mild atopic asthmatics (25,26), the numbers and activation status of mucosal T lymphocytes were assessed by immunostaining with monoclonal antibodies directed against T lymphocyte phenotypic and activation markers. Interestingly, the total number of both CD4 and CD8 T lymphocytes in the bronchial mucosa of these mild asthmatics was not significantly elevated as compared to normal controls; CD4 cells predominated over CD8 in both cases. In contrast, only cells in the biopsies from asthmatics showed evidence of IL-2 receptor expression, suggesting activation. Furthermore, in the biopsies from asthmatics, the numbers of activated T lymphocytes could be correlated with both the total numbers of eosinophils and the numbers of activated eosinophils. Finally, the degree of activation could be correlated with disease severity, as assessed by measurement of bronchial hyperresponsiveness. These observations provide circumstantial evidence supporting the hypothesis that activated CD4 T lymphocytes control the numbers and activation status of eosinophils in asthmatic bronchial inflammation, and that the degree of activation is one factor which determines disease severity. Using immunostaining and flow cytometry, it was shown that a proportion of CD4 T lymphocytes, but not CD8 cells, in the peripheral blood of patients with acute severe asthma are activated, as assessed by expression of IL-2 receptor, HLA-DR and VLA-1 (27). The degree of activation of these cells decreased after therapy to an extent that could be correlated with the degree of clinical improvement (28).

Some studies demonstrated an increase in the relative numbers of lymphocytes found in bronchoalveolar lavage (BAL) fluid obtained from patients with mild, stable asthma (29), whereas others showed similar numbers in asthmatics and normal controls (30). Studies on the activation status and the production of lymphokines by these cells are eagerly awaited. In a further study employing allergen bronchial challenge of sensitized atopic asthmatics (31), a selective increase in CD4 cells in BAL fluid was observed 48 hours after allergen challenge in those subjects who had previously been shown to develop a late phase reaction. These findings complement those of a decrease in CD4 T lymphocyte numbers in the peripheral blood following allergen inhalation by atopic asthmatics (32), and together suggest that a process of selective recruitment of CD4 T lymphocytes to the lung may occur in association with the late phase asthmatic reaction to allergen bronchial challenge. The possible relevance (or otherwise) of this model to the pathogenesis of "real" asthma is open to question. Similarly, in a study employing cutaneous allergen challenge of atopic subjects (33), activated CD4 T lymphocytes were selectively recruited during the course of the late phase reaction.

Despite the fact that sensitive ELISA and radioimmunoassays for many lymphokines are now available, measurement of lymphokine secretion *in vivo* is very difficult owing to their low concentrations and rapid metabolism. Furthermore, the concentrations of lymphokines in the peripheral blood and BAL fluid of asthmatics may only dimly reflect those concentrations released locally in the inflamed mucosa. In a study referred to above (28), serum concentrations of interferon-gamma were shown to be elevated in a group of acute severe asthmatics as compared to mild asthmatics and normal controls. Interferon-gamma secretion is characteristic of a "Th1 type" response, but since "Th2 type" lymphokines were not measured in this study it is impossible to assess the relative contributions of each type of response. Furthermore, Th1-type CD4 T lymphocyte activation might be a superimposed phenomenon in acute severe asthma owing, for example, to intercurrent infection.

One useful alternative to the direct measurement of lymphokine concentrations is the detection of the synthesis of their mRNA using the technique of *in situ* hybridization with lymphokine-specific cDNA probes or riboprobes. Although this is not a strictly quantitative technique, it does have the advantage that it can localize the secretion of lymphokines within cells and tissues. Using this technique it was recently demonstrated that IL-5 mRNA was elaborated by cells in the bronchial mucosa of a majority of mild asthmatics but not normal controls (34). The amount of mRNA detected correlated broadly with the numbers of activated CD4 T lymphocytes and eosinophils in biopsies from the same subjects, providing direct evidence supporting the hypothesis that activated CD4 T lymphocytes secrete IL-5 within the asthmatic bronchial mucosa which regulated the numbers and activation status of eosinophils. In a further study using *in situ* hybridization, the cutaneous inflammatory responses to challenge with allergen in atopic subjects and tuberculin in non-atopic subjects were compared (35). Both types of response (late phase allergic and DTH) were associated with an influx of activated CD4 T lymphocytes, but whereas mRNA molecules encoding IL-2 and interferon-gamma were abundant within the tuberculin reactions, very little mRNA encoding these lymphokines was observed in the late phase allergic reactions. Conversely, mRNA encoding IL-4 and IL-5 was abundant in the late phase allergic but not the tuberculin reactions. In effect, the profiles of lymphokine secretion in the allergic and tuberculin reactions closely paralleled those of Th2 and Th1 CD4 T lymphocytes, respectively. Furthermore, the relative numbers and types of granulocytes infiltrating these reactions reflected the different patterns of lymphokine release (36). The detection of mRNA does not necessarily equate with protein synthesis and it will need to be shown that translation and secretion of these lymphokines also occurs. Furthermore, as discussed above, T lymphocytes are not only the potential sources of these lymphokines. Finally, it must be borne in mind that the antigen specificity of the recruited T lymphocytes is unknown, and since the tuberculin response was elicited in non-atopic subjects, it is not certain whether the Th1 type response observed in the DTH reaction was antigen-specific or atopy-specific. Nevertheless, these observations provide direct evidence in support of the hypothesis that activated T lymphocytes, through their patterns of lymphokine secretion, regulate the types of granulocyte which participate in inflammatory reactions. Furthermore, they demonstrate that Th1 and Th2 CD4 T lymphocyte responses can be detected in humans under physiological conditions, and that the antigen specificity of the T lymphocytes might be one factor which determines which type of response is initiated.

References

1. Sanderson, C.J., Warren, D.J., and Strath, M. 1985. Identification of a lymphokine that stimulates eosinophil differentiation *in vitro*. J. Exp. Med. 162:60.
2. Campbell, H.D., Tucker, W.Q.J., Hort, Y., Martinson, M.E., Mayo, G., Clutterbuck, E.J., Sanderson, C.J., and Young, I.G. 1987. Molecular cloning, nucleotide sequence and expression of the gene encoding human eosinophil differentiation factor (interleukin 5). Proc. Natl. Acad. Sci. USA 84:6629.
3. Rothenberg, M.E., Owen, W.F., Silberstein, D.S., Soberman, R.J., Austen, K.F., and Stevens, R.L. 1987. Eosinophils cocultured with endothelial cells have increased survival and functional properties. Science 237:645.
4. Rothenberg, M.E., Petersen, J., Stevens, R.L., Silberstein, D.S., McKenzie, D.T., Austen, K.F., and Owen, W.F. 1989. IL-5 dependent conversion of normodense human eosinophils to the hypodense phenotype uses 3T3 fibroblasts for enhanced viability, accelerated hypodensity and sustained antibody-dependent cytotoxicity. J. Immunol. 143:2311.
5. Wang, J.M., Rambaldi, A., Biondi, A., Chen, Z.G., Sanderson, C.J., and Mantovani, A. 1989. Recombinant human interleukin-5 is a selective eosinophil chemoattractant. Eur. J. Immunol. 19:701.
6. Lopez, A.F., Sanderson, C.J., Gamble, J.R., Campbell, H.D., Young, I.G., and Vadas, M.A. 1988. Recombinant human interleukin-5 is a selective activator of eosinophil function. J. Exp. Med. 167:219.
7. Numao, T., Fukuda, T., Akutsu, I., Makino, S., Enokihara, H., and Honjo, T. 1989. Selective enhancement of eosinophil chemotaxis by recombinant human interleukin-5. J. Allergy Clin. Immunol. 83:298.
8. Rothenberg, M.E., Owen, W.F., Silberstein, D.S., Woods, J., Soberman, R.J., Austen, K.F., and Stevens, R.L. 1988. Human eosinophils have prolonged survival, enhanced functional properties and become hypodense when exposed to human interleukin-3. J. Clin. Invest. 81:1986.
9. Silberstein, D.S., Owen, W.F., Gasson, J.C., Di Persio, J.F., Golde, D.W., Bina, J.C., Soberman, R., Austen, K.F. and David, R. 1986. Enhancement of human eosinophil cytotoxicity and leukotriene synthesis by biosynthetic (recombinant) granulocyte-macrophage colony stimulating factor. J. Immunol. 137:3290.
10. Lopez, A.F., Williamson, D.J., Gamble, J.R., Begley, C.G., Harian, J.M., Klebanoff, S.J., Waltersdorph, A., Wong, G., Clark, S.C., and Vadas, M.A. 1986. Recombinant human granulocyte-macrophage colony stimulating factor stimulates *in vitro* mature human eosinophil and neutrophil function, surface receptor expression and survival. J. Clin. Invest. 78:1220.
11. Valerius, T., Repp, R., Kalden, J.R., and Platzer, E. 1990. Effects of interferon on human eosinophils in comparison with other cytokines. J. Immunol. 145:2950.
12. Raghavachar, A., Fleischer, S., Frickhofen, N., Heimpel, H., and Fleischer, B. 1987. T-lymphocyte control of human eosinophilic granulopoiesis. J. Immunol. 139:3753.
13. Stevens, R.L., and Austen, K.F. 1989. Recent advances in the cellular and molecular biology of mast cells. Immunol. Today 10:381.
14. Irani, A.A., Craig, S.S., De Blois, G., Elson, C.O., Schechter, N.M., and Schwartz, L.B. 1987. Deficiency of tryptase-positive, chymase-negative mast cell type in gastrointestinal mucosa of patients with defective T-lymphocyte funcion. J. Immunol. 138:4381.
15. Abe, T., and Nawa, Y. 1988. Worm expulsion and mucosal mast cell response induced by repetitive IL-3 administration in Strongyloides ratti infected nude mice. Immunology 63:181.

16. Sieff, C.A. 1987. Hematopoietic growth factors. J. Clin. Invest. 79:1549.
17. Moqbel, R., Hamid, Q., Sun Ying, Barkans, J., Hartnell, A., Tsicopoulos, A., Wardlaw, A.J., and Kay, A.B. 1991. Expression of mRNA and immunoreactivity for the granulocyte/macrophage-colony stimulating factor in activated human eosinophils. J. Exp. Med. 174:749.
18. Mosmann, T.R., and Coffman, R.L. 1989. Th1 and Th2 cells: Different patterns of lymphokine secretion lead to different functional properties. Annu. Rev. Immunol. 7:145.
19. Gajewski, T.F., Joyce, J., and Fitch, F.W. 1989. Anti-proliferative effect of interferon-gamma in immune regulation. III. Differential selection of Th1 and Th2 murine helper T-lymphocyte clones using recombinant IL-2 and recombinant interferon-gamma. J. Immunol. 143:15.
20. Fiorentino, D., Bond, H.W., and Mosmann, T.R. 1989. Two types of mouse T helper cells. IV. Th2 clones secrete a factor that inhibits cytokine production by Th1 clones. J. Exp. Med. 170:65.
21. Fiorentino, D.F., Zlotnik, A., Vieira, P., Mosmann, T.R., Howard, M., Moore, K.W., and O'Garra, A. 1991. IL-10 acts on the antigen-presenting cell to inhibit cytokine production by Th1 cells. J. Immunol. 146:3444.
22. Stevens, T.L., Bossie, A., Sanders, V.M., Fernandez-Botran, R., Coffman, R.L., Mosmann, T.R., and Vitetta, E.S. 1988. Regulation of antibody isotype secretion by subsets of antigen-specific helper T cells. Nature 334:255.
23. Quint, D.J., Bolton, E.J., MacNamee, L.A., Solan, R., Hissey, P.H., Champion, B.R., Mackenzie, A.R., and Zanders, E.D. 1989. Functional and phenotypical analysis of human T cell clones which stimulate IgE production *in vitro*. Immunology 67:68.
24. Paliard, X., de Waal Malefijt, R., Yssel, H., Blanchard, D., Chretien, I., Abrams, J., de Vries, J., and Spits, H. 1988. Simultaneous production of IL-2, IL-4 and interferon-gamma by activated human CD4+ and CD8+ T cell clones. J Immunol. 141:849.
25. Azzawi, M., Bradley, B., Jeffery P.K., Frew, A., Wardlaw, A.J., Knowles, G., Assoufi, B., Collins, J.V., Durham, S., and Kay, A.B. 1990. Identification of activated T lymphocytes and eosinophils in bronchial biopsies in stable atopic asthma. Am. Rev. Respir. Dis. 142:1407.
26. Bradley, B.L., Azzawi, M., Jacobson, J., Assoufi, B., Collins, J.V., Irani, AM.A., Schwartz, L.B., Durham, S.R., Jeffery, P.K., and Kay, A.B. 1991. Eosinophils, T-lymphocytes, mast cells, neutrophils and macrophages in bronchial biopsies from atopic asthmatics: Comparison with atopic non-asthma and normal controls and relationship to bronchial hyperresponsiveness. J. Allergy Clin. Immunol. 88:661.
27. Corrigan, C.J., Hartnell, A., and Kay, A.B. 1988. T-lymphocyte activation in acute severe asthma. Lancet i:1129.
28. Corrigan, C.J., and Kay, A.B. 1990. CD4 T-lymphocyte activation in acute severe asthma. Relationship to disease severity and atopic status. Am. Rev. Respir. Dis. 141:970.
29. Graham, D.R., Luksza, A.R., and Evans, C.C. 1985. Bronchoalveolar lavage in asthma. Thorax 40:717.
30. Wardlaw, A.J., Dunnette, S., Gleich, G.J, Collins, J.V., and Kay, A.B. 1988. Eosinophils and mast cells in bronchoalveolar lavage in mild asthma. Relationship to bronchial hyperreactivity. Am. Rev. Respir. Dis. 137:62.
31. Metzger, W.J., Zavala, D., Richerson, H.B., Moseley, P., Iwamota, P., Monick, M., Sjoerdsma, K., and Hunninghake, G.W. 1987. Local allergen challenge and bronchoalveolar lavage of allergic asthmatic lungs. Description of the model and local airway inflammation. Am. Rev. Respir. Dis. 135:433.
32. Gerblich, A.A., Campbell, A.E., and Schuyler, M.R. 1984. Changes in T-lymphocyte subpopulations after antigenic bronchial provocation in asthmatics. N. Engl. J. Med. 310:1349.
33. Frew, A.J., and Kay, A.B. 1988. The relationship between infiltrating CD4+ T lymphocytes, activated eosinophils and the magnitude of the allergen-induced late phase cutaneous reaction. J. Immunol. 141:4158.
34. Hamid, Q., Azzawi, M., Sun Ying, Moqbel, R., Wardlaw, A.J., Corrigan, C.J., Bradley, B., Durham, S.R., Collins, J.V., Jeffery, P.K., Quint, D.J., and Kay, A.B. 1991. Expression of mRNA for interleukin-5 in mucosal bronchial biopsies from asthma. J. Clin. Invest. 87:1541.
35. Kay, A.B., Sun Ying, Varney, V., Gaga, M., Durham, S.R., Moqbel, R., Wardlaw, A.J, and Hamid, Q. 1991. Messenger RNA expression of the cytokine gene cluster, IL3, IL4, IL5 and GMCSF in allergen-induced late-phase cutaneous reactions in atopic subjects. J. Exp. Med. 173:775.
36. Gaga, M., Frew, A.J., Varney, V.A., and Kay, A.B. 1991. Eosinophil activation and T lymphocyte infiltration in allergen-induced late phase skin reactions and classical delayed-type hypersensitivity. J. Immunol. 147:816.

Eosinophils, Allergic Diseases and Cytokines

Gerald J. Gleich*, Joseph H. Butterfield*, Kristin M. Leiferman*, Hirohito Kita*, John Abrams**

The eosinophilic leukocyte is now recognized as an important effector cell in numerous diseases, especially bronchial asthma. Here, we report on the relationships between cytokines, allergic diseases and eosinophils. First, because eosinophils are importantly influenced by cytokines, syndromes associated with eosinophilia were investigated to determine whether cytokine levels were elevated in bodily fluids. In two diseases, namely episodic angioedema associated with eosinophilia and in the capillary leak syndrome associated with interleukin (IL)-2 induced eosinophilia, increased serum concentrations of IL-5 were measured in affected patients. Further, in late inflammatory reactions induced in the lung by segmental challenge with antigen, eosinophils increased dramatically in bronchoalveolar lavage fluids obtained 48 hours after antigen challenge, and IL-5 was measurable in these fluids. Second, glucocorticoids are recognized as the most potent therapy for eosinophil associated diseases, and we present information indicating that glucocorticoids are able to inhibit the effects of cytokines on eosinophils. For GM-CSF, IL-3 and IL-5, the suppressive effects of glucocorticoids could be overridden by high levels of the cytokines, whereas in the case of interferon-γ, high levels of this cytokine did not overcome the effect of dexamethasone. Finally, evidence is presented that eosinophils themselves can produce cytokines. Overall, these results suggest that cytokines play important roles in the pathophysiology of eosinophil-associated diseases.

Over the past two decades, considerable new information has been acquired regarding the eosinophilic leukocyte and its constituents (1). In addition, the genes for all of the major eosinophil granule proteins have been cloned and, in some cases, localized to chromosomes (2-5). The eosinophil has been implicated in the pathophysiology of numerous diseases, including cutaneous diseases (6) and bronchial asthma (7,8). With the increasing recognition that the eosinophil is an effector cell for organ damage in several diseases, attention has been shifted from the role of the eosinophil itself to the mechanisms by which eosinophilia occurs. Because the eosinophil is strongly influenced by cytokines, especially interleukin (IL)-5 (9), our laboratory has begun investigations of the occurrence of these cytokines in disease.

Cytokines in Syndromes Associated with Eosinophilia

Episodic Angioedema and Eosinophilia

This syndrome, first recognized in 1984, is associated with episodic edema, urticaria, often striking weight gains, and marked eosinophilia (10). Because the eosinophilia is so striking and because it occurs in episodes, often with remarkable regularity, we measured IL-5 by an immunoenzymetric assay in the serum of four patients with episodic angioedema (11). This study revealed that IL-5 levels were measurable in the serum of all four patients; furthermore, the IL-5 levels were elevated during attacks and dropped spontaneously to undetectable or only slightly elevated levels between attacks. Because of these spontaneous variations in IL-5 levels, it was not possible to determine whether glucocorticoids suppressed these levels. Finally, because of the ability of IL-5 to upregulate eosinophil function (9,11), it seems likely that it is an important determinant of disease activity in the syndrome of episodic angioedema associated with eosinophilia.

IL-2 Induced Eosinophilia

Since the introduction of IL-2 as a therapy for malignant disease, eosinophilia following administration of IL-2 has been recognized (12).

* Departments of Immunology, Internal Medicine and Dermatology, Mayo Clinic and Mayo Foundation, Rochester, MN 55905, USA;
** DNAX Research Institute, Palo Alto, CA, USA.

Because cytokines might be responsible for the eosinophilia following IL-2 therapy, five patients with advanced malignancy, who were being treated with IL-2, were studied by measurement of: eosinophils in their peripheral blood, eosinophil granule major basic protein (MBP) levels in their sera, and IL-5 levels in their sera (12). This study showed that eosinophilia developed after the second course of IL-2 and reached impressive levels by the fourth course of IL-2, the four courses being given over a period of 1 month. Serum levels of MBP became elevated after the first course of IL-2 and remained elevated throughout the duration of the treatment. IL-5 levels were measurable in four of the five sera, and the rises and falls of IL-5 were temporally related to the administration of IL-2. In one patient, IL-5, as measured by the immunoenzymetric assay, was elevated even before IL-2 therapy, and did not show the rises and falls seen in the other patients. Nonetheless, in this patient study of the level of cytokines utilizing the eosinophil survival assay (13) revealed elevations of IL-5 and changes in the levels of IL-5 comparable to the other patients. This study found that IL-2 treatment induces IL-5, leading to marked peripheral blood eosinophilia and extravascular eosinophil degranulation. The release of toxic eosinophil granule products at extravascular sites and in the circulation may contribute to the pathophysiology of the capillary leak syndrome which complicates IL-2 therapy. Interestingly, the symptoms experienced by the patients receiving IL-2 are closely similar to those of patients with the syndrome of episodic angioedema associated with eosinophilia.

Pulmonary Late Inflammatory Reactions Following Antigen Challenge

The mechanisms of eosinophilia occurring in allergen-induced late inflammatory reactions in the lung were investigated by segmental antigen bronchoprovocation and bronchoalveolar lavage (BAL) (14). This study revealed striking elevations of eosinophils, eosinophil granule proteins, and IL-5 in the BAL fluids 48 hours after antigen challenge. When normal subjects were challenged with antigen, neither eosinophils nor soluble mediators of eosinophils increased. Thus, these data suggest that eosinophils are attracted to the airway during the late phase allergic reaction and that IL-5 may activate eosinophils, enhancing release of granule proteins and causing increased survival of eosinophils.

Glucocorticoids and Cytokines

Glucocorticoids are the most useful class of drugs for treating many eosinophil-related disorders, such as bronchial asthma. Glucocorticoids produce eosinopenia in normal persons, decrease circulating eosinophils in patients with eosinophilia, and reduce eosinophil influx at sites of inflammation. The mechanisms of these effects are still uncertain. However, Lamas et al. reported that the increased eosinophil survival mediated by granulocyte-macrophage colony-stimulating factor (GM-CSF) was specifically decreased by glucocorticoids (15). Therefore, we studied the effects of glucocorticoids on cytokine-induced survival of human eosinophils *in vitro*. We found that the potency of glucocorticoids in inhibiting the effects of cytokines paralleled the potency of glucocorticoids in other assays of their anti-inflammatory properties (16). Concentrations of dexamethasone at $1x10^{-6}$M potently inhibited the eosinophil survival mediated by IL-5, GM-CSF, IL-3 and interferon-γ (IFN-γ). The effects of dexamethasone, $1x10^{-6}$M, were reversed by high concentrations of IL-5 and GM-CSF, but even 1,000 U/ml of IFN-γ did not overcome dexamethasone inhibition, indicating a difference between the mechanism of eosinophil survival induced by IFN-γ and other cytokines. These results suggest that glucocorticoids exert direct inhibitory effects on eosinophil survival which may be important in the treatment of allergic and other eosinophilic disorders. Contrariwise, antagonism of the glucocorticoid effect by high concentrations of cytokine may be a mechanism for glucocorticoid resistance.

Eosinophil Production of Cytokines

Because eosinophils might be able themselves to elaborate cytokines, they were stimulated by incubation with the calcium ionophore, ionomycin, and the supernatants from the stimulated eosinophils were assayed for their cytokine content (17). This study revealed that cytokine activity measured by the eosinophil survival assay (13) was detected as early as 3 hours after stimulation with ionomycin and was inhibited by an immunomodulating agent, cyclosporin A. The survival enhancing activity was abolished completely by treatment with anti-IL-3 and anti-GM-CSF monoclonal antibodies. Moreover, IL-3 and GM-CSF were measurable in ionomycin-stimulated eosinophil supernatants by immunoassay, and eosinophils produced approximately half as much IL-3 and one-fifth as much GM-CSF as ionomycin-stimulated mononuclear cells. In a complimentary study, evidence has been obtained for the production of GM-CSF by eosinophils, utilizing analyses of expression of mRNA for GM-CSF and the immunoreactivity of stimulated eosinophils (18). The studies of human peripheral blood eosinophils, activated by the calcium ionophore A23187 or by IFN-γ and analyzed by in situ hybridization, revealed that these activated cells expressed mRNA for GM-CSF. Between 15 and 27% of eosinophils showed positive hybridization signals for GM-CSF mRNA following stimulation with A23187 or IFN-γ, and 4–6% showed hybridization after incubation with IL-3 or GM-CSF. In addition, these stimulated cells exhibited specific immunoreactivity with anti-GM-CSF polyclonal antibody, suggesting that the message was translated into a functional protein. The results of these two studies (17,18) complement each other and indicate that activated eosinophils express message for GM-CSF, produce immunoreactive GM-CSF which can be localized to the cell, and secrete both GM-CSF and IL-3 into the fluids surrounding them.

Conclusions

The results of these studies in three eosinophil-associated diseases (11,12,14), as well as prior observations of elevated IL-5 in the hypereosinophilic syndrome (19) and the eosinophilia-myalgiasyndrome (20), are in keeping with a critical role for IL-5 in these diseases. Similarly, the findings that (a) anti-IL-5 specifically abolishes the increased numbers of eosinophils in the peripheral blood and tissues of mice infected with a helminth (21) and that (b) selective production of IL-5 by peripheral blood cells from helminth-infected patients can be demonstrated (22), support the belief that IL-5 is also critical in helminth-associated eosinophilia. The importance of glucocorticoid inhibition of cytokine-mediated eosinophil viability is uncertain. However, the time-course of glucocorticoid-induced clinical improvement, which occurs over days, is consistent with the effect of glucocorticoids on eosinophil survival (16). Furthermore, the inhibition of eosinophil viability by glucocorticoids provides a useful tool for investigating the effects of cytokines on eosinophils. Finally, the ability of high levels of cytokines, save for IFN-γ, to override glucocorticoid effects suggests a mechanism to account for resistance to glucocorticoid therapy in disease. The finding that eosinophils produce IL-3 and GM-CSF indicates that in addition to the release of basic proteins and lipid mediators (1), GM-CSF and IL-3 production must be taken into consideration in diseases associated with eosinophilia and tissue damage. Furthermore, eosinophils are able to produce other cytokines such as tumor necrosis factor-α (23) and IL-1(24). The IL-3, IL-4, IL-5 and GM-CSF gene cluster is expressed in allergen-induced late phase reactions in atopic subjects (25), and, although the T lymphocyte is considered to be the major source of these cytokines, the results showing IL-3 and GM-CSF release from eosinophils suggest that they may be the source of these cytokines in disease.

References

1. Slifman, N.R., Adolphson, C.R., and Gleich, G.J. 1988. Eosinophils: Biochemical and cellular aspects. In: Allergy: Principles and practice. E. Middleton, Jr., C.E. Reed, E.F. Ellis, N.F. Adkinson, Jr., and J.W. Yunginger, eds. St. Louis, MO: C.V. Mosby, 3rd. Ed., Vol. 1, p. 179.
2. Barker, R.L., Gleich, G.J., and Pease, L.R. 1988. Acidic precursor revealed in human eosinophil granule major basic protein cDNA. J. Exp. Med. 168:1493.
3. Ten, R.M., Pease, L.R., McKean, D.J., Bell, M.P., and Gleich, G.J. 1989. Molecular cloning of the human eosinophil peroxidase. Evidence

for the existence of a peroxidase multigene family. J. Exp. Med. 169:1757.
4. Barker, R.L., Loegering, D.A., Ten, R.M., Hamann, K.J., Pease, L.R., and Gleich, G.J. 1989. Eosinophil cationic protein cDNA. Comparison with other toxic cationic proteins and ribonucleases. J. Immunol. 143:952.
5. Hamann, K.J., Barker, R.L., Loegering, D.A., Pease, L.R., and Gleich, G.J. 1989. Sequence of human eosinophil-derived neurotoxin cDNA: Identity of deduced amino acid sequence with human nonsecretory ribonucleases. Gene 83:161.
6. Leiferman, K.M., Peters, M.S., and Gleich, G.J. 1986. The eosinophil and cutaneous edema. J. Am. Acad. Dermatol. 15:513.
7. Frigas, E., and Gleich, G.J. 1986. The eosinophil and the pathophysiology of asthma. J. Allergy Clin. Immunol. 77:527.
8. Gleich, G.J. 1990. The eosinophil and bronchial asthma: Current understanding. Review article. J. Allergy Clin. Immunol. 85:422.
9. Sanderson, C.J., Campbell, H.D., and Young, I.G. 1988. Molecular and cellular biology of the eosinophil differentiation factor (interleukin-5) and its effect on human and mouse B cells. Immuno. Rev. 102:29.
10. Gleich, G.J., Schroeter, A.L., Marcoux, J.P., Sachs, M.I., O'Connell, E.J., and Kohler, P.F. 1984. Episodic angioedema associated with eosinophilia. N. Engl. J. Med. 310:1621.
11. Butterfield, J.H., Leiferman, K.M., Gonchoroff, N., Silver, J.E., Abrams, J., Bower, J., Gleich, G.J. 1992. Elevated serum levels of interleukin-5 in patients with the syndrome of episodic angioedema and eosinophilia. Blood 79:688.
12. van Haelst Pisani, C., Kovach, J.S., Kita, H., Leiferman, K.M., Gleich, G.J., Silver, J.E., Dennin, R., and Abrams, J.S. 1991. Administration of IL-2 results in increased plasma concentrations of IL-5 and eosinophilia in patients with cancer. Blood 78:1538.
13. Begley, C.G., Lopez, A.F., Nicola, N.A., Warren, D.J., Vadas, M.A., Sanderson, C.J., Metcalfe, D. 1986. Purified colony-stimulating factors enhance the survival of human neutrophils and eosinophils *in vitro*: A rapid and sensitive microassay for colony-stimulating factors. Blood 68:162.
14. Sedgwick, J.B., Calhoun, W.J., Gleich, G.J., Kita, H., Abrams, J.S., Schwartz, L.B., Volovitz,B., Ben-Yaakov, M., and Busse, W.W. 1991. Immediate and late allergic airway response to segmental antigen challenge: Characterization of eosinophil and mast cell mediators. Am. Rev. Respir. Dis. 144:1274.
15. Lamas, A.M., Leon, O.G., Klunk, D.A., and Schleimer, R.P. 1991. Glucocorticoids inhibit eosinophil responses to granulocyte-macrophage colony-stimulating factor. J. Immunol. 147:254.
16. Wallen, N., Kita, H., Weiler, D., and Gleich, G.J. 1991. Glucocorticoids inhibit cytokine-mediated eosinophil survival. J. Immunol. 147:3490.
17. Kita, H., Ohnishi, T., Okubo, Y., Weiler, D., Abrams, J.S., and Gleich, G.J. 1991. Granulocyte/macrophage colony-stimulating factor and interleukin 3 release from human peripheral blood eosinophils and neutrophils. J. Exp. Med. 174:745.
18. Moqbel, R., Qutayba, H., Ying, S., Barkans, J., Hartnell, A., Tsicopoulos, A., Wardlaw, A.J., and Kay, A.B. 1991. Expression of mRNA and immunoreactivity for the granulocyte/macrophage colony-stimulating factor in activated human eosinophils. J. Exp. Med. 174:749.
19. Owen, W.F., Rothenberg, M.E., Petersen, J., Weller, P.F., Silberstein, D.S., Stevens, R.L., Soberman, R.J., and Austen, K.F. 1989. Interleukin 5 and phenotypically altered eosinophils in the blood of patients with the idiopathic hypereosinophilic syndrome. J. Exp. Med. 170:343.
20. Owen, W.F., Petersen, J., Sheff, D., Folkerth, R.D., Anderson, R.J., Corson, J.M., Sheffer, A.L., and Austen, K.F. 1990. Hypodense eosinophils and interleukin 5 activity in the blood of patients with the eosinophilia-myalgia syndrome. Proc. Natl. Acad. Sci. USA 87:8647.
21. Coffman, R.L., Seymour, B.W.P., Hudak, S., Jackson, J., and Rennick, D. 1989. Antibody to interleukin-5 inhibits helminth-induced eosinophilia in mice. Science 245:308.
22. Limaye, A.P., Abrams, J.S., Silver, J.E., Ottesen, E.A., and Nutman, T.B. 1990. Regulation of parasite-induced eosinophilia: Selectively increased interleukin 5 production in helminth-infected patients. J. Exp. Med. 172:399.
23. Wong, D.T.W., Weller, P.F., Galli, S.J., Elovic, A., Rand, T.H., Gallagher, G.T., Chiang, T., Chou, M.Y., Matossian, K., McBride, J., and Todd, R. 1990. Human eosinophils express transforming growth factor α. J. Exp. Med. 172:673.
24. Del Pozo, V., DeAndres, B., Martin, E., Maruri, N., Zubeldia, J.M., Palomino, P., and Lahoz, C. 1990. Murine eosinophils and IL-1:

αIL-1 mRNA detection by in situ hybridization. J. Immunol. 144:3117.
25. Kay, A.B., Ying, S., Varney, V., Gaga, M., Durham, S.R., Moqbel, R., Wardlaw, A.J., and Hamid, Q. 1991. Messenger RNA expression of the cytokine gene cluster, interleukin 3 (IL-3), IL-4, IL-5, and granulocyte/macrophage colony-stimulating factor, in allergen-induced late-phase cutaneous reactions in atopic subjects. J. Exp. Med. 173:775.

Role of Inlammatory Cytokines in Allergy

Joost J. Oppenheim*, Ji Ming Wang*, Andrew W. Lloyd*, Arthur O. Anderson**

The properties of cytokines such as interleukin 1 (IL 1), tumor necrosis factor α (TNFα), interleukin 8 (IL 8) and related chemoattractant cytokines are reviewed. Administration of these cytokines has been shown to induce local acute and chronic inflammatory reactions. IL 1 and TNF amplify delayed hypersensitivity (type IV allergic) reactions is well established. Evidence is accumulating that IL 1, TNF, IL 8 and monocyte chemotactic and activating factor (MCAF/MCP-1) also participate in the late phase of acute allergic reactions. Mast cells can be activated by anti-IgE to produce a variety of cytokines including IL 1 and TNF. These cytokines have been detected in the late phase of allergic responses and can emulate such reactions. Conversely, antisera to these cytokines can inhibit these reactions. IL 8 acts as an inhibitor of histamine release, whereas MCAF is a potent histamine releasing factor for human basophils. Finally, histamine itself may serve as a downregulator of cytokine production by H2 receptor-bearing cells that participate in acute allergic responses.

Mediators of inflammation such as interleukin 1 (IL 1), tumor necrosis factor (TNF) and derivative cytokines such as IL 8 and homologous peptide chemoattractants have been shown to participate in various aspects of allergic reactions. Certainly the role of IL 1 and TNF in initiating and amplifying delayed type hypersensitivity reactions has been amply documented (1). For example, studies utilizing a suction blister technique revealed significantly elevated IL 1 levels in the epidermis overlying the site of a patch test in patients with type IV allergic contact dermatitis reactions to a variety of allergens (2). In addition, proinflammatory cytokines participate in acute allergic reactions and their sequellae to a surprising extent. In this paper we will briefly summarize the relevant information concerning the properties of these proinflammatory cytokines and their capacity to induce acute and chronic inflammatory responses. This will be followed by a brief review of data documenting the roles of these cytokines in the late phase of acute allergic states and their bidirectional interactions with histamine.

Properties of IL 1 and TNF

Interleukin 1 (IL 1) was first detected in 1972 as a monocyte-derived lymphocyte activating factor (LAF) with comitogenic effects on thymocytes. There are two types of IL 1, (α and β) which are 28% homologous. Both are made as larger intracellular precursors which are processed to the mature extracellular forms by unknown mechanisms. IL 1α and β have been reported to be inducible in virtually every cell type and to induce diverse effects on many cells and tissues. Many of the myriad biological activities of IL 1 occur through the induction of other cytokines such as IL 2, IFN's, CSF's, TNF, IL 6, PDGF, TGFβ, IL 8, and related cytokines as well as through up-regulation of cytokine receptors including receptors for IL 1 itself, CSF's, and IL 2. As such, IL 1 can be considered a "first order" cytokine that is involved in mobilizing and amplifying inflammatory host defenses and repair processes (3,4).

Two distinct receptors for IL 1 have been identified, type I and type II, both belonging to the immunoglobulin superfamily. The type I receptor is widely distributed on connective tissue and vascular endothelial cells, T lymphocytes and other cell types (5). Type I IL 1 receptors have a higher affinity for IL 1α than β and activate functional biological responses. The signalling mechanism for the type I receptor

* Laboratory of Molecular Immunoregulation, Biological Response Modifiers Program, National Cancer Institute, Frederick, MD, USA;
** USAMRIID, Building 1425, Ft. Detrick, Frederick, MD, USA.
Acknowledgements: We are grateful for the critical review of this paper by Drs. Reuben Siraganian, Ruth Neta, David Kelvin and Dan Longo and the preparation of the manuscript and disk by Ms. Roberta Unger.

involves activation of serine/threonine protein kinases, distinct from protein kinases C or A (6). These kinases activate or unmask transcription factors such as c-jun and nuclear factor kappa B which in turn cause altered gene expression (7). The smaller but related type II receptor is found on B lymphocytes and myeloid cells. Type II IL 1 receptors have a very small cytoplasmic portion, bind IL 1β somewhat better than IL 1α, and their role in signalling remains to be established.

Tumor necrosis factor (TNFα) was discovered in 1975 as a substance that appeared in serum concomitant with tumor necrosis induced by bacterial endotoxin. TNF was also discovered as a factor causing the cachexia of chronic infections (8). TNFα is cytotoxic for some tumor cells *in vitro*, but not for normal cells. TNFα exhibits 28% homology to TNFβ, a cytotoxin produced by T cells otherwise known as lymphotoxin (LT/TNFβ), which uses the same receptor as TNFα and was discovered in 1968. TNFα and β, although structurally completely unrelated to IL 1α and β, show remarkable overlap in their pleiotropic activities (9) and have few unique functional activities. TNF and IL 1 cooperate synergistically in inducing biological effects such as cachexia and endotoxin shock. TNF, like IL 1, also operates as a "first order" cytokine whose activities are often mediated through the production of other cytokines. Two distinct TNF receptors have been cloned. The smaller receptor (p55) transduces a TNF signal, since antibodies to it are agonistic (10). The TNF signal transduction mechanism is not known, but it activates serine/threonine kinases similar to those activated by IL 1 (7).

IL 8 and Homologous Chemoattractant Cytokines

IL 1, TNF and at times PDGF and IFNγ induce a family of small molecular weight (8000–10,000 kDa) "intercrine" cytokines which can be considered "second order" cytokines (11). These intercrines exhibit more specialized functions in inflammation and repair and appear to be less pleiotropic than the "first order" inflammatory cytokines. These cytokines can be assigned to two subfamilies: an intercrine α subset based on their location on human chromosome 4 (q12-21) and on the fact that the first two of their four cysteine groups are separated by one amino acid (C-X-C). The human intercrine α group includes IL 8, melanoma growth stimulating activity (MGSA/GRO), platelet factor 4 (PF4), β thromboglobulin (βTG), and IP 10. The human intercrine β subgroup, which is located on chromosome 17 (q11-32), has no intervening amino acid between the first two cysteins (C-C), and includes macrophage chemotactic and activating factor (MCAF/MCP1), RANTES, LD78, ACT 2, and I-309.

The production by LPS stimulated mononuclear cell cultures of neutrophil chemoattractants was initially attributed to IL 1. However, subsequent studies demonstrated that pure recombinant IL 1 did not have the capacity to chemoattract inflammatory cells. This led to the isolation, purification, sequencing and cloning of a neutrophil chemoattractant, that is now called IL 8 (as reviewed in 12). IL 8 is produced by many cell types in response to exogenous stimuli such as polyclonal mitogens, injurious stimuli, infectious agents as well as endogenous cytokines such as IL 1 and TNF (12). IL 8 is a chemoattractant for neutrophils, basophils and a small proportion (10%) of resting OKT4 and OKT8 lymphocytes. IL 8 additionally activates neutrophil enzyme release, influences the mobility of melanocytes and is a comitogenic stimulant of keratinocytes. Injections of IL 8 cause a rapid local neutrophilic infiltration without other systemic sequelae such as induction of acute phase proteins or fever. IL 8 and the other intercrines have not as yet been documented to induce other cytokines.

At the time of writing two distinct receptors for human IL 8 have been cloned (13,14). The IL 8 receptors have a seven-transmembrane-spanning region typical of G-protein receptors. The receptor is probably coupled to phosphoinositide hydrolysis and elevates diacylglycerol and cytosolic Ca++ levels, which lead to activation of protein kinase C (15). As implied by the name, MGSA was first discovered as a factor that accelerated the growth of melanoma cell lines and also as a product of oncogene transfected cell lines (GRO) (as reviewed in 11). MGSA/GRO competes for the IL 8 binding site on myelocytic cells and is also a potent chemoattractant, as well as an activator of neutrophils. Both MGSA and IL 8 have been extracted from psoriatic tissues. GRO is probably the human homologue of the murine macrophage inflammatory peptides (MIP2).

PF4 and βTG are both present in platelet granules and are released by inducers of platelet aggregation. Consequently, they become available at sites of injury, hemorrhage and thromboses. Both are reported to chemoattract and to stimulate fibroblasts, presumably for repair purposes. In addition a 70 amino acid breakdown product of βTG, known as neutrophil attracting peptide 2 (NAP2), is a chemoattractant and activator of neutrophils, albeit at 100-fold higher concentrations than IL 8. IP 10 is produced by macrophages in response to IFNγ. The function of IP 10 remains unclear, but antibodies to IP 10 react with many cell types present at the site of delayed hypersensitivity reactions. Thus, IP 10 can presumably be produced by many cell types and probably participates in type IV allergic responses.

MCAF, otherwise known as MCP1, is produced by monocytes, fibroblasts and endothelial cells in response to the usual exogenous stimuli, and to endogenous cytokines such as IL 1, TNF and PDGF (12). MCAF chemoattracts and activates monocytes to release enzymes and to become cytostatic for tumor cells. There are no detectable binding sites for MCAF on neutrophils, lymphocytes or other cell types except monocytes. MCAF has been detected at inflamed atheromatous lesions in blood vessel walls and induces macrophages to accumulate by 6–18 hours at sites of injection. Recently MCAF production by pulmonary alveolar macrophages was shown to occur during acute arthus reactions in rat lung (16).

RANTES is chemoattractant for monocytes as well as for memory T cells, and has also been detected at sites of atheromatous inflammation. Although MIP 1α, the murine homologue of LD78, is reported to inhibit hematopoietic stem cell replication, the activities of LD78 and ACT2 are at present still unknown (11). I-309 is also said to be a chemoattractant for monocytes. Overall, the intercrine family members appear to be very potent chemoattractants and activators of inflammatory cells and fibroblasts. However, their functional capabilities and pathophysiological roles are still inadequately defined.

Role of Cytokines in Local Acute and Chronic Inflammation

The best evidence for the central role of IL1, TNF and the IL 8 family in local inflammation has come from dissecting the effects of endotoxin (LPS). Injection of LPS, recombinant human IL 1, (rhuIL 1) or rhuTNF all induce neutrophil emigration into intradermal injection sites (17). LPS and IL 1 are considerably more potent inducers than TNF, but the response to LPS was slower and occurred 30 min later than those to IL 1 and TNF. However, co-injection of IL 1α or β together with TNF resulted in synergistic neutrophil accumulation in the skin of rabbits (18). Similarly, rabbits injected intradermally with IL 1α or β together with TNFα followed 18 hours later by intravenous injection of LPS developed a local inflammatory and thrombohemorrhagic Schwartzman reaction at the site of injection (19). This was not the case at sites injected with only IL 1 or TNF. This further supports the importance of synergistic interactions of IL 1 and TNF in acute inflammatory respones. On the other hand, local intradermal injection of actinomycin D, cycloheximide or puromycin inhibits neutrophil emigration in response to IL 1, TNF or LPS, but not to C5a-desarg, FMLP or LTB4 (20). The neutrophil response to the latter chemoattractants was also more rapid than to the cytokines. These kinetics and the dependence on mRNA transcription and translation suggest that the neutrophil effects of IL 1 and TNF may be indirect and mediated by another factor. IL 8 and related factors may be responsible, since they are chemoattractants for inflammatory cells. Furthermore, intracutaneous injection of IL 8 results in rapid neutrophil accumulation in rats (12) and man (21).

Chronic cytokine administration at local sites has been achieved by implanting cytokine in slow release polymers of ethylene vinyl acetate subcutaneously in mice (22). This revealed that IL 1α and β, and to a lesser extent TNFα, induce acute inflammatory reactions at the site of the polymer at 6 hours which resolve by 48 hours. However, these pellets containing IL 1β and IL 1α become surrounded by chronic granulomatous reactions by 7–21 days. This is characterized by macrophage-rich infiltrates, fibroplasia, and angiogenesis. This was not seen with TNF. Consequently, persistent slow local release of IL 1 results in typical delayed hypersensitivity granuloma formation. Overall, these studies reveal that IL 1, TNF, IL 8 and related cytokines participate in various types of local inflammatory reactions, in the case of IL 1 and TNF presumably by inducing other cytokines and inflammatory mediators.

Role of Cytokines in the Late Phase of Acute Allergic Reactions

Virtually all nucleated cells can be induced by appropriate injurious or activating stimuli to produce IL 1, TNF or IL 8. Mast cells are capable of producing a wide variety of cytokines including GM-CSF, IL 1, 3, 5, 6 and TNFα (23). IgE-dependent activation of peritoneal or cultured murine mast cells augments the levels of TNFα mRNA as well as production of TNFα (24). Such immunological activation of mast cell TNFα release may contribute to leukocyte infiltration in late phase reactions of asthma or other allergic diseases. This is supported by the observation that rabbit anti-TNF antiserum diminishes IgE and mast cell dependent cutaneous inflammation in mice. Furthermore, sequential skin biopsies of patients with respiratory allergies during the late phase of the reaction (between 20 min and 24 hours) to intradermally injected ragweed or dust mite allergens revealed the appearance of endothelial leukocyte adhesion molecules (ELAM 1) on endothelial cells (EC) (25). The expression of ELAM 1 occurred by 3–4 hours after intradermal challenge concurrently with the development of inflammatory infiltrates. The expressionof ELAM 1 on EC was inhibited by a combination of antisera to TNFα and IL 1, but not by antisera to each cytokine alone. This observation points out the central role of cytokine-induced adhesion proteins in promoting local inflammation. Thus, these locally derived cytokines cooperate in inducing the accumulation of inflammatory cells in cutaneous allergic reactions.

The inflammatory cytokines may also contribute to the broncho-constriction seen in the late phase of the asthmatic response (26). Intrapulmonary administration of IL 1 or TNF to mice with an ultrasonic nebulizer resulted in significant increases in airway resistance for 2–5 hours,with a maximum at 3 hours, after IL 1 inhalation. The number of neutrophils in bronchoalveolar fluids was markedly increased by 5 hours after exposure to IL 1 and airway resistance reverted to normal at 7 hours. The effects of TNFα were similar, but more rapid, and bronchoconstriction occurred by 1 hour. Although these effects of IL 1 and TNF are probably indirect, cytokine antagonists may prove therapeutically beneficial in asthma.

Bidirectional Cytokine-Histamine Interactions

A number of cytokines have been reported to influence histamine release from human bisophils. IL 1, IL 3, IL 5 and GM-CSF can prime human basophils to release more histamine and/or leukotriene C4 when subsequently incubated with secretagogues such as anti-IgE or C5a (27). Higher concentration of IL 3, GM-CSF and IL 8 have also been reported to cause weak histamine release by themselves (28). However, at lower ($< 10^{-6}$ M) concentrations, IL 8 actually inhibits basophil histamine release (29). On the other hand, platelet-derived connective tissue activating peptide III (CTAP III), which is the precursor molecule for βTG and NAP II, does have weak histamine releasing activity (29). Furthermore, MCAF is the most potent histamine releasing cytokine described so far (31). MCAF does not act as a primer of histamine release for other agonists, but rapidly releases more histamine from basophils previously primed with IL 3 or IL 5. MCAF acts as an agonist on basophils from most nonatopic as well as atopic subjects at 10^{-9} to 10^{-6} M concentrations, with peak activity at 10^{-7} M. Thus histamine release due to MCAF can contribute to disorders such as late phase allergic reactions, chronic urticaria, atopic dermatitis and asthma.

Recently histamine was reported to actually suppress the expression of mRNA for TNFα and its production by LPS stimulated human peripheral blood mononuclear cells (30). This could be inhibited only by H2 receptor antagonists such as cimetidine and ranitidine. This data suggests that mast cell-derived histamine may have a negative feedback effect on cytokine synthesis by H2 receptor bearing cells.

This includes mast cells themselves, synovial cells, chondrocytes, macrophages and other inflammatory cells. One can speculate that histamine may thus prevent the progression from acute to chronic inflammation in acute allergic reactions and down-regulates cytokine mediated inflammatory component of the late phase of allergic responses.

Rererences

1. Durum, S.K., and Oppenheim, J.J. 1989. Macrophage derived mediators: IL 1, TNF, IL 6, IFN and related cytokines. In: Fundamental immunology, 2nd ed. W.E. Paul, ed. New York: Raven, p. 639.
2. Larsen, C.G., Ternowitz, T., Larsen, F.G., and Thestrup-Pedersen, K. 1988. Epidermis and lymphocyte interactions during an allergic patch test reaction. Increased activity of ETAF/IL 1, epidermal derived lymphocyte chemotactic factor and mixed skin lymphocyte reactivity in persons with type IV allergy. J. Invest. Dermatol. 90:230.
3. Neta, R., and Oppenheim, J.J. 1988. Why should internists be interested in IL 1? Ann. Intern. Med. 109:1.
4. Dinarello, C.A. 1991. Interleukin 1 and interleukin 1 antagonism. Blood 77:1637.
5. Sims, J.E., Acres, R.B., Grubin, C. E., McMahan, C.J., Wignall, J. M., March, C.J., and Dower, S.K. 1989. Cloning the interleukin 1 receptor from human T cells. Proc. Natl. Acad. Sci. USA 86:8946.
6. Muegge, K., and Durum, S.K. 1990. Cytokines and transcription factors. Cytokines 2:1.
7. O'Neill, L.A.J., Bird, T.A., and Saklatvala, J. 1990. How does interleukin 1 activate cells? Immunol. Today 11:392.
8. Beutler, B., and Cerami, A. 1988. The biology of cachectin-TNF: A primary mediator of the host response. Annu. Rev. Immuno. 7:625.
9. Le, J., and Vilcek, J. 1987. Cytokines with multiple overlapping biological activities. Lab. Invest. 56:234.
10. Englemann, H., Holtmann, H., Brakebusch, C., Avni, S.Y., Sarov, I., Nophar, Y., Hadas, E., Leitner, O., and Wallach, D. 1990. Antibodies to a soluble form of a tumor necrosis factor (TNF) receptor have TNF-like activity. J. Biol. Chem. 265:14497.
11. Oppenheim, J.J., Zachariae, C.O.C., Mukaida, N., and Matsushima, K. 1991. Properties of the novel proinflammatory supergene "intercrine" cytokine family. Annu. Rev. Immunol. 9:617.
12. Matsushima, K., and Oppenheim, J.J. 1989. Interleukin 8 and MCAF: Novel inflammatory cytokines inducible by IL 1 and TNF. Cytokine 1:2.
13. Holmes, W.E., Lee, J., Kuang, W-J., Rice, G.C., and Wood, W.I. 1991. Structure and functional expression of a human IL 8 receptor. Science 253:1278.
14. Murphy, P.M., and Tiffany, H.L. 1991. Cloning of complementary DNA encoding a functional IL 8 receptor. Science 253:1280.
15. Baggiolini, M., Walz, A., and Kunkel, S.L. 1989. Neutrophil activating peptide 1/interleukin 8, a novel cytokine that activates neutrophils. J. Clin. Invest. 84:1045.
16. Brieland, J., Jones M., Clarke, S., Warren, J., and Fantone, J. 1991. Expression of MCP-1 by rat pulmonary alveolar macrophages during acute inflammatory lung injury. J. Leuk. Biol. Suppl. 2:59 (Abstr.).
17. Cybulsky, M.I., McComb, D.J., and Movat, H.Z. 1988. Neutrophil leukocyte emigration induced by endotoxin. J. Immunol. 140:3144.
18. Wankowicz, Z., Megyeri, P., and Issekutz, A. 1988. Synergy between TNFα and IL 1 in the induction of polymorphonuclear leukocyte migration during inflammation. J. Leuk. Biol. 43:349.
19. Movat, H.Z., Burrowes, C.E., Cybulsky, M.I., and Dinarello, C.A. 1987. Acute inflammation and a Schwartzman-like raction induced by IL 1 and TNF. Amer. J. Path. 129:463.
20. Cybulsky, M.I., McComb, D.J., and Movat, H.Z. 1989. Protein synthesis dependent and independent mechanisms of nutrophil emigration. Amer. J. Path. 135:227.
21. Leonard, E.J., Yoshimura, T., Tanaka, S., and Raffeld, M. 1991. Neutrophil recruitment by intradermally injected neutrophil attractant/activation protein-1. J. Invest. Dermatol. 96:690.
22. Dunn, C.J., Hardee, M.M., and Staite, N.D. 1989. Acute and chouronic inflammatory responses to local administration of recombinant IL 1α, IL 2β, TNFα, IL 2 and IFNγ in mice. Agents and Actions 27:290.
23. Gordon, J.R., Burd, P.R., and Galli, S.J. 1990. Mast cells as a source of multifunctional cytokines. Immunol. Today 11:458.
24. Gordon, J.R., and Galli, S.J. 1990. Mast cells as a source of both performed and immunologically inducible TNFα/cachectin. Nature 346:274.

25. Leung, D.Y.M., Pober, J.S., and Cotran, R.S. 1991. Expression of endothelial-leukocyte adhesion molecule-N in elicited late phase allergic reactions. J. Clin. Invest. 87:1805.
26. Aratani, H., Inoue, H., Okada, S., and Takashima, T. 1991. Effect of cytokine on pulmonary function in mice. Amer. Rev. Resp. Dis. 143: Pt. 2 A15.
27. Kaplan, A.P., Reddigari, S., Baeza, M., and Kuna, P. 1991. Histamine releasing factors and cytokine-dependent activation of basophils and mast cells. Adv. Immunol. 50:237.
28. White, M.V., Yoshimura, T., Hook, W., Kaliner, M.A., and Leonard, E.J. 1989. Neutrophil attractant/activation protein-1 (NAP-1) causes human basophil histamine release. Immunol. Lett. 22:151.
29. Kuna, P., Reddigari, S.R., Kornfeld, D., and Kaplan, A.P. 1991. IL 8 inhibits histamine release from human basophils induced by histamine releasing factors, CTAP III and IL 3. J. Immunol. 147:1920.
30. Vannier, E., Miller, L.C., and Dinarello, C.A. 1991. Histamine suppresses gene expression and synthesis of TNFα via histamine H2 receptors. J. Exp. Med. 174:281.
31. Kuna, P., Redigari, S.R., Rucinski D., Oppenheim, J.J., and Kaplan, A.P. 1992. J. Exp. Med. 175:489.

Priming of Effector Cells by Lymphokines

Clemens A. Dahinden, Stephan C. Bischoff, Shigeru Takafuji, Martin Krieger, Thomas Brunner, Alain L. de Weck*

The function of inflammatory effector cells involved in allergic inflammation is modulated by distinct sets of cytokines. We propose that the cytokine-induced potentiation and modulation of mediator release by mast cells, basophils, and eosinophils stimulated with appropriate agonists, may be of major importance for the development of allergic immediate and late phase reactions. A better knowledge about the mechanism of action of these modulatory cytokines should provide a basis for novel therapeutic interventions in allergic disease and other inflammatory disorders. Mast cells, basophils and eosinophils are major effector cell types in allergic inflammatory processes (1,2). Basophils and eosinophils are particularly involved in late phase reactions, as well as in certain types of delayed type hypersensitivity reactions (Figure 1). The involvement of basophils in late phase reactions has also been assumed to be based upon the mediator profile observed several hours after allergen challenge *in vivo* (3). The extent of mediator release by basophils may therefore be of special relevance to the severity of symptoms in allergic disease. Another interesting feature of human basophils is their exceedingly high capacity to form lipid mediators in response to soluble agonists (1). Eosinophils, on the other hand, may also contribute to lipid mediator formation (leukotriene C4: LTC4; platelet-activating factor: PAF), and promote tissue damage by the release of cationic proteins (4).

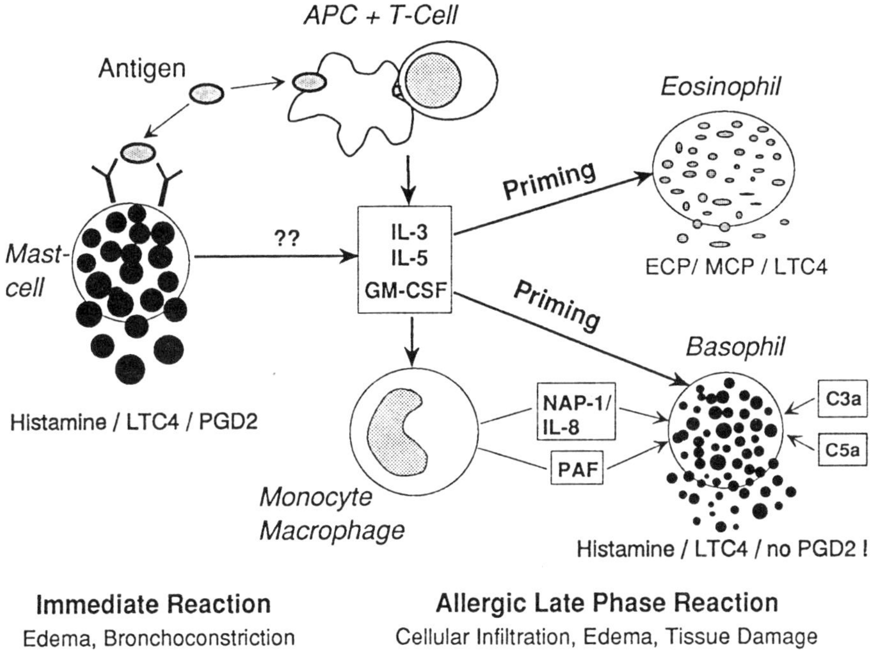

Figure 1. The pathogenesis of allergic immediate and late-phase reactions.

---

* Institute of Clinical Immunology, Inselspital, Bern, Switzerland.
Acknowledgements: This work was supported by the Swiss National Science Foundation, grant 31-27980.89.

Regulation of Mediator Release by Human Lung Mast Cells

It is unknown whether mediator release by mast cells can be regulated by certain cytokines as demonstrated in basophils and other inflammatory effector cells. We found that the c-kit ligand (KL), a recently identified stem cell growth factor (5), at concentrations of 10–100-times lower than required to promote cell proliferation, enhances the release of histamine and LTC4 in response to IgE receptor-crosslinking of human lung mast cells (6). KL does not induce mediator release by itself, but increases the sensitivity of mast cells to anti-IgE receptor stimulation. Furthermore, KL enhances the mediator release in response to maximally effective anti-IgE receptor antibody concentrations. By contrast, a large number of cytokines examined, including the mast cell growth factors/agonists in rodents, interleukin (IL)-3, IL-4, IL-9, and nerve growth factor (NGF) (references 7,8), are ineffective in this respect, suggesting a unique role of KL in regulating effector functions of human mucosal mast cells. In contrast to basophils, no IgE-independent agonists have been found yet, since C5a, C3a, FMLP, PAF, and IL-8 do not trigger lung mast cells for mediator release, even in the presence of KL (Figure 2).

Regulation of Mediator Release by Human Basophils

Crosslinking of high-affinity IgE receptors on basophils induces the release of histamine as well as leukotrienes (1,9–11). Divalent IgE receptor-crosslinking is sufficient, but large amounts of leukotrienes are only synthesized after multivalent IgE receptor-crosslinking (9,11). Relatively high concentrations of FMLP are also capable of inducing the release of both, preformed and newly synthesized mediators (9). By contrast, C5a, a complement-derived anaphylatoxin, is a potent histamine-releasing agent inducing a maximal release reaction already at 10^{-9} M (12). However, up to a C5a concentration of 10^{-7} M, no detectable amounts of LTC4 are generated (11,12). It is interesting that two chemotactic peptides, C5a and FMLP, both presumably acting through similar signal-transducing mechanisms, can induce a different mediator release pattern in basophils. Three basophil agonists, the cell-derived IL-8 and PAF, and the C-derived anaphylatoxin C3a, do not induce basophil mediator release by themselves up to concentrations of 10^{-6} M (= “incomplete agonists”). However, after preincubation with IL-3, IL-5, granulocyte/macrophage colony-stimulating factor (GM-CSF) or NGF (see below), basophils release histamine and leukotrienes in response to C3a, IL-8, and PAF (13–15). Of interest, cytokine-primed basophils optimally respond to C3a concentrations as low as 10^{-9} M, and PAF becomes a particularly potent inducer of LTC4 synthesis (14,15). Thus, the sequential action of a growth factor (IL-3, IL-5, GM-CSF, NGF) and cell-derived (IL-8, PAF) or humoral (C3a) products can induce efficient basophil mediator release (Figure 2).

Three hematopoietic growth factors, IL-3, GM-CSF, and IL-5, in a picomolar concentration range, profoundly modulate basophil mediator release in response to diverse agonists (11,12,16). Furthermore, NGF, a neurotrophic cytokine, also affects basophils at very low concentrations (1-4 pM of rhuNGF β) in a similar fashion (17). On a molar basis, IL3 and NGF are clearly the most potent cytokines, but at maximally effective concentrations all 4 growth factors are nearly equally effective. In particular, IL-3 can induce some histamine release by itself in rare cases, but in general, histamine release is minimal or absent, and leukotriene synthesis is never detected in response to any growth factors (11–18). The most prominent effect on basophils by these cytokines is seen when they are added at least 5 min before another agonist. In particular, these growth factors (a) enhance the releasability to all agonists, (b) change the mediator profile, e. g. allow LTC4 generation in response to C5a, which by itself induces histamine release only, (c) enhance the rate and extent of mediator release in particular with regard to LTC4 formation, (d) render basophils responsive to lower agonist concentrations, and (e) render basophils responsive to “incomplete agonists” such as IL-8, PAF or C3a (11-16).

Regulation of Mediator Release by Human Eosinophils

Of particular interest is the fact that the same set of cytokines profoundly modulates the function of basophils as well as eosinophils, both major effector cell types in allergic inflammatory processes (1,2,4,19). We recently found that IL3 and IL-5 also prime eosinophils to produce LTC4 in response to the soluble agonists FMLP, C5a, and PAF (20). In contrast to basophils, for which only a few minutes of cytokine preincubation are sufficient to potentiate mediator release, a preincubation time of approximately 90 min is required to modulate eosinophil function (20). A different target cell specificity is only found for NGF and tumor necrosis factor α (TNF), since NGF exclusively potentiates basophil function, while TNF enhances mediator release in eosinophils but not in basophils (own unpublished results).

Mechanisms Regulating Basophil Mediator Release

We previously found that the time interval and the sequence of addition of different basophil-activating molecules are critical for the final outcome of the release reaction as well as the profile of mediators formed (21,22). This, together with the clearly distinct influence on basophil function of response modifiers on the one hand, and the diverse triggering agents on the other, also suggests a different mechanism of action between these two classes of agonists.

Basophil Triggers

With the exception of IgE receptor-crosslinking, some, if not all, IgE-independent triggers, including the cytokine IL-8, interact with G-protein-coupled receptors (rhodopsine superfamily) (23), leading to activation of phospholipase C (PLC). PLC activation results in an IP_3-induced transient rise of intracellular calcium $[Ca^{2+}]_i$, and a diacylglycerol-induced activation of proteinkinase C (PKC). Indeed, we found that all agonists, including the incomplete agonists IL-8, PAF, and C3a, promote transient $[Ca^{2+}]_i$ rises (unpublished results). Calcium, but not PKC, seems necessary for basophil degranulation. For IL-8-related peptides such as NAP-2, connective tissue-activating peptide-III (CTAP-III), and platelet-factor-4, it has been found that the capacity to promote a $[Ca^{2+}]_i$ rise correlates with the affinity to the IL-8 receptor identified on basophils (24).

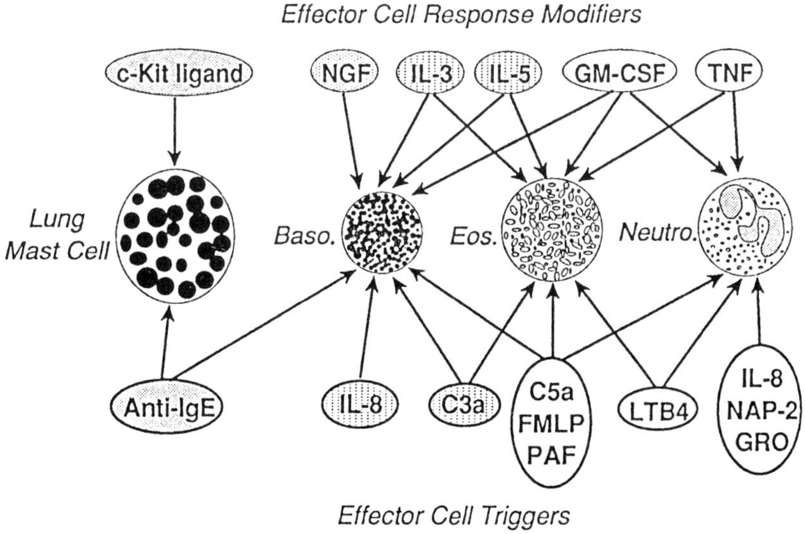

Figure 2. Cell agonists in allergic inflammation.

Basophil Response Modifiers

IL-3, GM-CSF, IL-5, and NGF neither induce a change of $[Ca^{2+}]_i$, nor alter the rise of $[Ca^{2+}]_i$ in response to the triggering agents. The presence of modulatory cytokines was also not required for the induction of $[Ca^{2+}]_i$ rise in response to basophil triggers, even incomplete agonists such as IL-8 or C3a (own unpublished results). By contrast, the modulatory cytokines seem to affect basophil function by stimulating a tyrosine kinase (or kinases). In this regard, it is interesting that a recently identified high-affinity binding component for NGF is the trk proto-oncogene, a tyrosine kinase receptor (25,26). IL-3, IL-5, and GM-CSF may activate basophils by the interaction of the ligand-receptor complexes with a common membrane protein (27). However, an association of the cytokine receptors with a tyrosine kinase has not yet been demonstrated. Nevertheless, it appears that tyrosine phosphorylation is critical but not sufficient for the induction of lipid mediator formation.

References

1. Charlesworth, E.N., Iliopoulos, O., MacDonald, S.M., Kagey-Sobotka, A., and Lichtenstein, L.M. 1989. Cells and secretagogues involved in the human late-phase response. Int. Arch. Allergy Appl. Immunol. 88:50.
2. Denburg, J.A., Otsuka, H., Ohnisi, M., Ruhno, J., Bienenstock, J., and Dolovich, J. 1987. Contribution of basophil/mast cell and eosinophil growth and differentiation to the allergic tissue inflammatory response. Int. Arch. Allergy Appl. Immunol. 82:321.
3. Naclerio, R.M., Proud, D., Togias, A.D., Adkinson, N.F., Meyers, D.A., Kagey-Sobotka, A., Plaut, M., Norman, P.S., and Lichtenstein, L.M. 1985. Inflammatory mediators in late antigen-induced rhinitis. N. Engl. J. Med. 313:65.
4. Gleich, G.J. 1990. The eosinophil and bronchial asthma: Current understanding. J. Allergy Clin. Immunol. 85:422.
5. Witte, O.N. 1990. Steel locus defines new multipotent growth factor. Cell 63:5.
6. Bischoff, S.C., and Dahinden, C.A. 1992. C-kit ligand: A unique potentiator of mediator release by human lung mast cells. J. Exp. Med. 175:237.
7. Rothe, M.J., Nowak, M., and Kerdel, F.A. 1990. The mast cell in health and disease. J. Am. Acad. Dermatol. 23:615.
8. Wasserman, S.I. 1990. Mast cell biology. J. Allergy Clin. Immunol. 86:590.
9. Dahinden, C.A., Kurimoto, Y., Baggiolini, M., Dewald, B., and Walz, A. 1989. Histamine and sulfidoleukotriene release from human basophils: Different effects of antigen, anti-IgE, C5a, f-Met-Leu-Phe and the novel neutrophil-activating peptide NAF. Int. Arch. Allergy Appl. Immunol. 90:113.
10. Hirai, K., Morita, Y., Misaki, Y., Ohta, K., Takaishi, T., Suzuki, S., Motoyoshi, K., and Miyamoto, T. 1989. Modulation of human basophil histamine release by hematopoetic growth factors. J. Immunol. 141:3958.
11. Kurimoto, Y., de Weck, A.L., and Dahinden. C.A. 1991. The effect of interleukin 3 upon IgE-dependent and IgE-independent basophil degranulation and leukotriene generation. Eur. J. Immunol. 21:361.
12. Kurimoto, Y., de Weck, A.L., and Dahinden, C.A. 1989. Interleukin 3-dependent mediator release in basophils triggered by C5a. J. Exp. Med. 170:467.
13. Dahinden, C.A., Kurimoto, Y., de Weck, A.L., Lindlay, I., Dewald, B., and Baggiolini, M. 1989. The neutrophil-activating peptide NAF/NAP-1 induces histamine and leukotriene release by interleukin 3-primed basophils. J. Exp. Med. 170:1787.
14. Bischoff, S.C., de Weck, A.L., and Dahinden, C.A. 1990. Interleukin 3 and GM-CSF render human basophils responsive to low concentrations of the complement component C3a. Proc. Natl. Acad. Sci. U.S.A. 87:6813.
15. Brunner, T., de Weck, A.L., and Dahinden, C.A. 1991. Platelet-activating factor induces mediator release by human basophils primed with IL-3, granulocyte-macrophage colony-stimulating factor, or IL-5. J. Immunol. 147:237.
16. Bischoff, S.C., Brunner, T., de Weck, A.L., and Dahinden, C.A. 1990. Interleukin 5 modifies histamine release and leukotriene generation by human basophils in response to diverse agonists. J. Exp. Med. 172:1577.
17. Bischoff, S.C., and Dahinden, C.A. 1992. The effect of nerve growth factor upon the release of inflammatory mediators by mature human basophils. Blood, in press.
18. MacDonald, S.M., Schleimer, R.P., Kagey-Sobotka, A., Gillis, S., and Lichtenstein, L.M. 1989. Recombinant IL-3 induces histamine release from human basophils. J. Immunol. 142:3527.

19. Fujisawa, T., Abu-Ghazaleh, R., Kita, H., Sanderson, C.J., and Gleich, G.J. 1990. Regulatory effect of cytokines on eosinophil degranulation. J. Immunol. 144:642.
20. Takafuji, S., Bischoff, S.C., de Weck, A.L., and Dahinden, C.A. 1991. Interleukin 3 and interleukin 5 prime normal human eosinophils to produce leukotriene C4 in response to soluble agonists. J. Immunol. 147:3855.
21. Bischoff, S.C., Baggiolini, M., de Weck, A.L., and Dahinden, C.A. 1991. Interleukin 8: Inhibitor and inducer of histamine and leukotriene release in human basophils. Biophys. Biochem. Res. Comm. 179:628.
22. Dahinden, C.A., Bischoff, S.C., Brunner, T., Krieger, M., Takafuji, S., and de Weck, A. L. 1991. Regulation of mediator release by human basophils: Importance of the sequence and time of addition in the combined action of different agonists. Int. Arch. Allergy. Appl. Immunol. 94:161.
23. Freissmuth, M., Casey, P.J., and Gilman, A.G. 1989. G protein control diverse pathways of transmembrane signaling. FASEB J. 3:2125.
24. Krieger, M., Brunner, T., Bischoff, S.C., von Tscharner, V., Walz, A., Moser, B., Baggiolini, M., and Dahinden, C.A. 1991. Activation of human basophils through the interleukin-8 receptor. Manuscript submitted.
25. Klein, R., Jing, S., Nanduri, E., O'Rourke, E., and Barbacid, M. 1991. The trk proto-oncogene encodes a receptor for nerve growth factor. Cell 65:189.
26. Hempstead, B.L., Martin-Zanca, D.R., Kaplan, D.R., Parada, L. F., and Chao, M. V. 1991. High-affinity NGF binding requires coexpression of the trk proto-oncogene and the low-affinity NGF receptor. Nature 350:678.
27. Hayashida, K., Kitamura, T., Gorman, D.M., Arai, K., Yokota, T., and Miyajima, A. 1990. Molecular cloning of a second subunit of the receptor for human granulocyte-macrophage colony-stimulating factor (GM-CSF): Reconstitution of a high-affinity GM-CSF receptor. Proc. Natl. Acad. Sci. U.S.A. 87:9655.

Interleukin 5 Receptor on Eosinophils

Kiyoshi Takatsu*, Satoshi Takaki*, Yoshiyuki Murata*, Masahiro Migita*, Seiji Mita*, Yasumichi Hitoshi*, Naoto Yamaguchi*, Shin Yonehara**, Toshio Kitamura***, Atsushi Miyajima***, Akira Tominaga*

Interleukin 5 (IL-5) is a T cell derived glycoprotein that stimulates eosinophil production and activation. Murine IL-5 (mIL-5), but not human IL-5 (hIL-5) is active on preactivated B cells to induce differentiation into Ig-producing cells. There are two classes of the mIL-5 binding sites, namely high and low affinity receptor, on eosinophils and B cells. The IL-5 signal can be transduced through the high affinity IL-5 receptors. The high affinity mIL-5 receptor consists of two different polypeptide chains: α and β. We isolated the mIL-5 receptor α chain cDNA that encodes the 60 kD protein of the low affinity IL-5 receptor. We also identified the β chain (130 kD protein) as the low affinity mIL-3 receptor-like protein, AIC2B, that can convert the low affinity receptor into the high affinity receptor. The β chain itself does not bind to IL-5. In the human, peripheral blood eosinophils expressed a single class of high affinity receptor. We cloned the hIL-5 receptor cDNA, by using the mIL-5 receptor α chain cDNA as a probe, that encodes the high affinity receptor of about 60 kD protein when expressed in COS7 cells. The expression of the hIL-5 receptor transcripts was observed in eosinophils. The predicted hIL-5 receptor protein has about 70% homology with the mIL-5 receptor α chain in the amino acid level, and each polypeptide is a membrane-penetrated glycoprotein that retains features common to the cytokine receptor superfamily. Murine interleukin 5 (mIL-5) is produced mainly by T cells as a glycoprotein with an Mr in the range of 45-60 kD (1). The study of mIL-5 originated in the search for one of the B cell growth and differentiation factors (T cell-replacing factor, TRF), that enhances antigen specific IgG antibody responses by B cells from antigen-primed mice (2). The cDNA cloning and the mAb against mIL-5 enabled us to identify this molecule as a cytokine that has pleiotropic activity on various target cells including B cells and eosinophils (3–5). A number of IL-5-dependent mouse B cell lines have now been isolated (6). These provide a convenient biological assay for this factor. IL-5 stimulates the production of eosinophils *in vitro* (7). An increased IL-5 production has been suspected in eosinophilia associated with malignant disease (8), helminth infections (7), and hypereosinophilic syndrome (9). However, there is a controversy whether human IL-5 (hIL-5) acts on human B cells (10). The pleiotropic activity of mIL-5 on target cells is directly dependent on initial binding to a specific cell-surface receptor. Like other cytokines, mIL-5 interacts with target cells with biphasic equilibrium binding kinetics, reflecting two classes of binding sites with high affinity and low affinity (11,12). The mIL-5 signal appears to be mediated through the high affinity mIL-5 receptor (11). Chemical cross-linking studies with the radiolabeled mIL-5 revealed that at least two different polypeptide chains (p60 and p130) may comprise the high affinity IL-5 receptor (12). Relatively little is known about the characteristics of hIL-5 receptor. Here, we summarize the structural and functional aspects of IL-5, and describe molecular structure of the high affinity mIL-5 receptor. Then, we report the molecular constitution of the hIL-5 receptor. Our results indicate that hIL-5 receptor appears to be expressed only on eosinophils and their precursors. Analysis of the sequence of hIL-5 receptor demonstrates that it is a member of a cytokine receptor supergene family.

* Department of Biology, Institute for Medical Immunology, Kumamoto University Medical School, 2-2-1 Honjo, Kumamoto 860;

** Tokyo Metropolitan Insitute of Medical Science, 3-12-22, Honkomagome, Bunkyo-ku, Tokyo 113, Japan;

*** DNAX Research Institute of Molecular and Cellular Biology, Palo Alto, CA, USA.

Acknowledgements: This study was supported by Grant-in-Aids for Scientific Research and for Special Project Research, Cancer Bioscience, from Ministry of Education, Science and Culture; by Special Coordination Funds for Promoting Science and Technology of the Science and Technology Agency, Japan; and by a Research Grant from the Tokyo Biochemistry Research Foundation. We are grateful to Drs. J.-I. Miyazaki (University of Tokyo) and A. Rolink (Basel Institute for Immunology) for providing pCAGGS vector and R52.120 mAb, respectively.

Structure and Function of IL-5

Both mIL-5 and hIL-5 have been characterized by cloning, sequencing and expression (Table 1) (3,5,13). Recombinant IL-5 produced in mammalian cells is about 45 to 60 kD, which changes from 22 to 30 kD after treatment with a reducing agent (14). Thus IL-5 is a disulfide-linked dimer that is unusual among the T cell-derived cytokines. This dimerization is essential for the biological activity of the IL-5 molecule. Monomeric mIL-5 produced by reduction and alkylation of IL-5 or by mutating the cystein residue to threonine were inactive on both an IL-5 dependent early B cell line and the murine eosinophils (15,16). McKenzie et al. found that two conserved cysteine residues cross-link the dimer in an anti-parallel arrangement (16). The heterogeneity of IL-5 in Mr is predominantly due to the heterogeneous addition of carbohydrate, which can be removed to leave a fully active molecule (17). Comparison of the cDNA sequence of mIL-5 with that of hIL-5 shows a sequence homology of 70% at the amino acid level. While mIL-5 and hIL-5 are equally active in human eosinophil assays, hIL-5 is 100-fold less active than mIL-5 in mouse cell assay (18). McKenzie et al. constructed human/mouse IL-5 hybrids to define the regions of the IL-5 molecules responsible for the species specificity (19). Their results clearly showed that the change of only eight residues in the C terminus region of hIL-5, to those of mIL-5, resulted in the hybrid producing biological activity comparable to mIL-5, suggesting that IL-5 may have two receptor binding sites located at the C terminus of each monomer.

A novel activity of eosinophil differentiation factor (EDF) which also has BCGFII activity has been initially reported by Sanderson et al. (7). The cloning of cDNA encoding the murine EDF revealed that the nucleotide sequence of the cDNA is completely identical to IL-5 cDNA (20). Murine IL-5 was also shown to maintain the viability and to induce the production of superoxide anion by mature eosinophils and to possess chemotactic activity for eosinophils (4,21). Transgenic mice carrying the mIL-5 gene exhibited the elevated levels of IL-5 in the serum (2–10 ng/ml) and increased the numbers of eosinophils in PBL more than 70-fold compared to those of age-matched control mice (22). Infiltration of eosinophils into various tissue was also obvious. Spleen had white patches consisting of the mass of eosinophils. Large parts of bone marrow were occupied by mature and immature eosinophils. Eosinophil infiltration was also observed in the muscle, and derangement sarcolemma and disappearance of striation were observed (22). Dent et al. also generated the IL-5 transgenic mice showing the massive eosinophilia (23). Passive administration of mAbs against mIL-5 or mIL-5 receptor caused the decrease in the levels of peripheral blood eosinophils in the IL-5 transgenic mice (24). It is clear that aberrant expression of the IL-5 gene induces accumulation of eosinophils.

Table 1. Structure, polypeptide, and target cells of IL-5

	Mouse	Human
1. Apparent m.w.	40-50 kD	30-40 kD
2. Number of amino acids	113	115
3. *N*-Glycosylation sites	3	5
4. Chromosome localization	11	5
5. Genomic structure	4 exons	4 exons
6. Producer cells	T cells	T cells
	Mast cells	Reed Sternberg cells
		EBV-transformed B cell
7. Target cells	Eosinophil	Eosinophils
	B cells	Basophils
	T cells	

Molecular Basis of the Murine High Affinity IL-5 Receptor

IL-5 Receptor Consists of Two Different Polypeptide Chains

IL-5 specifically interacts with IL-5 responsive early B cell lines, T88-M and Y16, with biphasic equilibrium binding kinetics, reflecting two classes of IL-5 binding sites with high affinity (dissociation constant, K*d* of ~150 pM) and low affinity (K*d* of ~20 nM) (11). Eosinophils purified from peritoneal cavity of the IL-5 transgenic mice also expressed IL-5 binding sites with both high and low affinity (24). Biological responsiveness to IL-5 depends on interactions with the high affinity form of the receptor. Chemical cross-linking of mIL-5 binding proteins revealed that the two polypeptide chains of about 60 kD and 120–130 kD are involved in the formation of the high affinity mIL-5 receptor (12). We prepared two mAbs H7 and T21 (25,26) specific for mIL-5-binding protein. The mAbs can immunoprecipitate the 60 kD protein (p60) from the membrane of mIL-5 receptor-positive cells (25), which can bind IL-5. Hereafter, we will refer to the p60 of H7 protein as the mIL-5 receptor α chain. The α chain is expressed on more than 70% of peritoneal B cells and on less than 10% of splenic B cells (26). Eosinophils also expressed the α chain, while neutrophils did not (24).

Molecular Cloning and Expression of the mIL-5 Receptor α Chain.

Four different cDNAs encoding the mIL-5 receptor α chain have been isolated by the expression cloning procedure with H7 mAb (27). The sequence of the cDNAs (pIL-5R.8 and pIL-5R.13) encoding the α chain indicates that it is a transmembrane protein with glycosylation of 415 amino acids, including an N-terminal signal peptide, a glycosylated extracellular domain, a single transmembrane segment, and a cytoplasmic tail (see below and Fig. 1) (27). The nucleotide sequences of pIL-5R.2 and pIL-5R.39 were identical to that of pIL-5R.8 except that they lacked small parts of the nucleotides (27). These deletions will cause altered translational reading frames, resulting in a lack in the transmembrane domain. The sequence analysis of the α chain cDNA reveals significant homology in the extracellular domain to several receptors for cytokines, growth hormone and prolactin (28). The extracellular region of the mIL-5 receptor α chain contains the homologous region of the cytokine receptor family that comprises four conserved cysteine residues in the amino-terminal half of the region and the tryptophan-serine-(X)-tryptophan-serine (WSXWS) motif located close to the transmembrane domain. In addition, this region was found to comprise three tandemly repeated sets of a fibronectin type III domain.

The cytoplasmic domain of the mIL-5 receptor does not contain the consensus sequences for either a tyrosine kinase domain or a catalytic domain of protein kinases. However, the

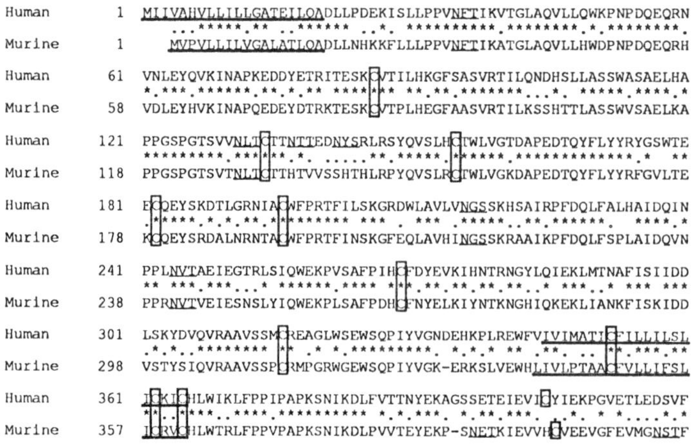

Figure 1. Alignment of amino acid sequences of the hIL-5 receptor and the mIL-5 receptor α chain. Astericks indicate identical amino acids, and horizontal lines mark gaps that were introduced to provide maximum alignment.

sequence from 367Leu to 380Asp in the IL-5 receptor following the transmembrane domain contains a proline cluster (27), which is well conserved among receptors GM-CSF, prolactin, and growth hormone. The cytoplasmic domain of the α chain has homology to a part of the actin-binding domain of human β-spectrin (29). Northern blot analysis revealed the presence of two mRNAs (~5.0-kb and 5.8-kb) whose expression was restricted to cell lines bearing the high affinity mIL-5 receptor (27). Analysis of the gene amplification of the α chain cDNA by PCR technique revealed that spleen cells, peritoneal exudate cells, and IL-5-dependent cell lines expressed transcripts corresponding to both membrane-bound form and soluble forms of the mIL-5 receptor α chain (27). COS7 cells transfected with the mIL-5 receptor α chain cDNA expressed at a density of 10^5 to 10^6 IL-5 binding sites per cell with low-affinity (K*d* of 6–9 nM). We then transfected the cDNA into IL-3-dependent cell line FDC-P1 (mIL-5 receptor α chain-negative) and established FDC-5R. FDC-5R expressed ~500 binding sites per cell for IL-5 with K*d* of 30 pM (high affinity) and 8,000 binding sites per cell with K*d* of 6 nM (low affinity) and became responsive to IL-5 for DNA synthesis (27). These results indicate that the mIL-5 receptor α chain cDNA encodes the low affinity mIL-5 receptor and that the α chain can associate with additional molecule(s) for the formation of the functional (high-affinity) mIL-5 receptor complex.

The mIL-5 Receptor β Chain (p130) is the IL-3 Receptor-Like Molecule, AIC2B

The anti-mIL-5 receptor mAb R52.120 described by Rolink et al. (30) down-regulated the number and K*d* of the high affinity IL-5 binding sites without affecting the levels of those with low affinity (31). Furthermore, R52.120 mAb inhibited the IL-3-driven proliferation of FDC-P1. Moreover, anti-mIL-3 receptor (anti-Aic-2) mAb (32) reacted with all five IL-5 responsive cell lines and down-regulated the expression of high affinity receptors (33). Both R52.120 and anti-Aic-2 mAbs immunoprecipitated similar doublet membrane proteins of 130–140 kD from Y16 or FDC-P1 cells, whereas they did not react with the recombinant α chain (31,33). These results suggest that the p130/p140 protein is indispensable together with the α chain for the formation of the high affinity mIL-5 receptor and appears to be involved in the mIL-3 receptor system. Anti-Aic-2 mAb recognizes the low affinity mIL-3 receptor (AIC2A) (34) and its homologue (AIC2B) (35). AIC2B is only 18 amino acid residues longer than AIC2A and has 91% amino acid sequence identity with AIC2A (35). The identity of the R52.120 protein with both AIC2A and AIC2B was verified using stable L cell transfectant. L cell transfectant expressing the mIL-5 receptor α chain alone (L-5R) expressed the low-affinity mIL-5 receptor. L-5R derived clones, transfected with AIC2A cDNA (L-5R-2A) and AIC2B cDNA (L-5R-2B), expressed almost equal amounts of the respective cDNA products. Only L-5R-2B reconstituted both high affinity (K*d* of 15 pM) and low affinity (K*d* of 2.2 nM) mIL-5 receptor (Fig. 2) (33). L cells transfected with AIC2A (L-2A) or AIC2B transfectants (L-2B) did not show any specific binding for IL-5 at concentraions up to 4 nM. When L-5R-2B was cross-linked with radiolabeled IL-5, two cross-linked complexes (p170 and p100) were detected. In contrast, we did not detect p170 cross-linked band in L-5R-2A or any cross-linked band in L-2B (33). These results clearly indicate that AIC2B hardly binds IL-5 by itself, but it contributes to the formation of the high-affinity mIL-5 receptor by interacting with the α chain. The dissociation of IL-5 from L-5R-2B was much slower than from L-5R, whereas association kinetics of IL-5 to both L-5R-2B and L-5R were almost similar. AIC2B may therefore stabilize the binding of IL-5 to the mIL-5 receptor. Recently Devos et al. independently clarified that AIC2B is a component of the high affinity IL-5R complex (36).

Characterization of the Human IL-5 Receptors on Eosinophils

Binding Characteristics of Human IL-5 Receptors

Peripheral blood eosinophils isolated from healthy volunteers and from a patient with id-

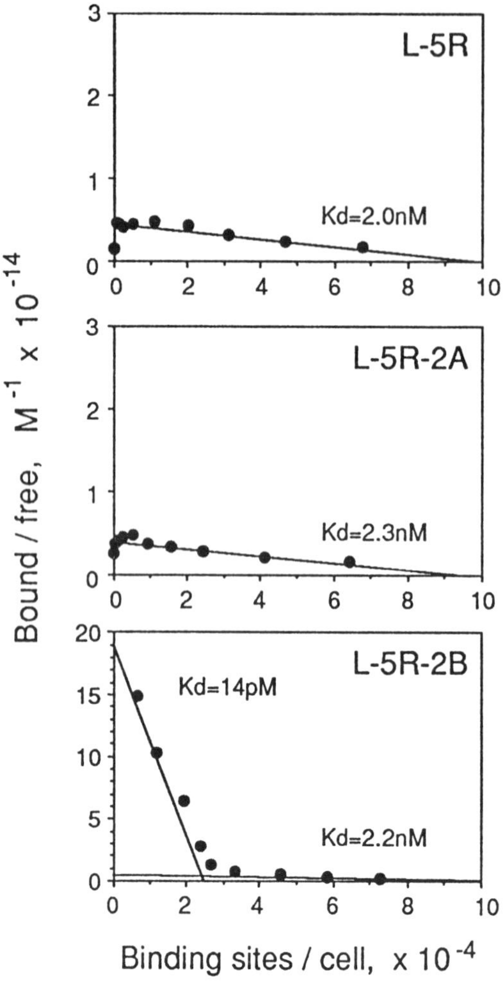

Figure 2. Scatchard plot analysis of 35S-labeled IL-5 binding to L cell transfectants (A) L-5R; (B) L-5R-2A; (C) L-5R-2B. (Taken from Takaki *et al.* (33).

iopathic eosinophilic syndrome responded to hIL-5 and mIL-5 for prolonged survival *in vitro* (37). Both ^{35}S-methionine labeled mIL-5 and ^{125}I-hIL-5 specifically bound to eosinophils. Scatchard plot analysis of the saturation binding data revealed that there is a single class (high affinity, K*d* of 170~330 pM) of the mIL-5 binding sites (260~380/cell) (37). Eosinophils from patients with eosinophilia and an eosinophilic subline of HL-60 gave similar estimates for the K*d* (38,39). Tonsillar B cells, peripheral blood neutrophils, Burkitt's lymphoma cell lines, ATL cell lines, ALL cell line, AMoL cell lines, erythroleukemia, and histiocytic leukemia cells did not express detectable numbers of IL-5 binding sites (37). Affinity cross-linking experiments revealed that IL-5 binds to 55–60 kD protein on eosinophils.

Isolation and Characterization of the Human IL-5 Receptor cDNA Clones

We constructed a cDNA library from peripheral blood eosinophils from healthy volunteers and the patient with eosinophilia. Using the ^{32}P-labeled *Hind*III-*Pst*I fragment of the mIL-5 receptor α chain cDNA as a probe, we isolated a clone (lh5R.12) by plaque hybridization (Murata et al., submitted). The entire nucleotide sequence of lh5R.12 cDNA contains one reading frame of 1260-bp that showed considerable similarity to coding sequence of the mIL-5 receptor α chain. lh5R.12 sequence can encode a polypeptide of 420 amino acids containing the N-terminal signal sequence, extracellular domain, a membrane-spanning segment, and intracellular domain. We also isolated a clone that encodes only the extracellular domain of this receptor molecule. Analysis of the predicted amino acid sequence indicated that the hIL-5 receptor has about 70% amino acid sequence homology with the mIL-5 receptor α chain (Fig. 1) and retains features common to the cytokine receptor superfamily. We also found fibronectin type III motifs not only in domains that belong to the cytokine receptor superfamily, but also in the N-terminal domain. RNA blot analysis demonstrated the presence of two species of mRNA transcripts (~5.3-kb and 1.4-kb) whose expression was restricted to human eosinophils and human erythroleukemic cell line TF-1 that expressed the high affinity hIL-5 receptor.

Binding and Biochemical Characteristics of the Recombinant Human IL-5 Receptor.

We inserted lh5R.12 cDNA fragments into the expression vector pCAGGS obtaining pCAGGS-h5R.12. COS7 transfectants with pCAGGS-h5R.12 specifically bound hIL-5 with an apparent K*d* of 590 pM (high affinity) (Fig. 3). Chemical cross-linking experiments of radiolabeled hIL-5 revealed that estimated molecular size of recombinant hIL-5 receptor would be about 60 kD. The results indicate

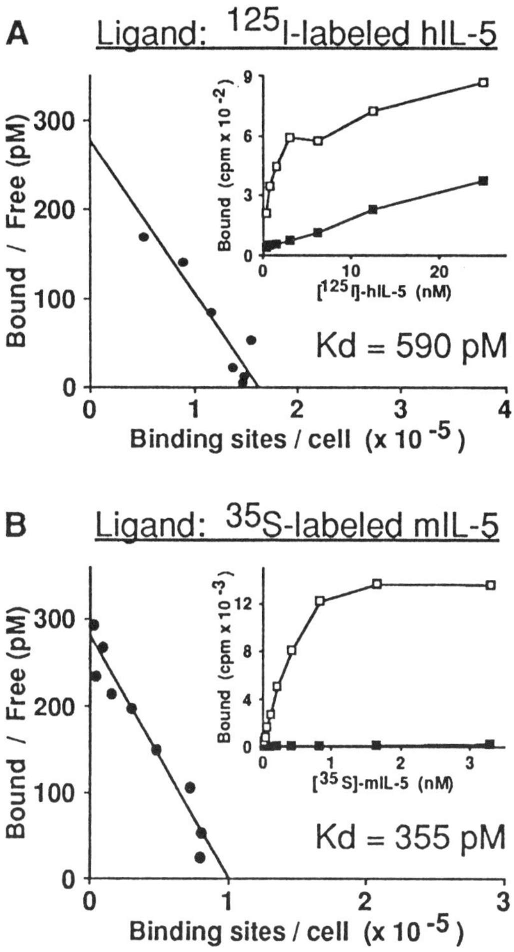

Figure 3. Scatchard plot analysis of radiolabeled IL-5 binding to the transfectants expressing the cloned hIL-5 receptor cDNA. The inset shows the direct binding data (❑, total binding; ■, non-specific binding). Points are means of duplicate determinations. Binding of 125I-hIL-5 (A) or 35S-labeled mIL-5 (B) to COS7 cells transfected with pCAGGS-h5R.12.

that both K*d* values and estimated molecular sizes of recombinant hIL-5 receptor are similar to those observed on eosinophils in peripheral blood (37). Cotransfection of pSV2-neo and pCAGGS-5R.12 into FDC-P1 induced the proliferation in response to hIL-5 for DNA synthesis. These results indicate that the hIL-5 receptor cDNA isolated in this study is a component of the functional hIL-5 receptor.

Interpretations

We identified the two polypeptide chains (α and β) involved in the construction of the high affinity mIL-5 receptor. The α chain binds mIL-5 with low affinity and associates with the β chain that is mIL-3 receptor-like protein, AIC2B resulting in the formation of the high affinity mIL-5 receptor (Fig. 4). Recently evidence has been presented that AIC2B appears to be a subunit of mGM-CSF receptor and essential for signal transduction (40). In mouse, AIC2B appears to be involved in both receptor systems for IL-5 and GM-CSF. If we consider that both IL-5 and GM-CSF support the growth and differentiation of eosinophils and have some different function, we have to ask how the signal of IL-5 is different from that of GM-CSF. The signals generated by both cytokines may be equivalent, and different functions of these cytokines are due to the various developmental stages of cells expressing the receptors. Alternatively, different signal transducing molecules, which generate a specific signal for each cytokine, are associated with respective ligand binding subunit (α chain) of each receptor. There is still the possibility that the ligand binding subunit of each receptor is involved in generating their respective signals. These possibilities are not mutually exclusive. It is noteworthy that AIC2B is not only the low affinity mIL-3 receptor (AIC2A)-like protein even in the cytoplasmic domain, but is also coexpressed with AIC2A in many cell lines (35). Furthermore, IL-3, IL-5, and GM-CSF induce phosphorylation of a similar set of proteins (41). In any case, therefore, part of the signal transducing machinery of IL-5 may be shared with GM-CSF, and even with IL-3. The predicted mature hIL-5 receptor has about 70% homology with that of the mIL-5 receptor α chain. The existence of the β chain of hIL-5 receptor is also suggested, because the mIL-5 receptor consists of α and β chain as described in the previous sections. Hayashida et al. (42) reported that the low-affinity hGM-CSF receptor together with the KH97 protein, encoded by a human cDNA homologous to mIL-3 receptor cDNA, forms the high affinity hGM-CSF receptor. Because the KH97 protein does not bind IL-3, the KH97 protein is the β chain of hGM-CSF receptor (42). In light of these studies, we interpret our results in two different

Recently, the existence of Th-1 and Th-2 subsets in man in certain disease situations has been demonstrated, with cytokine production patterns which are similar, but not identical to those found in the mouse. In general, the human counterpart of the murine Th-1 subset was demonstrated among T cell clones derived from donors with inflammatory diseases, whereas Th-2 like T cells were established from allergic patients (21). These findings indicate that human T cells can be primed *in vivo* to subsets with different cytokine production patterns under particular conditions.

It has been documented that prostaglandin E2 (PGE2) suppresses many functions of T cells in many experimental systems (22). The mechanism of action of PGE2 is thought to be mediated via the increase of intracellular second messengers such as cAMP. PGE2 suppressed the proliferation of SP-B21 cells induced by either anti CD3 Mab or TPA/A23187. However, the effects of PGE2 on cytokine production were more complicated. PGE2 suppressed anti CD3 Mab-induced production of GM-CSF, Th-1 cytokines IFN-γ and IL-2, and Th-2 cytokines IL-5 and IL-10, which is produced by human Th-1 and Th-2 like T cell clones (Yssel, H., et al., submitted for publication). It should be noted however that, among Th-2 cytokines, IL-4 is rather resistant to PGE2 (Table I). By contrast, PGE2 did not affect TPA/A23187-induced production of the above mentioned cytokines by SP-B21 clone with the exception of IL-5 which was elevated. In fact, TPA was shown to reverse the inhibitory effects of PGE2 on anti-CD3 induced cytokine production. Furthermore, the inhibitory action of PGE2 on anti CD3 Mab-induced cell proliferation of SP-B21 clone was effectively blocked by IL-2 in dose-dependent manner (Table I). Likewise, IL-2 restored the cell's abililty to produce most cytokines in response to anti CD3 Mab and in the presence of PGE2. However, IL-2 failed to restore PGE2-induced suppression of cell proliferation in the presence of TPA/A23187. Under the same conditions, IL-2 restored PGE2-induced elevation of IL-5 to normal level whereas other cytokines were not appreciably affected. These results indicate that PGE2 or other mediators produced by activated macrophages or mast cells can modulate T cell response. Therefore, the interplay between T cells and inflammatory cells through production of cytokines and lipid mediators may be the important elements in regulating inflammatory processes.

Regulation of Cytokine Genes on Chromosome 5 in Human T Cells

IL-3 gene is composed of 5 exons and 4 introns, whereas GM-CSF, IL-4 and IL-5 genes are composed of 4 exons and 3 introns (23). They are all located on human chromosome 5 (Fig. 3) and on murine chromosome 11. IL-3 and GM-CSF are only 9 and 14 kb apart in human and murine, respectively, and IL-4 and IL-5 genes are clustered within a several hundred kb region. Loss of the whole or the long arm of chromosome 5 has been observed in malignant cells of patients with acute lymphocytic leukemia. The 5′ flanking regions of IL-3 and GM-CSF genes share a short stretch of homologous sequences. Two homologous DNA motifs are at position -108 to -99 (5′-GGAGATTCCCA-3′, CLE1) and -94 to -88 (5′-TCAGGTA-3′, CLE2) in the murine GM-CSF gene (24). CLE1 is rela-

Table 1. Effects of PGE2 and IL-2 on cell proliferation and cytokine production from human T cell clone SP-B21.

Stimulus	Additions		Cytokine production [pg/ml]					Proliferation [cpm]
	PGE2 3*	IL-2 4*	IL-4	IL-5	IFN-g	GM-CSF	IL-10	
TPA 1* + A23187 2*	–	–	1559	4388	43000	70418	0	4882
	–	+	1626	4680	41398	70642	0	4480
	+	–	3146	14165	23000	27011	0	733
	+	+	1384	3143	22000	24978	0	301
anti CD3	–	–	650	2201	1153	3284	12689	9863
	–	+	1223	6969	841	5356	64458	23729
	+	–	0	0	0	0	0	145
	+	+	1070	2600	0	0	0	22401

1* TPA:1 ng/ml, 2* A23187:500 ng/ml, 3* PGE2:10 uM, 4* IL-2:100 units/ml tively well conserved among cytokines whereas CLE2, well conserved in IL-3, is not necessarily found in other cytokines. Downstream of CLE2 is a sequence motif that is referred to as a GC box, similar to the recognition site of transcription factor Sp1. Transfection experiments have established that the final target of the GM-CSF gene mediating the response to T cell activation signals is CLE2/GC box (24). The CLE2/GC-box contains at least two DNA binding motifs (25). One is the inducible NF-GM2 binding sequence GGTAGTTCCCC (positions -91 to -81) and the other is the GC-rich sequence CCCCGCC which can be recognized constitutively by non-inducible factors. NF-GM2, induced by TPA/A23187 stimulation, effectively competed with the NF-kB consensus sequence which suggests that NF-GM2 is an NF-kB-like protein (26). In addition to CLE2/GC box, an additional element (CLE0) at positions -40 to -54 of the GM-CSF gene is required for induction by TPA/A23187 in T cells (27). CLE0 shows homology to sequences in IL-4, IL-5 and G-CSF genes, and forms an inducible protein-DNA complex with NF-CLE0. These results indicated that multiple proteins, both inducible and constitutive, interact with the 5′ flanking region of the GM-CSF gene to initiate transcription. However, it is not known whether other cytokine genes are regulated by common transactivator(s) or unique ones specific for each. Likewise, it remains to be established whether NF-KB-like proteins can account for the coordinate regulation of cytokine genes (23,28).

Figure 3. Localization of several cytokine genes on human chromosome 5.

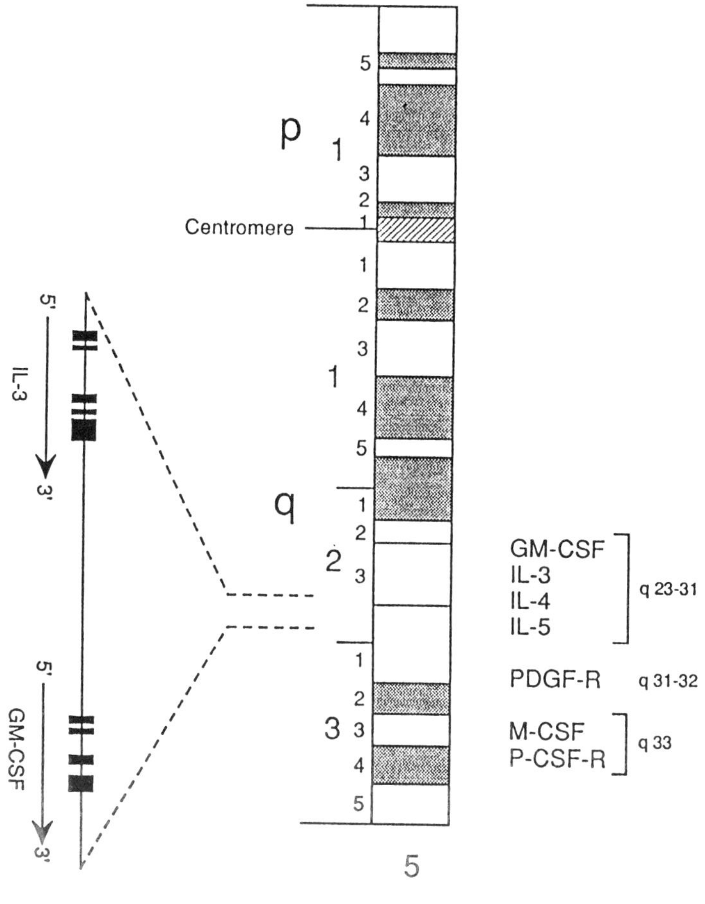

Growth Factor-Type and Cytokine-Type Receptors on Mast Cells

Cytokines are generally pleiotropic (23,29). This strongly indicated that the ligand-binding unit of the cytokine receptors may be coupled to multiple signal transduction components and there would be cross-communication among cytokine receptors. This notion was verified by the recognition that increasing numbers of cytokine receptors form a new cytokine receptor family based on their common sequence motif. Unlike EGF, PDGF and FGF receptors, none of the cytoplasmic domains of these cytokine receptors has tyrosine kinase activity. Among cytokines that stimulate mast cells, basophils and eosinophils, IL-3, IL-4, IL-5 and GM-CSF receptors are the members of cytokine receptor family, and Sl product interacts with proto-oncogene c-kit which is the member of growth factor receptor family having tyrosine kinase activity (30). Epithelial cells or fibroblasts may be regulated primarily by members of the growth factor receptor family whereas lymphocytes may be mainly regulated by members of the cytokine receptor family. It appears that proliferation and differentiation of many hemopoietic cells are controlled by two types of receptors, i. e., cytokine receptor family and growth factor receptor family. IL-3, IL-4, IL-5 and GM-CSF produced transiently by activated T cells and mast cells support inducible proliferation of hemopoietic cells (Fig. 4). In contrast, Sl product and M-CSF support constitutive proliferation of mast cells and macrophages by interacting with c-kit and c-fms, respectively. Probably, growth factor type receptor may be the cellular device to support proliferation and/or survival of hemopoietic cells which have the ability to migrate to various tissues outside of blood vessels during inflammation. The two types of receptor systems may be activated in a different manner under particular conditions. The balance that many occur between the activation of two systems may be important for determining the nature of the cellular responses for immune response and development.

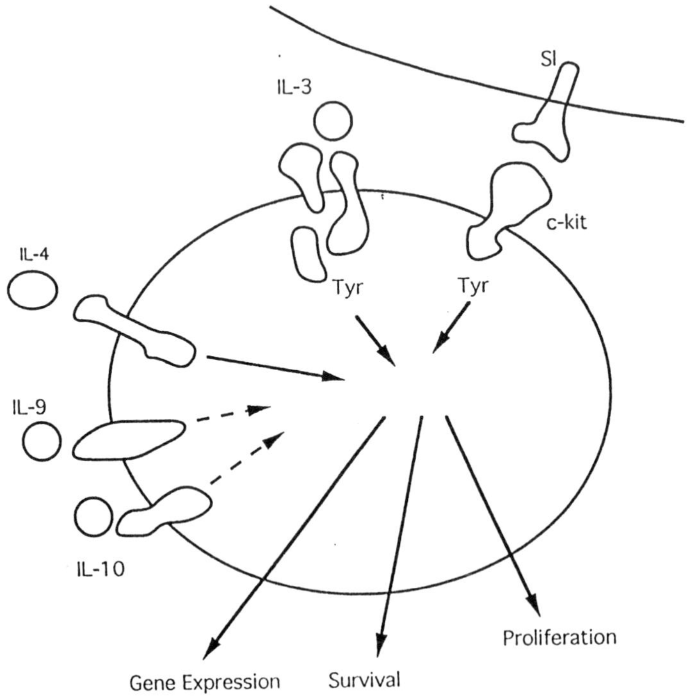

Figure 4. Multiple receptors that stimulate mast cell growth.

Structure of the Murine IL-3 Receptor

Murine IL-3 receptor exibits both high and low affinities. By using anti-Aic2 Mab, which partially blocks IL-3 binding, a mouse IL-3 receptor cDNA (AIC2A) that encodes a protein of 878 amino acids was isolated (31)(Fig.5). The AIC2A protein binds IL-3 with low affinity which is rapidly dissociated. The extracellular domain (417 amino acids) is divided into two segments each of which contains a common motif of the cytokine receptor family.(32). Although evidence indicates that IL-3 induces protein tyrosine phosphorylation, the cytoplasmic domain of the AIC2A protein does not have a tyrosine kinase activity. It is incapable of transducing proliferation signals when expressed in fibroblasts. Most likely, additional component(s) may be required to reconstitute functional high affinity receptor capable of transducing growth promoting signals. Using the same antibody, another cDNA (AIC2B) encoding a protein of 896 amino acids was isolated (33). AIC2B is 91% identical to the IL-3 receptor (AIC2A) but does not bind any cytokines examined including IL-3, IL-5 and GM-CSF. AIC2A and AIC2B proteins are encoded by two distinct genes which are closely linked on murine chromosome 15. These two genes probably arose by gene duplication and their expression is tightly coregulated.

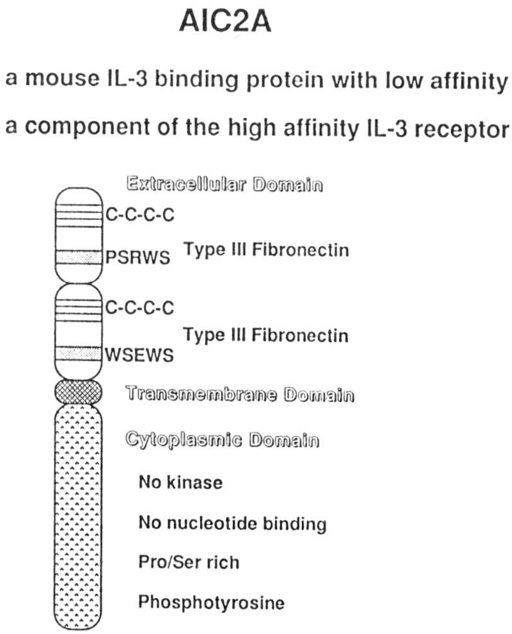

Figure 5. Structure of AIC2A protein

Structure of High-Affinity Human GM-CSF and IL-3 Receptors

A human cDNA (KH97) was isolated based on the homology with the AIC2A cDNA (34). This cDNA encodes a protein of 897 amino acids which is 56% identical to murine AIC2A and AIC2B and has features in common with the cytokine receptors. KH97 protein by itself is unable to bind human IL-3 or GM-CSF by. However, we speculated that KH97 protein may be the second component of the high affinity GM-CSF receptor. In fact, this was found to be the case. Cotransfection of fibroblasts with the KH97 clone and the cDNA encoding low-affinity human GM-CSF receptor (α chain) (Fig.6) resulted in the formation of a high-affinity GM-CSF receptor (34). This indicated that KH97 cDNA encodes the second component (β chain) of the GM-CSF receptor. IL-3 and GM-CSF share overlapping biological activities and induce similar intracellular signals. The fact that the human GM-CSF receptor is composed of two chains and the β chain is highly homologous to murine IL-3 receptor prompted us to reevaluate the structure of the IL-3 receptor. There are several indications that IL-3 and GM-CSF receptors share the same components in their ligand binding units. First, human GM-CSF partially but specifically inhibits the binding of human IL-3 and vice versa in certain human hemopoietic cells. Second, IL-1 upregulates the larger component of both IL-3 and GM-CSF receptors in a similar manner (35). Based on these observations, it was hypothesized that the IL-3 receptor is also composed of two chains one of which is shared with the GM-CSF receptor. In fact, the cDNA encoding the α subunit of the human IL-3 receptor was isolated by cotransfection of the GM-CSF receptor β cDNA with a cDNA library made from an IL-3 dependent cell line. Cloned IL-3 receptor α chain cDNA encodes a protein of

Table II. Development of mast cells in the skin grafts

Donors	Receipients	Mast cells /cm skin grafts[a]
W/W^v mice	+/+ mice [b]	414
W/W^v mice	nude mice [c]	487
Sl/Sl^d mice	+/+ mice [b]	3
Sl/Sl^d mice	nude mice [c]	1
Ws/Ws rats	nude rats [b]	495

a: Numbers of mast cells were counted in paraffin sections.
b: Skin pieces of embryos were grafted under the kidney capusule (11).
c: Skin pieces of adult mice were grafted on the back (3).

c-*kit* cDNA was determined by using a cDNA library prepared from the hippocumpus of Spargue-Dawley rats. The coding region of the c-*kit* gene showed 91% homology between rats and mice and 83% homology between rats and humans. The predicted amino acid sequence showed 92% homology between rats and mice and 84% homology between rats and humans (23). The c-*kit* cDNA of *Ws/Ws* and normal (+/+) control rats was obtained by reverse transcriptase modification of the polymerase chain reaction. When compared with authentic sequence, a deletion of 12 bases was found in the c-*kit* cDNA of *Ws/Ws* rats (Figure 1). This change was shown to be a result of the deletion of the genomic DNA. Four amino acids encoded by the deleted 12 bases (i. e., Val-Lys-Gly-Asn) were located at two amino acids downstream from autophosphorylation site in the c-*kit* kinase and were conserved not only in mouse and human c-*kit* kinases but also in mouse and human c-*fms* kinases (i. e., receptors of colony-stimulating factor-1) (Figure 1). Since the deleted four amino acids appear to have an important physiological role, the *Ws/Ws* rat is the first animal characterized with a mutant of the c-*kit* gene after the mouse (23).

Infection of *Nippostrongylus brasiliensis to Ws/Ws* Rats

The proportion of basophils is very small in leukocytes of mice and rats; basophils are hardly detectable in blood smears of these animals. We performed direct counts of basophils rather than differential counts of total leukocytes for the accurate determination of the basophil number. Since an appreciable volume of blood is necessary for the direct counts, rats are better than mice as experimental animals due to their bigger size. The number of basophils is known to increase markedly in rats infected with *N. brasiliensis* (24). We studied the effect of *N. brasiliensis* infection on numbers of basophils in *Ws/Ws* and control +/+ rats. Basophils started to increase from Day 7 after the infection and reached a peak value on Day 14; a 100-fold increase was observed. The basophil number decreased thereafter, and resumed the pre-infection levels on Day 28 after the infection. There was no significant difference between *Ws/Ws* and +/+ rats, suggesting that the stimulus through the c-*kit* receptor does not play an indispensable role for production of basophils.

The infection of *N. brasiliensis* is also known to induce a marked increase of mucosal type mast cells (MMC) in the small intestine (25–27). Although some MMC were present in the lamina propria of non-infected +/+ rats, no MMC were detectable in the lamina propria of *Ws/Ws* rats. When *N. brasiliensis* were infected, the number of MMC showed a 10-fold increase in +/+ rats, and MMC did develop in the lamina propria of *Ws/Ws* rats. The proportion of mast cells in S phase was determined by injecting bromodeoxyuridine 1 hour before sacrifice. The incorporated bromodeoxyuridine was demonstrated by immunohistochemistry. The proportion reached a maximum value on Day 14 and dropped to the pre-infection level on Day 21. No significant difference was detectable between +/+ and *Ws/Ws* rats. The number of MMC started to increase from Day 14 after the infection and attained a maximum value on Day 21 in both +/+ and *Ws/Ws* rats. Since practically no MMC were detectable in non-infected *Ws/Ws* rats, the relative number of MMC divided by the pre-infection value was greater in *Ws/Ws* rats than in +/+ rats. However, the absolute number of MMC in the lamina propria of *Ws/Ws* rats was about 10% that of +/+ rats on Day 21, and was comparable to the pre-infection value of +/+ rats.

Mast cells in intestinal epithelium are called globule leukocytes (28). Globule leukocytes were not observed in both +/+ and *Ws/Ws* rats before the infection of *N. brasiliensis*. On Days 14 and 21 after the infection, a considerable number of globule leukocytes were observed in both +/+ and *Ws/Ws* rats. Here again the number of globule leukocytes in *Ws/Ws* rats was about 10% that of +/+ rats. In spite of the apparent development of MMC and globule leukocytes in the intestine of *Ws/Ws* rats, mast cells did not develop in the skin of *Ws/Ws* rats. Mast cells in S phase were hardly detectable in the skin of +/+ rats.

Egg count per gram feces (EPG) was done to estimate the activity of worms. EPG became negative on Day 14 after the infection, and there was no significant difference between +/+ and *Ws/Ws* rats in the regression curve of EPG. Whether development of MMC and globule leukocytes is indispensable for expulsion of helminths has not been determined. The present experiment does not give any answers to this question, either. Even if the development of MMC and globule leukocytes is necessary, the small numbers of MMC and globule leukocytes as observed in the intestine of *Ws/Ws* rats (i.e., 10% those of +/+ rats) appear to be enough for the expulsion of *N. brasiliensis*.

The increase of MMC does not occur in nude athymic mice and rats infected with helminths (5,25–27), and the nunber of basophils does not increase in nude rats infected with *N. brasiliensis* (24). Therefore the production of MMC and basophils appears to be dependent on T cells.

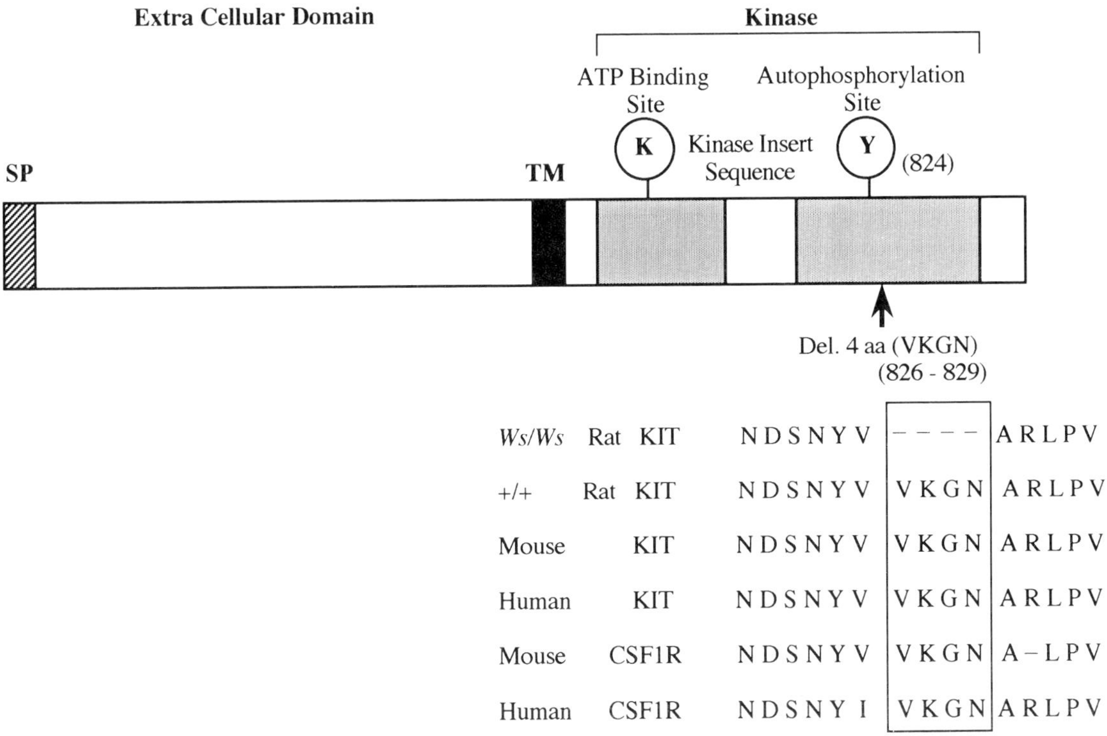

Figure 1. A schema of c-*kit* receptor tyrosine kinase and a comparison of amino acid sequences. Amino acid residues (820 through 834) of rat c-*kit* protein (KIT) are compared with homologous regions of mouse and human KIT and mouse and human c-*fms* proteins (CSF1R). The deletion of four amino acids (i.e., Val-Lys-Gly-Asn), residues 826 through 829 observed in KIT of *Ws/Ws* rats, is boxed. Dashed lines were introduced for optimal alignment. SP, signal peptide; TM, transmembrane portion.

Table III. Necessity of fibroblast-dependent and T-cell-dependent mechanisms for development of connective tissue-type mast cells, mucosal-type mast cells and basophils

Cell types	Necessity of each mechanism Fibroblast-dependent	T-cell-dependent
Connective tissue-type mast cells	Yes	No
Mucosal-type mast cells	Yes	Yes
Basophils	No	Yes

The T cell-dependent increase of MMC appears to be mediated by IL-3, IL-4, IL-9, and IL-10 (29–31), and the T cell-dependent increase of basophils at least by IL-3 (32,33). Although MMC does not develop in the intestine of *W/W*^{v} mice infected with *N. brasiliensis* (34), MMC did develop in the intestine of *Ws/Ws* rats infected with the helminth. Since the infusion of pharmacological doses of IL-3 resulted in the development of MMC in *W/W*^{v} mice (35), there is a possibility that sufficient amounts of T cell-derived cytokines are not produced in the *W/W*^{v} mice infected with *N. brasiliensis.*

The numbers of basophils were comparable between *Ws/Ws* and +/+ rats infected with *N. brasiliensis*, a 100-fold increase was observed in both animals. On the other hand, the numbers of MMC and globule leukocytes in the intestine of *Ws/Ws* rats was about 10% those of +/+ rats. This suggests that only a T cell-dependent mechanism is enough for production of basophils and that both T cell-dependent and fibroblast-dependent mechanisms are necessary for production of MMC (Table III). Since practically no mast cells were detectable in the skin of *Ws/Ws* rats infected with *N. brasiliensis*, the fibroblast-dependent mechanism mediated by the c-*kit* receptor appears to be indispensable for development of connective tissue-type mast cells (CTMC). Taken together, *Ws/Ws* rats infected with *N. brasiliensis* are a useful model to discriminate T-cell-dependent and fibroblast-dependent mechanisms for production of basophils, MMC and CTMC.

References

1. Kitamura, Y., Shimada, M., Hatanaka, K., and Miyano, Y. 1987. Development of mast cells from grafted bone marrow cells in irradiated mice. Nature 268:442.
2. Kitamura, Y., Go, S., and Hatanaka, K. 1978. Decrease of mast cells in *W/W*^{v} mice and their increase by bone marrow transplantation. Blood 52:447.
3. Kitamura, Y., Shimada, M., Go, S., Matsuda, H., Hatanaka, K., and Seki, M. 1979. Distribution of mast cell precursors in hematopoietic and lymphopoietic tissues of mice. J. Exp. Med. 150:482.
4. Kitamura, Y., and Go, S. 1979. Dcreased production of mast cells in *Sl/Sl*^{d} anemic mice. Blood 53:492.
5. Kitamura, Y. 1989. Heterogeneity of mast cells and phenotypic change between subpopulations. Ann. Rev. Immunol. 7:59.
6. Kitamura, Y., Nakayama, H., and Fujita, J. 1989. Mechanisms of mast cell defficiency in mutant mice of *W/W*^{v} and *Sl/Sl*^{d} genotype. In: Mast cell and basophil differentiation and function in health and disease. S.J. Galli, and K.F. Austen, eds. New York: Raven Press, p. 15.
7. Kitamura, Y., Yokoyama, M., Matsuda, H., Ohno, T., and Mori, K. J. 1981. Spleen colony forming cell as common precursor for tissue mast cells and granulocytes. Nature 291:159.
8. Sonoda, T., Katayama, Y., Hara, H., Hayashi, C., Tadokoro, M., Yonezawa, T., and Kitamura, Y. 1984. Proliferation of peritoneal mast cells in the skin of *W/W*^{v} mice. J. Exp. Med. 160:138.
9. Kuriu, A., Sonoda, S., Kanakura, Y., Jozaki, K., Yamatodani, A., and Kitamura, Y. 1989. Proliferative potential of degranulated murine peritoneal mast cells. Blood 74:925.
10. Jozaki, K., Kuriu, A., Waki, N., Adachi, S., Yamatodani, A., Tarui, S., and Kitamura, Y. 1990. Proliferative potential of murine peritoneal mast cells after degranulation induced by compound 48/80, substance P, tetradecanoy I-phorbol acetate, or calcium ionophore A23187. J. Immunol. 145:4252.
11. Niwa, Y., Kasugai, T., Ohno, K., Morimoto, M., Yamazaki, M., Dohmae, K., Nishimune, Y., Kondo, K., and Kitamura, Y. 1991. Anemia

and mast cell depletion in mutant rats that are homozygous at "White spotting (*Ws*)" locus. Blood 78:1936.

12. Russell, E.S. 1979. Hereditary anemia of the mouse: A review for geneticists. Adv. Genet. 20:357.
13. Chabot, B., Stephenson, D. A., Chapman, V. M., Besmer, P., and Bernstein, A. 1988. The proto-oncogene c-*kit* encoding a transmembrane tyrosine kinase receptor maps to the mouse *W* locus. 1988. Nature 335:88.
14. Geissler, E. N., Ryan, M. A., and Houseman, D. E. 1988. The dominant-white spotting (*W*) locus of the mouse encods the c-*kit* proto-oncogene. Cell 55:185.
15. Besmer, P., Murphy, P. C., George, P. C., Qui, F., Bergold, P. J., Lederman, L., Snyder, H. W., Brodeur, D., Zuckerman, E. E., and Hardy, W. D. 1986. A new acute transforming feline retrovirus and relationship of its oncogene v-*kit* with the protein kinase gene family. Nature 320:415.
16. Yarden, Y., Kuang, W. J., Yang-Feng, T., Coussens, L., Munemitsu, S., Dull, T. J., Chen, E., Schlessinger, J., Francke, U., and Ullrich, A. 1987. Human proto-oncogene c-*kit*: A new cell surface receptor tyrosine kinase for an unidentified ligand. EMBO J. 6:3341.
17. Qui, F., Ray, P., Brown, K., Barker, P.E., Jhanwar, S., Ruddle, F. H., and Besmer, P. 1988. Primary structure of c-*kit*: Relationship with the CSF-1/PDGF receptor kinase family—oncogenic activation of v-*kit* involves deletion of extracellular domain and C-terminus. EMBO J. 7:1003.
18. Williams, D. E., Eisenman, J., Baird, A., Rauch, C., Ness, K. V., March, C. J., Park, L. S., Martin, U., Mochizuki, D. Y., Boswell, H. S., Burgess, G. S., Cosman, D., and Lyman, S. D. 1990. Identification of ligand for the c-*kit* proto-oncogene. Cell 63:167.
19. Flanagan, J. G., and Leder, P. 1990. The *kit* ligand: A cell surface molecule altered in steel mutant fibroblasts. Cell 63:185.
20. Zsebo, K. M., Williams, D. A., Geissler, E. N., Broudy, V. C., Martin, F. H., Atkins, H. L., Hsu, R. Y., Birkett, N. C., Okino, K. H., Murdock, D. C., Jacobson, F. W., Langley, K. E., Smith, K. A., Takeishi, T., Cattanach, B. M., Galli, S. J., and Suggs, S. V. 1990. Stem cell factor is encoded at the *Sl* locus of the mouse and is the ligand for the c-*kit* tyrosine kinase receptor. Cell 62:213.
21. Huang, E., Nocka, K., Beier, D. R., Chu, T. Y., Buck, J., Lahm, H. W., Wellner, D., Leder, P., and Besmsr, P. 1990. The hematopoietic growth factor KL is encoded by the *Sl* locus and is the ligand of the c-*kit* receptor, the gene product of the *W* locus. Cell 63:225.
22. Galli, S. J., and Kitamura, Y. 1987. Animal model of human disease: Genetically mast cell-deficient W/W^v and Sl/Sl^d mice. Their value for the analysis of the role of mast cells in biologic responses *in vivo*. Am. J. Pathol. 127:191.
23. Tsujimura, T., Hirota, S., Nomura, S., Yamazaki, M., Tono, T., Morii, E., Kim, H. M., and Kitamura, Y. 1991. Characterization of *Ws* mutant allele of rat: 12 base deletion in tyrosine kinase domain of c-kit gene. Blood 78:1942.
24. Ogilvie, B. M., Askenase, P. W., and Rose, M. E. 1980. Basophils and eosinophils in three strains of rats and in athymic (nude) rats following infection with the nematodes *Nippostrongylus brasiliensis* or *Trichinella spiralis*. Immunology 39:385.
25. Befus, A. D., and Bienenstock, J. 1979. Immunologically mediated intestinal mastocytosis in *Nippostrongylus brasiliensis*-infected rats. Immunology 38:95.
26. Woodbury, R. G., Miller, H. R. P., Huntley, J. F., Newlands, G. F. J ., Palliser, A. C., and Wakelin, D. 1984. Mucosal mast cells are functionally active during spontaneous expulsion of intestinal nematode infections in rats. Nature 312:450.
27. Arizono, N., and Nakao, S. 1988. Kinetics and staining properties of mast cells proliferating in rat small intestine tunica musclalis and subserosa following infection with *Nippostrongylus brasiliensis*. APMIS 96:964.
28. Murray, M., Miller, H. R. P., and Jarrett, W. F. H. 1968. The globule leukocyte and its derivation from the subepithelial mast cell. Lab. Invest. 19:222.
29. Arai, K., Lee, F., Miyajima, A., Miyatake, S., Arai, N., and Yokota, T. 1990. Cytokine: Coordinators of immune and inflammatory responses. Ann. Rev. Biochem. 59:783.
30. Huntler, L., Moeller, J., Schmitt, E., Jagar, G., Reisbach, G., Ring, J., and Dormer, J. 1989. Thiol-sensitive mast cell line derived from mouse bone marrow respond to a mast cell growth-enhancing activity different from both IL-3 and IL-4. J. Immunol. 142:3440.
31. Thompson-Snipes, L., Dhar, V., Bond, M. W., Mosmann, T. R., Moore, K. W., and Rennick, D. M. 1991. Interleukin 10: A novel stimulatory factor for mast cell and their progenitors. J. Immunol. 142:507.

32. Saito, H., Hatake, K., Dvorak, A. M., Leiferman, K. M., Donnenberg, A. D., Arai, N., Ishizaka, K., and Ishizaka, T. 1988. Selective differentiation and proliferation of hematopoetic cells by recombinant human interleukins. Proc. Natl. Acad. Sci. USA 85:2288.
33. Mayer, P., Valent, P., Schmidt, G., Liehl, E., Bettelheim, P. 1989. Interleukin-3 is a differentiation factor for human basophils. Blood 73:1763.
34. Kojima, S., Kitamura, Y., and Takatsu, K. 1980. Prolonged infection of *Nippostrongylus brasiliensis* in genetically mast cell depleted *W/W^v* mice. Immunol. Lett.. 2:159.
35. Ody, C., Kindler, V., and Vassalli, P. 1990. Interleukin 3 perfusion in *W/W^v* mice allows the development of macroscopic hematopoietic spleen colonies and restores cutaneous mast cell number. J. Exp. Med. 172:403.

Ultrastructural Identification of Human Mast Cells Arising in *In Vitro* Culture Systems

Ann M. Dvorak, Teruko Ishizaka*

Isolated human lung mast cells co-cultured with 3T3 fibroblasts maintain their *in vivo* ultrastructural phenotype characterized by large numbers of scroll granules and lipid bodies. By contrast, human mast cells arising in co-cultures of human cord blood cells and 3T3 fibroblasts are distinguished by the presence of numerous crystal granules and the relative absence of lipid bodies, an ultrastructural phenotype analogous to that of human skin mast cells. The ultrastructural criteria for assignment of cells to the mast cell lineage differ from criteria for assignment of cells to the macrophage lineage, cells that also appear in co-cultures of cord blood cells and 3T3 fibroblasts. These criteria are reviewed here, as well as those for the identification of immature cells in the eosinophil and basophil lineages, lineages which also develop in human cord blood cells cultured with appropriate growth factors.

Human mast cells have been maintained in short-term cultures, either after IgE-mediated degranulation or not, following their isolation from human lung samples (1–3) or either with or without 3T3 fibroblasts cultured with them for longer terms (up to 1 month) (4,5). In the latter case, functional assays have shown either enhanced release or new generation of mast cell-derived mediators over that found in initially isolated human lung mast cells (5). More recently, a reliable culture system for the development of cells of the mast cell lineage in humans was described (6). In this case, human cord blood mononuclear cells were co-cultured with Swiss albino mouse skin-derived 3T3 fibroblasts, and mast cells were definitively identified by their unique crystal-containing granules (6,27). Additionally, these cells were shown to contain histamine, tryptase, chymase and Fcε receptors (6).

Numerous pitfalls are associated with the correct lineage assignment of cultured human mast cells. Electron microscopy is one important tool necessary for investigations designed to determine these assignments. A number of recent studies have suggested that human mast cells, either developing in or becoming established from variable sources in culture, have occurred (reviewed in 27). Some of these studies present certain morphological difficulties regarding these conclusions (reviewed in 27). We review here (a) the necessary morphological criteria for the identification of human mast cells arising in culture systems, (b) the morphological criteria for the identification of the most commonly misinterpreted cellular lineages including macrophages (7–9), eosinophils (7,9–12), and basophils (9,10,13,14), and (c) the morphological similarities of mast cells arising in co-cultures of cord blood cells and 3T3 fibroblasts (6,27) to human skin mast cells *in vivo* (15,16).

Isolated human lung mast cells maintain their *in vivo* phenotype in short-term cultures during recovery from IgE-mediated anaphylactic degranulation and in long-term co-cultures with or without 3T3 fibroblasts

Human lung mast cells *in vivo* (17,18), following isolation procedures (19), during short-term cultures (either unstimulated or during recovery from IgE-mediated anaphylactic de-

---

* Departments of Pathology, Beth Israel Hospital and Harvard Medical School, and the Charles A. Dana Research Institute, Beth Israel Hospital, Boston, Massachusetts 02215; the Division of Allergy, La Jolla Institute for Allergy and Immunology, La Jolla, California 92037.
Acknowledgements: Supported by U.S.P.H.S. grants CA-28834 and AI-10060. We thank Susan Kissell-Rainville and Patricia Estrella for technical assistance, and Peter K. Gardner for editorial assistance.

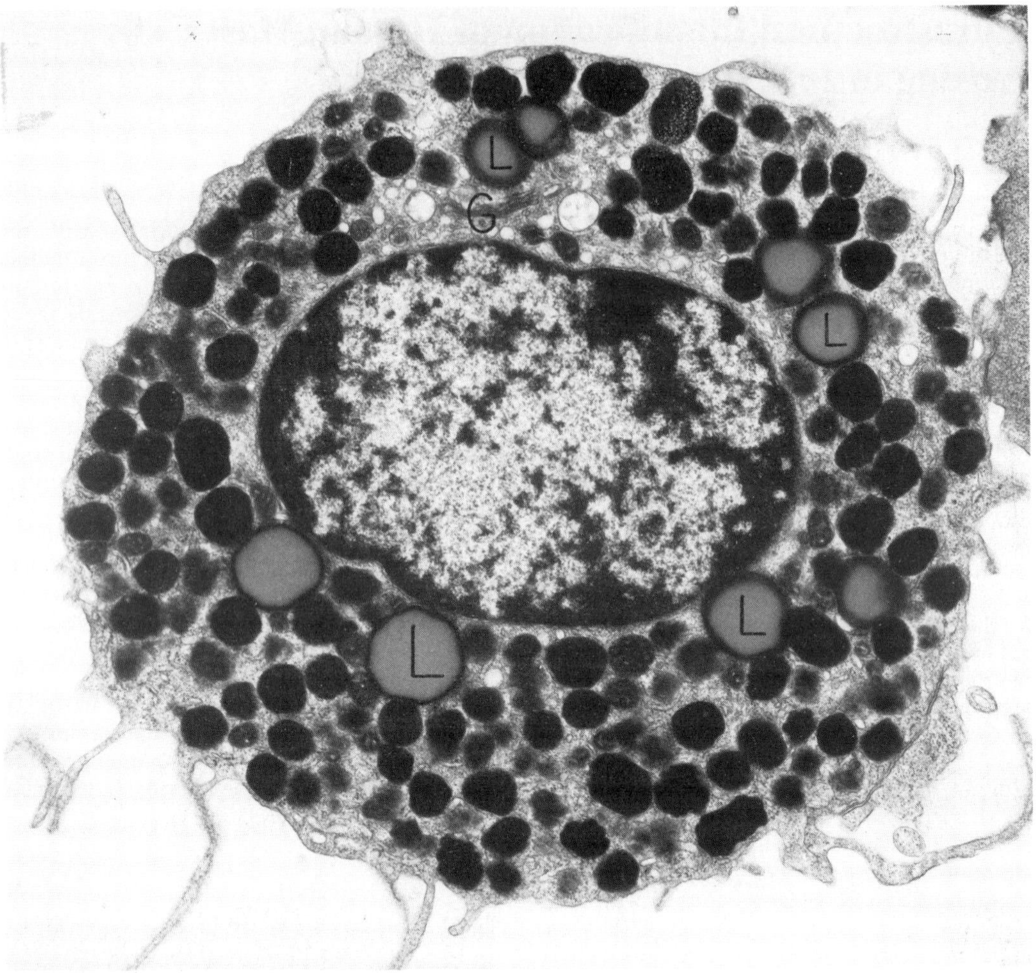

Figure 1. Isolated human lung mast cell co-cultured with 3T3 fibroblasts for one month shows a completely granulated mononuclear cell with narrow surface folds. A small Golgi apparatus (G), eight lipid bodies (L), and numerous dense granules are present. ×12,500.

granulation [1–3]), and during long-term co-cultures with (Fig. 1) or without 3T3 fibroblasts (4), maintain their ultrastructural phenotypic features despite the superimposed morphologies associated with functional states and recovery therefrom, as well as cell isolation and culture. For example, this cellular population frequently displays variable numbers of an intracytoplasmic organelle known to be involved with arachidonic acid metabolism: lipid bodies (Figs. 2, 3) (1–3,20–23). Also, the predominant granule pattern (scrolls: Figs. 2, 3) prevails, whether these cells are examined *in vivo*, *ex situ*, or *in vitro*. Particle granules and mixed granules are also evident, but true crystal granules are quite rare. Lipid bodies are not unique to mast cells. They can be present in a wide variety of mammalian cells (24,25). Lipid

Figure 2. Isolated human lung mast cell in culture for one month shows numerous lipid bodies (L) and granules completely filled with scrolls. ×23,500.

Figure 3. Isolated human lung mast cell in culture for one month shows a typical scroll granule and a lipid body (L) at high magnification. ×36,500.

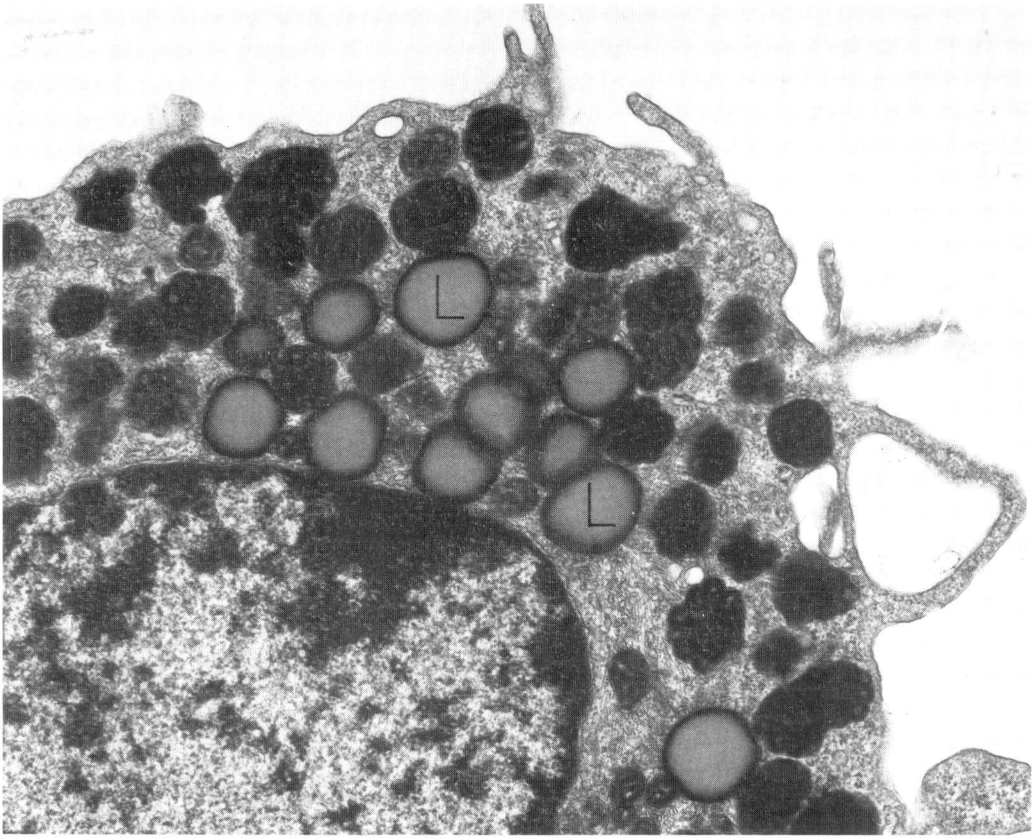
L
L

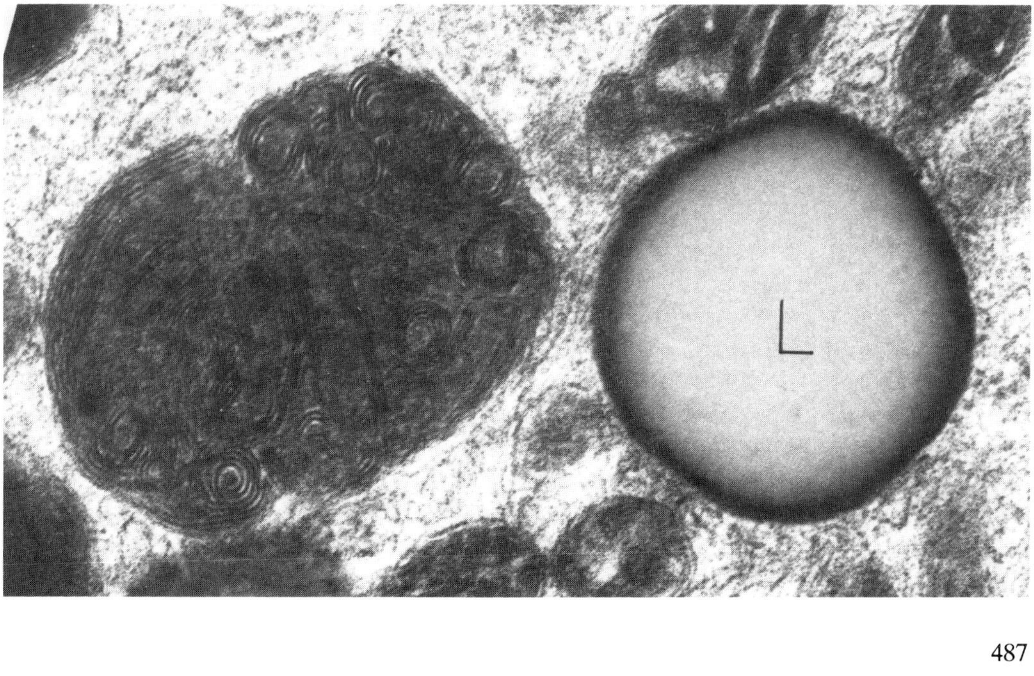
L

bodies are also not invariably present in human mast cells. For example, they are extremely rare in normal human skin mast cells *in vivo* (15). Scroll granules, present in quantity, are very suggestive for the identification of human mast cells. We have seen certain membranous arrays within human basophil granules that resemble human mast cell scroll granules. In general, they are more frequently seen in basophils accompanying malignant myelocytic proliferations than in peripheral blood basophils in either the blood vascular space, tissues, after isolation procedures, or arising *de novo* from human cord blood mononuclear cells cultured in various growth media or in rhIL-3 or rhIL-5 (9,10,13,14). Thus, classical scroll granules in quantity are more typical of the mast cell lineage than of the basophil lineage.

Human mast cells arising *de novo* in co-cultures of 3T3 fibroblasts and cord blood mononuclear cells resemble human skin mast cells *in vivo*

Human skin mast cells *in vivo* (15), following isolation procedures and short-term cultures, either unstimulated or after IgE-mediated degranulation (16), are distinguished by the small number of cytoplasmic lipid bodies present and by the predominance of crystal granules. Scroll and mixed granules are also noted; particle granules are, however, exceedingly unusual. Mature human mast cells, arising *de novo* in

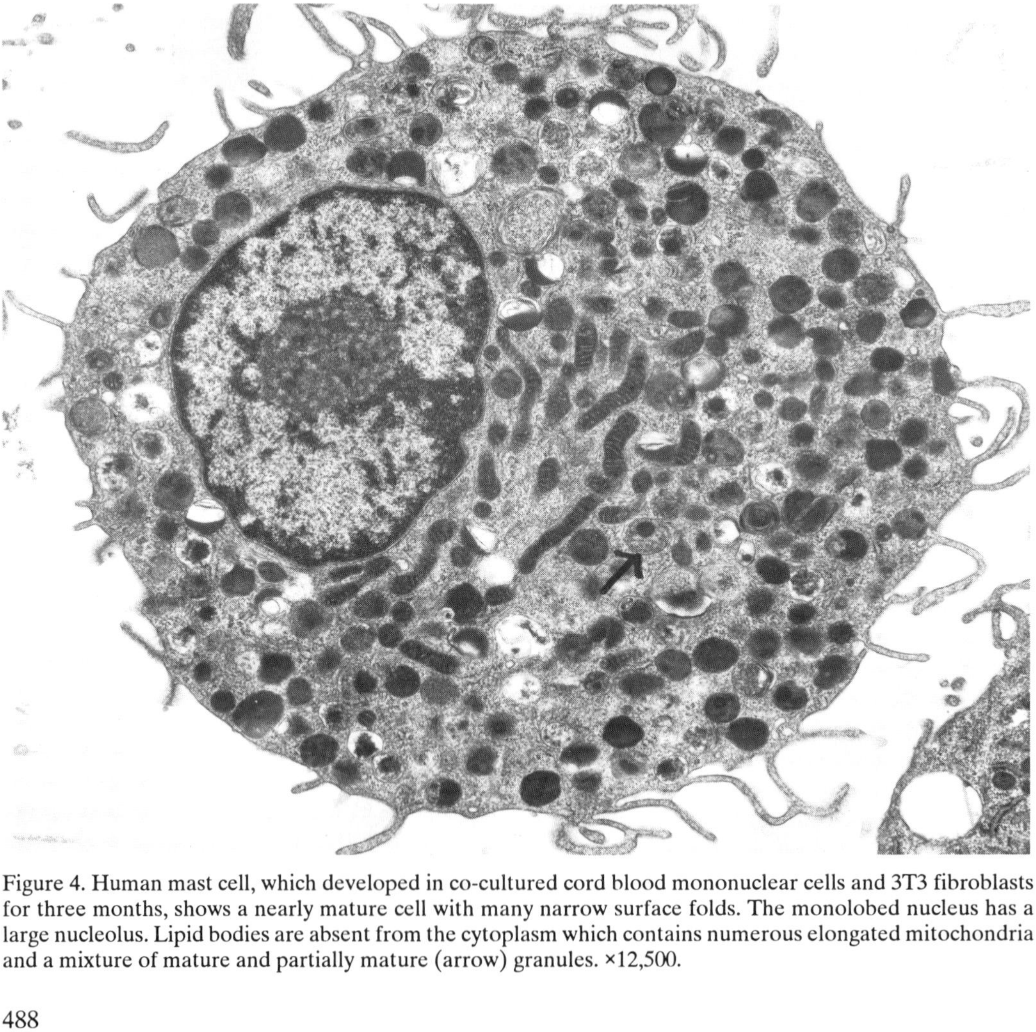

Figure 4. Human mast cell, which developed in co-cultured cord blood mononuclear cells and 3T3 fibroblasts for three months, shows a nearly mature cell with many narrow surface folds. The monolobed nucleus has a large nucleolus. Lipid bodies are absent from the cytoplasm which contains numerous elongated mitochondria and a mixture of mature and partially mature (arrow) granules. ×12,500.

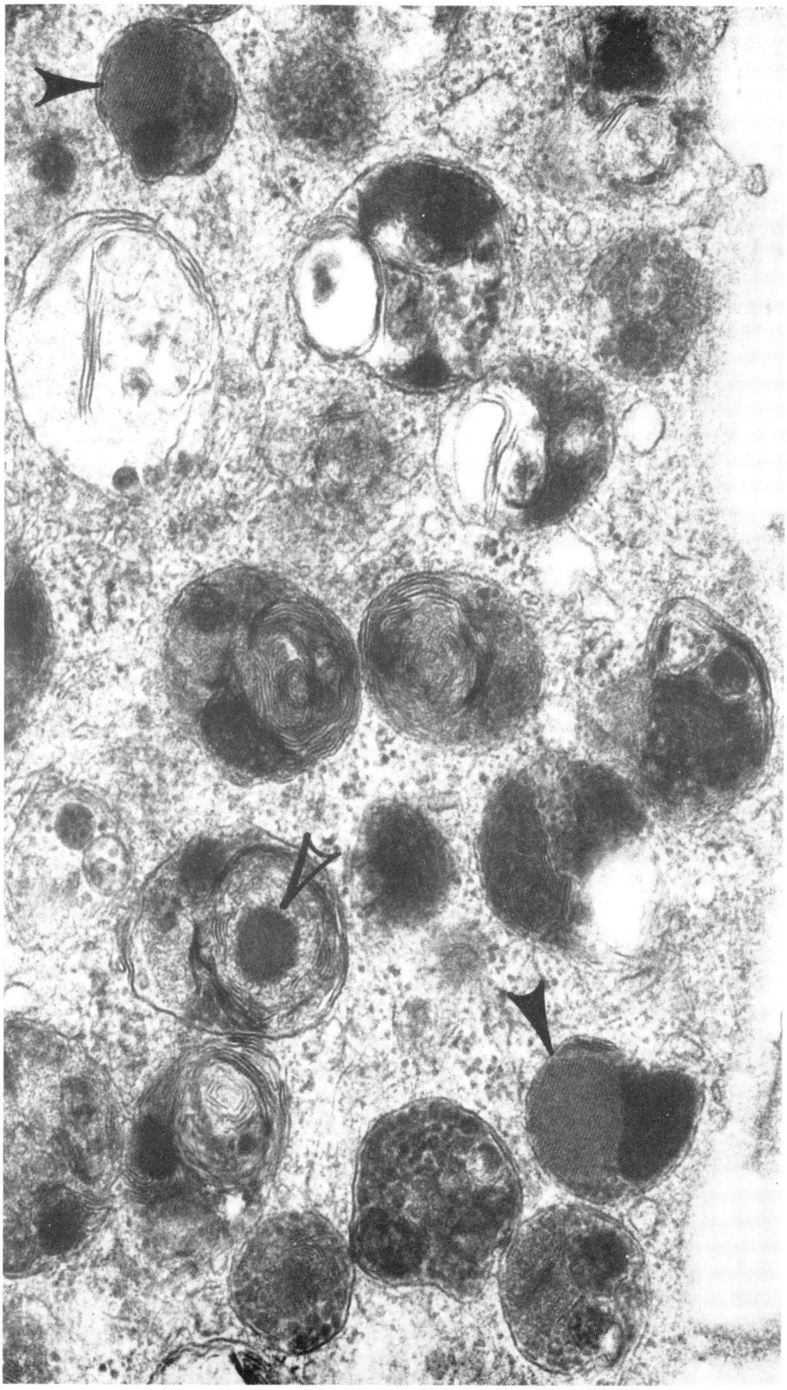

Figure 5. Higher magnification micrograph of a similarly developing mast cell shows typical immature developing granules with central dense nucleoid (open arrowhead), granules with variable mixtures of dense, vesicular, and membranous contents and classical crystal granules (closed arrowheads). x61,000.

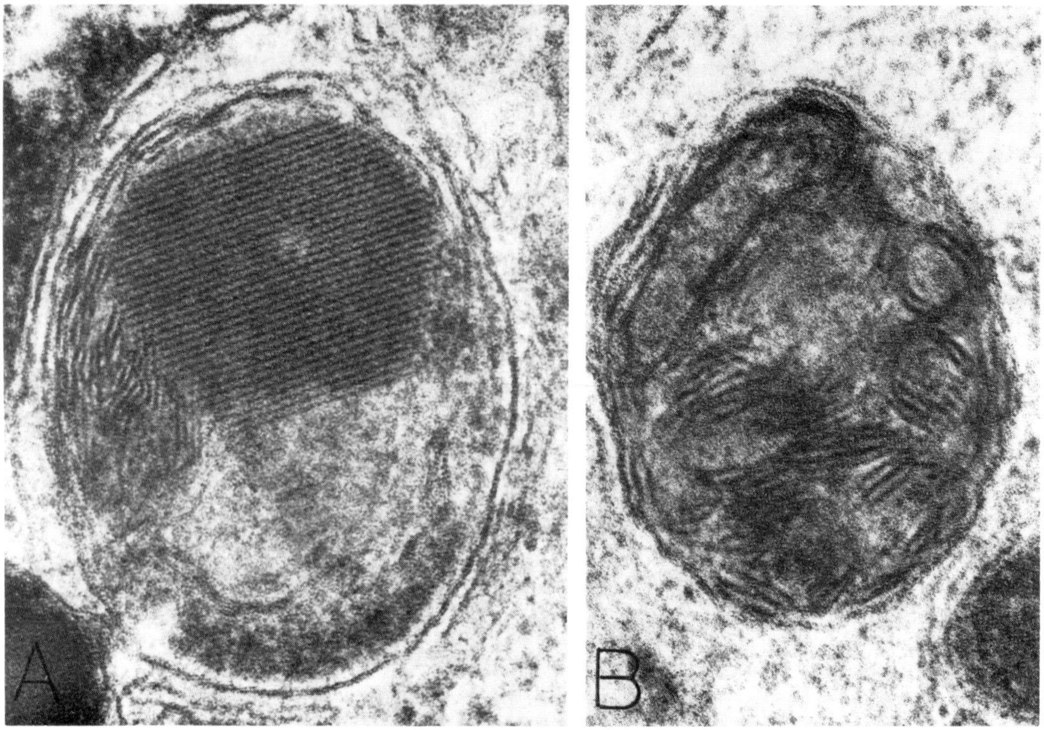

Figure 6. Typical crystal (A) and scroll (B) granules seen at high magnification in mast cells arising after three months of co-cultures of human cord blood cells and 3T3 fibroblasts. A. ×97,000; B. ×109,000.

co-cultures of 3T3 fibroblasts and cord blood cells examined by electron microscopy at 3 months, shared these features of human skin mast cells (27) (Fig. 4) (6). That is, lipid bodies were unusual, and crystal granules were plentiful (Figs. 5, 6A). Scroll (Fig. 6B) and mixed granules could be found, but particle granules were unusual. Additional features of a maturing lineage were noted. Thus, nuclear size, lobulation and chromatin condensation, nucleoli, cytoplasmic organelles associated with synthesis, and partially filled immature granules with condensing nucleoids existed in immature mast cells that were simultaneously present with mature mast cells in these co-cultures (27). Crystal granules (Fig. 6A) are specific to the mast cell lineage in humans (18,26). They have never been seen in human basophil (or eosinophil) granules, and we have never found them in macrophages, a cell lineage that is generally present in long-term cultures of either cord blood cells or isolated lung mast cells (4,7,9,10). Therefore, crystal granules are sufficiently unique that the identification of the mast cell lineage can be made with certainty when they are found.

Macrophages are ubiquitous in culture systems and can be identified with certainty

We regularly find macrophages (Figs. 7,8) in long-term cultures of human cord blood cells or isolated human lung mast cells (4,7,9,10). These cells are readily distinguished from cells in the mast cell lineage as follows. Mast cell crystal, scroll, mixed or particle granules are absent. Lipid bodies are sometimes present, often in quantity, and thus cannot be used to distinguish these two cellular lineages. Macrophage nuclei are generally more complex in their contours than are the monolobed mast cell nuclei, and macrophage nuclear chromatin is less con-

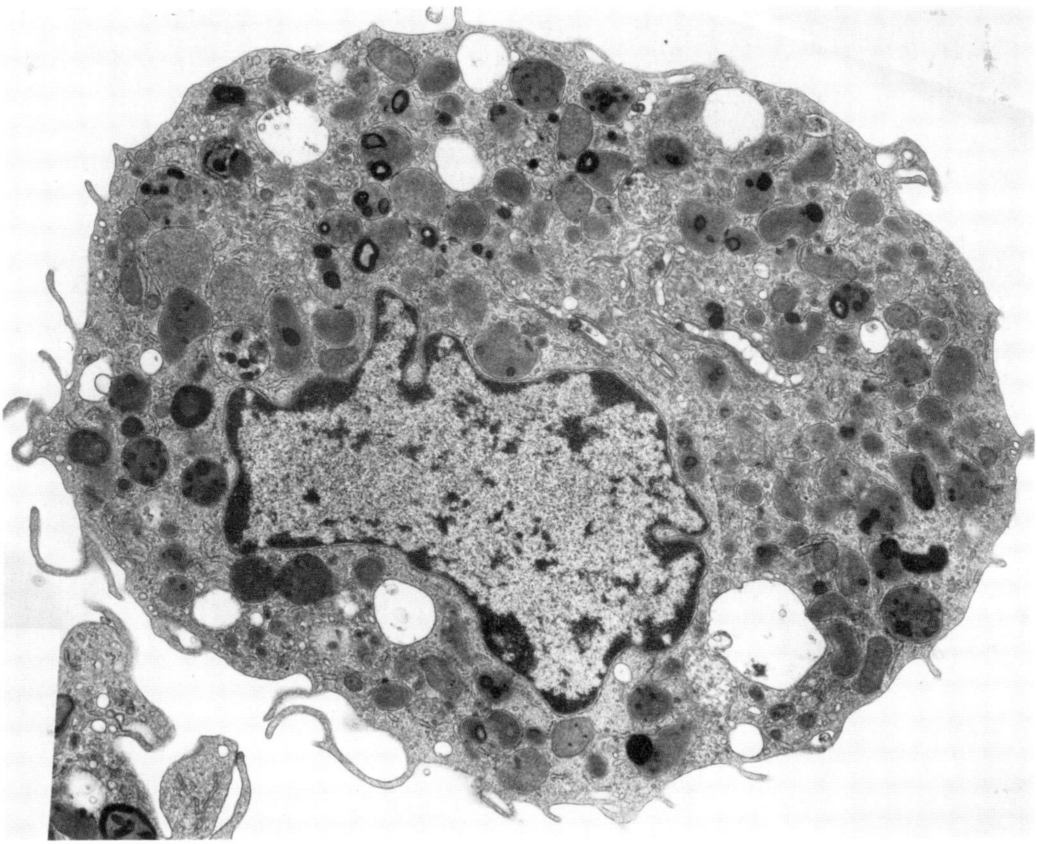

Figure 7. Human macrophage, from a six-week culture of cord blood mononuclear cells in 3T3 fibroblast supernatant, shows typical macrophage ultrastructural morphology. The monolobed nucleus has an irregular shape, and the chromatin is dispersed. The surface has focal narrow surface folds. The cytoplasm is filled with a mixture of electron-lucent vacuoles and membrane-bound dense bodies of variable size, shape, and contents. These are typical macrophage lysosomes and phagolysosomes. Other cytoplasmic organelles include a Golgi area, vesicles, short narrow strands of rough endoplasmic reticulum, and several mitochondria. ×11,500.

densed than the chromatin in mature mast cell nuclei. Macrophage and mast cell surfaces both have narrow folds; however, extensive involvement of macrophage surface folds with prominent underlying endocytotic structures is absent in mast cells. Macrophages generally have variable amounts of non-dilated cisterns of rough endoplasmic reticulum, whereas these structures are exceedingly rare in mature mast cells. Most conspicuously, however, macrophages contain numerous lysosomes and phagolysosomes (Figs. 7,8). Primary lysosomes are small, dense, membrane-bound granules of variable shape that generally reside in the Golgi area; they are also present in focal clusters throughout the cytoplasm. Secondary lysosomes are those which have acquired structures destined for destruction in them, whether it be from within (autophagosomes) or from the microenvironment (phagolysosomes). In the former case, effete mitochondria, cytoplasmic segments, membranes, etc., are contained within electron-dense structures; in the latter case, identifiable internalized materials prevail. Many times, the precise identity of materials in phagolysosomes or in autophagosomes is not possible in electron micrographs. Thus, variable mixtures of membranous arrays, vesicles, and densities constitute these electron-dense membrane-bound structures (Fig. 8). The com-

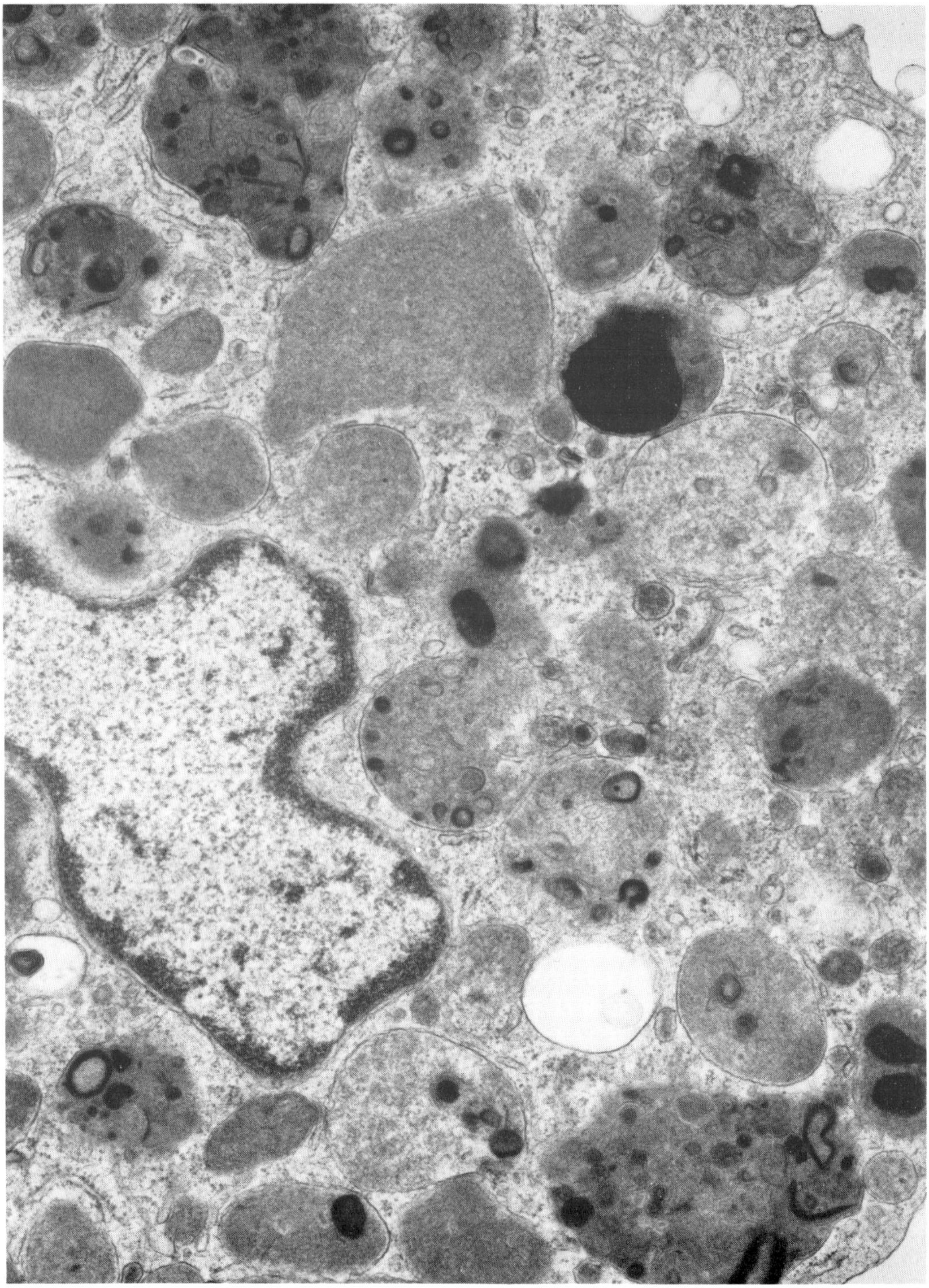

Figure 8. Higher magnification micrograph of a human macrophage from similar culture shows the heterogeneous size, shape, and contents of cytoplasmic phagolysosomes. ×25,000.

pelling findings which set these electron-dense granules apart from the secretory granules of mast cells are their extreme size, shape and content variabilities. Thus, the size range of macrophage lysosomes is great, whereas the size of mature mast cell granules is fairly uniform. While the shape of mast cell granules is variable, it is not generally as variable as that of macrophage lysosomes. For example, shape irregularities of mast cell granules are associated with the addition of unit progranules (18,22) and, therefore, are visibly related to this process as, for example, individual scrolls are added to scroll or mixed granules. The shape of macrophage lysosomes can be extra-ordinarily malformed by their residual internalized contents. These morphological guidelines should serve to assign the ubiquitous macrophages to their correct lineage and to avoid their incorrect assignment to the mast cell lineage in humans.

Eosinophil and basophil lineages are generally easy to distinguish from the mast cell lineage when mature cells predominate, but the discrimination of their myelocytic precursors can be difficult

Eosinophilic and basophilic myelocytes are of similar size to those of human mast cells (9–13). Their distinctive immature and mature granules and extensive arrays of dilated cisterns of rough endoplasmic reticulum serve to delineate these three lineages (all of which can have blue-to-purple granules in Giemsa-stained, plastic embedded light microscopic preparations) in electron microscopy samples (9–13,18).

References

1. Dvorak, A.M., Schleimer, R.P., Schulman, E.S., and Lichtenstein, L.M. 1986. Human mast cells use conservation and condensation mechanisms during recovery from degranulation. *In vitro* studies with mast cells purified from human lungs. Lab. Invest. 54:663.
2. Dvorak, A.M., Schleimer, R.P., and Lichtenstein, L.M. 1987. Morphologic mast cell cycles. Cell. Immunol. 105:199.
3. Dvorak, A.M., Schleimer, R.P., and Lichtenstein, L.M. 1988. Human mast cells synthesize new granules during recovery from degranulation. *In vitro* studies with mast cells purified from human lungs. Blood 71:76.
4. Dvorak, A.M., Furitsu, T., Estrella, P., and Ishizaka, T. 1991. Human lung-derived mast cells cultured alone or with mouse 3T3 fibroblasts maintain an ultrastructural phenotype that is different from that of human mast cells that develop from human cord blood cells cultured with 3T3 fibroblasts. Am. J. Pathol. 139:1909.
5. Levi-Schaffer, F., Austen, K.F., Caulfield, J.P., Hein, A., Gravallese, P.M., and Stevens, R.L. 1987. Co-culture of human lung-derived mast cells with mouse 3T3 fibroblasts: Morphology and IgE-mediated release of histamine, prostaglandin D_2, and leukotrienes. J. Immunol. 139:494.
6. Furitsu, T., Saito, H., Dvorak, A.M., Schwartz, L.B., Irani, A.-M.A., Burdick, J.F., Ishizaka, K., and Ishizaka, T. 1989. Development of human mast cells *in vitro*. Proc. Natl. Acad. Sci. U.S.A. 86:10039.
7. Dvorak, A.M., Furitsu, T., Letourneau, L., Ishizaka, T., and Ackerman, S.J. 1991. Mature eosinophils stimulated to develop in human cord blood mononuclear cell cultures supplemented with recombinant human interleukin-5. I. Piecemeal degranulation of specific granules and distribution of Charcot-Leyden crystal protein. Am. J. Pathol. 138:69.
8. Dvorak, A.M., Weller, P.F., Monahan-Earley, R.A., Letourneau, L., and Ackerman, S.J. 1990. Ultrastructural localization of Charcot-Leyden crystal protein (lysophospholipase) and peroxidase in macrophages, eosinophils and extracellular matrix of the skin in the hypereosinophilic syndrome. Lab. Invest. 62:590.
9. Dvorak, A.M., Saito, H., Estrella, P., Kissell, S., Arai, N., and Ishizaka, T. 1989. Ultrastructure of eosinophils and basophils stimulated to develop in human cord blood mononuclear cell cultures containing recombinant human interleukin-5 or interleukin-3. Lab. Invest. 61:116.
10. Dvorak, A.M., Ishizaka, T., and Galli, S.J. 1985. Ultrastructure of human basophils developing *in vitro*. Evidence for the acquisition of peroxidase by basophils and for different effects of human and murine growth factors on

human basophil and eosinophil maturation. Lab. Invest. 53:57.
11. Saito, H., Hatake, K., Dvorak, A.M., Leiferman, K.M., Donnenberg, A.D., Arai, N., Ishizaka, K., and Ishizaka, T. 1988. Selective differentiation and proliferation of hematopoietic cells induced by recombinant human interleukins. Proc. Natl. Acad. Sci. U.S.A. 85:2288.
12. Dvorak, A.M., Ackerman, S.J., and Weller, P.F. 1991. Subcellular morphology and biochemistry of eosinophils. In: Blood cell biochemistry, Vol. 2: Megakaryocytes, platelets, macrophages and eosinophils. J.R. Harris, ed. London: Plenum, p. 237.
13. Dvorak, A.M. 1988. Morphologic and immunologic characterization of human basophils, 1879 to 1985. Riv. Immunol. Immunofarmacol. 8:50.
14. Ishizaka, T., Dvorak, A.M., Conrad, D.H., Niebyl, J.R., Marquette, J.P., and Ishizaka, K. 1985. Morphologic and immunologic characterization of human basophils developed in cultures of cord blood mononuclear cells. J. Immunol. 134:532.
15. Dvorak, A.M., Kissell, S. 1991. Granule changes of human skin mast cells characteristic of piecemeal degranulation and associated with recovery during wound healing *in situ*. J. Leukocyte Biol. 49:197.
16. Dvorak, A.M., Massey, W., Warner, J., Kissell, S., Kagey-Sobotka, A., and Lichtenstein, L.M. 1991. IgE-mediated anaphylactic degranulation of isolated human skin mast cells. Blood 77:569.
17. Peters, S.P., Dvorak, A.M., and Schulman, E.S. 1989. Mast cells. In: Lung cell biology. D. Massaro, ed. [Vol. 41 in the series: Lung biology in health and disease. C. Lenfant, series ed.]. New York: Marcel Dekker, p. 345.
18. Dvorak, A.M. 1989. Human mast cells. In: Advances in anatomy, embryology, and cell biology, Vol. 114. F. Beck, W. Hild, W. Kriz, R. Ortmann, J.E. Pauly, and T.H. Schiebler, series eds. Berlin: Springer, p. 1.
19. Dvorak, A.M. 1989. Recovery of human lung mast cells from anaphylactic degranulation utilizes a mixture of conservation and synthetic mechanisms. In: Mast cell and basophil differentiation and function in health and disease. S.J. Galli, K.F. Austen, eds. New York: Raven, p. 119.
20. Dvorak, A.M., Dvorak, H.F., Peters, S.P., Schulman, E.S., MacGlashan, Jr., D,W,, Pyne, K., Harvey, V.S., Galli, S.J., and Lichtenstein, L.M. 1983. Lipid bodies: Cytoplasmic organelles important to arachidonate metabolism in macrophages and mast cells. J. Immunol. 131:2965 (republished, 1984, J. Immunol. 132:1586).
21. Dvorak, A.M., Hammel, I., Schulman, E.S., Peters, S.P., MacGlashan, Jr., D.W., Schleimer, R.P., Newball, H.H., Pyne, K., Dvorak, H.F., Lichtenstein, L.M., and Galli, S.J. 1984. Differences in the behavior of cytoplasmic granules and lipid bodies during human lung mast cell degranulation. J. Cell Biol. 99:1678.
22. Hammel, I., Dvorak, A.M., Peters, S.P., Schulman, E.S., Dvorak, H.F., Lichtenstein, L.M., and Galli, S.J. 1985. Differences in the volume distributions of human lung mast cell granules and lipid bodies: Evidence that the size of these organelles is regulated by distinct mechanisms. J. Cell Biol. 100:1488.
23. Dvorak, A.M., Schulman, E.S., Peters, S.P., MacGlashan, Jr., D.W., Newball, H.H., Schleimer, R.P., Lichtenstein, L.M. 1985. Immunoglobulin E-mediated degranulation of isolated human lung mast cells. Lab. Invest. 53:45.
24. Galli, S.J., Dvorak, A.M., Peters, S.P., Schulman, E.S., MacGlashan, Jr., D.W., Isomura, T., Pyne, K., Harvey, V.S., Hammel, I., Lichtenstein, L.M., and Dvorak, H.F. 1985. Lipid bodies: Widely distributed cytoplasmic structures that represent preferential nonmembrane repositories of exogenous [^{3}H]arachidonic acid incorporated by mast cells, macrophages, and other cell types. In: Prostaglandins, leukotrienes, and lipoxins. biochemistry, mechanism of action, and clinical applications. J.M. Bailey, ed. New York: Plenum, p. 221.
25. Weller, P.F., Ryeom, S.W., and Dvorak, A.M. 1991. Lipid bodies: Structurally distinct nonmembranous intracellular sites of eicosanoid formation. In: Prostaglandins, leukotrienes, lipoxins and PAF. J.M. Bailey, ed. New York: Plenum, p. 353.
26. Fedorko, M.E., and Hirsch, J.G. 1965. Crystalloid structure in granules of guinea pig basophils and human mast cells. J. Cell Biol. 26:973.
27. Dvorak, A.M., Furitsu, T., Kissell-Rainville, S., and Ishizaka, T. 1992. Ultrastructural identification of human mast cells resembling skin mast cells stimulated to develop in long-term human cord blood mononuclear cells co-cultured with 3T3 mouse skin fibroblasts. J. Leuk. Biol., in press.

Development of Human Mast Cells *In Vitro*

Teruko Ishizaka*, Takuma Furitsu*, Naoki Inagaki*, Yutaka Tagaya*, Hideki Mitsui*, Masao Takei*, Krisztina M. Zsebo**

In 1989, we succeeded in developing morphologically and functionally mature human mast cells *in vitro* in a long term co-culture of mononuclear cells of cord blood with 3T3 fibroblasts derived from Swiss albino mouse. Subsequent studies revealed that culture supernatants of 3T3 fibroblasts contained human mast cell growth factor(s). The major mast cell growth promoting activity in the culture supernatant of BALB/3T3 fibroblasts was recovered in the protein fraction precipitated between 50% and 70% saturated ammonium sulfate. In DEAE Sepharose column chromatography at pH 8.1, the factor was eluted from the column between 150 mM and 200 mM NaCl. The molecular size of the mast cell growth factor(s) estimated by gel filtration was between 70 kDa and 100 kDa. Human mast cells developed in suspension cultures of cord blood cells in the presence of partially purified human mast cell growth factors bore 1.5–4.2 x 10^5 FcεRI per cell but no FcεRII. The majority of the cultured mast cells could be stained with monoclonal Ab, YB5.B8 which selectively recognizes human mast cells surface components, but not with monoclonal Ab VIM12 specific for human basophil. Cultured mast cells contain histamine (1.4–6.3 μg/10^6 cells) and tryptase specific for human mast cells; some of the cells contain both human mast cell tryptase and chymase. When the cultured mast cells were sensitized with human IgE and then challenged with anti-IgE, sensitized cells released histamine and arachidonic acid, and generated prostaglandin D_2 (PGD_2) and leukotriene C_4 (LTC_4). While our studies were in progress, a new cytokine, c-kit ligand or stem cell factor (SCF) was characterized. It was found that 5 ng to 100 ng/ml of recombinant human SCF promoted the development of human mast cells in the long term cord blood cell culture. The results suggest that mouse c-kit ligand may represent the major human mast cell growth factor in the culture supernatant of BALB/3T3 fibroblasts.

In the murine mast cell system, several cytokines, such as interleukin 3 (1), 4 (2), 9 (3), 10 (4) and c-kit ligand (5–9), have been shown to promote differentiation and proliferation of mouse mast cells. Until recently, however, no one succeeded in reproducible growth of human mature mast cells having physiological functions, in spite of numerous attempts made by many investigators. Recombinant human IL-3 promotes a transient increase in selective differentiation of basophils (10,11), but failed to facilitate differentiation of mast cells. Our results revealed that none of recombinant IL-1, 2, 3, 4, 5, 6, 9, 10 and GMCSF and no combination of these cytokines promoted differentiation of human mast cells from the progenitors in cord blood. Thus, we explored the possibility that some feeder layers may facilitate the development of human mast cells. Finally, in 1989, we were able to develop human mast cells in a long term co-culture of mononuclear cells of cord blood with 3T3 fibroblasts derived from Swiss albino mouse (12). In this co-culture system, however, the development of mast cells was slow; mast cells were first detected in the culture after 8 weeks of co-culture. Human mast cells developed in the co-culture of cord blood cells and 3T3 fibroblasts for over 10 weeks were morphologically distinct from basophils developed in the culture, and the major-

* La Jolla Institute for Allergy and Immunology, La Jolla, CA, USA 92037;
** Amgen Center, Thousand Oaks, CA, USA 91320.
Acknowledgements: This work is supported by Health Human Service grant AI-10060 and a research contract with Gemini Science, Inc. This is Publication No.23 from La Jolla Institute for Allergy and Immunology. We would like to express our gratitude to Mrs. Melinda Kozloski, La Jolla Institute for Allergy and Immunology for her excellent technical assistance, to Dr. K. Ishizaka for his support and encouragement and Ms. Virginia Walborn, Scripps Memorial Hospital, for umbilical cord blood. Our special appreciation goes to Dr. Steven Gillis, Immunex Research and Development Corporation, for his generous supply of recombinant mouse c-kit ligand or mast cell growth factor (rm MGF).

Table I. Development of Human Mast Cells on ψCRE Fibroblasts[a)]

Culture period	Viable cells	Viability	Metachromatic granule containing cells		Tryptase (+) cells	Histamine content
			Basophils	Mast cells		
weeks	per well	%	%	%	%	ng/well
0	10^6	99	2.0	0	ND	0.7
2	4.2×10^5	90	2.8	1.2	1.8	14
4	3.7×10^5	94	3.8	7.4	8.1	34
6	3.0×10^5	92	0.4	24.2	27.6	72
8	3.0×10^5	93	0	28.6	30.5	123
10	2.0×10^5	95	0	26.0	29.7	118

a) Mononuclear cells of cord blood (10^6 cells per well) were co-cultured with yCRE fibroblasts

ity of the mast cells had ultrastructural characteristics of mature human mast cells (12). In this presentation, the progress made in the past 3 years on the development of human mast cells *in vitro* will be summarized.

Human Mast Cells

Selection of 3T3 Fibroblasts for the Development of Human Mast Cells and for Human Mast Cell Growth Factor(s)

In order to advance our studies further, we examined other 3T3 fibroblasts which could provide better support for the mast cell differentiation than those derived from Swiss albino mouse. When cord blood cells were co-cultured with a derivative of NIH/3T3 fibroblasts, ψCRE (13), mast cells were detected as early as after 2 to 3 weeks in culture, as determined by metachromatic staining and anti-human mast cell tryptase staining (14). The number of mast cells and histamine content per well reached maximum at around 8 weeks (Table I). Using ψCRE fibroblasts, we were able to demonstrate that direct contact with 3T3 fibroblasts was not essential for the differentiation of mast cell progenitors. As shown in Table II, the number of mast cells developed in the 3 week culture of cord blood cells in the presence of the culture supernatant of ψCRE fibroblasts, was comparable to that developed in the co-culture of the same cord blood cells with ψCRE fibroblasts. The results indicated that soluble factors released from 3T3 fibroblasts are sufficient for the differentiation of mast cells progenitors.

Properties of Human Mast Cell Growth Factor(s)

Based on the findings described above, we proceeded to characterize human mast cell growth factors. First, we selected the cell source of the growth factors and found that the culture supernatant of BALB/3T3 fibroblasts had the highest human mast cell growth promoting activity among several human and mouse fibroblasts tested (Table III). Thus, we fractionated concentrated culture supernatant of BALB/3T3 fibroblasts. It was found that the major mast cell growth promoting activity was recovered in the protein fraction precipitated between 50% and 70% saturated ammonium sulfate. In a DEAE Sepharose column equilibrated with 10 mM Tris, pH 8.1, the activity was eluted from the column between 150 mM and 200 mM sodium chloride (Fig. 1). The molecular size of human mast cell growth factor was estimated to be between 70 kDa and 100 kDa, as estimated by gel filtration through a Superose 12 column (Fig. 2).

Functions and Properties of Cultured Human Mast Cells

We established suspension cultures of cord blood cells in the presence of partially purified human mast cell growth factors. In this system, 1 to 1.2×10^5 mast cells per well could be re-

Table II. Development of Mast Cells by ψCRE Culture Supernatant

Culture	Mast cells developed from cord blood cells*	
	Cultured with culture-supernatant (2x)	Co-culture with ψCRE
	/well	/well
1	1.1×10^4	6.4×10^3
2	1.1×10^4	1.7×10^4
3	7.2×10^3	1.2×10^4
4	3.1×10^4	1.5×10^4
5	1.2×10^4	1.8×10^4
mean ± SD	$1.44 \pm 0.94 \times 10^4$	$1.37 \pm 0.47 \times 10^4$

* 1.5×10^6 cord blood cells were seeded per well and cultured for 3 weeks. Cord blood cells contained no mast cells.

covered after 8 weeks of culture of 1.5×10^6 cord blood cells. Purity of the mast cells was up to 50%. Using these mast cell preparations, we examined functions and properties of the cultured mast cells in detail. All of the cultured mast cells were stained with Toluidine blue at low pH. They are formaldehyde-sensitive cells, and were stained with Alcian blue but not with Safranine. Mast cells developed in the culture bore high affinity IgE receptor, i.e. FcεRI which was demonstrated by immunofluorescence, and by direct binding of ^{125}I-labeled human E myeloma protein. The number of FcεRI was in the range of 1.5 to 4.2×10^5 per cell. In contrast, the monoclonal antibody H107 (15), which is specific for low affinity IgE receptor FcεRII, failed to bind to cultured mast cells. The majority of the cultured mast cells were stained with monoclonal Ab, YB5.B8 (16,17) which selectively recognizes human mast cell surface components, but was not stained with monoclonal Ab VIM12 (18) which recognizes

Table III. Development of mast cells by culture supernatant of murine and human fibroblasts

Concentrated[a)] culture supernatant of	Mast cells developed	
	3 weeks	6 weeks
	per well	per well
BALB/3T3	7.0×10^4	9.3×10^4
ψCRE/3T3	2.6×10^4	1.4×10^4
MCR-9 (Human)	2.4×10^4	1.1×10^4
Detroit 551 (Human)	1.4×10^3	1.3×10^3

a) Culture supernatant of fibroblasts containing 5% fetal calf serum was concentrated 20 fold and added to cord blood cell culture (1.5×10^6 cells/well) at 10% (V/V)

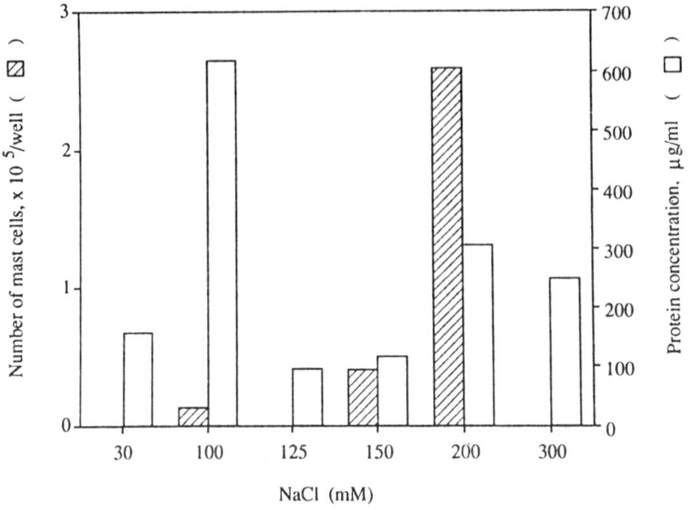

Figure 1: Fractionation on DEAE-Sepharose. 10 liters of serum free culture supernatant of BALB/3T3 fibroblast was concentrated 1000 fold, dialyzed against 10 mM Tris-HCl buffer (pH 8.1), and applied to a DEAE-Sepharose CL-6B (Pharmacia) column equilibrated with the same buffer. The column was eluted with a stepwise NaCl gradient in 10 mM Tris-HCl buffer (pH 8.1). Each fraction was concentrated into 3 ml, dialyzed against PBS and used for human cord blood cell culture at the final concentration of 2% (v/v).

human basophil surface markers. The granules of cultured mast cells contained 1.4-6.3 µg histamine per 10^6 cells, and tryptase specific for human mast cells (14). Some of the cells contained both human mast cell tryptase and chymase (19). When the cultured mast cells were sensitized with human IgE, sensitized cells released histamine and arachidonic acid, and generated prostaglandin D_2 (PGD_2) and leukotriene C_4 (LTC_4), upon challenge with anti-IgE (Table IV). The average amount of PGD_2 generated upon challenge with anti-IgE was 60.6 ± 8.9 pmol per 10^6 mast cells in nine separate experiments, while 50.2 ± 9.9 pmol of LTC_4 per 10^6 mast cells were generated in five experiments. These results indicate that mast cells developed in the long term culture of cord blood cells in the presence of partially purified human mast cell growth factor(s) are functionally mature human mast cells.

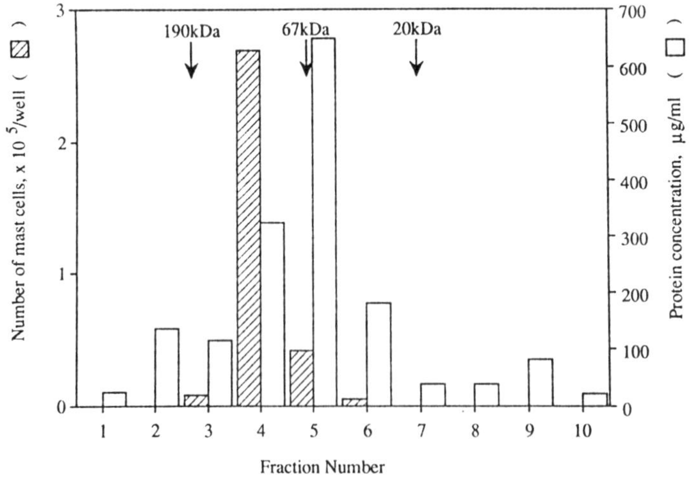

Figure 2: Gel filtration chromatography. Gel filtration chromatography was performed on a Superose 12 prep grade HR 16/50 column (Pharmacia, Uppsala Sweden) with a bed volume of 100 ml using a Beckman HPLC system. The column was equilibrated with PBS and calibrated with molecular weight markers; bovine serum albumin (M_r 67000), soybean tryψn inhibitor (M_r 20100) and cytochrome c (M_r 12600). One ml of concentrated serum-free conditioned medium was loaded with the flow rate of 1ml/min and 5 ml fractions were collected from 30 to 80 min. Pooled fractions were 10-fold concentrated, dialyzed against RPMI 1640 medium and used for human cord blood cell culture at the final concentration of 5% (v/v).

Table IV. Generation of PGD2 and LTC4 in cultured mast cells by anti-IgE

Mast Cells	Per cent histamine released	Mediators (pmol/10^6 cells)[a]		
		Histamine released	PGD_2[b] generated	LTC_4[c] generated
1	32.3	2,990	111	91
2	15.0	1,620	128	46
3	13.8	1,740	57	51

a) Numerals in the table represent net release or net generation of the mediators
b) PGD_2 and LTC_4 were measured by Radioimmunoassay (Amersham)

Differentiation of Human Mast Cell Progenitors by Recombinant c-kit Ligand

While our studies were in progress, a new cytokine, c-kit ligand was characterized, and several groups of investigators isolated cDNA clone encoding the cytokine from various cell sources (5–9). One group purified the cytokine from culture supernatant of BALB/3T3 fibroblasts (8). c-kit belongs to the family of cell-surface receptors that possess an intrinsic protein tyrosine kinase activity (20). The receptor tyrosine kinases are classified into three groups based on primary sequences. The first group is represented by epidermal growth factor receptor, while the insulin receptor represents the second group. Putative c-kit ligand receptor belongs to the third group. Since recombinant c-kit ligand has proven to be a potent stem cell growth factor (21) and promoted mast cell growth in the murine system (6), we wanted to determine whether recombinant human (rh) c-kit ligand or stem cell factor (SCF) from Amgen promotes the development of human mast cells in our cord blood cell culture. As shown in Table V, 5 ng to 100 ng/ml of recombinant human SCF promoted the development of human mast cells in the long term cord blood cell culture in a dose dependent manner. It was also found that the addition of either recombinant human IL-3 or IL-4 did not show any significant effect on the rh SCF-induced growth of human mast cells. Thus, rh c-kit ligand or SCF appears to be a unique human mast cell growth factor which promotes the differentiation of human mast cell progenitors in cord blood and supports the survival of mast cells. Our results also suggest that the decline of the other cells during a long term culture resulted in an increase in the proportion of viable mast cells in the culture. Thus it appears that rh SCF is a human mast cell differentiation factor rather than a proliferation factor. Since our human mast cell growth factor(s) are derived from mouse 3T3 fibroblasts, mononuclear cells from cord blood were also cultured in the presence of recombinant mouse (rm) c-kit ligand (mouse mast cell growth factor, MGF) from Immunex. As shown in Table VI,

Table V. Development of mast cells from cord blood cell[a]in the presence of partially purified HMGF or rhSCF

Culture with		Cells developed in the culture					
		Total cells	viability	basophils	mast cells	Tryptase (+)cells	mast cells
	weeks	/well	%	%	%	%	/well
HMGF (50-70%SAS-Fr)[b]	4	9.0×10^5	92	7.6	9.0	9.6	8.4×10^4
	13	4.0×10^5	98	0.4	26.6	28.8	1.1×10^5
rhSCF (100 ng/ml)	4	3.2×10^6	98	20.8	8.4	10.9	3.1×10^5
	13	6.0×10^5	98	5.0	44.2	41.4	2.6×10^5
rhSCF (20 ng/ml)	4	2.1×10^6	99	20.4	4.2	6.8	1.2×10^5
	13	1.0×10^5	97	2.0	37.0	35.2	3.6×10^4
rhSCF (5ng/ml)	4	7.0×10^5	97	18.2	5.2	7.2	4.3×10^4
	13	5.0×10^4	98	1.4	19.6	17.4	9.3×10^3
culture medium alone	4	2.0×10^5	98	14.2	0	0.3	NS[c]
	13	2.0×10^4	90	0	0	0	0

a) 1.5×10^6 mononuclear cells of cord blood were seeded per well.
b) Human mast cell growth factor enriched fraction obtained by precipitation of culture supernatant of BALB/3T3 fibroblasts with 50-70% saturated ammonium sulfate.
c) NS: not significant

Table VI. Development of mast cells from cord blood cells[h])in the presence of rm MGF[b)]

Cultured with	Cells developed in the culture[c)]				
	Total cells	viability	basophils	mast cells	
	/well	%	%	%	/well
rm MGF (100 ng/ml)	1.3×10^6	93	1.6	9.8	1.3×10^5
rm MGF (20 ng/ml)	3.5×10^5	91	6.5	3.0	1.1×10^4
rm MGF (5 ng/ml)	1.1×10^5	97	5.3	0.2	2.2×10^2
medium alone	4.4×10^4	94	8.8	0	0

a) 1.5×10^6 mononuclear cells of cord blood were cultured in the presence of rm SCF (MGF) for 4 weeks.
b) rm MGF; Recombinant mouse mast cell growth factor from Immunex.
c) Numerals in the table represent average of 4 wells.

a dose-dependent development of human mast cells was obtained within 4 weeks of culturing cord blood cells in the presence of rm MGF, comparable to that observed in the cultures with rh SCF. We also confirmed that even 100 ng/ml of rh SCF failed to facilitate differentiation of mouse mast cell progenitors in bone marrow, although rm MGF promotes differentiation of human mast cell progenitors. These results suggest that mouse c-kit ligand or MGF may represent the major human mast cell growth promoting activity in the culture supernatant of BALB/3T3 fibroblasts. In order to clarify the relationship between rm MGF and human mast cell growth factor(s) present in the culture supernatant of BALB/3T3 fibroblasts, experiments are underway to determine whether the monoclonal anti-mouse MGF, supplied by Immunex, could absorb human mast cell growth promoting activity in our partially purified growth factor preparations. We expect to have a definitive answer on the relationship between our mast cell growth factor and MGF in the near future.

Future Prospects

Since we identified mast cells and basophils as the target of IgE (22–25), I have been working with IgE, mast cells and basophils for many years. Rodent mast cells and basophils have provided us with a tremendous amount of fundamental information on the activation and the development of mast cells and basophils. However, we have to be cautious about the application of the information to human mast cells. We already have some evidence which suggests that some of the crucial biochemical events for the IgE-dependent activation of mast cells, as well as cytokines involved in the differentiation and proliferation of mast cells, are different depending upon animal species from which mast cells are derived. In order to apply basic findings to clinical studies, we have to establish *in vitro* systems with human mast cells and basophils. Since we were able to develop functional human basophils and mast cells *in vitro*, my ultimate goal to develop human basophil or mast cell lines having physiological functions may not be out of reach.

References

1. Rennick, D.M., Lee, F.D., Yokota, T., Arai, K., Cantor, H., and Nabel, G.J. 1985. A cloned MCGF cDNA encodes a multilineage hematopoietic growth factor: Multiple activities of interleukin 3. J. Immunol. 134:910.
2. Rennick, D.M., Young, G., Muller-Sieburg, C., Smith, C., Arai, N., Tanabe, Y., and Gemmell, L. 1987. Interleukin 4 (B-cell stimulatory factor 1) can enhance or antagonize the factor-dependent growth of hemopoietic progenitor cells. Proc. Natl. Acad. Sci. USA 84:6889.
3. Renauld, J-C, Goethals, A., Houssiau, F., Roost, E.V., and Van Snick, J. 1990. Cloning and expression of a cDNA for the human homology of mouse T cell and mast cell growth factor P40. Cytokine 2:9.
4. Thompson-Snipes, L.A., Dhar, V., Bond, M.W., Mossman, T.R., Moore, K.W., and Rennick, D.M. 1991. Interleukin 10: A novel stimulatory factor for mast cells and their progenitors. J. Exp. Med. 173:501.
5. Williams, D.E., Eisenman, J., Baird, A., Rauch, C., Ness, K.V., March, C.J., Park, L.S., Martin, W., Mochizuki, D.Y., Boswell, H.S., Burgess, G.S., Cosman, D., and Lyman, S.D. 1990. Identification of a ligand for the c-kit proto-oncogene. Cell 63:167.
6. Anderson, D.M., Lyman, S.D., Baird, A.E., Wignall, J.M., Eisenman, J., Rauch, C., March, C.J., Boswell, H.S., Gimpel, S.D., Cosman, D., and Williams, D.E. 1990. Molecular cloning of mast cell growth factor, a hematopoietin that

is active in both membrane bound and soluble forms. Cell 63:235.

7. Zsebo, K.M., Williams, D.A., Geissler, E.N., Broudy, V.C., Martin, F.H., Atkins, H.L., Hsu, R.Y., Birkett, N.C., Okino, K.H., Murdock, D.C., Jacobsen, F.W., Langley, K.E., Smith, K.A., Takeish, T., Cattanach, B.M., Galli, S.J., and Suggs, S.V. 1990. Stem cell factor is encoded at the *Sl* locus of the mouse and is the ligand for the c-kit tyrosine kinase receptor. Cell 63:213.
8. Huang, E., Nocka, K., Beier, D.R., Chu, T.Y., Buck, J., Lahm, H.W., Wellner, D., Leder, P., and Besmer, P. 1990. The hematopoietic growth factor KL is encoded by the *Sl* Locus and is the ligand of the c-kit receptor, the gene product of the W locus. Cell 63:225.
9. Martin, F.H., Suggs, S.V., Langley, K.E., Lu, H.S., Ting, J., Okino, K.H., Morris, C.F., McNiece, I.K., Jacobson, F.W., Mendiaz, E.A., Birkett, N.C., Smith, K.A., Johnson, M.J., Parker, V.P., Flores, J.C., Patel, A.C., Fisher, E.F., Erjavec, H.O., Herrera, C.J., Wypych, J., Sachdev, R.K., Pope, J.A., Leslie, I., Wen, D., Lin, C.H., Cupples, R.L., and Zsebo, K.M. 1990. Primary structure and functional expression of rat and human stem cell factor DNAs. Cell 63:203.
10. Saito, H., Hatake, K., Dvorak, A.M., Leiferman, K.M., Donnenberg, A.D., Arai, N., Ishizaka, K., and Ishizaka, T. 1988. Selective differentiation and proliferation of hematopoietic cells induced by recombinant human interleukins. Proc. Natl. Acad. Sci. USA 85:2288.
11. Valent, P., Schmidt, G., Besemer, J., Mayer, P., Zenke, G., Liehl, E., Hinterberger, W., Lechner, K., and Bettelheim, P. 1989. Interleukin-3 is a differentiation factor for human basophils. Blood 73:1323.
12. Furitsu, T., Saito, H., Dvorak, A.M., Schwartz, L.B., Irani, A.M.A., Burdick, J.F., Ishizaka, K., and Ishizaka, T. 1989. Development of human mast cells *in vitro*. Proc. Natl. Acad. Sci. USA 86:10039.
13. Danos, O., and Mulligan, R.C. 1988. Safe and efficient generation of recombinant retroviruses with amphotropic and ecotropic host ranges. Proc. Natl. Acad. Sci. USA 85:6460.
14. Schwartz, L.B. 1985. Monoclonal antibodies against human mast cell tryptase demonstrate shared antigenic sites on subunits of tryptase and selective localization of the enzyme to mast cells. J. Immunol. 134:526.
15. Noro, N., Yoshioka, A., Adachi, M., Yasuda, K., Masuda, T., and Yodoi, J. 1986. Monoclonal antibody (H107) inhibiting IgE binding to FcεRI(+) human lymphocytes. J. Immunol. 137:1258.
16. Ashman, L.K., Gadd, S.J., Mayrhofer, G., Spargo, L.D.J., and Cole, S.R. 1987. A murine monoclonal antibody to an acute myeloid leukemia associated cell surface antigen identifies tissue mast cells. In: Leukocyte typing III. A. Mc Michael, ed. Oxford: Oxford University Press, p. 726.
17. Mayerhofer, G., Gadd, S.J., Spargo, L.D.J., and Ashman, L.K. 1987. Specificity of a mouse monoclonal antibody raised against acute myeloid leukemia cells for mast cells in human mucosal and connective tissues. Immunol. Cell Biol. 65:241.
18. Knapp, W., Majdic, O., Stockinger, H., Bettelheim, P., Liszka, K., Koller, U., and Peschel, C. 1984. Monoclonal antibodies to human myelomonocyte differentiation antigens in the diagnosis of acute myeloid leukemia. Med. Oncol. & Tumor Pharmacother. 1:257.
19. Irani, A.M.A., Schecter, N.M., Craig, S.S., DeBlois, G., and Schwartz, L.B. 1986. Two types of human mast cells that have distinct neutral protease compositions. Proc. Natl. Acad. Sci. USA 83:4464.
20. Yarden, Y. 1988. Growth factor receptor tyrosine kinases. Ann. Rev. Biochem. 57:443.
21. Zsebo, K.M., Wypych, J., Mc Niece, I.K., Lu, H.S., Smith, K.A., Karkare, S.B., Sachdev, R.K., Yuschenkoff, V.N., Birkett, N.C., Williams, L.R., Satyagal, V.N., Tung, W., Bosselman, R.A., Mendiaz, E.A., and Langley, K.E. 1990. Identification, purification, and biological characterization of hematopoietic stem cell factor from buffalo rat liver condition medium. Cell 63:195.
22. Ishizaka, K., Tomioka, H. and Ishizaka, T. 1970. Mechanisms of passive sensitization. I. Presence of IgE and IgG molecules on human leukocytes. J. Immunol. 105:1459.
23. Ishizaka, K., and Tomioka, H. 1971. Mechanisms of passive sensitization. II. Presence of receptors for IgE on monkey mast cells. J. Immunol. 107:971.
24. Ishizaka, T., Tomioka H., and Ishizaka, K. 1972. Release of histamine and slow reacting substance of anaphylaxis (SRS-A) by IgE-anti-IgE reaction on monkey mast cells. J. Immunol. 108:513.
25. Ishizaka, T., DeBernardo, R., Tomioka, H., Lichtenstein, L.M., and Ishizaka, K. 1972. Identification of basophil granulocytes as a cite of allergic histamine release. J. Immunol. 108:1000.

Mucosal Cells and Nerves

John Bienenstock*

In many tissues in the body, mast cells seem to have closer anatomic proximity to nerves than would be found by chance alone. These associations should be viewed in the broader context of neuroimmune interactions. They should not be considered obligatory or essential, but part of an amplification and fine-tuning system. Data are reviewed in this paper which support the suggestion that mast cells communicate with, and are communicated by nerves. These associations and inter-communications are bi-directional in nature, and either may cause mast cell degranulation, or the inhibition of secretion by this cell type. Antigen induced mast cell secretion can, through axon-type reflexes, promote changes in target tissues, such as epithelial chloride ion secretion. Evidence is given for neuronal changes in the course of intestinal inflammation which parallel changes in mast cell numbers. Evidence for central nervous system regulation of peripheral mast cell degranulation is given in the form of data from Pavlovian conditioning experiments.

We should really review the subject of the interactions between mast cells and nerves in the broader context of interactions between the nervous and immune systems (1). Thus, there is considerable evidence for neuroimmune interactions ranging from morphological evidence of membrane-membrane contact between nor-adrenergic nerves and lymphocytes in the spleen (2), to the characterization of neuropeptide receptors on a number of immune cells, such as lymphocytes (3). What used to be considered the study of esoterica is slowly becoming more respectable, and is being drawn into the mainstreams of neuroscience and immunology. We do not believe that there is an obligatory mast cell-nerve association essential to the well being of the host, but rather that mast cells can and do communicate directly with the nervous system, and in this way, can amplify and fine-tune immune and inflammatory reactions, at sites where they are localized. Furthermore, this communication system is probably bi-directional and allows both the central and peripheral nervous systems to communicate with, and be communicated by, immune cells in the periphery, including those found in mucosal tissues (4,5).

Morphologic Associations

There are now a considerable number of reports in the literature showing morphologic associations both at the light- and electron-microscopic levels between mast cells and nerves (6). We have shown such associations in the normal rat intestine, as well as in the intestine inflamed by response to a nematode, Nippostrongylus brasiliensis. We have made similar observations in the human intestine (7). These observations, which suggest that mast cells and nerves may form a functional unit, have been confirmed by Arizono et al. (8) who extended them to other cell types such as eosinophils and plasma cells.

Ussing Chamber Experiments

Using the Ussing Chamber a variety of investigators have suggested that, both in the intestine as well as in the trachea, a unit consisting of mast cells and nerves can influence in a purposive manner a target tissue, in this case, epithelium by promotion of chloride ion secretion (9–11). Whether such events are valid axon reflexes or not may be a semantic argument. Evidence was recently obtained that mast cell deficient mice, w/w^v and sl/sl^d, have a very poor secretory response to antigen in sensitized animals but that this can be reconstituted in the w/w^v by a bone marrow infusion, indicating that it is likely that intestinal mast cells play a central

* Departments of Medicine and Pathology, McMaster University, Hamilton, Ontario, Canada.
Acknowledgements: The author gratefully acknowledges the grant support of the Medical Research Council of Canada in support of this research.

role in this system (12). It is however important to note that in the reconstituted w/w^{v} animals, there was nevertheless a response to antigen. This may be interpreted as a response by mast cell precursors or another cell type such as lymphocytes, eosinophils or macrophages responding to the antigen. The data nevertheless support the concept of a functional homeostatic unit between mast cells, nerves and intestinal epithelium (13). The work of Weinreich and Undem (14) also support these interactions. These investigators have explored the effect of antigen on para-sympathetic and sympathetic ganglia and have shown that excitatory post synaptic potentials (EPSPs) can be generated by antigen, and that these effects are complex and mediated by H1, H2 and H3 receptors. The role of other mediators is at this point not completely clarified in this system.

Electrical Stimulation

Recent work of Dimitriadou et al. (15) has shown that electrical stimulation of the trigeminal ganglion can cause mast cell granule changes on the ipsilateral, but not contralateral sides in the dura mater and tongue. These changes were observed both at the light- and electron-microscopic levels. The changes depended on the intensity of the current used to stimulate, and the length of the experiment. Some work has recently appeared suggesting that mast cell degranulation will only occur after prolonged antidromic electrical stimulation, and that mast cells are not necessarily involved in this so-called neurogenic inflammation (16). However, there is considerable literature on this subject to support mast cell-nerve involvement in neurogenic inflammation (17). The easiest way to explain these apparently disparate data is to suggest that mast cells are not necessarily involved in the development of vasodilatation and plasma extravasation, and that their involvement depends on the nature of the nervous stimulus. Coderre and co-workers (18) have shown that different, but not all, forms of nervous stimulation in the knee joints of rats will involve mast cells and vice versa. Not all nervous stimulation produces a "positive" action on mast cells as is shown by the work of Miura et al. (19). These workers used cats sensitive to ascaris which were treated with propanol and atropine. Antigen inhalation caused plasma histamine levels to rise and the pulmonary resistance to increase. Bilateral electrical stimulation of the vagus nerves abolished both the histamine increase and the pulmonary physiologic changes, indicating a non-adrenergic non-cholinergic (NANC) inhibitory system communicating with mast cells, and able to inhibit their degranulation.

Co-Culture Experiments Between Mast Cells and Nerves

A detailed discussion of this subject is outside the scope of the present paper but the reader is referred elsewhere to these experiments (5,20). We have shown selective associations between mast cells and nerves in co-culture. Mast cells exert tropic and trophic effects on sympathetic neurons from the superior cervical ganglion. These interactions, once formed, occur over a prolonged period of time, and we have observed electrophysiologic changes occurring in the mast cells as a consequence of them.

Nerve Growth Factor (NGF)

This factor, found in most external secretions, is known to be essential for the growth, differentiation and survival of sensory and sympathetic neurons, as well as having some central nervous system effects (21). It has been known for some years that injections of NGF into a neonatal animal will cause extensive mast cell hyperplasia, and we have confirmed these findings (5,22). In addition, using classic methyl cellulose hemopoietic colony assays with human peripheral blood, we have been able to show that NGF promotes colony growth, especially via T cells (23). There was some selectivity to the promotion of Eo colonies which contained either eosinophils or histamine containing basophils. More recently Tsuda and colleagues (24) have shown that NGF synergizes with GM-CSF and IL-5 to promote these types of effects. Most recently, Matsuda et al. (25) have repeated these types of observations in a murine system, showing that NGF induced significant mast cell growth in this system, in the presence of IL-3 and fibroblasts in co-culture, but not in the absence of a second factor. This suggests that NGF may have important local effects in tissues in which it is being locally synthesized. The best known situation in which this occurs is of course in nerve injury. The principal factor promoting up-regulation of mRNA for NGF and NGF receptor is IL-1, secreted by invading macrophages (26). In this respect, it is interesting that IL-1 is secreted by atopics sensitive to ragweed antigen after application of the antigen onto the skin, in a skin window technique (27). Furthermore, IL-1 causes up-regulation of message for pre-protachykinin in sympathetic ganglia, as well as synthesis of substance P (28). Marshall (29) has shown that the likely mechanism whereby NGF causes mast cell hyperplasia when injected into the rat is via degranulation of connective tissue type mast cells. The mucosal mast cell proliferation may be via action on the mucosal mast cells themselves without degranulation or via a second cell such as a T-cell. This work fits well with the current knowledge that mast cells are able to make a variety of cytokines which include IL-3, IL-4, IL-5, IL-6, GM-CSF and TNF alpha (30). We (31) recently showed that peritoneal mast cells synthesize and secrete leukaemia inhibitory factor (LIF), also known as cholinergic differentiation factor, a potent molecule also capable of causing increases in mRNA for preprotachykinin in superior cervical ganglia.

Neuronal Remodelling in the Intestine

Recent work by Stead et al. (32) has shown that in the course of intestinal inflammation in reaction to nippostrongylus, there are significant changes in the numbers of small nerve profiles stained with an antibody to growth associated protein (GAP 43) in cross sections of rat villi. This molecule is expressed primarily in the growth cones of developing or regenerating nerves. The numbers of small nerves increased and correlated with the numbers of mast cells ($r = 0.76$). The density of nerve profiles as measured by a computer assisted image analyzer still had not returned to normal by day 49 when mast cell numbers were normalized. We take this evidence as indicating that NGF could well be important in this regulation of local inflammatory events in the GI tract via its production in the course of local neuronal remodelling. These observations need to be repeated in other types of inflammation, but may be of great significance in understanding mucosal inflammatory diseases such as asthma and inflammatory bowel disease.

Pavlovian Conditioning

Lastly, for the sake of completeness, we wish to tangentially mention that classical Pavlovian conditioning experiments give evidence that exposure to the conditioning stimulus alone can cause mast cell degranulation. A conditional stimulus consisting of an odor associated with exposure to antigen caused elevations in blood histamine (33). We showed (34) that rats only responded to exposure with loud noise and flashing lights, by increases in serum rat mast cell protease II, if training with antigen injections had previously been coupled with the conditioning stimulus.

References

1. Stead, R.H., Bienenstock, J., and Stanisz, A.M. 1987. Neuropeptide regulation of mucosal immunity. Immunol. Rev. 100:333.
2. Felten, S.Y., and Olschowka, J. 1987. Noradrenergic sympathetic innervation of the spleen: II. Tyrosine hydroxylase (TH)-positive nerve terminals form synaptic like contacts on lymphocytes in the splenic white pulp. J. Neurosci. Res. 18:37.
3. Payan, D.G., Brewster, D.R., and Goetzl, E.J. 1983. Specific stimulation of human T lymphocytes by substance P. J. Immunol. 131:1613.
4. Carr, D.J.J., and Blalock, J.E. 1986. A molecular basis for bi-directional communication between the immune and neuroendocrine system. In: Progress in immunology, VI. B. Cinader, and R.G. Miller, eds. Orlando: Academic Press, p. 619.
5. Stead, R.H., and Bienenstock, J. 1990. Cellular interactions between the immune and peripheral nervous systems. In: Cell to cell interaction. M.M. Burger, M.M., B. Sordat, and R.M. Zinkernagel, eds. Basel: Karger, p. 170.

6. Stead, R.H., Tomioka, M., Quinonez, G., Simon, G.T., Felten, S.Y., and Bienenstock, J. 1987b. Intestinal mucosal mast cells in normal and nematode-infected rat intestines are in intimate contact with peptidergic nerves. Proc. Natl. Acad. Sci. USA 84:2975.
7. Stead, R.H., Dixon, M.F., Brawell, M.H., Riddell, R.H., and Bienenstock, J. 1989. Mast cells are closely apposed to nerves in the human gastrointestinal mucosa. Gastroenterology 97:575.
8. Arizono, N, Matsuda, S., Hattori, T., Kojima, Y., Maeda, T., and Galli, S.J. 1990. Anatomical variation in mast cell nerve associations in the rat small intestine, heart, lung, and skin: Similarities of distances between neural processes and mast cells, eosinophils, or plasma cells in the jejunal lamina propria. Lab. Invest. 62:626.
9. Castro, G.A., Harari, Y., and Russell, D. 1987. Mediators of anaphylaxis-induced ion transport changes in small intestine. Am. J. Physiol. 253:G540.
10. Baird, A.W., and Cuthbert, A.W. 1987. Neuronal involvement in type I hypersensitivity reactions in gut epithelia. Brit. J. Pharm. 92:647.
11. Perdue, M.H., and Bienenstock, J. 1991. Immunophysiology of the gut. Current Opinion in Gastroenterology 7:421.
12. Perdue, M.H., Masson, S., Wersheil, B.K., and Galli, S.J. 1991. Role of mast cells in ion transport abnormality associated with intestinal anaphylaxis. J. Clin .Invest. 87:687.
13. Bienenstock, J., MacQueen, G., Sestini, P, Marshall, J.S., Stead, R.H., and Perdue, M.H. 1991. Mast cell/nerve interactions *in vitro* and *in vivo*. Am. Rev. Respir. Dis. 143 Suppl:S55.
14. Weinreich, D., and Undem, B.J. 1987. Immunological regulation of synaptic transmission in isolated guinea pig autonomic ganglia. J. Clin. Invest. 79:1529.
15. Dimitriadou, V., Buzzi, M.G., Moskowitz, M.A., and Theoharides, T.C. 1991. Trigeminal sensory fiber stimulation induces morphological changes reflecting secretion in rat dura mater mast cells. J. Neurosci. 44:97.
16. Didier, A., Kowalski, M.L., Jay, J., and Kaliner, M.A. 1990. Neurogenic inflammation, vascular permeability, and mast cells: Capsaicin desensitization fails to influence IgE-anti-DNP induced vascular permeability in rat airways. Am. Rev. Respir. Dis. 141:398.
17. Foreman, J.C., and Jordan, C.C. 1984. Neurogenic inflammation. TIPS 5:116.
18. Coderre, T.J., Basbaum, A.I., and Levine, J.D. 1989. Neural control of vascular permeability: Interactions between primary afferents, mast cells, and sympathetic efferents. J. Neurophys. 62:48.
19. Miura, M., Inoue, H., Ichinose, M., Kimura, K., Katsumata, U., and Takishima, T. 1990. Effect of nonadrenergic noncholinergic inhibitory nerve stimulation on the allergic reaction in cat airways. Am. Rev. Respir. Dis. 141:29.
20. Blennerhassett, M.G., Tomioka, M., and Bienenstock, J. 1991. Formation of contacts between mast cells and sympathetic neurons *in vitro*. Cell Tissue Res. 265:121.
21. Levi-Montalcini, R. 1987. The nerve growth factor: Thirty-five years later. EMBO Journal 1145.
22. Aloe, L., and Levi-Montalcini, R. 1977. Mast cells increase in tissues of neonatal rats injected with the nerve growth factor. Brain Res. 133:358.
23. Matsuda, H., Coughlin, M.D., Bienenstock, J., and Denburg, J.A. 1988. Nerve growth factor promotes human hemopoietic colony growth and differentiation. Proc. Natl. Acad. Sci. USA 850:6508.
24. Tsuda, T., Wong, D., Dolovich, J., Bienenstock, J., Marshall, J., and Denburg, J.A. 1991. Synergistic effects of nerve growth factor and granulocyte-macrophage colony-stimulating factor on human basophilic cell differentiation. Blood 77:971.
25. Matsuda, H, Kannon, Y., Ushio, H., Kiso, Y., Kanemoto, T., Suzuki, H., and Kitamura, Y. 1991. Nerve growth induces development of connective tissue-type mast cells *in vitro* from murine bone marrow cells. J. Exp. Med. 174:7.
26. Lindholm, D., Heumann, R., Meyer, M., and Thoenen, H. 1987. Interleukin-1 regulates synthesis of nerve growth factor in non-neuronal cells of rat sciatic nerve. Nature 330:658.
27. Bochner, B.S., Charlesworth, E.N., Lichtenstein, L.M., Derse, C.P., Gillis, S., Dinarello, C.A., and Schleimer, R.P. 1990. Interleukin-1 is released at sites of human cutaneous allergic reactions. J. Allergy Clin. Immunol. 86:830.
28. Freidin, M., and Kessler, J.A. 1991. Cytokine regulation of substance P expression in sympathetic neurons. Proc. Natl. Acad. Sci. USA 88:3200.
29. Marshall, J.S., Stead, R.H., McSharry, C., Nielsen, L., and Bienenstock, J. 1990. The role of mast cell degranulation products in mast cell hyperplasia. I. Mechanism of action of nerve growth factor. J. Immunol. 144:1886.
30. Plaut, M., Pierce, J.H., Watson, C.J., Hanley-Hyde, J., Nordan, R.P., and Paul, W.E. 1989. Mast cell lines produce lymphokines in re-

these two very closely related inflammatory cell phenotypes, depending on factors not yet totally characterized (15,16). In addition to IL-3 and IL-5, granulocyte-macrophage colony-stimulating factor (GM-CSF) has major activity in both basophil and eosinophil differentiation, as well as more general hemopoietic stimulatory activity for other myeloid lineages (reviewed in 2,11). In conjunction with nerve growth factor (NGF), we have shown that GM-CSF synergizes in basophil differentiation (17). More recent evidence from other laboratories has related the importance of fibroblast-derived hemopoietic factors in the differentiation of human mast cells (18), and the potential contribution of steel locus factor (SLF), the ligand for the proto-oncogene c-kit (19), in the *in vivo* differentiation of mast cells (20).

Ex Vivo **Studies**

Based upon the above observations, we have explored the hemopoietic cytokine contributions of tissue structural cells derived from allergic-type inflamed tissues in the airways of humans. Using nasal polypepithelial cells or fibroblast lines (21,22), as well as bronchial or pulmonary epithelial cells and fibroblasts, we have found that GM-CSF is the principal hemopoietic cytokine, along with other pro-inflammatory cytokines such as IL-6 and IL-8, elaborated *in vitro* by primary lines established from these tissues (2–4). There is constitutive production of GM-CSF by both epithelial cells and fibroblasts; however, stimulation with IL-1 or neuropeptides such as substance P can upregulate GM-CSF production by these cells (4). This can be shown both in terms of expression of messenger RNA for GM-CSF as well as elaboration into cell culture supernatants (1–4; Ohtoshi et al., submitted). Monoclonal antibodies to these cytokines have been used to neutralize the presence of GM-CSF elaborated by tissue structural cells *ex vivo*, blocking their effects on differentiation of basophils and eosinophils, as well as their survival-prolonging activities upon eosinophils and other inflammatory cell types (23–25). The methods by which GM-CSF has been established as a cytokine produced by structural cells are summarized in Table I.

TABLE I. Airway Structural Cell Production of GM-CSF

Cell Source	Methods of Detection
Nasal polyp epithelial cells	Bioassay
Nasal polyp fibroblasts	Immunoassay
Bronchial epithelial cells	mRNA expression
Pulmonary fibroblasts	Immunostainng

Effects of Corticosteroids *In Vitro* and *Ex Vivo*

We have explored the anti-inflammatory effects of corticosteroids in the above systems. Budesonide at physiologic concentrations can inhibit both gene expression and production of GM-CSF as well as other pro-inflammatory cytokines elaborated by epithelial cells and fibroblasts from the airways (26). Moreover, corticosteroids have direct effects upon inflammatory effector cells themselves, such as eosinophils, down-regulating the irresponses to GM-CSF (25). Lastly, budesonide inhibits differentiation of basophil and eosinophil progenitors in both semi-solid and suspension culture systems using normal and leukemic cells (Denburg, in preparation).

In Vivo Studies

We have measured nasal lavage fluids from patients with polyposis to establish whether or not cytokines shown to be active *in vitro* are present *in vivo*. Indeed, by immunoassay as well as bioassay we can detect GM-CSF, IL-3 and IL-5 in the nasal lavage from patients with polyposis (1,2,27). Other cytokines such as IL-6, IL-8, TGF and TNF can also bedetected by immunoassay of nasal lavage fluids (1,2,27; un-

TABLE II. Nasal Lavage Fluid Cytokines in Polyposis

Cytokine	Method of Detection
IL-3	Immunoassay; bioassay
IL-5	Immunoassay; bioassay
IL-6	Immunoassay; bioassay
IL-8	Immunoassay
GM-CSF	Immunoassay; bioassay

published observations). Eosinophil survival-enhancing assays have proved to be most sensitive in detecting the levels and presence of IL-3, IL-5 and GM-CSF (25,28); however, differentiation assays using the leukemic cell line HL-60 have also proved useful in this regard (unpublished observations). Table II summarizes the cytokines measureable in nasal lavage and the methods used to detect them *in vivo*.

Effects of Cytokines on Inflammatory Cell Phenotype

Fibroblast and epithelial cells produce factors which control not only the differentiation and state of activation of cells from progenitors, but also the phenotype of an inflammatory effector cell population. For example, we have recently established that GM-CSF, derived from T-cells, fibroblasts or epithelial cells, can help promote phenotype switch of cultured human mast cells represented by the HMC-1 cell line (1). This has been measured by a change in the number of cells expressing the protease, chymase, in addition to expression of tryptase (1). Other factors derived from fibroblasts, and not requiring cell-cell contact, appear to be important in inducing differentiation into tryptase-type (MCT) and tryptase plus chymase-type (MCTC) human nasal mast cells (29,30) *in vitro* (1; unpublished observations). Whether these factors include SLF, GM-CSF or other novel cytokines remains to be determined. Another novel activity involved in inflammatory cell phenotype control appears to be derived from nasal polyp epithelial cells. This factor can induce differentiation of a subtype of cells found in the HL-60 cell line assay into monocyte-macrophages, characterized by the presence of CD14 on the surface of these cells (31). Such differentiation induction can also be shown to occur when one uses peripheral blood mononuclear cell populations; CD14 expression appears to occur in a subpopulation of basophilic differentiating HL-60 cell cultures, and may contribute interactively to this differentiative event (32).

Cytokines Elaborated by Inflammatory Effector Cells

Using immunohistological techniques, together with in situ hybridization for gene expression, we have recently been able to show that inflammatory effector cells themselves participate in an interactive cytokine network within the tissue microenvironment. Eosinophils express and produce transforming growth factor β (TGFβ) as well as GM-CSF (1,33); while not all eosinophils produce these molecules, it may be that activation phenotype is associated with cytokine expression and production. Recent studies have also shown the production of tumor necrosis factor (TNFα) by human mast cells *in vitro* and by cells within the nasal polyp microenvironment in tissue sections (unpublished observations). The abundance of mast cells in these tissues and their compartmentalization into epithelial and stromal types based on histochemical staining and protease content (29), makes attractive the hypothesis that mast cell-derived TNFα, together with potentially other cytokines, can contribute to the interactive network within the tissue microenvironment by analogy to work in murine systems (34).

It is becoming clear that cytokine networks involved in allergic inflammation are a feature of a tissue microenvironment in which the allergic reaction is taking place. Not only this, but positive and negative feedback signals from cytokines derived from structural cells to inflammatory cells and vice-versa probably determine the type and extent of reactions. Pharmacologic manipulation of allergic inflammation, such as through the use of corticosteroids, interrupts some of these circuits by down-regulating gene expression and production of cytokines from structural cells and, potentially, inflammatory effector cells themselves. To what extent the *in vitro*, *ex vivo* and *in vivo* studies outlined above help to unravel clinically relevant phenomena in allergy remains to be clarified.

References

1. Denburg, J.A., Finotto, S., Marshall, J.S., Kawabori, S., Jordana, M., and Dolovich, J. 1991. Mast cells, stromal cells and inflammation. In: The role of the mast cell in health and

disease. M. Kaliner, D.D.Metcalfe, eds. New York: Dekker, in press.

2. Denburg, J.A., Dolovich, J., and Harnish, D. 1989. Basophil, mast cell and eosinophil growth and differentiation factors in human allergic disease. Clin. Exp. Allergy. 19:249.
3. Denburg, J.A., Jordana, M., Gibson, P., Hargreave, F.H., Ohtoshi, T., Cox, G., Gauldie, J., and Dolovich, J. 1990. Cellular and molecular basis of allergic airway inflammation. In: Pharmacia Allergy Research Foundation award book. S.G.O. Johansson, ed. Uppsala: A.W. Grafiska, p. 15.
4. Denburg, J.A., Dolovich, J., Ohtoshi, T., Cox, G., Gauldie, J., and Jordana, M. 1990. The microenvironmental differentiation hypothesis of airway inflammation. Am. J. Rhinol. 4:29.
5. Denburg, J.A., Telizyn, S., Belda, A., Dolovich, J., and Bienenstock, J. 1985. Increased numbers of circulating basophil progenitors in atopic patients. J. Allergy Clin. Immunol. 76:466.
6. Otsuka, H., Dolovich, J., Befus, A.D., Telizyn, S., Bienenstock, J., and Denburg, J.A. 1986. Basophilic cell progenitors, nasal metachromatic cells and peripheral blood basophils in ragweed-allergic patients. J. Allergy Clin. Immunol. 78:365.
7. Otsuka, H., Dolovich, J., Befus, A.D., Bienenstock, J., and Denburg, J.A. 1986. Basophilic cell progenitors, peripheral blood basophils and nasal metachromatic cells in patients with allergic rhinitis. Am. Rev. Resp. Dis. 133:757.
8. Gibson, P., Dolovich, J., Girgis-Gabardo, A.. Morris, M.M., Anderson, M., Hargreave, F.E., and Denburg, J.A. 1990. The inflammatory response in asthma exacerbation: Changes in circulating eosinophils, basophils, and their progenitors. Clin. Exp. Allergy. 20:661.
9. Gibson, P.G., Manning, P.J., O'Byrne, P.M., Girgis-Gabardo, A., Dolovich,J., Denburg, J.A., and Hargreave, F.E. 1991. Allergen-induced asthmastic responses. Relationship between increases in airway responsiveness and increases in circulating eosinophils, basophils and their progenitors. Am. Rev. Resp. Dis. 143:331.
10. Valent, P., Schmidt, G., Besemer, J., Mayer, P., Zenke, G., Liehl, E.,Hinterberger, W., Lechner, K., and Bettelheim, P. 1989. Interleukin-3 is a differentiation factor for human basophils. Blood. 73:1763.
11. Denburg, J.A. 1990. Cytokine-induced human basophil/mast cell growth and differentiation *in vitro*. Springer Semin. Immunopathol. 12:401.
12. Sanderson, C.J., Warren, D.J., and Strath, M. 1985. Identification of a lymphokine that stimulates eosinophil differentiation *in vitro*: Its relationship to interleukin 3, and functional properties of eosinophils produced in culture. J. Exp. Med. 162:60.
13. Clutterbuck, E.J., and Sanderson, C.J. 1988. Human eosinophil hematopoiesis studied *in vitro* by means of murine eosinophil differentiation factor (IL-5): Production of functionally active eosinophils from normal human bone marrow. Blood 71:656.
14. Denburg, J.A., Silver, J.E., and Abrams, J.S. 1991. Interleukin-5 is a human basophilopoietin: Induction of histamine content and basophilic differentiation of HL-60 cells and of peripheral blood basophil-eosinophil progenitors. Blood 77:1462.
15. Denburg, J.A., Telizyn, S., Messner, H., Lim, B., Jamal, N., Ackermann,S.J., Gleich, G.J., and Bienenstock, J. 1985. Heterogeneity of human peripheral blood eosinophil-type colonies: Evidence for a common basophil-eosinophil progenitor. Blood 66:312.
16. Tanno, Y., Bienenstock, J., Richardson, M., Lee, T.G., Befus, A.D., and Denburg, J. 1987. Reciprocal regulation of human basophil and eosinophil growth by separate factors in cord blood cultures. Exp. Hematol. 15:24.
17. Tsuda, T., Wong, D.A., Dolovich, J., Bienenstock, J., and Denburg, J.A. 1991. Synergistic effects of nerve growth factor and granulocyte-macrophage colony-stimulating factor on human basophilic cell differentiation. Blood 77:971.
18. Furitsu, T., Saito, H., Dvorak, A.M., Schwartz, L.B., Irani, A.M., Burdick, J.F., Ishizaka, K., and Ishizaka, T. 1989. Development of human mast cells *in vitro*. Proc. Natl. Acad. Sci. USA 86:10039.
19. Zsebo, K.M., Williams, D.A., Geissler, E.N., Broudy, V.C., Martin, F.H., Atkins, H.L., Hsu, R.Y., Birkett, N.C., Okino, K.H., Murdock, D.C., Jacobson, F.W., Langley, K.E., Smith, K.A., Takeishi, T., Cattanach, B.M., Galli, S.J., and Suggs, S.V. 1990. Stem cell factor is encoded at the *S1* locus of the mouse and is the ligand for the c-*kit* tyrosine kinase receptor. Cell 63:213.
20. Tsai, M., Shih, L.-S., Newlands, G.F.J., Takeishi, T., Langley, K.E., Zsebo, K.M., Miller, H.R.P., Geissler, E.N., and Galli, S.J. 1991. The rat c-kit ligand, stem cell factor, induces the development of connective tissue-

type and mucosal mast cells *in vivo*. Analysis by anatomical distribution, histochemistry, and protease phenotype. J. Exp. Med. 174:125.
21. Ohnishi, M., Ruhno, J., Dolovich, J., and Denburg, J.A. 1988. Allergic rhinitis nasal mucosal conditioned medium stimulates growth and differentiation of basophil/mast cell and eosinophil progenitors from atopic Blood J. Allergy Clin. Immunol. 81:1149.
22. Ohnishi, M., Ruhno, J., Bienenstock, J., Dolovich, J., and Denburg, J.A. 1989. Hemopoietic growth factor production by human nasal polypepithelial scrapings: Kinetics, cell source and relationship to clinical status. J. Allergy Clin. Immunol. 83:1091.
23. Ohtoshi, T., Tsuda, T., Vancheri, C., Abrams, J.S., Gauldie, J., Dolovich, J., and Denburg, J.A. 1991. Human upper airway epithelial cell-derived granulocyte-macrophage colony-stimulating factor (GM-CSF) induces histamine-containing cell differentiation of human progenitor cells. Int. Arch. Allergy Appl. Immunol. 95:376.
24. Vancheri, C., Ohtoshi, T., Cox, G., Xaubet, A., Abrams, J.S., Gauldie,J., Dolovich, J., Denburg, J., and Jordana, M. 1991. Neutrophilic differentiation induced by human upper airway fibroblast-derived granuloctye/macrophage colony-stimulating factor (GM-CSF). Am. J.Respir. Cell. Mol. Biol. 4:11.
25. Cox, G., Ohtoshi, T., Gauldie, J., Denburg, J.A., Dolovich, J., and Jordana, M. 1991. Promotion of eosinophil survival by human bronchial epithelial cells and its modulation by steroids. Am. J. Resp. Cell. Mol. Biol. 4:525.
26. Ohtoshi, T., Xaubet, A., Andersson, B., Vanzeigleheim, M., Dolovich, J., Jordana, M., and Denburg, J.A. 1990. Nasal inflammation mediated by human structural cell derived GM-CSF: Effect of budesonide. J. Allergy Clin.Immunol. 85:297a (abstract).
27. Keith, P., Wong, D., Liehl, M., Ceska, J., Denburg, J.A., and Dolovich, J. 1991. *In vivo* assessment of airway inflammation in nasal polyposis: Presence of IL-8 and albumin in nasal lavage fluid. J. Allergy Clin. Immunol. 87:139 (abstract).
28. Walker, C., Virchow, J.-C. Jr., Bruijnzeel, P.L.B., and Blaser, K. 1991. T cell subsets and their soluble products regulate eosinophils in allergic and non-allergic asthma. J. Immunol. 146:1829.
29. Kawabori, S., Denburg, J.A., Schwartz, L.B., Irani, A.A., Wong, D., Jordana, G., Evans, S., and Dolovich, J. 1991. Histochemical and immunohistochemical characteristics of mast cells in nasal polyps. Amer.J. Resp. Cell. Mol. Biol. 6:37.
30. Finotto, S., Marshall, J., Jordana, M., Dolovich, J., and Denburg, J.A. 1991. Isolation and functional studies of human nasal polyp mast cell populations. J. Allergy Clin. Immunol. 87:20 (abstract).
31. Ohtoshi, T., Vancheri, C., Cox, G., Gauldie, J., Dolovich, J., Denburg, J.A., and Jordana, M. 1991. Monocyte-macrophage differentiation induced by human upper airway epithelial cells. Amer. J. Resp. Cell. Mol. Biol. 4:255.
32. Wong, D.A., Kawabori, S., Switzer, J., Valent, P., Bettelheim, P., Dolovich, J., Ishizaka, T., Jordana, M., and Denburg, J. 1990. Characterization of histamine-containing basophilic cells after *in vitro* induction of HL-60 cell line. J. Allergy Clin. Immunol. 85:173 (abstract).
33. Ohno, I., Cox, G., Lea, R., Dolovich, J., Clark, D., Gauldie, J., and Jordana, M. 1991. Synthesis and localization of GM-CSF in human airway tissues. Am. Rev. Resp. Dis. 143:A201.
34. Wershil, B.K., Wang, Z.S., Gordon, J.R., and Galli, S.J. 1991. Recruitment of neutrophils during IgE-dependent cutaneous late phase reactions in the mouse is mast cell-dependent. Partial inhibition of the reaction with antiserum against tumor necrosis factor-alpha. J. Clin.Invest. 87:446.

Section XV

Dermatoimmunology

Cytokines and Epidermal Langerhans Cells

J. Thivolet*

The effect of various cytokines on epidermal Langerhans cells (LC) is difficult to study, since LC cannot be maintained for a sufficiently long time in culture. The most studied cytokine is GM-CSF, which has been shown to increase (a) the survival of murine (but probably not human) LC in short-term cultures, (b) the antigen-presenting ability of human and murine LC, and (c) the down-regulation of CD1a on human LC. TNFα increases the viability of murine LC in culture without inducing up-regulation of class II-MHC antigens. Intradermal injection of TNFα in mice reduces the number of epidermal LC, thereby prevening induction of contact hypersensitivity. TNFβ reduces the antigen-presenting capacity of normal cultured and fresh psoriatic but not fresh normal LC. IL1 acts synergistically with GM-CSF in enhancing the antigen-presenting capacity of LC and also induces chemotactic migration of LC into the central cornea in mice. IFNγ increases class II-MHC antigen expression on human and murine LC and also modulates CD4 expression on human LC. IL4 and IFNγ induce the expression of CD23 (FcERII) on normal human LC. Resting LC do not release cytokines but upon stimulation *in vitro* or in the course of inflammatory dermatoses may release IL1, TNFα and INFγ.

* Clinique Dermatologique, Hopital E Herriot, Place d'Arsonval, 69437 Lyon Cedex 03, France.

cluding platelet basic protein, β-thromboglobulin, platelet factor 4, IFN-γ inducible protein and melanoma growth stimulating activity/growth related gene product (24,25). A variety of different cells are capable of producing IL-8 on stimulation. Recently, IL-8 was also isolated from psoriatic scales, and keratinocytes upon stimulation were found to express IL-8 specific mRNA (26). Accordingly, IL-8 may be involved in the attraction of neutrophils during the development of psoriatic skin lesions. Since IL-8 also appears to be chemotactic for epidermal cells it may have an important role in reepithelization during wound healing (27). The proinflammatory activities of IL-8 are mediated via high affinity cell surface receptors (24). IL-8 is chemotactic for neutrophils and lymphocytes, and induces adhesion molecule expression (MAC-1) contributing to the adhesion of neutrophils to endothelial cells (24). Recently, another mediator has been described which is related to the IL-8 family and is chemotactic for monocytes. Primarily isolated from monocytes, this monocyte chemotactic and activating factor (MCAF) was also found to be transcribed and released by keratinocytes (24).

Tumor Necrosis Factor α

Tumor necorsis factor α was characterized as a macrophage derived mediator responsible for hemorrhagic necrosis of tumors and cachexia in animals (28). Subsequently, it became clear that TNFα like IL-1 and IL-6 is produced by almost any cell and has a broad spectrum of biological activities. When exposed to tumor promoters, UV light, IL-1 or IL-6, keratinocytes express mRNA specific for TNFα and release TNFα activity (29). TNFα, like IL-1, is a pyrogenic cytokine and activates a variety of inflammatory cells such as neutrophils, eosinophils, macrophages, fibroblasts and others (10). Endothelial cells in response to TNFα proliferate, produce cytokines and express adhesion molecules such as ICAM-1 (10). Moreover, TNFα enhances MHC class I and II antigen expression on various cells, and costimulates T and B lymphocytes as well as hematopoietic stem cells (10, 28).

Within the epidermis TNFα appears to be relevant for several reasons. In addition to being able to produce TNFα, keratinocytes also express TNFα receptors and respond to TNFα with increased expression of ICAM-1, which is possibly of importance in T cell keratinocyte interactions (30). TNFα is also released in increasing amounts after UV exposure and appears to be involved in the development of apoptotic keratinocytes ("sunburn cells"). Accordingly, treatment of animals with a TNFα antiserum resulted in a significant reduction in sunburn cell formation (31). Futhermore, TNFα is one of the cytokines involved in Langerhans cell maturation (32). During the elicitation of contact hypersensitivity and the occurrence of cutaneous lesions in graft versus host disease, TNFα also seems to be one of the crucial mediators (33,34).

Colony Stimulating Factors

Colony stimulating factors induce hematopoietic stem cell proliferation and differentiation and induce non lineage specific CSF's such as IL-3 (multi CSF) and granulocyte/macrophage CSF (GM-CSF) as well as the more specific granulocyte CSF (G-CSF) and macrophage CSF (M-CSF) (35). It has been demonstrated that keratinocytes are able to release all four types of CSF, and their transcripts were detected in keratinocytes following stimulation (3). Although murine keratinocytes were clearly shown to produce IL-3, there is no clear evidence for human keratinocytes being able to secrete IL-3 (3). GM-CSF, together with IL-1 and TNFα, plays an important role in the maturation of Langerhans cells (32). Moreover, GM-CSF was found to be expressed in increased amounts in keratinocytes following UV exposure which would be sufficient to reverse myelosuppression (36).

Growth Factors

Growth factors were originally characterized according to their growth promoting capacity for specific cells. Keratinocytes have been found to synthesize and release a variety of growth factors including transforming growth factor (TGF) α and β, platelet derived growth factor (PDGF) and basic fibroblast growth factor (bFGF) (3). Accordingly, TGFα mRNA is expressed in the stratified epidermis and psoriatic plaques, and TGFβ transcripts have been found in normal and psoriatic epidermis (37,38). PDGF has been shown to be released by EC in response to TGFβ (39). Moreover, bFGF has recently been reported to be expressed in proliferating keratinocytes and to function as a growth factor for melanocytes (40).

Recently, it became evident that growth factors additionally appear to have several immunomodulating functions. TGFβ may inhibit IL-1 receptor expression and block the biological activity of IL-1, IL-2 and CSF's (41). PDGF has been recognized as a mitogen and chemoattractant for inflammatory cells and may stimulate MHC class II antigen expression (42). During inflammatory reactions the growth promoting and chemotactic activities of growth factors such as FGF, PDGF and TGF on endothelial cells may also be of particular importance (42,43).

Suppressor Factors

Cytokines which downregulate an ongoing immune- or inflammatory reaction have attracted increasing interest. In addition to the immunoinhibitory mediator TGFβ, a specific IL-1 receptor antagonist (IL-1ra) was recently identified which was also found to be expressed in keratinocytes (44,45). Moreover, IL-10 was identified as cytokine synthesis inhibitory factor (CSIF) blocking the production of IL-2, IL-3, IFN-γ, GM-CSF and TNFα (46). On UV irradiation or treatment with PMA, keratinocytes have been shown to release distinct inhibitory mediators which specifically block the activity of IL-1 and the induction of a contact hypersensitivity reaction (CHS) (19). Although the structure of these EC derived inhibitors has not yet have been defined, they seem to be distinct from known inhibitory cytokines (3,19). Within the epidermis these mediators appear to be of importance during UV mediated immunosuppression. Since they were also detected in the circulation of UV treated animals, these inhibitory mediators may also be involved in systemic immunosuppression (47).

Conclusion

The finding that keratinocytes are able to secrete cytokines may allow new insights into the pathomechanism of immune and inflammatory skin diseases. Further elucidation of cytokine interactions and their multiple functions will possibly help to define disease activity. Thus, understanding the cytokine-eicosanoide-hormone network may perhaps allow us to use some of these mediators, their analogues or antagonists, to develop new strategies to treat skin diseases.

References

1. Bos, J.D., Das, P.R., and Kapsenberg, M.L. 1989. The skin immune system (SIS). In: The skin immune system (SIS). J.D. Bos, ed. Boca Raton, Florida: CRC Press, p. 3.
2. Streilein, J.W. 1989. Skin-associated lymphoid tissue. In: Immune mechanisms in cutaneous disease. D.A. Norris, ed. New York and Basel: Marcel Dekker, p. 73.
3. Luger, T.A., and Schwarz, T. 1991. Epidermal cell-derived secretory regulins. In: Epidermal Langerhans cells. G. Schuler, ed. Boca Raton, Florida: CRC Press, p. 217.
4. Kupper, T.S. 1990. Role of epidermal cytokines. In: Immunophysiology. J.J. Oppenheim, and E. Shevach, eds. Oxford and New York: Oxford University Press, p. 285.
5. Köck, A., Schwarz, T., Micksche, M., and Luger, T.A. 1991. Cytokines and human malignant melanoma immuno- and growth-regulatory peptides in melanoma biology. In: Melanoma research: Genetics, growth factors, metastases, and antigens. L. Nathanson, ed. Boston: Kluwer Academic Publishers, p. 41.
6. Luger, T.A., Stadler, B.M., Katz, S.I., and Oppenheim, J.J. 1981. Epidermal cell (keratinocyte) derived thymocyte activating factor (ETAF). J. Immunol. 124:1493.
7. Hauser, C., Saurat, J.H., Schmitt, A., Jannin, F., and Dayer, J.M. 1986. Interleukin-1 is present in normal human epidermis. J. Immunol. 136:317.
8. Blanton, R.A., Kupper, T.S., McDougal, J.K., and Dower, S. 1989. Regulation of interleukin-1 and its receptor in human keratinocytes. Proc. Natl. Acad. Sci. USA 86:1273.
9. Durum, S.K., Oppenheim, J.J., and Neta, R. 1990. Immunophysiologic role of interleukin-

1. In: Immunophysiology: The role of cells and cytokines in immunity and inflammation. J.J. Oppenheim, E.M. Shevach, eds. New York: Oxford University Press, p. 210.
10. Dinarello, C.A. 1989. Interleukin-1 and its biologically related cytokines. Adv. Immunol. 44:153.
11. Dejana, E., Brevario, R., Erroi, A., Bussolino, F., Mussoni, L., Gramse, M., Pintucci, G., Casali, B., Dinarello, C.A., VanDamme, J., and Mantonvani, A. 1987. Modulation of endothelial cell function by different molecular species of interleukin-1. Blood 69:695.
12. Bateman, A., Singh, A., Kral, T., and Solomon, S. 1989. The immune-hypothalamic-pituitary-adrenal axis. Endocrine Reviews 10:92.
13. Köck, A., Schauer, E., Schwarz, T., and Luger, T.A. 1991. Human keratinocytes synthesize and release neuropeptides such as α-MSH and ACTH. In: Cellular and cytokine networks in tissue immunity. M. Meltzer, and A. Mantonvani, eds. New York: John Wiley & Sons Inc., p.105.
14. Wong, G.G., and Clark, S.C. 1989. Multiple actions of interleukin 6 within a cytokine network. Immunol. Today. 9:137.
15. Kirnbauer, R., Köck, A., Schwarz, T., Urbanski, A., Krutmann, J., Borth, W., Damm, D., Shipley, G., Ansel, J.C., and Luger, T.A. 1989. Interferon β2, B-cell differentiation factor 2, hybridoma growth factor (interleukin-6) is expressed and released by human epidermal cells and epidermal carcinoma cell lines. J. Immunol. 142:1922.
16. Krüger, J.G., Krane, J.F., Carter, D.M., and Gottlieb, A.B. 1989. Role of growth factors, cytokines, and their receptors in the pathogenesis of psoriasis. J. Invest. Dermatol. 94 (Suppl.):135S.
17. Neuner, P., Urbanski, A., Trautinger, F., Möller, A., Kirnbauer, R., Kapp, A., Schöpf, E., Schwarz, T., and Luger, T.A. 1991. Increased IL-6 production by monocytes and keratinocytes in patients with psoriasis. J. Invest. Dermatol. 97:27.
18. Armstrong, C.A., Koppula, S.V., Tara, D.C., Ansel, J.C. 1991. The effect of melanoma derived interleukin-6 on melanoma growth and development in a murine model. J. Invest. Dermatol. 96:548.
19. Schwarz, T., and Luger, T.A. 1989. Effect of UV irradiation on epidermal cell cytokine production. J. Photochem. Photobiol. 4:1
20. Urbanski, A., Schwarz, T. Neuner, P., Krutmann, J., Kirnbauer, R., Köck, A., and Luger, T.A. 1990. Ultraviolet light induces increased circulating interleukin-6 in humans. J. Invest. Dermatol. 94:808.
21. Linker-Israeli, M., Deans, R.J., Wallace, D.J., Prehn, J., Ozeri-Chen, T., and Klinenberg, J.R. 1991. Elevated levels of endogenous IL-6 in systemic lupus erythematosus. A putative role in pathogenesis. J. Immunol. 147:117.
22. Henney, C.S. 1989. Interleukin-7, effects on early events in lymphopoiesis. Immunol. Today 10:170.
23. Heufler, C., Young, D., Peschel, G., and Schuler, G. 1990. Murine keratinocytes express interleukin-7. J. Invest. Dermatol. 94:534A .
24. Matsushima, K., and Oppenheim, J.J. 1989. Interleukin-8 and MCAF, novel inflammatory cytokines inducible by IL-1 and TNF. Cytokine 1:2.
25. Westwick, J., Li, S.W., and Camp, R.D. 1989. Novel neutrophil-stimulating peptides. Immunol. Today 10:146.
26. Schröder, J.M., and Christophers, E. 1988. Identification of a novel family of highly potent neutrophil chemotactic peptides in psoriatic scales. J. Invest. Dermatol. 91:395.
27. Hein, R., Schröder, J.M., Christophers, E., and Krieg, T. 1990. NAP/IL-8, a human monocyte derived peptide is chemotactic for epidermal cells but not for human dermal fibroblasts. Arch. Derm. Res. 281:571A.
28. Beutler, B., and Cerami, A. 1990. Cachectin (tumor necrosis factor), an endogenous mediator of shock and inflammatory response. In: Immunophysiology; The role of cells and cytokines in immunity and inflammation. J.J. Oppenheim, and E.M.Shevach, eds. New York: Oxford University Press, p. 226.
29. Köck, A., Schwarz, T., Kirnbauer, R., Urbanski, A., Perry, P., Ansel, J.C., and Luger, T.A. 1990. Human keratinocytes are a source for tumor necrosis factor α: Evidence for synthesis and release upon stimulation with endotoxin or ultraviolet light. J. Exp. Med. 172:1609.
30. Trefzer, U., Brockhaus, M., Köck, A., Kapp, A., Schöpf, E., and Krutmann, J. 1991. The 55kD type I tumor necrosis factor receptor (TNFRI) plays a pivotal role in the regulation of human keratinocyte ICAM-1 expression. J. Invest. Dermatol. 96:543A.
31. Schwarz, T., Urbanski, A., Trautinger, F., Neuner, P., and Luger, T.A. 1991. Effect on UV light on cytokine production by epidermal cells. In: Basic mechanisms of physiological and aberrant lymphoproliferation in the skin. W.A. Van Vloten, and W.C. Lambert, eds.,

New York: Plenum Publishing Corporation, in press.
32. Koch, F., Heufler, C., Schneeweiss, D., Kaempgen, E., and Schuler, G. 1990. Tumor necrosis factor alpha maintains viability of murine epidermal Langerhans cell in culture, but in contrast to GM-CSF without inducing functional maturation. J. Exp. Med. 171:159.
33. Piguet, P.F., Grau, G.E., Allet, B., and Vasalli, P. 1987. Tumor necrosis factor/cachectin is an effector of skin and gut lesions of the acute phase of graft- vs. host- disease. J. Exp. Med. 166:1280.
34. Piguet, P.F., Grau, G.E., Hauser, C., and Vassalli, P. 1991. Tumor necrosis factor is a critical mediator in hapten-induced irritant and contact hypersensitivity reactions. J. Exp. Med. 173:673.
35. Cosman, D. 1988. Colony stimulating factors *in vivo* and *in vitro*. Immunol. Today 9:97.
36. Birchall, N., Gamba, C., and Kupper, T. 1988. Cutaneous UVB irradiation enhances recovery from bone marrow suppression. Clin. Res. 36:801A.
37. Gottlieb, A.B., Chang, G.K., Posnett, D.N., Fanelli, B., and Tam, J.P. 1988. Detection of transforming growth factor-α in normal, malignant, and hyperproliferative human keratinocytes. J. Exp. Med. 167:670.
38. Fisher, G., Elder, J., Voorhees, J., Kawalki, J., Petersen, C., Derynck, R., and Ellingsworth, L. 1988. Tranforming growth factor beta mRNA is expressed in normal and psoriatic epidermis and has similar biological effects on normal and psoriatic lesional cultured keratinocytes. Clin. Res. 36:645A.
39. Damm, D., Shipley, G., Hart, C., and Ansel, J.C. 1990. The expression and modulation of PDGF in normal human keratinocytes. In: Molecular and cellular biology of cytokines. J.J. Oppenheim, M.C. Powanda, M.J. Kluger, and C.A. Dinarello, eds. New York: Wiley-Liss, p.111.
40. Halaban, R., Langdon, R., Birchall, N., Cuono, C., Baird, A., Scott, G., Moellmann, G., and McGuire, J. 1988. Paracrine stimulation of melanocytes by keratinocytes through basic fibroblast growth factor. Ann. N .Y. Acad. Sci. 548:180.
41. Wahl, S.M., McCartney-Francis, N., and Mergenhagen, G. 1989. Inflammatory and immunomodulating roles of TGF-β. Immunol. Today 10:258.
42. Ross, R. 1989. Platelet-derived growth factor. Lancet. ii:1179.
43. Thomas, K.A. 1987. Fibroblast growth factors. FASEB J. 1:4334.
44. Eisenberg, S.P., Evans, R.J., Arend, W.P., Verderber, E., Brewer, M.T., Hannum C.H., and Thompson, R.C. 1990. Primary structure and functional expression from complementary DNA of a human interleukin-1 receptor antagonist. Nature 343:341.
45. Bigler, C.F., Weston, W.L., Norris, D.A., and Arend, W.P. 1991. Interleukin-1 receptor antagonist production by human keratinocytes. Clin. Res. 39:291A.
46. Moore, K.W., Vieira, P., Fiorentino, D.F., Trounstine, M.L., Khan, T.A., and Mosmann, T.R. 1990. Homology of cytokine synthesis inhibitory factor (IL-10) to the Epstein-Barr virus gene BCRFI. Science 248:58.
47. Schwarz, T., Urbanski, A., Kirnbauer, R., Köck, A., Gschnait, F., and Luger, T.A. 1988. Detection of a specific inhibitor of interleukin-1 in sera of UVB-treated mice. J. Invest. Dermatol. 91:536.

The Immunology of Mouse γδ Dendritic Epidermal T Cells: Still More Questions Than Answers

Robert E. Tigelaar, Julia M. Lewis*

Dendritic epidermal T cells (DETC) in adult mice express a monomorphic T cell receptor (TCR) composed of V5J1Cγ1 and V1D2J2Cδ chains devoid of junctional diversity. Identical TCRs are expressed on early fetal thymocytes, and transfer of fetal thymocytes into young *nude* mice, whose skin lacks DETC, leads to the appearance of Vγ5/Vδ1+ DETC in recipient skin. Recent studies indicate DETC can be activated by keratinocytes stressed *in vitro* by heat shock or *in vivo* by contact dermatitis reactions. Characterization of this potential physiologic ligand for DETC, together with identification of the relevant biologic function(s) of murine DETC, may clarify the relationships between these cells and human γδ cells.

TCRs on Recirculating T Cells

In man and rodents most recirculating T cells express either CD4 or CD8 and have TCRs composed of an α and a β chain. A minor proportion (< 10%) express TCRs which are γδ heterodimers; such cells are typically CD4- or CD8-. Enormous TCR diversity in both αβ and γδ cells is generated within their junctional regions, the consequence of variable exonucleolytic nibbling of the coding segment ends and insertion into these junctions of non-germline encoded (N) nucleotides. This TCR heterogeneity gives recirculating T cells the collective capacity to recognize a vast array of foreign antigens; at the same time the capacity to recirculate enhances the likelihood of a given T cell confronting its particular antigen.

Unique Features of Mouse DETC

Initially named Thy-1+ dendritic epidermal cells because of their characteristic morphology and phenotype (1,2), it soon became clear that normal mouse epidermis was populated by Ia-, CD4-, CD8-cells which could display functional properties of T cells, e.g., mitogen and IL-2 responsiveness, secretion of IL-2, and various forms of cytotoxicity (3,4). With the demonstration that the overwhelming majority of such cells from normal adult mice expressed a CD3-associated γδ TCR (5,6), they were renamed dendritic epidermal T cells, or DETC. The results of more precise characterization of the γδ TCRs on DETC were totally unanticipated. Not only did all of several independent DETC lines from AKR/J mice express TCRs with identical γ coding segments (V5J1Cγ1) and identical δ coding segments (V1D2J2Cδ), but the γ and δ junctional regions each were homogeneous and devoid of N nucleotides (7). Compatible results have been obtained on non-cultured DETC by both FACS and PCR analysis (8,9), and our own studies of epidermal sheets from various strains of mice have shown that > 95% of the CD3+ cells also stain with a monoclonal antibody (named 17D1) which reacts only with TCRs containing both Vγ5 and Vδ1 (10). Furthermore, in adult mice, the epidermis is the only site known to contain Vγ5/Vδ1+ T cells; they have not been found in adult thymus, lymph nodes or spleen (8), or from other epithelia populated preferentially with other distinct subsets of γδ cells, such as intestinal (Vγ7+) or reproductive (Vγ6/Vδ1+) epithelium (11,12).

* Departments of Dermatology and Immunobiology, Yale University School of Medicine, 333 Cedar Street, New Haven, Connecticut 06510 USA.
Acknowledgements: Supported by NIH grant AI27404.

Early Fetal Thymic Dependence of Vγ5/Vδ1+ DETC

The first fetal thymocytes to express a CD3/TCR complex (about fetal d14) express exclusively V5J1Cγ1/V1D2J2Cδ TCRs devoid of junctional diversity, i.e., identical to the monomorphic TCRs on DETC (13,14). The proportion of fetal thymocytes with DETC-type TCRs peaks about d17 and becomes undetectable by birth. Their TCR identity suggested early fetal thymocytes could serve as DETC precursors. Data showing this can occur has been obtained by capitalizing on the fact that the epidermis of young adult athymic nude mice lacks Thy-1+ CD3+ Vγ5/Vδ1+ cells; transfer of CD3+ Vγ5/Vδ1+ fetal thymocytes into newborn or adult nude recipients results in the gradual appearance of epidermal dendritic CD3+ Vγ5/Vδ1+ cells (10,15,16). While such data is consistent with the hypothesis that DETC are thymic dependent, they do not prove this path is followed by all DETC in normal mice. In fact, support for thymic independent differentiation has also been generated recently; grafts of d16 fetal skin containing scattered Thy-1+, but CD3- TCR-cells result in the gradual appearance of donor-type dendritic CD3+ Vγ5+ DETC (Stingl, personal communication). While additional studies are necessary before concluding that junctionally homogeneous Vγ5/Vδ1+ DETC can be thymic independent, it is clear that the differentiation path(s) used by DETC precursors have not been definitively established.

Antigen Recognition and Function of DETC

The monomorphism of DETC TCRs suggested that DETC recognize only one ligand, generating the hypothesis that DETC function in immune surveillance by recognizing a common self antigen, such as a stress-induced, or heat shock protein (HSP), expressed on the surface of damaged, altered or transformed epidermal cells (7,17). HSPs are widely conserved protein families normally expressed at low levels, but markedly upregulated after stimuli such as heat shock, oxidizing agents, heavy metal ions, nutrient deprivation, intracellular infection or malignant transformation (18). Recent data is consistent with the expression of the DETC TCR ligand on stressed epidermal cells (EC) (19,20). In our studies, a DETC line maintained *in vitro* with IL-2 was stimulated to proliferate and secrete IL-2 when confronted with either heat shocked or nutrient deprived EC (compared to baseline proliferation in response to freshly isolated EC). That this recognition was TCR-mediated was suggested by the capacity of anti-Vγ5/Vδ1 Fab fragments to block the response to stressed EC. That the DETC stimulation was not mediated solely by soluble factors was shown by the failure of supernatants from stressed EC to stimulate DETC proliferation. That stressed keratinocytes express the ligand was indicated by the vigorous DETC response to stressed EC depleted of both Thy-1+ and Ia+ cells. Data suggesting that DETC ligand expression may be confined to the epidermis, was obtained in experiments showing that heat shocked spleen cells or dermal fibroblasts did not stimulate DETC proliferation. Furthermore, equivalent proliferation was observed using stressed syngeneic or allogeneic (class I and class II MHC-disparate) EC, suggesting that if DETC TCR activation requires its ligand to be seen in the context of a restriction element, such a restriction element is distinct from the usual polymorphic class I and II MHC molecules used by αβ T cells. Such results obviously do not exclude the possibility that other less polymorphic MHC-like molecules expressed on keratinocytes serve such a role; class Ib molecules such as CD1 or TL, whose expression has been shown to be tissue restricted, represent a theoretically attractive alternative (21). Finally, that DETC may be activated *in vivo* by stressed or altered EC was suggested by two findings. First, Vγ5/Vδ1+ DETC density increased >2-fold following topical application of DNFB croton oil, and DETC morphology suggested their *in situ* division. Second, freshly isolated EC from skin painted 16 hours earlier with croton oil stimulated proliferation of the DETC line without requiring any additional *in vitro* stress such as heat shock.

While these studies are consistent with the hypothesis that DETC function in immune surveillance by recognition of a common stress-related self-antigen on altered epidermal cells, even future precise ligand identification by itself will not clarify the currently unknown *in vivo* physiologic and/or pathologic relevance of DETC. However, this situation is not unique to mouse DETC; our ignorance of biologically relevant function applies to all γδ cells, regardless of location or species. Historically, understanding of conventional T cell immunobiology proceeded in exactly the opposite direction from that for γδ cells. We were aware of the consequences of T cell absence or dysfunction (such as increased susceptibility to various infections) before we began to clarify the range of functional activities of conventional T cells (such as B cell help, suppression, cytotoxicity). And knowledge of functional diversity, along with the ability to routinely generate antigen-specific, MHC-restricted T cells preceded knowledge about the structure and molecular biology of the TCRs that recognized those antigens. In the case of γδ cells such as DETC, we are proceeding "backwards", i.e., having detailed knowledge of their TCRs but ignorant of the antigens which commonly trigger them, their full range of functional capabilities, or the biologic consequences of their selective absence or dysfunction. Speculation about an immune surveillance role for DETC has focussed on their effecting the removal of epidermal cells altered in such a way as to threaten the skin's functional integrity. DETC-mediated removal of altered cells could be direct via the known cytotoxic activity of activated DETC and/or indirect via secretion of lymphokines which could recruit and activate other more conventional pro-inflammatory cells. However, epidermal integrity/function can also be impaired by inadequately suppressed intracutaneous immune responses mediated by conventional T cells, and several correlative studies suggest DETC can indeed function as downregulators of immunologically mediated injury (22,23). Finally, if DETC can recognize ligands expressed on subtly altered cells in their microenvironment, then their potential participation as pathogenic effector cells in autoimmune disease should not be summarily dismissed. Recent studies of human skin indicate that human epidermis does not contain a regular dendritic network of γδ cells expressing a monomorphic TCR (20,24). A number of factors, whose discussion is beyond the scope of this review, could contribute to this lack of a precise human morphological and phenotypic equivalent of murine DETC. Such factors clearly include major differences between the two species in fetal thymic ontogeny and the nature of their hair coat, and may also include differences in epidermal expression of the adhesion molecules necessary for a subset of γδ cells to maintain an intraepidermal localization. However, before concluding that human skin lacks the biologically relevant counterpart of murine DETC, and that further detailed study of this subset of mouse T cells is thus unnecessary, considerably more data from studies in both species are needed .

References

1. Bergstresser, P., Tigelaar, R., Dees, J., and Streilein, J. 1983. Thy-1 antigen-bearing dendritic cells populate murine epidermis. J. Invest. Dermatol. 81:286.
2. Tschachler, E., Schuler, G., Hutterer, J., Leibl, H., Wolff, K., and Stingl, G. 1983. Expression of Thy-1 antigen by murine epidermal cells. J. Invest. Dermatol. 81:282.
3. Romani, N., Stingl, G., Tschachler, E., Witmer, M., Steinman, R., Shevach, E., and Schuler, G. 1985. The Thy-1-bearing cell of murine epidermis. J. Exp. Med. 161:1368.
4. Takashima, A., Nixon-Fulton, J., Bergstresser, P., and Tigelaar, R. 1988. Thy-1+ DEC in mice: precursor analysis and cloning of Con A-reactive cells. J. Invest. Dermatol. 90:671.
5. Stingl, G., Gunter, K., Tschachler, E., Yamada, H., Lechler, R., Yokoyama, W., Steiner, G., Germain, R., and Shevach, E. 1987. Thy-1+ DEC belong to the T-cell lineage. Proc. Natl. Acad. Sci. USA 84:2430.
6. Steiner, G., Koning, F., Elbe, A., Tschachler, E., Yokoyama, W.M., Shevach, E.M., Stingl, G., and Coligan, J.E. 1988. Characterization of TCRs on resident murine DETC. Eur. J. Immunol. 18:1323.
7. Asarnow, D.M., Kuziel, W.A., Bonyhadi, M., Tigelaar, R.E., Tucker, P.W., and Allison, J.P. 1988. Limited diversity of γδ antigen receptor genes of Thy-1+ dendritic epidermal cells. Cell 55:837.
8. Havran, W., Grell, S., O'Brien, R., Born, W., Tigelaar, R., and Allison, J. 1989. Limited diversity of TCR γ-chain expression of murine Thy-1+ DEC revealed by Vγ3-specific monoclonal antibody. Proc .Natl. Acad. Sci. USA 86:4185.

9. Asarnow, D., Goodman, T., Lefrancois, L., and Allison, J. 1989. Distinct antigen receptor repertoires of two classes of murine epithelium-associated T cells. Nature 341:60.
10. Tigelaar, R., Lewis, J., and Bergstresser P. 1990. TCR γ/δ^+ dendritic epidermal T cells as constituents of skin-associated lymphoid tissue. J. Invest. Dermatol. 94 Suppl.:58S.
11. Kyes, S., Carew, E., Carding, S., Janeway, C., Jr., and Hayday, A. 1989. Diversity in T-cell receptor γ gene usage in intestinal epithelium. Proc. Natl. Acad. Sci. USA 86:5527.
12. Itohara, S., Farr, A., Lafaille, J., Bonneville, M., Takagaki, Y., and Tonegawa, S. 1990. Homing of a γδ thymocyte subset with homogeneous T-cell receptors to mucosal epithelia. Nature 343:754.
13. Havran, W., and Allison, J. 1988. Developmentally ordered appearance of thymocytes expressing different TCRs. Nature 335:443.
14. Lafaille, J.J., DeCloux A., Bonneville, M., Takagaki, Y., and Tonegawa, S. 1989. Junctional sequences of T cell receptor γδ genes: Implications for γδ T cell lineages and for a novel intermediate of V-(D)-J joining. Cell 59:859.
15. Havran, W., and Allison, J. 1990. Origin of Thy-1^+ DEC of adult mice from fetal thymic precursors. Nature 344:68.
16. Payer, E., Elbe, A., and Stingl, G. 1991. Circulating $CD3^+$/TCR $V\gamma3^+$ fetal murine thymocytes home to the skin and give rise to proliferating DETC. J.Immunol. 146:2536.
17. Janeway, C.A., Jr., Jones, B., and Hayday, A. 1988. Specificity and function of T cells bearing γδ receptors. Immunol. Today 9:73.
18. Kaufmann, S.H.E. 1990. Heat shock proteins and the immune response. Immunol. Today 11:129.
19. Havran, W.L., Chien, Y.-H., and Allison, J.P. 1991. Recognition of self antigens by skin-derived T cells with invariant γδ antigen receptors. Science 252:1430.
20. Modlin, R.L., Lewis, J., Uyemura, K., and Tigelaar, R.E. 1991. T-lymphocytes bearing γδ antigen receptors in skin. Chem.Immunol., in press.
21. Wu, M., Van Kaer, L., Itohara, S., and Tonegawa, S. 1991. Highly restricted expression of the thymus leukemia antigens on intestinal epithelial cells. J. Exp. Med. 174:213.
22. Amornsiripanitch, S., Barnes, L.M., Nordlund, J.J., Trinkle, L.S., and Rheins, L.A. 1988. Immune studies in the depigmenting C57BL/Ler-vit/vit mice. J. Immunol. 140:3438.
23. Shiohara, T., Moriya, N., Gotoh, C., Hayakawa, J., Nagashima, M., Saizawa, K., and Ishikawa, H. 1990. Loss of epidermal integrity by T cell-mediated attack induces long-term local resistance to subsequent attack. J. Exp. Med. 171:1027.
24. Foster, C.A., Yokozeki, H., Rappersberger, K., Koning, F., Volc-Platzer, B., Rieger, A., Coligan, J.E., Wolff, K., and Stingl, G. 1990. Human epidermal T cells predominately belong to the lineage expressing α/β T cell receptor. J. Exp. Med. 171:997.

Does Allergy Play a Role in Atopic Eczema?

Johannes Ring*, Thomas Bieber**, Dieter Vieluf*, Bernhard Przybilla*

While the pathomechanisms of respiratory atopy are rather well established, the role of IgE-mediated hypersensitivity in the elicitation and maintenance of eczematous skin lesions in atopic eczema (AE) is still controversial. There is evidence for exogenous elicitation of AE by contact with aero or food allergens. Recent investigations suggest that Langerhans cells in the epidermis may play a role in mediating these reactions. Langerhans cells can bind IgE probably by different receptors. They may express *in vitro* low affinity IgE receptors (CD 23) whereby the cytokines interleukin 4 and gamma-interferon act synergistically. Furthermore, there is now evidence that epidermal Langerhans cells can also express the high affinity receptor for human IgE which, until recently, was only known to be present on mast cells and basophils. The clinical relevance of sensitizations against aero allergens may be evaluated by an "atopy patch test" which has to be further standardized before it can be recommended for clinical routine. Apart from a clear-cut role of allergic reactions in atopic eczema, other factors such as non specific skin irritability have to be considered. The influence of environmental pollutants upon the development and maintenance of atopic eczema has to be further studied. There is preliminary evidence for increased prevalence rates of AE in areas with high degrees of air pollution. Thus the question in the title can be answered: Yes, allergy does play a role in AE. However, this has to be determined by careful allergological and dermatological examination in each individual patient and critically differentiated from other, non-immunological factors.

While the pathomechanisms of allergic respiratory diseases are rather well established, the role of allergic reactions in the elicitation and maintenance of atopic eczema (AE) is still controversial (1,2,3,4,5,6). Many authors regard the highly elevated serum levels of IgE antibodies as epiphenomenon relevant for the respiratory symptoms but not for the skin lesions. In an attempt to answer the question in the title of this paper, one has to first define the relevant terms. A distinction must then be made between the "prevalence" or "coincidence" of atopic diseases, including AE, and the etiopathophysiology, namely the relevance of certain allergic reactions for the actual eczematous skin lesions. Allergy is used here to designate immunologically mediated hypersensitivity leading to disease, and atopy designates the tendency to develop certain diseases (allergic rhinoconjunctivitis, extrinsic bronchial asthma, atopic eczema) on the basis of a hypersensitivity of the skin and mucous membranes against environmental substances. It usually occurs in predisposed families and is associated with increased IgE-production and/or non-specific reactivity (5).

Different Hypersensitivity Reactions in Relation to Atopic Eczema

Among the six types of allergic reactions (modified according to the classification of Coombs and Gill [7]) only type I, namely the IgE-mediated sensitization, is clearly associated with AE (Table 1). The role of other types of allergic reactions, such as cytotoxic antibodies, immune complexes (8), IgG4-antibodies or pseudo-allergic mechanisms is still controversial. Preliminary data from placebo-controlled oral provocation tests suggest that food additives may elicit eczematous skin lesions (9). Pathogenic photo-reactions may also play a role in a sub-

* Haut-Klinik and Allergie-Abteilung, Universitäts Krankenhaus Eppendorf, Universität Hamburg Martinistraβe 52, 2000 Hamburg 20, Germany;

** Dermatologische Klinik and Poliklinik, Ludwig Maximilians Universität München, Frauenlobstraβe 9, 8000 München 2, Germany.

Acknowledgements: This work has been supported in part by grants from the Bundesministerium für Forschung and Technologie (07ALL03) and from the Wilhelm-Sander Stiftung.

Table 1. Atopic eczema, allergy and pseudo-allergy:coincidence or relevance?

Type of Allergy	Coincidence	Relevance
I	+++	+–++
II	0	0
III	±	?
IV	<–++	?
V	0	0
VI	± (auto-anti IgE)	?
Pseudo-allergy		
Acetylsalicylic acid	±	±
Additives	+	+?
Radiographic-contrast media	0	0
Local anesthetics	0	0
Photosensitization	+	+?

group of patients. However, the exact mechanisms are not known (10).

Allergic Contact Dermatitis and Atopic Eczema

Numerous reports describe a decreased cell-mediated immunity in patients with AE which is correlated with a decreased frequency of allergic contact dermatitis (4). Most of these studies however, are retrospective and lack adequate control groups. In a study of 12,000 patients undergoing patch tests we found that the frequency of positive contact allergic reactions (40%) in patients with AE was equal to that seen in other patients

Table 2. Positive patch test reaction and atopy

	Atopics (n=2021)	Non-atopics (n=9837)
5 positive (total)	40.4	39.7
Single allergens (%)		
Nickel sulfate	15.2*	10.0
Potassium dichromate	5.9*	4.3
Thiuram mix	4.2*	2.6
Fragrance mix	9.5	9.2
Cobalt chloride	5.5	4.7
Lanolin	2.9	4.3*
Caine mix	2.2	4.5*
Clioquinol	1.1	2.8*

* Significantly more frequent in comparing the two groups

(Table 2). However, there were significant differences in the analysis of single allergens: Patch test reactions to nickel sulfite, cobalt chloride, potassium dichromate and thiurammix were significantly more frequent while, on the other hand, reactions against substances such as lanolin and caines were significantly less frequent in atopics (11).

Immunoglobulin E and IgE Receptors

Few diseases are characterized by such elevated serum concentrations of IgE antibodies as in AE. These antibodies are specifically directed against environmental substances. Many authors, however, regard this as epiphenomenon. On the other hand, there are many clinical examples of clear-cut evidence showing exacerbations of eczematous skin lesions after contact with certain aero (e.g. cat epithelium, house dust mite, pollen) or food allergens (12,13). Some of the most obvious cases, as when direct contact of a protein allergen has elicited an eczematous skin eruption, have been known for a long time as "protein contact dermatitis" (14). A variety of hypotheses may help to explain the participation of IgE antibodies in the induction of eczema (Table 3). Vasoactive mediators secreted by mast cells or basophils in the skin may produce itch, contact urticaria or a "late-phase-reaction", with consequent eczematous skin changes, after allergen contact (6). Eosinophils also seem to be involved in the inflammatory response in AE. Products such as major basic protein (MBP) (15), or eosinophil cationic protein (ECP), which have been found to be elevated in AE, may be released. (16). Lymphocytes may act directly by producing certain cytokines or chemotactic factors. The basic mechanisms for the regulation of IgE production are not well established. The regulatory components include T cells, cytokines (especially interleukin 4) and IgE receptors (or the respective binding factors) (17,18). Receptors for IgE have been demonstrated on human T cells in culture after *in vitro* stimulation with specific allergen (19). In patients with AE, elevated numbers of $Fc_{\epsilon}RII$-positive B cells have been observed (together with P. Rieber and J. Prinz, unpublished results).

Langerhans Cells and Atopic Eczema

Recent investigations have stressed the role of dendritic epidermal Langerhans cells, which have been found to carry IgE, in patients with severe AE (20,21) as well as in patients with other, IgE related, inflammatory skin diseases (Bieber et al., in preparation). There was a positive correlation between the number of IgE-positive Langerhans cells in the epidermis and the serum IgE concentrations. After topical treatment with corticosteroids, the number of IgE-positive Langerhans cells decreased significantly (21). The nature of the IgE binding site on Langerhans cells is the focus of much current allergy research: It is well known that Langerhans cells can be induced to express a low affinity IgE receptor (CD 23) when incubated with interleukin 4 and interferon-gamma (in a synergistic manner) in culture. Other cytokines, such as interleukin 1, interleukin 2, GM-CSF, were without effect (22). However, monoclonal antibodies against the CD 23 marker *in situ* revealed that the distribution of the receptor was not equivalent to the detected IgE on the Langerhans cell surface. Therefore, another IgE binding site, such as an IgE binding protein or the classical high affinity IgE receptor or a totally new structure, has been speculated on. Shortly before the congress in Kyoto (October 13–18, 1991), in cooperation with a number of other laboratories, we were able to detect the high affinity receptor using a DNA probe and *in situ* hybridization as well as mRNA of the human α chain, and a specific monoclonal antibody against the human α chain (23). Similar findings, independent of ours, have been observed by the group of Stingl et al. (23 b). This unexpected new finding opens a new dimension of allergy research and possible new ways of understanding the pathophysiology of AE: IgE bearing Langerhans cells might not only act as antigen presenters, as has been shown by several groups, but also in a proinflammatory way in the epidermis when the high affinity IgE receptor has been in contact with the allergen.

Clinical Relevance of IgE Mediated Reactions in Atopic Eczema

One way to prove the clinical relevance of an IgE mediated sensitization is the "Epicutaneous test with allergens known to induce an IgE mediated sensitization and the evaluation of an eventually occurring eczematous skin reaction", a procedure which we have called "atopy patch test" (24). With this procedure, we found positive reactions to at least one allergen, most frequently against house dust mite, in 36% of the tested patients. In this context, the possible role of microbial allergens present on the skin surface deserves further interest (25,26). Stapholococcal proteins might not only act as allergens (IgE antibodies have been detected) but also as inducers of IgE receptor expression. The relation between food allergy and AE has been very controversial over the years (4). The double blind placebo-controlled food challenge study performed by Sampson et

Table 3. Atopic eczema: Hypothetical role of IgE in induction of eczematous skin lesions

Cells	Mediators/Function	Consequences
Mast cells, Basophils	Histamine, eicosanoids PAF, etc.	itch, "invisible" contact urticaria Late phase reaction
Langerhans Cells	Ag presentation cytokines?	DTH? regulatory role?
Lymphocytes	cytokines (e.g. HRF, IL-4)	mediator release IgE production
Eosinophils	MBP, EOP, ECP, etc.	inflammation

al. represented the major step forward (13). In this study, 56% of the mostly juvenile patients showed positive reactions to various foods. We have found similar results in adults with severe AE (27). Furthermore, we were able to provoke eczematous skin lesions under placebo-controlled conditions by application of various food additives in patients with severe AE (9). The most frequently observed elicitors of these reactions were colorings, benzoates and sulfites. These reactions may be regarded as possibly pseudo-allergic in origin.

Non-specific Skin Hyperreactivity

Despite the role stressing allergic reactions in the pathophysiology of AE, it is important to remember that in many patients with AE, allergy does not seem to play the major role in the disease. In these patients, other factors have to be considered, such as impaired skin function, bacterial colonization, psychosomatic interactions, etc., which may give rise to non-specific hyperreactivity of the skin (4). Among the many disturbances in skin functions, "dry skin" is a major characteristic of AE. This implies not only the increased transepidermal loss but also an increased roughness as well as a decrease in epidermal lipid content sometimes together with lowered sebaceous activity (28). It is well known that fewer patients with AE suffer from acne vulgaris than controls and that the sebaceous gland secretion is reduced. This "unspecific hyperreactivity" of the skin may be measured by using modern techniques such as laser-doppler flowmetry or evaporimetry over skin sites pretreated with mild irritants (i.e. sodiumauryl sulfate) (4).

Environmental Pollution and Atopic Eczema

In this context, it seems interesting to discuss briefly the studies showing a higher prevalence of AE in preschool children in areas with high environmental pollution (29). In many studies, a possible effect of environmental pollutants upon the development of allergic reactions has been discussed, both in the sense of an adjuvant activity upon IgE production (30) as well as in a complex interaction at the allergen level and the effector pathways (31). The emerging new discipline dealing with the influence of toxic substances upon induction, elicitation and maintenance of allergic reactions has been named "allerotoxicology" (31) and represents one of the most fascinating current fields of research. In our own study there was no significant correlation between SO_2 and NO_x air concentrations and prevalence of atopic diseases. However, cigarette smoke proved to be a critical parameter: Offspring of mothers who smoked during pregnancy and/or lactation had a significantly elevated risk of developing atopic diseases as compared to other children (32). Similar findings have been observed by others (33). The possible role of automobile exhaust deserves further studies (Behrendt, personal communication).

Conclusion

It is now clear that at least in some patients with AE, IgE-mediated reactions play a pathophysiological role in maintaining the skin disease. However, it is also important to keep in mind that there are many patients in whom other factors such as irritants, psychosomatic influences, etc., are of major importance. Follow-

Table 4. IgE mediated atopic diseases and non-allergic differential diagnoses

IgE-mediated	Diseases	No relevant allergy detectable
Extrinsic allergic	Asthma	Intrinsic (cryptogenic)
Allergic	Rhinitis	Vasomotoric
Allergic (type 1)	Conjunctivitis	Keratoconjunctivitis vernalis ?
'Extrinsic'	Atopic eczema	'Intrinsic (cryptogenic)'

ing the suggestion of Wüthrich, we would recommend that AE be classified into an "extrinsic, allergic" and "intrinsic, cryptogenic" form (Table 4) as with other atopic diseases. Diagnostic and therapeutic consequences make a careful allergy diagnosis mandatory in patients with severe AE not responding to mild topical treatment. It is critical to differentiate coincidence and relevance of a given allergic sensitization in each individual patient: Each positive test reaction has to be evaluated carefully with regard to the possible clinical relevance of the eczematous skin lesions.

References

1. Wüthrich, B. 1975. Zur Immunpathologie der Neurodermitis constitutionalis. Bern, Stuttgart, Wien: Huber
2. Rajka, G. 1990. Essentials on atopic dermatitis. Berlin: Springer.
3. Hanisfin, J.M. 1982. Atopic dermatitis. J. Amer. Acad. Derm. 8:1.
4. Ruzicka, T., Ring, J., and Przybilla, B. (eds). 1991. Handbook of atopic eczema. Berlin: Springer.
5. Ring, J. 1988. Angewandte Allergologie. 2 Auflage. München: MMV-Vieweg.
6. Ring, J., and Dorsch, W. 1985. Altered releasability of vaso-active mediator secreting cells in atopic eczema. Acta Derm. Venereol. (Stockh) 114:9.
7. Coombs, R.R.A., and Gell, P.G.H. 1963. The classification of allergic reactions underlying disease. In: Clinical aspects of immunology. P.G.H. Gell and R.R.A. Coombs, eds. Philadelphia: Davis, p. 317.
8. Brostoff, J., Carini, C., Wraith, D.G., and Johns, P. 1979. Production of IgE complexes by allergen challenge in atopic patients and the effect of sodium cromoglycate. Lancet I:1268.
9. Vieluf, D., Przybilla, B., Traenckner, I., and Ring, J. 1990. Provocation of atopic eczema (AE) by oral challenge test (OCT) with food additives (FA). J. Allergy Clin. Immunol. 85:206.
10. Przybilla, B. 1990. Lichttherapie bei atopischem Ekzem. In: Fortsch. prakt. Dermatol. Venerol. Bd. XII. O. Braun-Falco and J. Ring, eds. Berlin, Heidelberg, New York, London, Paris, Tokyo: Springer, p. 140.
11. Enders, F., Przybilla, B., Ring, J., Burg, G., and Braun-Falco, O. 1989. Epikutantestung mit einer Standardreihe. Ergebnisse bei 12026 Patienten. Hautarzt 39:779.
12. Platts-Mills, T.A.E., Mitchell, E.B., Rowntree, S., Chapmann, M.D., and Wilkins, S.R. 1983. The role of dust mite allergens in atopic dermatis. Clin. Exp. Dermatol. 8:223.
13. Sampson, H.S., and MacCaskill, C.C. 1985. Food hypersensitivity and atopic dermatitis: evaluation of 113 patients. J. Pediatr. 107:669.
14. Hiorth, N., and Roed-Peterson, J. 1976. Occupational protein contact dermatitis in food handlers. Contact Dermatitis 2:28.
15. Leiferman, K.M., Ackerman, S.J., Sampson, H.A., Haugen, H.S., Venencie, P.Y., and Gleich, G.J. 1985. Dermal deposition of eosinophil-granule major basic protein in atopic eczema. N. Engl. Reg. Allergy Proc. 9:411.
16. Jakob, T., Hermann, K., and Ring, J. 1991. Eosinophil cationic protein in atopic eczema. Arch. Dermat. Res. 283:5.
17. Ishizaka, K., Iwata, M., Carzui, C., and Takeashi, T. 1989. A new approach to suppressing the IgE antibody response to allergen. In: Progress in allergy and clinical immunology. W.J. Pichler et al., eds. Toronto, Lewiston, Bern, Göttingen, Stuttgart: Hogrefe and Huber, p 129.
18. Coffman, R.L., and Carty, J. 1986. A T cell activity that enhances polyclonal IgE production and its inhibition by interferon-gamma. J. Immunol. 136:949.
19. Prinz, J.C., Enders, N., Rank, G., Ring, J., and Rieber, E.P. 1987. Expression of Fcα receptors on activated human T lymphocytes. Eur. J. Immunol. 17:757.
20. Bruijnzeel-Koomen, C., van Wichen, L., Toonstra, J., and Berrens Bruijnzeel, P. 1986. The presence of IgE molecules on epidermal Langerhans cells form patients with atopic dermatitis. Arch. Dermatol. Res. 278:199.
21. Bieber, T., Dannenberg, B., Prinz, J.C., Rieber, E.P., Stolz, W., Braun-Falco, O., and Ring, J. 1989. Occurrence of IgE-bearing epidermal Langerhans-cells in atopic eczema: A study of the time course of the lesions and with regard to the IgE serum level. J. Invest. Dermatol. 92:215.
22. Bieber, T., Rieger, A., Neuchrist, C., Prinz, J.C., Rieber, E.P., Boltz-Nitulecsu, G., Scheiner, O., Kraft, D., and Ring, J. 1989. Induction of Fcα R2/CD23 on human epidermal Langerhans cells by human recombinant Interleukin 4 and Interferon J. Exp. Med. 170:309.

23a. Bieber, T.C., de la Salle, A., Wollenberg, R., Chizzonite, J., Hakimi, J., Ring, J., Hanau, D.,

and de la Salle, H. 1991. Constitutive expression of the high affinity receptor for IgE ($FC_\epsilon RI$) on human Langerhans cells. Abstract. Congress of "Arbeitsgem. Dermat. Forschung" (ADF), Graz (Austria).
23b. Rieger, A., Wang, B., Kilgus, O., Ochiai, K., Kinet, J.P., and Stingl, G. 1991. Evidence for FcαR1-expression by epidermal Langerhans cells. Abstract. Congress of "Arbeitsgem. Dermat. Forschung" (ADF), Graz (Austria).
24. Ring, J, Kunz, B, Bieber, T, Vieluf, D, and Przubilla, B. 1989. The "Atopy Patch Test" with aeroallergens in atopic eczema. J. Allergy Clin. Immunol. 82:195.
25. Leyden, J.J., Marples, R.R., and Kligman, A.M. 1974. Staphylococcus aureus in the lesions of atopic dermatitis. Br. J. Dermatol. 90:525.
26. Waersted, A., and Hjorth, N. 1985. Pityrosporum orbiculare: a pathogenetic factor in atopic dermatitis of the face, scalp and neck. Acta Derm. Venereol. (Stockholm) (Suppl.) 114:146.
27. Ring, J., Bieber, T., Vieluf, D., Kunz, B., and Przybilla, B. 1991. Atopic eczema Langerhans cells and allergy. Int. Archs. Allergy Appl. Immun. 94:194.
27a. Ramb-Lindhauer, C.H., Feldmann, A., Rotte, M., and Neumann, C.H. 1990. Characterization of grass pollen reactive T-cell lines derived from lesional atopic skin. Arch. Dermatol. Res. 283:71.
27b. Tanaka, Y., Tanaka, M., Anan, S., and Yoshida, H. 1989. Immunohistochemical studies on dust mite antigen in positive reaction site of patch test. Acta Dermat. Venerol. (Stockholm) (Suppl.) 144:93.
28. Wirth, H., Gloor, M., and Stoika, D. 1981. Sebaceous glands in uninvolved skin of patients suffering from atopic dermatitis. Arch. Dermatol. Res. 270:167.
29. Ring, J. (ed). 1991. Epidemiologie allergischer Erkrankungen: Nehmen Allergien zu? München: MMV-Vieweg.
30. Muranaka, M., Suzuki, S., Koizumi, K., Takafuji, S., Miyamoto, T., Ikemori, R., and Tokiwa, H. 1986. Adjuvant activity of diesel exhaust particles of the production of IgE antibody in mice. J. Allergy Clin. Immuno. 77:616.
31. Behrendt, H., Friedrichs, K.H., Kainka-Stänike, F., Darsow, U., Becker, W., and Tomingas, R. 1991. Allergens and pollutants in the air: a complex interaction. In: New trends in allergy, III. J. Ring and B. Przybilla, eds. Berlin, Heidelberg, New York: Springer, p. 467.
32. Kunz, B., Ring, J., and Dirschedl, P. 1989. Effect of maternal smoking during pregnancy on the development of atopic diseases in the child. J. Invest. Dermatol. 92:465.
33. Zetterström, O. Osterman, K., Machedo, L., Johannson, S.G.O. 1981. Another smoking hazard: raised IgE concentration and increased risk of occupational allergy. Br. Med. J. 283:1215.

Current Topics on Atopic Dermatitis

Hikotaro Yoshida, Yoichi Tanaka, Keisuke Maeda, Sadao Anan*

In order to better understand the pathogenesis of atopic dermatitis (AD), some immunohistochemical studies were done. The skin materials for this study were biopsy specimens taken from dermatitic lesions of AD patients and positive patch test sites to mite antigen (MA). Anti-MA serum was prepared by immunizing rabbits with MA using Freund's complete adjuvant. By double-labelling immunofluorescence studies, we observed the presence of IgE molecules and MA on the surface of OKT6 positive cells both in the epidermis and dermis of AD lesions. Furthermore, it was found that about 13% of OKT6 positive cells bore IgG4 molecules. Immunoelectron microscopic study revealed that the membrane of the intermediate cells and T lymphocytes in the dermis were stained by peroxidase reaction products of MA. This was observed in the lesion of the patients with positive IgE-RAST to MA, but not in healthy controls or in patients with negative IgE-RAST to MA. From these findings, it may be hypothesized that immune responses of immunoglobulins and MA on the surface of OKT6 positive cells play a very important role in the pathogenesis of AD.

It has been widely accepted that dust mite antigen and mite-specific IgE are essential to provoke the lesion of atopic dermatitis (AD). We (1) previously reported that serum levels of mite specific IgG, IgG4 and IgE were significantly higher than those in healthy subjects. In this study, we investigated the importance of mite antigen and mite-specific immunoglobulins in the pathogenesis of AD.

Materials and Methods

Antigens

Antigen solutions of Dermatophagoides pteronyssinus (DP) and D. farinae (DF) were prepared from full-grown mite cultures by the method of Miyamoto et al. (2). The antigen material was defatted in anhydrous acetone and homogenized with phosphate buffered saline (0.005 M phosphate buffer pH 7.2 containing 0.15 M NaCl). After centrifugation at 15,000 g for 20 minutes, the supernatants were dialyzed against distilled water, and freeze-dried. The antigens obtained from whole cultures of DP and DF were denoted DP-WCE and DF-WCE respectively. Mite-free culture medium extract (CME) was also prepared by the same procedure.

Antisera and Affinity Purified Antibodies

Antisera to DP-WCE and DF-WCE were obtained by immunizing New Zealand white rabbits with both antigens using complete Freund's adjuvant. Each antiserum was absorbed with CME. For specific purification, 10 mg of each extract was bound to Sepharose activated with CNBr. One hundred milliliter of anti-DP-WCE or anti-DF-WCE antisera were passed over an affinity column containing DP-WCE or DF-WCE immunosorbent. The bound antibody was eluted with 0.1 M glycine-HCl, pH 2.5 dialyzed with PBS, and stored in a cold room at -20°C in closed vessels and labelled affinity purified anti-DP (1 mg/ml) and anti-DF (1 mg/ml) antibodies. On immunodiffusion with these antibodies, both showed several cross-reactive precipitation lines against DP-WCE, DF-WCE and house dust extract. But no reaction was seen against extracts from whole culture of Tyrophagus putrescetiae and Glycyphagus privatus (3). Crossed immunoelectrophoresis demonstrated up to 27 precipitates for the DP-WCE and 28 for the DF-WCE respectively (3).

Patch Tests

White petrolatum containing 0.1% sodium lauryl sulfate (SLS) was used as the vehicle according to the SLS provocative patch test described by Kligman (4). Patch testing with 0.1% (w/w) DP-WCE and 0.1% (w/w) DF-

* Department of Dermatology, Nagasaki University School of Medicine, Nagasaki, Japan.

WCE, in the vehicle was performed with Fin Chambers on the clinically normal skin of the back. As for the controls, 0.1% (w/w) CME in SLS-containing white petrolatum and vehicle alone were patch-tested. The test reactions were read after 48 hrs and evaluated according to the criteria of the ICDRG.

Patients and Control Subjects

The following groups were patch tested. Twenty patients with AD (aged 2–25 years, mean 14.9 years; serum IgE titer 20–12,306 U/ml, mean 1,858.9 U/ml) and 20 healthy volunteers without history of atopy (aged 21–25 years, mean 22.5 years; serum IgE titer 20–297 U/ml, mean 107.1 U/ml). The IgE titer was measured using the radioimmunosorbent test (RIST, Pharmacia, Uppsala, Sweden). All subjects gave their informed consent.

Histopathology

Some biopsies were taken from dermatitic lesions and positive patch test sites after 48 hrs. Biopsy specimens were prepared for routine histological examination and processed as described below. Further, to examine the time-course of the reaction, skin biopsies were done at the sites of patch testing of an AD patient after 1 hr, 6 hrs, 24 hrs and 48 hrs. About one half of each biopsy specimen was prepared for routine histological examination, while the remaining half of each of the specimens was processed for immunohistochemical and immunoelectron microscopical studies as described below.

Processing of Skin Biopsies

Biopsy specimens were fixed using 4% paraformaldehyde in 0.1 M phosphate buffer (PB), pH 7.4 for 6 hrs at 4°C for immuno-double labelling and immunoelectron microscopy, washed in 10–20 % sucrose in PBS overnight and span-frozen and stored at -80°C. The 5 μm frozen sections were used for both immuno-double labelling studies and immunoelectron microscopic study. Anti-mite antibody was prepared by mixing equal volumes of affinity purified anti-DP (1 mg/ml) and anti-DF (1 mg/ml) antibodies.

Immuno-double Labelling Study-1: Frozen sections were then incubated with the anti-mite antibody (1:50 in PBS) for 30 min at 37°C, followed by FITC conjugated anti-rabbit IgG (TAGO Inc., Burlingame, CA, USA, 1:50 in PBS) for 30 min at 37°C. Afterwards, the sections were treated with monoclonal OKT6 (Ortho Diagnostic Systems Inc., Raritan, NJ, USA, 1:100 in PBS) for 30 min at 37°C, followed by incubation with rhodamine conjugated anti-mouse IgG (TAGO, 1:100 in PBS) for 30 min at 37°C. Between each step, the sections were washed in three changes of PBS for 15 min. The stained sections were examined under a Zeiss fluorescent microscope with an appropriate FITC and rhodamine filter setting.

Immuno-Double Labelling Study-2: To examine coexistent IgE and mite antigen, immuno double-labelling studies were performed with anti-IgE (TAGO, 1:50 in PBS) and anti-mite antibody (1:50 in PBS) as described above.

Immuno-double labelling study-3: To see the IgG4 molecules on the surface of OKT6 positive cells, immuno-double labelling studies with OKT6 and anti-IgG4 were performed.

Immunoelectron microscopy: The other part of the cryostat sections were used for immunoelectron microscopic study with anti-mite antibodies. The sections were incubated with the anti-mite antibody (1:100 in PBS) for 12 hrs at 4°C and washed 6 times for 10 min in 10% sucrose in PBS. Subsequently, the sections were incubated with peroxidase conjugated anti-rabbit IgG (TAGO, 1:100 in PBS) for 6 hrs at 4°C. After washing in 10% sucrose in PBS, the sections were postfixed in 1% glutalaldehyde in 0.1 M PB (pH 7.4) for 10 min at 4°C. Following PBS rinse and preincubation in 3,3-diaminobenzidene (DAB) solution for 30 min at room temperature, the sections were postfixed again using 2% OsO4 in PB, dehydrated in graduated alcohols and resin embedded using the inverted capsule method. The ultrathin sections with slight electron staining were observed with JOEL electron microscope.

Results

Results of the patch tests with mite antigen are illustrated in Table I. Of twenty patients with AD, 14 showed positive reactions (70%) to the DP-WCE, 13 were positive (65%) to the DF-WCE. In the mite RAST-positive AD group (2 or more of the RAST scores were regarded as

Table I. Results of patch tests with mite antigen in patients with atopic dermatitis (n=20).

	Patch test with DP-WCE Positive	Patch test with DP-WCE Negative
RAST[a] positive for DP	13	1
RAST negative for DP	1	5
	Patch test with DF-WCE Positive	**Patch test with DF-WCE Negative**
RAST positive for DF	12	1
RAST negative for DF	1	6

[a] RAST assays were performed according to the producer (Pharmacia). Results were expressed in the RAST score system, 0, 1, 2, 3 and 4. Score 2 or more was regarded as positive.

positive), the percentage of patients with positive reaction both to DP-WCE and to DF-WCE was more than 90%. It is much higher than that of the mite RAST negative group (approximately 15%). None of the 20 non-atopic groups reacted to any mite antigens. Mite-free culture medium extract alone elicited no reaction in any groups. The positive reaction site showed edematous erythema with red papules and vesicles. Histologically, acanthosis, spongiosis and dermal infiltrates consisting of lymphocytes and eosinophils were observed. These reactions resembled AD lesions both clinically and histopathologically.

By use of immuno-double labelling study, it could be demonstrated that the mite antigen invaded percutaneously and was located on the dendritic OKT6 positive cells (Langerhans cell, LC) in the dermis of positive patch test sites. Such mite antigen-bound LCs were particularly distributed around clusters of lymphocytes, which were predominantly composed of Leu3a$^+$ cells. And many double-labelling dendritic cells with anti-mite antibody and anti-IgE were observed. These cells were possibly LCs. In the double-labelling study-3, it was found that about 13% of OKT6 positive cells bore IgG4 molecules. Immunoelectron microscopic study showed that some macrophages in the dermis exhibited positive labelling with anti-mite antibody on the cytoplasmic membrane and contained positively labelled small particles in the cytoplasm. And the apposition of macrophages to lymphocytes was often observed. Some mast cells labelled with anti-mite antibody were seen and these cells were activated morphologically.

As to the time-course for the patch test reaction, a slight erythema was shown as early as 24 hrs after patch testing. At 48 hrs, definite erythema with many papules and edema was observed. Histologically, only mild changes were seen after 1 hr. The dermal infiltration of lymphocytes slightly increased after 6 hrs. After 24 hrs, the lymphocytic infiltration was becoming prominent and an influx of eosinophils was observed in the dermis. After 48 hrs, spongiotic changes, irregular acanthosis and exocytosis of lymphocytes were seen in the epidermis. In the dermis, the lymphocytes accumulated and some clusters were observed and many eosinophils were scattered throughout the upper dermis. Immunohistochemically, mite antigens were seen only slightly in the epidermis at 1 hr to 6 hrs. However, after 24 hrs, many mite antigen-bearing LCs were observed both in the epidermis and in the dermis. After 48 hrs, they were seen exclusively in the dermis.

Discussion

AD has clinical and histological features of delayed-type hypersensitivity. However, it was still unclear whether delayed-type reaction to mite antigen could be induced in the patients with AD. Some reports (5,6) demonstrated a substantial lymphocyte proliferation response to mite antigen in AD. Moreover, several workers (7–11) have shown that eczematous reactions were provoked by patch testing with mite antigen in AD. In this study, we confirmed this by use of the modification of SLS provocative patch testing described by Kligman (4). We succeeded in reproducing an eczematous reaction by patch testing with mite antigen in the majority of patients with AD. Mitchell et al. (7) and Gondo et al. (10) applied mite antigen in abraded skin sites and Bruynzeel-Koomen et al. (11) made the application after stripping the skin by adhesive tape. Abrasion, stripping and SLS application may simulate naturally occurring conditions by scratching and sweating in AD. These results suggested that house dust mite may contribute to the pathogenesis of AD.

The histological picture of the patch test was consistent with that of AD. An infiltrate of eosinophils was observed to a higher degree than the typical lesions of AD. A similar finding was earlier reported by Mitchell et al. (7) and Bruynzeel-Koomen et al. (11). Bruynzeel-Koomen et al. (11) suggested that eosinophils might play an important role in patch test reactions to mite antigen in AD.

Our immunohistochemical study demonstrated the penetrating route of mite antigen and the response of immuno-competent cells thereafter. It was shown that applied mite antigen entered percutaneously and bound to LCs. Gondo et al. (10) observed percutaneous entry of mite antigen in the dermis by conjugating ferritin to mite antigen. Silberberg-Sinakin et al. (12) observed LC-bound ferritin in the skin after intradermal challenge with ferritin. Shelley and Juhlin (13) demonstrated the selective uptake of some contact allergen by LCs. And it can be hypothesized by our findings of the time-course reaction that LCs may trap mite antigen in the epidermis, migrate to the dermis, and present the antigen in close contact with lymphocytes. It is well known that LCs belong to the macrophage-monocyte series and LCs have a capacity for antigen-presenting and migrating. Silberberg-Sinakin et al. (14) reported that after DNCB challenge in passively sensitized Guinea pigs, LCs in the epidermis decrease after 6 hrs and increase in the dermis, and the apposition of LCs to lymphocytes was seen mainly in the dermis at 3 or more hours after challenge. Lipsky et al. (15) found that physical interactions between antigen-bearing macrophages and lymph node lymphocytes from animals specifically immunized to that antigen were markedly apparent. It is still unknown whether the interaction between LCs and lymphocytes occurs in the dermis or in the lymph node or in both. Our results suggest that it may occur in the dermis and induce the proliferation of lymphocytes.

The fact that some OKT6 positive cells bear IgG4 molecules in the lesional skin of AD is extremely interesting. At present we cannot explain the role of IgG4 molecules. However, it may show clearly that IgG4 also participates in the development of the AD lesion.

In 1986, Bruynzeel-Koomen et al. (17) demonstrated that IgE molecules were seen on epidermal LCs in AD lesions. We confirmed their finding by use of the immuno-double labelling method. This finding has considerable importance because it suggests an integration of immediate-type and delayed-type reactions in AD. Furthermore, we observed numerous dendritic cells bearing IgE molecules and mite antigen in the patch test site. These dendritic cells seemed to be LCs. And, furthermore, the positive ratio of the mite antigen patch testing in the mite IgE-RAST positive AD group was much higher than in the IgE-RAST negative AD group. These results suggest that IgE might be involved in contact hypersensitivity to mite allergen in AD. Our results suggest the importance of IgE molecules and LC in the pathogenesis of AD. However the functional role of IgE on LCs is still unknown. It now seems necessary to elucidate whether applied mite antigen may bind to IgE molecules on LCs, and whether these LCs are activated, release cytokines and can induce proliferation of T cells. Taken together, our results indicate that mite antigen contact induced an allergic contact sensitivity to it, and that IgE might participate in this reaction. We speculate that the reaction might be compatible with the IgE-mediated contact hypersensitivity described by Ray et al. (18).

References

1. Anan, S., Akahoshi, Y., Yoshimura, S., Ushijima, N., and Yoshida, H. 1982. Measurement of IgG, IgE and IgG subclass antibodies to mite (Dermatophagoides farinae) allergen in patients with atopic dermatitis by using indirect enzyme-linked immunosorbent assay. Jpn. J. Allergol. 31:244.
2. Miyamoto, J., Ishii, A., and Sasa, M. 1975. A successful method for mass culture of the house dust mite, Dermatophagoides pteronyssinus (Troussart, 1897). Jpn. J. Exp. Med. 45:133.
3. Tanaka, Y., Tanaka, S., Anan, S., and Yoshida, H. 1989. Immunohistochemical studies on dust mite antigen in positive reaction site of patch test. Acta Derm. Venereol.(Stockh) Suppl. 144:93.
4. Kligman, A.M. 1966. The provocation patch test in allergic contact sensitization. J. Invest. Dermatol. 46:573.
5. Elliston, W.L., Heise, E.A., and Huntley, C.C. 1982. Cell-mediated hypersensitivity to mite antigens in atopic dermatitis. Arch. Dermatol. 118:26.
6. Rawle, F.C., Mitchell, E.B., and Platts-Mills, T.A.E. 1984. T cell responses to the major

allergen from the house dust mite Dermatophagoides pteronyssinus, antigen P1: Comparison of patients with asthma, atopic dermatitis, and perennial rhinitis. J. Immunol. 133:195.
7. Mitchell, E.B., Crow, J., Chapman, M.D., Jouhal, S.S., Pope, F.M., and Platts-Mills, T.A.E. 1982. Basophils in allergen-induced patch test sites in atopic dermatitis. Lancet I:127.
8. Young, E., Bruynzeel-Koomen, C., and Berrens, C. 1985. Delayed type hypersensitivity in atopic dermatitis. Acta Derm. Venereol. (Stockh.) Suppl.114:77.
9. Reitamo, S., Visa, K., Kahonen, K., Kayhko, K., Stubb, S., and Salo, O.P. 1986. Eczematous reactions in atopic patients caused by epicutaneous testing with inhalant allergens. Br. J. Dermatol. 114:303.
10. Gondo, A., Saeki, N., and Tokuda, Y. 1986. Challenge reactions in atopic dermatitis after percutaneous entry of mite antigen. Br. J. Dermatol. 115:485.
11. Bruynzeel-Koomen, C.A.F.M., Van Wichen, D.F., Spray, C.J.F., Venge, P., and Bruynzeel, P.L.B. 1988. Active participation of eosinophils in patch test reactions to inhalant allergens in patients with atopic dermatitis. Br. J. Dermatol. 118:229.
12. Silberberg-Sinakin, I., Thorbecke, G.J., Bear, R.L., Rosenthal, S.A., and Berezowsky, V. 1976. Antigen-bearing Langerhans cells in skin, dermal lymphatics and in lymph nodes. Cell. Immunol. 25:137.
13. Shelley, W.B., and Juhlin, L. 1977. Selective uptake of contact allergens by the Langerhans cell. Arch. Dermatol. 113:187.
14. Silberberg-Sinakin, I., Baer, R.L., Rosenthal, S.A., Thorbecke, G.J., and Berezowsky, V. 1975. Dermal and intravascular Langerhans cells at sites of passively induced allergic contact sensitivity. Cell. Immunol. 18:435.
15. Lipsky, P.E., and Rosenthal, A.S. 1975. Macrophage-lymphocyte interaction. Antigen-mediated physical interactions between immune Guinea pig lymph node lymphocytes and syngeneic macrophages. J. Exp. Med. 141:138.
16. Unanue, E.R., and Cerottini, J.C. 1970. The immunogenicity of antigen bound to the plasma membrane of macrophages. J. Exp. Med. 131:711.
17. Bruynzeel-Koomen, C., van Wichen, D.F., Toonstra, J., Berrens, L., and Bruynzeel-Koomen, P.L.B. 1986. The presence of IgE molecules on epidermal Langerhans cells in patients with atopic dermatitis. Arch. Dermatol. 278:199.
18. Ray, M.C., Tharp, M.D., Sullivan, T.J., and Tigelaar, R.E. 1983. Contact hypersensitivity reactions to dinitrofluorobenzene mediated by monoclonal IgE anti-DNP antibodies. J. Immunol. 131:1096.

Autoimmune Bullous Diseases of the Skin

Jean-Claude Bystryn*

The skin can be the target of autoimmune reactions to endogenous antigens which are normal components of skin. These reactions often manifest themselves by bullous eruptions, and can be some of the most severe diseases which afflict the skin. The immunological aspects of these diseases are discussed below.

Antigens of Skin

Skin is a highly antigenic organ. Endogenous antigens of skin to which immune reactions can develop can be classified into two basic categories according to whether they are normal or modified components of skin. The normal antigens are components of skin present in most individuals. The modified antigens arise in only some individuals as a result of injury to skin, of bacterial or viral infection, malignant transformation, or from conjugation to foreign or altered chemicals. All primary autoimmune skin diseases appear to be directed to normal rather than to modified skin antigens. There are probably more normal antigens in skin capable of inducing autoimmune responses than in any other organ in the body. Such antigens are present in all of the major anatomical structures of skin: the nuclei and cytoplasm of keratinocytes, the basement membrane zone and the intercellular substance, the stratum corneum, and in melanocytes. Surprisingly, autoimmune responses to antigens in the dermis proper appear to be rare. The two most important classes of endogenous antigens, from the perspective of autoimmune bullous diseases, are those present in the intercellular substance and in the basement membrane zone. While autoantibodies can develop to other endogenous skin antigens they do not cause bullous diseases.

General Characteristics of Skin Antigens Associated with Autoimmune Bullous Diseases

The antigens which are the targets of autoimmune bullous diseases share several common features: (A) They are skin specific. They are present in normal stratified squamous epithelia of man and other mammals, but not in other tissues. (B) They are expressed in the extracellular space, either in the intercellular substance between keratinocytes or in the basement membrane zone. This characteristic probably accounts for their involvement in clinical diseases, as they are available to interact *in vivo* with autoimmune reactions directed to them. (C) Multiple distinct antigens are expressed in the intercellular substance and in the basement membrane zone; and within each of these structures different antigens can be expressed in different layers of the epidermis. This apparently accounts for some of the clinical manifestations of autoimmune skin diseases.

Autoimmune Bullous Diseases Associated with Immune Reactions to Intercellular(ic) Antigens

Pemphigus is the most serious autoimmune bullous disease, and one of the most severe skin diseases known. Prior to the introduction of corticosteroid therapy, over 80% of individuals afflicted with this disease died within 18 months. It results from an autoantibody response to IC antigens. The disease is characterized by flaccid bullae which arise from normal skin. The bullae are within the epidermis, nor-

* Department of Dermatology, New York University School of Medicine, 560 First Avenue, New York, NY, USA 10016.
Acknowledgements: Supported in part by USPHS research grants AR39749 and AR 27663 from the Skin Cancer Foundation, the Evans Foundation, and the Rudolph Baer Foundation.

mally just above the basal cell layer, within the intercellular substance. Adjacent epidermal cells lose their adhesion and come apart, resulting in a cavity within the intercellular substance which gradually enlarges to form clinical bullae. There is very little inflammatory cell infiltrate suggesting that cellular immune responses do not play a major role in pathogenesis. The disease normally begins with chronic, painful erosions, in the oral cavity. In days to months bullae appear on the skin. While these lesions arise from normal appearing skin, the skin is not normal. Rubbing normal-appearing skin adjacent to a pemphigus lesion leads to the separation of the epidermis from the dermis. The bullae break within a few days leaving a sharply outlined, painful, superficial erosion. Without treatment the lesions gradually increase in size and number, until a considerable portion of the skin surface area is destroyed. At this point the disease resembles an extensive burn. As with burns, patients with pemphigus develop metabolic imbalance and infections. Untreated, the mortality of pemphigus is over 80%. One of the triumphs of medicine has been to reduce the mortality of this disease to below 10% by using high doses of corticosteroid.

There are two forms of pemphigus, which are distinguished by the level within the epidermis where the bulla occurs. In pemphigus vulgaris, bullae arise deep in the epidermis just above the basal cell layer. In pemphigus foliaceus, the bullae arise high up in the epidermis, just below the stratum corneum. The majority of patients with active pemphigus have circulating antibodies to intercellular (IC) antigens. These antibodies along with complement are also fixed in the IC substance of the epidermis of patients with the disease, at the site of the earliest lesion that can be seen by electron microscopy. There is usually a correlation between the titer of the antibodies and the activity of the disease. Incubating skin in organ culture with pemphigus antibodies causes a split in the epidermis identical to that seen in pemphigus. Passive administration of pemphigus antibodies to neonatal mice causes skin bullae which clinically, histologically, and immunologically are similar to those of pemphigus. Thus, pemphigus is an autoimmune disease resulting from an antibody response to normal intercellular antigens. It is believed these antibodies bind to the surface of keratinocytes, causing the synthesis and/or release of proteases, which in turn dissolve the intercellular cement substance leading to loss of adhesion (acantholysis) between adjacent epidermal cells and to clinical bullae. Alternatively, the acantholysis might simply result from the antibodies binding to and inactivating the binding sites.

The antigens which are the target of autoantibody responses in pemphigus are called "pemphigus" antigens. There is a family of pemphigus antigens as evidenced by serological analysis. This is confirmed by the observation that different pemphigus antigens are stratified in different layers of the epidermis.

More recently, some of these pemphigus antigens have been defined at the molecular level. The antibodies in pemphigus vulgaris react to a 210 kD complex, composed of a 130 kD polypeptide (the actual antigen to which the pemphigus sera react) bound to plakoglobin (an 85 kD protein which is a structural component of desmosomes). The antibodies in pemphigus foliaceus react to a 260 kD complex composed desmoglein (a 160 kD protein which forms part of the adhesion site of desmosomes) also complexed to plakoglobin. Thus, the pemphigus antigens which have been best characterized to date, appear to be external components of desmosomes, the adhesive structure that holds keratinocytes together. More recently, additional pemphigus antigens with molecular weights ranging from 45 to 85 kD have been identified. These appear to be fragments of the larger molecules described above which carry the actual epitopes recognized by pemphigus sera.

The expression of pemphigus antigens is varied over the epiderm and within the epidermis. This appears to account for some of the clinical features of the disease. For example, the expression of pemphigus vulgaris antigens is particularly high on the scalp, face and upper torso but low on the extremities. This parallels, and may account for, the clinical distribution of lesions in this form of the disease. As another striking example, pemphigus vulgaris antigens are expressed strongly in oral mucosa whereas the pemphigus foliaceus antigens are expressed poorly in this area. This may account for the fact that oral lesions are common in pemphigus vulgaris but very rare in pemphigus foliaceus. Another difference between both forms of pemphigus is that the lesions are localized deep within the epidermis in pemphigus vulgaris but higher up in the epidermis in pemphigus foliaceus. Two observations may explain the location of lesions in the superficial layers of the epidermis in pemphigus foliaceus: One is that some patients with this disease have antibodies directed to antigens localized strictly in the superficial layers of the epidermis. Another is that many patients with pemphigus foliaceus lack the antigens normally recognized by pemphigus antibodies in the deeper layers of their epidermis. Both of these abnormalities would result in immune reactions occurring in the superficial layers of the epidermis, the location where the lesions are rare in this form of the disease. A number of other antigens are present on the surface of keratinocytes, such as HLA and ABO blood antigens; but these do not appear to be involved in clinical bullous diseases.

Autoimmune Diseases Associated with Immune Reactions to Basement Membrane Zone (BMZ) Antigens

The other major group of autoimmune bullous diseases involves autoantibody response to normal antigens in the BMZ. The BMZ is a complex structure composed of four anatomical structures: the cell membrane of basal keratinocytes, an underlying electron lucent zone (the lamina lucida), an electron dense zone (the lamina densa), and a fibrous zone consisting of the uppermost layer of the dermis (the sublamina densa zone). Distinct antigens are present within each of these zones. A critical advance in the past several years has been the identification of the antigens present in each zone and the appreciation that each is usually localized to a single zone. This has greatly furthered our understanding of the pathogenesis of diseases involving the BMZ, simplified the differential diagnosis of these diseases, and has led to the recognition of previously unknown diseases involving this structure.

The bullous diseases which result from autoantibody responses to BMZ antigens are bullous pemphigoid, herpes gestationis, cicatrizing pemphigoid, epidermolysis bullosa acquisita (EBA), and perhaps linear IgA bullous dermatosis. It is thought that each of these diseases involves an autoantibody response to a distinct set of antigen(s). In two of these diseases, bullous pemphigoid and EBA, the target antigens have been identified. These two diseases will be discussed further.

Bullous Pemphigoid (BP)

This is the most common of the autoimmune bullous diseases involving BMZ antigens. BP is characterized by tense bullae which arise from abnormal appearing skin. The skin at the base of the bullae is red and indurated and resembles urticaria. The bullae arise at the dermal-epidermal junction, within the lamina lucida. There is an inflammatory cell infiltrate within the upper layers of the dermis. The disease normally begins with pruritic, urticarial plaques that resemble ordinary hives. Eventually bullae appear on top of the urticarial plaques. As with pemphigus, BP evolves in days to months, with new lesions appearing and old lesions extending. Unlike pemphigus, however, lesions can heal spontaneously and the course of the disease is cyclical rather than continually progressive. As a result mortality in untreated disease is much less, averaging approximately 10%. The treatment of bullous pemphigoid is similar to that of pemphigus. It involves administration of high doses of systemic corticosteroid, with or without adjuvant therapy with cytotoxic drugs, gold, or dapsone. The majority of patients with active bullous pemphigoid have circulating antibodies to BMZ antigens. There is usually a correlation between the titer of the antibodies and the activity of the disease. These antibodies together with complement are also fixed *in vivo* at the BMZ. Under immunoelectronmicroscopy, the deposits are seen in the lamina lucida, at the exact site of the earliest lesion that can be seen by electronmicroscopy. These observations suggest that bullous pemphigoid is an autoimmune disease mediated by antibodies to a lamina lucida antigen. However, reproducible induction of the disease by passive transfer of pemphigoid antibodies remains to be done.

As with pemphigus, a family of BP antigens can be defined by serological analysis. These can be classified into major and minor antigens based on the frequency with which individuals with BP develop antibodies to the respective antigen. One of the major BP antigens has been identified as a glycoprotein with a MW of approximately 230 kDs which is synthesized by basal keratinocytes. A minor antigen has been identified as a protein with a MW of 160 kds. Most patients with BP have antibodies to the 230 kd, a minority to the 160 kD antigen, and some have antibodies to both antigens. It is thought that these antibodies bind to the antigens which are present in the lamina lucida, and fix complement which both injures basal keratinocytes and attracts inflammatory cells. Proteases released by the inflammatory cells and possibly from injured basal cells in turn are thought to cause the actual bullae.

The distribution of pemphigoid antibodies over the epiderm is also variable. The major BP antigens are expressed most strongly on flexural surfaces of the body (where lesions of the disease are most common) and are poorly expressed on the scalp, face and extensor surface of the extremities (where lesions of pemphigoid are less common). This correlation between the expression of the antigen and that of skin lesions suggests that the unique distribution of skin lesions in bullous pemphigoid is due to regional variations in the expression of BP antigens. The pattern of expression of PV and BP antigens varies, indicating that the expression of each antigen is under separate control.

Herpes Gestationis (HG) and Cicatrizing Pemphigoid (CP)

These two diseases resemble bullous pemphigoid histologically and immunologically in that in both the lesions arise within the lamina lucida, and patients have circulating and tissue-fixed antibodies to antigens in the lamina lucida. However, each disease differs from BP clinically. Herpes gestationis occurs only in pregnant women. Cicatrizing pemphigoid has a predilection to recur at the same site which leads to scarring, and frequently involves the mucosal surface of the eyes and mouth leading to blindness. The target antigens in CP have MWs of approximately 230 and 160 kD, and appear similar to those involved in BP. However, the frequency of antibody responses to the different antigens differ. In CP most antibodies are directed to the 160 kd antigen, whereas in BP most antibodies are directed to the 230 kd antigen. This, together with the fact that the 160 kd antigen appears to be expressed lower down in the lamina lucida, may account for the differences in the clinical manifestations of the two diseases. The antigen(s) involved in herpes gestation has has not yet been identified.

Epidermolysis Bullosa Acquisita (EBA)

This is an autoimmune disease to the BMZ which has recently been recognized as a distinct entity because it is associated with an antibody response to a unique BMZ antigen. The classic manifestations of EBA are trauma induced erosions and bullae on the extensor surface of the digits, the elbows, and knees. More recently it has become appreciated that this condition can also be associated with a generalized bullous eruption which clinically resembles bullous pemphigoid. As with bullous pemphigoid, the majority of patients with this disease have circulation antibodies to basement zone antigens. However, EBA can be clearly differentiated from BP because the initial lesions in EBA occur below the lamina densa, whereas in BP they are in the lamina lucida. The antibodies in EBA are directed to a protein complex of 290 kD, composed of two 145 kd chains. The EBA antigen is localized in the lamina densa and the sublamina densa zone, the site of the earliest lesion of the disease. This antigen is type VII collagen, a component of the microfibrils which bind the upper dermis to the lamina densa.

Use of Immunological Abnormalities in Autoimmmune Diseases for Diagnosis

The fact that most autoimmune bullous diseases involving the skin are associated with circulating and tissue-fixed antibodies to distinct components of skin permits the use of immunological techniques to diagnose these diseases. For example, detection of intercellular antibodies in the blood by indirect immunofluorescence or (when the antibodies are fixed to the epidermis of a patient with the disease) by direct immunofluorescence, permits a diagnosis of pemphigus to be made. The detection of circulating BMZ antibodies in the blood or fixed to tissue suggests that the patient has bullous pemphigoid, herpes gestationis, cicatrizing pemphigoid, or EBA. EBA can be differentiated from the first three conditions by the fact that the antibodies in this condition will react to the floor of skin which has been split with 1 M sodium chloride (which splits the skin in the middle of the lamina lucida) whereas the antibodies in bullous pemphigoid will bind to the roof of the blister. Identification of the actual antigen to which these antibodies are directed by immunoprecipitation or western blotting technique improves the accuracy of the diagnosis.

Conclusion

The skin is the target of several autoimmune diseases which are directed to antigens which are normal components of the skin. These diseases can be differentiated according to the antigen which is the target of the autoimmune process. A great deal has been learned about the pathogenesis of these diseases. However, nothing is known about the causes which trigger the development of the autoimmune process.

Section XVI

Pathogenesis and Treatment of Collagen Diseases

TNFα in Rheumatoid Inflammation and its Potential as a Therapeutic Target

Fionula M Brennan*, Deena L Gibbons*, Andrew P Cope*, Richard Williams**, Max Field**, Ravinder N Maini**, Marc Feldmann*

Over the last few years we have investigated which cytokines are produced spontaneously by cells isolated from the rheumatoid arthritis (RA) joint, and have identified TNFα as a pivotal molecule in contributing to the pathogenesis of the disease. This is based upon the observation that the spontaneous production of IL-1 and GM-CSF by RA synovial cells in culture is dependent on the presence of TNFα. Furthermore TNFα is also involved in the regulation of HLA class II expression and possibly cell adhesion molecule expression on these cells. This hypothesis was further substantiated by the observation that pretreatment of DBA/1 mice with monoclonal anti-mouse TNF antibodies dramatically reduced the cartilage and bone resorption induced by collagen type II immunization. These observations suggest that TNFα is a possible target for therapy in RA. One possible therapeutic agent is recombinant soluble TNF receptor. These molecules are natural inhibitors of TNFα, exist in normal plasma, and are found at increased levels in inflammatory disease such as RA. We have found that in RA synovial cells there is over-expression of the TNF receptor on the cell surface and that shed TNF receptor is produced spontaneously by these cells in culture. Therefore, despite the inflammation, regulatory mechanisms do exist but are insufficient to control the pathological effects of TNFα. Studies are currently in progress to ascertain whether recombinant soluble TNF receptor in the RA synovial cultures will neutralize TNFα-mediated effects, and as such be a possible therapeutic agent for the treatment of RA.

Rheumatoid Arthritis (RA) is a chronic inflammatory disease with autoimmune features in which the joints are infiltrated by activated T cells, macrophages and plasma cells (1). The pathology of the joint lesion is complex, with progressive fibrotic growth of the inflamed synovial lining layer in association with destruction of articular cartilage and subchondral bone. The pathogenesis of RA is currently under intensive investigation from many different points of view. Over the last few years, following developments in cDNA cloning and expression of cytokines it has been possible to develop assays both specific and sensitive enough to investigate the role of these inflammatory and regulatory mediators in the pathogenesis of RA. Using a combination of cDNA probes, immunoassays and bioassays, we have documented the expression of cytokines in samples taken from the RA synovial joint and their continuous production in the absence of extrinsic stimulation in cultures of RA joint cell mixtures (Table 1). Thus cytokines such as interleukin 1 (IL-1α & IL-1β), tumor necrosis factor (TNFα), interleukin 6 (IL-6), granulocyte macrophage colony stimulating factor (GM-CSF) transforming growth factor β (TGFβ) and interleukin 8 (IL-8) are produced at high levels (2,3,4,5,6). In contrast, the production of T cell cytokines such as interferon gamma (IFNγ), interleukin 2 (IL-2) and lymphotoxin (LT), while readily detectable at the mRNA level, is low at the protein level (7,8). The demonstration of the cytokines TNFα and IL-1 in RA samples is of importance, as both are potent inducers of degradative enzymes such as collagenase from fibroblasts (9,10) and in bone culture systems they induce bone resorption (11,12).

We have defined using this *in vitro* culture system that TNFα has a pivotal role in the cytokine interactions in the RA joint, as it induces IL-1 (13) and GM-CSF (4) production (Figure 1a & 1b) and expression of HLA class II and cell adhesion molecules (unpublished observation), all of which are important factors contributing to the joint destruction in RA.

* Charing Cross Sunley Research Centre, 1 Lurgan Avenue, Hammersmith, London W6 8LW, UK.
** Kennedy Institute of Rheumatology, 6 Bute Gardens, Hammersmith, London, W6 7DW.
Acknowledgements: Grant Support: Arthritis & Rheumatism Council, Medical Research Council, Wellcome Trust.

Table 1. Summary of cytokines produced spontaneously by RA synovial cells

Cytokine	mRNA	Protein
IL-1α	Yes	Yes
IL-1β	Yes	Yes
TNFα	Yes	Yes
LT	Yes	No (+/–)
IL-2	Yes	No (+/–)
IL-3	No	No
IL-4	?	No
IFNγ	Yes	No (+/–)
IL-6	Yes	Yes
GM-CSF	Yes	Yes
IL-8/NAP-1	Yes	Yes
RANTES	Yes	?
G-CSF	Yes	?
M-CSF	No	?
TGFβ	Yes	Yes
EGF	Yes	Yes
TGFα	No	No
PDGF-A	Yes	Yes
PDGF-B	Yes	Yes

These observations have been extended to investigate the role of TNFα in contributing to an animal model of arthritis (type II collagen induced arthritis in DBA/1 mice). It was found that both pretreatment of the mice with monoclonal anti-TNF antibody prior to collagen type II injection (14), or treatment of the mice once arthritis was established (unpublished observation) significantly reduced the severity of the arthritis and in particular the cartilage and bone destruction.

Although TNFα is produced spontaneously by RA cells in culture, little is known regarding the factors which lead to its production and which (if any) control mechanisms are present. Investigation of control mechanisms of TNFα have demonstrated that in common with other cytokines it is complex and occurs at multiple levels. Instances of transcriptional and post transcriptional regulation (15) as well as translational activation have been documented (16). Control mediated by prostaglandin E2 (17) and glucocorticoids (18) allows feedback between TNFα-producing and TNFα-responsive cells in different organ systems. Recently, with the description of cytokine binding proteins in urine and plasma of normal individuals attention has focussed on the role of such binding proteins in cytokine homeostasis. These proteins have been isolated from urine, purified to homogeneity, and are now known to be the shed versions of the surface TNF receptors (19). This binding protein inhibits binding of TNFα to mouse fibroblasts (TNFβ to a lesser extent) (19,20,21), and inhibits PGE2 release from dermal fibroblasts (22) and the further induction of HLA class I on human Colo 205 tumor cells induced with TNFα. A second TNFα binding protein has also been purified from urine and it is thought that these two proteins represent the soluble forms of the two molecular species of the cell surface TNF receptors (23). The presence of binding proteins in urine is not unique for TNFα as those for IL-2 (26), IL-6 and IFN-γ (27), IL-4 (28) and IL-7 (29) have been described. It is speculated that such proteins may be important regulators for many cytokines, and that inflammatory diseases such as RA result from a lack of these inhibitory molecules (or an imbalance), rather than purely from an increase in cytokine production.

In support of this hypothesis is our observation that in culture both osteoarthritic and RA synovial cells spontaneously produce TNF binding proteins capable of inhibiting TNFα bioactivity (24). However, insufficient TNF binding proteins are produced to effectively neutralize TNFα in the RA cultures. To date, it is not known what the cellular source of this inhibitor is in these cultures, but preliminary evidence shows that these TNF binding proteins have biochemical and immunological similarities to shed TNF receptor. Both binding proteins are produced spontaneously in culture by mononuclear cells isolated from either the synovial fluid or synovial membrane of RA patients. Interestingly the soluble p75 TNF receptor is found at higher levels than the p55 TNF receptor in both RA and OA synovial cultures. Both binding proteins are also found at elevated levels in both the plasma and synovial fluid of RA patients where there appears to be an association with disease activity. In order to study the regulation of the TNFα by its shed receptor, both TNF receptors 55kD

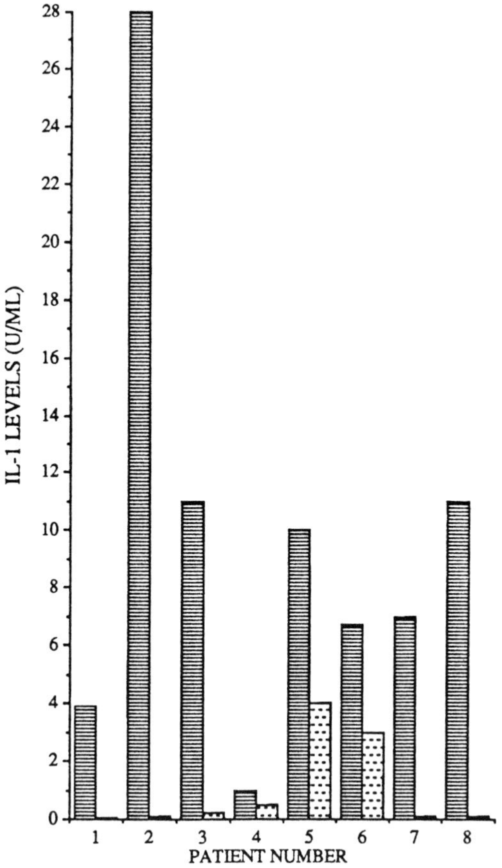

Figure 1a. Anti-TNFa inhibits IL-1 production in RA synovial joint cells in culture.
RA synovial joint cells were cultured for five days in the presence (lineal columns) or absence (dotted columns) of neutralising antibodies to TNFα. IL-1 levels were measured using the co-mitogenic mouse thymocyte bioassay. Data adapted from Brennan et al. 1991 (13).

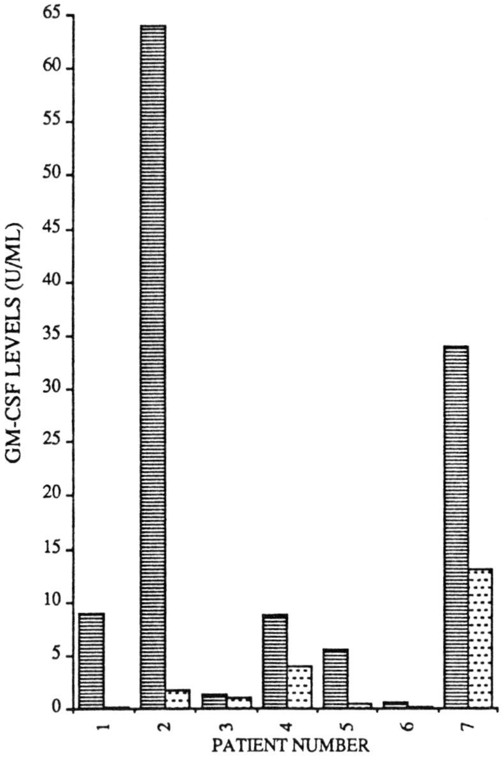

Figure 1b. Anti-TNFa inhibits GM-CSF production in RA synovial joint cells in culture.
RA synovial joint cells were cultured for five days in the presence (lineal columns) or absence (dotted columns) of neutralising antibodies to TNFα. GM-CSF levels were measured using the Mo7E bioassay. Data from Haworth et al. 1991 (4).

(25) and 75kD have been cloned and variants of each receptor encoding a soluble receptor expressed. The efficacy of recombinant soluble p55 and/or p75 receptor to block TNFα mediated effect in RA synovial cultures is currently being assessed.

The expression and distribution of the p55 and p75 TNF receptor on RA and OA synovial cells has been determined by flow cytometry using monoclonal antibodies specific for the p55 and p75 TNF receptor. Both the p55 and p75 TNF receptor are significantly elevated on RA synovial mononuclear cells compared to matched or normal peripheral blood (26). The p75 TNF receptor is increased predominantly on the lymphocyte population, and found to be mainly T lymphocytes by double staining techniques. It is not known at this stage what the functional relevance of increased TNF receptor expression on these T lymphocytes is, since the effects of TNFα on T cells are not fully understood. The p55 TNF receptor is predominantly increased on the 'non-lymphocyte' population on synovial membrane cells isolated from both RA and OA joints. These cells are predominantly of macrophage and fibroblast origin. These observations have been confirmed by immunostaining of synovial membrane biopsies. In addition to increased TNF receptor protein expression, there is abundant mRNA for both receptors (shown using specific cDNA probes by Northern blotting hybridization and *in situ* analysis) suggesting *de novo* synthesis.

These studies have shown therefore, that in RA there is disregulation of both TNF and its receptor. It is clear that the relationship between TNFα production, surface receptor expression and shed receptor formation is of key importance in understanding TNFα homeostasis. The ultimate aim will be to determine whether recombinant shed TNF receptor will inhibit TNFα activity *in vivo*, and as such be a novel therapeutic agent in the treatment of RA.

References

1. Feldmann, M. 1989. Molecular mechanisms involved in human autoimmune diseases: Relevance of chronic antigen presentation, class II expression and cytokine production. Immunology 2:66.
2. Buchan, G., Barrett, K., Turner, M., Chantry, D. Maini, R.N., and Feldmann, M. 1988. Interleukin-1 and tumor necrosis factor mRNA expression in rheumatoid arthritis: Prolonged production of IL-1a. Clin. Exp. Immunol. 73:449.
3. Hirano, T., Matsuda, T., Turner, M., Miyasaka, N., Buchan, G., Tang, B., Sato, K., Shimizu, M., Maini, R., Feldmann, M., and Kishimoto, T. 1988. Excessive production of interleukin 6/B cell stimulatory factor-2 in rheumatoid arthritis. Eur. J. Immunol. 18:1797.
4. Haworth, C., Brennan, F.M., Chantry, D., Turner, M., Maini, R.N., and Feldmann, M. 1991. Expression of granulocyte-macrophage colony stimulating factor (GM-CSF) in rheumatoid arthritis: Regulation by tumor necrosis factor α. Eur. J. Immunol., 21:2575.
5. Brennan, F.M., Zachariae, C.O.C., Chantry, D., Larsen, C.G., Turner, M., Maini, R.N., Matsushima, K., and Feldmann, M. 1990 Detection of interleukin-8 biological activity in synovial fluids from patients with rheumatoid arthritis and production of IL-8 mRNA by isolated synovial cells. Eur. J. Immunol. 20:2141.
6. Brennan, F.M., Chantry, D., Turner, M., Foxwell, B., Maini, R.N., and Feldmann, M. 1990. Detection of transforming growth factor-β in rheumatoid arthritis synovial tissue: Lack of effect on spontaneous cytokine production in joint cell cultures. Clin. Exp. Immunol. 81:278.
7. Buchan, G.S., Barrett, K., Fujita, T., Taniguchi, T., Maini, R.N., and Feldmann, M. 1988. Detection of activated T cell products in the rheumatoid joint using cDNA probes to interleukin 2, IL-2 receptor and interferon γ. Clin. Exp. Immunol. 71:295.
8. Brennan, F.M., Chantry, D., Jackson, A.M., Maini, R.N., and Feldmann, M. 1989. Cytokine production in culture by cells isolated from the synovial membrane. J. Autoimmunity 2: (Suppl) 177.
9. Dayer, J.M., Beutler, B., and Cerami, A. 1985. Cachectin/tumor necrosis factor stimulates collagenase and prostaglandin E_2 production by human synovial cells and dermal fibroblasts. J. Exp. Med. 162:2163.
10. Saklatavala, J., Sarsfield, S.J., Townsend, Y. 1985. Pig interleukin-1. Purification of two immunologically different leucocyte proteins that cause cartilage resorption, lymphocyte activation and fever. J. Exp Med. 162:1208.
11. Thomas, B.M., Mundy, G.R., and Chambers, T.J. 1987. Tumor necrosis factor α and β induce osteoblastic cells to stimulate osteoclast bone resorption. J. Immunol. 138:775.
12. Gowen, M., Wood, D.D., Ihrie, E.J., McGuire, M.K.B., and Russell, R.G. 1983. An interleukin-1 like factor stimulates bone resorption *in vitro*. Nature 306:378.
13. Brennan, F.M., Chantry, D., Jackson, A., Maini, R.N., and Feldmann, M. 1989. Inhibitory effect of TNFα antibodies on synovial cell interleukin-1 production in rheumatoid arthritis. Lancet ii:244.
14. Williams, R., Williams, D., Maini, R.N., and Feldmann, R. N. 1991. Attenuation of murine collagen-induced arthritis by anti-tumor necrosis factor antibody. Submitted manuscript.
15. Sariban, E., Imamura, K., Luebbers, R., and Kufe, D. 1988. Transcriptional and post-transcriptional regulation of tumor necrosis factor gene expression in human monocytes. J. Clin. Invest. 81:1506.
16. Han, J, and Beutler, B. 1990. The essential role of the UA-rich sequence in endotoxin-induced cachectin/TNF synthesis. Eur. Cytokine Net. 1:71.
17. Kunkel, S.L., Spengler, M., May, M.A., Spengler, R., Larrick, J., and Remick, D. 1988. Prostaglandin E2 regulated macrophage-derived tumor necrosis factor gene expression. Proc. Natl. Acad. Sci. 263:5380.
18. Beutler, B., Krochin, N., Milsark, I. W., Luedke, C., and Cerami, A. 1986. Control of cachetin (tumor necrosis factor) synthesis: Mechanisms of endotoxin resistance. Science 232:977.

19. Seckinger, P., Vey., Turcatti, G., Wingfield, P., and Dayer, J.-M. 1990. Tumor necrosis factor inhibitor: Purification NH2-terminal amino acid sequence and evidence for anti-inflammatory and immunomodulatory activities. Eur. J. Immunol. 20:1167.
20. Olsson, I., Lantz, M., Nilsson, E., Peetre, C., Thysell, H., Grubb, A., and Adolf, G. 1989. Isolation and characterisation of a tumor necrosis factor binding protein from urine. Eur. J. Haematol. 42:270.
21. Engelmann, H., Aderka, D., Rubenstein, M., Rotman, D., and Wallach, D. 1989. A tumor necrosis factor-binding protein purified to homogeneity from human urine protects cells from tumor necrosis factor toxicity. J. Biol. Chem. 264:11974.
22. Seckinger, P., Zhang, J-H., Hauptmann, B., and Dayer, J.-M. 1990. Characterisation of a tumor necrosis factor-α (TNFα) inhibitor: Evidence of immunological cross-reactivity with the TNF receptor. Proc. Natl. Acad. Sci. 87:5188.
23. Engelmann, H., Novick, D., and Wallach, D. 1990. Two tumor necrosis factor-binding proteins purified from human urine. J. Biol. Chem. 265:1531.
24. Brennan, F.M., Katsikis, P., Chantry, D., Wallach, D., and Feldmann, M. 1991. TNF binding proteins are produced spontaneously in synovial cell cultures derived from patients with RA and OA. In preparation.
25. Gray, P., Barrett, K., Chantry, D., Turner, M., and Feldmann, M. 1990. Cloning of human tumor necrosis factor receptor cDNA and expression of recombinant soluble TNF-binding protein. Proc. Natl. Acad. Sci. 87:7380.
26. Marcon, L., Fritz, M. E., Kurman, C., Jensen, J. C., and Nelson, D.L. 1988. Soluble Tac peptide is present in the urine of normal individuals and at elevated levels in patients with adult T cell leukaemia. Clin. Exp. Immunol 73:29.
27. Novick, D., Engelman, H., Wallach, D., and Rubinstein, M. 1989. Soluble cytokine receptors are present in normal human urine. J. Exp. Med. 170:1410.
28. Fernandez-Botran, R., and Vitetta, E.S. 1990. A soluble, high affinity, interleukin-4 binding protein is present in the biological fluids of mice. Proc. Natl. Acad. Sci. 87:4202.
29. Goodwin, R.G., Friend, D., Ziegler, S.F., Jerzy, R., Falk, B.A., Cosman, D., Dower, S.K., March, C.J., Namen, A.E., and Park, L.S. 1990. Molecular cloning of the human and murine interleukin-7 receptors: Demonstration of a soluble form and homology to a new receptor superfamily. Cell 60:941.

Pathogenesis of Rheumatoid Inflammation

John J. Cush, Peter E. Lipsky*

Rheumatoid arthritis (RA) is a chronic systemic disease characterized by persistent inflammation of the synovium, local destruction of bone and cartilage and a variety of systemic manifestations. As a result of an unknown inciting stimulus, the rheumatoid synovium becomes the focus of an acute and ultimately chronic inflammatory process. The persistence of immunologic activity within the joint is considered to be the driving force that eventually results in damage to articular cartilage, bone and periarticular structures. During the evolution of this inflammatory process, the rheumatoid synovial membrane is histologically transformed by an increase in the number of synovial lining cells and the intense infiltration of mononuclear cells, primarily lymphocytes, plasma cells and mononuclear phagocytes. Characteristically, the rheumatoid synovium exhibits a great deal of histologic variability. The variable distribution and progressive nature of the synovitis have made it difficult to characterize rheumatoid inflammation completely. It is apparent, however, that infiltration with large numbers of mononuclear cells is one of the characteristic and pathogenically important features of this process.

Histopathology

As rheumatoid synovitis evolves over time, the histopathology varies according to the stage of disease. The histopathologic findings in early RA (onset phase) are generally different than that observed in late RA (chronic phase) (1,2). Examination of synovial tissue obtained during the first 2 months of RA reveals prominent capillary or venular abnormalities (3) (i. e., endothelial cell injury, vascular obliteration, congestion and edema) associated with modest increases in the number of synovial lining cells and scant perivascular accumulations of inflammatory cells. In the first several weeks of rheumatoid inflammation, it is not uncommon to find neutrophils infiltrating the synovial tissues. However, as the disease evolves, lymphocytes and other mononuclear cells become the predominant cells infiltrating the sublining layers. The chronic phase of rheumatoid inflammation is characterized by a further increase in the number of synovial lining cells, focal or segmental vascular changes, and intense mononuclear cell infiltration. The development of lymphoid follicles with germinal centers becomes evident with chronicity.

Within the rheumatoid synovium, lymphocytes aggregate in the perivascular regions of the sublining layers. In these areas, the majority of cells are T cells and the majority of these are of the CD4(+) "helper/inducer" phenotype (4–6). In areas away from the perivascular dense lymphoid aggregates, the majority of cells are CD8(+) T cells. In the perivascular aggregates, many of the CD4(+) T cells are found in close proximity to HLA-DR(+) macrophages and dendritic cells (6). This histopathologic picture is reminiscent of the pathology observed in delayed-type hypersensitivity reactions to a known antigen (7). It has therefore been postulated that the rheumatoid synovium is a tissue in which there is ongoing presentation of antigen to CD4(+) T cells. However, the nature of this putative antigen is currently unknown.

The rheumatoid synovium also contains numerous lymphoblasts and plasma cells that are often arranged in nodular aggregates with germinal centers. Presumably, the small lymphoblasts migrate into the synovium and differentiate into immunoglobulin and RF secreting plasma cells (8). In the chronic phase of RA, granulation tissue, or pannus, eventually develops within the joint tissues. Pannus is a highly vascularized connective tissue that is composed of a variety of cell types including lymphocytes, macrophages, histiocytes, fibroblasts and mast cells, and is frequently found

* Harold C. Simmons Arthritis Research Center, University of Texas Southwestern Medical Center at Dallas, Dallas, TX 75235, USA.

encroaching upon articular cartilage and tendon sheaths. It remains unclear whether pannus is the residuum of aggressive, antecedent inflammation or whether it is an invasive tissue, capable of eroding articular and periarticular structures (1,8).

The histologic changes seen in the synovial tissue are not specific for rheumatoid inflammation, and have been observed in other conditions, including gout, septic arthritis, systemic lupus erythematosus, and Reiter's syndrome (9). The features that are unique to rheumatoid synovitis are the intensity of the mononuclear cell infiltration, especially that of CD4(+) T cells, and the presence of lymphoid follicles and plasma cells secreting large amounts of immunoglobulin and the autoantibody, rheumatoid factor.

Endothelium and Rheumatoid Inflammation

The prominent microvascular abnormalities observed in rheumatoid synovitis most commonly involve the capillaries and post-capillary venules, such that the endothelial cells assume the morphologic characteristics of high endothelial venules (10), as well as exhibiting endothelial cell injury, vascular obliteration by inflammatory cells or thrombi, and neovascularization. These vascular changes are associated with the infiltration of inflammatory cells, but the mechanisms by which inflammatory cells migrate into and accumulate within the rheumatoid synovium have not been fully elucidated. It is clear, however, that the endothelial cells in the rheumatoid synovium express a variety of adhesion molecules that are involved in binding circulating neutrophils and mononuclear cells, thereby facilitating their entry into tissues. Expression of these adhesion molecules is enhanced by a variety of proinflammatory cytokines produced in the rheumatoid synovium including interleukin 1 (IL-1), tumor necrosis factorα (TNFα), and gamma interferon (IFNγ), as well as other inflammatory mediators produced by the synovium (11–13). IL-1 and TNFα stimulate the vascular endothelium to express the adhesion ligand endothelial leukocyte adhesion molecule 1 (ELAM-1), and thereby induce increased adhesiveness for neutrophils (12). IL-1, TNFα, and IFNγ also increase the expression of intercellular adhesion molecule 1 (ICAM-1), that serves as an adhesion ligand for circulating mononuclear cells (13), whereas IL-1 and TNFα enhance the expression of vascular cell adhesion molecule (VCAM), an adhesion molecule for lymphocytes. Thus, under the influence of a variety of effector molecules produced by activated mononuclear cells, synovial cells and endothelial cells, there is an increase in the binding of circulating cells to the endothelial cells of the post-capillary venules and migration through the vascular endothelium into the inflammatory site.

T Lymphocytes and Rheumatoid Inflammation

The nature of the cells circulating in the blood and infiltrating the synovial fluid and synovium have been analyzed in detail (Table 1). Peripheral blood T cells of RA patients exhibit abnormalities that tend to correlate with disease activity. Although normal numbers of CD3(+) and CD4(+) T cells are usually found (4), slightly decreased numbers of circulating CD8(+) lymphocytes may be observed in the most active RA patients (14,15). The number of circulating "memory" (CD29 bright or CD45RO+) and "naive" (CD45RA+) CD4(+) T cells is usually normal (16). Although the frequency of each of these subsets is usually normal, there is evidence that patients with active RA have increased numbers of circulating activated T cells. Thus, in

Table 1. Phenotype of Lymphocyte Subsets Found in Excess in the Rheumatoid Synovium

T-Cell Differentiation Antigens
CD3 "dim"
CD4 "dim"
CD4+CD45RO+
CD4+CD29 "bright"
Activation Antigens
CD3+HLA-DR+
CD9+
CD49a+CD29+
Adhesion Molecules
CD11a/CD18 "bright"
CD54+

patients with active disease, the density of CD3 and CD4 expression on T cells is reduced in a manner similar to that observed after *in vitro* mitogenic stimulation (4,18). Moreover, increased numbers of cells expressing activation antigens, such as HLA-DR, CD9, CD71 and 4F2, can be found, particularly in patients with active disease (4,18,19).

Nearly all of the synovial tissue CD4(+) T cells are of the "memory" phenotype, CD29 bright, CD45RO+, and CD45RA dim (16,17). By contrast, the synovium is nearly devoid of "naive" CD4+/CD45RA "bright" lymphocytes. In most studies, the frequency of CD8(+) synovial T cells is not different than that found in normal or rheumatoid peripheral blood (17). The synovium also contains a large number of activated T cells, as indicated by the decreased density of CD3 and CD4 and the enrichment of cells expressing HLA-DR, DQ, and DP antigens (4,20,21). Other activation markers are similarly augmented, including CD9 and CD49a/CD29 or VLA-1, a late activation antigen expressed only after persistent proliferation (4,20). Notably absent in the rheumatoid synovium are activated T cells expressing IL-2 receptors (CD25) and transferrin receptors (CD71) (4,16,18). A number of adhesion receptors and ligands, including LFA-1 (CD11a/CD18) and ICAM-1 (CD54), have also been shown to be expressed at increased density on synovial tissue lymphocytes (4,16,19).

Despite the expression of activation antigens and other features of an activated phenotype by T cells in the joint, the functional status of the cells in rheumatoid synovium has been debated (5,20-23). Morphologically, many of the lymphocytes are small and without the characteristics of lymphoblasts (6). Moreover, few of them express IL-2 receptors (CD25) or transferrin receptors (CD71) (20), and their *in vitro* responses to antigens and mitogens are diminished (20,22). In addition, the amounts of T cell derived cytokines, such as IL-2 and gamma interferon, produced by the rheumatoid synovium is less than might be expected for a T cell driven response (23). Despite these findings, it is clear from the phenotype of cells in the synovial tissue that they are not resting T cells. Moreover, an excess of T cell cytokines are clearly produced within the synovium (Table 2). Whether the activated T cells within the synovial tissue have migrated from the blood to the synovial tissue or alternatively, whether they are cells that have proliferated locally within the synovial tissue has not been resolved. The finding that circulating T cells are also activated could support the former interpretation, whereas the observation that many synovial, but not blood, T cells express VLA-1 that is upregulated only after many rounds of proliferation, supports the conclusion that the expansion of T cells has occurred within the rheumatoid synovium.

RA has been associated with the expression of certain class II molecules of the major histocompatibility complex. Thus, individuals with RA are more likely to express one of a number of HLA-DR molecules (Dw4, Dw14, Dw15, Dw16, and DR1) that are identical in the third hypervariable region of the β chain, a portion of the molecule that plays a major role in determining the capacity of T cells to recognize specific antigenic epitopes (24,25). This association strongly implies a role for recognition of a specific antigen by MHC restricted T cells in the development of rheumatoid inflammation. Attempts to identify the antigen driving rheumatoid inflammation, however, have not yielded definitive results, although several potential candidate antigens have been implicated, including altered autoantigens (such as IgG or collagen), viruses (such as Epstein-Barr virus, parvovirus, or the retrovirus HTLV-1) and heat shock proteins (20). Attempts to determine whether the T cells in the rheumatoid synovium are oligoclonal or polyclonal have also not generated consistent results (25–28). Analysis of the T cell receptor rearrangement (TCR) patterns of 87 T cell clones derived from the synovial tissues of 4 HLA-DR4 (+) RA patients with active synovitis in our own institution has not provided evidence of oligoclonality within the rheumatoid synovium (28). Whether there exists a small, but definite population of clonal T cells, that drives rheumatoid inflammation remains unresolved.

B Lymphocytes and Rheumatoid Inflammation

The autoimmune hallmark of RA is the autoantibody, rheumatoid factor (RF), which can be demonstrated in about 80% of affected individuals. Increased serum levels of IgM-RF has been associated with the presence of rheumatoid nodules, extra-articular manifestations of RA (i.e., vasculitis, Felty's syndrome), severe erosive disease, and poor outcome, suggesting an important role for IgM-RF in the pathogenesis of RA (20,29,30). This conclusion has been supported by the finding of excessive production of intraarticular immunoglobulin and RF and the associated immune complex formation and complement activation (20).

Circulating B cells in patients with RA demonstrate phenotypic evidence of *in vivo* activation, including the expression of an increased density of HLA-DR molecules (20). Moreover, B cell hyperactivity in patients with active RA is indicated by the presence of circulating cells spontaneously secreting RF (29,30). In addition, several studies have demonstrated an increased number of CD5(+) B cells in the circulation of RA patients (30). CD5 is found on all mature T cells and a subset (15–20%) of B cells. In some mouse strains with spontaneous autoimmunity, CD5(+) B cells account for much of the autoantibody production, whereas in humans, these cells do not appear to be uniquely capable of autoantibody formation. The presence of increased numbers of CD5(+) B cells in the circulation of patients with RA and those with Sjogren's syndrome probably reflects the presence of activated B cells, since CD5 has the characteristics of an activation antigen in man, rather than a lineage specific B cell marker (20). Moreover, the number of CD5(+) B cells does not correlate with serum RF titers or disease activity in patients with RA. Finally, this subset does not seem to be solely responsible for RF production in seropositive patients with active RA.

In contrast to the peripheral blood and synovial fluid, the synovial tissues contains large numbers of B cells and plasma cells that express CD20 and PCA-1 respectively (17). These cells are found in the perivascular regions, often arranged in nodular aggregates with germinal centers. Immunoglobulin and IgM-RF is spontaneously secreted by cells of the rheumatoid synovium. Thus, cells eluted from the synovial tissue of seropositive, but not seronegative, patients, have been shown to secrete large amounts of IgM-RF spontaneously in culture (31).

Cytokines as Effector Molecules in Rheumatoid Inflammation

Many of the manifestations of RA can be ascribed to the action of a host of cytokines and other secretory products synthesized within the rheumatoid synovium. Cytokines are peptides, secreted by a variety of activated inflammatory cells that regulate the function of numerous different cell types in an autocrine, paracrine and/or endocrine fashion. The multiple overlapping biologic activities of these cytokines make it difficult to ascribe a particular *in vivo* effect to an individual cytokine. Nonetheless, the numerous cellular participants in rheumatoid synovitis are likely to communicate and effect surrounding cells via their secreted cytokines. The enhanced production of cytokines in patients with RA has been the subject of a number of recent reviews (11–13,20). The cellular sources and actions of the cytokines produced in the rheumatoid synovium are summarized in Table 2.

Many of the features of rheumatoid arthritis can be accounted for by the activity of the cytokines produced locally. Thus, within the inflamed synovium, increased vascular adhesiveness for circulating mononuclear cells and their subsequent chemotaxis is promoted by IL-1, TNFα, IFNγ, TGFβ and IL-8. The expression of class I and class II MHC molecules is induced by IFNγ, GM-CSF, and TNFα. Activation and proliferation of T cells is primarily related to the action of IL-2, although IL-1, IL-6, and TNFα may amplify responses. The differentiation of B cells into immunoglobulin secreting cells locally within the synovium is also driven primarily by IL-2, although other cytokines, including IL-1, IL-6, IFNγ, and TNFα may enhance immunoglobulin synthesis. The local activationof macrophages is induced by a number of cytokines, including IFNγ, GM-CSF, M-CSF, and IL-2. Local proliferation of synovial cells is stimulated by a variety of cytokines, including IL-1, PDGF, IGF-1, FGF and TGFβ, and neovascularization, a common feature of the inflamed synovium, is driven by TNFα, FGF, TGFβ and PDGF. Finally, activation of chondrocytes and osteoblasts is induced by IL-1 and TNFα with the resultant loss of cartilage and bone matrix.

Table 2. Cytokines Detected in the Synovial Fluid or Tissue of RA Patients

Cytokine	Probable Source*
Interleukin-1 (IL-1)	Mo, MP, FB, EC
Interleukin-2 (IL-2)	TL
Interleukin-6 (IL-6)	TL, MP, FB, BL
Interleukin-8 (IL-8)	MP, EC, FB
Tumor Necrosis Factorα (TNFα)	TL, Mo, MP
Interferonγ (IFNγ)	TL
Granulocyte-Macrophage Colony-Stimulating Factor (GM-CSF)	FB, EC, TL
Macrophage Colony-Stimulating Factor (M-CSF)	FB, EC, Mo, MP, SV
Epidermal Growth Factor (EGF)	MP, SV
Fibroblast Growth Factor (FGF)	Plt, MP, EC
Insulin-Like Growth Factor (IGF-1)	MP
Platelet-Derived Growth Factor (PDGF)	EC, Plt, MP
Transforming Growth Factor β (TGFβ)	FB, MP, Mo, TL, EC

*Mo = monocyte; MP = macrophage; FB = fibroblast; EC = endothelial cell; TL = T lymphocyte; BL = B lymphocyte; SV = synoviocyte; Plt = Platelets

Overriding the chronic inflammation in the synovial tissue is an additional inflammatory process in the synovial fluid. Although a variety of inflammatory mediators, including complement cleavage products, lipoxygenase and cyclooxygenase pathway metabolites of arachidonic acid, histamine, serotonin, and platelet activating factor contribute to this inflammatory response, cytokines produced in the synovium also play a central role in the induction of this process. Thus, TNFα and IL-1 increase the adhesiveness of post-capillary venules for neutrophils by induction of adhesion molecules, whereas IL-8 and TNFα are chemotactic for neutrophils. Finally, IL-8, TNFα and GM-CSF activate various aspects of neutrophil function.

Some of the extra-articular manifestations of RA may also be accounted for by the systemic effects of locally produced cytokines with IL-1 and TNFα inducing fever and constitutional symptoms and IL-1, TNFα, and IL-6 stimulating the production of acute phase reactants by the liver. Thus, many of the systemic features of RA may result from dissemination of cytokines produced within the inflamed synovium.

Conclusion

A considerable body of evidence exists to support the conclusion that activated T cells in the synovium play a primary role in perpetuating chronic inflammation. Much has been learned about the nature of rheumatoid inflammation by observing the effects of specific therapies. Thus, the amelioration of disease by depletion or interference with the function of immunocompetent T cells with total lymphoid irradiation, thoracic duct drainage, or monoclonal antibodies to CD4 or CD5 (20,22) has indicated the central role of T cells in the pathogenesis of RA. In addition, an unfortunate experiment of nature has confirmed the central role of CD4(+) T cells in rheumatoid inflammation. Thus, the loss of functionally competent CD4(+) T cells in RA patients who have become infected with the human immunodeficiency virus (HIV) has resulted in the clinical remission of chronic rheumatoid inflammation (32).

Improvement of joint inflammation observed with the above therapies often occurs without alterations in serum rheumatoid factor titers. This dichotomy underscores the primary role of T cells in the perpetuation of chronic rheumatoid inflammation, although perhaps not the ongoing production of RF. Some of the extra-articular manifestations of RA appear not to be effected by these forms of therapy, suggesting a central role for RF-containing immune complexes in their pathogenesis. Although synovial inflammation in RA is unlikely to be driven by immune complexes, the local production of RF and immunoglobulin, the associated complement activation and the deposition of immune complexes contributes to the severity of the inflammation (33). The deposition of immune complexes and associated complement activation are also likely to contribute to the progressive intraarticular damage observed. This hypothesis is supported by studies demonstrating the proinflammatory effects of rheumatoid factors *in vivo* (34) and the destructive synergistic effects of antibodies to type II collagen in rats with adjuvant arthritis (35), suggesting that locally generated immune complexes can amplify and aggravate the course of chronic cell mediated inflammation.

An understanding of the immunopathogenic mechanisms responsible for rheumatoid inflammation suggests new approaches to the control of disease activity. Such therapies include approaches aimed at blocking the specific immunologic response that might underlie the chronic inflammation or less specific interventions to inhibit particular phases of the cascade of events set in motion by the initiating stimulus. These therapeutic interventions may be tailored to the stage of disease, genetic background of the individual or the characteristics of the synovitis in a particular patient. Such approaches may lead to more rapid disease control, far more clinical remissions and improvement in the morbidity and mortality associated with this disease.

References

1. Bromely, M., and Woolley, D.E. 1984. Histopathology of the rheumatoid lesion: Identification of cell types at sites of cartilage erosion. Arthritis Rheum. 27:857.
2. Schumacher, H.R., and Kitridou, R.C. 1972. Synovitis of recent onset: A clinicopathologic study during the first month of disease. Arthritis Rheum. 15:465.
3. Rothschild, B.M., and Masi, A.T. 1982. Pathogenesis of rheumatoid arthritis: A vascular hypothesis. Sem. Arthritis Rheum. 12:11.
4. Cush, J.J., and Lipsky, P.E. 1988. Phenotypic analysis of synovial tissue and peripheral blood lymphocytes isolated from patients with rheumatoid arthritis. Arthritis Rheum. 31:1230.
5. Janossy, J., Panayi, G., Duke, O., Bofill, M., Poulter, L.W., and Goldstein, G. 1981. Rheumatoid arthritis: A disease of T-lymphocyte/macrophage immunregulation. Lancet i:839.
6. Kurosaka, M., and Ziff, M. 1983. Immunoelectron microscopic study of the distribution of T cell subsets in the rheumatoid synovium. J. Exp. Med. 158:1191.
7. Klareskog, L., Forsum, U., Scheynius, A., Kabelitz, D., and Wigzell, H. 1982. Evidence insupport of a self-perpetuating HLA-DR-dependent delayed-type cell reaction in rheumatoid arthritis. Proc. Natl. Acad. Sci. 79:3632.
8. Fassbender, H.G. 1984. Is pannus a residue of inflammation? Arthritis Rheum. 27:956.
9. Goldenberg, D.L., and Cohen, A.S. 1978. Synovial membrane histopathology in the differential diagnosis of rheumatoid arthritis, gout, pseudogout, systemic lupus erythematosus, infectious arthritis, and degenerative joint disease. Medicine 57:239.
10. Oppenheimer-Marks, N., and Ziff, M. 1986. Binding of normal human mononuclear cells to blood vessels in rheumatoid arthritis synovial membrane. Arthritis Rheum. 29:789.
11. Lipsky, P.E., Davis, L.S., Cush, J.J., and Oppenheimer-Marks, N. 1989. The role of cytokines in the pathogenesis of rheumatoid arthritis. Springer Semin. Immunopathol. 11:123.
12. Pober, J.S. 1988. Cytokine-mediated activation of vascular endothelium: Physiology and pathology. Am. J. Pathol. 133:426.
13. Mantovani, A., and Dejana, E. 1989. Cytokines as communication signals between leukocytes and endothelial cells. Immunol. Today 10:370.
14. Bertouch, J.V., Roberts-Thomson, P.J., Brooks, P.M., and Bradley, J. 1984. Lymphocyte subsets and inflammatory indices in synovial fluid and blood of patients with rheumatoid arthritis. J. Rheumatol. 11:754.
15. Goto, M., Miyamoto, T., and Nishioka, K. 1987. 2 dimensional flow cytometric analysis of activation antigens expressed on the synovial fluid T cells in rheumatoid arthritis. J. Rheumatol. 14:230.
16. Cush, J.J., and Lipsky, P.E. 1990. Dual immunoflourescence analysis of lymphocyte subsets eluted from rheumatoid synovium. FASEB J. 4:1855.
17. Nakao, H., Eguchi, K., Kawakami, A., Migita, K., Otsubo, T., Ueki, Y., Shimomura, C., Tezuka, H., Mastsunaga, M., Maeda, K., and Nagataki, S. 1989. Increment of Ta1 positive cells in peripheral blood from patients with rheumatoid arthritis. Arthritis Rheum. 16:907.
18. Smith, M.D., and Roberts-Thomson, P.J. 1990. Lymphocyte surface marker expression in rheumatic diseases: Evidence for prior activa-

tion of lymphocytes *in vivo*. Ann. Rheum. Dis. 49:81.
19. Potocnik, A.J., Kinne, R., Menninger, H., Zacher, J., Emmrich, F., and Kroczek, R.A. 1990. Expression of activation antigens on T cells in rheumatoid arthritis patients. Scand. J. Immunol. 1:213.
20. Cush, J., and Lipsky, P.E. 1991. Cellular basis for rheumatoid inflammation. Clin. Orthop. Rel. Res. 265:9.
21. Jahn, B., Burmester, G.R., Stock, P., Rohwer, P., and Kalden, J.R. 1987. Functional and phenotypical characterization of activated T cells from intra-articular sites in inflammatory joint diseases: Possible modulation of the CD3 antigen. Scand. J. Immunol. 26:745.
22. Cush, J.J., and Lipsky, P.E. 1987. The immunopathogenesis of rheumatoid arthritis: The role of cytokines in chronic inflammation. Clin. Aspects Autoimmunity 1:2.
23. Firestein, G.S., and Zvaifler, N.J. 1990. How important are T cells in chronic rheumatoid synovitis? Arthritis Rheum. 33:768.
24. Winchester, R.J., and Gregersen, P.K. 1988. The molecular basis of susceptibility to rheumatoid arthritis: The conformational equivalence hypothesis. Springer Semin. Immunopathol. 10:119.
25. Duby, A., Sinclair, A.K., Osborne-Lawrence, S.L., Zeldes, W., Kan, L., and Fox, D.A. 1989. Clonal heterogeneity of synovial fluid T lymphocytes from patients with rheumatoid arthritis. Proc. Natl. Acad. Sci. 86:6206.
26. Savill, C.M., Delves, P.J., Kioussis, K., Walker, P., Lydyard, P.M., Colaco, B., Shipley, M., and Roitt, I. 1987. A minority of patients with rheumatoid arthritis show a dominant rearrangement of T-cell receptor β chain genes in synovial lymphocytes. Scand. J. Immunol. 25:629.
27. Stamenkovic, I., Stegagno, M., Wright, K.A., Krane, S.M., Amento, E.P., Colvin, R.B., Duquesnoy, R.J., and Kurnick, J.T. 1988. Clonal dominance among T-lymphocyte infiltrates in arthritis. Proc. Natl. Acad. Sci. 85:1179.
28. Cush, J., Duby, A.D., Lightfoot, E., and Lipsky, P.E. 1990. The search for oligoclonal T cells in rheumatoid synovium. Arthritis Rheum. 33 [Suppl]:S16.
29. Olsen, N.J., and Jasin, H.E. 1985. Synthesis of rheumatoid factor *in vitro*: Implications for the pathogenesis of rheumatoid arthritis. Sem. Arthritis Rheum. 15:146.
30. Petersen, J. 1988. B lymphocyte function in patients with rheumatoid arthritis: Impact of regulatory T lymphocytes and macrophages – modulation by antirheumatic drugs. Danish. Med. Bull. 35:140.
31. Wernick, R.M., Lipsky, P.E., Marban-Arcos, E., Maliakkal, J.J., Edelbaum, D., and Ziff, M. 1985. IgG and IgM rheumatoid factor synthesis in rheumatoid synovial membrane cell cultures. Arthritis Rheum. 28:742.
32. Epinoza, L.R., Aguilar, J.L., Berman, A., Gutierrez, F., Vasey, F.B., and German, B.F. 1989. Rheumatic manifestations associated with human immunodeficiency virus infection. Arthritis Rheum. 32:1615.
33. Klareskog, L., Homdahl, R., Nordling, C., Tarkowski, A., and Rubin, K. 1987. Synovial class II antigen expression and immune complex formation in rheumatoid arthritis. Acta Med. Scand. Suppl. 715:85.
34. Rawson, A.J., Hollander, J.L., Quismorio, F.P., and Abelson, N.V. 1969. Experimental arthritis in man and rabbit dependent upon serum anti-immunoglobulin factors. Ann. N. Y. Acad. Sci. 168:188.
35. Taurog, J.D., Kerwar, S.S., McReynolds, R.A., Sandberg, G.P., Leary, S.L., and Mahowald, M.L. 1985. Synergy between adjuvant arthritis and collagen-induced arthritis in rats. J. Exp. Med. 162:962.

Pathogenetic and Etiologic Implications of Autoantibodies in Collagen Diseases

Eng M. Tan*

In the collagen-vascular diseases now more commonly known as the systemic autoimmune diseases, there is an immunological response which is characterized by the production of autoantibodies reactive with antigens which are intracellular in location. The most commonly encountered autoantibodies are directed against antigens present in the nucleoplasm, nucleolus and cytoplasm in that order of frequency. Autoimmune diseases such as systemic lupus erythematosus (lupus), scleroderma, Sjogren's syndrome, dermatomyositis and polymyositis, each have their own characteristic profiles of autoantibodies which have the following features: Some antibodies are uniquely associated with a disease, some antibodies are present in higher frequency in one disease compared to others, and distinct clusters of different antibodies are segregated in some diseases. Because the target antigens in the systemic autoimmune diseases are intracellular in location, autoantibodies are not able to react with these "sequestered" antigens unless there is previous cell injury. Thus, it must not be automatically assumed that autoantibodies participate in tissue injury. Autoantibodies should be considered to be the immunological footprints of a previous biologic event. Important insights have been provided by the characterization of the molecular and functional properties of these intracellular antigens. Many of the antigens are subunit components of larger subcellular particles and the epitopes of the antigens recognized by autoantibodies appear to be the active sites, catalytic centers or functioning regions of these subcellular particles. The new structural and functional knowledge of the nature of intracellular antigens suggests that the immunogen driving the autoimmune response is an activated or functioning subcellular particle. Future research in this area should be targeted at identifying the stimuli which drive the activation of highly specific subcellular particles.

Overview of the Nature of Autoantibodies to Intracellular Antigens

Autoantibodies to the intracellular antigens are found in a number of systemic autoimmune diseases, especially systemic lupus erythematosus (lupus), drug-induced lupus (DIL), mixed connective tissue disease (MCTD), scleroderma or systemic sclerosis, Sjogren's sydnrome, dermatomyositis and polymyositis (for a comprehensive review, see Ref. 1). The systemic autoimmune diseases previously called collagen-vascular diseases have one distinctive feature in common: the presence of autoantibodies to antigens which are intracellular in location. By far the most common autoantibodies which have been detected and characterized have been antibodies directed against nucleoplasmic, nucleolar and cytoplasmic antigens in that order of frequency. Antinuclear antibodies (ANAs) (a term used to include both anti-nucleoplasmic and anti-nucleolar antibodies) and anti-cytoplasmic antibodies have become important aids to the clinician in the differentiation of systemic autoimmune diseases. This development in the clinical utility of autoantibodies has been related to the ability to define the immunologic specificity of autoantibodies. In the approach to interpretation of the clinical significance of autoantibodies, it might be useful to keep in mind the following considerations:

A: Autoantibodies, such as antinuclear antibodies (ANAs) or anti-cytoplasmic antibodies are generic terms which describe the complete repertoire of all antinuclear and anti-cytoplasmic antibodies. Because many different dis-

* W. M. Keck Autoimmune Disease Center, The Scripps Research Institute, 10666 N. Torrey Pines Road, La Jolla, California 92037, U.S.A.
Acknowledgements: Supported by NIH grants AR32063 and AI32834.

eases are capable of making autoimmune responses to these antigens, a positive autoantibody, whether anti-nuclear or anti-cytoplasmic, does not by itself denote any particular autoimmune disease. And:

B: Each autoimmune disease possesses a distinctive profile of autoantibodies. There are some autoantibodies which are associated predominantly with only one disease. These autoantibodies are relatively disease-specific. Examples of such disease-specific autoantibodies are: (a): Lupus: antibodies to native DNA and antibodies to Sm antigen; (b): Scleroderma: antibodies to Scl-70 and the nucleolar antigens RNA polymerase 1 and fibrillarin; (c): CREST (*c*alcinosis, *R*aynaud's phenomenon, *e*sophageal dysmotility, *s*clerodactyly, *t*elangiectasia): antibodies to centromere/kinetochore antigens; and (d): Dermatomyositis and polymyositis: antibodies to transfer RNA synthetases, called Jo-1, PL-7 and PL12.

Another feature is the occurrence of autoantibodies as clusters so that one autoantibody is often associated with another. Antibodies to DNA are frequently associated with antibodies to histones, antibodies to Sm with antibodies to nuclear RNP (U1-RNP) and antibodies to SS-B/La with antibodies to SS-A/Ro. These linkages of antibodies are mechanistically related to the fact that the linked antibodies are directed at antigens which are complexed to each other *in vivo*. DNA and histones are present together as nucleosomes, Sm and U1-RNP are present together as nuclear particles called small nuclear ribonucleoproteins (snRNPs) and SS-B/La and SS-A/Ro are also complexed as intracellular particles. Linked sets of antibodies are also observed in scleroderma, where the autoantibody response appears to be directed at antigens which at certain phases of the cell cycle are all localized in the nucleolus. These antigens are DNA topoisomerase 1, RNA polymerase 1, fibrillarin and PM-Scl (see Table 5).

Are Autoantibodies to Intracellular Antigens Involved in Pathogenesis?

The much quoted statement of Ehrlich that an autoimmune response is a state of "horror autotoxicus" has given rise to the widely held concept that autoantibodies are pathogenic and therefore play a role in causing tissue injury. The statement implies that when autoantibodies react with self-antigens, the resulting antigen-antibody reaction would initiate a series of events including activation of inflammatory pathways which result in tissue damage and injury. This scenario of events is applicable in the situation where antibodies have access to their cognate antigens. This line of reasoning may not be applicable to the situation where autoantigens are present intracellularly, as in the case of autoantibodies directed at nucleoplasmic, nucleolar or cytoplasmic antigens. These intracellular antigens are normally inaccessible to circulating autoantibodies when cell membranes are intact as in healthy cells. In most situations, these intracellular antigens have not been demonstrated in the extracellular milieu. An exception has been the demonstration that macromolecular DNA can be detected in the circulation in certain patients with SLE. In some body fluids, histones have also been detected (2). However, for other intracellular autoantigens, there have been no systematic studies to determine if these antigens can be detected in extracellular fluids. Until such time as more information is available on this question, it would be inappropriate to consider (with the exception of antibodies to DNA and histones), that autoantibodies to intracellular antigens are playing a role in pathogenesis. What needs to be kept in mind is that in the systemic autoimmune diseases, the targets of the autoantibodies are antigens which are normally intracellular in location and are therefore inaccessible to circulating antibody.

The Immunogen is a Component of a Subcellular Particle

An important picture has emerged from studies showing that autoantibodies in diseases like SLE are directed against multiple intracellular antigens (3). This has been described as a polyclonal response indicating that many different clones of B cells were stimulated to produce antibodies. The data have also been informative from the antigen side of the immune response. The Sm immune response is directed against several different proteins present in the

Table 1. Functions of Certain Intracellular Autoantigens.

Antigen	Function of Antigen	Autoantibodies Detected in
Sm	Splicing of pre-mRNA	Lupus
U1-RNP	Splicing of pre-mRNA	Lupus, MCTD
SS-B/La	Processing of RNA pol III transcripts	Lupus, Sjogren's syndrome
Ribosomal (r) RNP (P proteins)	Involved in protein biosynthesis by ribosomes	Lupus
PCNA	DNA replication and repair	Lupus
Scl-70	Relaxation of supercoiled DNA. DNA synthesis and transcription	Scleroderma
Centromere/ Kinetochore	Cell division (mitosis)	Scleroderma subset (CREST)
RNA pol I	Transcription of ribosomal DNA	Scleroderma
Fibrillarin (U3 RNP)	Processing of RNA pol I transcripts	Scleroderma
NOR-90	Promoter of RNA pol I transcription	Scleroderma
Transfer (t) RNA synthetases	Involved in protein biosynthesis	Dermatomyositis, Polymyositis

snRNP particles, including proteins described as B', B, D and E proteins which represent core components of the snRNP particles. The autoantibody reponse in mixed connective tissue disease is also polyclonal since it can be shown that antibodies are directed against the A and C proteins of the U1-RNP particle and also against a 70 kilodalton protein. When the antibody response to individual proteins was further studied, it was demonstrated that several regions of each protein were targets of antibodies with different specificities. This complexity of the immune response is difficult to explain in the context of a hypothesis advanced by some investigators, that autoantibodies were originally stimulated by a foreign antigen and that the resultant antibodies cross-reacted with self-antigens. This is in essence the basis of the molecular mimicry hypothesis. The molecular mimicry hypothesis is untenable in the face of the demonstrated complexity of the autoimmune response, not only in SLE, but in many other systemic autoimmune diseases such as scleroderma, dermatomyositis and polymyositis. On the other hand, the polyclonality of the autoimmune response can be better understood if it is considered that the immunogen is a subcellular particle consisting of many subunits some of which are proteins and some nucleic acids, and that the subunits of the particle can be separate targets of the autoimmune response.

Autoepitopes Are Active Sites, Catalytic Centers or Functioning Regions of Immunogenic Subcellular Particles

There is increasing evidence pointing to the fact that autoantibodies are capable of inhibiting the functions of their cognate antigens. This has been demonstrated for anti-Sm and anti-U1-RNP which inhibit the splicing of precursor messenger RNA. Autoantibodies to tRNA synthetases are identified by their ability to inhibit the function of these synthetases, which charge specific tRNAs with their cognate amino acids. Autoantibody to RNA polymerase 1 from patients with scleroderma are capable of inhibiting 28S and 18S RNA synthesis when microinjected into Xenopus laevis (frog) oocytes. The special significance of these observations is that experimentally-induced antibodies produced by immunizing animals with purified an-

Table 2. Autoantibodies in Systemic Lupus Erythematosus.

Antibody Reactive with	Prevalence (%) of Antibody	Nature of Antigen
Native DNA	40	Double-strand DNA
Denatured DNA	70	Single-strand DNA
Histones	70	All Histone classes H1, H2A, H2B, H3 and H4
Sm	30	Proteins called B,D,E,F and G complexed with small nuclear RNAs (snRNA) U1,U2,U4-U6, U5
Nuclear RNP (U1 RNP)	32	Proteins called A,C and 70 kDa complexed with snRNA U1
SS-A/Ro	35	Proteins of 60 and 52 kDa complexed with RNAs called Y1, Y3,Y4 and Y5
SS-B/La	15	Phosphoprotein of 48 kDa complexed with RNA polymerase III transcripts
Ku	10	Protein doublet of 70 and 80 kDa shown to bind directly to DNA
Ribosomal (r)RNP (Ribosomal P proteins)	10	Phosphoproteins of 38,16 and 15 kDa associated with large ribosomal subunit
Ki/SL	6	Protein of 32 kDa of unknown function
PCNA (proliferating cell nuclear antigen)	3	Protein of 36 kDa which is auxiliary protein of DNA polymerase DDD

Table 3. Autoantibodies in Drug-Induced Lupus.

Antibody Reactive with	Prevalence (%) of Antibody	Nature of Antigen
Native DNA	<10	Double-strand DNA
Denatured DNA	80	Single-strand DNA
Histones	>95	Individual Histone H1, H2A, H2B, H3,H4 IgG antibody to H2A-H2B complex is strongly associated with clinically active disease
Other nuclear antigens	<10	Refer to Tables 1, 5 and 6

tigens were incapable of inhibiting the known function of the immunizing antigen. Experimentally-induced antibodies, although just as immunologically reactive with the immunizing antigen, recognized epitopes which were not the functional sites of the antigen.

The facts that many autoantibodies inhibit function and are likely to be reactive with determinants which are active sites of these antigens further suggest that activated subcellular particles might be implicated in the immunogenic stimulus. An important focus of

Table 4. Autoantibodies in Mixed Connective Tissue Disease.

Antibody Reactive with	Prevalence (%) of Antibody	Nature of Antigen
Native DNA	<10	Double-strand DNA
Denatured DNA	<10	Single-strand DNA
Histones	<10	All Histone classes
Sm	<10	Refer to Table 1
Nuclear RNP	>95	Proteins called A, C and 70 kDa complexed with snRNA U1
Other nuclear antigens	<10	Refer to Tables 1, 5 and 6

further research in this area would be to elucidate mechanisms which might be activating certain subcellular particles in an aberrant fashion or in a manner which is discordant with the normal function of the cell. Of great interest have been recent studies which showed that chemicals such as mercuric chloride injected into certain strains of mice can induce an autoantibody response to a nucleolar antigen called fibrillarin. Autoantibodies to fibrillarin are detected in some patients with scleroderma (see Table 5).

The known functions of certain intracellular autoantigens are described in Table 1. Sm and U1-RNP, which are targets of autoantibodies in patients with SLE are components of intranuclear subcellular particles which are engaged in the important cellular function of splicing of precursor messenger RNA. Autoantibodies from patients with lupus have been used to

Table 5. Autoantibodies in Scleroderma.

Antibodies Reactive with	Prevalence (%) of Antibody	Nature of Antigen
Scl-70	40-70% in diffuse scleroderma	100 kDa topoisomerase I. Degradation product of 70 kDa (Scl-70) is a major antigenic fragment
Centromere/ kinetochore	80% in CREST	Proteins of 17,80 and 140 kDa at centromeric regions of chromosomes
RNA polymerase I	4%	Multiple proteins of 210 to 11 kDa which are subunits of RNA pol I
PM-Scl	3%	Multiple proteins of 110 to 20 kDa which are subunits of particle of unknown function
Fibrillarin	8%	34 kDa protein-a component of U3 ribonucleoprotein
To/Th	Rare	40 kDa protein complexed with 7-2 and 8-2 RNA
NOR-90	Rare	Protein doublet of 90 kDa associated with nucleolus organizer region (NOR)
Mitochondrial 70 kDa	8%	70 kDa protein of adenosineII tri-phosphatase complex

Table 6. Autoantibodies in Sjogren's Syndrome.

Antibody Reactive with	Prevalence (%) of Antibody	Nature of Antigen
Native DNA	<10	Double-strand DNA
Denatured DNA	<10	Single-strand DNA
Histones	<10	All Histone Classes
SS-A/Ro	70-80	60 and 52 kDa without anti 60 kDa limited to Sjogren's syndrome
SS-B/La	60-70	Phosphoprotein of 48 kDa com-plexed with RNA polymerase III transcripts
Other nuclear antigens	<10	Refer to Tables 1, 5 and 6

Table 7. Autoantibodies in Dermatomyositis and Polymyositis.

Antibodies Reactive with	Prevalence of Antibody	(%) Nature of antigen
Jo-1	25	Protein of 55/60 kDa – histidyl tRNA synthetase
PL-7	4	Protein of 80 kDa – threonyl tRNA synthetase
PL-12	Rare	Protein of 110 kDa – alanyl tRNA synthetase
Mi-2	5	Proteins 53 and 61 kDa of unknown function
SRP (signal recognition par-ticle	Rare	Protein of 54 kDa complexed with 7SL RNA
PM-Scl	8	See Table 5

Note absence of detectable antibodies to DNA, Histones and other antigens associated with lupus and scleroderma.

demonstrate inhibition of this function in an *in vitro* system. Inhibitory activities of autoantibodies have been demonstrated for the majority of the antigens described in Table 1. In addition to splicing, these antigens are involved in RNA processing, protein biosynthesis, DNA replication and repair and in transcription of ribosomal genes.

Autoantibody Profiles in Autoimmune Diseases

In this section, the autoantibodies present in different systemic autoimmune diseases are presented in Tables 2 to 7. These tables are intended to be a practical reference guide for the clinician seeking to interpret the significance of a particular autoantibody and also provides some essential information concerning the molecular nature and function of the antigens. The diseases represented include lupus, drug-induced lupus, mixed connective tissue disease, scleroderma, Sjogren's syndrome, dermatomyositis and polymyositis.

For detailed information on antigen-antibody systems, see the references provided.

References

1. Tan, E.M. 1989. Antinuclear antibodies: Diagnostic markers for autoimmune diseases and probes for cell biology. Adv. Immunol. 44:93.

2. Waga, S., Tan, E.M., and Rubin, R.L. 1987. Identification and isolation of soluble histones from bovine milk and serum. Biochemical J. 244:676.
3. Tan, E.M., Chan, E.K.L., Sullivan, K.F., and Rubin, R.L. 1988. Antinuclear antibodies (ANAs): Diagnostically specific immune markers and clues towards the understanding of systemic autoimmunity. Clin. Immunol. Immunopathol. 47:121.
4. Hargraves, M.M., Richmond, H., and Morton, R. 1948. Presentation of two bone marrow elements: The "tart" cell and the "L.E." cell. Mayo Clinic Proc. 27:25.
5. Tan, E.M., Carr, R.I., Schur, P.H., and Kunkel, H.G. 1966. DNA and antibody to DNA in the serum of patients with systemic lupus erythematosus. J. Clin. Invest. 45:1732.
6. Tan, E.M., and Kunkel, H.G. 1966. Characteristics of a soluble nuclear antigen precipitating with sera from patients with systemic lupus erythematosus. J. Immunol. 96:464.
7. Lerner, M.R., and Steitz, J.A. 1979. Antibodies to small nuclear RNAs complexed with proteins are produced by patients with systemic lupus erythematosus. Proc. Natl. Acad. Sci. USA 76:5495.
8. Conner, G.E., Nelson, D., Wiesniewolski, R., Lahita, R.G., Blobel, G., and Kunkel, H.G. 1982. Protein antigens of the RNA-protein complexes detected by anti-Sm and anti-RNP antibodies found in serum of patients with systemic lupus erythematosus and related disorders. J. Exp. Med. 156:1475.
9. Busch, H., Reddy, R., Rothblum, L., and Choy, Y.C. 1982. SnRNAs, SnRNPs and RNA processing. Annu. Rev. Biochem. 51:617..
10. Mattioli, M., and Reichlin, M. 1971. Characterization of a soluble nuclear ribonucleoprotein antigen reactive with SLE sera. J. Immunol. 107:1281.
11. Northway, J.D., and Tan, E.M. 1972. Differentiation of antinuclear antibodies giving speckled staining patterns in immunofluorescence. Clin. Immunol. Immunopathol. 1:140.
12. Ben-Chetrit, E., Chan, E.K.L., Sullivan, K.F., and Tan, E.M. 1988. A 52 kD protein is a novel component of the SS-A/Ro antigenic particle. J. Exp. Med. 167:1560.
13. Gottlieb, E., and Steitz, J.A. 1989. Function of the mammalian La protein: Evidence for its action in transcription termination by RNA polymerase III. EMBO J. 8:851.
14. Ben-Chetrit, E, Fox, R.I., and Tan, E.M. 1990. Dissociation of immune responses to the SS-A/Ro 52 kD and 60 kD polypeptides in systemic lupus erythematosus and Sjogren's syndrome. Arthr. Rheum. 33:349.
15. Reeves, W.H. 1985. Use of monoclonal antibodies for the characterization of novel DNA-binding proteins recognized by human autoimmune sera. J. Exp. Med. 161:18..
16. Mimori, T., and Hardin, J.A. 1986. Mechanisms of interaction between Ku protein and DNA. J. Biol. Chem. 261:10375.
17. Francoeur, A.M., Peebles, C.L., Heckman, K.J., Lee, J.C., and Tan, E.M. 1985. Identification of ribosomal protein autoantigens. J. Immunol. 135:2378.
18. Elkon, K.B., Parnassa, A.P., and Foster, C.L. 1985. Lupus autoantibodies target ribosomal P proteins. J. Exp. Med. 162:459.
19. Bonfa, E., Golombek, S.J., Kaufman, L.D., Skelly, S., Weissbach, H., Brot, N., and Elkon, K.B. 1987. Association between lupus psychosis and anti- ribosomal P protein antibodies. N. Eng. J. Med. 317:265.
20. Tan, E.M., Cohen, A.S., Fries, J.M., et al. 1982. The 1982 revised criteria for the classification of systemic lupus erythematosus. Arthr. Rheum. 25:1271.
21. Fritzler, M.J., and Tan, E.M. 1978. Antibodies to histones in drug-induced idiopathic lupus erythematosus. J. Clin. Invest. 62:560.
22. Totoritis, M.C., Tan, E.M., McNally, E.M., and Rubin, R.L. 1988. Association of antibody to histone complex H2A-H2B with symptomatic procainamide-induced lupus. N. Eng. J. Med. 318:1431.
23. Sharp, G.C., Irwin, W., Tan, E.M., Gould, G., and Holman, H.R. 1972. Mixed connective tissue disease: An apparently distinct rheumatic disease syndrome associated with a specific antibody to an extractable nuclear antigen (ENA). Amer. J. Med. 52:148.
24. Kasukawa, R. 1987. Preliminary diagnostic criteria for classification of mixed connective tissue disease. In: Mixed connective tissue disease and antinuclear antibodies. R. Kasukawa and G.C. Sharp, eds. Amsterdam: Excerpta Medica, p. 41.
25. Douvas, A.S., Achten, M., and Tan, E.M. 1979. Identification of a nuclear protein (Scl-70) as a unique target of human antinuclear antibodies in scleroderma. J. Biol. Chem. 254:10514.
26. Guldner, H.H., Szostecki, C., Vosberg, H.P., Lakomek, H.J., Penner, E., and Bautz, F.A. 1986. Scl-70 autoantibodies from scleroderma patients recognize a 95 kD protein identified as DNA topoisomerase 1. Chromosoma 94:132.
27. Shero, J.H., Bordwell, B., Rothfield, N.F., and Earnshaw, W.C. 1986. Autoantibodies to to-

mark of acute rheumatic attacks previously recognized for 300 years appeared also to be related to molecular mimicry mechanisms with the demonstration that sera from children with acute chorea contained antibodies capable of reacting with antigens present within caudate or subthalamic nuclear cytoplasmic antigens in the very regions of the central nervous system presumably involved in generating the characteristic movement disorder itself (7). An example of anti-neuronal antibody present within the serum of a child affected with Sydenham's rheumatic chorea is shown in Figure 1. The element of molecular mimicry in this instance was convincingly demonstrated by abolition of anti-neuronal antibody staining of neuronal cytoplasm after absorption of rheumatic patients' sera with highly purified preparations of Group A streptococcal membranes but not by control membranes taken from other Group D streptococcal organisms (7).

More recently the molecular mimicry hypothesis for acute rheumatic fever has been extended even more with the demonstration by Baird et al. (13) of cross reacting epitopes involving a limited sequential region of M-proteins M1, M5 and M18 and antigens shared by chondrocytes, cartilage and synovium. This work demonstrated the presence of M-protein-specific, joint cross-reactive antibodies in sera from patients with acute rheumatic fever. Moreover, inhibition of positive immunofluorescence reactions was demonstrated using pepsin fragments of M-proteins. Because it appears likely that part of the pathogenesis of the acute arthritis noted in association with acute rheumatic fever may be secondary to deposition of cross-reactive anti-synovial and cartilage antibodies and activation of the complement system, these same workers demonstrated that M-protein-specific human antibodies from patients with acute rheumatic fever actually activated complement *in vitro* and released measurable C5a (13). These observations would support a direct cross-reactive mechanism between autologous anti-M-protein antibodies and self constituents of synovium, cartilage and possibly other joint structures as a basic mechanism in the production of the arthritis during an acute episode of rheumatic

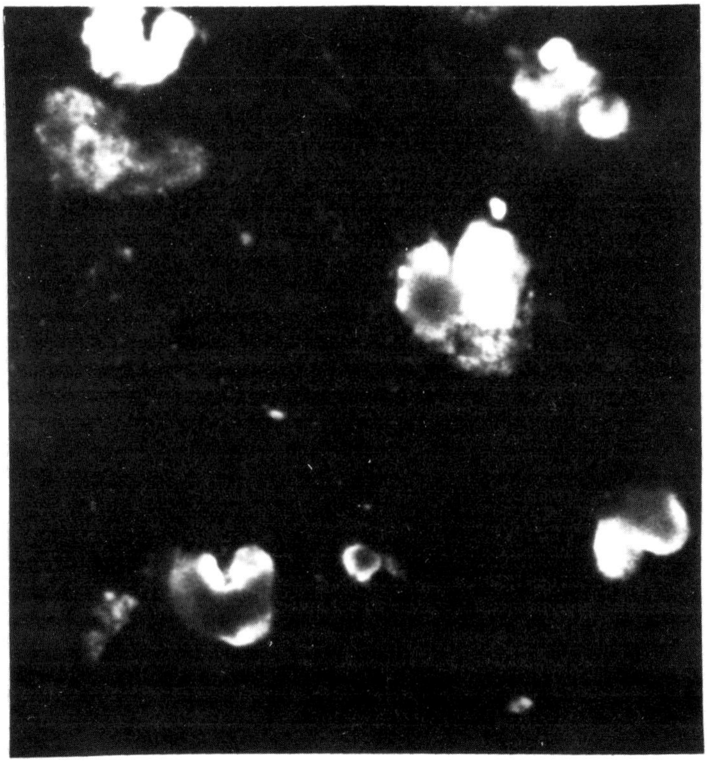

Figure 1. Example of anti-neuronal antibody from serum of child with Sydenham's chorea staining cytoplasmic constituents of human caudate nucleus neurons. Central dark area of neuron cells represents nuclei. The positive neuronal cytoplasmic staining was completely eliminated by absorption of patient serum with Group A streptococcal membranes.

fever. Supporting the direct complement activating hypothesis in such patients are the previous much older observations of complement profiles within rheumatic fever synovial fluid suggestive of direct conventional and alternative pathway activation (16).

Clearly there is considerable evidence for a number of humoral mechanisms of molecular mimicry between the Group A streptococcus and many human tissues affected in acute rheumatic fever. Additional evidence for similar mechanisms of cell-mediated immune reactions being instrumental in both the acute as well as the chronic lesions of rheumatic heart disease has also been reported as well. A number of observations using material from both acute and chronic rheumatic fever patients have supported similar cross-reacting epitopes between the streptococcus and human tissues as being involved in T cell-mediated immune reactions in acute rheumatic fever and chronic rheumatic heart disease (17,18).

Molecular Mimicry and Spondyloarthropathy

Another major area of human medicine in which molecular mimicry has been implicated is that of ankylosing spondylitis and the reactive arthritides such as Reiter's syndrome. After the original reports in 1973 of association of HLA-B27 antigen and ankylosing spondylitis (AS) by Brewerton et al. (19) and Schlosstein and coworkers (20), many clinical, epidemiologic and immunochemical studies have been directed at what this striking correlation between one of the HLA Class I molecules and spondyloarthropathies really means. A number of hypotheses have been advanced which might explain this association. One theory which initially gained a great deal of attention centered around what was called the Geczy phenomenon, based on reports that HLA B27 molecules or other determinants genetically associated with HLA B27 might function as cell surface receptors for bacterial components (21,22). This hypothesis postulated that after HLA B27 receptors were modified by bacterial components, they could then themselves become targets for autologous host antibodies against bacteria and eventually translate into a disease state (22). Other investigators have encountered difficulty in reproducing the Geczy phenomenon (23), despite confirmation by van Rood and coworkers (24).

More recently direct cross-reactivity between bacterial components and HLA B27 antigens has been identified using both rabbit antisera (25) and monoclonal antibodies (26,27). The report by Schwimmbeck et al. (28) provided direct evidence that primary amino acid sequences encompassing the hexamer QTDRED showed exact homology at positions 72-77 in HLA B27.1 and residues 188-193 in the enzyme *Klebsiella* nitrogenase. In this paper, elevations of antibodies reacting with both the peptide from HLA B27.1 as well as the Klebsiella peptide were noted in HLA B27(+) patients with AS as well as those with reactive arthritis and Reiter's syndrome. Our own studies of similar patients confirmed elevations of antibodies to the B27.1 peptide AKAQTDREDLRTLLRY in 23% of 60 male Norwegian patients with AS but not among Norwegian controls (29). All patients showing anti-B27.1 antibody were B27 positive; however, anti-*Klebsiella* peptide CNSRQTDREDELI antibody was neither significantly elevated nor correlated with anti-B27.1 antibody in the AS patients studied.

An attempt was made to examine HLA B27.1 and *Klebsiella* nitrogenase cross reactive epitopes within synovial tissues of patients with AS or reactive arthritis using immunoperoxidase staining and both anti-B27.1 and anti-*Klebsiella* peptide antisera (30). Definite cross-reacting epitopes were identified within synovial lining cells, vascular endothelium and infiltrative synovial inflammatory cells. These observations appeared to support a molecular mimicry mechanism since inflamed synovial tissues clinically affected by the disease showed strong levels of cross-reacting antigenic epitopes.

Additional studies of autoantibodies possibly representing similar molecular mimicry were completed in 160 spondyloarthropathy patients using serum antibody to a peptide representing the putative gene product of plasmid pHS-2 isolated from arthritogenic *Shigella flexneri* strains (31). Antibody levels to B27 and the pHS-2 peptide were significantly correlated ($p<0.001$) in 134 B27(+) patients. Leucine appeared to represent a critical residue in the actual epitope responsible for this cross reaction.

Further fascinating data relevant to the HLA B27-AS and spondyloarthropathy association have also recently been reported by Hammer et al. (32) in studies of rats transfected with the human HLA B27 gene. The transfected animals which expressed high levels of the transferred gene product developed a disease characterized by many of the histologic and pathologic features of a spondyloarthropathy. Our own studies of serum samples from these same rats (kindly provided by Dr. Taurog) have indicated that a small proportion of the transfected animals show serum antibody reacting with HLA B27 peptide; however, of great interest was that the presence of serum antibody in these B27-transfected rats did *not* appear to correlate directly with their development of clinical disease. These latter observations suggest that presence of a major degree of expression of the HLA B27 gene product rather than merely generation of antibody to B27 epitopes may be one of the most fundamental pathologic processes responsible for AS and the spondyloarthropathies.

Other Examples of Possible Molecular Mimicry

Several other examples of molecular mimicry possibly initiating autoimmune human diseases of unknown etiology are found in the case of myasthenia gravis (MG) (33) and with respect to various heat shock proteins, mycobacterial antigens and diseases such as RA (34,35). A large proportion of patients with MG show antibody to components of the acetylcholine receptor (AchR). Schwimmbeck et al. (33) employed synthetic peptides to identifiy antibodies in MG sera reacting with the AchR α-subunit residues 160-167. This subunit demonstrated specific immunological cross-reaction with a shared homologous region on herpes simplex virus glycoprotein D, residues 286-293, using both direct binding and inhibition studies. These observations suggested that herpes simplex virus might be associated with activation of the disease itself in some instances.

In the case of heat shock proteins, molecular mimicry between certain mycobacterial proteins and cartilage proteoglycans has been emphasized by Cohen (34). In Lewis rats, cross reactivity appears to evolve into a T-cell dependent autoimmune disorder in many ways simulating the histologic picture and chronicity of RA (35). In the case of various heat shock proteins, the complete significance of such components on autoimmunity and the immune system still continues to evolve. In some respects many similar components could also act somehow as superantigens and possibly by-pass conventional mechanisms of T and B cell activation.

Much remains to be learned concerning whether basic mechanisms of molecular mimicry can by themselves actually induce autoimmune or various connective tissue disease. How reactivity to an external antigen such as the β-hemolytic streptococcus or pHS-2 Shigella-related peptide can eventually evade normal mechanisms of tolerance and by so doing induce human disease now still remains to be determined.

References

1. Oldstone, M.B.A. 1987. Molecular mimicry and autoimmune disease. Cell 50:819.
2. Oldstone, M.B.A., and Notkins, A.L. 1986. In: Concepts in viral of pathogenesis (Vol. 2). A.L. Notkins, and M.B.A. Oldstone, eds. Berlin and New York: Springer.
3. Zabriskie, J.B., and Freimer, E.H. 1966. An immunological relationship between the group A streptococcus and mammalian muscle. J. Exp. Med. 124:661.
4. Van de Rijn, I., Zabriskie, J.B., and McCarty, M. 1977. Group A streptococcal antigens. Cross reactivity with myocardium, purification of heart-reactive-antibody and isolation and characterization of streptococcal antigen. J. Exp. Med. 146:579.
5. Kaplan, M.H. 1963. Immunologic relation of streptococcal and tissue antigens. I. Properties of antigen in certain strains of group A streptococci exhibiting an immunologic cross-reaction with human heart tissue. J. Immunol. 90:595.
6. Goldstein, I., Halpern, B. and Robert, L. 1967. Immunological relationship between streptococcus A polysaccharide and the structural glycoproteins of the heart valves. Nature 213:44.

7. Husby, G., van de Rign, I., Zabriskie, J.B., Abdin, Z.H., and Williams, R.C., Jr. 1976. Antibodies reacting with cytoplasm of subthalamic and caudate nuclei neurons in chorea and acute rheumatic fever. J. Exp. Med. 144:1094.

8. Kasp-Groschowska, E., and Kingston, D. 1977. Streptococcal cross-reacting antigen and the bundle of His. Clin. Exp. Immunol. 27:43.

9. Dale, J.B., and Beachey, E.H. 1982. Protective antigenic determinant of streptococcal M protein shared with sarcolemmal membrane protein of human heart. J. Exp. Med. 156:1165.

10. Kraus, W., Dale, J.B., and Beachey, E.H. 1990. Identification of an epitope of type 1 streptococcal M protein that is shared with a 43-KDa protein of human myocardium and renal glomeruli. J. Immunol. 145:4089.

11. Dudding, B.A., and Ayoub, E.M. 1968. Persistence of streptococcal group A antibody in patients with rheumatic valvular disease. J. Exp. Med. 128:1081.

12. Krisher, K., and Cunningham, M.W. 1985. Myosin: A link between streptococci and heart. Science 227:413.

13. Baird, R.W., Bronze, M.S., Kraus, W., Hill, H.R., Veasey, L.G., and Dale, J.B.. 1991. Epitopes of group A streptococcal M protein shared with antigens of articular cartilage and synovium. J. Immunol. 146:3132.

14. Zabriskie, J.B., Hsu, K.C., and Seegal, B.C. 1970. Heart-reactive antibody associated with rheumatic fever: Characterization and diagnostic significance. Clin. Exp. Immunol. 7:147.

15. Ayoub, E.M., Taranta, A., and Bartley, T.D. 1974. Effect of valvular surgery on antibody to the group A streptococcal carbohydrate. Circulation 50:144.

16. Svartman, M., Potter, E.V., Poon-King, T., and Earle, D.P. 1975. Immunoglobulins and complement components in synovial fluid of patients with acute rheumatic fever. J. Clin. Invest. 56:111.

17. Gowrishankar, R., and Agarwal, S.C. 1980. Leucocyte migration inhibition with human heart valve glycoproteins and group A streptococcal ribonucleic acid proteins in rheumatic heart disease and post-streptococcal glomerulonephritis. Clin. Exp. Immunol. 39:519.

18. Gray, E.D., Wannamaker, L.W., Ayoub, E.M., El Kholy, A., and Abdin, Z.H. 1981. Cellular immune responses to extracellular streptococcal products in rheumatic heart disease. J. Clin. Invest. 68:665.

19. Brewerton, D.A., Caffrey, M., Hart, F.D., James, D.C.D., Nicholls, A., and Sturrock, R.D. 1973. Ankylosing spondylitis and HL-A27. Lancet 1:904.

20. Schlosstein, L., Terasaki, P.I., Bluestone, R., and Pearson, C.M. 1973. High association of an HL-A antigen, W27, with ankylosing spondylitis. N. Engl. J. Med. 288:704.

21. Seager, K., Bashir, H.V., Geczy, A.F., Edmonds, J., and De Vere-Tyndall, A. 1979. Evidence for a specific B27-associated cell surface marker on lymphocytes of patients with ankylosing spondylitis. Nature 277:68.

22. Geczy, A.F., Alexander, K., Bashir, H.V., Edmonds, J.P., Upfold, L., and Sullivan, J. 1983. HLA-B27, Klebsiella, and ankylosing spondylitis: Biological and chemical studies. Immunol. Rev. 70:23.

23. Cameron, F.H., Russel, P.J., Easter, J.F., Wakefield, D., and March, L. 1987. Failure of *Klebsiella pneumoniae* antibodies to cross-react with peripheral blood mononuclear cells from patients with ankylosing spondylitis. Arthritis Rheum. 30:300.

24. Van Rood, J.J., van Leeuwen, A., Ivanyi, P., Cats, A., Breur- Vriesandorp, B.S., Dekker-Saeys, A.J., Kijistra, A., and van Kregten, E. 1985. Blind confirmation of Geczy factor in ankylosing spondylitis. Lancet 2:943.

25. Welsh, J., Avakian, H., Cowling, P., Ehringer, A., Wooley, P., Panayo, G., and Ebringer, R. 1980. Ankylosing spondylitis, HLA-B27 and *Klebsiella*. I. Cross-reactivity studies with rabbit antisera. Br. J. Exp. Pathol. 61:85.

26. Chen, J.H., Kono, D., Yong, Z., Park, M.S., Oldstone, M.B.A., and Yu, D.T.Y. 1987. A *Yersinia pseudotuberculosis* protein which cross-reacts with HLA-B27. J. Immunol. 139:3003.

27. Raybourne, R.B., Bunning, V.K., and Williams, K.M. 1988. Reaction of anti-HLA-B monoclonal antibodies with envelope proteins of *Shigella* species. Evidence for molecular mimicry in the spondyloarthropathies. J. Immunol. 140:3489.

28. Schwimmbeck, P.L., Yu, D.T.Y., and Oldstone, M.G.A. 1987. Autoantibodies to HLA-B27 in the sera of HLA-B27 patients with ankylosing spondylitis and Reiter's syndrome. Molecular mimicry with *Klebsiella pneumoniae* as potential mechanism of autoimmune disease. J. Exp. Med. 166:173.

29. Tsuchiya, N., Husby, G., and Williams, R.C. Jr. 1989. Studies of humoral and cell-mediated immunity to peptides shared by HLA-27.1 and

Klebsiella pneumoniae nitrogenase in ankylosing spondylitis. Clin. Exp. Immunol. 76:354.
30. Husby, G., Tsuchiya, N., Schwimmbeck, P.L., Keat, A., Pahle, J.A., Oldstone, M.B.A., and Williams, R.C., Jr. 1989. Cross-reactive epitope with Klebsiella pneumoniae nitrogenase in articular tissue of HLA-27+ patients with ankylosing spondylitis. Arth. & Rheum. 32:437.
31. Tsuchiya, N., Husby, G., Williams, R.C., Jr., Stieglitz, H., Lipsky, P.E., and Inman, R.D. 1990. Autoantibodies to the HLA-B27 sequence cross-react with the hypothetical peptide from the arthritis-associated Shigella plasmid. J. Clin. Invest. 86:1193.
32. Hammer, R.E., Maika, S.D., Richardson, J.A., Tang, J.P., and Taurog, J.D. 1990. Spontaneous inflammatory disease in transgenic rats expression HLA-B27 and human β_2M: An animal model of HLA-B27-associated human disorders. Cell 63:1099.
33. Schwimmbeck, P.L., Dyrberg, T., Drachman, D.B., and Oldstone, M.B.A. 1989. Molecular mimicry and myasthenia gravis: An autoantigenic site of the acetylcholine receptor α-subunit that has biologic activity and reacts immunochemically with herpes simplex virus. J. Clin. Invest. 84:1174.
34. Cohen, I.R.. 1988. The self, the world and autoimmunity. Sci. Am. 258:34.
35. Van Eden, W., Holochitz, J., Nevo, Z., Frenkel, A., Klajman, A., and Cohen, I.R. 1985. Arthritis induced by a T-lymphocyte clone that responds to *Mycobacterium tuberculosis* and to cartilage proteoglycans. Proc. Natl. Acad. Sci. USA 82:5117.

F(ab′)2 Preparations from RA Patients Bind to IgG-Free Staphylococcal Protein A

Tohru Abe, Osamu Hosono, Jun Koide, Hiromi Sekine, Tsutomu Takeuchi*

Binding of $F(ab')_2$ preparations from patients with RA to IgG-free Staphylococcal protein A was examined on ELISA. Five of 16 RA patients showed significant binding to IgG-free Staphylococcal protein A. The protain A binding was further confirmed by immunoblotting. The $F(ab')_2$ preparations of high protein A-binding activity from RA patients gave a specific reaction with IgG-free protein A on nitrocellulose paper. These results indicate the presence of anti-protein A antibodies in patients with RA. Those RA patients with anti-protein A antibodies were more active cases as judged by the Lansbury's activity index. RA patients with anti-protein A antibodies had significantly higher levels of serum rheumatoid factor (RAHA).

Rheumatoid arthritis (RA) is a chronic destructive arthritis characterized by persistent inflammation of the synovium. Such inflammation results from immune-mediated mechanism involving rheumatoid factor (RF) (1). Thus, RF has an important role in the pathogenesis of RA. Since RF is also present in low titer in healthy individuals, RF has an important physiological role in the immune response (2). We have been working on RF for the past few years and have hypothesized that RF arises as anti-idiotypic antibodies against anti-protein A antibodies, and perturbation of the idiotypic network with microbial pathogens bearing the idiotype results in the modulation of RF production (3,4). In this study, we examined anti-protein A antibodies in sera from five of 16 RA patients by ELISA and immunoblotting.

Materials and Methods

Patients

Sixteen patients with RA were studied. There were 13 females and three males, with a mean age of 51 years. The diagnosis of RA was made according to the 1987 revision of diagnostic criteria for RA (5). All of the RA patients were sero-positive and were receiving a non-steroidal anti-inflammatory drug (NSAID). None had received an immuno-suppressant.

Purification of IgG, IgG Fragment, Protein A and Chicken Anti-SPA

These were performed by affinity-chromatography. IgG contamination of protein A was determined by RIA.

Preparation of Patients' IgG and IgG Fragments

IgG was isolated by DE-52 ion-exchange chromatography. The $F(ab')_2$ and pFc of IgG were prepared by pepsin digestion and Fc by papain digestion.

Binding of the $F(ab')_2$ Preparations from RA Patients to Protein A

ELISA was used to estimate binding.

SDS Slabgelelectrophoresis and Western Immunoblot Analysis

For protein analysis, SDS-PAGE was used according to the method of Laemelli (6) and the reactivity of protein A with $F(ab')_2$ preparations was analyzed using an immunoblot method (7).

* The Second Department of Internal Medicine, Saitama Medical Center, Saitama Medical School, Saitama Japan.
Acknowledgements: This study was supported in part by a research grant from the Intractable Disease Division, Public Health Bureau, Ministry of Health & Welfare.

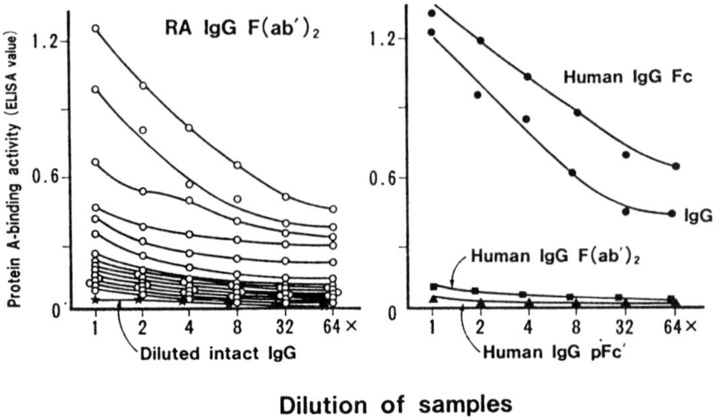

Figure 1. The protein A binding activity of the $F(ab')_2$ preparations of IgG from RA patients. The binding activity of the $F(ab')_2$ preparations to protein A was examined by ELISA by coating wells with IgG-free protein A (O) IgG $F(ab')_2$ (100 μg/ml) from patients with RA; (●) intact IgG (5000× of 100 μg/ml) diluted to give the same activity as the $F(ab')_2$ preparations in the anti-Fc coated plates in Fig. 1; (▲) pFc′.

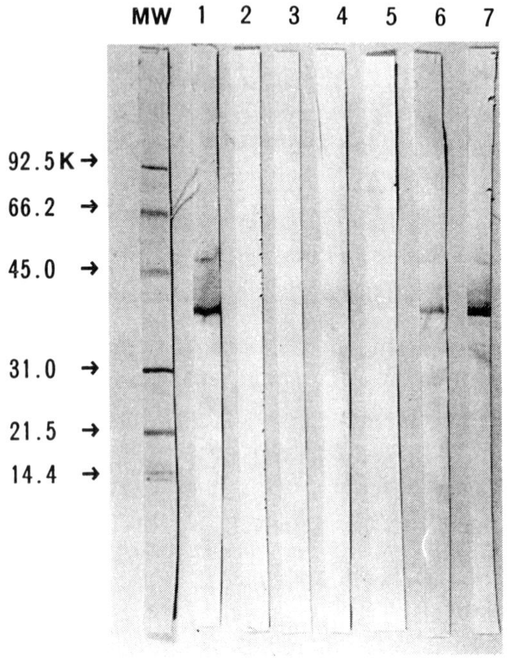

Figure 2. Western immunoblot analysis of anti-protein A antibodies. After the electrophoresis of protein A and its transfer to nitrocellulose paper, the paper was reacted with the indicated samples and developed with BCIP. MW, molecular weight stardard. Lane 1, intact IgG as a positive control; Lane 2, pFc′ fragment from human IgG; Lane 3, $F(ab')_2$ preparation from human IgG; Lanes 4 and 5, $F(ab')_2$ preparation from two RA patients without protein A binding activity as determined by ELISA; Lanes 6 and 7, $F(ab')_2$ preparations from two RA patients with high protein A-binding activity as determined by ELISA.

Results

Detection of Protein A Binding Activity to the $F(ab')_2$ Preparations of IgG from RA Patients by ELISA

Protein A binding activity was determined by ELISA. The $F(ab')_2$ preparations were conclusively proved not to be contaminated by Fc, intact IgG molecules or RF activity. As shown in Fig. 1, some $F(ab')_2$ preparations of IgG from RA patients showed significantly higher binding activity to protein A. The results indicate that some RA patients have anti-protein A antibody in their sera.

Demonstration of Anti-Protein A Antibody by Immunoblotting

To rule out the possibility of non-specific binding in ELISA, the presence of anti-protein A antibody was further investigated by Western immunoblot analysis. As shown in Fig. 2, using intact IgG as positive control (lane 1) resulted in two major bands between 40 and 50 KDa, corresponding to the molecular size of protein A. pFc′ fragments (lane 2) and $F(ab')_2$ preparations from human IgG (lane 3), and two RA patients without protein-A binding activity on ELISA, failed to react with protein A (lane 4 and 5). In contrast, the $F(ab')_2$ preparations from two RA patients with high protein A-binding activity on ELISA (lane 6 and 7) reacted with protein A on nitrocellulose paper. The results confirmed the presence of anti-protein A antibody.

Exclusion of Binding of the F(ab′)2 Preparations to Protein A via the Alternative Binding Sites

Protein A interacts with immunoglobulins via two non-immune mechanisms. The alternative binding is F(ab′)2-mediated. Accordingly, it is necessary to exclude binding of F(ab′)2 preparations via the alternative binding site. As shown in Fig. 3, five of 16 preparations showed significant binding to protein A (open bar). To exclude binding of the F(ab′)2 preparations via the non-immune alternative binding site, the antigenic site for anti-protein A antibody on protein A was blocked by chicken anti-SPA and then the binding of the F(ab′)2 preparations was determined. Two samples (nos. 4 and 11) showed binding to chicken anti-SPA-blocked protein A. However, the binding of the five preparations (nos. 1–5) to chicken anti-SPA-blocked protein A was not considered to be significant. This indicates that the binding was not via the alternative binding site.

Comparison of the Characteristics of 16 RA Patients with or without Anti-Protein A Antibody

As shown in Table 1, RA patients with anti-protein A antibody had more active disease. The serum level of RF was significantly higher in patients with anti-protein A antibody than in those without anti-protein A antibody.

Discussion

In this study, we showed the presence of anti-protein A antibody in sera from five of 16 (31.3%) RA patients using a sensitive ELISA. Because these findings are based on immunological interaction by sensitive ELISA, care was taken to detect trace contamination or non-specific interactions. In particular, it was essential to prove the absence of intact IgG molecules and/or Fc fragments in the F(ab′)2 preparations from RA patients. In addition, IgG contamination of commercial protein A was assiduously avoided in these experiments. In our study, IgG pFc′ did not bind to protein A. SPA binds to sites at the Cr2–Cr3 interface region, as does monoclonal IgG RF. But IgG pFc′is a Cr3 domain dimer equivalent to the c-terminal half of Fc. These facts were considered to explain why IgG pFc′ did not react with protein A. It is known that protein A has a weaker non-immune alternative binding site to F(ab′)2 outside the antigenic site for anti-protein A antibody. Recently Sasso et al. reported that specificity of the protein A alternative binding site is highly restricted to VH III-bearing molecules (8,9). We had to exclude binding of the F(ab′)2 preparations to protein A via the alternative binding site. Since the present result is not a direct demonstration, the specificity of the protein A binding sites should be examined in future studies. The significance of positive anti-protein A antibody in more active RA patients remains unsolved and needs further clarification. Our study included sero-positive RA patients only. No statement can, therefore, be made regarding anti-protein A antibody in sero-negative RA patients and in other kinds of inflammatory arthritis. In this respect, studies of sero-negative RA patients will be of great interest. Furthermore, studies on the serial determination of anti-protein A antibody are in progress. Such studies will certainly disclose the inciting stimuli and mechanism of RF production. To the

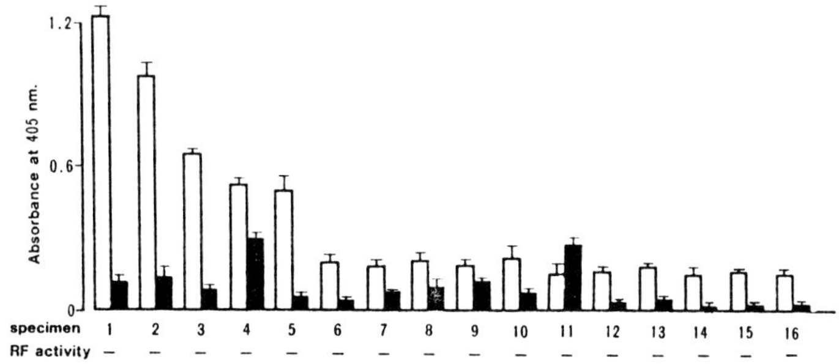

Figure 3. Binding of the F(ab′)2 preparations from patients with RA to IgG-free protein A-coated Immulon titre plates (open bar), and to plates in which the antigenic site for anti-protein A antibodies was blocked by chicken anti-SPA before the binding of the F(ab′)2 preparations was determined (closed bar). Error bars indicate absorbance at 405 nm of duplicate wells.

Impact of Biotechnology on Allergy Research: Can Structural and Functional Studies on Components of the Immunoglobulin (Ig)E Receptor/Effector System Assist the Design of Rational IgE Antagonists?

Birgit A. Helm*, Yan Ling*, Nicholas Rhodes*, Eduardo A. Padlan**

In order to inhibit the clinical manifestations characteristic of immediate and delayed hypersensitivity, the prevention of mediator release from mast cells and basophils is highly desirable. Strategies that block the initial binding of IgE to its high affinity receptor present on these cells are explored. This approach appears preferable to the interference with the triggering mechanism since IgE-mediated target cell activation shares common pathways of signal transmission with other important cell-surface receptors. In order to identify the sites in IgE which bind to the receptors, a family of overlapping IgE-derived peptides was synthesized by recombinant DNA technology and peptide chemistry. All truncated peptides which are smaller than the Fc fragment prepared by papain digestion have a lower affinity for the receptors and are therefore unsuitable as inhibitors of the allergic response. We propose that development of potential IgE antagonists may benefit from a detailed understanding of the structural requirements and the identification of the amino acid residues involved in the complementary interaction of the ligand and the receptors. A strategy combining chemical screening and activity measurements with genetic engineering techniques and protein chemistry, model building and structural studies using X-ray crystallography and N. M. R. may be decisive in the eventual design of a clinically effective inhibitor of the allergic response.

The central role of immunoglobulins of the IgE isotype in immediate hypersensitivity responses has been extensively documented since their identification as the mediator of the allergic response in 1966 (1). The antibody binds via residues located in the Fc portion of the IgE molecule to high-affinity receptors (FcεR1) expressed on the surface of tissue mast cells and blood basophils and also to low-affinity receptors (FcεR2) on various inflammatory cells including monocytes, macrophages, eosinophils and platelets. Thus, although the blood levels of IgE are lower than those of any other Ig class, cell-bound IgE is extensively distributed on cells of the mucosal lining of the gut, lung, and the skin and these are the major target organs in immediate hypersensitivity reactions. The binding of multivalent antigen to the V-region of receptor occupied IgE causes the cross-linking of adjacent receptors, and cells respond with the secretion of potent mediators that cause the clinical symptoms of allergy. Available medications can partially inhibit IgE-mediated target cell exocytosis in certain populations of mast cells, while other therapeutic attempts are aimed at attenuating the physiological effects of mediator release. Unfortunately, the mode of action of most IgE antagonists is ill defined, and undesirable side-effects are common. The development of more rational inhibitors of the allergic response is clearly highly desirable since at least 20% of the human population is afflicted by some type of allergy and the incidence of the disorder is increasing world-wide.

---

* Krebs Institute for Biomolecular Research, Department of Molecular Biology and Biotechnology, University of Sheffield, Sheffield S10 2UH., U.K.;

** Laboratory of Molecular Biology, National Institute of Diabetes and Digestive and Kidney Diseases, National Institutes of Health, Bethesda, MD. 20892, USA.

Acknowledgements: This work was supported by grants from the University of Sheffield Research Stimulation Fund, the MRC (G8825490CB), the NIH, the SERC Protein Engineering LINK Programme (GR/G/53378), and the Diagnostics Products Corporation (DPC), Witney, Oxon. Y.L. is a recipient of a DPC European Research Institute Special Fellowship.

A better understanding of the "Natural History of IgE" should expedite the development of rational IgE antagonists. Over the past decade modern molecular biology has had a significant impact on allergy research culminating in the cloning and expression of several key components of the IgE receptor/effector system (reviewed in Ref. 2). Biotechnological advances made these proteins amenable to detailed analysis by combining genetic engineering techniques with protein chemistry, and structural and immunological investigations. A combined application of these techniques may help to answer the question why certain innocuous substances like cereal grains, nuts, grass pollens, or house dust mites, give rise to an IgE response in some individuals but not in others. The possibility that a variety of allergens share common epitopes is currently investigated through the synthesis of allergen by recombinant DNA techniques (3,4). The outcome of such studies may lead to the identification of a limited number of allergenic epitopes, and this in turn could facilitate the design of peptide vaccines which could be used to desensitize susceptible individuals. An improvement in our knowledge of the regulation of IgE synthesis should assist the development of strategies which will modulate or selectively inhibit the isotype specific immune response. The recent demonstration of isotype specific extra-cellular sequences on membrane-bound, but not secreted antibody, points to the potential utility of antibodies raised against these so-called "migis" peptides in the regulation of antibody secretion from IgE-bearing cells (5). Similarly, understanding the mechanism(s) by which anti-IgE auto-antibodies, observed in the serum of many allergic patients, can aggravate or attenuate IgE activity could lead to new therapeutic strategies (6).

The identification of the nature and sequence of events that trigger the IgE-mediated, allergen-induced, activation of FcεR1 may assist the design of rational inhibitors capable of preventing target cell exocytosis. Figure 1 demonstrates the central role of mast cell and basophil mediators, which are released following FcεR1 triggering, in the selective activation of inflammatory cells: Lymphokines interleukin (IL)3, IL4, IL5, IL6 and granulocyte-macrophage colony stimulating factor (GM-CSF) have been shown to be involved in IgE-regulation, mast-cell differentiation, and the regulation of FcεR2 expression. Thus, eosinophil-mediated cytotoxicity requires accessory mast cells and their mediators, while the mast-cell derived chemotactic factor of anaphylaxis (ECF-A) plays a role in the up-regulation of FcεR2 expression on eosinophils. It is interesting to note in this context that eosinophils are often found closely associated with mast cells in tissues after immediate hypersensitivity reactions. In addition, IgE-activated eosinophils generate platelet activating factor (PAF), eosinophil peroxidase, and oxygen metabolites, while macrophages secrete a variety of lysosomal enzymes, IL1, PAF, and oxygen metabolites, and the latter, in turn, can induce secretion from mast cells (reviewed in Ref. 2). The initial prevention of the FcεR1-mediated activation of target cells is therefore highly desirable and should inhibit, or at least attenuate, the recruitment, priming and activation of monocytes, macrophages, eosinophils, natural killer cells and platelets. This should reduce the clinical manifestations characteristic of both immediate and delayed hypersensitivity.

The binding of IgE to both receptors is a reversible process, it sensitizes, but does not activate target cell degranulation unless the ligand is aggregated. The early demonstration that an Fcε fragment, prepared from myeloma IgE, can inhibit the binding of allergen specific IgE to cells bearing FcεR1, raised the hope that it might be possible to block the allergic reaction with an IgE-derived peptide. Since the IgE/FcεR1 interaction is highly specific, an identification of the structural variables and the nature of the amino acid (a.a.) residues comprising the complementary binding site(s) on ligand and receptor may provide the basis for the development of blocking agents that will not only inhibit but, in order to be clinically effective, must also reverse target cell sensitisation.

Similarly, the elucidation of the mechanisms of mast cell and basophil triggering following antigen recognition may facilitate the development of agents that can specifically inhibit mediator release from these cells. For such drugs to be useful, it is essential that they selectively inhibit IgE-mediated cell activation, since the FcεR1-mediated target cell activation appears to share common pathways of signal transmission with many G protein linked cell surface receptors (7), and an interference with the action of other biologically important receptors could be associated with severe side effects.

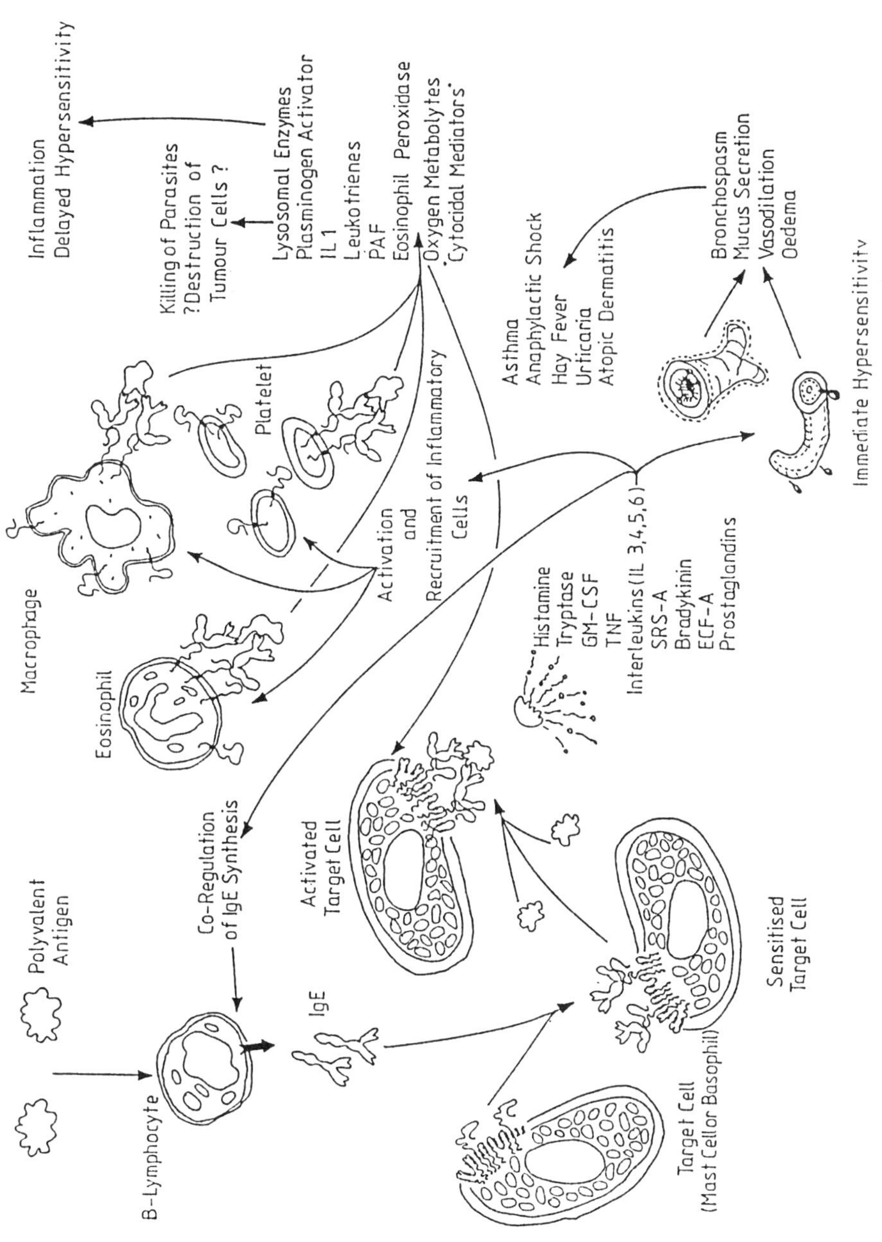

Figure 1: Consequences of IgE-mediated target cell activation in immediate and delayed hypersensitivity. IgE binds with high affinity to Fc-receptors on mast cells and basophils. The initial ligand-receptor interaction does not activate any post-receptor response. The crosslinking of receptor bound IgE by allergen initiates target cell secretion resulting in the release of pharmacologically active substances that cause the clinical manifestations associated with type 1 hypersensitivity. They also contribute to the late response through the recruitment, priming and activation of inflammatory cells, which bear and will up-regulate low-affinity IgE-receptors in response to the secretion of mast-cell mediators. Similarly, activated inflammatory cells will secrete mediators that can induce secretion of mast cell mediators. A prevention of the initial IgE-mediated mast cell triggering event is therefore highly desirable (reviewed in Ref. 2).
(Drawing by J.L. Davies, University of Sheffield).

Mapping the FcεR1 Binding Site on Human IgE

The demonstration that an IgE fragment prepared by papain cleavage from an unusual human (h) myeloma protein can competitively inhibit the binding of antigen specific IgE to mast cells and basophils led to the quest for progressively smaller peptides. Early studies employing proteolysis, however, produced only a limited number of fragments, and none but the papain Fcε fragment, encompassing a.a. 227-547 of hIgE could block target cell sensitisation with antigen-specific IgE (8,9). Following these early observations, several attempts were made to map the sites in IgE which interact with Fcε-receptors. In order to overcome the limitations imposed by proteolysis, IgE-derived fragments were generated by chemical synthesis or recombinant DNA techniques.

Our own approach, based on the observation that carbohydrate is not a critical determinant involved in IgE/FcεR1 interaction and that the association/dissociation kinetics of IgE-Fc expressed in *E. coli* are indistinguishable from those of native IgE (10), utilised recombinant (r) DNA techniques to express an overlapping family of IgE-Fc derived fragments. To map the minimum binding sequence necessary for FcεR1 interaction, gene deletions were introduced at both the 5′ and 3′ end of the ε-chain gene, the truncated fragments were expressed in *E. coli*, and evaluated *in vivo* and *in vitro* for their capacity to engage FcεR1 and/or inhibit the binding of native IgE. The outcome of these studies, summarised in Figure 2, suggests that FcεR1 interaction requires sequences C- and N-terminal to Val336, since ε-chain sequences comprising the separate sequences (a.a. 218-336 and 340-547) are inactive (11). This confirms earlier studies, which showed that the products of pepsin cleavage, which generates a covalently linked $(Fab)_2$ fragment (a.a. 1-336) and a peptide comprising (most of) the non-covalently associated Cε3-4 (a.a. 337-547) are inactive (8,9). Of the peptides investigated, the shortest recombinant fragment capable of blocking hIgE/FcεR1 interaction comprises a.a. 301-376 which spans the inter-domain region between Cε2 and Cε3. Cε4-derived residues do not contribute to the interaction since this do-

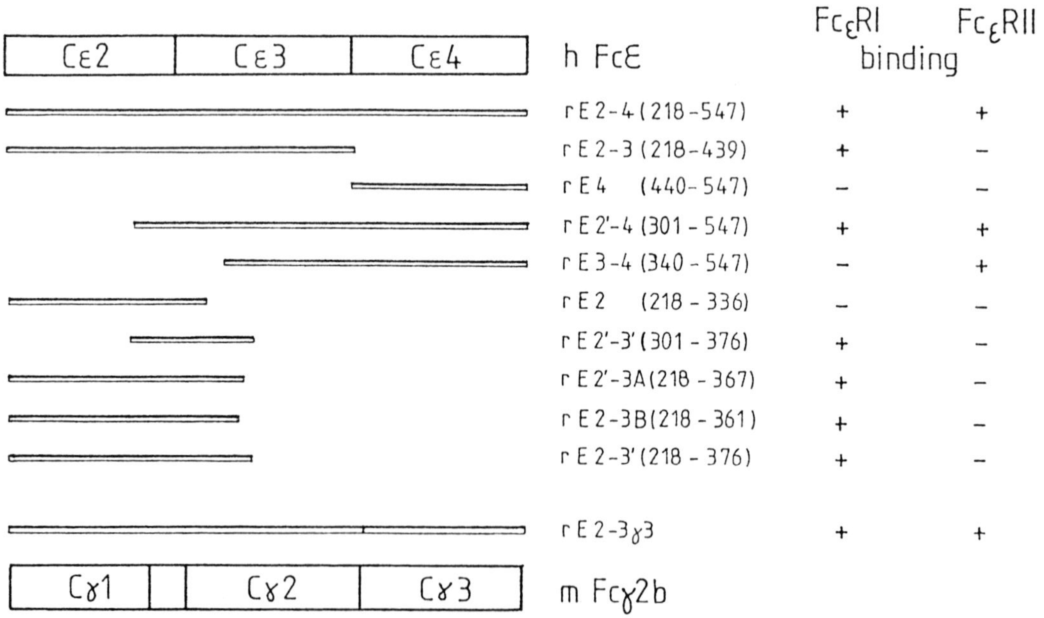

Figure 2: Recombinant ε-chain and chimaeric ε/γ fragments employed in the delineation of high-and low-affinity receptor binding sites on the human ε-chain. The peptides were generated by subcloning restriction fragments into suitable vectors (11,32).

main can be replaced by the homologous Cγ3 domain, and it is possible to delete a major part of Cε3 (up to a.a. 361) without losing FcεR1 binding capacity (12).

Baird *et al.* investigated the interaction of mouse (m) IgE with FcεR1 employing a set of chimaeric hIgG1 and constant mε-chain region domains, and arrived at similar conclusions since substitution of mCε4 by hCγ3 does not affect FcεR1 interaction, but exchange of mCε3 by hCγ2 or replacement of mCε1-2 by hCγ1 and the inter-domain Cγ hinge leads to loss of FcεR1 binding (13). At present, the contribution of the Cε2 domain to FcεR1 interaction must be considered as unresolved. Eshhar and collaborators (14) proposed that the binding site for FcεR1 in mIγE is located in the Cεe3 domain. Their approach at mapping ligand FcεR1 interaction employs exon shuffling combined with domain deletion and utilises the observation that rodent IgE can engage the human receptor, but hIgE cannot bind to rodent FcεR1. Again, these investigators rule out a contribution of Cε4 specific residues, but their results indicate that except for the two penultimate residues in Cε2, the second constant domain is not required for FcεR1 binding (14). The outcome of further studies using truncated rFcε chain peptides, currently in progress in our laboratory, should shed light on the the importance of Cε2 specific residues for receptor interaction.

In addition to studies with rIgE and its fragments, a number of IgE-derived peptides were synthesized by solid phase peptide chemistry. These were either assayed directly for their capacity to block the binding of native IgE, or antibodies were raised against such sequences and assessed in inhibition assays. Figure 3 shows the sequences of peptides used in such studies in the context of a recently developed 3-dimensional model of human IgE. Most of these peptides comprise linear sequences located in the Cε3 domain of human or rodent IgE, some correspond to Cε4-derived sequences, although the latter, as shown in a number of independent studies (12,13,14), are not essential for either FcεR1 or FcεR2 binding. We reevaluated the blocking capacity of a pentapeptide comprising either the native hIgE sequence of a.a. 330-334, or with Asn332 substituted by Asp (15), but in our hands, both peptides are inactive in *in vitro* competition assays, confirming earlier *in situ* observations (11). Similarly, we failed to observe significant activity with a peptide corresponding to a.a. 345-352. Claims that this sequence might comprise the class-specific effector determinant residues emerged as a result of a comprehensive study, which employed a series of overlapping hCε3-derived peptides in the mmolar concentration range to inhibit the sensitization of peripheral blood basophils with antigen-specific IgE (16). The authenticity of the synthetic peptides used in our study was confirmed by mass spectrometry, and shows that the lack of activity of these peptides in our hands cannot be attributed to incomplete unblocking of protective side chains, which can be a significant problem in the synthesis of larger peptides.

Can IgE-Derived Peptides be Used in the Treatment of Allergy?

Although full activity can be observed with small ligand derived peptides where the active site is made up of a single continuous sequence, reduced activity is commonly observed with truncated proteins (17). With the exception of IgE-Fc, all IgE-derived peptides are less active than the native molecule when employed in competition assays, the reported efficacy is in the μ-mmolar range, and the *in vivo* half life of some is of the order of minutes, rather than days (16,18). The shortest recombinant peptide known to engage FcεR1 *in vivo* displays only some 2% of the activity of native IgE in *in vitro* competition studies, although its *in situ* half life compares favorably with that of the native ligand (11,12). Its lower activity is due to an increased dissociation rate from the receptor (12). This points to the involvement of more than one non-contiguous site on both ligand and receptor in the complementary interaction, and it would be surprising if substantially truncated receptor-derived IgE-binding peptides retained full activity.

Several considerations render it improbable that IgE-derived peptides will be of use in the therapy of allergic disorders: IgE-receptor interaction is a reversible process, and receptor-bound peptide will be in dynamic equilibrium with cell-bound and circulatory IgE. *In vivo*, both form part of a plasma pool which will

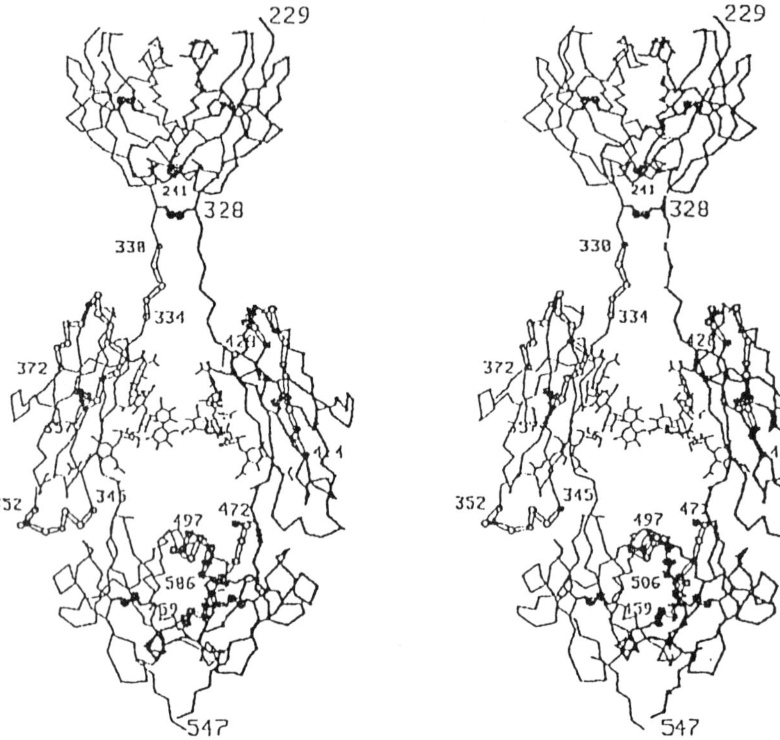


```
301-376 a                                                                                  SQKHWLSDRTYTCQVTYQGHTFEDS
250-546 b                         TIQLLCLVSGYTPGTINITWLEDGQVM-DVDLSTASTTQEGELASTQSELTLSQKHWLSDRTYTCQVTYQGHTFEDS
Human IgE Fc   RDFTPPTVKILQSSCDGGGHFPPTIQLLCLVSGYTPGTINITWLEDGQVM-DVDLSTASTTQEGELASTQSELTLSQKHWLSDRTYTCQVTYQGHTFEDS
Rat IgE Fc     VNITKPTVDLLHSSCDPNA-FHSTIQLYCFVYGHIQNDVSIHWLMDDRKIYETHAQNVLIKEEGKLASTYSRLNITQQQWMSESTFTCKVTSQGENWYAH

345-352 c                        PFDLFIRK
330-334 d           DSDPR
340-546 e                    LSRPSPFDLFIRKSPTITCLVVDLAPSKGTVNLTWSRASGKPVNHSTRKEEKQRNGTLTVTSTLPVGTRDWIEGETYQCRVTHPH
328-546 f         CADSNPRGVSAYLSRPSPFDLFIRKSPTITCLVVDLAPSKGTVNLTWSRASGKPVNHSTRKEEKQRNGTLTVTSTLPVGTRDWIEGETYQCRVTHPH
301-376 a      TKKCADSNPRGVSAYLSRPSPFDLFIRKSPTITCLVVDLAPSKGTVNLTWSRASG
250-546 b      TKKCADSNPRGVSAYLSRPSPFDLFIRKSPTITCLVVDLAPSKGTVNLTWSRASGKPVNHSTRKEEKQRNGTLTVTSTLPVGTRDWIEGETYQCRVTHPH
Human IgE Fc   TKKCADSNPRGVSAYLSRPSPFDLFIRKSPTITCLVVDLAPSKGTVNLTWSRASGKPVNHSTRKEEKQRNGTLTVTSTLPVGTRDWIEGETYQCRVTHPH
Rat IgE Fc     TRRCSDDEPRGVITYLIPPSPLDLYENGTPKLTCLVLDLE-SEENITVTWVRERKKSIGSASQRSTKHHNATTSITSILPVDAKDWIEGEGYQCRVTHPH
357-372 g                                     KLTCLVVDLE-SEKNITVTWV
414-428 h                                                                                   SILPVDAKDWIEGEG

340-546 e      LPRALMRSTTKTSGPRAAPEVYAFATPEWPGSRDKRTLACLIQNFMPEDISVQWLHNEVQLPDARHSTTQPRKT--KGSGFFVFSRLEVTRAEWEQKDEF
328-546 f      LPRALMRSTTKTSGPRAAPEVYAFATPEWPGSRDKRTLACLIQNFMPEDISVQWLHNEVQLPDARHSTTQPRKT--KGSGFFVFSRLEVTRAEWEQKDEF
250-546 b      LPRALMRSTTKTSGPRAAPEVYAFATPEWPGSRDKRTLACLIQNFMPEDISVQWLHNEVQLPDARHSTTQPRKT--KGSGFFVFSRLEVTRAEWEQKDEF
Human IgE Fc   LPRALMRSTTKTSGPRAAPEVYAFATPEWPGSRDKRTLACLIQNFMPEDISVQWLHNEVQLPDARHSTTQPRKT--KGSGFFVFSRLEVTRAEWEQKDEF
Rat IgE Fc     FPKPIVRSITKAPGKRSAPEVYVFLPPE-EEEKDKRTLTCLIQNFFPEDISVQWLQDSKLIPKSQHSTTTPLKYNGSNQRFFIFSRLEVTKALWTQTKQF
459-472 i                           VYVFLPPE-EEEKDKR
491-503 j                                                                   LQDSKLIPKSQHS

340-546 e      ICRAVHEAASPSQTVQRAVSVNPGK
328-546 f      ICRAVHEAASPSQTVQRAVSVNPGK
250-546 b      ICRAVHEAASPSQTVQRAVSVNPGK
Human IgE Fc   ICRAVHEAASPSQTVQRAVSVNPGK
Rat IgE Fc     TCRVIHEALREPRKLERTISKSLG-
```

Figure 3: (A) Sequences of recombinant and synthetic peptides in the context of a recently developed model structure of hIgE. Stereo-representation of the a-carbon backbone of a model of the Fc of human IgE (23) showing peptides 330-334, 345-352, and 357-372 in the heavy chain on the left and the peptides 414-428, 459-472, and 497-506 on the right chain. The sulphur atoms in the intradomain disulphide bridges are indicated by small circles, those in the interdomain disulphide links are depicted by larger open circles. The carbohydrate between the two Cε3 domains are drawn with thin lines. (B) Linear sequences alignment of above peptides.
a: ref 11,12; *b*: ref 29; *c*: ref 16; *d*: ref 15; *e*: ref 11; *f*: Helm, B.A., unpublished observations; *g*: ref 30; *h,i,j*: ref 31.

constantly exchange with receptor-bound ligand until native IgE and "blocking" peptide become represented on the surface of target cells relative to their molar ratios and relative affinities. Degranulation studies show that only a few molecules of receptor-bound, antigen-specific IgE have to be cross-linked to cause target cell exocytosis, and such peptides, even when administered at high molar excess, may not be able to prevent the eventual sensitisation with allergen-specific IgE (19). Furthermore, in common with other IgE-derived peptides that have a deleted Cε4 domain, the rE2'-3' peptide is initially monomeric, but has a tendency to aggregate, and the resultant polymers, which can trigger FcεR1 activation, could elicit anaphylaxis if administered *in vivo* (2).

Development of New Approaches Towards the Discovery of Potential IgE Antagonists

The rational design of IgE antagonists should be greatly assisted by a detailed understanding of the structural requirements and the nature of the a.a. residues that are essential for the binding of IgE to the receptors. A determination of the minimum sequence requirements necessary for ligand/receptor interaction should considerably expedite the identification of effector determinant residue(s) by site-specific mutagenesis, although the initial selection of such residues is complicated by the absence of structural data.

At present, no high resolution structure is available for any part of the IgE molecule or its receptors. Earlier structural models were based on the sequences homology that exist with IgG-Fc and projected an arrangement whereby Cys241 in one ε-chain pairs with Cys328 in the opposite chain (20,21). A number of biochemical observations, including the postulated requirement of covalent inter-ε-chain linkage for biological activity were not satisfied by the "crossed" inter-ε-chain disulphide bond model (22). In order to identify the nature and biological importance of the inter-ε-chain Cys residues, we introduced site-specific mutations into the Cε2 domain of hIgE. The development of a new technique, which involved the introduction of an additional cyanogen bromide cleavage site between the Cys residues under consideration, facilitated the rapid identification of a parallel inter-chain disulphide bond arrangement in IgE(ND). Additional support for such a linkage was obtained by sequence determination of disulphide linked dimers isolated from the Cε2 domain of IgE(PS), (for the strategy see Figure 4). Contrary to earlier claims, we also demonstrated that none of the Cys residues in IgE are essential for biological activity: Substitution of Cys residues involved in inter-ε-chain disulphide bond formation by Ser, computed to mimic reduction, does not destroy receptor binding, although reductive alkylation, or the replacement of Cys328 by Met, thought to simulate alkylation, is associated with loss of receptor binding. Taken together, these observation clearly indicate that covalent dimerization is not essential for IgE/receptor binding, but point to the sensitivity of the interaction to structural perturbations in this region (23).

A revised model structure, based on these observations, was developed (23). The new model takes into account that the inter-ε-chain disulphides in human IgE, like those in IgG, are parallel, and proposes the presence of an exposed and probably flexible hinge segment, consisting of residues 329-335, in the inter-domain region between Cε2 and Cε3. The shortest linear IgE-derived peptide sequence that can act as a molecular decoy in competition studies with hIgE for FcεR1 binding sites comprises this sequence and the effector determinant residues in IgG-Fc have been mapped to this region: Residues in positions 234-237 (homologous to 332-335 in hIgE) are essential for Fcγ1 and FcγIII recognition (24,25). This suggests that the mast cell binding site in IgE may be found in the structural equivalent of the accessible and flexible hinge region of other antibodies, and not, as previously suggested, in a cleft formed by the C-terminal Cε2 and N-terminal Cε3 domains. Mutagenesis studies, currently in progress in our laboratory, point to the importance of residues in this inter-domain segment for high-affinity receptor binding. The identification of effector determinant residues in IgE and/or its receptors, together with the demonstration that a single ε-chain may form the site of attachment to FcεR1, may facilitate the development of small oligopeptide D-

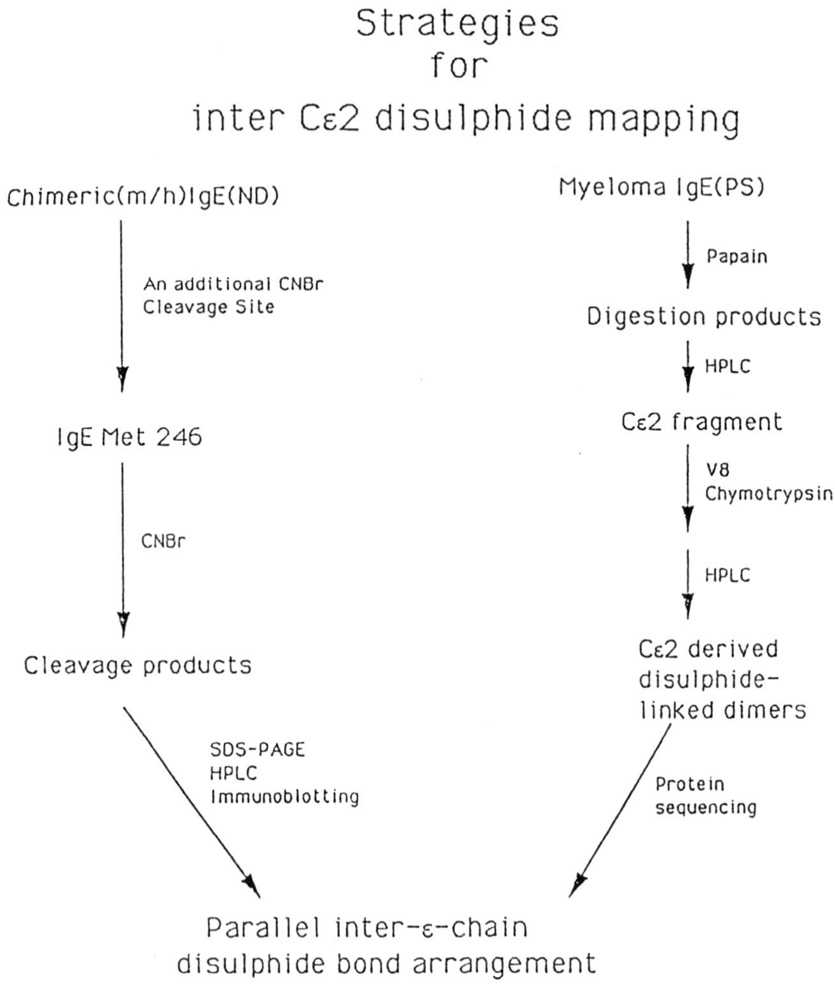

A

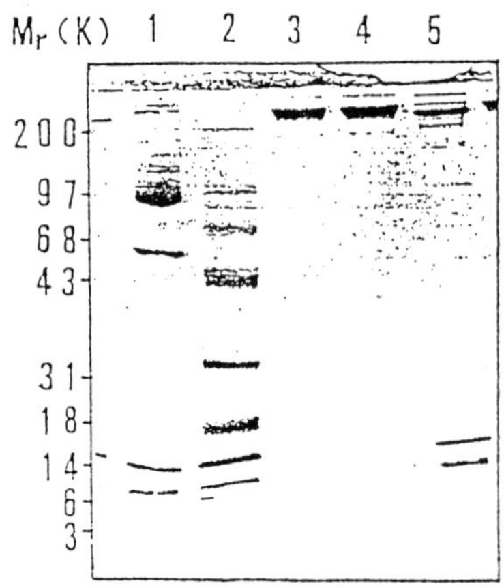

B

Identification of the inter-ε-chain disulphide bond arrangement in human myeloma IgE PS

Disulphide-linked peptides in the Cε2 domain of human myeloma IgE PS

A	peptide A1	FPPTIQLL-LVSGY	(a.a. 247-260)
	peptide A2	TYT-QVTY	(a.a. 309-316)
B	peptide B	FTPPTVKILQSS-D	(a.a. 229-242)
C	peptide C	STKK-AD	(a.a. 324-330)

amino acid analogues of the effector determinant residue(s) with an N-terminal carboxymethyl moiety and a C-terminal benzyl ester, since *in situ* studies with analogous peptides, based on the identification of the effector determinant residues between HIV-1 and CD4, appear to be promising forerunners to an effective inhibitor of HIV-1 infection (26) (although no kinetic data are currently available regarding the affinity of analogous CD4-derived peptides for HIV). A similar strategy could be developed to block the site of attachment of IgE to FcεR1 following the identification of the IgE-binding site on this receptor. In the short term, such peptides may form the basis for the development of a new family of anti-allergic drugs. In the medium to long term, other prospects hold: The availability of theoretically unlimited quantities of ligand and receptor proteins made available through recombinant DNA technology will facilitate the screening of vast quantities of natural products. As with other receptor antagonists (27), serendipity may well lead to the discovery of natural inhibitors of the allergic reaction, and a determination of their structure could form the starting point for the development of rational IgE antagonists.

Such a quest should benefit from structural input, and a high resolution 3D image to define the complementary sites between the partners of the interaction is clearly desirable. It would be presumptuous to forecast a positive outcome of crystallization trials currently in progress. If, as predicted, the mast cell binding site in IgE is located in a flexible interdomain segment, the growth of ordered crystals may be difficult to achieve, and in crystals of IgG, the homologous region is disordered and invisible. Meanwhile, the development of 3D structural models of the ligand-receptor complex by molecular graphics, taking into account the molecular recognition forces between ligand, receptor and solvent (28) may further our understanding of the interaction and assist the development of analogues. Our capacity to genetically manipulate both partners of the interaction provides an important means to assess the projections made by molecular modelling through mutagenesis and ligand binding studies, which in turn may yield useful information for the design of more active ligands.

References

1. Ishizaka, K., Ishizaka, T., and Hornbrook, M.M. 1966. Physicochemical properties of human reaginic antibody. J. Immunol. 97:840.
2. Helm, B.A., Ling, Y., Mackie, S., and Padlan, E.A. 1991. Protein engineering of IgE antibodies and its applications. In: Molecular diagnostics: Research towards application. M. Walker, and R. Rapley, eds. Oxford: Blackwell Scientific Publishers, in press.
3. Donovan, G.R., and Baldo, B.A. 1990. Crossreactivity of IgE antibodies from sera of subjects allergic to both ryegrass pollen and wheat endosperm proteins: Evidence for common allergenic determinants. Clin. and Exp. Allergy 20:501.
4. Mohapatra, S.S., Hill, R., Astwood, J., Ekramoddoullah, A.K.M., Olsen, E., Silvanovitch, A., Hatton, T., Kisil, F.T., and Sehon, A. 1990. Isolation and characterisation of a cDNA clone encoding an IgE-binding protein from

Figure 4: Strategies used in the identification of the inter-ε-chain disulphide bond arrangement in human IgE (23)

Panel A: SDS-PAGE (4–20% gradient) run under non-reducing conditions. Lane 1: IgE Met246 after CNBr cleavage; lane 2 standard proteins; lanes 3 and 4: uncleaved controls for native IgE and Met246; lane 5: native IgE after CNBr cleavage.

Panel B: Following chymotrypsin and V8 protease digestion of isolated Cε2 dimers derived from IgE PS, three disulphide-linked peptides (A,B,C) were identified. Upon reductive carboxymethylation (^{14}C-iodoacetamide, Amersham), peptide A gives rise to two peptides A1 and A2 comprising a.a. 247-260 and 309-316 which correspond to sequences surrounding Cys 254 and 312 involved in intra-Cε2 disulphide linkage. Reductive carboxymethylation of peptide B yields sequence B spanning a.a. 229-242, and that of peptide C sequence C corresponding to a.a. 324-330. Peptide B and C encompass sequences surrounding the C- and N-terminal Cys residues involved in inter-ε-chain disulphide bond formation.

Kentucky Bluegrass (*Poa pratensis*) pollen. Int. Arch. Allergy Appl. Immunol. 91:362.

5. Davis, F.M., Gossett, L.A., and Chang, T. 1991. An epitope on membrane bound but not secreted IgE: Implications in isotype-specific regulation. Biotechnology 9:53.
6. Iwamoto, I., Nawata, Y., Koike, T., Tanaka, M., Tomioka, H., and Yoshida, S. 1989. Relationship between anti-IgE autoantibody and severity of bronchial asthma. Int. Arch. Allergy Appl. Immnunol. 90:414.
7. Bourne, H.R. 1986 One molecular machine can transduce diverse signals. Nature 321:814.
8. Stanworth, D.R., Humphrey, J.H., Bennich, H., and Johansson, S.G.O. 1968. Inhibition of Prausnitz-Küstner reaction by Proteolytic cleavage fragments of a human myeloma protein of immunoglobulin E class. Lancet 2:17.
9. Ishizaka, K., Ishizaka, T., and Lee, E.H. 1970. Biologic function of the Fc fragments of E myeloma protein. Immunochemistry 7:687.
10. Ishizaka, T., Helm, B.A., Hakimi, J., Niebl, J., Ishizaka, K., and Gould, H.J. 1986. Biological properties of a recombinant human immunoglobulin ε-chain fragment. Proc. Natl. Acad. Sci. USA 83:8323.
11. Helm, B. A., Marsh, P., Vercelli, D., Padlan, E., Gould, H., and Geha, R. 1988. The mast cell binding site on human immunoglobulin E. Nature 331:180.
12. Helm, B. A., Kebo, D., Vercelli, D., Glovsky, M. M., Gould, H., Ishizaka, K., Geha, R., and Ishizaka, T. 1989b. Blocking of passive sensitization of human mast cells and basophil granulocytes with IgE antibodies by a recombinant ε-chain fragment of 76 amino acids. Proc. Natl. Acad. Sci. USA. 186:9465.
13. Weetall, M., Shopes, R., Holowka, D., and Baird, B. 1990. Mapping the site of interaction between murine IgE and its high affinity receptor with chimaeric Ig. J. Immunol. 145:3849.
14. Nissim, A., Jouvin, M.H., and Esshar, Z. 1991. Mapping of the high affinity Fcε receptor binding site to the third constant region domain of IgE. EMBO 10:101.
15. Hamburger, R.N. 1975. Peptide inhibition of the Prausnitz-Küstner reaction. Science 189:389.
16. Nio, N., Seguro, K., Aryoshi, Y., Nakanishi, K., Kita., A., Ishii, K., and Nakamura, H. 1989. Inhibition of histamine release by synthetic human IgE peptide fragments: Structure-activity studies. Peptide Chemistry, p. 203.
17. Gershoni, J.M., and Aronheim, A. 1988. Molecular decoys: Ligand-binding recombinant proteins protect mice from curarimimetic neurotoxins. Proc. Natl. Acad. Sci. USA. 85:4087.
18. Hamburger, R.N., Hahn, G.S., Daigle, A.E., Rangus, K.F., and Thayer, T.O. 1989. Results of clinical trials of the IgE pentapeptide. In: Progress in allergy and clinical immunology, W.J. Pichler, ed. Toronto: Hogrefe & Huber, p. 109.
19. Jarrett, E., Mackenzie, S., and Bennich H.H. 1981. Parasite-induced non-specific IgE does not protect against allergic reactions. Nature 283:302.
20. Padlan, E. A., and Davies, D. R. 1986. A model of the Fc of immunoglobulin E. Mol. Immunol. 23:1063.
21. Pumphrey, R. 1986. Computer models of the human immunoglobulins. Immunol. Today 7:206.
22. Helm, B.A. Short, N.J., and Geha, R.S. 1989a. The mast cell binding site on human IgE. In: Progress in allergy and clinical immunology, W.J. Pichler, ed. Toronto: Hogrefe & Huber, p. 96.
23. Helm, B.A., Ling, Y., Teale, C., Padlan, E.A., and Brüggemann, M. 1991. The nature and biological importance of the inter-ε-chain disulphide bonds. Eur. J. Immunol. 21:1543.
24. Duncan, A. R., Woof, J. M., Partridge, L. J., Burton, D. R., and Winter, G. 1988. Localisation of the binding site of the human high-affinity receptor on IgG. Nature 332:563.
25. Jefferis, R., Lund, J., Pound, P., Jones, P., and Winter, G. 1991. Mouse FcγRll interacts with two topograpically distinct sites within the CH2 domain of immunoglobulin G. FASEB Abstract 6343.
26. Finberg, R.W., Diamond, D.C., Mitchell, D.B., Rosenstein, Y., Soman, G., Norman., T.C., Schreiber, S.L., and Burakoff, S. 1990. Prevention of HIV-1 infection and preservation of CD4 function by the binding of CPfs to gp120. Science 249:287.
27. Lotti, V.J., and Chang, R.S.L. 1989. A new potent and selective non-peptide gastrin antagonist and brain choleocystokinin receptor ligand: L 365,260. Eur. J. Pharmacol. 162:273.
28. Lewis, R.A., and Dean, P.M. 1989. Automated site-directed drug design: The formation of molecular templates in primary structure generation. Proc. R. Soc. Lond. B 236:141.
29. Liu, F.T., Albrandt, K.A., Bry, C.G., and Ishizaka, T. 1984. Expression of a biologically ac-

tive fragment of human ε-chain in *E. coli*. Proc. Natl. Acad. Sci. USA 81:5369
30. Robertson, M.W., and Lui, F.T. 1988. IgE structure-function relationship defined by sequence directed antibodies induced by synthetic peptides. Mol. Immunol. 25:103.
31. Burt, D.S., and Stanworth, D.S. 1987. Inhibition of binding of rat IgE to mast cells by synthetic peptides. Eur. J. Immunol. 17:437.
32. Vercelli, D., Helm, B., Marsh, P., Padlan, E., Geha, R., and Gould, H. 1989. The B-cell binding site on human immunoglobulin E. Nature 338:649.

The High Affinity Receptor for IgE (FcεRI): New Developments

Jean-Pierre Kinet*

Over the last few years, much progress has been made in our understanding of the molecular structure of the high affinity receptor for immunoglobulin E (FcεRI). The cloning of the three subunits α, β and γ has been accomplished in rat, mouse and most recently in human. Gene transfer into receptor-negative cells has led to the structural and functional reconstitution of the complete tetrameric complex $\alpha\beta\gamma_2$. Our laboratory has provided new insights into the signal transduction mechanisms used by this multimeric receptor to activate mast cells and basophils. Receptor engagement immediately activates a set of kinases tyrosine and threonine/serine kinases which in turn phosphorylate the receptor on β (tyrosine and serine) and γ (tyrosine and threonine), and various substrates such as phospholipase Cγ-1. Receptor phosphorylation is specific to "activated" receptor and is immediately reversible upon receptor disengagement.

The high affinity receptor for IgE, a tetrameric complex $\alpha\beta\gamma_2$, is an essential element in the initiation of the allergic reaction (1,2). Receptor-bound IgE molecules react with allergens to induce a redistribution of the cell surface receptors. In turn, this redistribution is responsible for cell degranulation and the release of mediators of the allergic response, such as histamine. This FcεRI-mediated cellular activation affects only mast cells and basophils, which are the only cell types known to express the receptor. Since FcεRI is critical to the initiation of IgE-induced allergic diseases, understanding its structure and its function may help in the development of new therapeutic strategies.

Structure of Human FcεRI

Complementary DNAs have been isolated for α, β, and γ chains in mouse, rat and human (1,2). The molecular cloning of these subunits has permitted the reconstitution of surface-expressed receptor complexes following transfection into various cell lines. One of the surprising findings from these studies was the differential requirements for surface expression among the different species. Cotransfection of the three chains α, β and γ was required to promote efficient surface expression of the rat or mouse receptor. In contrast, surface expression of human αγ complexes was achieved by cotransfecting α and γ without suggesting that β may not be necessary for the stable expression of a high affinity receptor. This result (and our inability to clone human β) had raised the interesting possibility that αγ complexes might exist naturally in human cells. We have now cloned the gene and cDNA encoding human β (3). The corresponding mRNAs are expressed in basophils of ten individuals tested, making the existence of different receptor phenotypes (containing β or not) unlikely. Therefore, it appears that the human receptor, like its rodent counterpart, is a tetrameric hetero-oligomer composed of an α chain, a β chain and two disulfide-linked γ chains.

The Receptor Binding Site

We have engineered a construct of the human α containing only the extracellular segment of α. This truncated α chain is secreted in soluble and active form by transfected cells (4). The affinity of the construct for IgE is characteristic of receptors on intact cells. The other subunits, the receptor membrane attachment and the sugar moiety do not seem to play any role in high affinity binding. Therefore, the extracellular domain of α, which is solely responsible for the receptor high affinity binding site, should be a suitable reagent for crystallographic analy-

* Molecular Allergy and Immunology Section, National Institutes of Allergy and Infectious Diseases, NIH, Twinbrook II Building, 12441 Parklawn Drive, Rockville, MD 20852, USA.

sis. If successful, such an analysis should give us a more detailed knowledge of the receptor binding site. This could be the first step in the development (for example by molecular design) of therapy for IgE-mediated allergy based upon the interaction of IgE/FcεRI binding.

The Kinase and Phosphatase Connection

It has been assumed that the cytoplasmic domains of β and γ play an important role in coupling FcεRI to signal transduction pathways. However until now this role had remained largely undefined. We have now found that FcεRI engagement induces immediate (within 5 seconds) *in vivo* phosphorylation on β (tyrosine and serine) and γ (tyrosine and threonine) via at least two different non-receptor kinases (5). In addition, the activated kinases are able to discriminate between engaged and non-engaged receptors. When only a fraction of the receptors are engaged with antigen, the adjacent and non-engaged receptors are not phosphorylated. Furthermore we have shown that kinase activation and the resulting receptor phosphorylation require continuous receptor engagement. Receptor dephosphorylation occurs within 5 seconds of receptor disengagement, presumably due to the action of undefined phosphatases. The dephosphorylated receptors can then be rephosphorylated following further stimulation.

We propose that cycles of kinase and phosphatase activation are initiated and maintained by receptor engagement. As a consequence, the receptor would become phosphorylated and dephosphorylated in a continuous manner. This model would explain the rapid receptor dephosphorylation following receptor disengagement and the absence of increase in receptor phosphorylation over time. The β and γ phosphorylation/dephosphorylation would then serve as a way to couple/uncouple the receptor to other components of the signalling machinery.

References

1. Kinet, J.-P. 1990. The high affinity receptor for immunoglobulin E. Current Opinion in Immunology 2:499.
2. Ravetch J.V., and Kinet, J.-P. 1991. Fc receptors. Ann. Rev. Immunol. 9:457.
3. Kuster, H., Zhang, L., Brini, A., MacGlashan, D.M.J., and Kinet, J.-P. The gene for the human high affinity receptor β chain. Submitted.
4. Blank, U., Ra, C., and Kinet, J.-P. 1991. Characterization of truncated α chain products from human, rat and mouse high affinity receptor for immunoglobulin E. J. Biol. Chem. 266:2639.
5. Paolini. R., Jouvin, M.-H., and Kinet, J.-P. Phosphorylation and dephosphorylation of the high affinity receptor for immunoglobulin E immediately following receptor engagement and disengagement. Nature, in press.

Immunogenic Peptides and Perspectives for the Treatment of Autoimmune Diseases

Jorge R. Oksenberg, Lawrence Steinman*

Much information has accumulated on the nature of trimolecular interactions (Major histocompatibility complex determinant-antigen-T cell receptor) which lead to the activation of self reactive T lymphocytes. Based on this knowledge, the application of selective immunotherapies that target either class II MHC molecules, T cell receptor variable gene products, or the interaction between them, is given consideration in disease-like multiple sclerosis and rheumatoid arthritis.

Autoimmune diseases are characterized by a breakdown in the mechanisms mediating tolerance to self components. Consequently, the immune system of an individual is triggered to mount a pathological response against self-antigens. This response can be generalized in diseases like systemic lupus erythematosus, or targeted to a particular compartment or organ in diseases like Graves disease, multiple sclerosis, myasthenia gravis or rheumatoid arthritis. The pace of research on the pathogenesis and treatment of autoimmune diseases has intensified in the past five years. The cloning and sequencing of autoantigens, the structural analysis of the MHC, the genetic analysis of the T cell receptor (TCR) and our understanding of lymphokine physiology, all contributed substantially to our present view of disease mechanisms. In addition many lessons have been learned from experimental animal models, like experimental allergic encephalomyelitis (EAE) and the non-obese diabetic (NOD) mouse.

In order to stimulate a T cell response, protein antigens must be processed by antigen presenting cells into peptides that bind to major histocompatibility complex (MHC) class I and class II molecules (1,2). In fact, a correlation between the stability of empty MHC molecules and their ability to bind extracellular peptides *in vivo*, was recently proposed as the basis for their association with certain autoimmune diseases (3).

Competitive Binding of Peptides to the MHC

MHC molecules must bind self peptides in order to activate T cells responsible for autoimmune disease. Therefore, by inhibition of this binding it should be possible to block the stimulation of autoaggressive immuno-pathogenic T cells. Exogenous peptides have been proposed as potential candidates to mediate such inhibition. In the EAE system, the detailed study of the molecular interactions between MHC-TCR and the myelin basic protein (MBP) epitope Ac (acetylated)1-11 led to attempts to use *in vivo* competition between self-peptides in order to modulate the induction of autoreactivity (4) (Tables 1 and 2). AcN1-11 is a strong pathogenic peptide for PL/J and (PLSJ)F1 mice, and T cells that can recognize this self-antigen mediate encephalomyelitis in these strains of mice. Non-encephalitogenic but immunogenic MBP peptides 1-20 and Ac 9-20 suppressed proliferation to the encephalitogenic peptide AcN1-11 both *in vivo* and *in vitro*. The peptides 1-20 and Ac9-20 significantly prevented EAE induction at a 3:1 co-immunization ratio with AcN1-11 (5). In reviewing representative sections of 20 mice treated with competitors (N1-20 and AcN9-20), which did not show any clinical signs of EAE, no perivascular cuffs or submeningeal cell infiltrates were evident (4,5).

---

* Department of Neurology and Neurological Sciences, Stanford University School of Medicine, Stanford, California, 94305-5235, USA.
Acknowledgements: This work was supported by a grant of the National Institute of Health ROI NS28759, the Allan Trust and the Rosenthal Foundation.

Table 1. Discrete T-cell epitopes of MBP in mice (4,5,29).

Peptide	Encephalito-genicity	Class II restriction	TCR V usage
Ac1-9	+	I-$A\alpha^uA\beta^u$	$V\alpha4.3$ and $V\beta8$ predominantly
Ac1-11	+	I-$A\alpha^uA\beta^u$	$V\alpha4.3$ and $V\beta8$ predominantly
Ac1-20	+	I-$A\alpha^uA\beta^u$	$V\beta8$ predominantly
1-20	+	I-$A\alpha^uA\beta^u$	$V\beta8$ predominantly
5-16	–	I-$A\alpha^uA\beta^u$ I-$A\alpha^sAb^u$	$V\beta8$ predominantly
17-27	?	I-$A\alpha^sAb^s$	Not determined
35-47	+	I-$E\alpha^uEb^u$ I-$E\alpha^uEb^s$	Not $V\beta8$
89-100	–	I-$A\alpha^sAb^s$	Not determined
89-101	+	I-$A\alpha^sAb^s$	$V\beta17$ predominantly
96-109	+	I-$A\alpha^sAb^s$	Not determined
92-103	+	I-$A\alpha^sAb^s$	Not determined

Table 2. Peptide Therapy on H-2^u mice.

Peptide	Sequence	Encephalitogenic capabilities	Stimulates encephalito-genic T cells	Binding to I-A^u
Ac1-9	Ac-ASQKRPSQR	Induces disease	+++	+
Ac1-11	Ac-ASQKRPSQRHG	Induces disease	+++	+
Ac1-11[4A]	Ac-ASQ*A*RPSQRHG	Inhibits disease	+++	+++
1-20	ASQKRPSQRHG SKYLATAST	Inhibits disease	–	+
Ac9-20	Ac-RHGSKYLATAST	Inhibits disease	–	+
1-11	Ac-ASQKRPSQRHG	–	–	?
Ac-2-11	Ac-SQKRPSQRHG	–	–	?
Ac1-11 [3A,4A]	Ac-AS*AA*RPSQRHG	–	–	+++

Additional studies have revealed that a single amino acid substitution in the Ac1-11 sequence, alanine for lysine at position 4, yields a peptide that binds with greater affinity than does Ac1-11 to I-A^u. This peptide is also able to powerfully stimulate *in vitro* encephalitogenic T cell clones responsive to Ac 1-11. This peptide was predicted to be a strong inducer of disease. Surprisingly, mice co-immunized with Ac1-11 [4a] were protected from EAE (6) (Table 2).

From these results, it is clear that a variety of synthetic peptides can have regulatory effects on the autoimmune phenomenon. This raises the possibility of therapy using designer peptides, competing for the antigen binding site. However, attempts to reverse established disease have been unsuccessful so far. Furthermore, the information about immunodominant epitopes in human diseases like multiple sclerosis (MS) reveals a complicated picture (Table 3). In addition, we are not yet able to accurately predict which peptide will be an effective therapeutic agent, and which epitope should be blocked. Characterization of natural peptides bound by class I molecules shows that they are smaller than expected, about nine aa, (peptides of 12 to 15 aa are frequently used in *in vitro* experiments), matching more precisely the crystallography data currently available (7). From sequencing both peptide mixtures and individual peptides bound by particular MHC molecules, conserved motifs of anchoring residues one at the C terminus and the other close to N terminus, distinguish sets of binding peptides for different class I molecules (8). The extension of these findings to class II molecules may lead to a more rational design of therapeutic blocking peptides. In addition, since it is possible that a given MHC molecule has a single functional antigen-binding site, peptides from unrelated antigens can compete with self-peptides for T cell activation. For example, it was possible to block the proliferative response of acetylcholine receptor α subunit-T cell clones and lines by the I-A^b restricted synthetic peptide (T,G)-A—L, but not by the I-A^k restricted polypeptide (H,G)-A—L (9). Results with other substances like Copolymer I (Cop I) appear promising. Cop I decreased the exacerbation rate and slowed disease progression, particularly in relapsing-remitting MS patients (10). The proposed mechanism of action of Cop I may be exerted by MHC blockade or generation of antigen specific suppressor cells.

Vaccination with TCR Peptides

Cohen and associates have shown that it is possible to use autoimmune T cell clones or lines as vaccines to prevent or reverse autoimmune disease (11). In the EAE system for example, animals inoculated with MBP reactive T cells remained free of disease for prolonged times, and disease could not be induced with MBP in adjuvant. The detailed knowledge of the TCR repertoire involved in EAE (5) allowed the development of even more selective vaccination therapies based on TCR-peptides. Recently, EAE in the Lewis rat was prevented by immunization with a nonapeptide spanning the V-D-J region of Vβ8:p72-86 (12) and a 21 amino acid sequence that included the second complementarity determining region (CDR2), Vβ8:39-59, predicted to be immunogenic for T cells (13). Moreover, TCR peptides were used to treat established disease in rats. Injection of TCR Vβ8p:39-59 (DMGHGKRLIHY-SYDVNSTEKG) without adjuvant, to animals with clinical signs of EAE reduced disease severity and speeded recovery. The apparent mechanisms may be active by stimulating anti Vβ8+ T cells and by inducing antibodies raised naturally in response to encephalitogenic Vβ8 cells (14). The application of these therapies in man will depend upon increased knowledge of the TCR repertoire utilized by pathogenic T cells.

T Cell Receptor Gene Usage in Multiple Sclerosis

Several groups have analyzed the distribution of rearranged TCRs in T lymphocytes reactive to MBP. Some of these studies indicate that these T cells may rearrange a restricted number of TCR Vα and Vβ genes (Table 3). Hafler and colleagues studied 83 T cell lines in man that react to MBP peptide 84-102 (15, 16). In one patient who was HLA-DR2/DR7, 24 of 31 clones used Vβ 17. Other clones from other DR2 patients used Vβ 1, 3, 4, 5, 6, 7, 8, 12, 14 and 17. In a study by Martin et al., four cytotoxic T cell clones from MS patients with different immunogenetic backgrounds, specific for the p89-99 core sequence of the 87-106 epitope of MBP, expressed different Vβ-Dβ-Jβ gene rearrangements (17). Kotzin, Vandenbark, Hashim and colleagues suggested that the TCR family Vβ5.2 is preferentially used in the context of HLA-DR2, in response to different BP epitopes (18,19). The experimental observation that MBP reactive cells can be cloned from peripheral blood from both MS patients and controls complicates the evaluation of their relevance in disease (20). To overcome this problem, Allegretta et al. used a somatic mutation marker, hypoxantine guanine phosphoribosyltransferase (HRPT) to select for activated PBLs. Although interpatient variability was seen, mutant clones were more frequent in patients and 4% of these reacted to MBP, where no such clones were observed in controls (21).

Recently we have used the PCR method to specifically amplify TCR Vα sequences from transcripts derived from MS brain lesions in three patients (22). In each of the three MS brains, a limited number of rearranged TCR Vα transcripts was detected. No Vα sequences could be found in three control brains without inflammation. Sequence analysis of 25 cDNA clones from MS white matter plaques with Vα 12.1-Jα-Cα rearrangements demonstrated only two Jα sequences, reinforcing further the notion of a limited heterogeneity of TCR transcripts in MS brain. The extension of this study

Table 3. Discrete T-Cell Epitopes of MBP in Multiple Sclerosis.

Epitope	Class II restriction	TCR usage	Comments	Ref.
84-102 142-168	DR2,DQw1 DRw11	Vβ17 and Vβ12 Vβ17 infrequent	Over 15000 short term T cell lines were established. The epitope 142-168 was recognized in MS patients and controls	15, 16
87-106	DR2, 4 DR2(1501) DR4,13	Vβ6.6-Jβ2.3 Vβ5.2-Jβ2.4 Vβ-Jβ1.6/1.4	One epitope is recognized in the context of four different HLA molecules and different TCRs	17
Several	HLA-DR2	Vβ5.2 (predominant)	HLA-DR2 as a permissive restriction element for a variety of epitopes	18, 19
1-44 45-89 90-170	HLA-DR	Heterogeneous	MBP specific lines could be isolated with comparable efficiency from MS patients and controls	20
90-170 149-162 149-171	HLA-DR	Heterogeneous	Predominant Vβ gene usage among each individual. No correlation with the epitope or HLA restriction molecule	28

by us and others, may result in the elucidation of genetic susceptibility patterns where particular TCR V genes are expressed in regions of demyelination. Certain V genes might be expressed in the brains of individuals who possess particular HLA class II genes. As sequences become available from T cell clones reactive to other myelin proteins like PLP, MAG and MOG, correlations may emerge between T cell clones with defined specificities and particular T cell receptor rearrangements in diseased areas of MS brain. These findings may lead to an understanding of how the trimolecular complex (MHC-antigen-TCR) triggers the autoimmune response in MS, and might have therapeutic implications, given the success of reversing or preventing EAE with reagents targeting TCR V genes, either using monoclonal antibodies or synthetic peptides. A pilot trial of treatment of MS with TCR peptides is underway.

Anti CD4 Monoclonal Antibodies (mAbs)

The CD4 surface protein is associated with "helper/inducer" T cell functions. Anti-CD4 therapy is the most extensively studied antibody used in the treatment of experimental autoimmunity. Anti CD4 mAbs have been employed successfully by our group (23) and by Brostoff and Mason (24) for reversal of EAE. One drawback of this approach is that administration of anti CD4 antibody might generate general immunosuppression and might induce tolerance to dangerous pathogens. Though restoration of tolerance to self antigens is advantageous in autoimmunity, it could have deleterious consequences when given to individuals with chronic or persistent infection, such as toxoplasmosis (25). Despite these considerations, Phase I clinical trials with chimeric anti CD4 are now underway in Stanford Medical Center with patients with the chronic progressive form of MS. Opportunistic infections have not occurred in the first 25 patients treated with the anti-CD4 antibody. Construction of hybrid chimeric antibodies, humanizing murine mAbs, may avoid the stimulation of human anti mouse responses, while retaining and even increasing the potency of the antibody (26).

Conclusions

The experimental data suggests that specific immunotherapy of autoimmune diseases utilizing simple protocols of peptides or antibodies directed at single or multiple sites in the trimolecular complex appears to be a formidable challenge. Many practical issues must be addressed like the development of appropriate carriers in order to extend the half-life time of peptides *in vivo*, or the design of antibodies that do not elicit anti-idiotypic responses. Furthermore, beyond these practical concerns basic questions remain unanswered regarding genetic susceptibility and environmental influences on the development of autoimmunity. In established disease, the pathological immune response may involve multiple epitopes or even multiple antigens, and it is likely that an individual's HLA background shapes the TCR repertoire. Consequently, specific therapy will be customized to a certain extent. A valid interpretation of the currently available experimental data stresses the complexity of the autoimmune reaction, forecasting the likely success of less specific modes of immunotherapy. Therapies aiming to block the MHC-peptide-TCR interaction may be more complicated to implement in human systems than anticipated. Nevertheless, the design of treatment-protocols should be pursued vigorously in light of the success of these approaches obtained on experimental systems (4–6, 11–14, 26–30).

References

1. Moller, G. 1987. Antigenic requirements for activation of MHC restricted responses. Immunol. Rev. 98:1.
2. Bjorkman, P.J., Saper, M.A., Samraoui, B., Bennet, W.S., Strominger, J.L., and Wiley, D.C. 1987. The foreign antigen binding site and T cell recognition regions of class I histocompatibility antigens. Nature 329:512.
3. Benjamin, R.J., Madrigal, J.A., and Parham, P. 1991. Peptide binding to empty HLA-B17 molecule of viable human cells. Nature 351:74.
4. Zamvil, S.S., and Steinman, L. 1990. The T lymphocyte in experimental allergic encephalomyelitis. Annu. Rev. Immunol 8:579.
5. Steinamn, L. 1991. The development of rational strategies for selective immunotherapy against autoimmune demyelinating disease. Adv Immunol. 49:357.
6. Wraith, D.C., Smilek, D.E., Mitchell D.J., Steinman, L., and McDevitt H.O. 1989. Antigen recognition in autoimmune encephalomyelitis and the potential for peptide-mediated immunotherapy. Cell 59:247.
7. Schumacher, T.N.M., M. de Bruijn, M.L., Vernie, L.N., Kast, W.M., Melief, C.J., Neefjes, J.J., Ploegh, H.L. 1991. Peptide selection by MHC class I molecule. Nature 350:703.
8. Parham, P. 1991. Oh to be twenty seven again. Nature 351:523.
9. Brocke, S., Dayan, M., Steinman, L., Rothbard, J., and Mozes, E. 1990. Inhibition of T cell proliferation specific for acetylcholine receptor epitopes related to myasthenia gravis with antibody to T cell receptor or with competitive synthetic polymers. International Immunol. 2:735
10. Bornstein, M.B., Miller, A., Slagle, S., Drexler, E., Keilson, M., et al. 1987. A pilot trial of Copolymer I in exacerbating-remitting multiple sclerosis. N. Engl. J. Med. 317:408.
11. Lider, O. Reshef, T., Beraud, E., Ben-Nun, A., and Cohen, I.R. 1981. Anti-idiotypic network induced by T cell vaccination against experimental autoimmune encephalomyelitis. Science 239:181.
12. Howell, M.D., Winters, S.T., Olee, T., Powell, H.C., Carlo, D.J., and Brostoff, S.W. 1989. Vaccination against experimental allergic encephalomyelitis with T cell receptor peptides. Science 246:668.
13. Vandenbark, A.A., Hashim, G., and Offner, H. 1989 Immunization with a synthetic T cell receptor V region peptide protects against experimental autoimmune encephalomyelitis. Nature 341:541.
14. Ofner, H., Hashim, G., and Vandenbark, A.A.1991. T cell receptor peptide therapy triggers autoregulation of experimental encephalomyelitis. Science 251:430.
15. Ota, K., Matsui, M., Milford, E., Macking, G., Weiner, H.L., and Hafler, D.A. 1990. T cell recognition of an immunodominant myelin basic protein epitope in multiple sclerosis. Nature 346:183.
16. Wucherpfennig, K., Ota, N., Endo, N., Seidman J.G., Rosenzweig, A., Weiner, H.L., and Hafler, D.A. 1990. Shared human T cell receptor Vβ usage to immunodominant regions of myelin basic protein. Science 248:1016.
17. Martin, R., Howell, M.D., Jaraquemada, D., Flerlage, M., Richert, J., Brostoff, S., Long, E.O., McFarlin, D.E., and McFarland, H.E. 1991. A myelin a basic protein peptide is recognized in the context of four HLA-DR types associated with multiple sclerosis. J Exp. Med. 173:19.

18. Chou, Y.K., Henderikx, P., Vainiene, M., Whitman, R., Bourdette, D., Chou, C.H.J., Hashim, G., Offner, H., and Vandenbark, A.A. 1991. Specificity of human T cell clones reactive to immunodominant epitopes of myelin basic protein. J. Neurosc. Res. 28:280.
19. Kotzin, B., Satyanarayanas, S., Chou, Y.K., Lafferty, J., Forrester, J.M., Better, M., Nedwin, G.E., Offner, H., and Vandenbark, A.A. 1991. Preferential V beta usage in myelin basic protein reactive T cell clones from patients with multiple sclerosis. Proc. Natl. Acad. Sci. USA 88:9161.
20. Pette, M., Fujita, K., Kitze, B., Whitaker., J.N., Albert, E., Kappos, L., and Wekerle, H. 1990. Myelin basic protein-specific T lymphocyte lines from MS patients and healthy individuals. Neurology 40:1770.
21. Allegretta, M., Nicklas, J.A., Sriram, S., Albertini, R.J. 1990. T-Cells responsive to myelin basic protein in patients with multiple sclerosis. Science 47:718.
22. Oksenberg, J.R., Stuart, S., Begovich, A.B., Bell, R.B., Erlich, H.A., Steinman, L., and Bernard, C.C.A. 1990. Limited heterogeneity of rearranged T-cell receptor V alpha transcripts in brains of multiple sclerosis patients. Nature 345:344.
23. Waldor, M.K., Hardy, R., Herzenberg, L.A., Herzenberg, L.A., Lanier, L., Sriram, S., Lim, M., and Steinman, L. 1983. Reversal of EAE with monoclonal antibody to a T cell subset marker (L3T4). Science 227:415.
24. Brostoff, S.W., and Mason D.W. 1984. Experimental allergic encephalomyelitis: Successful treatment *in vivo* with a monoclonal antibody that recognizes T helper cells. J. Immunol. 133:1938.
25. Vollmer, T., Waldor, M.K., Steinman, L., and Conley, F. 1987. Depletion of T4+ lymphocytes reactivates toxoplasmosis in the central nervous system. J. Immunol. 138:3737.
26. Alpers, S., Sakai, K., Seinman, L., Oi, V.T. 1990. Mechanisms of anti CD4 mediated depletion and immunotherapy. A study using a set of chimeric anti-CD4 antibodies. J. Immunol. 144:4587.
27. Smilek, D.E., Lock, C.B., and McDevitt, H.O. 1990. Antigen recognition and peptide mediated immunotherapy in autoimmune disease. Immunol. Rev. 118:37.
28. Ben Nun, A., Liblau, R., Cohen, L., Lehman, D., Tournier-Lasserve, E., Rosenzweig, A., Jinwu, Z., Raus, J.C.M., and Bach, M. 1991. Restricted T cell receptor usage by myelin basic protein-specific T-cell clones in multiple sclerosis: Predominat genes vary in individuals. Proc. Natl. Acad. Sci. USA 88:2466.
29. Acha-Orbea, H., Mitchell, D.J., Timmerman, L., Wraith, D.C., Tausch, G.S., Waldor, M.K., Zamvil, S.S., McDevitt, H.O., and Seinman, L. 1988. Limited heterogeneity of T cell receptors from lymphocytes mediating autoimmune encephalomyelitis allows specific immune intervention. Cell 54:263.
30. Bell, R.B., and Steinamn, L. 1991. Trimolecular interactions in experimental autoimmunee demyelinating disease and prospects for immunotherapy. Seminars in Immunol. 3:408.

Synthesis of Allergens by Recombinant DNA Technology

Wayne R. Thomas, Kaw-Yan Chua*

In recent years cDNA encoding many of the major allergens has been cloned and used to provide invaluable information for the characterisation of allergens and synthesis of peptides. The clones also provide an opportunity to express the cDNA or modified cDNA in foreign hosts to produce practical quantities of clonally pure allergen or modified allergen. Most of the allergens expressed in bacteria to date have been expressed in a form showing strong reactivity with IgE. Some allergens such as *Der p* I have shown reduced reactivity, and strategies will be described which have developed products with improved IgE reactivity, approaching that of the natural allergen. T cell studies will increasingly benefit from the synthesis of recombinant products especially since the natural conformation is not an absolute requirement.

Importance of Sequence Analysis

The first step in the synthesis of an allergen or modified allergen by recombinant technology is sequence analysis. cDNA sequences can be used to define a prototype of an allergen, compare it with related allergens and locate homologies which can point to biological function and structure. An example of this is with *Der p* I from the house dust mite (1). The sequence revealed conserved residues forming the catalytic cleft of a family of thiol proteases which include actinidin and papain whose x-ray crystallographic structure has been determined. This also told us our cDNA clone lacked an N-terminal preproenzyme sequence of approximately 100 residues which we have now cloned both for *Der p* I and *Der f* I (2) and which could be important for folding. The sequence also supported evidence showing carbohydrate in purified *Der p* I. Both *Der p* I and *Der f* I retain the Asn X Ser/Thr motif at residues 52–54, although 5/9 bp of the codons have been changed only conserving those required to preserve the site. Further information from DNA analysis was that Southern hybridisation revealed hybridisable fragments of 2 Kb (1) indicating only one gene.

Other allergens have also shown homologies: *Bet v* I has homology to a disease resistance gene (3), *Dol m* V to a pathogenesis protein (4), *Fel d* I to uterglobulin (5), and *Candidia albicans* 40 Kd allergen to alcohol dehydrogenase (6), while *Chi t* I is chironomid haemoglobin (7). Recently *Bet v* II was found to be profilin (8), a conserved protein associated with actin, and *Der f* and *p* III are serine proteases (9). Homology between *Mus m* I and rat alpha 2 u globulin has also led to peptide studies with T cell clones (10). Sequence homology is useful in considering cross reactivity. One example is the group V-like grass allergens where sequences of rye (11) and Kentucky blue grass (12) show strong homology and also with the N-terminal of timothy group V (13). In keeping with Western data (11,13,14) the sequences show a family of molecules. A family has also been found for *Amb a* I (15,16), so decisions have to be made about which sequence to express.

Synthesis of Recombinant Allergens

Many allergens have been cloned, and most show high IgE binding activity (Table 1). Constructs of *Amb a* I and *Der p* I have had low IgE binding, but now better expressions of

* The Western Australian Research Institute for Child Health, GPO Box D184, Perth, Western Australia 6001.
Acknowledgements: This work was supported by grants from the National Health and Medical Research Foundation, the Asthma Foundation of Western Australia, and Immulogic Pharmaceutical Corporation, Cambridge.

Table 1. IgE binding of recombinant allergens

Good	Poor
Der p II	*Der p* I
Der f II	*Der f* I
Lol p I	*Amb a* I
Lol p (V)	*Fel d* I (?)
Amb a V	
Poa p IX (V)	
Bet v I	
Bet v II	
Amb a II	
Car b I	
HDM 14K	

Der p I have been developed. *Dol m* V (4) and *Bet v* I and II (17) have been expressed by the plasmid pKK223-3. The birch allergens had IgE reactivity in 100 different sera, reacting to all with antibody to the natural allergens. Studies with *Der p* II (18) similarly have shown that the allergen produced as a fusion with glutathione-S-transferase from the pGEX vector has most of the IgE binding activity of the natural *Der p* II. Another allergen, KGB 7.2, was expressed as a fusion with beta galactosidase in pWR 590 (14). The fusion was insoluble, but when isolated in 0.1% SDS could bind IgE in all 5 allergic sera tested and stimulated lymphocyte proliferation.

Much of our work on the synthesis of allergens has been performed with *Der p* I. Fusions from pGEX with mature allergen sequences react with IgE in about 50% of sera. Full preproenzyme sequences have been cloned although evaluation of the synthesis from these molecules is very incomplete. In the attempt to circumvent problems with folding, a series of cDNA fragments was constructed to express large peptides which could be used for epitope analysis. Perhaps certain structures expressed by themselves would have high antigenicity. IgE reactivity with fusion peptides was found across the whole molecule but only for sera which also reacted with the whole recombinant molecule. Reactions to peptides 53–99, 57–130, 98–140 and 101–150 were often as strong as those to the whole recombinant (19). The region containing these peptides interestingly corresponds largely to an outside loop connecting the domains. Although experiments with the expression from the preproenzyme continue, there is evidence that it is not required for folding. DNA encoding the mature *Der p* I was cloned into a metallothionein cassette in a yeast vector pYELC5 where it was expressed at 40 mg/ml of insoluble protein with an extra 5 N terminal residues from the vector (20). This protein was soluble in urea and remained in solution when dialysed against a physiological buffer. Some of this could be isolated by affinity chromatography and used to show IgE reactivity to 9/11 sera and removed much of IgE to native *Der p* I by absorption. Attempts are now being continued to develop more practical methods. Perhaps the area to benefit most from recombinant allergens is T cells. Since they recognize processed peptides the need for correct folding is less important.

Complexities and Conclusions

The obvious advance from molecular cloning has been the generation of sequences to define allergens and to synthesize peptides for T cell studies. A related use has been the provision of allergen to maintain and verify T cell clones. The introduction of recombinant allergens for diagnosis awaits the demonstration that cocktails or panels of pure allergens will be useful. Since the battery of recombinant allergens is increasing, advances in this area can be expected. Similarly, purified allergens are required for the measurement of lymphokines in T cell studies. New initiatives in genetically modified allergen can also be expected. There are, of course, some problems such as suitable expression systems for multichain allergens. Problems of secondary modification of protein remain and are highlighted by the *Phl p* V which has a large number of hydroxyprolines (13). This also shows the continued need for amino acid sequencing because the prolines of the equivalent sequence from rye grass are not modified (11). An important problem is presented by the sequence polymorphisms. Even for different *Der p* I cDNA from a commercial culture different clones contain a number of changes which could affect T cell epitopes and the relationship of these to ones in the environment needs to be determined.

References

1. Chua, K.Y., Stewart, G.A., Thomas, W.R., Simpson, R.J., Dilworth, R.J., Plozza, T.M., and Turner, K.J. 1988. Sequence analysis of cDNA coding for a major house dust mite allergen, *Der* p I, homology with cysteine proteases. J. Exp. Med. 167:175.
2. Dilworth, R.J., Chua, K.Y., and Thomas, W.R. 1991. Sequence analysis of cDNA coding for a major house dust mite allergen *Der f* I. Clin. Exp. Allergy 21:25.
3. Breiteneder, H., Pettenburger, K., Bito, A., Valenta, R., Kraft, D., Rumpold, H., Scheiner, O., and Breitenbach, M. 1989. The gene coding for the major birch pollen allergen *Bet v* I is highly homologous to a pea disease resistance response gene. EMBO J. 8:1935.
4. Fang, K.F.S., Vitale, P., Fehler, P., and King, T.P. 1988. cDNA cloning and primary structure of a white-faced hornet venom allergen. Proc. Nat. Acad. Sci. 85:895.
5. Morgenstern, J.P., Griffith, I.J., Brauer, A.W., Pollock, J., Rogers, B.L., Yu, X-B., Burke, C.M., Chapman, M.D., and Kuo, M-C. 1991. Determination of the amino acid sequence and cDNA cloning of the major allergen of the domestic cat *Fel d* I J. Allergy Clin. Immunol. 87:327.
6. Shen, H-D., Choo, K-B., Lee, H-H., Hsieh, J-C., Lin, W-L., Lee, W-R., and Han, S-H. 1991. The 40 kilodalton allergen of *Candida albicans* is an alcohol dehydrogenase: molecular cloning and immunological analysis using monoclonal antibodies. Clin. Exp. Allergy 21:675.
7. Baur, X., Aschauer, H., Majur, G., Dewair, M., Preling, H., and Steigemann, W. 1986. Structure, antigenic determinants of some clinically important insect allergens: *Chironomid hemoglobins*. Science 351:233.
8. Valenta, R., Duchene, M., Pettenburger, K., Sillaber, C., Valent P., Bettelheim, P., Breitenbach, M., Rumpold, H., Kraft, D., and Schiener, O. 1991. Identification of profilin as a novel pollen allergen; IgE-autoreactivity in sensitised individuals. Science 253:557.
9. Stewart, G.A., Thompson, P.J., and Simpson, R.J. 1989. Protease antigens from the house dust mite. Lancet II:154 and Lancet 2:462 (correction).
10. Gurka, G., Ohman, J.L., and Rossenwasser, L.J. 1989. Allergen specific human T cell clones. J. Allergy Clin. Immunol. 83:945.
11. Singh, M.B., Hough, T., Theerakulpisut, P., Avjioglu, A., Davies, S., Smith, P.M., Taylor P., Simpson, R.J., Ward, L.D., McCluskey, J., Puy, R., and Knox, R.B. 1991. Isolation of cDNA encoding a newly identified major allergenic protein of rye-grass pollen: Intracellular targetting to the amyloplast. Proc. Natl. Acad. Sci. 88:1384.
12. Silvanovich, A., Astwood, J., Zhang, L., Olsen E., Kisch, F., Sehon, A., Mohapatra, S., and Hill, R. 1991. Nucleotide sequence analysis of three cDNAs coding for *Poa p* IX isoallergens of Kentucky blue grass pollen. J. Biol. Chem. 266:1204.
13. Matthiesen, F., and Lowenstein, H. 1991. Group V allergens in grass pollens. I. Purification and characterization of the group V allergen from *Phleum pratense* pollen *Phl p* V. Clin. Exp. Allergy. 21:297.
14. Yang, M., Olsen, E., Dolovich, J., Sehon, A.H., Mahapatra, S.S. 1991. Immulogic characterisation of a recombinant Kentucky blue grass (*Poa pratensis*) allergenic peptide. J. Allergy Clin. Immunol. 87:1096.
15. Bond, J.F., Garman, R.D., Keating, K.M., Briner, T.J., Rafnar, T., Klapper, D.G., and Roges, B.L. 1991. Multiple *Amb a* I allergens demonstrate specific reactivity with IgE and T cells from ragweed-allergic patients. J. Immunol. 146:3380.
16. Rafnar, T., Griffith, I.J., Kuo, M-C., Bond, J.F., Rogers, B.L., Klapper, D.G. 1991. Cloning of *Amb a* I (antigen E), the major allergen family of short ragweed pollen. J. Biol. Chem. 266:1229.
17. Valenta, R., Duchene, M., Vrtala, S., Birkner, T., Ebner, C., Hirschwehr, H., Brietenbach, M., Rumpold, H., Scheiner, O., and Kraft, D. 1991. Recombinant allergens for immunoblot diagnosis of tree pollen allergy. J. Allergy Clin. Immunol. 88:889.
18. Chua, K.Y., Dilworth, R.J., and Thomas, W.R. 1990. Expression of *Dermatophagoides pteronyssinus* allergen *Der p* II in *Escherichia coli* and binding studies with human IgE. Int. Arch. Allergy Appl. Immunol. 91:124.
19. Greene, W.K., Cyster, J.G., Chua, K-Y., O'Brien, R.M., and Thomas, W.R. 1991. IgE and IgG binding peptides expressed from fragments of cDNA encoding the major house dust mite allergen *Der p* I. J. Immunol. 147:3768.
20. Chua, K-Y., Kehal, P.K., Thomas, W.R., Vaughan, P.R., and Macreadie, I.G. 1992. High frequency binding of IgE to the *Der p* I allergen expressed in yeast. J. Clin. Allergy Immunol. 89:95.

Anti-IgE Autoantibodies: A Functional Comparison with Heterologous Antibodies

Beda M. Stadler, Sylvia Miescher, Monique Vogel, Kazuhito Furukawa, Ivan Aebischer, Martin R. Stämpfli, Mirjam E. Holzner, Yu Yan, Qiu Gang*

Several new approaches have enabled a clearer characterization of the epitope specificity as well as the biological function of anti-IgE autoantibodies. We have produced recombinant IgE peptides consisting of whole immunoglobulin domains. Such immunoglobulin domains were very useful for determining IgE binding sites for Fcϵ receptor I or II as well as for epitope mapping of monoclonal anti-IgE and anti-IgE autoantibodies. Our recent progress in understanding the events that lead to isotype switching at the molecular level also provides new tools to study *in vitro* IgE de novo synthesis by measuring IgE mRNA levels rather than the IgE protein itself. Finally, it is hoped that with the antibody repertoire cloning technique it will be possible to generate human recombinant autoantibodies that react directly with IgE. Depending on the clones obtained it will be possible to define functional subtypes of anti-IgE autoantibodies that may eventually be used for therapy of allergic diseases.

During the last 20 years, many different groups have reported the presence of anti-IgE autoantibodies in sera of patients with different diseases (1–5). More recently we have invested much effort to determine precisely anti-IgE autoantibodies and to study their biological activities (6–9). From this work it can be concluded that anti-IgE determinations are at best crude estimations, and also that their levels are usually lower than IgE serum levels (10). The important question in this context that remains to be solved is whether such autoantibodies against IgE play a role *in vivo*. In this respect it has become clear that autoantibodies must be classified into different subtypes. We have tried to classify autoantibodies according to their epitope specificity. Still, this approach neglects the question whether the isotype itself of the autoantibodies may play a crucial role.

In Vivo Role of Anti-IgE Autobodies

Occurrence and Clinical Correlation of Anti-IgE Autoantibodies

The fact that one may detect anti-IgE autoantibodies in patient's sera is not yet an argument that such antibodies also play a role *in vivo*. However, in some bee venom allergic individuals with low IgE levels we have found elevated anti-IgE autoantibody levels (Y. Yan et al., manuscript submitted). This may suggest that IgE was effectively present but immunologically hidden within immunocomplexes consisting of IgE and anti-IgE antibodies (9). Or one may also speculate that these autoantibodies did not effectively neutralize the IgE, as the patients still suffered from their allergies. Similarly, we have found elevated anti-IgE levels in non-atopic asthmatic children (10). When comparing the estimated levels of anti-IgE/IgE immunocomplexes in the atopic and the nonatopic child populations, we even found identical levels of immunocomplexes, again suggesting that IgE has been hidden immunologically but not neutralized.

In Vitro Effects of Anti-IgE Autoantibodies

Many findings obtained during the last years with anti-IgE autoantibodies have not been explained. For example, we found autoantibodies to IgE that removed IgE from the surface of CD23 positive cells (11). But we also found anti-IgE preparations that enhanced the binding of IgE to CD23 positive cells. Mediator release from human basophils shows clear evidence of antibodies that are either anaphylac-

* Institute of Clinical Immunology, University of Bern, Inselspital, 3010 Bern, Switzerland.
Acknowledgement: This work was supported in part by Swiss National Science Foundation grant numbers 31-27567.89 and 32-28660.90.

togenic or may even inhibit sensitization with IgE or subsequent triggering with other anti-IgE antibodies (7,8). Such *in vitro* data imply that there is a need to define more precisely the different types of anti-IgE autoantibodies. By using different *in vitro* models we intended, therefore, to address the question of whether the different functional types of autoantibodies may be defined via their epitope specificity.

In Vitro Systems for Evaluating Anti-IgE Autoantibody Activities

Production of Recombinant IgE Peptides

Either synthetic or recombinant IgE peptides have been produced by different laboratories. To preserve the immunogenicity of IgE peptides we have generated whole immunoglobulin domains by recombinant technology instead of linear sequences. The reason for this approach was our intention to use these peptides for specificity mapping of anti-IgE autoantibodies. As B cells will only recognize native antigen the chance for an antibody interaction with a linear peptide would be minimal or even accidental. Our constructs of IgE peptides include either all four epsilon heavy chain domains, or the CϵH2 to CϵH4, the CϵH3 to CϵH4 or the CϵH4 domain alone. As discussed below, these recombinant peptides maintained most but not all antigenic properties of native IgE.

Monoclonal Anti-IgE Antibodies

As monoclonal antibodies against IgE may be a good model for anti-IgE autoantibodies, we tested whether the recombinant epsilon peptides would be recognized by a large panel of IgE specific monoclonal antibodies. We found monoclonal antibodies against each of the four epsilon domains. Still, there were also antibodies, e. g. BSW17 (12), which recognized only the CϵH3 to CϵH4 peptide and not the longer ones or CϵH4 suggesting that some antibodies recognize delicate conformational structures that are not present in some recombinant peptides even though the same domain was present. Interestingly, some antibodies that recognized such sensitive quaternary structures also did not recognize 100% of a purified myeloma IgE protein when used in radioimmunoassays. This now opens the possibility that IgE assays can be produced that will discriminate between "denatured" and "native" IgE. Natural anti-IgE autoantibodies seemed to recognize preferentially the CϵH3 or the CϵH4 domains. But as long as it is not known whether the CϵH1 and CϵH2 domains are in their native structure such observations may only be an artifact.

IgE Receptor Binding Assays

Using the RPMI 8866 cell line we studied IgE binding to the low affinity IgE receptor CD23 (13). Here we could clearly show that the CϵH3 domain was involved in binding to CD23. More interestingly, the amount of IgE that was needed for cold competition of IgE binding was related directly to the immunogenicity of IgE as determined by monoclonal antibodies that recognized the sensitive quaternary structures on IgE, suggesting that denatured IgE would not bind to CD23. Furthermore, as the recombinant proteins are not glycosylated it seems that sugar moieties do not play a role in the interaction with this receptor.

By using monoclonal antibodies against the CϵH3 domain we could also completely inhibit the binding of IgE to CD23. In contrast, antibodies against the CϵH2 domain enhanced binding of IgE to CD23 positive cells. Thus, by using the recombinant IgE peptides and characterized human monoclonal antibodies against IgE we were able to exactly reproduce our previous finding with natural autoantibodies. They also fell into two different classes, namely antibodies that could remove IgE from the surface of CD23 positive cells or bind more to the cell surface.

The binding of IgE to the FcϵRI on human basophils seems more complex than the interactions with CD23. Among a panel of approximately 20 anti-IgE monoclonal antibodies, we have so far found only one antibody that was not capable of triggering histamine release (BSW17). This antibody recognizes IgE within the CϵH3 domain. Interestingly, other antibodies that also recognize the CϵH3 domain are capable of triggering histamine release. BSW17 is probably not anaphylactogenic because it prevents the binding of IgE to human basophils. Again our preliminary findings show that the amount of IgE that is needed to sensitize is directly related to the amount of immunogenic IgE and not to the protein concentration. This indicates that some of the antibodies that recognize delicate quaternary structures may actually recognize a heat labile epitope that characterized IgE and may be involved in binding to FcεRI.

IgE Class Switching

There is evidence in the literature (14) and from our studies that anti-IgE autoantibodies may also be involved as a feedback regulatory moiety in the synthesis of IgE. Until recently the major problem was the necessary addition of antibodies against IgE. This would mean that for studying the effect of the anti-IgE one would have to rule out that the added anti-IgE will not mask IgE and prevents its determination. Now the question of the effect of autoantibodies on IgE synthesis can be addressed by determining the IgE mRNA levels. Earlier we showed that human PBL produce a truncated genomic transcript soon after stimulation and that the coding mRNA is only found later on in culture concomitantly with the measurable IgE protein in the supernatant (15). This 1.75 Kb truncated mRNA has attracted some interest since it may be involved in isotype switching. So far we have only been able to switch cells to IgE synthesis if this genomic transcript was found beforehand in the cells. Recently, we have also found two macrophage cell lines that express this genomic epsilon mRNA. The sequence of this macrophage mRNA was identical with the 1.75 Kb RNA in normal human B cells (16). Future studies will show whether the production of this mRNA in macrophages is only a curiosity or whether differences in the promotor region may be found between the different cell types.

Repertoire Cloning

It has become clear that autoantibodies exhibit different biological activities. Now it is possible to find all the types of anti-IgE antibodies as autoantibodies that have previously been obtained by immunizing animals with IgE. Thus, the total measurement of anti-IgE autoantibody levels may not be very meaningful as one should also have the information on the biological properties of the different autoantibodies. Presently we are using the methodology of repertoire cloning to produce a whole variety of different recombinant autoantibodies.

We have generated a combinatorial library of light and heavy chain immunoglobulins that can be expressed in E. coli to produce Fab antibodies. Approximately 80% of the clones produce variable amounts of Fab antibodies that are presently being screened for specificity. It is hoped that this approach will deliver several answers. One can plausibly argue that individuals will show different profiles of autoantibodies concerning their epitope specificity and it may be possible to compare the frequency of autoantibodies to the frequency of antibodies against strong immunogens and eventually other autoantibodies. Finally, this recombinant technology will allow us to produce larger amounts of recombinant autoantibodies that may eventually be of therapeutic use.

Conclusions

Our *in vitro* data have demonstrated that autoantibodies can perform most of the biological functions *in vitro* that have been described previously by using heterologous antibodies including monoclonal anti-IgE antibodies. This demonstrates that autoantibodies are as potent as heterologous anti-IgE antibodies. The difficulty now remains to establish whether, e.g., an anaphylactogenic autoantibody will perform its anaphylactogenic activity *in vivo* or whether its activity will be inhibited by the presence of other anti-IgE autoantibodies that are, e.g., blocking anti-IgE autoantibodies. Thus, it may be that the epitope specificity of anti-IgE autoantibodies, i.e., the profile or phenotype, is more relevant than the absolute amounts. If it could be established whether the biological function relates to the epitope specificity of an anti-IgE antibody, then one may be able to construct assays to measure only relevant anti-IgE autoantibodies in serum. A major handicap in determining anti-IgE antibodies in serum is that immunological assays still have to be used. If anti-IgE antibodies bind to solid phase IgE which are then developed by monoclonal anti-IgG antibodies, sufficient controls can usually be established to be sure that an antibody has been measured. But this type of assay still cannot distinguish between panspecific anti-immunoglobulin antibodies and isotype specific anti-IgE antibodies. Also, the antibody that attaches to the IgE may be within an immunocomplex. Thus, our studies indicate that the measurement of denatured versus native IgE may be just as important as the measurement of neutralizing versus inert anti-IgE antibodies that will not block the biological activity of IgE.

References

1. Carini, C., Fratazzi, C., and Barbato, M. 1988. IgG autoantibody to IgE in atopic patients. Ann. Allergy 60:48.
2. Koike, T., Tsutsumi, A., Nawata, Y., Tomioka, H. and Yoshida, S. 1989. Prevalence and role of IgG anti-IgE autoantibody in allergic disorders. Monogr. Allergy 26:165.
3. Magnusson, C.G., and Vaerman, J.P. 1986. Autoantibodies of the IgM class against a human myeloma protein IgE (DES). I. Occurrence. Int. Arch. Allergy Appl. Immunol. 79:149.
4. Marshall, J.S., Prout, S.J., Jaffery, G., and Bell, E.B. 1987. Induction of an auto-anti-IgE response in rats. II. Effects on mast cell populations. Eur. J. Immunol. 17:445.
5. Paganelli, R., Quinti, I.D., Offizi, G.P., Papetti, C., Nisini, R., and Aiuti, F. 1988. Studies on the *in vitro* effects of auto-anti-IgE. Inhibition of total and specific serum IgE detection by a human IgG autoantibody to IgE. J. Clin. Lab. Immunol. 26:153.
6. Stadler, B.M., Nakajima, K., Yang, X., and de Weck, A.L. 1989. Potential role of anti-IgE antibodies *in vivo*. Prog. Int. Arch. Allergy Appl. Immunol. 88:206.
7. Stadler, B.M., Gauchat, D., Vassella, C., Nakajima, K., Qiu G., and Gauchat, J.-F. 1989. Anti-isotype regulation: Cytokines and anti-IgE autoantibodies. In: Cytokines regulating the allergic response, 2. ed.. C. Sorg ed. Basel: Karger, p. 37.
8. Stadler, B.M., Qiu, G., Vogel, M., Jarolim, E., Miescher, S., Aebischer, I., and de Weck, A.L. 1990. IgG anti-IgE autoantibodies in immunomodulation. In molecular and cell networks in allergy and clinical immunology. Int. Arch. Allergy. Appl. Immunol. Karger Verlag, in press.
9. Vassella, C.C., de Weck, A.L., and Stadler, B.M. 1990. Natural anti-IgE antibodies interfere with diagnostic IgE determination. Clin. Exp. Allergy 20:295.
10. Ritter, C., Bättig, M., Kraemer, R., and Stadler, B.M. 1991. IgE hidden in immune complexes with anti-IgE autoantibodies in children with asthma. J. All. Clin. Immunol., in press.
11. Nakajima, K., de Weck, A.L., and Stadler, B.M. 1989. Effect of anti-IgE antibodies on IgE binding to CD23. Allergy. 44:187.
12. Knutti-Müller, J.M., Stadler, B.M., Magnusson, C.M., and de Weck, A.L. 1986. Human IgE synthesis *in vitro*. Detection with monoclonal antibodies. Allergy 41:457.
13. Delespesse, G., Hofstetter, H., and Sarfati, M. 1989. Low-affinity receptor for IgE (FcεRII, CD23) and its soluble fragments. Int. Arch. Allergy Appl. Immunol. 90 Suppl 1:41.
14. Sherr, E.H., and Saxon, A. 1987. A mechanism for the suppression of ongoing IgE synthesis. Int. Arch. Allergy Appl. Immunol. 82:14.
15. Qiu, G., Gauchat, J.-F., Vogel, M., Mandallaz, M., de Weck, A.L., and Stadler, B.M. 1990. Human IgE mRNA expression by peripheral blood lymphocytes stimulated with interleukin 4 and pokeweed mitogen. Eur. J. Immunol. 20:2191.
16. Gauchat, J.-F., Lebman, D.A., Coffman, R.L., Gascan, H., and de Vries, J.E. 1990. Structure and expression of germline epsilon transcripts in human B cells induced by interleukin 4 to switch to IgE production. J. Exp. Med. 172:463.

Development of New Vaccines

Ruth Arnon*

Two new approaches for vaccine development are described. The first is based on synthetic peptides which comprise relevant epitope(s) of the disease-causing agent. The second approach is based on recombinant DNA technology, employing synthetic oligonucleotides which code for relevant peptide epitopes. The peptides corresponding to the regions 8–20 and 50–64 of the B subunit, of *Cholera toxin*, when conjugated to tetanus toxin, induced neutralizing antibodies against the native toxin as well as against the homologous heat labile toxin of toxigenic *E. coli*. In the case of *Shiga toxin*, several peptides from the amino- and carboxy-termini of the B-chain, in macromolcular conjugates or polymers, led to efficient systemic and local immunity, manifested in both neutralizing antibodies and *in vivo* protection of the mice and rats against the detrimental effects of the toxin. Expression of these peptides as recombinant products led to similar protective effects. A peptide corresponding to the sequence 91–108 of *influenza haemagglutinin*, conjugated to tetanus toxoid, elicited antibodies which reacted with several strains of H3 influenza virus and neutralized their biological functions. Mice immunized with this conjugate were partially protected against infection. Furthermore, coupling of muramyl-dipeptide (MDP) to this conjugate led to a synthetic vaccine with built-in adjuvanticity. A synthetic recombinant vaccine, in which this epitope was expressed in *Salmonella flagellin*, induced partial protection by intranasal immunization without the aid of adjuvant.

This presentation describes two new approaches for vaccine preparation, namely the use of synthetic peptides which constitute relevant protective epitopes, and employment of synthetic oligonucleotides coding for such peptides as synthetic "genes" in recombinant DNA-technology. In earlier studies we demonstrated that synthetic antigens containing immunoreactive region(s) of a protein can give rise to a specific, and often conformation-dependent, immune response towards the intact protein (1). When the protein in question was a component of a virus, e. g. the coat protein of MS-2 coliphage, the antibodies induced by a synthetic peptide fragment were capable of neutralizing the viability of the phage (2). These findings paved the way for the use of synthetic peptides as the basis for vaccine design (3), as demonstrated in the following for three systems: the influenza virus and the bacterial toxins of Cholera and Shigella.

Vaccines Based on Synthetic Peptides

Cholera Toxin

The toxin of *Vibrio cholerae* is composed of two subunits, A and B. Subunit A activates adenylate cyclase, which triggers the biological activity, whereas subunit B is responsible for binding to cell receptors. The B subunit expresses most of the immunopotent determinants, and antibodies against it are capable of neutralizing the biological activity of the intact toxin. We have synthesized nine peptides, corresponding to various regions of the B subunit and coupled them to tetanus toxoid (TT). All the conjugates elicited antibodies against the respective homologous peptides, some of which reacted also, to different extents, with the intact B subunit and with the native cholera toxin (4). Of most interest among these peptides were CTP 1 (residues 8 to 20) and CTP 3 (residues 50 to 64), which elicited antibodies that inhibited the biological activities of cholera toxin (i. e., the fluid accumulation in ligated small intestinal loops, as well as the induction of adenylate cyclase). The inhibitory effect of the antipeptide sera manifested in these assays reached inhibition values of 60 to 70% (5). It is noteworthy that the synthetic peptides as such did not cause any

---

* Department of Chemical Immunology, The Weizmann Institute of Science, Rehovot, Israel.
Acknowledgements: This work was supported in part by Grant No. 2860/88 from the Israel Council for Research and Development, and Grant No. DAMD 17-90-Z-0015 from the U.S. Army.

toxic or other biological side effect, which is a crucial consideration in the evaluation of their possible suitability for vaccine preparation.

In view of the high level of sequence homology between the B subunits of the cholera toxin (CT) and the heat labile toxin of *E. coli* (LT), and the immunological relationship between the two toxins (6), we studied the cross-reactivity of the synthetic peptides with LT. This is of importance since the LT of pathogenic strains of *E. coli* is the causative agent of diarrhea in many tropical countries and due to its wide spread, it presents probably a more serious health problem than cholera. Indeed, the antiserum elicited by CTP 3 and to a lesser extent by CTP 1 were cross-reactive with native LT of multiple strains of human and porcine *E. coli*. Moreover, these antisera, which are inhibitory towards CT, were found equally effective in neutralizing the biological activity of the *E. coli* LT (7). This indicates that synthetic peptides may serve as a basis for a general vaccine against the coli-cholera family of diarrheal diseases.

Shiga Toxin

Vaccination against *Shigella* species, to prevent shigellosis, presents a number of problems, and as a consequence no efficient shigella vaccine is available as yet. In addition to the invasive properties of the organism, the various species of *Shigella* produce a protein toxin, which experimentally reproduces the major features of the infection (8). Shiga toxin (ST), isolated from *Shigella dysenteriae 1* strains, is one of the most potent of the lethal microbial toxins. Similarly to CT it consists of A and B subunits. Antibodies raised against the B subunit were shown to neutralize the cytotoxic effects of the toxin (9), and hence this subunit was the subject of our investigation.

According to the amino acid sequence (10), as well as the hydrophilicity and surface residues patterns, we synthesized several peptides of the B chain, corresponding to its amino and carboxy terminal regions, and conjugated them to macromolecular carriers. Rabbit antisera raised against all the conjugates or against polymerized peptides were highly reactive with the respective homologous peptides and cross-reacted with the native Shiga toxin. More significantly, the antisera showed considerable neutralizing capacity (60%–80%) against all three biological effects of the toxin, namely cytotoxicity towards HeLa cells, enterotoxic activity as measured by fluid secretion into ligated intestinal loops of rats, as well as the neurotoxic lethal effect in mice (11). Not only were antisera induced by the various peptides capable of neutralizing the different activities of the toxin, but active immunization of mice and rats with the peptide conjugates led to partial protection against the detrimental effects of the Shiga toxin. Thus, for example, in mice immunized with the conjugates of the peptides and exposed to lethal dose of toxin, the results show up to 80% long-term survival.

In shigellosis, like in all other enteric diseases, the intestinal area is the site of the first encounter with the infectious agent, as well as where the toxin is secreted and exerts its detrimental effect. Hence, we investigated whether local immunity by intragastric immunization will lead to neutralization of the toxic effect *in-situ*. The local immunity in the gut is usually assessed in animal models, either rabbits or rats, by determination of the IgA level. Indeed, we have shown that oral immunization of rats with the synthetic peptide conjugates by intragastric feeding, following priming by parenteral immunization, led to elevation of specific IgA antibodies (12). Furthermore, the immunized rats manifested significant protection against the enterotoxic effect of Shiga toxin. These findings indicate that synthetic peptides vaccines are capable of inducing both systemic and local immunity.

Influenza

The presently available influenza vaccines consist of either attenuated or inactivated viral particles. Their effectiveness is only partial and of short duration, mainly due to the frequent antigenic variation of the external glycoproteins of the virus (13), each new strain presenting a new challenge to the host immune system. The two major antigenic components of influenza virus are the haemagglutinin and the nucleoprotein. The haemagglutinin (HA), towards which the neutralizing anti-viral antibodies are directed, occurs as trimeric spikes projecting from the viral proteolipid envelope. It is quantitatively the most important glycoprotein in the viral surface, and undergoes frequent genetic variations, denoted "shifts" and "drifts".

We have studied several synthetic peptides of the HA molecule, all of which proved immunoreactive (14,15). The most effective peptide consisted of 18 amino acid residues corresponding to the sequence 91–108 of the HA molecule. This region, which is common to at least twelve H3 strains, although not overlapping with any of the antigenic sites proposed by Wiley et al. (16), was computer-predicted to be immunologically reactive. Hence, we deliberately chose it for our study since, being part of a conserved sequence, we believed that it would lead to a broad specificity immune response. Indeed, a conjugate of this peptide with tetanus toxoid elicited in both rabbits and mice antibodies that reacted with the synthetic peptide, as well as with the intact influenza virus of several type A H3 strains. These antibodies caused haemagglutination inhibition and also interfered with the *in vitro* growth of the virus in tissue culture. Furthermore, mice immunized with the peptide conjugate were partially protected against challenge infection with several H3 strains of the virus (14).

The above results were achieved by immunization in complete Freund's adjuvant (CFA), which is a very effective adjuvant evoking high level and long lasting immunity, but is not suitable for human use. To explore the possibility of replacing the CFA by a less harmful substance, we have employed the synthetic adjuvant MDP (N-acetyl-muramyl-L-alanyl-D-isoglutamine) (17). Our findings show that in a conjugate with the 91–108 peptides, this adjuvant was similar to CFA in the induction of antibodies specific towards the peptide. As for the cross-reactivity with the intact virus, although the antibody level was rather low, immunization with this covalent conjugate led to a high protection level against *in vivo* viral challenge, even higher than that induced in the presence of CFA (18). It should be emphasized that this conjugate of the synthetic peptide and MDP with tetanus toxoid is water soluble and was administered in a physiological aqueous solution and hence constitutes a synthetic vaccine with built-in adjuvanticity, which could be suitable for use in humans.

Synthetic Recombinant Vaccines Based on Oligonucleotides

An alternative approach to the chemical synthesis of vaccines is the use of genetic engineering. This technology is used for insertion of genes into expression vectors, for the biosynthesis of intact proteins. We attempted to bridge the synthetic and recombinant DNA approaches with regard to the three systems investigated in our laboratory, namely, the cholera toxin peptide CTP 3, the N-terminal and C-terminal regions of the Shiga toxin, as well as the epitope 91–108 of influenza haemagglutinin. Our working hypothesis was that the expression of such peptides by recombinant bacteria may lead to appropriate agents for induction of immunity towards the intact toxins or infectious virus.

In the case of cholera toxin, two plasmids containing a synthetic "gene" coding for CTP 3 (residues 50 to 64 in the amino acid sequence of cholera toxin B subunit), were prepared and inserted in phase into the gene coding for *E. coli* β-galactosidase. The resulting fusion protein, which was expressed by the two vectors, reacted with antibodies against β-galactosidase, as well as with antibodies against CTP 3 and, though to a much lesser extent, with antibodies against intact CT. Immunization with the fusion protein by itself did not lead to a significant titer of antibodies recognizing CT. However, when followed by a booster injection of a minute amount of CT, or the *E. coli* LT, too small to provide any immune response by itself, it led to a substantial level of neutralizing antibodies (19).

In the case of the Shiga toxin, several plasmids were prepared, with insertion of synthetic oligonucleotides coding for two N-terminal peptides (corrsponding to residues 9–21 and 19–31, respectively), and/or the carboxy terminal peptide (residues 54–67) in the amino acid sequence of the B subunit. These vectors were used for transfection of either *E. coli* K12, or the non-virulent mutant of *Salmonella dublin*, SL 1438. The bacteria expressed the respective peptides as fusion proteins either with β-galactosidase (in *E. coli*) or in flagellin (in *Salmonella*). Rabbits immunized with the partially

Allergy Treatment with a Peptide Vaccine

D. R. Stanworth*

In their contributions to this volume, Ruth Arnon describes the development of peptide vaccines for protection against viral and bacterial infective agents, and Dr Oksenberg details attempts to develop immunogenic peptides for the treatment of autoimmune diseases. In contrast, I describe the work we have been undertaking in our Unit towards the development of a peptide vaccine capable of abrogating IgE-mediated allergies of the asthma-hay fever type.

Our early PK-inhibition studies, using cleavage fragments of the first myeloma form of IgE to be discovered (1), demonstrated the presence of Fc receptors for this immunoglobulin on mast cells, while more recently we have exploited both synthetic peptides representative of short chain Fc sequences, and antibodies raised against these, to probe in much more detail into the molecular pathology of IgE. For instance, we employed this approach to demonstrate that rat IgE binds to the Fc(ε)RI receptor on rat peritoneal mast cells via sites within both the CH3 and CH4 domains (2,3) and obtained experimental evidence to suggest that such sites located in only one of the two identical Fc limbs of the immunoglobulin molecule are involved in mast cell binding. Whereas an analogous approach, employing synthetic peptides representative of human IgE Fc sequences and antibodies raised against these, has revealed that the immunoglobulin binds to the low affinity Fc(ε)RII on human B lymphocytes via sites restricted to the CH3 domain (4), possibly explaining the weaker binding affinity for this receptor.

Just one of the human IgE Fc peptides thus examined, comprising the CH4 domain sequence 497–506, proved capable of stimulating human tonsillar B cells which had not been prior treated with phorbol ester. And, significantly, this peptide alone of the many tested was shown by FACS analysis to behave like IL-4 in up-regulating the expression of the Fc(ε)RII on B cells. It is probably not fortuitous therefore that this same human Cε4 domain sequence has been shown, from studies to be outlined in the next section, to be responsible for providing a direct triggering signal to mast cells during their immunological stimulation.

Identification of a Mast Cell Trigger Site Within the CH4 Domain of Human IgE

It was assumed that histamine releasing polypeptides, such as melittin and ACTH 1–24, act directly on mast cells by short-circuiting the two stage IgE antibody-antigen (allergen) stimulatory process (illustrated in Fig. 1). Consequently by performing structure-activity studies on melittin cleavage fragments and ACTH analogues, employing purified rat peritoneal mast cells *in vitro*, it proved possible to predict the likely amino acid sequence of a mast cell trigger site within the Fc region of human IgE. Only one stretch within the CH4 domain of the human IgE myeloma protein "ND" appeared to possess all the primary structural credentials necessary for mast cell triggering as thus defined.

Octa-, nona- and decapeptides comprising this sequence were synthesised, initially by a classical procedure, and shown to initiate mediator release from rat peritoneal mast cells in a manner which closely resembled the natural immunological stimulatory process (5). Later, by exploitation of the more recent solid phase technology, we were able to synthesise a whole range of peptide analogues, thus permitting more detailed structure-activity studies (6), resulting in the delineation of the optimal mast cell trigger sequence (that is, the decapeptide Lys-Thr-Lys-Gly-Ser-Gly-Phe-Phe-Val-Phe). A study of the effect of a selection of these ε-chain peptides on

* Rheumatology and Allergy Research Unit, Department of Immunology, University of Birmingham, Birmingham B15 2TJ, United Kingdom.

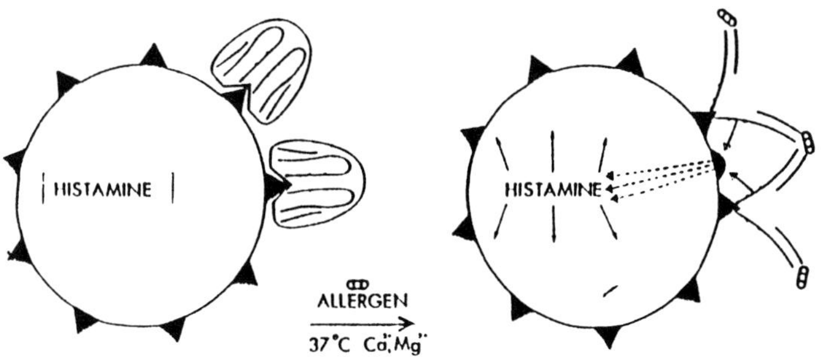

Figure 1. Postulated manner in which a conformational change brought about within mast cell bound IgE antibody molecules, as a result of bridging by specific allergen, could lead to the triggering of release of histamine and other mediators (reproduced from Ref. 14).

the rotational properties of band 3 protein in a model rbc membrane system, involving measurement of flash-induced transient dichroism of the target probe eosin maleimide (7), suggested that ampiphilic peptides like the mast cell triggering decapeptide insert into lipid bilayers via their hydrophobic regions; thus leaving their cationic regions available for interaction with oppositely charged groups within the effector cell membrane.

Interestingly, the neuropeptide substance P which is released from nerve endings in response to antidromic stimuli where it is thought to induce histamine release from neighboring mast cells, possesses similar overall structural features (as discussed in Ref. 8). It is important to note, therefore, that it has been suggested (9,10) that ampiphilic peptides like substance P are capable of activating mast cell G proteins directly, as a consequence of their capacity to insert into the plasma membrane in the manner already described! This raises the possibility, as I discussed elesewhere (11), that IgE-mediated mast cell exocytosis likewise involves the direct activation of G proteins by the ampiphilic trigger sequence we have identified within the CH4 domains of the IgE antibody molecule.

Immunological Intervention in the IgE-Mediated Triggering of Mast Cells as a Basis for a Novel Form of Allergy Therapy

Like others, we have considered the possibility of using synthetic ε-chain peptides, representative of sites within the Fc(ε)RI binding region of IgE, to block the interaction of the anaphylactic antibody with the high affinity receptor on mast cells and basophils. And, indeed, in the study referred to in the introduction (2), four out of the seven synthetic rat Fc ε-chain peptides tested brought about a substantial inhibition of ^{125}I-labelled rat immunocytoma IgE to purified rat peritoneal mast cells *in vitro*. But, the relatively high concentrations of peptide needed to achieve such levels of inhibition, under favorable *in vitro* experimental conditions, suggest that such an approach would unlikely prove to be a viable proposition *in vivo*! Moreover, even the preferential occupancy of the Fc(ε)RI receptors on mast cells by intact IgE (a possible therapeutic approach which I conjectured on in a review article way back in 1971) would seem to be a "non-starter"; in the light of the later findings of Jarrett et al. (12), which revealed that the huge increase in level of circulating IgE brought about by infecting mice with a parasite failed to render the animals refractory to subsequent passive cutaneous sensitization with murine IgE antibody.

Another possible therapeutic approach which we have investigated was an attempt to design an analogue form of the IgE triggering peptide sequence (delineated as described in the previous section) capable of antagonising its stimulatory effect on mast cells. This assumes that the trigger peptide behaves like a peptide hormone (such as LHRH), which acts on a specific receptor on the mast cell surface, and therefore ought to be capable of being antagonized by a derivative in which an essential amino acid is replaced by an irrelevant one. But none of the wide range of candidate peptides we produced for such a role turned out to be capable of inhibiting allergen-induced histamine release from IgE antibody-sensitized rat mast cells *in vitro*.

It was against this background that we decided to look into the possibility of immunologically intervening in the IgE mediated mast cell triggering event. As reported in *The Lancet* in 1990 (13), we raised an antibody (polyclonal) against the human ε-chain decapeptide in rabbits, and showed that incubation of antiserum containing this with the trigger peptide substantially reduced (by over 70%) its capacity to induce histamine release from purified rat peritoneal mast cells *in vitro*. Furthermore, this inhibitory activity was confirmed from inhibition-PCA testing in rats, a significant reduction in the blueing response being observed when the rabbit anti-peptide antiserum was administered before (2 min) or at the same time as challenge with allergen (ovalbumin), or 72 hr after passive cutaneous sensitization of normal rats with ovalbumin sensitized rat's serum.

These preliminary *in vitro* and *in vivo* inhibition findings encouraged us to go on to look at the effect of actively immunising experimentally sensitised rats with the human ε-chain decapeptide. Immunization of groups (5) of experimentally-sensitized rats (outbred, Wistar) with peptide protein (KLH or PPD) conjugate was shown to protect them against fatal (or near fatal) systemic anaphylactic responses to subsequent intravenous injection of allergen (ovalbumin); in contrast to non-peptide immunized groups of sensitized rats. Furthermore, in later studies (also reported in 13) it was shown that immunization of rats with peptide-protein conjugate before or after experimental sensitization to ovalbumin brought about a highly significant reduction in histamine release into the animals' circulations, when measured 10 min after intravenous allergen challenge. And, moreover, both pre- and post-mmunization with peptide caused some reduction in the animals' levels of serum IgE antibody against the experimental allergen (ovalbumin).

Further peptide-immunization studies, employing the same experimental design in allergic rats, have shown that similar protection against the effects of allergen (ovalbumin) challenge could be accomplished by pre- or post-immunization with a rat ε-chain (CH4 domain) peptide which was a structural analogue of the human Cε4 domain mast cell trigger peptide, whereas immunization with a non-mast cell triggering analogue of this rat ε-chain peptide, in which the key lysine residue in position 1 was replaced by a glycine residue, afforded no protection whatsoever. These findings suggest that it should be possible likewise to protect allergic patients from the consequences of subsequent natural exposure to allergen, by active immunization with the homologous human ε-chain decapeptide. In other words, the human ε-chain decapeptide-protein (e.g. KLH) conjugate would be expected to be immunogenic in humans, particularly as this CH4 domain located sequence does not appear to be antigenically detectable in native human IgE.

Future Horizons

The results of the experimental animal studies outlined in the previous section suggest that a human ε-chain decapeptide could form the basis of a novel vaccine for the treatment of IgE-mediated allergies of the asthma-hay fever type. This claim is strengthened by the results of our more recent studies, for instance, in which relatively long lasting protection in allergic rats has been achieved by active immunization with protein-carrier together with an adjuvant (i. e. $Al(OH)_3$) which would be acceptable in humans. Furthermore, preliminary immunization studies in monkeys (cynomolgous) have revealed that the same immunogenic form of the peptide is capable of inducing the production of protective anti-peptide antibodies, as indicated by the demonstration that they are capable of markedly reducing allergen-induced histamine release from IgE antibody-sensitized rat mast cells *in vitro*.

It is also worth mentioning that we have shown in other recent studies that it is possible to produce a relatively high degree of protection in experimentally sensitized rats, against the consequences of subsequent allergen challenge as measured by histamine released into their blood, as a result of passively immunizing them (48 hr earlier) with a murine monoclonal antibody directed against the human ε-chain mast cell trigger peptide. The 'humanization' of this antibody might well offer an opportunity of providing temporary protection to allergic individuals, for instance, to patients who are going to be exposed very rarely to a drug (e.g. a particular antibiotic) or a local anaesthetic to which it is suspected they could be hypersensitive. Further experimental studies now in progress are being aimed at defining the optimal conditions for long term protection in primates and to confirming that this approach will, unlike conventional hyposensitization, be applicable as anticipated to "across the board" treatment of IgE-mediated allergies, irrespective of the nature of the offending allergens which will not even need to be identified.

References

1. Stanworth, D.R., Humphrey, J.N., Bennich, H., and Johansson, S.G.O. 1968. Inhibition of Prausnitz-Küstner reaction by proteolytic cleavage fragments of a human myeloma protein of class E. Lancet ii:17.
2. Burt, D.S. and Stanworth, D.R. 1987. Inhibition of binding of rat IgE to rat mast cells by synthetic IgE peptides Eur. J. Immunol. 17:437.
3. Burt, D.S., Hastings, G.Z, Healy, J. and Stanworth, D.R. 1987. Analysis of the interaction between rat immunoglobulin E and rat mast cells using anti-peptide antibodies. Molec. Immunol. 24:379.
4. Stanworth, D.R., and Ghaderi, A.A. 1990. The role of high and low affinity IgE receptors in cell signalling processes. Molec Immunol. 27:1291.
5. Stanworth, D.R, Kings, M., Roy, P.D., Moran, J.M, and Moran, D.M. 1979. Synthetic peptides comprising sequences of human immunoglobulin E heavy chain capable of releasing histamine. Biochem. J. 180:665.
6. Stanworth, D.R., Coleman, J.W., and Khan, Z. 1984. Essential structural requirements for triggering of mast cells by a synthetic peptide comprising a sequence in the Cε4 domain of human IgE. Molec. Immunol. 21:243.
7. Dufton, M.J., Cherry, R.J., Coleman, J.W., and Stanworth, D.R. 1984. The capacity of basic peptides to trigger exocytosis from mast cell correlates with their capacity to immobilize band 3 proteins in erythrocyte membranes. Biochem. J. 223:67.
8. Stanworth, D.R. 1984. The role of non-antigen receptors in mast cell signalling processes. Molec. Immunol. 21:1183.
9. Mousli, M., Blueb, J.-L., Bronner, C., Ronot, B., and Landry, Y. 1990. G protein activation: A receptor-independent mode of action for cationic ampiphilic neuropeptides and venom peptides Trends in Pharmacol. Sci. 11:358.
10. Regoli, D., and Nantel, F. 1990. Receptor independent action of bradykinin. Trends in Pharmacol. Sci. 11:400.
11. Stanworth, D.R. 1991. Allergy treatment with a peptide vaccine. Proc. European Academy of Allergology and Clinical Immunology meeting (Zurich, May, 1991), in press.
12. Jarrett, E., McKenzie, S., and Bennich, H. 1980. Parasite-induced non-specific IgE does not protect against allergic reactions. Nature 283:302.
13. Stanworth, D.R., Jones, V.M., Lewin, I.V., and Nayyar, S. 1990. Allergy treatment with a peptide vaccine. Lancet 336:1279.
14. Stanworth, D.R. 1971. Immunoglobulin E (reagin) and allergy. Nature 233:310.

Inflammation and Asthma

Michael A. Kaliner*

The cardinal signs of inflammation are redness, swelling, cellular inflammation and pain (or increased irritability). Over the past decade, since the late phase allergic reaction was recognized to be a sequela of mast cell activation (1,2), a great deal of attention has been directed at the role that airway inflammation plays in asthma. Most attention has been directed at cellular infiltration of the airway mucosa and movement of inflammatory cells into the epithelial lining fluid where it can be recovered by bronchoalveolar lavage (BAL). A great volume of data has suggested that increased inflammation concomitantly increases airway reactivity, and that aiming therapy at the inflammation reduces airway responsiveness. However, relatively little interest has been shown toward airway edema and its role in asthma. In this review, data for each of the signs of inflammation, their pathogenesis, and roles in asthma will be briefly discussed. In the end, vascular permeability and its contribution to acute airflow obstruction as well as death from asthma will be underscored. A working definition of asthma could be the following: "A disease of reversible airflow obstruction manifested as wheezing and caused by various combinations of airway mucosal edema and inflammation, increased secretions, and smooth muscle contraction. Asthmatics exhibit airway hyperreactivity, and the clinical course is quite variable" (modified from Reference 3). This definition stresses the four causes of airflow obstruction, as well as emphasizing the influence of airway hyperresponsiveness. Part of the intention of this review will be to integrate how inflammation participates in both airflow obstruction and airway hyperresponsiveness.

Airway Edema

In the classical description of the pathology of fatal bronchial asthma, Dunnill noted the presence of edema of the mucosa in 18 of 20 cases (4). The overlying mucosal denudation was attributed to the force of the mucosal edema, and the contribution of the plasma exudate to the excessive fluid in the bronchial lumen was discussed. The presence of large amounts of plasma proteins in the airway fluid has been confirmed many times (reviewed in 5), and was carefully documented in a recent study of broncho-lavage after allergen challenge (6). In the human nasal mucosa, a careful study of the dynamics of the formation of respiratory epithelial lining fluid was recently published (7) which documents that a mammoth movement of plasma-protein rich fluid occurs within minutes of allergen exposure of allergic individuals. The microvascular permeability leading to the plasma exudate causes both mucosal edema and a marked increase in nasal secretions. There is speculation on the precise causes for the plasma protein exudation, but after allergen exposure, mast cell mediators are the most likely cause (Table 1). However, mast cell mediator release also causes secondary reflexes, which might also participate in the microvascular permeability. The capacity of histamine antagonists to effectively reduce the acute response to allergen suggests that histamine release is an important factor in nasal allergic reactions. There is however a contribution from reflexely stimulated submosal glands, account-

Table 1 Mediators Thought to Cause Microvascular Permeability in Asthma

Mast Cell Mediators:
Histamine
Bradykinin
Leukotrienes
Several Prostaglandins
Chymase
Platelet Activating Factor
Reactive Oxygen Species
Neuropeptides:
Substance P
NeurokininA
Calcitonin Gene Related Peptide

* Allergic Diseases Section, National Institute of Allergy and Infectious Diseases, National Institutes of Health, Bethesda Maryland, 20892, USA.

ing for about 20% of the proteins secreted into nasal epithelial fluid.

In animal models, the process of microvascular permeability in the airways has been carefully studied and involves the following events: release of the vasoactive substance, development of intercellular openings between post-capillary venule endothelial cells, escape of plasma protein rich fluid into the tissues surrounding the venule, movement of water into the tissues and the formation of mucosal edema. In the conducting airways, the responding post-capillary venules are part of an extensive plexus of sub-basement membrane vessels which probably act to warm and humidify inspired air. These vessels leak fluid into the area just deep to the basement membrane, which is precisely the area in which edema is found in asthmatic lungs. The edema may be cleared by two mechanisms: lymphatic clearance or epithelial secretion into the lumen. Lymphatic clearance undoubtedly contributes to the removal of the plasma exudation, but this process is slow and unproven. On the other hand, the process of paracellular transport of edema fluid between epithelial cells and into the bronchial or nasal lumen has been well documented. This process occurs within seconds of the formation of edema and may participate in the development of increased luminal fluid, which is a major factor in the airflow obstruction of asthma. Thus, the evidence that airway edema plays an important role in asthma is based upon morphologic evidence of its presence, proof that plasma proteins are increased in luminal fluid, and an understanding of the processes involved in the dynamics of both microvascular permeability and the movement of the edema fluid into the lumen.

A protective role of this process in asthma has been suggested (8). The edema fluid that transverses the epithelium into the respiratory lining fluid would provide volume for increased mucociliary clearance, albumin to nonspecifically absorb proteins, IgG (and other plasma immunoglobulins) to interact with pathogens, inflammatory mediators (bradykinin, anaphylatoxins) to amplify the reaction, and enzyme inhibitors to limit the tissue destruction induced by pathogenic products. It seems more likely, however, that the process itself may be a useful primitive host defense mechanism. But in asthma, the edema and increased lining fluid are certain to be detrimental, contributing to airflow obstruction and the increased secretions thought to actually be responsible for death in many severe asthmatics. The admixture of plasma proteins with mucus and dead and dying cells must contribute to the increased viscosity of secretions.

Vasodilation

Inflammatory responses always initiate concomitant hyperemia due to vasodilation. This response can be seen in the skin or nasal mucosa after applying inflammatory mediators. Several mediators which cause increased blood flow also cause increased vascular permeability (PAF, bradykinin, leukotrienes, histamine), while others primarily increase blood flow (PGE, VIP, CGRP). Addition of agents which increase blood flow to those causing vascular permeability potentiates the permeability (reviewed in 9). However, increased vasodilation by itself does not lead to increased vascular permeability (10). Thus, increasing the blood flow through the mucosa does not by itself lead to plasma protein exudation but, in the presence of vasoactive amines, will potentiate the action of the amines.

Inflammation

The association of asthma with airway inflammation has been recognized since the first recognition of eosinophils in the airways and sputum of asthmatics was noted. The classical descriptions of asthma pathology note the presence of eosinophils and neutrophils both in the lamina propria and airway lumen of asthmatics (11). However, the understanding of the potential contribution of inflammatory events in asthma took a giant leap forward with the use of bronchoalveolar lavage and bronchial biopsy of mild, ambulatory asthmatics. The presence of eosinophils in the bronchial wall, in the absence of diseases associated with hypereosinophilia, is pathognomonic of asthma. Some reputable investigators now describe asthma as "chronic eosinophilic bronchitis" (12). Biopsies of mild asthmatics have confirmed the presence of eosinophils in the mucosa, often found beneath the basement membrane and in the epithelium (reviewed in 13). Not only are eosinophils present, but their granule derived proteins may be found in both the tissue and in BAL. Another consistent finding is the presence of activated mucosal mast cells in the airways, along with an increased number of mast cells. The relationship between mast cell degranulation and severe asthma was noted many years ago (reviewed in 11). The finding of increased mast cell mediators in BAL confirms the presence of ongoing mast cell activation even in apparently healthy asthmatics (reviewed in 13). Lymphocytes also appear to be increased in asthma, with increased numbers having been noted both in the epithelium and in the lamina propria (14). These lymphocytes have been noted to express the cell surface marker for IL2, suggesting that they have been activated (15). It has been suggested that these activated lymphocytes might be producing cytokines which participate in the airway hyperreactivity and cellular infiltration in asthma. Other changes which have been noted by biopsy include a thickening of the basement membrane due to the deposition of collagens and fibronectin. Myofibroblasts along the basement membrane are increased in conjunction with this thickening and may be responsible (16). Mucous gland and goblet cell hyperplasia are also constant features.

Pain or Increased Irritability

The airways of asthmatics express increased irritability in response to diverse nonspecific stimuli. As the airways have few pain fibers, this increased reactivity is taken to be the equivalent of the pain noted with cutaneous inflammation. The underlying causes for bronchial hyperresponsiveness have not been identified with precision, although many contributing factors have been suggested (17,18). While the underlying hyperresponsiveness seen in all asthmatic patients is unexplained, increases in hyperresponsiveness in relationship to allergen challenge, natural allergy exposure, late phase allergic reactions, viral infections, exposure to noxious fumes, inhalation of chemical sensitizers, and a variety of other stimuli have been documented. One of the features of these diverse provocations which all lead to airway reactivity is the development of cellular infiltrates. Precisely how mast cell activation, eosinophil infiltration, lymphocyte activation, and the other events which are associated with increased reactivity actually cause the change is not clear. One recent study in a monkey model of asthma suggested that mast cell activation and elaboration of tumor necrosis factor led to the generation of adhesion molecules which then facilitated eosinophil infiltration and the generation of increased airway reactivity. Pretreatment with antibodies directed at TNF prevented the response (19). Compelling arguments, however, can also be raised for the role of neutral endopeptidase, increased or decreased amounts of neuropeptides, and specific actions of mediators derived from mast cells, lymphocytes or eosinophils.

Conclusions

The cardinal features of inflammation are present in asthma, and are important in the disease. Cellular infiltration and activation participates in the airflow obstruction as well as increasing airway reactivity. Edema is a major contributor to airflow obstruction and leads to increased airway fluid, which is often the cause of death in acute asthma. Vasodilation is part of asthma, and has been suggested as an important part of exercise induced asthma. Therapy aimed at reducing inflammation in asthma will become increasingly important, not only to reduce airflow obstruction but also to reduce airway reactivity. Currently there is a great deal of attention being directed at reducing the cellular infiltration in asthma, particularly the eosinophilia. In the future, therapy aimed at reducing airway edema may also be available, and will likely produce important new therapeutic advantages.

References

1. Tannenbaum, S., Oertel, H., Henderson, W., and Kaliner, M. 1980. The biologic activity of mast cell granules. I. Elicitation of inflammatory responses in rat skin. J. Immunol. 125:325.

2. Lemanske, R.F., and Kaliner, M. 1982. Mast cell-dependent late phase reactions. Clin. Immunol. Rev. 1:547.
3. Kaliner, M., Eggleston, P., and Mathews, K. 1987. Rhinitis and asthma. JAMA 258:2851.
4. Dunnill, M.S. 1960. The pathology of asthma, with special reference to changes in the bronchial mucosa. J. Clin. Path. 13:27.
5. Perrson, C.G.A. 1988. Plasma exudation and asthma. Lung 166:1.
6. Fick, R.B., Metzger, W.J., Richerson, H.B., Zavala, D.C., Moseley, P.L., Schoderbek, W.E., and Hunninghake, G.W. 1987. Increased bronchovascular permeability after allergen exposure in sensitive asthmatics. J. Clin. Invest. 63:1147.
7. Raphael, G.D., Igarashi, Y., White, M.V., and Kaliner, M.A. 1991. The pathophysiology of rhinitis. V. Sources of protein in allergen-induced nasal secretions. J. Allergy Clin. Immunol. 88:33.
8. Perrson, C.G.A., Erejefalt, I., Alkner, U., Baumgarten, C., Greiff, L., Gustafsson, B., Luts, A., Pipkorn, U., Sundler, F., Svensson, C., and Wollmer, P. 1991. Plasma exudation as a first line respiratory mucosal defense. Clin. Exp. Allergy 21:17.
9. Cheung, K.F., Rodgers, D.F., Barnes, P.J., and Evans, T.W. 1990. The role of increased airway microvascular permeability and plasma exudation in asthma. Eur. Respir. J. 3:329.
10. Mullol, J., Raphael, G.D., Lundgren, J.D., Baraniuk, J.N., Merida, M., Shelhamer, J.H., and Kaliner, M.A. 1991. Comparison of human nasal mucosal secretion *in vivo* and *in vitro*. J. Allergy Clin. Immunol., in press.
11. Kaliner, M.A., Blennerhassett, J., and Austen, K.F. 1976. Bronchial asthma. In: Textbook of immunopathology. P.A. Meischer, and H.J. Muller-Eberhard, eds. New York: Grune & Stratton, p. 387.
12. Frigas, E., and Gleich, G.J. 1986. The eosinophil and the pathophysiology of asthma. J. Allergy Clin. Immunol. 77:527.
13. Djukanovic, R., Roche, W.R., Wilson, J.W., Beasley, C.R.W., Twentyman, O.P., Howarth, P.H., and Holgate, S.T. 1990. Mucosal inflammation in asthma. Amer. Rev. Resp. Dis. 142:434.
14. Jeffery, P.K., Wardlaw, A.J., Nelson, F.C., Collins, J.V., and Kay, A.B. 1989. Bronchialbiopsies in asthma. An ultrastructural, quantitative study and correlation with hyperreactivity. Amer. Rev. Resp. Dis. 140:1745.
15. Azzawi, M, Bradley, B., Jeffery, P.K., Frew, A.J., Wardlaw, A.J., Knowles, G., Assoufi, B., Collins, J.V., Durham, S., and Kay, A.B. 1990. Identification of activated T lymphocytes and eosinophils in bronchial biopsies in stable atopic asthma. Amer. Rev. Resp. Dis. 142:1407.
16. Brewster, C.E.P., Howarth, P.H., Djukanovic, R., Wilson, J., Holgate, S.T., and Roche, W.R. 1990. Myofibroblasts and subepithelial fibrosis in bronchial asthma. Am. J. Respir. Cell. Mol. Biol. 3:507.
17. Boushey, H.A., Holtzman, M.J., Sheller, J.R., and Nadel, J.A. 1980. Bronchial hyperreactivity. Amer. Rev. Resp. Dis. 121:389.
18. Barnes, P.J. 1989. New concepts in the pathogenesis of bronchial hyperresponsiveness and asthma. J. Allergy Clin. Immunol. 83:1013.
19. Wegner, C.D., Gundel, R.H., Reilly, P., Haynes, N., Letts, L.G., and Rothlein, R. 1990. Intercellular adhesion molecule-1 (ICAM-1) in the pathogenesis of asthma. Science 247:456.

Platelets and Eosinophils in Asthma

J. Morley*

Asthma has been defined as a disease that is characterised by variable airway obstruction (1). In asthma, airway obstruction is usually associated with hyperreactivity of the airways, and intermittent symptoms can largely be attributed to changed responsivity of the airways to neurotransmitters and inflammatory autocoids. Attempts to understand the mechanisms underlying airway hyperreactivity in asthma have been hampered by an inability of many investigators to appreciate the distinction between hyperreactivity and the process of airway smooth muscle contraction. Failure to demonstrate hyperreactivity *in vitro* can be presumed to have contributed to this situation and has caused attention to be directed to those autocoids which are potent spasmogens of airway smooth muscle. For instance, much effort was expended in defining the chemical characteristics of smooth muscle spasmogens, such as the peptido-leukotrienes, whose capacity to effect protracted contraction of airway smooth muscle was considered significant (2). The idea that mediators might act selectively to evoke hyperreactivity of the airways was not generally accepted, since it was anticipated that a range of inflammatory mediators would induce mucosal oedema and thereby obstruct the airway lumen physically. On theoretical grounds, it could be argued that non-selective hyperreactivity of airways would be an inevitable consequence of this process (3). This situation was changed by platelet activating factor, which could be shown to induce airway hyperreactivity upon intravenous infusion in the guinea-pig and rabbit (4) by a process dependent upon platelet activation (5), whereas plasma protein extravasation in response to PAF is independent of platelet activation (6). The emergence of PAF into asthma research (7) revived interest in the concept of chemical mediation of airway hyperreactivity in asthma and, because of the capacity of PAF to activate platelets and eosinophils, contributed to a reappraisal of cellular events in asthma.

Platelets and Asthma

An involvement of platelets in asthma pathology was indicated by the finding that thrombocytopenia occurred during allergic reactions to inhaled allergens in asthma patients (8). This finding is consistent with the occurrence of platelet activation and aggregation when sensitised laboratory animals are exposed to antigen. In the rabbit, this phenomenon was analysed in some detail to reveal that antigen interacts with basophils to yield a labile lipid which was a potent stimulus to platelet activation (9). It follows that platelet activation in asthma might reasonably be anticipated to occur; but it was not until allergic reactions in asthma were shown to be accompanied by elevation of platelet factor 4 (10) that attention was redirected to this blood element. Although the occurrence of platelet activation in asthma has since been disputed (11), there is now consensus that platelet activation occurs in asthma; indeed, it has been proposed that platelet dysfunction should be considered characteristic of allergic asthma (12), and measures of platelet activation can be used as an index of allergic status (13). To those who had followed these events over the decade, it was therefore not surprising that platelet aggregates were detected in biopsied material from asthmatic airways (14). These observations do not however resolve the question as to what role should be given to platelet activation in asthma pathology.

Three possibilities might be considered. Firstly, platelet activation may be an essential pre-requisite to some critical and characteristic event in asthma pathology. Since certain adhesion molecules are shared by platelets and leucocytes (15), it is possible to conceive of schemes whereby leucocyte accumulation is preceded by, and subservient to, platelet accumulation and extravasation (16). Observation of platelet extravasation into lung tissue (17)

* Preclinical R & D, Sandoz Pharma Ltd. CH-4002, Basel, Switzerland.

and airway lumen (18) gives some credence to such a concept. However, protagonists have presumed that development of airway hyperreactivity will be secondary to cellular inflammation, thereby considerably weakening their thesis, since prostacyclin has proved inconsequential as an inhibitor of asthmatic bronchospasm (19). In view of the evidence distinguishing airway hyperreactivity from cellular inflammation (20), it cannot be concluded that cellular inflammation is not impaired by prostacyclin, and this issue remains unresolved. Notwithstanding that caveat, it must be acknowledged that an experimental analysis of *in vivo* interaction between platelets and neutrophils in response to intravenous injection of PAF did not indicate a primary role for platelets in the process of margination (21). A second possibility is that platelet activation is incidental to release or generation of a critical mediator of asthma pathology. It is in this context that PAF has achieved significance, for it could be reasoned that, were generation of PAF to account for the changed airway responsivity that characterises asthma, then incidental exposure of platelets to this material during transit through the lung would account for activation of platelets. Since inflammatory leucocytes generate PAF in substantial quantity (22), this thesis is superficially attractive. The concept that PAF release explains platelet activation in asthma accords with existing evidence (12) and has not been refuted. However, the corollary that PAF accounts for airway hyperreactivity in asthma now seems unlikely: firstly because of an inability of prostacyclin to modify asthma symptoms (19) and secondly because PAF induces a pattern of airway hyperreactivity inappropriate to asthma (23). A dearth of reports describing efficacy of PAF antagonists in asthma might be considered silent testimony to this opinion. The third possibility, that these modest changes of platelet function are unrelated to asthma but rather reflect events in atopy or inflammatory lung disease, has been given insufficient attention despite supportive evidence (12,13).

Eosinophils and Asthma

The other element of asthma pathology that is brought into focus by PAF is the eosinophil. Unlike the platelet, the eosinophil was recognised as an obvious and characteristic feature of the asthmatic lung in death (24) and subsequently in less severe stages of asthma (25,14). It is ironic therefore that the potential of this cell to account for asthma pathology was disregarded for so long and obfuscation of reality undoubtedly retarded asthma research for many years. However, in the last decade it has become apparent that the eosinophil is the most plausible candidate to account for desquamation of airway epithelium, though whether this is attributable to secretion of toxic, highly basic proteins (26) or to secretion of protease (27) has yet to be resolved. It is apparent therefore that proposal of PAF as a putative mediator of asthma (7) did not bring the eosinophil into prominence, but by providing a mechanism to account for eosinophil accumulation in the airways, study of PAF did reinforce the attention that has been directed to this cell type in recent years.

Prior to 1986, there were concepts to account for eosinophil accumulation in tissues, but available materials to test these concepts were most notable for a lack of efficacy. Hence, the demonstration that PAF was a potent and selective agent of eosinophil recruitment into the lung was a major advance (28), especially as PAF provided a relatively modest stimulus (if compared to allergen in actively sensitised animals) and therefore was useful for evaluation of anti-asthma drugs (29). However, from the outset it was clear that the modest accumulation achieved by administration of PAF precluded explanation of eosinophil accumulation as secondary to platelet activation, as some were to propose (16,17). The possibility of priming should be considered, for it has been demonstrated that actively sensitised animals, in which antigen depots induce persisting immunological reactions, responded to PAF almost as effectively as to antigen (30). It has been suggested that PAF may act as a priming agent, but priming effects of PAF on eosinophils *in vivo* are slight or undetectable in the guinea-pig; moreover, the evidence that eosinophil accumulation is absolutely dependent upon an intact population of T-lymphocytes (31) makes such a concept implausible. Consistent with this opinion is the finding that whereas potent PAF receptor antagonists are ineffectual as inhibitors of allergic inflammation in the airways, cyclosporin A is highly effective (32). Direct evidence favors interleukins

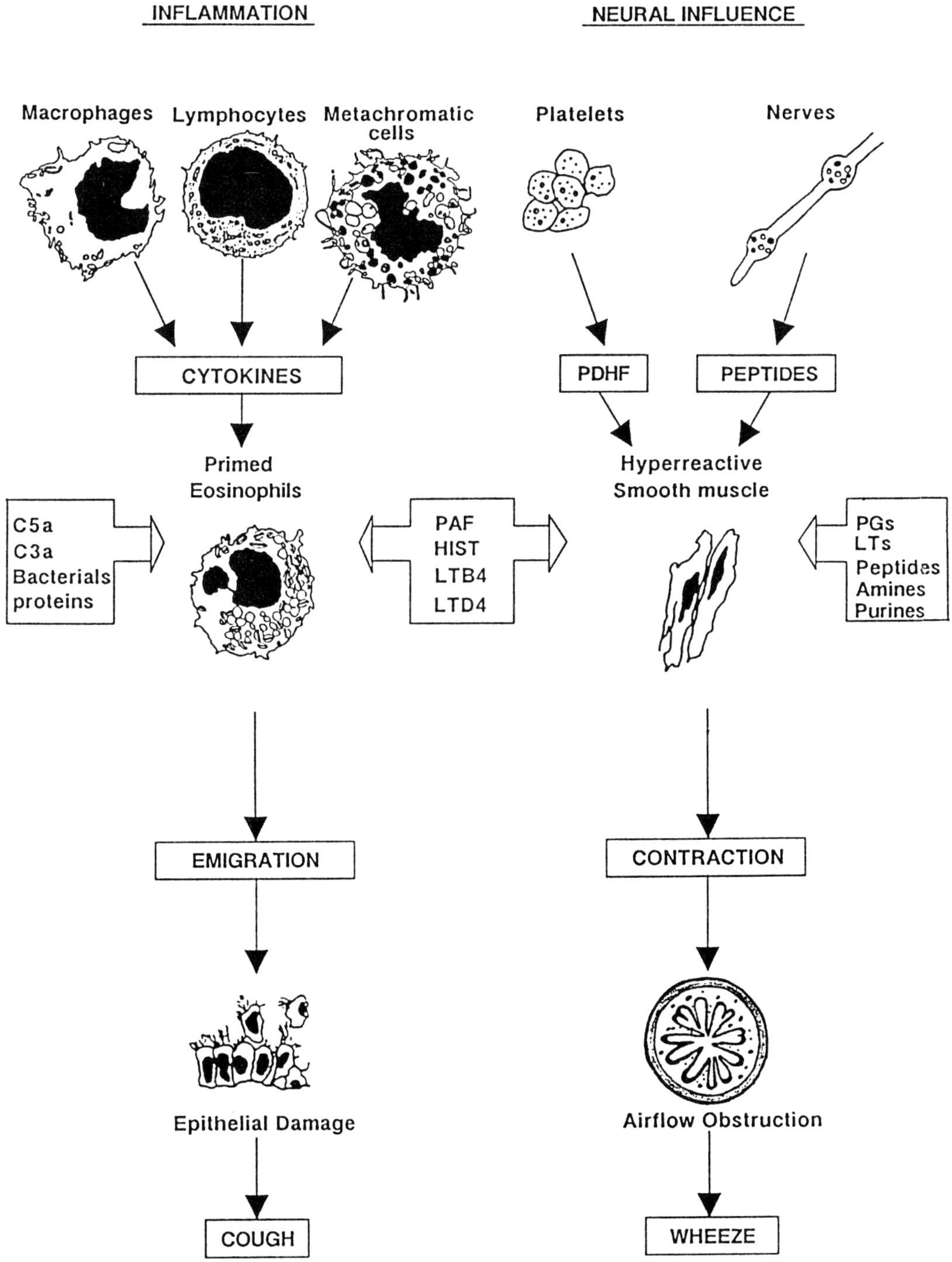

Figure 1. Schematic representation of parallel processes in asthma pathology (from 20 with permission).

Beta Receptor Decrease: A Consequence of Atopy?

A. Oehling, María L. Sanz, P. M. Gamboa, C. G. de la Cuesta*

In Szentivanyi's studies of 1968 (1) and the very few studies subsequently published (2–7), there seemed to be sufficient evidence that asthmatic patients presented a decrease in beta-adrenergic receptors. The theory was that the asthmatic or atopic patients could be considered as such precisely because of this decrease in beta-receptors. "Atopic status" was determined as a consequence of a deficit in beta-receptors. We began to consider this little-studied phenomenon about 5 years ago in order to understand it further. Our team, Gamboa and colleagues (8), had already shown in a previous study that the degree of variation in the decrease of beta-receptors depended on the parenchyma involved and the condition of the patients (Table 1). Thus, in rhinitic allergic patients there was a decrease of 24% in beta-receptors with respect to controls, whereas in asthmatic patients in an active phase, the decrease was 36% (Table 2). However, inactive patients only showed a deficit of 7%. In subsequent studies (9) and in view of the results obtained, we decided to study the possible modifications in the number of beta-receptors in asymptomatic patients after the bronchial provocation test with antigens. We worked with asthmatic patients with intense sensitization to Dermatophagoides pt. shown by skin tests, specific IgE and a strong positive histamine release test. Assays and determinations were carried out in basal conditions after 30 minutes (Fig. 1) and subsequent measurements, and we were able to show that a significant decrease in beta-receptors of 30.4% took place 24 hours (Fig. 2 & 3) after the specific bronchial provocation. This led us to conclude that the decrease in beta-receptors was a conseqence of the antigen-antibody reaction. The delay in its detection could be due to the existence of a latent period before the antigen-antibody reaction is detected by the lymphocytes in peripheral blood.

Table I. Beta-receptor number in allergic patients.

	n	x	S.D.	P
Symptomatic asthma	25	336(-33%)	116	< 0.01*
Asymptomatic asthma	21	555	280	ns
Symptomatic rhinitis	51	360(-29%)	185	< 0.05*
Asymptomatic rhinitis	43	536	230	ns
Controls	30	598	100	

* With respect to controls.

Table II. Beta-receptor numbers in allergic symptomatic and asymptomatic patients.

	n	x	S.D.	P
Symptomatic patients	51	360(-40%)	185	< 0.001*
Asymptomatic patients	43	536(-10%)	230	< 0.01**
Control	30	598	100	

* in relation to control group.
** in relation to symptomatic patients.

* Clinica Universitaria, Faculty of Medicine, University of Navarra, 31080-Pamlona, Spain.

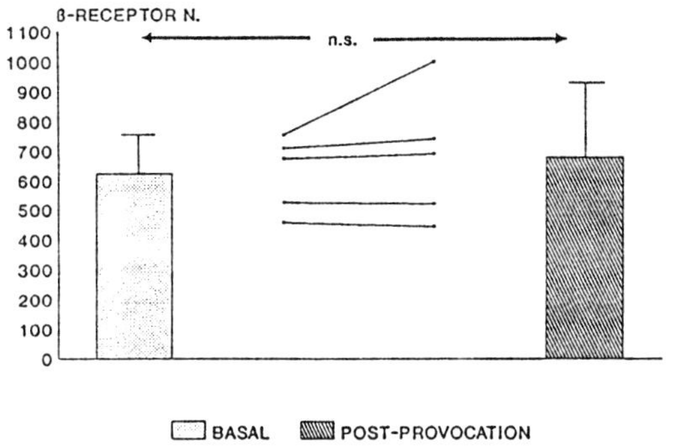

Figure 1. Specific Bronchial Provocation Test (30 min.)

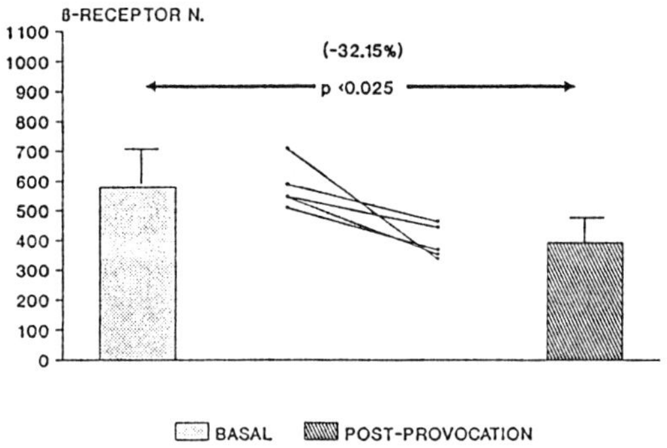

Figure 3. Metacholine Provocation Test.

Subsequently, we decided to study these phenomena more deeply and therefore selected a larger group: 93 allergic patients with monosensitization to Dermatophagoides pt., and 30 healthy subjects (Fig. 4). We studied beta-receptors in the controls, and in 27 patients with nasal symptomatology, 27 asthmatic patients in the asymptomatic phase, and 27 patients with evident asthmatic symptomatology (10). As can be seen in Figure 4, patients with nasal symptomatology had a decrease of 40.28%. We can see that in this more numerous group, the decrease in beta-receptors is even greater, whereas the analysis of serum IgE levels showed no correlation between beta-receptors and IgE levels.

Regarding these beta-receptors in clinical cases produced by antigens with a higher degree of antigenicity and aggressiveness, we studied a group of 67 patients with pollinic rhinoconjunctivitis due to sensitization against gramineous pollen (11) (Fig. 5). Patients were divided into 2 gropus: 30 asymptomatic pollinics and 27 with exclusively nasal symptoms. Another group was formed of 10 pollinic and asymptomatic patients whose beta-receptors were determined both during and outside the pollenation season. The study showed that the symptomatic group presented a decrease of 30.42% in beta-receptors with respect to controls (Fig. 6). It should be noted that, although atopic, they did not behave as such according to Szentivanyi's theory. The group of asymptomatic patients studied during and outside of pollen season presented a decrease of 13,2% in beta-2-receptors during pollination.

In view of the results, we decided to study these problems further, to see whether this alteration could be due to the changes which take place in the membrane lipids, as well as to the release of mediators, all seen in relation to the antigen-antibody reaction. There are some

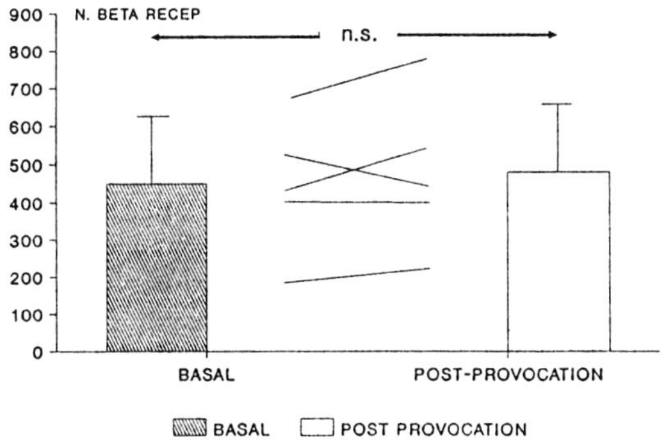

Figure 2. Specific Bronchial Provocation Test (24 hours)

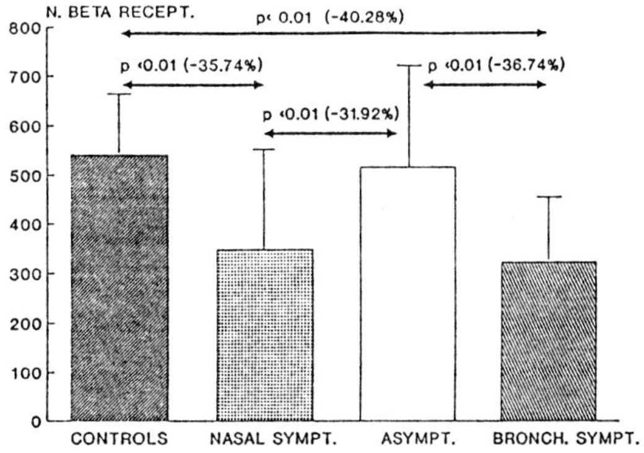

Figure 4. Number of Beta Receptors.

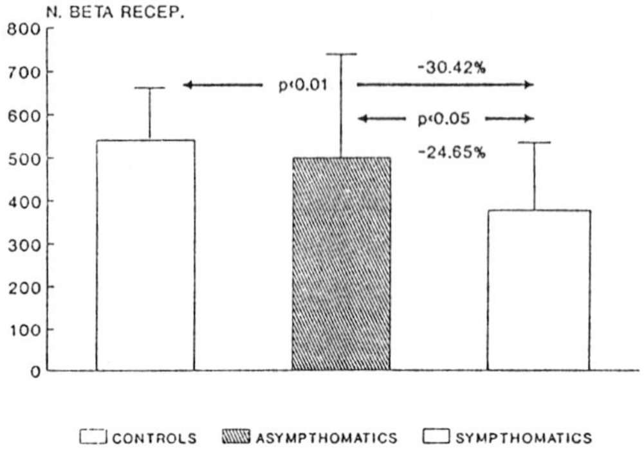

Figure 5. Number of Beta Receptors.

papers that endorse this hypothesis (12–14). We therefore decided to study the possible variations in the number of adrenergic beta-receptors in lymphocitary cells, isolated after *in vitro* stimulation with different mediators such as histamine, leukotrien D4, and platelet activating factor (PAF). We were also interested to know whether the activator of the phospholipasa A2 (Mellitine) was capable of modifying the number of beta-receptors after its *in vitro* incubation with isolated lymphocitary cells. Seventy-five patients were selected, 40 of whom presented sensitization against house dust mite Dermatophagoides pt. and 35 against gramineous pollen Phleum pratensis. For each one beta-receptors on isolated cells were determined in basal conditions and after the exposure to antigen *in vitro*. Healthy patients were stimulated with the allergen against which they were sensitized, either Phleum pratensis pollen or Dermatophagoides pt.

As shown in Figure 7, the results demonstrate that in the group of allergic subjects, there was a significant statistical reduction of 23.24% in beta receptors after the *in vitro* antigen-specific stimulus. No significant differences were noted in the control group. This also corroborates how under *in vitro* conditions the antigenic challenge is capable of modifying the number of beta-receptors, and shows that their decrease is a consequence of the antigen-antibody reaction.

When studying the group of allergic patients, we observed that, according to the antigen against which they are sensitized, the number of beta-receptors decreased significantly after the antigenic stimulus, even though this reduction was greater for Phleum (28.92%) (Fig. 8). This fact could be due to the greater antigenic power of the pollinic allergen.

As far as clinical diagnosis is concerned, we observed that there was a significant reduction in beta-receptors in both rhinitics and asthmatics, although rhinitic patients presented a more notable decrease (Fig. 9). As mentioned before, we thought it appropiate to study the possible modifications in the levels of beta-receptors in lymphocytes, depending on the *in vitro* addiction of mediators. The first group was composed of 15 healthy people and presented a decrease of 14.69% in beta-receptors after *in vitro* stimulation with histamine with respect to basal conditions. Therefore, histamine release by target cells seems to play the role of modulator of beta-adrenergic receptors (Fig. 10).

Leukotriens are mediators that constitute the slow-reacting substances of anaphilaxis. These mediators come from the arachidonic acid liberated from the membrane lipids, as a consequence of the action of phospholipase A2

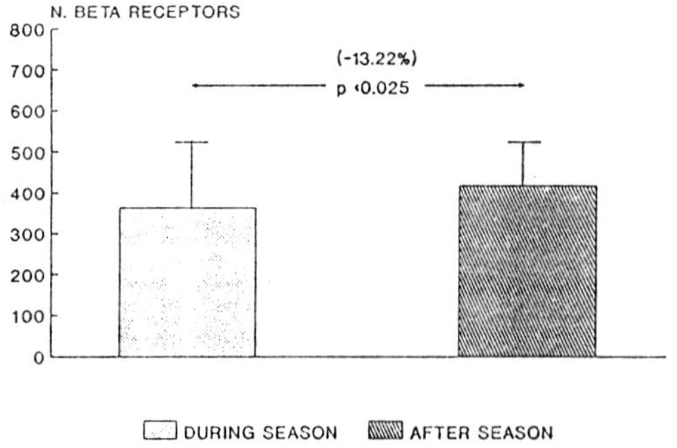

Figure 6. Number of Beta Receptors during and after Pollen Season.

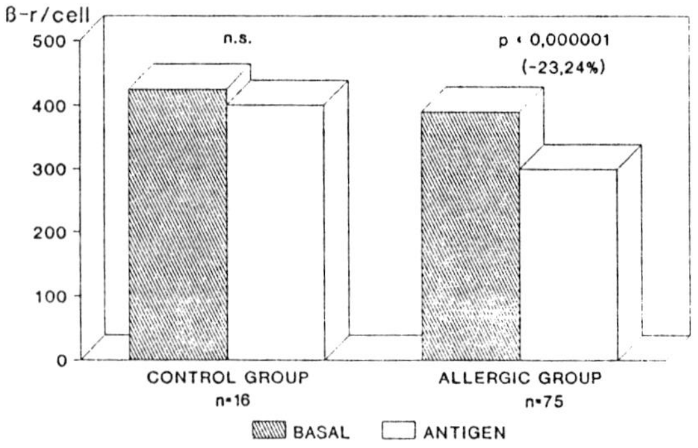

Figure 7. Number of β-Receptors in Control and Allergic Patients.

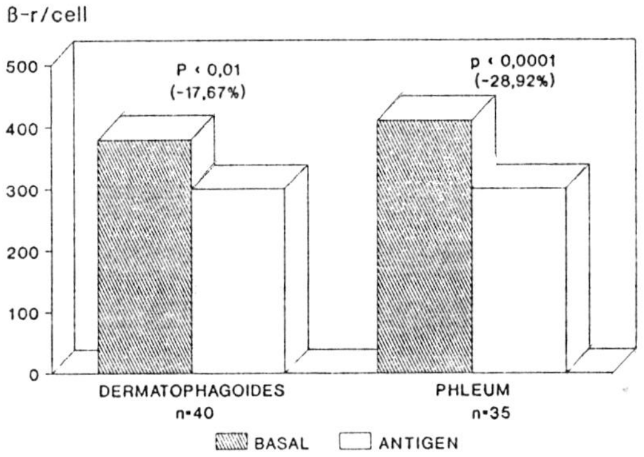

Figure 8. Number of β-Receptors in Allergic Patients Depending of the Antigen.

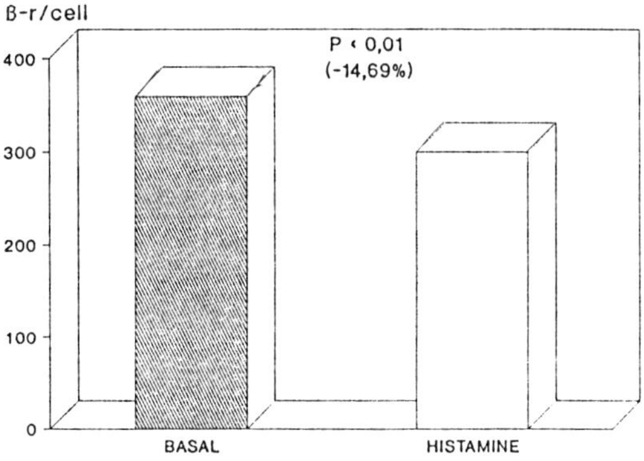

Figure 10. Number of β-Receptors in Healthy individuals after "In Vitro" Histamine Stimulation.

in activated cells, following the lipoxigenase way. We selected Leukotrien D4 due to its powerful *in vivo* bronchoconstrictive action (Fig. 11). Stimulation with this *in vitro* mediator on isolated lymphocytes in a group of healthy individuals, produced a statistically significant decrease in beta-receptors (15%). And so this leukotrien could also play an important modulating role in beta-receptors, even though its constant of affinity is not modified.

PAF aceter has been considered by some authors to be the most important mediator, capable of initiating a late response. In our study, no statistically significant differences were observed after the *in vitro* stimulation with a platelet activating factor (Fig. 12).

Lastly, we determined the effect of *in vitro* activation of lymphocytes with an activator of phospholipase A2 (Mellitine) and the possible modifications on beta-receptors (Fig. 13). The stimulus of these cells with Mellitine leads to a significant decrease in beta-receptors (21.13%). This confirms the regulating role of phospholipase 2 in the adreno-receptor system. Therefore, the reduction of these receptors is the consequence and not the cause of the activity of atopic diseases.

From a hypothetical point of view and taking into account what has been thus far explainded, the bridging of the membrane IgE antibodies by the allergen initiates the activation of the membrane, allowing the calcium channels to open, and the subsequent intracellular increase of this cation, which in turn activates phospholipase A2, a calcium-dependent enzyme. This last activation procures the metabolism of phospholipids including phosphatidilcoline and phosphatidiletanolamine, essential components of the beta-adrenergic receptor. In its turn, the activation of phospholipase A2 also

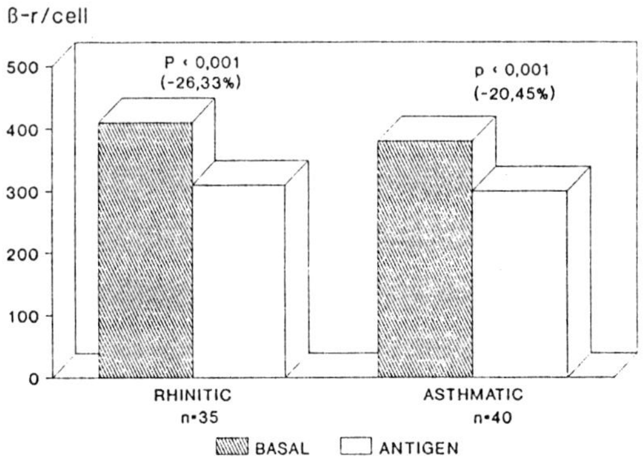

Figure 9. Number of β-Receptors in Asthmatic and Rhinitic Patients.

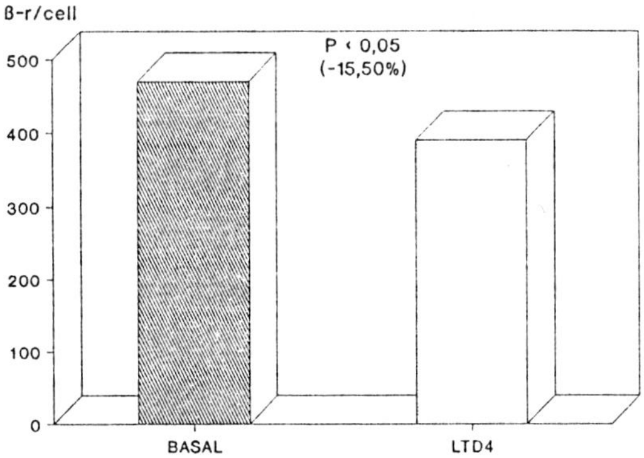

Figure 11. Number of β-Receptors in Healthy Individuals after "In Vitro" Leucotriene D4 Stimulation.

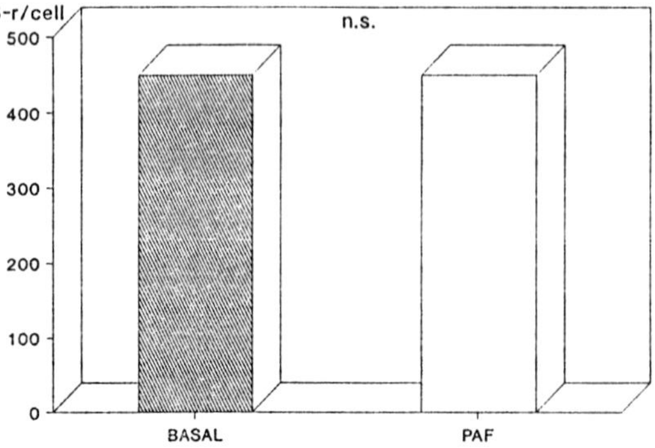

Figure 12. Number of β-Receptors in Healthy Individuals after "In Vitro" Platelet Activator Factor Stimulation.

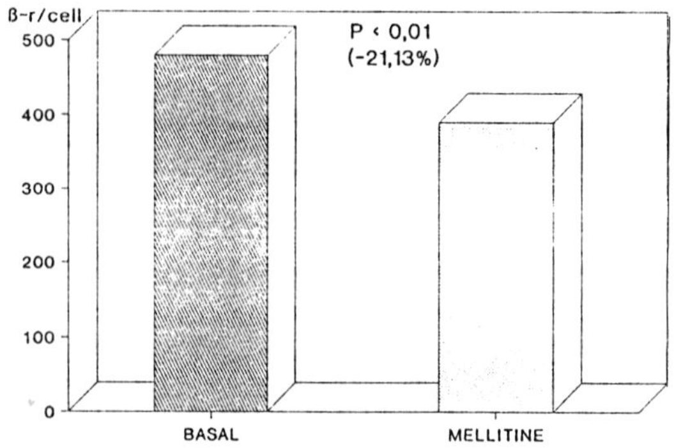

Figure 13. Number of β-Receptors in Healthy Individuals after "In Vitro" Mellitine Stimulation.

originates the synthesis of arachidonic acid and the synthesis of mediators, which at the same time produces the modulation of beta-adrenergic receptors.

References

1. Szentivanyi, A. 1968. The beta-adrenergic theory of the atopic abnormality in bronchial assthma. J. Allergy Clin. Immunol. 203-232.
2. Szentivanyi, A., Heim, O., and Schultz, P. 1979. Changes in adrenoceptor densities in membranes of lung tissue and lymphocytes from patients with atopic diseases. A. N.Y. Acad. Sci., 332:295.
3. Szentivanyi, A., and Szentivanyi, J. 1983. Some selected aspects of the immunopharmacology of adrenoceptors. In: Advances in immunopharmacology (Vol. II). J.W. Hadden (Ed). New York: Pergamon, p. 269.
4. Sano, Y., Watt, G., and Townley, R.G. 1983. Decreased mononuclear cell beta-adrenergic receptors in bronchial asthma. Parallel studies of lymphocytes and granulocyte desensitization. J. Allergy Clin. Immunol.72:495.
5. Kariman, K. 1980. Beta-adrenergic receptor binding in lymphocytes from patients with asthma. Lung 158:41.
6. Brooks, S.M., Mc Gowan, K., Bernstein, L., and Altenau, P. 1979. Relationship between numbers of beta adrenergic receptors in lymphocytes and disease severity in asthma. J. Allergy Clin. Immunol. 63:401.
7. Bittera, I., Gyurkovits, K., Falkay, G., Eck, E., and Koltai, M. 1988. Beta-adrenergic respiratory receptors of lymphocytes in children with allergic respiratory disease. Pedit. Pulmonol. 5:69.
8. Gamboa, P.M., Oehling, A., Sanz, M.L., and Castillo, J.G. 1987. Decrease of beta-receptors in asthmatic and rhinitic patients. Allergol. Immunopathol. 15:65.
9. Gamboa, P.M., De La Cuesta, C.G., Sanz, M.L., Garcia, B.E., and Oehling, A. 1990. Decrease of beta-receptors after the antigen-specific bronchial test in bronchial asthma. Allergol. Immunopathol. 3:115.
10. Gamboa, P.M., Sanz, M.L., De La Cuesta, C.G., and Garcia, B.E. 1991. Number of beta-receptors in patients allergic to Dermatophagoides pteronyssinus. J. Invest. Allergol. Clin. Immunol. 1(1):59.
11. Gamboa, P.M., Sanz, M.L., De La Cuesta, C.G., Garcia, B.E., Castillo, J.G., and Oehling, A. 1991. Number of beta-receptors in rhinitis pollinic patients. J. Invest. Allergol. Clin. Immunol. 1(2):113.
12. Agrawal, D.K., and Townley, R.G. 1987. Effect of plateleet-activating factor on beta-adrenoceptors in human lung. Res. Commun. 143:1.
13. Omini, C., Abbrachio, M.P., Coen, E., Daffonchio, L., Fano, M., Cattabeni, F. 1985. Involvement of arachidonic acid metabolites in beta-adrenoceptor desensitization: Functional and biochemical studies. Eur. J. Pharmacology. 106:601.
14. Safko, M.J., Chan, S.C., Cooper, K.D., Hanifin, J.M. 1981. Heterologons desensitization of leukocytes: A possible mechanism of beta-adrenergic blockade in atopic dermatitis. J. Allergy. Clin. Immunol. 68:218.

The Relationship of Viral Respiratory Infections to Bronchial Responsiveness and Asthma

William W. Busse*

Viral respiratory infections provoke wheezing in many patients with asthma. The mechanisms by which viral respiratory infections increase asthma are numerous and not fully established. Nonetheless, there is increasing evidence that one mechanism of virus-induced asthma is a promotion of the allergic response. This effect is noted on a number of IgE-dependent mechanisms. Some respiratory viruses can stimulate the development of IgE-antibodies and also promote other elements of the allergic reaction, particularly the development of the late asthmatic reaction. Thus, there is mounting evidence that an important contribution of viral respiratory infections to asthma is enhanced airway injury which is mediated, in part, by the ability of these illnesses to upregulate the inflammatory function of cells involved in the allergic reaction.

Respiratory infections have an important relationship to asthma as many patients wheeze with these illnesses. Epidemiological studies have shown that viral, not bacterial respiratory infections cause asthma to become more severe (1–4). The mechanisms of virus-induced asthma are multifactorial and not fully established. Nonetheless, present data and focus suggest that viral respiratory infections enhance the potential for airway inflammation, a factor similar to the pathogenesis of asthma. Thus, virus-induced asthma is not only relevant as a clinical problem but also provides insight to mechanisms of asthma.

Mechanisms of Virus-Induced Airway Hyperresponsiveness

A number of mechanisms have been identified to explain how viral respiratory infections enhance airway responsiveness and provoke an attack of asthma (Table 1). No single, unifying cause has yet been established; rather the virus-effects are multiple, interrelated and interactive. Most intriguing, however, is the possible inter-relationship that viral illnesses have on IgE-dependent allergic reactions.

The Role of Virus-Specific IgE Antibody Responses

Welliver et al. (5) evaluated 79 children with documented respiratory syncytial virus (RSV) infection for IgE-specific antibody to the infecting virus. The patterns of clinical illness were divided into four groups: (a) upper respiratory tract illness; (b) pneumonia without wheezing; (c) pneumonia and wheezing; and (d) wheezing (bronchiolitis). A striking and intriguing association appeared: IgE titers to RSV were highest in patients with airway obstruction, e.g. pneumonia/wheezing or bronchiolitis. Furthermore, patients with the highest RSV-IgE titers also had the lowest arterial pO2 values, possibly reflecting the greatest degree of airway obstruction. A similar pattern of response to parainfluenza virus (PV) was found (6). Together these studies indicate that some respiratory viruses stimulate IgE-specific antibody responses and the degree to which this occurs is associated with the clinical manifestations of airway disease.

Generation of Chemical Mediators

Welliver and colleagues also measured nasal secretions for mast cell mediators (5). Histamine was greater in children with bronchiolitis (lower airway disease) than subjects who did

* University of Wisconsin Medical School, University of Wisconsin, Hospital, 600 Highland Avenue, H6/360, Madison, WI, USA, 53792.
Acknowledgements: Support for work on this manuscript has come from grants NIH AI-20487, AI-26609, AI-15231, and General Clinical Research Grant RR-03186.

TABLE 1. Mechanisms of Virus-Induced Asthma

1. Sensitization of rapidly adapting afferent vagus sensory fibers.
2. Damage to airway epithelium
   (a) Loss of relaxing factor
   (b) Inactivation of enkephalinase, substance P degrading enzyme
3. Beta-adrenergic blockade
4. Production of virus-specific IgE antibody
5. Development of late asthmatic reactions to inhaled antigen
6. Enhanced leukocyte inflammatory function

not experience wheezing. Leukotriene C4 (LTC4) was also measured in children with either bronchiolitis or upper respiratory illness to RSV (7). LTC4 was detected twice as frequently in patients with bronchiolitis as those with upper airway disease alone, and the concentration of LTC4 was greater in children with bronchiolitis. Thus, although certainly not conclusive, these data suggest that inflammatory mediator release, or their generation, is greater in patients with obstructive airway illnesses during viral respiratory infections.

The Effect of Viral Respiratory Infections on Airway Hyperresponsiveness and the Development of Late-Phase Asthmatic Reactions

Many patients experience increased airway responsiveness during respiratory infections. To more precisely evaluate the effects of a respiratory infection on airway responsiveness, we experimentally infected selected subjects with rhinovirus (RV) and determined its effect on airway reactivity to histamine and to an IgE-dependent stimulus, antigen (8). Patients selected for study were evaluated on three separate occasions: at baseline, during acute infection, and recovery. All ten patients had an RV infection at the time of study. During the acute RV respiratory infection, airway responsiveness to histamine significantly increased (Figure 1). Likewise, acute airway reactivity to inhaled antigen was increased. The change in airway responsiveness to histamine and antigen was similar, suggesting that the respiratory infection effects on the immediate response to antigen related to alterations in overall bronchial reactivity. The patients were also evaluated for the development of a late allergic reaction (LAR) to antigen. Prior to RV inoculation, only one of the ten patients had an LAR to inhaled antigen (Figure 2). However, during the acute respiratory infection, eight of ten patients experienced late-phase airway obstruction; many of these patients persisted in having a LAR to an antigen inhalation challenge when retested 4 weeks later. These observations indicate that RV respiratory infection not only increases airway responsiveness but also changes the pattern of the airway response to inhaled antigen.

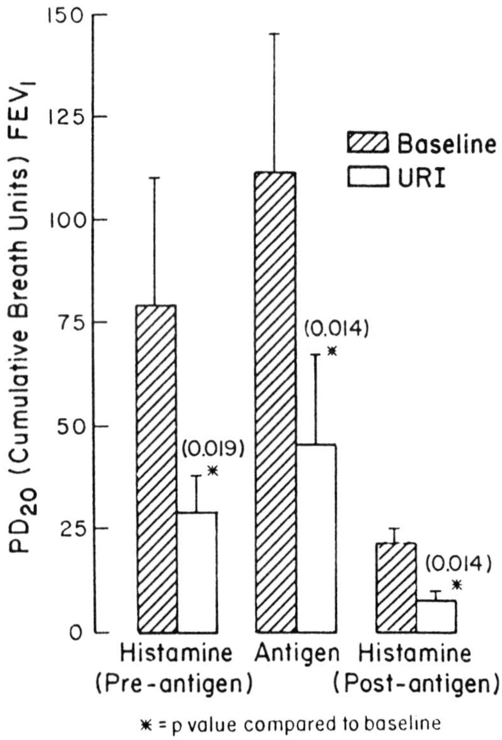

Figure 1. The effect of an acute rhinovirus respiratory infection on airway reactivity to histamine and antigen along with reactivity to histamine following antigen challenge. Values are mean ± SEM, n = 10. URI: upper respiratory infection. (Reprinted with permission from J. Clin. Invest., 1989, 83:1.)

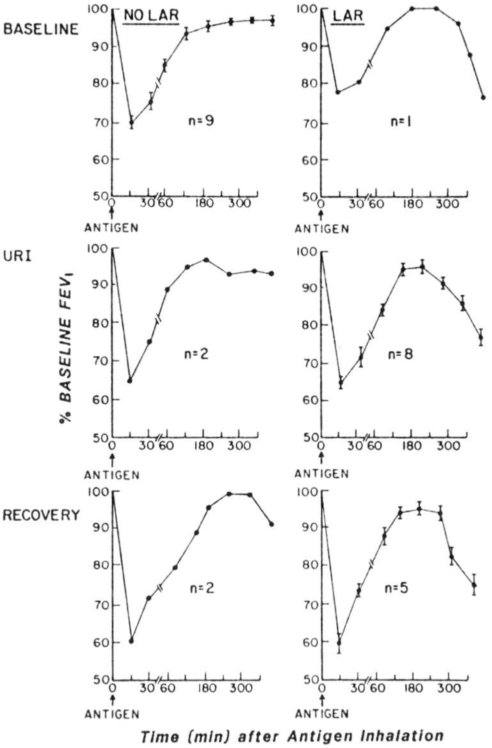

Figure 2. The pattern of airway response to inhaled ragweed antigen in patients prior to, during and following an acute rhinovirus infection. (Reprinted with permission from J. Clin. Invest., 1989, 83:1.)

Mechanisms in the Development of a Late-Phase Asthmatic Reaction During Respiratory Infections

Virus-associated airway hyperresponsiveness is a multifactorial process involving a complex interplay of IgE-dependent reactions, epithelial damage, autonomic nervous system dysfunction, and enhanced inflammation (9). In addition, individual patient features, such as inborn lung function and a family history of atopy, also contribute to the outcome in specific patients (10).

To begin to unravel the mechanisms by which a respiratory viral infection increases the potential for late-phase asthma, it is helpful to examine steps involved in the airways' response to antigen. From this analysis, a number of sites emerge as being potentially susceptible to respiratory virus effects and eventually influence the development of late-phase asthma. In IgE-mediated reactions, the tissue response, be it the skin, nose, or airway, is influenced by IgE sensitization of mast cells and basophils, release of bronchospastic and inflammatory mediators from sensitized cells, and the response of the target organ, which, in asthma, is bronchial smooth muscle. There are no available data to suggest that the concentration of IgE antibody necessarily determines either the intensity or likelihood of a late reaction (8,11). Therefore, other parameters involved in the LAR must be evaluated.

To evaluate the effects of respiratory viruses on another facet of the allergic response (mediator release) basophil histamine secretion has provided a model for study. We, and others, have found increased IgE-dependent basophil histamine release following an *in vitro* incubation with live respiratory viruses (12,13); this enhanced response may result, in part, from interferon production during the virus-leukocyte incubation (12,13). Thus, the possibility exists that respiratory virus interacts with lymphocytes, or monocytes, and stimulates cytokine generation which then influences the immediate hypersensitivity response. In the studies which showed increased bronchial reactivity to histamine and the development of late-phase asthma during an RV infection, basophil histamine release was also found to be enhanced (8). Although this associaon does not indicate a "cause-and-effect" relationship between enhanced leukocyte secretion and changes in airway reactivity to the development of an LAR, they do imply that the *in vivo* viral infection had effects upon human basophil function similar to that found with *in vitro* exposure to respiratory viruses. Thus, such *in vitro* models may have clinical relevance.

Since the role of basophils in allergic disease and asthma is not fully established, it is difficult to fully ascertain the importance of *in vitro* and *in vivo* studies with basophils. Nonetheless, present evidence indicates that basophils are present in increased concentrations during late phase reactions in the skin, nose and lower airway (14–16). Therefore, if virus infections enhance the basophil's ability to release histamine (and other mediators), this could lead to greater inflammation and obstruction during the respiratory illness. This, at present, is conjectural but intriguing. Other cells, i.e. neutrophils and eosinophils in particular, are associated with airway inflammation during LARs. When we incubated isolated neutrophils with influenza virus, their ability to generate superoxide (atoxic oxygen species) was significantly enhanced (17). A similar effect was noted with eosinophils. This becomes another example of how respiratory viruses enhance the inflammatory function of leukocytes to promote airway injury and the likelihood for late phase obstruction.

To integrate these findings into understanding the development of late-phase asthma, we hypothesize the following series of events. During initiation of the allergic response in the airway, inflammatory cells (neutrophils, eosinophils, and basophils) are recruited to the airway and, when activated, release inflammatory mediators. The amount of inflammatory mediators released determines the intensity of the response and possibly whether a LAR occurs. If an allergic reaction occurs during a viral respiratory infection, leukocytes recruited to the airway are "primed" and consequently produce greater inflammation when activated. Thus, because the cells recruited to the lung during the respiratory illness are "upregulated" leukocytes, the likelihood for airway injury and the development of a late asthmatic reaction increases.

Conclusion

There are a number of other mechanisms which contribute to virus-induced asthma including beta-adrenergic dysfunction, epithelial injury, and potentiation of neurogenic inflammation (9). However, all the mechanisms involved in the development of airway hyperresponsiveness, airway obstruction, recurrent wheezing with viral respiratory infections have yet to be fully appreciated. Nonetheless, current evidence indicates that viruses, or products of virus infected cells, influence the inflammatory property and potential of many cells. Precisely how these virus-effects translate into increased airway injury, responsiveness, and obstruction will require further work. Current evidence, however, indicates that virus-dependent effects on immune cells may increase their inflammatory potential; in this manner, the mechanisms of virus-asthma are similar to concepts of asthma in general: airway inflammation is a pivotal factor. As the mechanisms of virus-induced asthma are established, so will there be an improved understanding of asthma pathogenesis and its treatment.

References

1. McIntosh, K., Ellis, E.F., Hoffman, L.S., Lybass, T.G., Eller, J.J., and Fulginiti, V.A. 1973. The association of viral and bacterial respiratory infections with exacerbations of wheezing in young asthmatic children. J. Pediatr. 83:578.
2. Minor, T.E., Dick, E.C., DeMeo, A.N., Ouellette, J.J., Cohen, M., and Reed, C.E. 1974. Viruses as precipitants of asthmatic attacks in children. JAMA 227:292.
3. Minor, T.E., Dick, E.C., Baker, J.W., Ouellette, J.J., Cohen, M., and Reed, C.E. 1976. Rhinovirus and influenza A infections as precipitants of asthma. Am. Rev. Respir. Dis. 113:149.
4. Hudgel, D.W., Lanston, E. Jr., Selner, J.C., and McIntosh, K. 1979. Viral and bacterial infections in adults with chronic asthma. Am. Rev. Respir. Dis. 120:393.
5. Welliver R.C., Wong, D.T., Sun, M., Middleton, E. Jr., Vaughan, R.S., and Ogra, P.L. 1981. The development of respiratory syncytial virus specific IgE and the release of histamine in nasopharyngeal secretions after infection. N. Engl. J. Med. 305:841.
6. Welliver, R.C., Wong, D.T., Middleton, E. Jr., Sun, M., McCarthy, R.N., and Ogra, P.L. 1982. Role of parainfluenza virus-specific IgE in pathogenesis of croup and wheezing subsequent to infection. J. Pediatr. 101:889.
7. Volovitz, B., Welliver, R.C., DeCastro, G., Krystofik, D.A., and Ogra, P.L. 1988. The release of leukotriene in the respiratory tract during infection with respiratory syncytial virus: Role in obstructive airway disease. Pediatr. Res. 24:504.
8. Lemanske, R.F., Jr., Dick, E.C., Swenson, C.A., Vrtis, R.F., and Busse, W. 1989. Rhinovirus upper respiratory infection increases airway reactivity in late asthmatic reactions. J. Clin. Invest. 83:1.
9. Frick, W.E., and Busse, W.W. 1988. Respiratory infections: their role in airway responsive-

ness and pathogenesis of asthma. Clin. Chest Med. 9:539.

10. Morgan, W.J. 1990. Viral respiratory infection in infancy: Provocation or propagation? Sem. Respir. Med. 11:306.
11. Lemanske, R.F., Jr., and Kaliner, M.A. 1988. Late-phase allergic reactions. In: Allergy: Principles and practice. E. Middleton, Jr., C.E. Reed, E.F. Ellis, N.F. Adkinson, Jr., and J.W. Yunginger, eds. St. Louis, MO: C.V. Mosby, p. 224.
12. Ida, S., Hooks, J.J., Siraganian, R.P., and Notkens, A.L. 1979. Enhancement of IgE-mediated histamine release from human basophil by viruses: Role of interferon. J. Exp. Med. 145:892.
13. Busse, W.W., Swenson, C.A., Borden, E.C., Treuhauft, M.W., and Dick, E.C. 1983. The effect of influenza A virus on leukocyte histamine release. J. Allergy Clin. Immunol. 71:382.
14. Bascom, R., Wachs, M., Naclerio, R.M., Pipkorn, U., Galli, S.J., and Lichtenstein, L.M. 1988. Basophil influx occurs after nasal antigen challenge: Effects of topical corticosteroid treatment. J. Allergy Clin. Immunol. 81:580.
15. Charlesworth, E.N., Kagey-Sobotka, A., Schleimer, R.P., Norman, P.S., and Lichtenstein, L.M. 1991. Prednisone inhibits the appearance of inflammatory mediators and the influx of eosinophils and basophils associated with the cutaneous late-phase response to allergen. J. Immunol. 146:671.
16. Liu, M.C., Hubbard, W.C., Proud, D., Stealey, B.A., Galli, S.J., Kagey-Sobotka, A., Bleecker, E.R., and Lichtenstein, L.M. 1991. Immediate and late inflammatory responses to ragweed antigen challenge of the peripheral airways in allergic asthmatics. Am. Rev. Respir. Dis. 144:51.
17. Busse, W.W., Vrtis, R.F., Steiner, R., and Dick, E.C. 1991. *In vitro* incubation with influenza virus primes human polymorphonuclear leukocyte generation of superoxide. Am. J. Respir. Cell Mol. Bio. 4:347.

TABLE II. Diagnosis and Therapy for Allergic Asthma

A. Diagnosis of Immunologic Features of Asthma

Demonstration of IgE antibody by skin tests to	*Correlation of respiratory symptoms with*
Pollens	Pollenation season
Mold spores	Mold spore aerobiology
House dust mite	Correlation of symptoms with exposure and improvement with avoidance
Animal danders	Correlation of symptoms with exposure and improvement with avoidance

B. Immunologic Therapy for Asthma

1. Environmental control:
   Feasible for animal dander, house dust mite, occupational asthma.
2. Allergen immunotherapy
   A. Trial indicated for unavoidable allergen.
   B. Indicated when allergic rhinitis makes environmental allergen obvious.
   C. More likely effective in younger populations.
   D. Demonstrated effectiveness by 1 year in order to justify continuation.
   E. Efficacy of therapy would most likely be advanced by polymerized allergens.

TABLE III. Diagnostic and Therapeutic Approaches to Allergic Bronchopulmonary Aspergillosis (ABPA)

A. Diagnosis of ABPA

Clinical and laboratory:	Asthma, x-ray infiltrates in lungs, eosinophils
Serologic:	Increase in total IgE, IgE and IgG antibody against *Aspergillus fumigatus* (Af)
	Precipitins against Af
	Decline in total IgE with corticosteroid therapy

B. Therapy for ABPA

1. No avoidance programs are feasible. Exacerbations are not related to high level exposure to fungal spores.
2. Allergen immunotherapy is not indicated.
3. Antifungal agents are of no value.
4. Control of ABPA is by systemic corticosteroids for induction of remission, treatment of exacerbations and control of Stage IV (corticosteroid dependent stage).

antigenic load from Af plus the multiple immune responses of the host to Af antigens leads to the immunopathologic changes in the bronchi and then the lung parenchyma. This inflammatory reaction can be arrested by oral corticosteroid therapy and elimination of Af by control of asthma and elimination of the mucous which serves as a culture medium for Af. The result is a remission of ABPA and the future control and well being of the patient depend on the degree of irreversible pulmonary damage that has already occurred (13). These diagnostic and therapeutic features of ABPA are summarized in Table III.

Occupational Asthma

Asthma related to occupational exposures can be the most complex and perplexing diagnostic problems in the field of allergy and immunolo-

TABLE IV. Guidelines to Consider in Diagnosis and Management of Immunologic Occupational Asthma

Diagnostic Evaluation of Immunologic Factors in Occupational Asthma: Summary Statements

1. This is one of the most difficult diagnostic areas in the field of Allergy-Immunology.
2. Correlation of asthma with work exposure is very important but may be extremely difficult.
3. The work environment may be extremely complex with various protein antigens, chemical antigens and irritants. Environmental assessment is essential.
4. Coincidental adult onset asthma may be impossible to exclude.
5. For foreign proteins, diagnostic evaluation of IgE antibody mediated factors is the same as in Table II.
6. For allergic chemicals, the current status is that the immunologic evaluation is research rather than standard clinical practice.

Immunologic Management of Occupational Asthma

1. Allergen immunotherapy in the presence of continued occupational exposure is contraindicated except in very rare cases.
2. The principle of immunologic management is avoidance of exposure by internal job transfer, cessation of work or careful control of respiratory exposure at the work site.

gy. The possible etiologic relationships to the work environment may be clear and easily documented such as exposure to animal dander in an animal handler. Alternatively, there may be no clear relation to the work environment and no foreign proteins to evaluate. The more complex industrial exposures to chemical irritants and allergenic chemicals become, at times, an intense research experience to demonstrate causal immunologic relations. Furthermore, other cases labelled as occupational asthma may actually be other diseases such as (a) bronchitis due to cigarette smoking, (b) coincidental adult onset asthma, (c) compensation neurosis labelled asthma and variants of all of these problems. These complex features are summarized in Table IV. As noted in Table IV, asthma due to immunologic reactivity to allergenic chemicals is best considered as a phase of research activity at this time. Currently, trimellitic anhydride is the major model of this type of allergic asthma (14).

References

1. Busse, W.W. 1990. Respiratory infections: Their role in airway responsiveness and the pathogenesis of asthma. J. Allergy Clin. Immunol. 85:671.
2. Barnes, P.J. 1987. Neuropeptides in the lung: Localization, function, and pathophysiologic implications. J. Allergy Clin. Immunol. 79:285.
3. Ishizaka, K., Ishizaka, T., and Terry, W.D. 1967. Antigenic structure of gamma E globulin and reaginic antibody. J. Immunol. 99:849.
4. Pruzansky, J.J., and Patterson, R. 1966. Histamine release from leucocytes of hypersensitive individuals. I. Use of several antigens. J. Allergy 38:315.
5. Orange, R.P., and Austen, K.F. 1971. Chemical mediators of immediate hypersensitivity. In: Immunobiology. R.A. Good, and D.W. Fisher, eds. New York: Sinauer Associates, p. 115.
6. Samuelson, B., and HammarstrU S. 1980. Nomenclature for leukotrienes. Prostaglandins 19:645.
7. Grammer, L.C., Zeiss, C.R., Suszko, I.M., Shaughnessy, M.A., and Patterson, R. 1982. A double-blind placebo controlled trial of polymerized whole ragweed for immunotherapy of ragweed allergy. J. Allergy Clin. Immunol. 69:494.
8. Yunginger, J.W., and Gleich, G.J. 1973. Seasonal changes in IgE antibodies and their relationship to IgG antibodies during immunotherapy for ragweed hay fever. J. Clin. Invest. 52:1268.
9. Melam, H., Pruzansky, J.J., and Patterson, R. 1970. Correlation between clinical symptoms, leukocyte sensitivity, antigen binding capacity and Prausnitz-Kustner activity in the longitudinal study of ragweed pollinosis. J. Allergy 46:292.

sible for asthmatic patients, and children in particular (6). Education of asthmatic patients is very important in this field so that the patients can alter their own treatment without permanent dependency on their physician. Education also leads to an improved control of asthma as well as a reduced number of attacks, particularly the life-threatening ones. This may be achieved by a permanent and co-ordinated relationship between specialists (pneumologist, allergologist, physical medicine, etc.), general practitioners, medical co-workers (nurses, physiotherapists, health education teachers, psychologists) and the asthmatic patient (5).

The First Asthma Assessment

(A): Establish the severity of asthma. The first visit is particularly important in order to perform a check-up of the patient and to establish a management plan for the future. After a detailed history and the classical physical examination, a measurement of the respiratory function and of the reversibility of the airways obstruction must be performed in order to ascertain the precise respiratory function at the start of the treatment. A chest X-ray completes the examination. We establish the severity of asthma according to the Aas score.

(B) Attempt to identify the cause of asthma. Asthma is a complex disease in which allergic and non allergic triggers interact. The identification of triggers causing asthma is an important step in the management of asthmatics. The objective of non-pharmacologic treatment is, in the short term, to reduce the triggers precipitating symptoms by the use of avoidance measures. The allergy investigation may be performed at this visit. One can start with a "yes or no" immunological test such as the Phadiatop®, then the skin testing by the allergologist and, enventually, the measurement of specific IgE antibodies. Sinus X-rays and, if necessary, a CT-scan complete the check-up.

(C) Propose a management plan with a pharmacologic treatment. Anti-asthma drugs can be classified into two groups (7,8): either preventive and anti-inflammatory drugs or bronchodilatators. Preventive and anti-inflammatory drugs help to give a better control of asthma and bronchial hyperreactivity (9,10): First line drugs include the inhaled corticosteroids (11,12); second line drugs include cromoglycate and nedocromil; and third line drugs involve ketotifene. There is a trend to use anti-inflammatory drugs very early in the course of asthma. Bronchodilators relieve bronchospasm, but do not appear to control asthma in the long term. In this case the first line drugs are the inhaled β2-mimetics; and the second line drugs involve xanthines, oral β2-agonists and inhaled anticholinergics. There is a trend to reduce the use of xanthines (13). Recent, highly controversial studies have suggested that the regular use of β2-agonists may worsen asthma (14), but precise data backing this proposal are still lacking. Concerning the choice of drugs and therapeutic strategy, much national consensus has been reached within certain countries (15–17), although international consensus on the management of asthma has yet to be achieved. However, there is no such thing as the "miracle pill" to treat asthma, and the available drugs must be used correctly with reference to the severity and the type of bronchial obstruction:

In mild asthma (FEV1 > 80% of predicted value) inhaled β2-agonists (spray or powders) are used p.r.n. according to the needs and symptoms. Long acting theophyllines BID or OD have been proposed for some years but there is a trend to avoid these drugs at this stage. In moderate asthma, if bronchodilators are needed more than once a day, it is usually recommended that anti-inflammatory drugs be started using low-doses of inhaled steroids (i. e. a daily dose of under 400 µg/d for beclomethasone dipropionate, and budesonide or flunisolide). Cromolyn Sodium (particularly in children) or Nedocromil sodium are particularly useful in mild to moderate asthma. Finally, Ketotifen may be used in long term administration. In moderately severe forms (FEV1 60–80%): If the control of asthma is inadequate (symptoms and/or regular use of over four to six puffs of inhaled β2-agonists), the dosage of inhaled corticosteroids should be increased to an equivalent dose of 1,000 µg of BDP. At these levels, systemic side effects may be seen in a minority of highly susceptible patients. The use of a spacer improves the administration of inhaled corticosteroids and reduces their side effects. In severe asthma uncontrolled by inhaled anti-inflammatory drugs, long-term bronchodilator treatment should be supplemented by using inhaled long-acting β2-agonists (formoterol and salmeterol), and, if necessary, theophyllines, in which case plasma levels of theophylline should be serially controlled. Ipratropium bromide may be used if it has been shown to be effective during a respiratory function test. In some very severe cases, there is a permanent airflow obstruction requiring the addition of intermittent oral steroids, from 2 to 3 g yearly, as well as nebulized β2-agonists. In patients with very severe asthma (permanent airflow obstruction and FEV1 or PEFR under 50–60% of predicted values) long term oral corticosteroids may be necessary. Alternative anti-inflammatory drugs such as methotrexate or even cyclosporine are tested but they should not be given except during controlled drug trials. These proposals should be adjusted to individual patients and at each visit, in order to achieve the best control with the lowest rate of side effects.

(D) Start the education of the patient. The first consultation ends with the patient having the following information: What asthma is; what allergy is; what the etiologies and mechanisms are. This could be achieved by the use of videotapes, slides or booklet distribution. Peak flow monitoring may be proposed at this visit.

At this stage, details of the treatment should be discussed: preventive measures, allergen avoidance, pollutant avoidance (passive smoking, occupational factors), and different forms of treatment available. Asthmatic patient information involves explanations regarding the different ways of administring drugs, in particular the inhaled route, the use of sprays and alternative devices, and the differences between the doses of inhaled and systemic drugs. The side effects and means of their prevention should then be indicated.

The Following Visits

The goal of the regular examination of asthmatic patients is to maintain the control of asthma and to improve patient compliance to drug regimens. One way of achieving this is by an educational program. The first step of this program is to teach the patients how to perform a self-assessment of the disease. This is possible with the use of "the symptoms score": The asthmatic patient registers his daily symptoms in a diary (including information on crisis, cough, dyspnea, severity, nocturnal asthma, EIA, etc.). The symptoms score is evaluated on a scale from 0 to 5. One must emphasize that the ability to perceive the condition of dyspnea varies from patient to patient, some of whom request an emergency admission for slight levels of dyspnea, while others fail to notice even severe levels. Some sudden deaths in asthmatic patients may be due to this self-misperception of dypsnea.

The next step of this program is to teach the patients how to perform regular peak-flow measurements and to register the results on their diary card (18). Each patient with severe or chronic asthma should use a peak-flow meter morning and night. Peak-flow measurements demonstrate asthma variability, show the stable or unstable character of such a case of asthma, and thus indicate the improvement or worsening of bronchial obstruction. Daily variability is assessed according to the formula:

$$\frac{\text{Highest PEF} - \text{Lowest PEF}}{\text{Highest PEF}} \times 100$$

These results may be expressed as a percentage of the patient's personal highest score.

A third step in this program could involve non-pharmacological treatment, making use of either (a) specific immunotherapy or (b) physiotherapy: Specific immunotherapy (SIT) remains very controversial. Too much used in certain countries, it has been prohibited in others such as the United Kingdom. Its goal is to reduce hypersensitivity (or even curing it altogether) to a level compatible with the individual's ecosystem through repeated injections of the allergenic substance responsible for the affection. The efficacy of SIT in asthma was contested some years ago. Significant progress has been made since then, but, using potent extracts, allergen injections did result in a greater number of severe systemic reactions. It is therefore essential to consider several factors in order to appreciate the respective values of allergen avoidance and SIT in comparison with other available therapeutic methods (19,20): (a) the potential severity of the asthma to be treated; (b) the efficacy of available treatments; (c) the cost and duration of each type of treatment; and (d) the risk incurred by the patient due to the allergic disease and the treatments.

There are individual forms of treatment within a general SIT program depending on the allergen: (a) house dust mite asthma, (b) allergy to animal proteins, (c) allergy to molds, and (d) other extracts. (A) House dust mite asthma: House dust immunotherapy should not be used any more. The efficacy of mite SIT in asthma has been assessed in many controlled studies. Standardized extracts are effective but expose 5–30% of the patients to systemic reactions according to the protocol. With other extracts the results are more disparate. The indications of SIT in mite allergy have been examined. In a study of 225 patients followed-up for one year, Bousquet et al. found that patients with multiple allergen sensitivities and/or non-allergic triggers did not benefit from SIT. This treatment was more effective in children and young adults than later in life, and was seldom effective when FEV1 was under 70% of predicted values (after an adequate pharmacological treatment). Moreover, most patients with FEV1 under 70% of predicted values presented asthma during SIT. Thus, although it is suggested that patients with FEV1 over 70% of predicted values should only receive SIT, definite indications will not be available until the NIH sponsored study on mite allergy has been published. Studies of BHR are still unclear. The duration of SIT with mite extracts is still a subject of debate but may require life-long treatment. (B) Allergy to animal proteins: Although the Position Papers of the European Academy of Allergy and Clinical Immunology and WHO/IUIS have recommended that allergen avoidance be preferred to SIT in animal dander allergy, SIT may be considered, especially for occupational exposure, since it was shown to be effective. (C) Allergy to molds: Molds are major allergens in asthma but they often induce polysensitizations, and most extracts are not yet standardized. SIT together with standardized extracts of Alternaria and Cladosporium was proven to be effective. However, with many mold species or with extracts of unknown quality SIT should not be administered. (D) Immunotherapy with other extracts or other routes: Although SIT may be administered by oral or sub-lingual routes, there is no controlled study showing that it is effective in asthma. Specific immunotherapy with extracts of undefined allergens (bacteria, foods, Candida albicans, insect dusts, etc.) should be avoided. In summary, the decision to start a hyposensitization is dependent on five conditions: (a) the right choice of treatment, (b) the right allergenic extract, (c) the right protocol, (d) the right ethical code, and (e) the right price.

The second non-pharmacological form of treatment (the third step of our program) involves physiotherapy: In our clinic, we believe that asthmatic patients themselves should play an active role in bringing about their own cure, for example by modulating their breathing pattern, rather than passively waiting for their doctor to supply drugs. Physiotherapy can be introduced in three different steps in bronchial asthma: (a) during an asthmatic crisis, (b) in "classical" classroom training, and (c) in a program of "outdoor training": (A) During an asthmatic crisis, individual re-education includes: Emergency physiotherapy (involving the application of precise advice on how to cope with the crisis), stress management (by meditation or by relaxation techniques which induce a rapid decrease in tension), "awareness training" (developing an increased awareness of one's own body, in particular the thorax and the diaphragm, using both gentle and stretching techniques), and learning about the natural defense mechanisms of the body (including muscle contraction, as certain specialized techniques allow the patient to eliminate those contractions centered around the thorax and the back). (B) The "classical classroom" re-education aims at an improvement in effective ventilation, teaching the asthmatic subject to clear his bronchi, if necessary to correct a thoracic-vertebral deformity which is often present, to increase muscular tone necessary for efficient ventilation, and to decrease tension which gives rise to respiratory distress. (C) However one must also give "outdoor" re-education to asthmatic patients. That is, they should be encouraged to take part in a field of sports which does not give rise to an asthmatic attack and which, in the case of children, is associated with play activity. Here, there is obviously a wide range of possible choices. One must simply avoid those sports which may precipitate an asthmatic attack (all sports which require a sudden violent effort such as rugby, tennis and sprinting). However, other sporting activities are highly beneficial (swimming, supervised climbing, cross-country skiing, and cycling). A great variety of sports may therefore be undertaken as long as the following two conditions are fulfilled: (a) the asthmatic patient is prepared to train for this new activity; and (b) prophylactic medication is taken half an hour beforehand. Under these conditions, respiratory re-education allows an asthmatic to overcome what could be a potential handicap, that is, there is a "minus" side, but there is also a "plus" side, and the patients are also encouraged to maximize physical and personal development which will, we hope, eventually result in a completely normal, personal, professional, social and family life. This is not idle fantasy: In the world today there are many asthmatics who, with proper training, are capable of winning an Olympic gold medal.

References

1. Burr, M.L. 1987. Is asthma increasing? J. Epidemiol. Community Health 41:185.
2. Bousquet, J., Hatton, F, and Michel, F.B. 1987. Asthma mortality in France. J. Allergy Clin. Immunol. 80:389.
3. Buist, S. 1989. Asthma mortality: What we have learned? J. Allergy Clin. Immunol. 84:275.
4. Bousquet, J, Chanez, P., Lacoste, J.Y., et al. 1990. Assessment and clinical relevance of eosinophil inflammation in asthma. N. Engl. J. Med. 323:1031.
5. Parker, S.R., Mellins, R.B., and Sogn, D.D. 1990. Asthma education: A national strategy. NHLBI workshop summary. Am. Rev. Respir. Dis. 140:848.
6. Executive summary: Guidelines for the diagnosis and management of asthma. 1991. US Department of Health and Human Services, Publication No 91-3042A.
7. Barnes, P.J. 1989. A new approach to the treatment of asthma. N. Engl. J. Med. 321:1517.
8. Jenne, J.W, and Murphy, S. (Eds.). 1987. Drug therapy for asthma: Research and clinical practice. In: Lung biology in health and disease, Vol. 31. New York: Marcel Dekker.
9. Haathela, T., Järvinen, M., Kava, T., et al. 1991. Comparison of a β-agonist, terbutaline, with an inhaled corticosteroid, budesonide, in newly detected asthma. N. Engl. J. Med. 325:388.
10. Kerrebijn, K.F., van Essen-Zandvliet, E.E.M., and Neijens, H.J. 1987. Effects of long-term treatment with inhaled corticosteroids and beta-agonists on bronchial responsiveness in children with asthma. J. Allergy Clin. Immunol. 79: 653.
11. Salmeron, S., Guérin, J.C., Godard, P., et al. 1989. High doses of inhaled corticosteroids in unstable chronic asthma. Am. Rev. Respir. Dis. 140:167.
12. Toogood, J.H. 1989. High dose inhaled steroid therapy for asthma (Symposium). J. Allergy Clin. Immunol. 83:528.
13. Lam, A., and Newhouse, M.T. 1990. Management of asthma and chronic airflow obstruction. Are methylxanthines obsolete? Chest 98:44.
14. Pearce, N., Crane, J., Burgess, C. Jackson, R., and Beasley, R. 1991. Beta-agonists and asthma mortality. Clin. Exp. Allergy 21:401.
15. Hargreave, F.E., Dolovich, J., and Newhouse, M.T. 1989. The assessment and treatment of asthma: A conference report. J. Allergy Clin. Immunol. 85:1098.
16. British Thoracic Society [Research Unit of the Royal College of Physicians, King's Fund Centre, National Asthma Campaign]. 1990. Guidelines for management of asthma in adults. 1: Chronic persistent asthma. Br. Med. J. 301:651.
17. Warner, J.O., Götz, M., Landau, L.I., et al. 1989. Management of asthma: A consensus statement. Arch. Dis. Child. 64:1065.
18. Harm, D.L., Kotses, H., and Creer, T.L. 1985. Improving the ability of peak expiratory flow rates to predict asthma. J. Allergy Clin. Immunol. 76:688.
19. Bousquet, J., Hejjaoui, A., and Michel, F.B. 1990. Specific immunotherapy in asthma. J. Allergy Clin. Immunol. 86:292.
20. Thompson, R.A., Bousquet, J., Cohen, S.L., et al. 1990. Current status of allergen immunotherapy (hyposensitization). Shortened version of a WHO/IUIS Report. Lancet I:259.

Section XIX

Improving the Quality of Life in Asthma in the 1990's

Future Trends in Asthma Therapy

Terumasa Miyamoto*

There is every indication that the prevalence of asthma is increasing in the world. In Japan, the prevalence of asthma was about 1% in children and adults among the general population about 30 years ago. A recent survey disclosed, however, that it is now at 3 to 4%. In spite of extensive research and a better understanding of asthma, it cannot be considered under control. Because of the increasing prevalence of asthma and associated mortality, we must do our best to control it.

Avoidance of Allergens

In addition to the treatment of asthma, it is quite important to find its causes and avoid them to prevent this disease. This is essential for the prohylaxis of allergic diseases. Most cases of asthma may be caused by a number of factors; however, one or two may be particularly important and worth avoiding. Among various precipitating factors, house dust mites are the most important. Therefore vigorous house dust mite avoidance measures should be exerted. House dust mites can be reduced by careful cleaning, avoiding carpets, using bare wood floors, etc. Even if intensive anti-dust mite precautions are taken, complete avoidance is not possible, although an intensive program might not be indicated for all patients, particularly those with very mild symptoms. Thus chemical acaracides of low toxicity to humans may be a more desirable and more practical method of controlling the house dust mite population.

Medical Therapy

There are various drugs used in the treatment of asthma, including β-agonists, xanthine derivatives, anticholinergics, steroids, so-called anti-allergics, immunomodulating agents, etc., as well as immunotherapy.

β-Agonists

β-agonists are effective bronchodilators irrespective of the cause and have been used widely. Many diffrent β-agonists are available. In chronic asthma, the regular inhalation of β-stimulant has become popular for prophylactic purposes. Nevertheles, the regular use of β-agonists should be employed cautiously so as to avoid abuse, although recently advented β-agonists have a much lower incidence of side reactions. There has been a search for β-agonists which are more selective for β_2-receptors. The most important future advance will be the introduction of inhaled β_2-agonists with a long duration of action. Salmeterol appears to have a bronchodilator effect in excess of 12 hours, and to be particularly effective in preventing nocturnal asthma. At this moment, it is difficult for me to imagine that some future drug might be a more effective bronchodilator than the β_2-agonists, although many drugs have been investigated and are, in some respects, promising bronchodilators, a topic which will be touched on below.

Xanthine Derivatives

The bronchodilator effect of theophylline may not be as potent as the β-agonists, but slow-release theophylline preparations are currently available and widely used. Long acting preparations are more useful in round-the-clock (RTC) therapy than short acting ones. In addition, the "morning dip" may be controlled by a long acting preparation. There have been no newly developed xanthine derivatives as bronchodilators. New derivatives with a wide range of effective serum levels with fewer side reactions are expected in the future.

Anticholinergic Drugs

The development of atropine-like drugs, such as ipratropium bromide and exitropium

* National Sagamihara Hospital, 18-1, Sakuradai, Sagamihara-shi, Kanagawa-ken 228, Japan.

bromide, which have fewer side effects than atropine, has revived interest in anti-asthmatic drugs. While these medications have proved useful in some patients, their main value appears to be in treating chronic airway obstructive diseases in which the only reversible element is vagal tone. Consequently, anticholinergics may be more useful in combination with β-agonists in management of asthma, but may not be significantly effective when used alone.

Other Bronchodilators

Recently, drugs which activate a potassium channel were found to inhibit spontaneous tone in guinea pig trachea *in vitro*. Therefore, it may be that such drugs reduce airway hyperreactivity. Clinical studies are needed before the efficacy is determined. Vasoactive intestinal peptide (VAP), the E-series prostaglandins, adenyl cyclase activator, phosphodiesterase inhibitors, etc., are found to be, in some respects, promising bronchodilators. Furthermore, airway epithelium releases a relaxant factor, although it has not yet been identified. Consequently, drugs which enhance its production or mimic its effects may be used in the treatment of asthma in the future.

Steroids

There is no doubt that steroids, which were introduced in the 1950s, are the most effective drugs for the treatment of asthma, and that every stage of asthma responds well to their administration. The mode of action of steroids is not fully understood in asthma but their anti-inflammatory action, anti-eosinophil action, and their enhancing effect on β-receptor responsiveness are thought to be factors contributing to their effectiveness. As asthma is an inflammatory airway disease, it is necessary to control inflammation or inflammatory cell infiltration. Consequently, the anti-inflammatory action of steroids is quite meaningful in the treatment of asthma. Various side-effects are still a major problem with the use of systemic steroids. The introduction of the inhalation of steroids with high topical potency revolutionized the treatment of asthma. In fact, steroid inhalation is quite effective clinically and, in most cases, much more useful than any other preparation. Since the target organ of asthma is the airway, inhalation is a reasonable way to control asthma. Steroid inhalation should be used for even mild asthma as steroids suppress every stage of inflammation with only minimum side effects. Further development of steroids with higher topical potency and which are metabolized locally will be sought to improve inhalation.

So-Called Anti-Allergic Drugs

The advent of Intal in 1968 was an epoch-making event in the treatment of asthma. Intal is a potent mast cell stabilizing agent, with no bronchodilator effect. Intal does not prevent antigen-antibody combination or fixation of antibody to the mast cell but does prevent mast cell degranulation. The action of Intal was quite unique and its clinical efficacy has been greatly appreciated not only by children but also by adults. Intal has been used for prophylaxis of asthma. The action of Nedocromil is similar to that of Intal but is more active on mucosal mast cells and appears to be superior to that of Intal in clinical profile.

It is well known that various chemical mediators are involved in asthma and that inflammatory changes due to the actions of various chemical mediators are quite important in asthma. Consequently, the efficacy of steroids is also appreciated from the standpoint of anti-inflammatory agents. Not only have steroids and Intal attracted attention, but new agents (such as chemical mediator release inhibitors, antagonists of chemical mediators such as leukotriene antagonists, thromboxane antagonists, PAF antagonists, etc., inhibitors of chemical mediator synthesis such as leukotriene or thromboxane inhibitors, calcium channel modulators, H_1 antihistamines, etc.) also attracted medical attention. In fact, some are quite effective in comparison with inactive placebo carried out under double blind studies. Most show progressive effectiveness as prophylactics during therapy. Since there are so many chemical mediators involved in asthma, drugs with multiple actions to antagonize inflammatory mediators or inhibit inflammatory mediator synthetase are expected to be more effective. For instance, simultaneous inhibitors of both cyclogenesase and lipoxygenase pathways might be more useful. Inhibition of the release of neuropeptides, such as substance P, neurokinin A, and calcitonin gene-related peptide would also be useful.

Other Drugs

Immunomodulator drugs such as cyclosporin A or a new generation of related drugs with much lower nephrotoxicity should have a role in controlling asthma. Similarly, methotrexate, cyclophosphamide or related drugs could be useful in the management of severe chronic asthmatic patients. Gold preparation has proven effective in the treatment of asthma. Further development of such drugs with fewer side effects are also expected.

Immunotherapy

Immunotherapy was first introduced in the treatment of asthma in the early part of this century and is still used although criticism has occasionally been raised because of the lack of significant clinical effectiveness and its side effects. Purified allergen should be used instead of crude allergen to improve clinical efficacy. Recent studies on oral immunotherapy appear promising. Further studies are in progress.

Future Prospects

Future development in asthma therapy should be directed towards the inflammatory mechanisms, and more specific therapy could be developed. The possibility of a "cure" for asthma seems remote at this moment but, when the fundamental abnormalities are clarified or the mechanisms of outgrowing asthma are known, a cure for asthma may be possible. We should dedicate our efforts to the complete cure of asthma.

Improving the Quality of Life with Asthma in the 1990's: Asthma Management – Current Perspectives

Michael A. Kaliner*

Asthma should no longer be equated with bronchospasm; instead, the airflow obstruction in asthma is due to combinations of mucosal edema and inflammation, increased secretions, and muscle contraction. The appreciation of the importance of these various factors in airflow obstruction and the role that inflammation plays in asthma dictates a new, logical approach to the treatment of asthma employing two parallel modalities, each of which is equal in importance. (A) Symptomatic drugs which act to relieve the airflow obstruction but have no effects on the underlying causes of the disease (e.g. bronchodilators such as beta adrenergic agonists, theophylline and anticholinergic compounds): These agents are used only as needed, and only for as long as needed. The regular use of symptomatic agents will be limited or used only symptomatically on an as needed basis until the underlying disease process is controlled. (B) Specific treatments aimed at preventing or reversing the underlying causes responsible for the disease: There are four specific treatments available today: allergen avoidance, allergy immunotherapy, cromolyn or nedocromil, and inhaled corticosteroids. Management of asthma in the 1990's requires that *all* patients receive specific treatments intended to reduce the underlying disease processes and that the use of symptomatic treatment be employed only as necessary. Experience dictates that specific treatments should be initiated on every patient as the first-line of therapy, while symptomatic treatments should be considered second-line approaches.

Pathogenesis of Asthma

A working definition of asthma (modified from Reference 1) could be formulated thus: "A disease of reversible airflow obstruction manifested as wheezing and caused by various combinations of airway mucosal edema and inflammation, increased secretions, and smooth muscle contraction. Asthmatics exhibit airway hyperreactivity, and the clinical course is quite variable." While the primary pathologic changes causing airflow obstruction in asthma have been documented for some time (2), it is our new appreciation of the importance of airway inflammation and its effects on airway hyperresponsiveness that have altered our approach to the treatment of asthma so radically. The lungs of asthmatics who have died in status asthmaticus have the following changes: epithelial denudation, goblet cell hyperplasia, basement membrane thickening due to the deposition of sub-basement membrane collagen, eosinophil and neutrophil infiltration of the lamina propria, muscle hyperplasia and contraction, and glandular hyperplasia and hypersecretion. The airway lumen contains excessive secretions, eosinophils, neutrophils, Creola bodies, Curschmann's spirals, and Charcot-Leyden crystals. Recent studies describing airway mucosal biopsies obtained from asthmatics have confirmed that (a) edema and denudation of the mucosa, (b) eosinophil, lymphocyte and neutrophil infiltration, (c) basement membrane thickening due to the deposition of sub-basement membrane collagen and (d) mast cell hyperplasia and degranulation are found even in mild ambulatory asthmatic patients (3,4).

These observations indicate that the airways of asthmatics exhibit a striking degree of inflammation as well as other changes even when the patient feels well. There is currently some uncertainty regarding the genesis of this inflammation. Most likely, mast cell initiated late phase reactions cause a significant portion of this inflammation. The late phase reaction was initially appreciated after antigen inhalation challenge in atopics and is due to the effects of mast cell mediators (5). Mediators such as in-

* Allergic Diseases Section, Laboratory of Clinical Investigation, National Institute of Allergy and Infectious Diseases, National Institutes of Health, Building 10, Room 11C205, Bethesda, Maryland 20892, USA.

flammatory factors of anaphylaxis, neutrophil chemotactic factors such as leukotriene B4, platelet activating factor, and others cause the infiltration of neutrophils and eosinophils at the site of mast cell degranulation. Recent evidence that mast cells induce the expression of adhesion molecules on the surface of endothelial cells (6), and that this expression is increased in asthma (7), supports this concept. Mast cells have also recently been found to synthesize and release several important cytokines capable of causing or facilitating inflammatory responses. These cytokines include IL-3, IL-4, IL-5, TNF, interferon gamma, and others (8,9). Thus, newly appreciated mast cell mediators appearing several hours after antigen exposure may also contribute to late phase responses. Moreover, basophil infiltration and release of mediators may also contribute to the late response. Current work suggests that basophils infiltrate the skin and nasal mucosa during the late response, and there is at least some suggestion that basophils are found in bronchoalveolar lavage fluid from asthmatics undergoing late phase reactions. In human nasal and cutaneous models of the late response, there is substantial evidence that mast cells (or perhaps basophils) are reactivated during the response and that one of the targets for allergy immunotherapy is the late reaction (5). In addition, many CD4+ lymphocytes have been found both in the airway lamina propria and in the epithelium (10). These cells are capable of synthesizing and secreting a number of pro-inflammatory molecules and participating in both the inflammatory and reactivity changes noted in asthma. Preliminary data has also suggested that alveolar macrophages can be activated *in vivo* by antigen inhalation challenge with the release of pro-inflammatory cytokines (such as IL-1).

Another newly appreciated aspect of asthma pathogenesis is the contribution of sensory nerve related neuropeptides such as substance P (SP). Stimulation of airway sensory nerves as might occur during allergic inflammation or as a consequence of mast cell activation, would result in the secretion of several neuropeptides into the mucus membrane. These peptides include SP, neurokinin A (NKA), calcitonin gene related peptide (CGRP) and gastrin releasing peptide (GRP). These agents would cause vascular permeability (SP, CGRP), vasodilation (CGRP, SP), mucus secretion (GRP, S NKA), and muscle contraction (SP, NKA) (11). Vascular permeability with subsequent edema formation and increased airway secretion of an albumin-rich exudate is certainly an important contributing factor in asthma, and may be caused by these neuropeptides in addition to the vasoactive amines secreted by mast cells.

Therapeutic Targets

One of the major new insights gained about the treatment of asthma has been in the relationship between allergen-induced late phase reactions and increased airway reactivity. It has been observed and confirmed that allergen challenge in the laboratory, as well as natural seasonal allergen exposure, lead to increased airway reactivity, and that conversely, reduction in allergen exposure reduces airway reactivity (5). It is therefore appropriate to include airway reactivity as one of the targets in the treatment of asthma. Thus, rather than treat asthma simply to reduce airflow obstruction, a new concept has evolved to actually aim therapy at the underlying causes of the disease, including airway hyperresponsiveness. For example, it has been shown that avoidance of allergens in dust allergic asthmatic children results in improvement both in airflow obstruction and in airway reactivity (12,13). These data confirm the findings that allergen exposure increases airway reactivity and suggest that reduction in allergic reactions should benefit asthmatics. Allergen avoidance, like the avoidance of non-steroidal inflammatory agents in aspirin-sensitive asthmatics, is a useful component of the specific treatment of asthma. This recognition also implies that physicians caring for asthmatics need to be trained to recognize potential allergens in their evaluation.

There is little controversy regarding the role of immunotherapy in the treatment of allergic rhinitis caused by pollens and dust. The controversy relates to immunotherapy of asthma. There are many studies published on this topic, and one can find both positive and negative studies in the literature. The problems responsible for the various outcomes in these studies relate to asthma itself, a disease which is far more complex than rhinitis. The recent literature suggests that, if one chooses relatively "pure" allergic asthmatics, such as can be found in cat allergen-induced asthma, the data are relatively clear. Immunotherapy with purified cat allergen improves asthma in cat allergic asthmatics (14,15). Other articles have specifically employed airway reactivity as the endpoint for immunotherapy and have also shown improvement. Thus, immunotherapy may be used appropriately in allergic asthmatics as a specific treatment to reduce underlying allergies, anticipating that with time this treatment will reduce both asthma and the allergen-induced component of increased airway reactivity. Moreover, immunotherapy is the only modality available today which has a long lasting response, reducing the needs for all other medications when effective.

Cromolyn is an agent whose precise mode of action remains unclear, but which has the ability to reduce mast cell reactivity. Nedocromil is a newly available agent which like cromolyn has anti-inflammatory properties, including the capacity to reduce mast cell degranulation. Given prophylactically, cromolyn and nedocromil can prevent allergen induced early asthmatic responses, late asthmatic responses, and the increased airway reactivity that ordinarily results from these challenges (16). While there is some controversy about the capacity of cromolyn to reduce airway reactivity, in general, studies conducted over a longer period of time (greater than 4–6 weeks) show improvement in airway reactivity. Indeed, a recent study by Petty (17) was performed in chronic adult asthmatics and demonstrated impressive improvements not only in airway reactivity but also symptom scores. Nedocromil appears to be even more impressive in its anti-inflammatory properties and in its capacity to reduce airway reactivity.

Corticosteroids have many actions which make them useful in treating asthma. Among the actions which are most relevant are: reduced microvascular permeability, reduced mucus secretion, reduced prostaglandin production, enhanced beta adrenergic responses, reduced mast cell number and reactivity *in vivo*, reduced late phase responses, and reduction in airway reactivity (reviewed in reference 18). Thus, topical corticosteroids have a wide range of potential therapeutic targets in asthma therapy. World-wide, inhaled corticosteroids are becoming increasingly more popular for asthma therapy, although certain questions regarding minimal effects on growth in children and subtle adrenal suppression are still of some concern. The recent Asthma Education Program developed by the National Heart, Lung and Blood Institute advocates the use of cromolyn (or nedocromil) early in asthma treatment, but recommends that inhaled corticosteroids may be useful in moderate to severe asthmatics (19).

The Era of Symptomatic Treatment

One can divide asthma therapy in the United States into the era of symptomatic control from 1970–1990. In this period of time, beta adrenergic agents specific for the beta-2 receptor were developed, modified, and made available for convenient and effective bronchodilation. Theophylline was formulated into extremely convenient, timed-release preparations which, when combined with accurate and convenient measurements of serum theophylline levels, led to the great popularity of this compound in the United States. Indeed, theophylline products became the foundation for the treatment of asthma. It was commonly taught that chronic asthma was best controlled employing theophylline as the foundation of clinical control, to which beta agonists were added if additional bronchodilation was necessary. Late in the era, ipratropium become available, both for bronchodilation and to inhibit mucus secretion. The focus on the symptomatic control of asthma with these three agents was very successful for the management of most patients, although both hospitalization and death rates increased. Recent publications have suggested the possibility that the use of inhaled beta adrenergic agents might "mask" underlying airways inflammation by keeping airways open, even in the presence of increasing inflammation. There is increasing evidence that the excessive use of chronic beta adrenergic therapy may be potentially harmful to a small number of subjects, primarily those using more than the approved amount of bronchodilator or who are using these agents without the concomitant use of specific treatments as well.

A New Era: The Era of Specific Treatment

Beginning about 1990, a new era in asthma therapy began in the United States (and was well underway in other parts of the world). This era is based upon the use of specific therapy as the foundation for asthma treatment, and includes the conceptual corollary that the use of symptomatic agents is restricted to an "as needed basis". Thus, patients are started on one or more specific treatments depending upon the specific pattern of their diseases and are also given symptomatic agents *as needed*. The specific treatments are intended to reduce the underlying cause of the disease, and, if successful, to reduce the need for concomitant symptomatic treatments. Treatment of an allergic asthmatic might include both allergen avoidance recommendations, consideration of immunotherapy, and inhaled anti-inflammatory agents, either cromolyn or corticosteroids. In addition, patients would receive bronchodilators until control of the underlying processes is satisfactory. The first choice of symptomatic therapy would be an inhaled beta adrenergic agonist, and theophylline would be added only if additional control was required.

What are the expectations for this new approach? The long term use of cromolyn, inhaled corticosteroids, allergen avoidance and immunotherapy will reduce both airway hyperreactivity and asthma symptoms, and thereby reduce the need for bronchodilators (symptomatic drugs) in most patients. This is the expectation for the bulk of the asthmatic population, not necessarily the severe asthmatic who may require oral corticosteroids on a daily basis. With the recent concerns about the safety of inhaled beta adrenergic agents, we are all starting to use these bronchodilators more cautiously. Our current approach (1991) is to prescribe inhaled beta adrenergics to be used only as often as needed, as indicated by the use of home peak flow monitoring. We now use beta adrenergics on a regular basis only in conjunction with concomitant anti-inflammatory agents. We are entering a period when various anti-inflammatory agents which have been found to be useful in treating diseases such as rheumatoid arthritis are also being studied in the treatment of severe asthma, and even medications like furosemide appear to have some possible use as well. The pharmaceutical companies are examining the usefulness of leukotriene antagonists, PAF blockers, 5-lipoxygenase inhibitors, and mucolytics in asthma therapy. It is certain to be a time of change. However, the greatest advance has been the change in the aim of therapy. Until very recently, we simply tried to control the symptoms of asthma. Now, it is conceivable that, for the majority of asthmatics, we should be aiming at reducing the disease itself. This very basic conceptual change will have profound effects on asthma therapy and perhaps on the morbidity and mortality of the disease as well.

References

1. Kaliner, M.A., Eggleston, P.A., and Mathews, K.P. 1987. Rhinitis and asthma. J. Amer. Med. Assoc. 258:2851.
2. Kaliner, M.A., Blennerhassett, J., and Austen, K.F. 1976. Bronchial asthma. In: Textbook of immunopathology. P.A. Meischer and H.J. Muller-Eberhard, eds. New York: Grune and Stratton, p. 387.
3. Laitinen, L.A., Heino, M., Laitinen, A., and Haahtela, T. 1985. Damage of the airway epithelium and bronchial reactivity in patients with asthma. Am. Rev. Respir. Dis. 131:599.
4. Beasley, R., Roche, W.R., Roberts, J.A., and Holgate, S.T. 1989. Cellular events in the bronchi in mild asthma and after bronchial provocation. Am. Rev. Respir. Dis. 139:806.
5. Lemanske, R.F., and Kaliner, M.A. 1988. Late phase allergic reactions. In: Allergy: Principles and practice (Third Ed.). E. Middleton, C.E. Reed, E.F. Ellis, N.F. Adkinson, and J.W. Yunginger, eds. St. Loius, MO: C.V. Mosby, p. 224.
6. Klein, L.M., Lavker, R.M., Matis, W.L., and Murphy, G.F. 1989. Degranulation of human mast cells induces an endothelial antigen central to leukocyte adhesion. Proc. Natl. Acad. Sci. USA 86:8972.
7. Wegner, C.D., Grundel, R.H., Reilly, P., Haynes, N., Letts, L.G., and Rothlein, R. 1990. Intercellular adhesion molecule-1 (ICAM-1) in the pathogenesis of asthma. Science 247:456
8. Plaut, M, Pierce, J., Watson, C., Hanley-Hide, J., Nordan, R., and Paul, W. 1989. Mast cell lines produce lymphokines in response to cross-linkage or to calcium ionophores. Nature 339:64.

9. Burd, P.R., Rogers, H.W., Gordon, J.R., Martin, C.A., Jayaraman, S., Wilson, S.D., Dvorak, A.M., Galli, S.J., and Dorf, M.E. 1989.Interleukin-3-dependent and independent mast cells stimulated with IgE and antigen express multiple cytokines. J. Exp. Med. 170:245.
10. Jeffery, P.K., Wardlaw, A.J., Neslon, F.C., Collins, J.V., and Kay, A.B. 1989. Bronchial biopsies in asthma. Amer. Rev. Resp. Dis. 140:1745.
11. Baraniuk, J.N., and Kaliner, M.A. 1990. Neuropeptides in the upper and lower respiratory tracts. In: Immunology and allergy clinics of North America, Vol. 10, No. 2. C.W. Bierman, and T.H. Lee, eds. Philadelphia: W.B. Saunders, p. 383.
12. Platts-Mills, T.A.E., Tovey, E.R., Mitchell, E.B., Moszoro, H., Nock, P., and Wilkins, S.R. 1982. Reduction of bronchial hypereactivity during prolonged allergen avoidance. Lancet 2:675.
13. Murray A.B., and Feguson, A.C. 1983. Dust-free bedroom in the treatment of asthmatic children with house dust or house dust mite allergy: A controlled trial. Pediatrics 71:418.
14. Ohman, J.L., Findlay, S., and Leitermann, K.M. 1984. Immunotherapy in cat-induced asthma. Double-blind trial with evaluation of *in vivo* and *in vitro* responses. J. Allergy Clin. Immunol. 74:230.
15. Van Metre, T.E., Marsh, D.G., Adkinson, N.F., Kagey-Sobotka, A., Khattignavong, A., Norman, P.S., and Rosenberg, G.L. 1988. Immunotherapy for cat asthma. J. Allergy Clin. Immunol. 82:1055.
16. Cockcroft, D.W., and Murdock, K.Y. 1987. Comparitive effects of inhaled salbutamol, sodium cromoglycate, and becloethasone diproprionate on allergen-induced early asthmatic responses, late asthmatic responses, and increased responsiveness to histamine. J. Allergy Clin. Immunol. 79:734.
17. Petty, T.L., Rollins, D.R., Cristopher, K., Good, J.T., and Oakley, R. 1989. Cromolyn sodium is effective in adult chronic asthmatics. Am. Rev. Respir. Dis. 139:694.
18. Peden, D.B., and Kaliner, M.A. (1991). The mechanisms of action of steroids in asthma. Immunol. Allergy Clin. N. A., in press.
19. Guidelines for the diagnosis and management of asthma. 1991. Ped. Asthma Allergy. Immunol. 5:57.
20. Furakawa, C.T., DuHamel, T.R., Weimer, L., Shapiro, G.G., Pierson, W.E., and Bierman, C.W. 1988. Cognitive and behavioral findings in children taking theophylline. J. Allergy. Clin. Immunol. 81:83.

Cellular Mechanisms of Glucocorticoid Action: Implications for Future Therapy

Stephen J. Lane, Tak H. Lee*

Glucocorticosteroids (GCS) are the most effective treatment for bronchial asthma. However, their mechanism of action is unknown. GCS bind to intra-cytoplasmic phospho-receptors (GR) which have highly conserved functional domains. The GCS-GR complex then translocates to the nucleus where it binds glucocorticoid response elements (GRE) in the promoter region of GCS responsive genes causing them to be induced or repressed. Subtle differences in this mechanism may explain the resistance to GCS seen in asthma. We have shown that monocytes from asthmatic subjects secrete a 3 Kd peptide which is pro-inflammatory *in vitro* for granulocytes. This activity is inhibited by hydrocortisone, methylprednisolone and dexamethasone in steroid-sensitive (CS) asthmatic subjects, with respective IC50s being 600 nM, 70 nM and 0.5 nM. In contrast, there was much reduced inhibition seen in the steroid-resistant (CR) group. Steroid resistance is not due to altered pharmacokinetics in CR subjects. Peak serum levels of prednisolone were 645 ± 43 and 676 ± 52 ng/ml in the CS and CR groups, respectively ($p = 0.92$). Estimated clearances of prednisolone were 155 ± 8 and 157 ± 7 ml/minute per 1.73 square meters in CS and CR patients, respectively. This defect is not caused by corticosteroid receptor characteristics. The Kd for dexamethasone was 2.45 ± 0.58 nM (mean ± SEM, $n = 6$) in the CS group and 1.6 ± 0.35 nM (mean ± SEM, $n = 6$) in the CR group of patients ($p = 0.14$). The Ro in the CS group was 3605 ± 984 binding sites per nucleus (mean ± SEM, $n = 6$) and 4757 ± 692 binding sites per nucleus (mean ± SEM, $n = 6$) in the CR group ($p = 0.23$). GCS-resistance seen in CR asthma may arise from subtle differences in the regulation of gene expression. Increasing knowledge of the cell types involved in asthma, coupled with recent knowledge on the mechanism of GCS action, will allow a rational approach to elucidating the cause of non-responsiveness to GCS.

Synthetic glucocorticosteroids (GCS) are the most effective treatment for bronchial asthma; however their mechanism of action is unknown. In addition, a certain proportion of asthmatics, i. e. 5%, appear to be insensitive to their effects (1). As molecular biological techniques continue to unravel the mechanism of steroid action, subtle differences in these patients may account for this resistance. Furthermore, there is now considerable information on the affected cell types in asthma and the target genes involved in the corticosteroid response.

The Glucocorticoid Receptor

GCS act through a 300 Kd glucocorticoid receptor (GR) phosphoprotein complex which has been shown by immunocytochemical techniques to be located mainly in the cytoplasm in nearly all human cell types (2).They are characterized by a receptor density of 2,000-30,000 binding sites per cell with dissociation constants for natural glucocorticoids (cortisol and corticosterone) that fall within the the normal range of plasma concentration for free hormone, i. e. c.30 nM (3). Upon binding GCS, the GR undergoes dephosphorylation, dissociates two 90 Kd associated heat shock proteins (HSP), forms dimers, and translocates to the nucleus in a temperature-dependent fashion (4). Here the GR binds to sequences of DNA known as glucocorticoid response elements (GRE) in the promoter region of glucocorticoid responsive genes (see below). The stability of the GR complex is affected by different factors (3). *In vitro*, activation and degradation of receptors are inhibited by molybdate and stabilised by phosphorylated-sugars. *In vivo* GCS treatment decreases receptor levels by increasing degradation or by decreasing synthesis depending on the cell type. Conversely, adrenalectomy increases receptor density. Receptor levels show cell cycle specificity and are doubled in HeLa cells in G1 phase.

* Department of Allergy and Allied Respiratory Disorders, U.M.D.S., Guy's Hospital, London SE1 9RT, U.K.

The GR belongs to a highly conserved superfamily of hormone receptor proteins characterised by a remarkable overall structural unity with impressive functional diversity (5). This group includes the receptors for the sex steroids, thyroid hormone, vitamin D3 and the retinoids. The use of GR cDNA expression vectors has revealed that these hormone receptors are structurally organised into five homologous domains, each responsible for different functions and each with different degrees of conservation within the superfamily. These are glucocorticoid and HSP90 binding, dimerization of the GR, nuclear localization of GR, DNA binding of the GR to GRE and transactivation of gene expression (6).

DNA binding is encoded by a central domain which is the most highly conserved region of the receptor. This is a cysteine-rich 70 amino acid sequence which folds into two zinc finger motifs, each of them with a zinc atom tetrahedrically co-ordinated to four cysteines. A Gly-Ser sequence in the root of the N-terminal zinc finger determines hormone response specificity and binds to the major groove on the GRE (7). The GR sub-family, which includes the androgen and progesterone receptors, has this amino acid sequence whereas the estrogen receptor sub-family has not (8).The C-terminal finger binds to a sugar-phosphate flanking sequence of the GRE and is possibly involved in receptor dimerization (9).

The steroid binding domain located at the C-terminal end of the GR is the next most conserved region of the receptor (10). This region binds the ligand in a hydrophobic pocket and participates in several other functions including dimerization, nuclear translocation, and is the binding site for HSP90. It also contains a 30 amino acid residue which is involved in hormone-dependent transcriptional activation. Another transactivating domain has been identified at the N-terminal domain which is independent of hormone binding (11).The N-terminal domain is the least conserved and possesses a marked cell-type and promoter specificity. It is also the immunogenic site of the receptor. The nuclear translocation domain is a short sequence which resembles that of the SV40 T antigen (12). It is interesting that, although nuclear translocation is a pre-requisite for activation, studies utilising GCS resistant cell lines have indicated that other interactions are necessary for optimal transactivating efficiency.

Glucocorticoid Response Elements and Trans-Activation

GR receptor dimers bind to specific elements of DNA called GREs and directly either induce or repress gene transcription. Most GREs consist of two half site hexamers separated by three base pairs, with a sequence resembling the consensus sequence GGTACAnnnTGTTCT (where n is any nucleotide) (13). Binding of the GR to this sequence usually results in promoter enhancement. The regulatory diversity of this interaction, however, is limited as it only involves a single factor. They are denoted "simple" GREs in order to distinguish them from the recently characterized "composite" GREs. Composite GREs do not contain the above consensus sequence and depend on protein-protein interactions between the GR and other transcriptional factors to achieve combinatorial regulation.In a recent study, Diamond showed that their activity depended upon the binding not only of GR but also of other non-receptor transcription factors, e. g. the activating protein 1 (AP-1), which is a dimer of two proto-oncogene products, c-fos and c-jun (14). The GR-GRE receptor complex was inactive in the absence of AP-I activity. The presence of the c-jun/c-jun homodimer conferred promoter enhancement while the c-jun/c-fos heterodimer conferred promoter repression. It is therefore fascinating that the c-fos and c-jun non-receptor products conferred GCS responsiveness by novel protein-GRE binding. Because of their regulatory versatility, it seems likely that composite GREs will prove to be the prevalent mode for regulation by steroids. In addition, protein-protein interaction independent of GR-DNA binding has recently been described as important in regulating positive or negative promoter function (15). This novel regulation involves down modulation of the trans-activating function of pre-existing unbound and DNA-bound AP-1. It is evident that positive or negative regulation of gene expression is a complex and versatile system. Its efficiency is governed by (a) *in vivo* hormone binding to GR which alters the kinetics of the subsequent GR-GRE interaction (16); (b) protein-protein interaction of the GR with other non-receptor transcriptional factors (17); (d) GR-DNA interactions which depend on the nature and quantity of GRE response elements (14); (d) dimerisation of the GR (18); and (e) as yet undefined GRE-chromatin interactions which determine the tissue and cell specifities of the glucocorticoids (19).

Anti-Inflammatory Models of Glucocorticoids

The anti-inflammatory mechanism of GCS is not known. One postulated mechanism is by production of lipocortins (20). GCS up-regulate lipocortin expression at the transcriptional and post-transcriptional levels.In some *in vitro* systems lipocortins appear to mediate GCS-induced suppression of eicosanoid and prostanoid generation from arachidonic acid breakdown by non-competitive inhibition of phospholipase (PL) A2 activity (20). However a recent study by Almawi has shown that although mitogen driven lymphocyte proliferation was inhibited by dexamethasone, this effect was independent of arachidonic acid breakdown, suggesting that the anti-inflammatory mechanism of the lipocortins is distinct from PLA_2 inhibition (21). In addition, work by Dennis et al. has demonstrated that the effect of the lipocortins can be overcome by increasing the concentration of phospholipid substrate and has questioned the physiological role of the lipocortins in non-competitive inhibition of PLA2 (22).

Walker et al. showed that lectin induced lymphocyte proliferation was bimodally distributed in terms of its suppression by GCS in a small number of normal subjects (23). Those subjects who exhibited GCS-resistance (CR) had higher levels of IL-2 in the cell free supernatants. This study raises the possibility that the resistance to GCS seen in various disease states may be an important primary phenomenon. Almawi has demonstrated that this effect could be abrogated by a combination of recombinant cytokines, i. e. rIL-1 + rIL-6 + rIFN-gamma and that the required anti-proliferative concentrations of GCS parallel the concentrations required for the blockade of various cytokines (24). These results indicate that inhibition of cytokine gene expresson is the most likely mechanism by which GCS exert their effect in this system. Whether they act directly on cis-regulating elements or indirectly by the generation of trans-activating cytokine transcription inhibitory factors, is not known. A fascinating finding is that numerous copies of the GRE consensus sequence have now been localized in the promoter region of several GCS responsive cytokine genes, i. e. IL-1, IL-2, IL-3, IL-5, IL-6, TNF, IFN (25). This finding supports the view that GCS may act by directly repressing the expression of these genes by acting on cis regulating elements. Indeed, in gene transfer experiments, dexamethasone-activated GR appeared to directly repress IL-6 gene expression by occlusion of both the GRE and the basal IL-6 promoter elements (26).

GCS can also regulate cytokine gene expression at post-transcriptional levels. They can alter the stability and thus steady-state levels of specific mRNAs. Kern et al. have demonstrated that IL-1 beta gene transcription was unaffected by 10 μM dexamethasone in LPS stimulated human adhered monocytes using nuclear transcription run-off assays (27). Post-transcriptionally dexamethasone prolonged the IL-1 half-life, moderately inhibited the translation of its precursors and profoundly inhibited its release into the extracellular fluid.

Other mechanisms postulated for the anti-inflammatory action of GCS include blockade of activation associated increases in transmembrane ionic fluxes (28), modulation of protein kinase C activity/function (29) and alteration in membrane phospholipid profile (30). Using mitogen and allo-antigen driven proliferation assays of human PBMC, Almawi et al. have ruled out blockade of activation-induced elevation in [Ca++] (31) and interference with protein kinase C activation and translocation from cytosolic to membrane bound compartments, as mechanisms by which GCS inhibit PBMC proliferation.

Corticosteroid-Resistant Bronchial Asthma

There is now abundant evidence implicating cells of the monocyte-macrophage series in the pathogenesis of bronchial asthma by their capacity to secrete bioactive mediators, cytokines and to present antigen (32). Monocytes in patients with bronchial asthma exhibit a number of other functional abnormalities which may be important in the elucidation of the mechanism of corticosteroid action in this disease (32). Corticosteroid responsiveness in asthma is defined as an increase in FEV1 of greater than 30% during a 14 day course of 40 mg prednisolone (CS) (1,33). Corticosteroid resistance in asthmatic subjects (CR) was defined as an improvement in the FEV1 of less than 15% after a similar course of prednisolone. The mechanism of corticosteroid resistance in bronchial asthma is not known. Wilkinson et al. have shown that monocyte primed super-natants from asthmatic subjects secrete a 3 Kd peptide which is pro-inflammatory *in vitro* for neutrophils and eosinophils (33). This activity is inhibited in a dose response and rank order fashion by hydrocortisone, methyl-prednisolone and dexamethasone in CS asthmatic subjects, with respective IC50s (concentration of steroid producing 50% inhibition of activity) being 600 nM, 70 nM and 0.5 nM. In contrast there was much reduced inhibition in the CR group (34). The elucidation of the nature of this peptide is clearly important in the mechanism of steroid resistance. We have recently shown that steroid resistance is not due to altered pharmacokinetics in CR subjects (35). Peak serum levels of prednisolone following the administration of 40 mg/1.73 square meters body surface area (rounded to the nearest 5 mg) were 645 ± 43 and 676 ± 52 ng/ml in the CS and CR groups, respectively ($p = 0.92$). Estimated clearances of prednisolone were 155 ± 8 and 157 ± 7 ml/minute per 1.73 square meters in CS and CR patients, respectively. In addition, there was no difference between each of the asthmatic groups studied and normal subjects. This defect is not caused by corticosteroid receptor characteristics (34). Nuclear binding studies with [^{3}H] dexamethasone have been performed to determine the dissociation constant (Kd) and receptor numbers (Ro) in the monocytes of these two groups of subjects. The Kd for dexamethasone was 2.45 ± 0.58 nM (mean ± SEM, $n = 6$) in the CS group and 1.6 ± 0.35 nM (mean ± SEM, $n = 6$) in the CR group of patients ($p = 0.14$). The Ro in the CS group was 3605 ± 984 binding sites per nucleus (mean ± SEM, $n = 6$) and 4757 ± 692 binding sites per nucleus (mean ± SEM, $n = 6$) in the CR group ($p = 0.23$). It is likely that CR is an important primary phenomenon, and recent work by Brown et al., demonstrating that cutaneous vasoconstrictor responses in asthmatics correlated with the airways response to oral GCS, suggests that it may not be a cell specific phenomenon (36). CR may arise from reduced binding affinity of the GR to the GRE, altered regulation of composite GREs, abnormalities of subsequent transactivation or as a result of/or failure of induction/suppression of specific genes. Recent studies using subtractive hybridization have indicated that the number of genes regulated by GCS in any given cell type is low, i.e. < 10 out of 3000 (4). By this technique subtle differences in gene expression between these two groups of patients may be elucidated. In addition comparison of the GR cDNA between CS and CR asthmatic subjects may reveal nucleotide sequence abnormalities in the domain encoding regions between these two groups of patients.

Conclusions

In summary, the increasing knowledge of the mechanism of action of GCS coupled to novel findings relating to the cellular basis of CR bronchial asthma will allow us to apply powerful molecular biological techniques in order to elucidate the mechanism(s) involved and design specific therapies in this difficult group of patients.

References

1. Carmichael, J., Paterson, I.C., Diaz, P., Crompton, G.K., Kay, A.B., and Grant, I.W.B. 1981. Corticosteroid resistance in chronic asthma. Br. Med. J.282:1419.
2. Hollenberg, S.M., Weinberger, C., Ong, E.S., Cerrelli, G., Oro, A., Lebo, R., Thompson, E.B., Rosenfeld, M.G., and Evans, R.M. 1985. Primary structure and expression of a functional human glucocorticoid receptor cDNA. Nature 318(6047):635.
3. Munck, A., Mendel, D.B., Smith, L.I., and Orti, E. 1990. Glucocorticoid receptors and actions. Am. Rev. Respir. Dis. (suppl.) 141,2:2.
4. Miesfeld, R.L. 1989. The structure and function of steroid receptor proteins. Critical Reviews in Biochemistry and Molecular Biology 24:101
5. Evans, R.E. 1988. The steroid and thyroid hormone receptor superfamily. Science 240:889.

6. Wahli, W., and Martinez, E. 1991. Superfamily of steroid nuclear receptors: Positive and negative regulators of gene expression. FASEB J. 5:2243.
7. Archer, T.K., Hager, G.L., and Omichinski, J.G. 1990. Sequence-specific DNA binding by glucocorticoid "zinc-finger peptides". Proc. Natl. Acad. USA 87:7560.
8. Green, S., Kumar, V., Thenlaz, I., Wahli, W., and Chambron, P. 1988. The N-terminal DNA binding zinc finger of the estrogen and glucocorticoid receptors determines target gene specificity. EMBO J. 7:3037.
9. Chalepakis, G., Postma, J.P.M., and Beato, M. 1988b. A model for hormone receptor binding to the mouse mammary tumour virus regulatory element based on hydroxyl radical footprinting. Nucl. Acids. Res. 16:10237
10. Carlstedt-Duke, J., Stromstedt, P.E., Persson, B., Cederlund, E., Gustafsson, J.A., and Jornvall, H. 1988. Identification of hormone interacting amino acid residues within the steroid binding domain of the glucocorticoid in relation to other steroid hormone receptors. J. Biol. Chem. 263:6842.
11. Hollenberg, S.M., and Evans, R.M. 1988. Multiple and cooperative trans-activation domains of the human glucocorticoid receptor. Cell 5:899.
12. Kaderon, D., Richardson, W., Markham, A.F., and Smith, A.E. 1984. Sequence requirements for nuclear localisation of SV40 large T-antigen. Nature 311:33.
13. Beato, M. Gene regulation by steroid hormones. 1989. Cell 56:335.
14. Diamond, M.I., Miner, J.N., Yoshinaga, S.K., Yamamoto, K.R. 1990. Transcription factor interactions: Selectors of positive or negative regulation from a single DNA element. Science 249:1266.
15. Jonat, J., Rahmsdorf, H.J., Park, K.K., Cato, A.C.B., Gebel, S., Ponta, H., and Herrlich, P. 1990. Antitumor promotion and antiinflammation: Downmodulation of AP-1 (fos/jun) activity by glucocorticoid hormone. Cell 62:1189.
16. Schauer, M., Chalepakis, G., Willman, T., and Beato, M. 1989. Binding of hormone accelerates the kinetics of glucocorticoid and progesterone receptor binding to DNA. Proc. Natl. Acad. Sci. USA 86(4):1123.
17. Ptashne, M. 1988. How transcriptional activators work. Nature 335:683.
18. Kumar, V., and Chambron, P. 1988. The estrogen receptor bind tightly to its responsive element as a ligand induced homodimer. Cell 55:145.
19. Yamamoto, K.R. 1985. Steroid receptor regulated transcription of specific genes and specific gene networks. Annu. Rev. Genet. 19:209.
20. Wallner, B.P., Mattaliano, R.J., Hession, C., Cata, R.L., Tizard, R., Sinclair, L.K., Foeller, C, Chow, E.P., Browning, K.L., Ramachandran, K.L., and Pepinsky, R.B. 1986. Cloning and expression of human lipocortin-1, a phospholipase A2 inhibitor with potential anti-inflammatory activity. Nature 320;:7.
21. Almawi, W.Y., Wallner, B.P., Hadro, E.T., and Strom, T.B. 1991. Glucocorticosteroid-mediated suppressive effect is associated with lipocortin induction but not via blockade of arachidonic acid release/metabolism. J.Immunol., in press.
22. Davidson, F.F., and Dennis, E.A. 1989. Biological relevance of lipocortins and related proteins as inhibitors of phospholipase A2. Biochem. Pharmacol. 38:3645.
23. Walker, K.B., Potter, J.M., and House, A.K. 1987. Interleukin 2 synthesis in the presence of steroids: A model of steroid resistance. Clin. Exp.Immunol. 68(1):162.
24. Almawi, W., Lipman, M.L., Stevens, A.C., Zanker, B., Hadro, E.T., and Strom, T.B. 1991. Abrogation of glucocorticosteroid-mediated inhibition of T cell proliferation by the synergistic action of IL-1, IL-6 and IFN-gamma. J. Immunol. 146:3523.
25. Almawi, W.Y., Sewell, K.L., Zanker, B., Hadro, E.T., and Strom, T.B. 1990. Mode of action of the glucocorticosteroids as immunosuppressive agents. Prog. Leukocyte Biol. 10A:321.
26. Ray, A., LaForge, K.S., and Sehgal, P.B. 1990. On the mechanism for efficient repression of the interleukin-6 promoter by glucocorticoids: Enhancer, TATA box and RNA start site. Mol. Cell Biol. 10(11):5736.
27. Kern, J.A., Lamb, R.J., Reed, J.C., Daniele, R.P., and Nowell, P.C. 1988. Dexamethasone inhibition of interleukin beta production by human monocytes. J. Clin. Invest. 81:237.
28. Dennis, G., June, C.H., Mizuguchi, J, Ohara, J., Witherspoon, K., Finkelman, F.D., McMillan, V., and Mond, J.J. 1987. Glucocorticoids suppress calcium mobilisation and phospholipid hydrolysis in anti-Ig stimulated B cells. J. Immunol. 139:2516.
29. Kido, H., Fukusen, N., and Katunuma, N. 1987. Inhibition by 1-(5-isoquinoline-sulphonyl)-2-methylpiperazine, an inhibitor of

Mechanism of Action

Over 200 papers have attempted to define how cromolyn sodium works; yet, the exact mechanism of action is still not understood. Cromolyn sodium stabilizes mast cells, preventing release of proinflammatory mediators, regardless of whether the stimulus is immunologic (related to IgE-antigen) or nonimmunologic (cold air, exercise). The drug most likely stabilizes mast cells by preventing the influx of calcium ions into the cells. However, its protective effect on mast cells is species-specific (effective in rats, primates, and humans, but not in guinea pigs) and tissue- specific (effective in lung but not in basophils or skin). Cromolyn sodium is very effective in blocking mediator release from mast cells obtained by bronchoalveolar lavage (5). In human bronchial challenge studies, cromolyn sodium protects the airways after inhalation of specific allergens (preventing both early and late-phase reactions), further demonstrating its role in stabilizing mast cells. Besides protecting against allergen challenge, cromolyn sodium blocks acute airway obstruction following inhalation of cold air, hyperventilation, exercise, or sulfur dioxide. The nature of this action could be the blocking of reflex neural activity, possibly by decreasing the number of impulses arising from stimulated C-fiber nerve endings in the lung (6). Cromolyn sodium also inhibits the activation of other cells, including peripheral blood leukocytes (7), monocytes (8), and macrophages (9). In addition, cromolyn sodium reduces platelet-activating factor, a substance that induces immediate and delayed inflammatory responses in the skin of nonatopic adults (10). However, cromolyn sodium does not block the action of other mediators of type I immediate hypersensitivity (11). Airway hyperreactivity correlates with several aspects of asthma, including: recurrence and severity, degree of difference between morning and evening peak flows (12), and the number of medications required for asthma control (13). Long-term use of cromolyn sodium decreases nonspecific airway reactivity which becomes more pronounced during the pollen season. This effect can be clearly seen in allergic subjects (14) but the effect is not limited to atopic patients (15). Because the late response correlates with increased bronchial hyperreactivity and is definitely related to the worsening of asthma, cromolyn sodium's role in preventing the late response may explain why it can successfully control or improve chronic asthma.

Clinical Trials in Asthma

Hundreds of published studies describe the clinical use of cromolyn sodium for the treatment of asthma. Studies have been performed with the powdered (Spinhaler capsule) form, the nebulized solution, and the metered-dose inhaler, and I have included each of these treatment forms in my summary of clinical trials. A success rate of 65% for both adults and children has been reported (16). Historically, however, many of the original studies did not include a placebo control, and trials before 1970 used a combination of cromolyn sodium plus 0.1 mg isoproterenol, although the addition of the latter appears to make little difference in the efficacy of the drug (17).

Spinhaler Capsules

The cromolyn sodium 20 mg Spinhaler form is no longer commonly used. For completeness, and to give a better historical perspective, however, I have included clinical trials using this formulation.

Studies in Adults: In 1969, a 4-week double-blind placebo-controlled study (18) of 252 children and adult asthmatics demonstrated, by subjective and objective measurements, that the use of Spinhaler QID was significantly better than placebo. A year-long double-blind placebo-controlled parallel study in England (19) of adult asthmatics with severe disease also demonstrated a significant effect. Allergic and non-allergic asthmatics fared equally well.

Studies in Children: Two placebo-controlled trials, one a 4-week crossover with 54 children (20) and another an 8-week crossover with 38 children (21) demonstrated significant efficacy and safety. In the former study, 20% of the children continued open-labeled cromolyn sodium for 12 months and demonstrated significant improvement in their asthma control over the previous year.

Nebulizer Solution

Cromolyn sodium has been available as a 1% nebulizer solution since 1982. Each unit-dose glass ampule contains 20 mg of cromolyn sodium in 2 ml of sterile water without preservatives. The solution is delivered to the lungs by using a nebulizer. The use of a face mask instead of a mouth piece allows delivery of the medication to the upper airways, giving an added benefit to patients with allergic rhinitis. The nebulizer solution is compatible with beta-agonists, enabling simultaneous administration (22-23). Studies have mostly been confined to children under 4 years of age. Eleven of 17 children improved in a 2-month double-blind placebo-controlled crossover trial (24) while 16 of 19 children ages 5–9 improved in a similar study (25). In a 12-week double-blind comparative trial (26), 68 chronic adult asthmatics received cromolyn sodium (by Spinhaler or nebulizer) QID. Use of the active drug resulted in significant improvement in day- and night-time asthma, cough, and spirometry. Physicians and patients judged cromolyn sodium to be more effective than placebo (61% vs. 27%).

Metered-Dose Inhaler (MDI)

This form of cromolyn sodium became available in 1986. Each activation of a 1-mg dose delivers 800 μg of drug to the patient. MDIs with concentrations of 1, 2, and 5 mg/puff are available in some countries outside the United States. Most of the studies summarized here, however, were done using the 1-mg dose.

Studies in adults: Most adult studies have used 2 mg (2 puffs) QID. Rubin et al. (27) studied 31 subjects in a double-blind crossover trial and showed a significant decrease in asthma symptoms and in as-needed bronchodilator use in the cromolyn sodium-treated group. Cordier (28) studied 29 adults in a similar way and obtained the same positive result.

Studies in children: In a double-blind 12-week placebo-controlled crossover study of 46 children, Geller-Bernstein (29) demonstrated significant improvement in asthma severity and objective measurements by 3 weeks in the cromolyn sodium-treated group. In a brief (1 week) double-blind study of 83 asthmatics (35 adults and 48 children) Selcow (30) demonstrated a positive effect for the cromolyn sodium-treated group.

Cromolyn Sodium versus Theophylline

The first trial comparing theophylline and cromolyn sodium as first-line agents for the treatment of asthma was a 4-week study conducted in London and Denver (31). Peak-flow measurements and use of extra medication were similar for both drugs, but theophylline showed significant difference in symptom-free days. However, theophylline-treated patients had more side effects. The study created a great deal of controversy: If the data had been evaluated after 4 weeks, rather than after 1 week, cromolyn sodium might have been superior overall since it may take four weeks to reach full effectiveness. An 8-week double-blind crossover study of preschool children, using cromolyn sodium nebulizer solution or short-acting liquid theophylline, showed that cromolyn sodium was significantly more effective in controlling symptoms, with the theophylline-treated group having significant side effects (32). Furukawa (33) in a 3-month double-blind placebo-controlled parallel group study (using Spinhaler and sustained-release theophylline) demonstrated equal effectiveness as measured by daily symptoms, physician evaluation, and use of as-needed bronchodilator medication. Cromolyn sodium had fewer side effects and most patients were able to taper the drug to BID dosing.

Cromolyn Sodium versus Steroids

Although some studies have shown that cromolyn sodium can reduce steroid-dependency (34–35), others have not (36–39). Lowhagen and Rak (39) treated 40 adult asthmatics with cromolyn sodium, inhaled steroid (budesonide), the combination, or placebo in an 8-week double-blind study. Both cromolyn sodium and budesonide (each alone) decreased histamine reactivity, but the combination provided no additional benefit over each drug used alone.

Conclusion

Over many years, large numbers of patients (children and adults) have relied on cromolyn sodium in their asthma management regimen. There is no longer any doubt that this drug deserves a prominent place in the treatment of mild-to-moderate asthma. Recently, an Expert Panel, assembled by the National Heart, Lung, and Blood Institute (NHLBI) reached a consensus on asthma management, based on new knowledge and new understanding of the asthma disease process. Guidelines of this Panel, soon to be published, emphasize the use of "antiinflammatory agents" to treat all asthma patients not controlled by occasional use of beta-agonists. Currently, cromolyn sodium and inhaled corticosteroids are the two agents the Panel recognizes as providing this disease-modifying, antiinflammatory function. The Guidelines, combined with cromolyn sodium's long history of safe and effective use, confirm the role of cromolyn sodium as basic preventive therapy for many patients with asthma.

References

1. Hollman, A. 1991. Plants in cardiology: Amiodarone, nifedipine, sodium cromoglycate. Br. Heart J. 65:57.
2. Allansmith, M.R., Petty, T.L., and Schwartz, H.J., eds. 1987. Cromolyn sodium: Clinical considerations. Princeton, N.J.: Excerpta Medica.
3. Settipane, G.A., Klein, D.E., Boyd, G.K., Sturam, J.H., Freye H.B., and Weltman, J.K. 1979. Adverse reactions to cromolyn. JAMA 23:811.
4. Sheffer, A.L., Rocklin, R.E., and Goetzl, E.J. 1975. Immunologic components of hypersensitivity reactions to cromolyn sodium. N. Engl. J. Med. 293:1220.
5. Flint, K.C., Leung K.B.P., Pearce, F.L., Hudspith, B.N., Brostoff, J., and Johnson, N.M. 1985. Human mast cells recovered by bronchoalveolar lavage: Their morphology, histamine release and the effects of sodium cromoglycate. Clin. Sci. 68:427.
6. Dixon, M., Jackson, D.M., and Richards, I.M. 1980. The action of sodium cromoglycate on "C" fibre endings in the dog lung. Br. J. Pharmacol. 70:11.
7. Kay, A.B., and Barnes, P.J. 1985. Pharmacological modulation of the asthmatic response. In: Current perspectives in the immunology of respiratory diseases. A.B. Kay, E.J. Goetzl, eds. Edinburgh: Churchill Livingstone, p. 30.
8. Moqbel, R., Durham, S.R., Carroll, M., McDonald, A.J., Walsh, G.M., McKay, J., Shaw, R.J., and Kay, A.B. 1985. Enhanced neutrophil and monocytotoxicity after exercise-induced asthma. Thorax 40:218.
9. Holian, A., Hamilton, R., and Scheule, R.K. 1991. Mechanistic aspects of cromolyn sodium action on the alveolar macrophage: Inhibition of stimulation by soluble agonists. Agents Actions 33(3/4):318.
10. Basran, G.S., Page, C.T., Paul, W., and Morley, J. 1983. Cromoglycate inhibits the responses to platelet-activating factor (PAF-acether) in man: An alternative mode of action for DSCG in asthma? Eur. J. Pharmacol. 86(1):143.
11. Suschitzky, J.L., and Sheard, P. 1984. The search for antiallergic drugs for the treatment of asthma — Problems in finding a successor to sodium cromoglycate. Progr. Med. Chem. 21:2.
12. Ryan, G., Latimer, K.M., Dolovick, J., and Hargreave, F.E. 1982. Bronchial responsiveness to histamine: Relationship to diurnal variation of peak flow rate, improvement after bronchodilator in airway calibre. Thorax 37:423.
13. Juniper, E.F., Frith, P.A, and Hargreave, F.E. 1981. Airway responsiveness to histamine and methacholine: Relationship to minimum treatment to control symptoms of asthma. Thorax 36:575.
14. Rak, S., Millqvist, E., and Lowhagen O. 1983. Therapeutic modification of non-specific hyperreactivity by sodium cromoglycate (SCG). J. Allergy Clin. Immunol. 71:149.
15. Numeroso, R., Torre, F.D., Radaelli, C., Scarpazza, G., and Ortolani, C. 1983. Effect of long-term treatment with sodium cromoglycate on non-specific bronchial hyperreactivity in nonatopic patients with chronic bronchitis. Respiration 44:109.
16. Bernstein, I.L. 1985. Cromolyn sodium and cromolyn-like drugs. In: Bronchial asthma: Mechanisms and therapeutics, 2nd ed. E.B. Weiss, M.S. Segal, M. Stein, eds. Boston: Little Brown & Co., pp. 724.
17. Shapiro, G.G., and Konig, P. 1985. Cromolyn sodium: A review. Pharmacotherapy 5:156.
18. Bernstein, I.L., Siegel, S.C., Brandon, M.L., Brown, E.B., Evans, R.R., Feinberg, A.R., Friedlaender, S., Krumholz, R.A., Hadley, R.A., Handelman N.I., Thurston, D., and Yamata, M. 1972. A controlled study of cromolyn sodium sponsored by the drug committee of the American Academy of Allergy. J. Allergy Clin. Immunol. 50:235.
19. Bromptom Hospital/Medical Research Council Collaborative Trial. 1972. Long-term study

of disodium cromoglycate in treatment of severe extrinsic or intrinsic bronchial asthma in adults. Br. Med. J. 4:383.
20. McLean, W.L., Lozano, J., Hannaway, P., Sakowitz, S., and Mueller, H.L. 1973. Cromolyn treatment of asthmatic children. Am. J. Dis. Child 125:332.
21. Hyde, J.S., Isenberg, P.D., and Floro, L.D. 1973. Short- and long-term prophylaxis with cromolyn sodium in chronic asthma. Chest 63:875.
22. Lesko, L.J., and Miller, A.K. 1984. Physical-chemical compatibility of cromolyn sodium nebulizer solution— bronchodilator inhalant solution admixtures. Ann. Allergy 53:236.
23. Emm, T., Metcalf, J.E., Lesko, L.J., and Chai, M.F. 1991. Update on the physical-chemical compatibility of cromolyn sodium nebulizer solution: Bronchodilator inhalant solution admixtures. Ann. Allergy 66(2):185.
24. Hiller, E.J., Milner, A.D., and Lenney, W. 1977. Nebulized sodium cromoglycate in young asthmatic children. Arch. Dis. Child 52:875.
25. Mellon, M.H., Harden, K., and Zeiger, R.S. 1982. The effectiveness and safety of nebulizer cromolyn solution in the young childhood asthmatic. Immunol. Allergy Pract. 4:168.
26. Petty, T.L., Rollins, D.R., Christopher, K., Good, J.T., and Oakley, R. 1989. Cromolyn sodium is effective in adult chronic asthmatics. Am. Rev. Respir. Dis. 139:694.
27. Rubin, A.E., Alroy, G., and Spitzer, S. 1983. The treatment of asthma in adults using sodium cromoglycate pressurized aerosol: A double-blind controlled trial. Curr. Med. Res. Opin. 8:553.
28. Cordier, R. 1984. Sodium cromoglycate delivered by pressurized aerosol in the treatment of adult asthma. Clin. Trials J. 21:483.
29. Geller-Bernstein, C., and Levin, S. 1983. Sodium cromoglycate pressurised aerosol in childhood asthma. Curr. Ther. Res. 34:345.
30. Selcow, J., Blumenthal, R., Spector, S., and Zeiger, R. 1986. A multicenter study to evaluate the clinical benefits of cromolyn sodium aerosol (1 mg) in the treatment of asthma. J. Allergy Clin. Immunol. 77(1):149.
31. Hambleton, G., Weinberger, M., Taylor, J., Cavanaugh, M., Ginchansky, E., Godfrey, S., Tooley, M., Bell, T., and Greenberg, S. 1977. Comparison of cromoglycate (cromolyn) and theophylline in controlling symptoms of chronic asthma: A collaborative study. Lancet 1:381.
32. Newth, C.J.L., Newth, C.V., and Turner, J.A.P. 1982. Comparison of nebulised sodium cromoglycate and oral theophylline in controlling symptoms of chronic asthma in pre-school children: A double blind study. Aust. N.Z. J. Med. 12:232.
33. Furukawa, C.T., Shapiro, G.G., Kraemer, M.J., Pierson, W.E., and Bierman, C.W. 1984. A double-blind study comparing the effectiveness of cromolyn sodium and sustained-release theophylline in childhood asthma. Pediatrics 74:453.
34. Chai, H., Molk, L, Falliers, C.J., and Miklich, D. 1971. Steroid-sparing effects of disodium cromoglycate (DSC) in children with severe clinical asthma. In: New concepts in allergy and clinical immunology. U. Serafini, ed. Amsterdam: Excerpta Medica, p. 385.
35. Friday, G.A., Facktor, M.A., Bernstein, R.A., and Fireman, P. 1973. Cromolyn therapy for severe asthma in children. J. Pediatr. 83:299.
36. Toogood, J.H., Jennings, B., and Lefcoe, N.M. 1981. A clinical trial of combined cromolyn/beclomethasone treatment for chronic asthma. J. Pediatr. 67:317.
37. Hiller, E.J., and Milner, A.D. 1975. Betamethasone 17 valerate aerosol and disodium cromoglycate in severe childhood asthma. Br. J. Dis. Chest 69:103.
38. Dawood, A.G., Hendry, A.T., and Walker, S.R. 1977. The combined use of betamethasone valerate and sodium cromoglycate in the treatment of asthma. Clin. Allergy 7:161.
39. Lowhagen, O., and Rak, I. 1984. Effect of sodium cromoglycate and budesonide on bronchial hyperreactivity in non-atopic asthmatics. Respiration 46(Suppl 1):105.

Pathogenesis of Allergic Airway Disease and its Pharmacological Modulation

Stephen T. Holgate, Peter Bradding, Alan Roberts, Peter H. Howarth, Ratko Djukanovik*

The efficacy of bronchodilator drugs in relieving attacks of asthma led to a concept of a disease in which contraction of airway smooth muscle ("bronchospasm") was the central abnormality. However, pathologists have long recognized that death from asthma is almost always accompanied by widespread airway inflammation with occlusion of both large and small airways with tenacious secretions comprising mucus, serum proteins and cell debris. It is only recently that these aspects of asthma could be investigated in the living patient through the application of fibreoptic bronchoscopy, lavage and biopsy.

Evidence for Airway Inflammation in Clinical Astha

Endobronchial mucosal biopsies in asthma have provided uncontroversial evidence for a specific type of airway inflammation underlying disordered airway function in both classical allergic and in non-allergic asthma (1). Characteristic features include loosening of the ciliated pseudostratified epithelium (2), deposition of interstitial collagens beneath the basement membrane (3), expression of leucocyte adhesion molecules and their complementary receptors on post-capillary venule endothelial cells (4), and above all, widespread infiltration of the submucosa and epithelium with activated T-cells (5), degranulating mast cells, eosinophils (6) and monocytes (7). A targeted inflammatory attack on the epithelium by mast cells and eosinophils leads to loss of desmosomal attachment of suprabasal cells to each other and to the basal cells with a consequent loss of the permeability barrier (2). In an attempt to diminish the tissue damaging effects of this, myofibroblasts proliferate under the epithelium to lay down a swathe of cross-linked collagen comprising Types I, III and V together with fibronectin (8). These events can be accounted for by the release of mediators from activated mast cells and eosinophils. Tryptase, the major neutral protease of the mucosal-type mast cell (MC_T) is able to hydrolyze desmosomal links within the epithelium to increase permeability. Eosinophils, both through their epitheliotoxic arginine-rich proteins and through a cognate interaction with epithelial cells, to metalloproteases such as gelatinase, also lead to epithelial disruption and disturbance of selective permeability characterization (9). A consequence of this targeted attack on the epithelium is an increased expression of molecules pertinent to maintaining the inflammatory response, including the MHC Class II molecule HLA-DRA (10), heat shock (stress) proteins, lipocortin 1β, endothelin (11), GM-CSF and IL-8.

In vivo Models of Mast Cell and Eosinophil Activation

Most persistent asthma in children is found in association with atopy, a genetic trait leading to enhanced production of IgE against common environmental allergens. Sensitization to allergens such as those derived from domestic mites and cats occurs early in life and is a major determinant for the later development of asthma. Once sensitized, challenge of the airways with high concentrations of allergen causes two phases of airway obstruction designated the early (EAR) and late (LAR) reactions in par-

* Medicine 1, Level D, Centre Block, Southampton General Hospital, Southampton, and University of Southampton, UK.

allel with an acquired increase in bronchial responsiveness.

Local challenge of an asthmatic airway via the fibreoptic bronchoscope demonstrates marked airway narrowing within 5 minutes being largely the result of contraction of the underlying circular and spiral smooth muscle. The mediators most likely to account for this response are histamine (H_1), prostaglandin D_2 and its metabolite 9α, 11βPGF$_2$ (TP_1) and leukotrienes C_4, D_4 and E_4 (LTD receptor) derived from mast cells. In addition to releasing bronchoactive autocoids, mast cell tryptase (and possibly other proteases) is released as a complex with heparin proteoglycan with consequent cleavage of matrix and intercellular adhesion proteins (13).

Fibreoptic bronchoscopy has shown that the LAR occurs secondary to eosinophil and T-cell recruitment. Macroscopically the airway becomes red and swollen with free fluid exuded onto the airway surface. The recruitment of inflammatory leukocyte involves the selective expression of specific adhesion molecules. In the case of the eosinophil the upregulation of intercellular adhesion molecule (ICAM-1) on endothelial cells is associated with eosinophil recruitment following allergen challenge in an Ascaris-sensitized monkey model of allergic airway inflammation (14). A similar upregulation of ICAM-I is also observed 4 hours after local allergen challenge of asthmatic airways, implicating a similar mechanism. Upregulation of VCAM with its capacity to interact with VLA-4 ligand on eosinophils is also thought to be involved in the selective recruitment of this cell in asthma (15). ICAM-1 is also able to interact with the LFA-1 (Cd11a/CD18) integrin on T-cells and helps explain why these cells are also selectively recruited during the late phase of allergic inflammation.

Once present in the airway wall eosinophils come under the influence of chemoattractants which also serve to prime these cells for mediator secretion. Examples include interleukin-5 (IL-5) and platelet activating factor (PAF). In the presence of IL-3 or IL-5 eosinophils also become responsive to IL-8 (NAP-1), a cytokine normally associated with neutrophil chemoattraction (16). The autocoids responsible for the target tissue responses observed during the LAR include the sulphidopeptide leukotriene and possibly PAF, two mediators with powerful effects on the microvasculature.

Induction Mechanisms of the Allergic Tissue Response

Response of the immune system to specific allergens first involves the processing and presentation of allergen along with MHC Class II molecules to CD_4^+ T-cells. Studies involving either lavage or biopsy show upregulation of HLA-DR on T-cells, macrophages and epithelial cells (10). Although part of the enhanced MHC Class II molecule expression may be "non-specific", in the case of T-cells, dendritic cells and macrophages, it is related to increased capacity to present antigen along with the amplification cytokines such as IL-β (macrophage), IL-6 (dendritic cell) and IL-2 (T-cell).

Evidence for T-cell upregulation in asthma and following challenge has been received elsewhere in these proceedings. Our own experience following local allergen challenge indicates an early (within 15 min) and selective T-cell recruitment into the airway wall, both from the circulation and from the airway lumen (17). What is not known is how this process occurs so quickly and is relatively selective for the TH_2 subtype with its capacity to elaborate IL-3, IL-4, IL-5, GM-CSF and IL-10, cytokines involved in the selective recruitment mast cells (IL-3, IL-10), eosinophils (IL-4, IL-5, GM-CSF) and B-cell isotype switching to IgE synthesis (IL-4).

The Role of the Mast Cell as a Primary Source of Cytokines

While there is increasing evidence for specific involvement of the TH_2-CD_4^+ lymphocyte in allergic tissue responses including asthma, activation of these cells with release of cytokines with a delay of 4–6 hours does not explain the early cellular events of the LAR nor how T-cells are recruited so rapidly into the airways. Using monoclonal antibodies (3H4 and 4D9) directed to different epitopes on IL-4, we have recently shown that in biopsies of both nasal and bronchial mucosa in rhinitis and asthma, 80–100% of IL-4 immunoreactivity localizes to cells staining positively for tryptase, i. e. mast cells (18). Further studies have shown similar localization of

IL-5 and IL-6 to mast cells. Recently almost all the mast cells purified from either human skin and lung have been shown to be IL-4+ and, following cross-linkage of cell bound IgE, this cytokine is released. Since IL-4 increases the expression of VCAM on endothelial cells (19) and is an enhancing factor for TH_2 lymphocyte proliferation, a mechanism is provided for the early cellular events observed in asthmatic airways following allergen. Inhibition of IgE-triggered release of mast cell-derived cytokine also provides for the first time a potential mechanism linking sodium cromoglycate's capacity to inhibit the mast cell-associated EAR with attenuation of the LAR and the attendant increase in bronchial responsiveness.

Clinical Implications of Viewing Asthma in Inflammatory Disease

Inhaled β_2-adrenoceptor agonists lead the world sales in anti-asthma drugs and yet the widespread use of these drugs as a primary treatment modality in all but the mildest diseases is being seriously challenged (20). The positioning of these drugs in the anti-asthma armamentarium is not made easier by the recent introduction of the potent and long-acting inhaled β-agonists: salmeterol and formoterol. When administered as a single dose both of these drugs provide bronchodilatation and functional antagonism for 12 hours or more and also protect the airways against the EAR, LAR and acquired increase in bronchial responsiveness (21). The question arises, therefore, as to whether or not they also confer an "anti-inflammatory" action. In a 6 week placebo-controlled trial, when compared to placebo, we failed to show any effect of salmeterol 50 μg bd on mast cell, eosinophil or T-cell markers in BAL or biopsies, indices of T-cell activation (IL-2r and HLA-DR) or mast cell mediators, despite producing impressive improvement in asthma symptoms, peak expiratory flow and use of rescue β-agonist mediation (22).

Contrasting with the findings observed with salmeterol, a similar 6 week trial involving the inhaled corticosteroid beclomethasone diproprionate resulted in similar clinical improvement but also marked reductions in mast cell numbers and their mediators, eosinophils and indices of T-cell activation when assessed in biopsies and lavage (23). These data argue strongly in favor of using disease modifying drugs such as sodium cromoglycate and topical corticosteroids early in the course of the disease as first line therapies with the short-acting inhaled β_2-agonists reserved as rescue medication and the long-acting β_2-agonists as supplemental treatment for those in whom disordered airway function and symptoms persist despite adequate use of the anti-inflammatory medications. Thus, direct observation made on the cellular and mediator mechanisms of asthma have provided a scientific basis for some of the new treatment strategies being introduced for the long-term management of this disease (24).

References

1. Djukanovic, R., Roche, W.R., Wilson, J.W., Beasley, C.R.W., Twentyman, O., and Holgate, S.T. 1990. Mucosal inflammation in asthma. Am. Rev. Respir. Dis. 142:434.
2. Montefort, S., and Holgate, S.T. 1991. Adhesion molecules and their role in inflammation. Respir. Med.85:91.
3. Roche, W.R., Beasley, R., Wililams, J.H., and Holgate, S.T. 1989. Subepithelial fibrosis in the bronchi of asthmatics. Lancet i:520.
4. Montefort, S., Roche, W.R., Howarth, P.H., Djukanovic, R., Carroll, M., Gratziou, C., Smith, L., Britten, K., Lee, T.H., and Holgate, S.T. 1991. Bronchial mucosal intercellular adhesion molecule-1 (ICAM-1) and endothelial leucocyte adhesion molecule-1 (ELAM-1) expression in normals and asthmatics. J. Allergy Clin. Immunol. 87:Abstr 285.
5. Azzawi, M., Bradley, B., Wardlaw, A.J., Frew, A.J., Kay, A.B., and Jeffrey, P.K. 1990. Identification of activated T-lymphocytes and eosinophils in bronchial biopsies in stable atopic asthma. Am. Rev. Respir. Dis. 142:1407.
6. Djukanovic, R., Wilson, J.W., Britten, K.M., Wilson, S.J., Walls, A.F., Roche, W.R., Howarth, P.H., and Holgate, S.T. 1990. Quantitation of mast cells and eosinophils in the bronchial mucosa of symptomatic atopic asthmatics and healthy control subjects using immunohistochemistry. Am. Rev. Respir. Dis. 142:863.
7. Lee, T.H., Poston, R., Godard, P., and Bousquet, J. 1991. Macrophages and allergy asthma. Clin. Exp. Allergy (Suppl 1) 21:22.

8. Brewster, C.E.P., Howarth, P.H., Djukanovic, R., Wilson, J., Holgate, S.T., and Roche, W.R. 1990. Myofibroblasts and subepithelial fibrosis in bronchial asthma. Am. Rev. Respir. Cell Mol. Biol. 3:507.
9. Herbert, C.A., Edwards, D., Boot, J.R., and Robinson, C. 1991. *In vitro* modulation of the eosinophil-dependent enhancement of the permeability of the bronchial mucosa. Br. J. Pharmacol. 104:391.
10. Poulter, L.W., Power, C., and Burke, C. 1990. The relationship between bronchial immunopathology and hyperresponsiveness in asthma. Eur. Respir. J. 3:792.
11. Springall, P.R., Howarth, P.H., Counitian, H., Djukanovic, R., Holgate, S.T., Polak, J.M. 1991. Endothelin immunostaining of airway epithelium in asthmatic patients. Lancet 337:697.
12. Holgate, S.T. 1990. Mediator and cellular mechanisms in asthma. The Phillip Ellman Lecture, RCP 1990. J. Roy. Coll. Phys. 24:304.
13. Walls, A.F., He, S.H., and Holgate, S.T. 1992 . Human mast cell tryptase and chymase can increase vascular permeability in skin (Abstr.). Clin. Exp. Allergy, in press.
14. Wegener, C.D., Gundel, R.H., Reilly, P., Haynes, N., Letts, G.Z., and Rothleirn, R. 1990. ICAM-1 in the pathogenesis of asthma. Science 247:416.
15. Walsh, G.M., Mermod, J.J., Hartnel, A., Kay, A.B., and Wardlaw, A.J. 1991. Human eosinophil but not neutrophil adherence to IL-1 stimulated HUVEC is $\alpha_4 B_1$ (VLA-4)-dependent. J. Immunol. 146:3419.
16. Warringa, R.A.J,. Koenderman, L., Kok, P.T.M., and Bruiznzeel, P.L.B. 1991. Modulation andinduction of eosinophil chemoxtaxis by granulocyte-macrophage colony-stimulating factor and interleukin-3. Blood 77:2694.
17. Gratziou, C., Carroll, M., Walls, A., and Howarth, P.H. 1992. Early changes in T-lymphocytes recovered by BAL following local allergen challenge of asthmatic airways. Am. Rev. Respir. Dis., in press.
18. Bradding, P., Fether, I.H., Howarth, P.H., Mueller, R., Roberts, J.A., Britten, K., Bews, J.P.A, Hunt, T.C., Okayama, Y., Heusser, C.H., Bullock, G.R., Church, M.K., and Holgate, S.T. 1991. Interleukin-4 is localised and released by human mast cells. Submitted to J. Exp. Med.
19. Masinovsky, B., Urdal, D., and Gallatin, W.M. 1990. IL-4 acts synergistically with IL-1 to promote lymphocyte ahesion to microvascular endothelium by induction of vascular adhesion molecule-1. J. Immunol. 145:2886.
20. Sears, M.R., Taylor, D.R., Print, C.G., Lake, D.C., et al. 1990. Regular inhaled beta agonist treatment in bronchial asthma. Lancet 336:1391.
21. Twentyman, O.P., Finnerty, J.P., Harris, A., Palmer, J., and Holgate, S.T. 1990. The long acting β_2-agonist salmeterol protects against allergen-induced inflammatory events in asthma. Lancet 336:1338.
22. Howarth, P.H. 1991. The investigation of the non-bronchodilator properties of asthma therapies *in vivo*. Eur. Respir. J. 4:3995.
23. Djukanovic, R., Wilson, J.W., Britten, K.M., Wilson, S.J., Walls, A.F., Roche, W.R., Howarth, P.H., and Holgate, S.T. 1992. The effect of inhaled corticosteroid on airway inflammation and symptoms of asthma. Am. Rev. Respir. Dis. 669-674.

20 Years of Anti-Allergic Drugs in Japan in Treatment of Asthma

Sohei Makino*

In allergic asthma antigen challenge causes the release of bronchoconstricting mediators and chemotactic mediators to eosinophils, inducing immediate bronchoconstriction, late-phase airway narrowing and post-late-phase airway hyperresponsiveness. Among agents which have anti-allergic effects, inhibitors of chemical mediator release from mast cells (ICMR), including DSCG, tranilast, ketotifen, azelastin and 10 other agents, have been used for the treatment of asthma for the past 20 years. The effectiveness of these ICMR has been proven by multi-institutional double-blind clinical trials. Since the effect of these ICMR becomes apparent 4 to 10 weeks after the start of the drug administration, their main effects are considered to be the suppression of eosinophil migration which causes airway hyperresponsiveness by damaging the alignment of the bronchial epithelial cells, not direct inhibition of bronchoconstricting mediators. The contribution of these ICMR to the treatment of asthma for the past 20 years since the introduction of DSCG was assessed by questionnaires to 12 experts who had seen asthmatic patients for more than 20 years. All of them replied that ICMR was useful for the treatment of asthma. It is expected that preventive therapy with anti-allergic drugs including ICMR should contribute more to the treatment of asthma in the future.

The incidence of asthma has increased in Japan for the past 30 years, being 0.5 to 1 percent in the 1960s and around 3 percent in 1989 in the population at large. This increase is more evident in infantile asthma. Other atopic diseases including allergic rhinitis, atopic dermatitis and allergic conjunctivitis have also increased. The reasons for this increase are not clear; however, the increase of mites in house dust has been considered to be one of the main causes. The treatment of asthma has also improved for the past 2 to 3 decades. Selective beta-2 adrenergic stimulants, oral or aerosols, slow-releasing theophylline preparations, beclomethason inhalation, and disodium cromoglycate and other oral anti-allergic drugs have been introduced. Among these anti-asthma drugs the use of anti-allergic drugs has increased markedly, consisting of approximately one fourth of the total in 1990 in Japan. Anti-allergic drugs have been used widely for the treatment of atopic diseases other than asthma (1).This increase of the use of anti-allergic drugs seems to be related to the recent understanding of bronchial asthma as an inflammatory disease of the airway.

Roles of Mast Cell-Derived Chemical Mediators for Airway Narrowing and Airway Hyperresponsiveness in Asthma

Chronic symptomatic asthma is characterized by enhanced airway responsiveness and inflammation of the bronchial mucosa associated with infiltration of eosinophils and lymphocytes. Approximately 70% of these patients have IgE antibody to environmental antigens including house dust mites. The inhalation of specific antigen causes the release of not only smooth muscle-constricting and vasoactive mediators, including histamine, leukotriene (LT) C4/D4/E4, prostaglandin D2 and thromoxane A2, but also of chemotactic meditators for eosinophils, including palatelet-activating factor (PAF) and LT B4. Infiltrated eosinophils release LT C4 and PAF, and basic proteins in specific granules including major basic protein, eosinophil peroxidase and eosinophil cationic protein. The toxic eosinophil granule proteins are considered to induce the damage of the bronchial mucosa, resulting in airway hyperresponsiveness. Eosinophil-induced airway hyperrepsonsiveness is thought to induce repeated episodes of dyspenea and wheezes.

* Department of Medicine and Clinical Immunology, Dokkyo University, Tochigi, Japan.

ICMR (Inhibitor of Chemical Mediator Release) Anti-Allergic Drugs in the Treatment of Asthma

Anti-allergic drugs may be defined as agents which suppress allergic reaction without suppressing the function of effector cells of the organs directly. A possible classification of anti-allergic drugs is as follows:

(a) Inhibitors of Chemical Mediator Production and Release: inhibitors of chemical mediator release (DSCG-like ICMR anti-allergic drugs), inhibitors of 5-lipoxygenase, inhibitors of thromboxane A2 synthetase, inhibitors of phospholipase A2, corticosteroids, Beta-2 stimulants;
(b) Receptor Antagonists for Chemical Mediators: H1-histamine antagonists, PAF antagonists, thromboxane A2 antagonists, leukotriene C4/D4 antagonists;
(c) Suppressants for Inflammatory Cell Activation and Migration: corticosteroids, T-cell suppressants, cyclosporin A, FK507, anti-eosinophil serum, anti-ICAM-1 serum.

In the treatment of asthma anti-allergic drugs are considered to be agents which suppress antigen-induced asthmatic response by (a) suppressing release or production of chemical mediators from mast cells, (b) blocking the combination of chemical mediators to the specific receptors on target cells in the airway and (c) modulating the activities of mast cells and other inflammatory cells in the airway as shown previously. At present 3 types of anti-allergic drugs have been used for the treatment of asthma, namely, (a) ICMR anti-allergic drugs, (b) H1-anti-histamines and (c) corticosteroids. H1-antihistmines are widely used for alllergic diseases, but their effect on asthma is only partial. Corticosteroids including oral prepareation and inhalation preparation are widely used to suppress the inflammation of the airway. A number of T-cell suppressants have been examined in preliminary trials in Japan as in other countries. DSCG-like ICMR anti-allergic drugs have been widely used for the treatment of asthma in Japan. At present 13 of ICMR anti-allergic drugs are available for clincial use. Only DSCG is given by inhalation and the others are given by oral route. ICMR anti-allergic drugs can be catergorized with or without H1-anti-histamine effect. DSCG, tranilast, repirinast, amlexanox, ibudilast, tazanolast and pemirolast do not have anti-histamine effects, while ketotifen, azelastine, oxatomide and terfenadine do have anti-histamine effects. These ICMR anti-allergic drugs *in vitro* suppress chemical mediator release from mast cells, lung tissue, and basophils by the stimulation of specific antigen or Ca Inophore A. They suppress antigen-induced immediate and late-phase airway narrowing in allergic asthmatic patients. They suppress exercise-induced airway narrowing, showing that these drugs stabilize mast cells, and not only antigen stimulation but also non-specific stimulation.

Mechanism of Effectiveness of ICMR Anti-Allergic Drugs in Asthma

DSCG and other ICMR anti-allergic drugs suppressed not only immediate bronchoconstriction but also late-phase airway narrowing. Late phase airway narrowing is closely associated with the infiltration of eosinophils in the airway, suggesting eosinophil infiltrated in the airway would cause late-phase airway narrowing, thus furthermore suggesting that DSCG suppressed LAR by suppressing esosinophil migration. Since post-late-phase airway hyperresponsiveness has been observed following late-phase airway narrowing, it is considered possible that eosinophil infiltration causes airway hyperresponsiveness as proposed in the beginning of this paper. ICMR anti-allergic drugs would suppress eosinophil infitration by suppressing the release of chemoatic mediators for eosinophils, resulting in suppression of airway hyperresponsivenss. In fact Diaz and Kay reported that 28 day's adminitration of DSCG decreased the number of eosinophils in bronchoalveolar lavage fluid. It is considered possible that ICMR anti-allergic drugs suppress antigen-induced airway hyperesponsivenss by suppressing eosinophil migration in the airway. Conforming to this hypothesis, there are reports that long-term administration of DSCG or ketotifen suppresses the enhancement of airway hyperresponsiveness during pollen seasons or reduces airway responsveness to inhaled acetylcholine and histamine as compared to the control period.

Usefulness of ICMR Anti-Allergic Drugs in Asthma

Multicenter Double-Blind Studies (3–16)

The effectiveness of ICMR-anti-allergic drugs was evaluated by multi-instituional double-blind clinical studies. In these clinical trials the subjects were patients with allergic asthma who had chronic symptoms enough to evaluate the improvement by the drugs. For patients who were kept on corticosteroids, mostly more than 5 mg of oral prednisolone or more than 8 puffs of beclomethasone inhalation per day, the effectiveness of these drugs was rated as very useful, useful, fairly useful, and not useful. Among 13 double-blind studies, 5 studies had inactive placebo, and the rest of the trials had active placebo or other established ICMR anti-allergic drugs. In the trials on adult asthmatic patients, the percentage of subjects who judged the drug very useful or useful was 15% in placebo and 34% in active ICMR drugs on avarage. The difference was statistically significant at the 1% level. The percentage judging their treatment as very useful, useful and fairly useful was 28% in inactive placebo and 74% in active drugs on the avarage. The difference was statistcally significant at the 1% level. These results of double-blind clinical trials clearly showed that ICMR anti-allergic drugs are effective for the treatment of asthma.

Comments of Expert Panel

In order to evaluate the usefulness of ICMR anti-allergic drugs in the practice of an allergy clinic, comments were collected from 12 experts who had seen more that 50 asthmatic patients for more than 20 years: 7 internists and 5 pediatricians.

In the treatment of asthma, ICMR anti-allergic drugs were judged as "very useful" by 1, "useful" by 4 and "fairly useful" by 2 internists. The judgements of 5 pediatricians were "very useful" by 1 and "useful" by 4, suggesting that these drugs are more effective in infantile asthma. The reasons for these judgments were (a) decrease of asthmatic symptoms, (b) avoidance of anti-asthma drugs and (3) low incidence of side-effects.

The place of anti-allergic drugs in the treatment of asthma

In mild sporadic asthma occasional bronchospasm is treated by the inhalation of beta-2 stimulant aerosols. In chronic asthma, routine prescription in my department is as follows: 500 to 700 mg of slow-releasing theophyllines, and oral and or aerosol beta-2 stimulants as bronchodilators, and ICMR anti-allergic drugs and beclomethasone inhalation.ICMR anti-allergic drugs are mainly indicated for patients with allergic asthma, but they are also reported in non-allergic asthma.In conclusion the strategy for preventive therapy of asthma is (a) continuous use of ICMR-anti-allergic drugs and beclomethasone inhalation for the prevention of inflammation of airway and (b) continuous or temporary use of slow-releasing theophylline preparations and beta-2 stimulants, depending on the severity of the asthmatic symptoms.

References

1. Makino, S. 1990. Preventive therapy in Japan. In: Preventive therapy in asthma. J. Moley, ed. London: Academic Press, p. 231.
2. Makino, S. 1990. Eosinophils in airway hyperresponsiveness. In: Inflammatory cells and mediators in bronchial asthma. D.K. Agrawal and R.G. Townley, ed. Boca Raton, Florida: CRC Press, p. 115.
3. Yamamura, Y. 1979. Evaluation of effectivenss of N-5′ in bronchial asthma (multi-center double-blind study). Igaku-no-Ayumi (Tokyo) 108:252.
4. Kumayai, A., Takahashi, T., Sdhidad, T., Tomioka, H., Mitui, S., Makino, S. et al. 1980. Clinical evaluation of HC-20-511 (ketotifen), a new oral anti-anaphylactic compound, in asthma (multi-center double-blind study in comparison with placebo). Clin. Eval. (Tokyo) 8:353 (with English abstract).
5. Yakura, T., Shida, T., Yamamura, Y., Mitsui, S., Makino, S., et al. 1982 . Clinical evaluation of

effectiveness of an anti-allergic agent, N-5′, to bronchial asthma (multi-center double-blind trial in comparison to disodium cromoglycate and palcebo). Shinryo-to-Shinyaku 19:529.
6. Kumagayi, A., Takahashi, T., Shida, T., Tomioka, H., Makino, S. et al. 1982. Clinical evaluation of HC20-511 (ketotifen), a new oral anti-anaphylactic compound, in bronchial asthma (multi-center double-blind study in comparison with disodium cromoglycate). Clin. Eval. (Tokyo) 10:737 (with English abstract).
7. Kawakami, Y., Takahashi, T., Shida, T., Yakura, T., Makino, S., et al. 1984. Clinical evaluation of an oral antiallergic agent, KW-4354 (Oxatomide), in adult bronchial asthma: Results of a double blind study with disodium cromoglycate and placebo served as control. Yakuri-to-Chiryo (Tokyo) 84:2505.
8. Kishimoto, S., Miyamoto, T., Shida, T., Igarashi, T. 1986. Effectiveness of amoxanox (AA-673) tablets on bronchial asthma (a multi-center double-blind study in comparison to tranilast) Igakuno-ayumi (Tokyo) 138:1005.
9. Takahashi, T. 1986. Clinical evaluation of KC404, a new anti-asthmatic agent, in the treatment of brocnhial asthma (multi-center double-blind study in comparison with tranilast). Clin. Eval. (Tokyo) 14:373.
10. Shida, T.,Miyamoto, T., Kishimoto, S., Makino, S., et al. 1986. Clinical effects of DSCG aerosol preparation on asthmatic adult patients (Comparatrive study in comparison to DSCG powder preparation) Shinryou-to-shinyaku (Tokyo) 23:1963.
11. Miyamoto, T., Takahashi, T., Shida, T., Kabe, J., Makino, S., et.al. 1986. Clincial evaluation of new antiallergic agent, MY-5116, to adult bronchial asthma. Shinryou-to Shinyaku (Tokyo) 23:251.
12. Makino, S., Ishizakid, T., Nagano, H., Tomioka, H., Shida, T. 1986. Clinical evaluation if E-0659 (azelastine) on bronchial asthma (multi-center double-blind study with ketotifen). Rinshou-to Kenkyuu (Fukuoka) 63:609.
13. Nagano, H., Hirose, T., Takishima, T., Kobayashi, S., Makino, S, et al. 1988. Clinical evaluation of mequitazine (L ~209) on bronchial asthma (Multicenter double-blind study with ketotifen). Rinshou-Iyaku (Tokyo) 4:1013.
14. Makino, S., Miyamoto, T., Kabe, J., Shida, T., Nakajima, S. 1988. Clinical evaluation of terfenadine in bronchial asthma: Comparison with ketotifen in a multi-center double-blind study. Rinshou-iyaku (Tokyo) 4:1678.
15. Yoshida, N.,Tomioka, H.,Takishima, N., Kobayashi, S., Makino, S., Miyamoto, T., Takahashi, T., Shida, T., Kishimoto, S., Nagano, H. 1989. Clinical evaluation of an orally antiallergic agent, TBX, in adult bronchial asthma: A multi-center double-blind study in comparison with tranilast. Yakuri-to-Chiryo (Tokyo) 17:933.
16. Miyamoto, T., Takahashi, T., Shida, T, Takishima, T, Makino, S., et al. 1989. Clinical evaluation of tazanolast (WP-833), a new anti-allergic agent in the treatment of bronchial asthma: A multi-center double-blind comparative study in comparison with tranilast. Rinshou-Iyaku (Tokyo) 5:501 (with English abstract).

Section XX

Pediatric Allergy

Viral Infections and Allergy in Children

Oscar L. Frick*

Because infections are so commonly associated with asthma and allergies and because both Co-chairmen of this symposium on pediatric allergy have research interests in viral infections, I shall confine my contribution to viral infections and allergy in children.

Dr. Ellis is a pioneer with his superb study in 1971 (1) of young asthmatic children at National Jewish Hospital in Denver in which he showed that 42% of asthma attacks were associated with proven viral infections, especially with RSV and parainfluenza-3, but there was no correlation with bacterial infections. These findings were confirmed by Minor et al. (2) in older school children and adults but more with rhinovirus and influenza A & B.

Our own interest was piqued when we studied prospectively 24 infants born into bilaterally allergic families that had a significantly higher incidence of allergic symptoms in 5 organ systems compared to 28 well, non-allergy-prone babies (3). Several laboratory tests for allergy (RAST, leukocyte histamine release and lymphoproliferation) became positive to a panel of allergens and this onset of symptoms and laboratory signs started within 4–6 weeks after a URI, especially RSV or PI-3, similar to those that Dr. Ellis found. Ours was a time coincidence between viral infection and onset of allergic sensitization.

We confirmed our observations in an atopic dog model (4) where puppies given live viral vaccine (distemper-hepatitis) followed by pollen-immunization developed canine IgE-antipollen antibodies within weeks. As adults, they had bronchospasm on inhalation of pollen extracts (5). Last year, we developed a dog model of food allergy (6) using a similar protocol of viral vaccine followed by food antigen injection; such animals developed diarrhea after blinded food challenges.

Welliver in Buffalo, N.Y., showed IgE anti-RSV (7) and anti-PI–3 (8) antibodies in nasal secretions of infants who developed bronchiolitis and wheezing with URI, and less so in infants who had only rhinitis or pneumonia without wheezing.

Our interest has focussed on a molecular mimicry between the bronchorelaxing neuropeptide, VIP (vasointestinal peptide) and parainfluenza-3 (PI-3) hemagglutinin L. Galinski et al. (9) cloned the gene and published the nucleotide and amino acid sequence of this protein in 1988. We were interested because PI-3 was one of the viruses affecting atopic infants' sensitization. The amino terminal 11 amino acids of VIP are analogous to those in the 1899–1914 segment of PI-3 hemagglutinin L. Therefore, we felt that PI-3 virus might compete with VIP for VIP-receptor and impede or augment its function.

In T and B-lymphocytes, VIP down-regulates lymphoproliferation and immunoglobulin synthesis, respectively. In this study, Stanisz et al. (10) found that over a concentration of 10^{-11} to 10^{-7} M, VIP and ST (SOM) inhibited CONA-induced lymphoproliferation of mouse spleen and Peyer's patch lymphocytes while substance P augmented such action. Therefore, in our study (11), we incubated human blood lymphocytes with either PHA or ConA concomitantly in presence or absence of VIP or PI-3 HA or together, and added ^{3}H-thymidine on day 3.

VIP markedly inhibited PHA-induced lymphoproliferation from 10^{-5} to 10^{-16} M, with a nadir at 10^{-7} M. Co-incubation of VIP with PI-3 HA reversed this VIP-induced inhibition and actually augmented lymphoproliferation. Similarly, either VIP or PI-3 HA alone inhibited ConA-induced lymphoproliferation; there was no inhibition when both VIP and PI-3 HA were co-incubated with ConA.

We interpreted these results that VIP and PI-3 HA competed for the same or adjacent overlapping receptors on T-lymphocytes, stimulation of which inhibited lymphoproliferation. Thus, virus by mimicry appeared to compete with VIP for its receptor and vice versa.

We wondered if virus would compete with VIP also for antigen-induced lymphoprolifera-

* University of California, San Francisco, CA 94143, USA

tion. Dr. Sreedharan synthesized the 14 amino acid PI-3 hemagglutinin peptide for us to determine if we were working with the correct part of the viral HA protein. I boosted myself with tetanus toxoid and up to 2 to 6 weeks later harvested my blood lymphocytes for lymphoproliferation assay with tetanus toxoid or Candida antigens on day 7.

With tetanus toxoid 1:10, VIP caused a small, but not significant, inhibition of lymphoproliferation. Virus peptide alone caused significant inhibition at 10^{-3} and 10^{-5} M concentrations, and not quite significant at 10^{-1} M. However, in co-culture with both VIP and peptide 10^{-1} and 10^{-3} M there was significant reversal of inhibition of lymphoproliferation with tetanus.

Finally with Candida 20 µg-induced lymphoproliferation, viral peptide at 10^{-3} and 10^{-5} M caused significant inhibition, which was reversed when co-cultured in presence of VIP 10^{-7} M. These antigen-specific lymphoproliferations were inhibited by VIP or viral peptide alone and reversed when both agents were present suggesting a competition between these for a common or closely associated receptor.

Recently, Sreedharan et al. (12) cloned and published the amino acid sequence and structure of VIP receptor on lymphocytes. In this hydrophobicity plot, the receptor has seven hydrophobic domains which are probably intramembranous, similar to that of other G-protein activation receptors. This represents a proposed structure with an extracellular amino terminal, seven intramembranous portions allowing three extracellular and three intracellular loops with 2 cysteines forming a disulfide bridge between extracellular loops 1 and 2; N-glycosylation sites of N-asparagine are in red dots. We are now trying to locate which part of this molecule binds VIP and our PI-3 peptide to prove our cross-binding hypothesis at the molecular level.

If the VIP-receptor in lymphocytes and in bronchial smooth muscle are the same, and such competition between VIP and parainfluenza-3 virus is common, then this might help explain partly why increased bronchial hyperirritability occurs after a virus infection where the virus blocks the VIP-relaxing mechanism in smooth muscle and inhibition of antibody synthesis, possibly in a jump in logic. This we are investigating in stimulation of IgE antibody production.

I turn now to the possible development of vaccines against RSV and parainfluenza-3 for infants, especially those from allergy-prone families. You may recall that there was a tragedy about 20 years ago with a killed RSV vaccine which was tried in 4 centers; 45% of the vaccinated infants had to be hospitalized with severe Hecht's pneumonia, similar to that with killed measles vaccine, and two died (13). In an RSV-infected cotton rat model (14), the same formalin-killed RSV vaccine caused similar pneumonia with immune complex deposition. This dampened enthusiasm for an RSV vaccine for a score of years.

Carolyn Hill recently reviewed prospects for an RSV vaccine (15). In 1985, Huang and Collins (16) characterized 10 viral proteins in RSV-4 in envelope, 2 of which were major glycoproteins F & G crucial for RSV immunity. F protein is a 70 Kd Fusion protein that fuses viral envelope with host cell membrane to promote cell-to-cell spread and syncytial formation. G protein is a 90 Kd large surface glycoprotein that promotes attachment of virus to host cells. Small infants have protective antibodies from mother to these two proteins, but these wane at 3–6 months, when infants become most susceptible. Ward et al. (17) found that antibody levels to F Fusion protein were higher in women whose babies were not infected with RSV; also, infants with severe RSV pneumonia had significantly lower anti-G protein titers, suggesting that F & G proteins were protective.

Genes for F & G proteins of RSV have been inserted in several viral vectors. Adenovirus is a particularly good vector, for it colonizes both respiratory and GI mucosa and stimulates mucosal immunity. This vector is particularly effective by intranasal route. Collins et al. (18) used such an adenoviral recombinant F protein vaccine that protected cotton rats from RSV infection. The F protein of both A and B strains of RSV results in good cross-strain immunity, whereas G protein cross-reacts only about 5%. This vaccine is now being tried in primates and will subsequently be applied in humans.

Prospects for a parainfluenza vaccine were reviewed by Beishe and Newman (19). With the cloning and sequencing of the parainfluenza-3 (9) and more recently parainfluenza-2 (20), subcellular fractions or peptides are being tried to induce immunity. The fusion F protein of PI-2 has been cloned and sequenced as a 59 Kd glycoprotein.

However, so far, the most successful PI-3 vaccine (21) has been derived from cold-adapted PI-3 in which virus was repeatedly passaged in African green monkey kidney cells at lower and lower temperatures for 18 to 45 passages. There were also several acquired genetic defects in the virus that prevented reversion back to the wild state. In weanling hamsters, wild type PI-3 grow well in nasal turbinates and lungs, but progressive cold passaged-attenuated viruses had progressively less growth in either tissue. In low seropositive children, the cold passage 18 attenuated PI-3 was shown to cause no symptoms and caused a significant rise in antibody titers, thus the attenuated virus was still antigenic. Such a clinical trial is underway now in seronegative children to assess for protection against natural PI-3 infection.

Finally, I shall conclude with a few words on Rhinoviruses. These were important triggers of asthma in older children and adults in the Minor et al. studies (2). There are over 100 strains of rhinoviruses, so vaccines are difficult to make. Rhinoviruses have a series of highly exposed peptide loops with great variability among serotypes; they also have a conserved series of amino acids in a "recessed groove", probably the conserved binding site of HRV. Greve et al. (22) and Staunton et al. (23) found that 90% of rhinovirus strains bind to a major 95 Kd Human Rhinovirus Receptor (HRVR) which has been cloned and sequenced and was found to be identical to intercellular adhesion protein, ICAM-1. Binding of rhinoviruses was inhibited by antibodies to ICAM-1.

Both IL-1 and Interferon-γ stimulate expression of ICAM-1 on human fibroblasts and other cells (24), but there is some discordance. Stimulation of fibroblast with IFN-γ causes increased binding of HRV and LFA-1 on T-lymphocytes. However, stimulation of fibroblasts with IL-1 only increased binding of HRV and not LFA-1 on T-cells. ICAM-1 thus appears to have two adjacent binding sites for LFA-1 on the D-1 domain and HRV on the D-2 domain which overlap. Binding of HRV to ICAM-1 on human fibroblasts can inhibit subsequent attachment of LFA-1 bearing T-cells in a molecular mimicry. It is also possible that after virus-binding the receptor-RSV complex is shed or internalized and unavailable for LFA-1 binding. Springer (25) suggested that rhinoviruses use ICAM-1 stimulation which produces increased cytokines which then increase nasal secretions that carry rhinoviruses to facilitate spread by sneezing to other persons. A subfraction of ICAM-1 might be a useful immunization agent for an anti-rhinovirus vaccine.

Finally, it was recently recognized that rhinoviruses in infants can cause a severe pertussis-like cough and vomiting and serious pneumonia with profound respiratory distress that may require intubation and mechanical ventilation (26). Up-regulation of ICAM-1 has been found to attract eosinophils in monkeys and secondary bronchial hyperreactivity and thus, asthma (27). These activities were blocked with a monoclonal anti-ICAM-1 antibody. Therefore, this might explain why rhinovirus infection might be a risk factor (28) for the development of asthma in infants.

In conclusion, I have reviewed (a) some of the associations of virus infections, first with asthma itself, then with allergic sensitization, and where parainfluenza-3 virus may compete with VIP – the neuro-inhibitor peptide – for its receptor and (b) implications for asthma and antibody-formation. Then, I reviewed the prospects for vaccines for RSV, parainfluenzae, and rhinoviruses, all of which may be important in allergic sensitization of children.

References

1. McIntosh, K., Ellis, E.F., Hoffman, L.S., et al. 1973. The association of viral and bacterial respiratory infections with exacerbations of wheezing in young asthmatic children. J. Pediatr. 82:578.
2. Minor, T.E., Dick, E.C., DeMeo, A.N., et al. 1974. Viruses as precipitants of asthmatic attacks in children. JAMA 227:292.
3. Frick, O.L., German, D., and Mill, J. 1979. Development of allergy in children. I. Association with virus infections. J. Allergy Clin. Immunol. 63:228.
4. Frick, O.L., and Brooks, D.L. 1983. Immunoglobulin E antibodies to pollens augmented in dogs by viral vaccines. Am. J. Vet. Res. 44:440.
5. Chung, K.F., Becker, A.B., Lazarus, S.C., Frick, O.L., Nadel, J.A., and Gold, W.M. 1985. Antigen-induced airway hyperresponsiveness in pulmonary inflammation in allergic dogs. J. Appl. Physiol. 58:1347.
6. Frick, O.L., Barker, S., and Parker, J. 1990. The atopic dog as a model for food allergy. Clin. Exper. Allergy. 20, Suppl. 1:54.

7. Welliver, R.C., Wong, D.T., DSun, M., et al. 1981. The development of respiratory syncytial virus-specific IgE and the release of histamine in nasopharyngeal secretions after infection. N. Engl. J. Med. 305:841.
8. Welliver, R.C., Wong, D.T., Middleton, E.Jr., et al. 1982. Role of parainfluenza virus-specific IgE in pathogenesis of croup and wheezing subsequent to infection. J. Pediatr. 101:889.
9. Galinski, M.S., Mink, M.A., and Pons, M.W. 1988. Molecular cloning and sequence analysis of the human parainfluenza 3 virus gene encoding the L protain. Virology 165:499.
10. Stanisz, A.M., Befus, D., and Bienenstock, J. 1986. Differential effects of vasoactive intestinal peptide, Substance P, and somatostatin on immunoglobulin synthesis and proliferations by lymphocytes and Peyer's patches, mesenteric lymph nodes and spleen. J. Immunol. 136:152.
11. Frick, O.L., and Barker, S. 1990. Parainfluenza-3 hemagglutinin attenuates VIP-induced inhibition of PHA-induced human lymphoproliferation. J. Allergy Clin. Immunol. 87:260.
12. Sreedharan, S.P., Robichon, A., Peterson, K.E., and Goetzl, E.J. 1991. Cloning and expression of the human vasoactive intestal peptide receptor. Proc. Nat. Acad. Sci. USA 88:4986.
13. Kim, H.W., Canchola, J.G., Brandt, C.D., et al. 1969. Respiratory syncytial virus disease in infants despite prior administration of antigenic inactivated vaccine. Am. J. Epidemiol. 89:422.
14. Prince, G.A., Jesnsen, A.B., Hemming, V.G., et al. 1986. Enhancement of respiratory syncytial virus pulmonary pathology in cotton rats by prior intramuscular inoculation of formalin-inactivated virus. J. Virol. 57:721.
15. Hall, C.B. 1991. Vaccines for respiratory syncytial virus: From Ghosts to genetic genies. Sem. Ped. Infect. Dis. 2:191.
16. Huang, Y.T., Collins, P.L., and Wertz, G.W. 1985. Characterization of 10 proteins in human respiratory syncytial virus: Identification of a fourth envelope-associated protein. Virus Res. 2:157.
17. Ward, K.A., Lambden, P.R., Ogilvie, M.M., et al. 1983. Antibodies to RSV peptides and their significance in human infection. J. Gen. Virol. 64:1867.
18. Collins, P.L., Davis, A., Lubeck, M., et al. 1989. Evaluation of the protective efficacy of recombinant vaccinia viruses and adenoviruses that express respiratory syncytial virus glycoproteins. In: Modern approaches to new vaccines including prevention of AIDS. Cold Spring Harbor Laboratory, p. 26.
19. Belshe, R.B., and Newman, F.K. 1991. Prospects for vaccines for parainfluenza virus. Sem. Ped. Infect. Dis. 2197.
20. Varsanyi, T.M., Kovamees, J., and Norrby, E. 1991. Molecular cloning and sequence analysis of human parainfluenza type 2 virus mRNA encoding the fusion protein. J. Gen. Virol. 72:89.
21. Crookshanks-Newman, F.K., and Belshe, R.B. Protection of weanling hamsters from experimental infection with wild-type parainfluenza virus type (para 3) by cold-adapted mutants of para 3. J. Med. Virol. 18:131.
22. Greve, J.M., Davis, G., Meyer, A.M., et al. 1989. The major human Rhinovirus receptor is ICAM-1. Cell 56:839.
23. Staunton, D.E, Merluzzi, V.J., Rothlein, R., et al. 1989. A cell adhesion molecule, ICAM-1, is the major surface receptor for Rhinoviruses. Cell 56:849.
24. Piela-Smith, T.H., Aniero, L., and Korn, J.H. 1991. Binding of Human Rhinovirus and T Cells to intracellular adhesion molecule-1 on human fibroblasts: Discordance between effects of IL-1 and IFN-γ. J. Immunol. 147:1831.
25. Springer, T.A. 1990. Adhesion receptors of the immune system. Nature 346:425.
26. Schmidt, H.J., and Fink, R.J. 1991. Rhinovirus as a lower respiratory tract pathogen in infants. Ped. Infect. Dis. J. 10:700.
27. Wegner, C.D., Gundel, R.H., Reilly, P., et al. 1990. Intracellular adhesion molecule-1 (ICAM-L) in the pathogenesis of asthma. Science 247:456.
28. Lemanske, R.F., Dick, E.C., Swenson, C.A., et al. 1989. Rhinovirus upper respiratory infection increases airway hyperreactivity and late asthmatic responses.

Immunodeficiency and Allergy

Rebecca Buckley*

Studies over the past two decades in rodents and, more recently, in man have revealed a fundamental role for T cells and their cytokines in the initiation and regulation of IgE synthesis. Since a number of human immunodeficiency diseases with partial T cell immunodeficiency are characterized by excessive IgE production, this has raised the possibility that the human atopic diseases might represent a form of immunodeficiency. Supporting this postulate is the increased incidence of viral diseases in asthma and, particularly, in atopic dermatitis. The demonstration that IL-4 is essential for IgE production is the most significant advance enabling the study of this hypothesis. The availability of a reproducibly positive *in vitro* system for studying IL-4-induced human IgE synthesis has already permitted initial exploration of this. B cells from normal and atopic subjects have been shown to respond with similar IgE production when stimulated with recombinant IL-4 *in vitro*, raising the strong possibility that excessive IgE production *in vivo* is caused by differences in other cell types and the cytokines they produce. Further study should permit elucidation of the mechanism of deficient IgE regulation in humans who produce excessive IgE and enable identification of safe and effective antagonists to IL-4 which could be used clinically.

Circumstantial Evidence from Clinical Observations in Man

The most compelling evidence supporting an association between immunodeficiency and allergy comes from the consistent finding of an increased incidence of atopic disease and/or excessive IgE antibody production among patients with certain primary immunodeficiency syndromes (1,2,3). This has been most apparent in patients with the Wiskott-Aldrich syndrome, who have atopic dermatitis, sometimes asthma, positive skin and RAST tests to allergens, an elevated serum IgE concentration, and partial impairments in both T and B cell functions (2,4). Another striking example is the "hyper-IgE syndrome" (3): a condition characterized by a lifelong history of severe staphylococcal skin and lung abscesses, a pruritic eczematoid dermatitis not typical of atopic dermatitis, extreme hyperimmunoglobulinemia E, persistent eosinophilia of blood, sputum and tissues and abnormal humoral and cellular anamnestic immune functions (3,5). Imbalances of CD4 and CD8+ subsets of human blood T lymphocytes have been reported in both acute and chronic graft-versus-host disease (GVHD) (6). During this period, marked elevations of serum IgE concentrations have been noted by several groups (7). Finally, patients with the acquired immune deficiency syndrome (AIDS) have been noted to have a high frequency of allergic reactions (8). These findings suggest that not only genetic defects in T cell function but also certain acquired immunodeficiency states are characterized by a deficiency of T cells important in the downregulation of IgE synthesis. The most convincing observations relating to the question of a possible underlying immunodeficiency in allergic individuals are those of the tendencies of patients with atopic dermatitis to develop recurrent localized and/or disseminated cutaneous viral infections with herpes simplex viruses and to have an increased incidence of molluscum contagiosum lesions (9). However, despite many investigations of immune function in atopy, only a few reproducible aberrations have been found. Among these are consistently higher serum IgE concentrations in groups of atopics when compared to groups of normals and delayed cutaneous anergy to ubiquitous antigens (10). In addition, peripheral blood lymphocytes from eczema patients have been reported to have significantly decreased cell-mediated lympholysis (CML) (11) and natural killer (NK)

---

* Duke University Medical Center, Durham, North Carolina 27710, USA.
Acknowledgements: Supported by Grant #AI28414 from the National Institutes of Allergy and Infectious Diseases.

cell functions (12). However, both the delayed cutaneous anergy and the decreased NK function were found to correlate with disease activity and were thus suspected to be secondary abnormalities.

Studies of Human IgE Regulation

Although many lymphocyte-derived soluble factors with either enhancing or suppressing effects on IgE synthesis have been described in experimental animals over the past 2 decades (13,14), recent studies in both mice and humans have demonstrated that the only one essential for the induction of IgE synthesis is interleukin 4 (IL-4) (15,16,17,18). In early studies of IL-4-induced murine IgE synthesis, this activity was found to be profoundly inhibited by the addition of interferon gamma (IFN-γ) (19). Subsequently, IFNγ, interferon alpha and prostaglandin E2 were all shown by Pene et al. (16) to inhibit IL-4-induced human IgE synthesis *in vitro*. In an effort to identify the cellular sources of these various cytokines, Mosmann and Coffman (20) examined the types of cytokines produced by cloned murine T helper cells. They were able to identify two patterns of cytokine production that distinguished some clones from others and named the two types TH1 and TH2 cells. TH1 clones produced IL-2 and IFNγ, whereas TH2 clones produced IL-4 and IL-5; both types produced some cytokines, such as IL-3. This led to speculation that excessive IgE production might be due to a predominance of TH2 type cells, whereas low IgE-producing animals would have a dominance of TH1 type cells. Unfortunately, human T helper cell clones have not demonstrated distinctive patterns of cytokine production similar to those reported in the mouse, as most clones studied produced not only IL-4 but also IL-2 and IFNγ (21).

Until recently, direct examination of cellular regulatory events in human IgE antibody synthesis had been hampered by a lack of a reproducible system for inducing IgE antibody synthesis *in vitro*. The fact that pokeweed mitogen (PWM) and other polyclonal B cell activators, such as Staphylococcus Cowan 1 organisms, failed to stimulate IgE production by human blood B cells in *in vitro* culture severely compromised studies of human IgE regulation for over a decade (22,23). In addition, the picogram quantities of IgE detected in human mononuclear (MNC) culture supernatants that were initially thought to represent synthesized IgE, eventually were shown to be largely from preformed IgE (24). A third technical problem was uncovered three years ago when it was discovered in the author's laboratory that Iscove's modified Dulbecco's medium, containing human transferrin, bovine insulin and serum albumin, oleic, palmitic and linoleic acids, when supplemented with 10% fetal calf serum (C-IMDM), but not RPMI 1640, would support the induction of nanogram quantities of IgE synthesis by human blood MNC by very small concentrations (2.5–5 ng/ml) of recombinant human IL-4 (rhIL-4) (17). This has aided these studies immensely by providing a reproducibly positive *in vitro* system for inducing true human IgE synthesis.

Using the above-mentioned optimized culture system, we sought to clarify whether a difference could be shown in B cell IgE responses to rhIL-4 when atopic and normal donors' cells were compared. In our initial as well as all subsequent studies, atopic and non-atopic donors' cells were found to produce similar quantities of IgE when stimulated with rhIL-4 at all doses evaluated (18). Moreover, the IgE produced was in easily measured high nanogram concentrations (17,18). Thus, B cells from normal donors responded similarly to those from atopic donors, suggesting that B cells from the latter are no more sensitive than those of normals to IL-4's effects (18). In cell separation studies, we also demonstrated that irradiated or non-irradiated T cells from atopic and nonatopic donors could support to a similar extent rhIL-4-induced IgE synthesis by purified human B cells from either source (18).

Since B cell responses to IL-4 appear similar in atopic and non-atopic subjects, investigations have turned to T cells and the cytokines they produce in an effort to explain excessive IgE production in atopy. Studies by the author and many others of blood MNC from patients with atopic dermatitis using monoclonal antibodies to CD3, CD4 and CD8 surface glycoproteins (25) have revealed normal percentages of T cells and the major T cell subsets. However, it has been reported that patients with atopic dermatitis have a significantly lower percentage of T cells with the CD4+ CD29+

(memory helper) phenotype when compared with normals (26). In addition, recent studies by the author and her associates (27) have demonstrated a deficiency of CD3+ T cells bearing the CD45RO isoform (memory T cell phenotype) in all patients with the hyper-IgE syndrome studied. In mice this isoform is present on TH1 but not TH2 cells (28). Whether this will ultimately be shown to have relevance to hyper IgE syndrome patients' abnormal anamnestic humoral and cellular responses and/or to their excessive IgE production is unknown. Speculation that the elevated IgE in these and other humans may be due to excessive IL-4 production has been difficult to prove, because IL-4 has not been measurable in their body fluids by the assays available. However, recent studies from the author's laboratory have demonstrated that blood B cells from hyper IgE patients are relatively refractory to stimulation with recombinant IL-4 *in vitro*, suggesting that they may have already been stimulated with excessive endogenous IL-4 *in vivo* (29). Studies by Maggi et al. (30) demonstrated that T cell clones derived from residual CD4+ blood T cells from stage IV AIDS patients exhibited increased helper activity for IgG and IgE synthesis as well as increased IL-4 and decreased IFN-γ production when compared to T cells from normal controls. The explanation for the selective survival of CD4+ T cells with this functional capacity in AIDS patients is unknown.

Possibly related to the reports of lower NK activity and to the elevated serum IgE concentrations of patients with atopic dermatitis is the finding by Reinhold et al. (31) of decreased IFNγ production following stimulation of eczema patients' blood MNC with PHA, ionomycin and phorbol esters, anti-CD3 or IL-2. This has not been confirmed in other laboratories as yet. Conflicting findings have also been reported regarding IFNγ production by noncloned T cells from patients with the hyper IgE syndrome. Del Prete et al. (32) and Paganelli et al. (33) reported reduced IFNγ production by stimulated blood MNC from four and five patients with the hyper IgE syndrome, respectively. However, neither Vercelli et al. (34) nor the author found deficient IFNγ production by MNC from larger groups (7 and 11, respectively) of such patients following stimulation with mitogens or phorbol esters plus calcium ionophores (33,32,34).

Several laboratories have recently found that allergen specific human T helper cell clones isolated from the blood of allergic donors produce more IL-4 and less IFNγ than similar allergen-specific clones from nonatopic donors and than T cell clones (from either atopic or nonatopic donors) that have specificity for antigens from bacteria or fungi (35). These lymphokine profiles were stable and were neither dependent on the dose of allergen nor the atopic or nonatopic state of the donor of the antigen-presenting cells. Thus, it is possible that the genetic difference between atopic and normal individual dictates the type of T cell (high versus low IL-4 producing and/or low versus high IFNγ producing) that responds to allergens.

References

1. Buckley, R.H., and Becker, W.G. 1978. Abnormalities in the regulation of human IgE synthesis. Immunol. Rev. 41:288.
2. Buckley, R.H., and Fiscus, S.A. 1975. Serum IgD and IgE concentrations in immunodeficiency disease. J. Clin. Invest. 55:157.
3. Buckley, R.H., and Sampson, H.A. 1981. The hyperimmunoglobulinemia E syndrome. In: Clinical immunology update. E.C.Franklin, ed. New York: Elsevier North-Holland, p. 147.
4. Waldmann, T.A., Polmar, S., and Balestra, S. 1972. Immunoglobulin E in immunologic deficiency diseases. II. Serum IgE concentration of patients with acquired hypogammaglobulinemia, myotonic dystrophy, intestinal lymphangiectasia and Wiskott-Aldrich syndrome. J. Immunol. 109:304.
5. Sheerin, K.A., and Buckley, R.H. 1991. Antibody responses to protein, polysaccharide, and X174 antigens in the hyperimmunoglobulinemia E (Hyper IgE) syndrome. J. Allergy Clin. Immunol. 87:803.
6. Reinherz, E.L., Parkman, R., Rappaport, J., Rosen, F.S., and Schlossman, S.F. 1979. Aberrations of suppressor T cells in human graft-versus-host disease. N. Engl. J. Med. 300:1061.
7. Heyd, J., Donnenberg, A., Burns, R., and Santos, G. 1988. Immunoglobulin E levels following allogeneic, autologous and syngeneic bone marrow transplantation: An indirect association between hyperproduction and acute graft-v-host disease in allogeneic BMT. Blood 72:442.

8. Seligmann, M., Chess, L., Fahey, J., Fauci, A.S., Lachmann, P.J., L'Age Stehr, J., Ngu, J., Pinching, A.J., Rosen, F.S., Spira, R.J., and Wybran, J. 1984. AIDS-immunologic reevaluation. N. Engl. J. Med. 311:1285.
9. Buckley, R.H. 1985. Atopic dermatitis. In: Allergy. A.P. Kaplan, ed. New York: Churchhill Livingstone, p. 417.
10. McGeady, S.J., and Buckley, R.H. 1975. Depression of cell-mediated immunity in atopic eczema. J. Allergy Clin. Immunol. 56:393.
11. Leung, D.Y.M., Wood, N., Dubey, D., Rhodes, A., and Geha, R. 1983. Cellular basis of defective cell-mediated lympholysis in atopic dermatitis. J. Immunol. 130:1678.
12. Jensen, J.R., Sand, T., Jorgensen, A., and Thestrup-Pedersen, K. 1984. Modulation of natural killer cell activity in patients with atopic dermatitis. J. Invest. Dermatol. 82:30.
13. Tada, R. 1975. Regulation of reaginic antibody formation in animals. Progr. Allergy 19:122.
14. Ishizaka, K. 1984. Regulation of IgE synthesis. Ann. Rev. Immunol. 2:159.
15. Paul, W.E., and Ohara, J. 1987. B cell stimulatory factor-1/interleukin 4. Ann. Rev. Immunol. 5:429.
16. Pene, J., Rousset, F., Briere, F., Chretien, I. Bonnefoy, J., Spits, H., Yokota, T., Arai, N., Arai, K., Banchereau, J., and DeVries, J. 1988. IgE production by normal human lymphocytes is induced by interleukin 4 and suppressed by interferons and prostaglandin E2. Proc. Nat. Acad.Sci. 85:6880.
17. Claassen, J.L., Levine, A.D., and Buckley, R.H. 1990. A cell culture system that enhances mononuclear cell IgE synthesis induced by recombinant human interleukin-4. J. Immunol. Meth. 126:213.
18. Claassen, J.L., Levine, A.D., and Buckley, R.H. 1990. Recombinant human IL-4 induces IgE and IgG synthesis by normal and atopic donor mononuclear cells: Similar dose response, time course, requirement for T cells, and effect of pokeweed mitogen. J. Immunol. 144:2123.
19. Coffman, R.L., and Carty, J. 1986. A T cell activity that enhances polyclonal IgE production and its inhibition by interferon-γ. J. Immunol. 136:949.
20. Mosmann, T.R., and Coffman, R.L. 1989. TH1 and TH2 cells: Different patterns of lymphokine secretion lead to different functional properties. Ann. Rev. Immunol. 7:145.
21. Paliard, X., de Wall Malefijt, R., Yssel, H., Blanchard, D.,Chretien, I., Abrams, J., De Vries, J., and Spits, H. 1988. Simultaneous production of interleukin 2, interleukin 4 and interferon gamma by activated human CD4+ and CD8+ T cell clones. J. Immunol. 141:849.
22. Fiser, P.M., and Buckley, R.H. 1979. Human IgE biosynthesis *in vitro*: Studies with atopic and normal blood mononuclear cells and subpopulations. J. Immunol. 123:1788.
23. Sampson, H.A., and Buckley, R.H. 1981. Human IgE synthesis *in vitro*: A reassessment. J. Immunol. 127:829.
24. Gamkrelidze, A., and Bjorksten, B. 1990. The determination of IgE synthesis *in vitro*. Methodological aspects. J. Immunol. Meth. 130:9.
25. Buckley, R.H. 1988. Immunologic deficiency and allergic disease. In: Allergy, Principles and practice. E. Middleton, Jr., Reed, E.D., Ellis, N., Adkinson, Jr., and J. Yunginger, eds. St. Louis: C.V. Mosby.
26. Schauer, R., Jung, T., Heymanns, J., and Rieger, C. 1991. Imbalance of CD4+ CD45R+ and CD4+ CD29+ T helper cell subsets in patients with atopic diseases. Clin. Exp. Immunol. 83:25.
27. Buckley, R.H., Schiff, S.E., and Hayward, A.R. 1991. Reduced frequency of CD45RO+ T lymphocytes in blood of hyper IgE syndrome patients. J. Allergy Clin. Immunol. 87:313.
28. Luqman, M., Johnson, P., Trowbridge, I., and Bottomly, K. 1991. Differential expression of the alternatively spliced exons of murine CD45 in TH1 and TH2 cloned lines. Eur. J. Immunol., 21:17.
29. Claassen, J.L., Levine, A.D., Schiff, S.E., and Buckley, R.H. 1991. Mononuclear cells from patients with the hyper IgE syndrome produce little IgE when stimulated with recombinant interleukin 4 *in vitro*. J. Allergy Clin. Immunol. 88.
30. Maggi, E., Macchia, D., Parronchi, P., Mazzetti, M., Ravina, A., Milo, D., and Romagnani, S. 1987. Reduced production of interleukin-2 and interferon gamma and enhanced helper activity for IgE synthesis by cloned CD4+ T cells from patients with AIDS. Eur. J. Immunol. 17:1685.
31. Reinhold, U., Wehrmann, W., Kukel, S., and Kreysel, H.W. 1990. Evidence that defective interferon-gamma production in atopic dermatitis patients is due to intrinsic abnormalities. Clin. Exp. Immunol. 79:374.
32. Del Prete, G., Tiri, A., Maggi, E., De Carli, M., Macchia, D., Parronchi, P., Rossi, M., Pietrogrande, M., Ricci, M., and Romagnani, S. 1989. Defective *in vitro* production of gamma interferon and tumor necrosis factor alpha by circulating T cells from patients with the hyper

immunoglobulin E syndrome. J. Clin. Invest. 84:1830.

33. Paganelli, R., Scala, E., Capobianchi, M., Fanales-Belasio, E., D'Offizi, G., Fiorilli, M., and Aiuti, F. 1991. Selective deficiency of interferon-gamma production in the hyper IgE syndrome. Relationship to *in vitro* IgE synthesis. Clin. Exp. Immunol. 84:28.
34. Vercelli, D., Jabara, H., Cunningham-Rundles, C., Abrams, J., Lewis, D., Meyer, J., Schneider, L., Leung, D., and Geha, R. 1990. Regulation of immunoglobulin IgE synthesis in the hyper IgE syndrome. J. Clin. Invest. 85:1.
35. Wierenga, E.A., Snoek, M., De Groot, C., Chretien, I., Box, J., Hansen, H., and Kapsenberg, M. 1990. Evidence for compartmentalization of functional subsets of CD4+ T lymphocytes in atopic patients. J. Immunol. 144:4651.

The Present Status of Pediatric Allergy in Oriental Countries

Montri Tuchinda*

Allergy is one of the most common causes of acute and chronic childhood diseases. It is responsible for a wide range of problems for children and the family. Allergic problems are similar to those caused by diseases, but may differ among countries depending on geographical, psycho-social, educational and economic aspects. The present status of pediatric allergy in the oriental countries is summarized here. The status of pediatric allergy is relatively well developed in oriental countries in comparison with Western countries. There is fairly accurate knowledge of atmospheric aeroallergens and their annual distribution in many countries. Studies from many countries in this region indicate that house dust mite is the most important indoor allergen. Although no data are available for the exact prevalence of each allergic disease in children in every country, detailed studies of asthma are available in nearly every country. Basic and clinical research, public education and immunotherapy are carried out in most countries, and many well trained pediatric allergists are available. There are allergology societies in all countries and they have now united to form "The Asian Pacific Federation of Allergology and Immunology Societies" to promote the exchange of knowledge in allergy and immunology among the countries of this region.

China

China is the largest country in the world with a population of more than one billion. The first allergy clinic was established in 1956 in Capital Hospital. Now there are many other allergy clinics and laboratories in the provinces and municipalities with several hundred clinic personnel. Modern research works dealing with both basic and clinical aspects of allergy are currently available in China. The prevalence of allergic disease in Chinese children is unknown, but a survey of 6,563 adults with various occupations in the Beijing area revealed a prevalence for total allergic diseases of 37.7%. Urticaria was the most common with 20.6%, drug allergy accounted for 7.9%, asthma 5.3%, allergic eczema 5.2%, allergic rhinitis 3.4%, and food allergy 3.4%. Surveys for atmospheric pollen and mold in the Beijing area have been carried out since 1958. The important pollens are *Astemisia* (sagebrush) which peaks in September, *Humulus* (hops) in August, *Broussonetia* (paper mulberry) in May and *Eraxinus* (ash) in March. The important mold spores and the peak count were *Alternaria* in June, Rust in June, and Smut in September. The house dust mite is the most important indoor allergen. *D. pteronyssinus* was the most common species. South China had a higher prevalence than the north because humidity and temperature are more favorable for its growth there. Besides the mite, other important indoor allergens in China include house dust, cotton, kapok, silk, various animal danders and hair, and various kinds of feathers. Immunotherapy is widely practised in China. About 150 different kinds of allergenic extracts are made locally for specific diagnosis and treatment (1).

Hong Kong

The prevalence of allergic diseases in children in Hong Kong is unknown, but asthma is common. Most cases are of the extrinsic type and boys are more affected than girls. The most common allergen is the house dust mite (*D. pterronyssinus*), which gives positive skin tests in about 80% of asthmatic children. There is a very low prevalence of positive skin tests to molds and pollens. Pets (cats and dogs), present in 40% of homes in Hong Kong, appear to be

* Department of Pediatrics, Faculty of Medicine, Siriraj Hospital, Mahidol University, Bangkok 10700, Thailand.

potentially important. About 50% of skin tests in asthmatic patients have shown positive results to pets (2).

India

The incomplete statistics have revealed that as many as 10% suffer from respiratory allergic disorders (3). About 10–12% of children visiting the Pediatric Outpatient Department suffer from asthma, and higher percentage of patients have allergic rhinitis (4). Analysis of skin prick test reactions to various allergens in asthmatic children in Bombay revealed that 81% of cases gave positive reactions to insects (cockroaches, mites, moths, etc.), 72% to dust (house dust, wheat dust, cotton dust, old paper dust), 41% to mold, 38% to pollens and 62% to food allergens (5). The most common air borne pollens found in metropolitan and urban areas are *Amaranthaceae, Compositae, Moraceae, Pinaceae, Casurinaceae*. Tree pollens had peaks between February to April, while the herb and weed pollens had peaks between August and October (6). Surveys of atmospheric mold spores have revealed that the important fungal spores are *Alternaria, Cladosporium, Drechaslera, Aspergillus, Penicillium, Curvularia, Nigrospora, Epicoccum, Mucor*, etc. The most dominant are *Alternaria* in the north and *Cladosporium* in the south. Fungal spores are found throughout the year and there is no definite peak as in pollens. Pediatric allergy training centers are limited in India. The Post-Graduate Institute of Medical Education and Research at Chandigarh, established in 1972, is one of the leading, with modern technology, treatment methods and research. Immunotherapy is practised in some Indian centers.

Indonesia

A survey of the prevalence of allergic diseases in children in an urban area near central Jakarta revealed that 8.2% had asthma, 10.2% had allergic rhinitis, and 25% had atopic diseases. Skin prick tests to 10 common allergens in 2,850 adult asthmatics revealed positive reactions to the mite (*D. pteronyssinus*) in 94.6% of the cases, house dust in 88.4%, dog fur in 80.6%, bird feathers in 78.3%, cat fur in 76.7%, kapok in 71.3%, *Aspergillus fumigatus* in 45%, and pollen in 39.5% (7). Training in pediatric allergy is given at the Department of Child Health, Dr.Cipto Mangunkusumo Hospital, Faculty of Medicine, University of Indonesia in Jakarta. Research in pediatric allergy concerns mainly clinical aspects.

Japan

The field of allergy has interested Japanese doctors for a long time. A survey of the population at large in the late 1950's revealed a prevalence of asthma of about 1–1.2%. In 1988 the prevalence was 3.14% (8). At the present time, the prevalence of asthma in children is about 4.4%, allergic rhinitis 4.2% and allergic dermatoses about 5.7%. The airborne pollen in Japan was investigated nationwide from 1975–1977. The pollen species that have been reported every year are cedar, cypress, pine, birch, beech, grass, ragweed, mugwort, and Japanese hops (9). Institutional therapy for children with severe asthma is available in Japan. There are 65 facilities in Japan, most of them belonging to national or municipal hospitals. The main objectives of this therapy are to teach the patients how to cope with attacks, and promote functional and mental recuperation through training therapy. Approximately 2,300 patients receive this type of treatment yearly, the majority being of elementary and junior high school age. The period of hospitalization is usually 1–2 years. The government supports these institutions and provides all medical services free of charge (10). Public education about asthma, including camps, is popular in Japan. Many training centers for pediatric allergy are available. Approximately 100 fellows are trained in pediatric allergy each year. Immunotherapy is well accepted.

South Korea

The field of pediatric allergy is well established in Korea, where there are about 150 pediatric allergists. Modern investigations as well as research, both basic and clinical, are carried out in many centers in Korea. A sur-

3. Viswanathan, R. 1964. Definition, incidence, etiology and natural history of asthma. Indian. J. Chest Dis. 6:109.
4. Kumar, L. 1981. Allergy in north India. Indian J. Pediat. 48:653.
5. Therwani, A.V., Desai, A.G., and Bhave, S.Y. 1985. An analysis of skin prick test reaction in asthmatic children in Bombay, Indian J. Chest & All. Sci. 27:219.
6. Singh, A.B. 1984. Aerobiological studies in India in relation to allergy. Indian J. Pediat. 51:345.
7. Mahdi, D.H., and Mahdi, H. 1988. Skin prick test in Indonesian bronchial asthma patients. Proceedings of the First West Pacific Allergy Symposium. Korea, p.102.
8. Nakagawa, T., and Miyamoto, T. 1988. Prevalence of asthma in Japanese population at large. Proceedings of the Second West Pacific Symposium on Clinical Allergy, p. 15.
9. Kishikawa, R., and Nagano, H. 1982. Airborne pollen in Japan. Arerugi. 31:1222.
10. Nishimuta, T. 1990. Special therapy in an institutional hospitals. Acta Paediatr. Japan. 32:201.
11. Lee, H.R., Hong, D.S., and Sohn, K.C. 1983. Survey on allergic diseases in children. J. Korean Med. Asso. 26:11.
12. Kang, S.Y., Chang, S.I., Min, K.U., and Kim, Y.Y. 1988. Japanese cedar pollinosis in Chedu Island. Proceedings of the First West Pacific Allergy Symposium, p. 67.
13. Azizi, H.O. 1990. Respiratory symptoms and asthma in primary school children in Kuala Lumpur. Acta Paediatr. Japan 32:183.
14. Ho, T.M., and Nadchatram, M. 1984. Distribution of house dust mites in a new settlement scheme in Jenka, Pahang, Malaysia. Tropical Biomedicine 1:49.
15. Noche, M.L., Villa-Real, M.J.R., and Co, B.G. 1990. Clinical profile of asthma among Philippino children. Philippine J. Pediat. 39:205.
16. Lim, F.C., Payawal, P.C., and Laserna, G. 1978. Studies on atmospheric pollens in the Philippines. Ann. Allergy 40:117.
17. Teo, Y., Quak, S.H., Low, P.S., and Wong, W.B. 1988. Childhood asthma in Singapore changing trend. Presented at 22nd Singapore-Malaysia Congress of Medicine.
18. Lee, B.W., Teo, J., and Vallayapphan, K. 1989. Role of atopy in childhood asthma. J. Singapore. Paed. Soc. 31:53.
19. Hsieh, K.H., and Shen, J.J. 1988. Prevalence of childhood asthma in Taipei, Taiwan and other Asian Pacific countries. J. Asthma 25:73.
20. Hsieh, K.H. 1984. A study of intracutaneous skin tests and radioallergosorbent tests on 1,000 asthmatic children in Taiwan. Asian Pacific J. Allerg. Immunol. 2:56.
21. Chang, Y.C., and Hsieh, K.H. 1989. The study of house dust mites in Taiwan. Ann. Allergy 62:101.
22. Boonyarittipong, P., Tuchinda, M., and Vanaprapa, N. 1990. Prevalence of allergic diseases in children in Bangkok. J. Pediat. Soc. Thailand 29:24.
23. Tuchinda, M., Habanananda, S., Vareenil, J., Srimaruta, N., and Piromrat, K. 1987. Asthma in Thai children: A study of 2,000 cases. Ann. Allergy 59:207.
24. Tuchinda, M., Theptaramond, Y., and Limsathayourat, N. 1983. A ten-year surveillance of atmospheric pollens and molds in Bangkok area. Asian Pacific J. Allerg. Immunol. 1:7.

Clinical Pharmacology of Drugs Used to Treat Asthma

Elliot F. Ellis*

New insights into the pathogenesis of asthma based upon bronchoalveolar lavage and biopsy studies have focused on the role of inflammation as a major contributor to the obstructive airway disease process. Drugs for treatment of asthma are being looked upon in terms of whether they function principally as bronchodilators, anti-inflammatory agents or perhaps both (Table 1).

Beta-Adrenergic Agents

This class of drugs has its origins in the earliest days of asthma therapeutics dating back centuries. In terms of mechanism of action, beta adrenergic drugs induce bronchial smooth muscle relaxation, an effect mediated by changes in intracellular 3',5' cyclic AMP concentration. Inhibition of antigen induced mediator release from mast by beta agonist cells has been shown in *in vitro* systems. Recently, a new long acting beta adrenergic agent, salmeterol, has been shown to inhibit both early and late inflammatory responses. These latter two actions suggest that, although bronchodilation is the major therapeutic effect of the beta adrenergic agents, they possess some anti-inflammatory properties as well. Clinically, adrenergic drugs, preferably administered by the aerosol route, are the first choice for relief of acute bronchoconstriction. Unfortunately, their duration of action is short, not much more than 4 hours. The development of new compounds with duration of action of up to 12 hours should remedy this shortcoming. There are, however, some problems associated with the use of adrenergic drugs. Development of tolerance is a long recognized phenomenon in adrenergic pharmacology. There are approximately 40 publications on this phenomenon, 2/3 of which confirm its existence and 1/3 do not. Tolerance (also subsensitivity or down regulation) expresses itself as (a) a diminished bronchodilator response to adrenergic drug administration as a result of chronic use and (b) perhaps more significant, a shortened duration of action. Administration of beta adrenergic agents is associated with an increase of airway hyperresponsiveness to methacholine and histamine which fortunately appears to be of an evanescent nature. Most worrisome are recent reports linking regular use of beta adrenergic drugs with poorer control of asthma compared to prn use and increasing asthma mortality associated with overuse.

Drugs for Treatment of Asthma

Bronchodilator	Anti-inflammatory	Both
Adrenergics	Cromolyn	? Theophyline
Theophylline	Nedocromil	
Ipatroprium	Corticosteroids	

Theophylline

Despite much research, the mechanism of action of the xanthines, principally theophylline, in asthma is still not fully understood. Theophylline functions as a non-specific airway smooth muscle relaxant. As a group the methylxanthines have long been known to inhibit cyclic nucleotide phosphodiesterases which are the only enzymes known to inactivate both cyclic AMP and cyclic GMP. The initial hypothesis that theophylline acted in concert with adrenergic agents to increase intracellular cyclic AMP concentration was very attractive but doubt was cast upon the role of theophylline in this regard for two reasons. First, concentrations of theophylline that are required to inhibit phosphodiesterase activity were far in excess of that achievable *in vivo* and secondly, other phosphodiesterase inhibitors such as papavarine had little effect on asthma. However, recently it has been shown that phosphodiesterase found in human bronchioles is

* Nemours Children's Clinic, P.O. Box 5720, Jacksonville, FL 32247, USA.

actually composed of four different forms or isozymes with different sensitivities to pharmacologic inhibitors. Animal experiments have shown that *in vitro* bronchodilator effects of both xanthines and non-xanthine phosphodiesterase inhibitors correlate with the inhibition of a particular isozyme of cyclic AMP phosphodiesterase. Experiments with canine tracheal muscle strips have shown a strong correlation between mechanical relaxation and pharmacologic inhibition of two forms of phosphodiesterase, one with more specificity for cyclic AMP and the other with more specificity for cyclic GMP. The concentrations of theophylline that inhibited these isozymes by 50% were within the therapeutic range of the drug in humans. Previous studies have discounted the previously postulated role of catecholamine release as the mediator of the bronchodilator effect of theophylline. Adenosine antagonism also has been proposed as a mechanism of theophylline's bronchodilator effect. However, since both enprofylline (a theophylline derivative) and theophylline exert similar bronchodilator effects, despite enprofylline's lack of activity as an adenosine antagonist, adenosine antagonism is unlikely as an important factor in theophylline's anti-asthma effect. Theophylline's popularity as an asthma therapeutic agent has waxed and waned in the approximately 50 years since it was introduced into clinical medicine. The drug clearly has beneficial effects in asthma including the following: (a) increase in the number of asymptomatic days, (b) decrease in prn use of inhaled $beta_2$ agonists and corticosteroids for acute symptoms, (c) improvement in exercise tolerance in a serum concentration dependent manner, (d) suppression of nocturnal symptoms and (e) steroid sparing effect in steroid dependent subjects. There are a number of current controversies in regard to the drug. First of all, its use in acute asthma has been questioned. For years, in hospital emergency departments it has been customary (in addition to administering beta adrenergic agents) to start an infusion of aminophylline. Recently a number of studies has shown that if the patient has an optimal response to repeated administration of inhaled beta agonists, the addition of theophylline adds nothing but adverse effects. However, if the patient does not receive an optimal response to $beta_2$ agonists and needs to be hospitalized, available data indicate that theophylline is useful in terms of shortening the duration of illness. While conventionally thought of as a bronchodilator, there is published evidence for and against theophylline's anti-inflammatory properties. The medical literature is very contradictory on this point but publications supporting at least a modest anti-inflammatory effect outnumber those discounting an anti-inflammatory effect by a ratio of 2:1. That theophylline has an effect on behavior is of no surprise since it is closely related to caffeine, a drug with very substantial behavioral effects. The original reports that theophylline had an adverse effect on learning have not been confirmed by more recent and better controlled studies.

Anticholinergic Agents

The anticholinergic bronchodilators are antagonists of the muscarinic effects of acetylcholine. The prototype is atropine which is highly specific for muscarinic receptors. While this class of compounds has been used since the 17th century for relief of airway obstruction, it has only been within the past several decades that interest in the use of anticholinergic bronchodilators has been renewed, largely as a result of the development of synthetic congeners of atropine that are relatively free of many of atropine's adverse effects. Atropine and its congeners cause bronchodilatation both in normal subjects and in subjects with airway obstruction. As compared to the adrenergic agents, the onset of bronchodilator action occurs somewhat slower than with the adrenergic agents and peak effect is delayed by up to two hours. Peak effect occurs between 30 minutes and two hours. The effect is, however, more sustained than with the adrenergic drugs. In the United States, the congener of atropine that is used clinically, ipratropium bromide, has a variable bronchodilator effect in patients with chronic asthma. Some asthmatics will have a favorable response to the addition of inhaled ipratropium while others will respond little, if at all. On the other hand, in acute asthma, there is evidence that the addition of anticholinergic therapy to conventional adrenergic therapy produces a significant amount of further improvement in FEV_1. Where anticholinergic agents fit into the day-to-day management of patients with asthma who are being treated with other drugs is still an unresolved question.

Cromolyn

The mechanism of action of cromolyn has been extensively studied since the drug was introduced. Its effect generally has been described as "stabilization of mast cell membranes". Numerous experiments have shown that cromolyn blocks mast cell activation in several different *in vitro* systems. This effect appears to be mediated by cromolyn's action in binding to specific mast cells surface proteins and thus regulating calcium flux. Recently, cromolyn has been shown to inhibit the activation of a variety of human inflammatory cells including neutrophils, eosinophils, and monocytes. The drug also appears to have a direct dampening effect on non-myelinated irritant nerve receptors. Many clinical studies with cromolyn have shown that it reduces signs and symptoms of chronic asthma. The drug seems to be more useful in mild asthma than in patients with severe, intractable disease. While originally thought to be most efficacious in patients with allergen induced asthma, cromolyn clearly has an ameliorating effect on non-allergic asthma as well. Administration of cromolyn immediately prior to an antigen challenge prevents acute bronchoconstriction and also inhibits the development of the late phase response. Not only does cromolyn block allergen induced bronchoconstriction, it also prevents airway obstruction in asthmatics in response to sulphur dioxide, cold air and exercise. Cromolyn, however, is less effective in blocking exercise induced bronchoconstriction than the beta agonists. Perhaps cromolyn's most outstanding property is the fact that it is, for all practical purposes, devoid of any significant adverse effects. Nedocromil, a pyranoquinolone dicarboxylate acid, is chemically unrelated to cromolyn. Nedocromil is very similar to cromolyn in terms of its action on mast cells and inhibition of the activity of inflammatory cells. In the human, nedocromil has been shown to inhibit allergen induced bronchoconstriction and to prevent the late phase response to allergen challenge. Whether or not nedocromil is superior to cromolyn as a therapeutic agent in asthma remains to be proven.

Corticosteroids

Corticosteroids, long known to be the most effective agents for treatment of asthma, are receiving increasing attention as a result of the recognition of the role of inflammation in chronic asthma. Corticosteroids have multiple mechanisms of action in asthma. The more important ones include interference with inflammatory cell traffic, impairment of mediator synthesis and release, enhancement of beta adrenergic receptor activity and decrease in microvascular permeability. In regard to asthma management, the early use of systemic corticosteroids during an exacerbation of asthma has clearly been shown in both children and adults to decrease the morbidity of the attack, to reduce emergency department visits and hospitalization, to prevent relapse and shorten the duration of the symptomatic illness. The availability of a new generation of surface active inhaled agents that can be given in microgram doses has favorably influenced treatment of patients with moderate to severe asthma. Unfortunately, many of the physicians in the United States suffer from steroidophobia and the inhaled corticosteroids presently only have a 7% share of the asthma medication market. While greatly reducing the risk of adverse effects associated with use of systemic steroids, as with the latter, the adverse effect of inhaled agents are also dose related. Doses above 1000 µg/day (and even less in some studies) have been shown to be associated with hypothalamic-pituitary-adrenal axis suppression. In addition, dose dependent depression of linear growth in children has been reported recently as has dose dependent purpura and dermal thinning in adults, and cataracts both in children and adults. Several new inhaled corticosteroids with even greater topical potency and less systemic bioavailability than the presently available agents are under development.

Anti-Allergic Drugs in Pediatric Allergy

Keun Chan Sohn*

A large number of studies have documented the efficacy of anti-allergic drugs, and their effectiveness would be predicted on the basis of their ability to inhibit release of mediators. The basic concept of prophylactic therapy, its indication, and recent trends in anti-allergic drugs are discussed. The present chapter describes the current status of anti-allergic drugs, especially in the viewpoint of pediatric practice.

The concept of anti-allergic drugs was introduced in 1967 when Roger Altounyan described the drug Intal (disodium cromoglycate, DSCG) and its experimental use in the treatment of asthma (1). Originally, it was hypothesized that DSCG inhibited mast cell activation; however, the exact mode of action of this drug continues to elude investigators (2). DSCG has been effective in controlling the acute and latent reactions in asthma; however, the site of action is still unknown. Despite our lack of knowledge on the exact mechanisms by which DSCG works, its use in many countries has gained wide acceptance as investigators acknowledge its effectiveness in children and adults alike. The success of DSCG in the therapy of asthma and other allergic disease has produced an extensive search for other anti-allergic drugs.

Basic Concept of Prophylactic Anti-Allergic Drugs

In 1962 the American Thoracic Society defined asthma as "a disease characterized by an increased responsiveness of the trachea and bronchi to various stimuli and manifested by a widespread narrowing of the airways, that changes in severity, either spontaneously or as a result of therapy." Asthma or reversible obstructive airway disease was then defined by physiologic changes in flow rates and this formed the basis of treatment for the next two decades. Bronchoconstriction was managed pharmacologically by drugs that decreased smooth muscle contraction and release of mediators from mast cells, or basophils. This emphasis seemed to lead to improved treatment of asthmatic patients, but increasing rates of both hospitalization and mortality strongly suggested that a reevaluation was critical (3). Current concepts of the IgE-mediated reaction contain the classical early phase characterized by mediator release from mast cells and subsequent smooth muscle contraction and increased vascular permeability. The late phase, initiating only after several hours and often lasting days, is characterized by the presence of both mediators and cellular infiltrates, which lead to significant inflammation (4,5). This late phase is associated with bronchial hyperresponsiveness, as assessed by either histamine or metacholline challenge. As a result of this information, clinicians now understand asthma as an inflammatory disease. These opinions have encouraged investigators to discover new drugs to control asthmatic symptoms.

Anti-Allergic Drugs

The current concept of asthma suggests that appropriate drug treatment should be directed not only toward improving airway caliber, but also toward preventing the release or the direct tissue effects of inflammatory mediators. The beta-adrenergic agents, theophylline and corticosteroids, are the drugs generally accepted for the relief of acute attacks. If the attacks occur less than once a month, medication can be administered only when needed. However, some patients require prophylactic treatment including: (a) those with frequent attacks (more than

* Department of Pediatrics, National Medical Center, Seoul, Korea.

once per month), (b) those whose asthma is less frequent but severe enough to require emergency room care or hospital admission, and (c) those whose asthmatic attacks interfere with daily activities such as sleep, school and play (6).

DSCG, the first compound to be described as a prophylactic agent for use in allergic asthma has been shown to inhibit both early (immediate) and late asthmatic reactions following antigen bronchial challenge. This would suggest a reduction in non-specific bronchial hyperreactivity with the use of DSCG. After numerous studies, this agent has been proved to have significant potential as a prophylactic agent for chronic asthmatic patients with bronchial hyperreactivity (7,8).

Prophylactic treatment is a useful treatment mode for patients assigned to any of the categories. Long-term use of prophylactic drugs has resulted in the conversion of severe asthmatics to the moderate category and moderate asthmatics to the mild category (7).

DSCG has been the subject of extensive investigation (9). It has emerged from these trials in a favorable position as a first choice for treatment of asthma and allergic rhinitis. It also appears to have an important role in treatment of both allergic seasonal and vernal keratoconjunctivitis. While there has been considerable interest in its use for treatment of food allergy, DSCG can be of benefit in atopic dermatitis related to food allergy (10). Recently topically applied DSCG solution on atopic dermatitis in young children has also been investigated with good results (11). Certain problems do arise with DSCG therapy, however, that limit its widespread use as the drug of choice for chronic asthma. Occasionally, patients have complained of throat irritation, coughing, and wheezing, which probably is related to the inhalation of the powder rather than the active medication. Also, compliance in children is not quite adequate with this type of inhalation. Thus, new oral anti-allergic drugs were developed based on their ability to inhibit release of mediators. For asthmatic patients who have other concomitant allergic diseases, such as allergic rhinitis and atopic dermatitis, oral drugs may be much more convenient and reasonable therapeutic agents. Prophylactic anti-allergic agents can be divided into two groups based on their anti-histaminic action, namely agents with and without anti-histaminic action. The latter includes DSCG, tranilast, amlexanox and repirinast; the former includes Ketotifen, azelastine and oxatomides.

The ability of Ketotifen to restore beta-adrenergic responsiveness, which leads to reduced bronchial hyperresponsiveness, and its inhibitory effect on platelet-activating factor, stand out as the most promising anti-allergic properties of the drug. The metabolism of Ketotifen in children is faster than in adults and children need full adult doses (12).

The Use of Anti-Allergic Drugs

An anti-allergic drug is used as a rule for the prophylactic treatment during non-attack, but it is usually administered with symptomatic drugs when the attack has slightly improved. Adequate control of bronchospasm with bronchodilators should be achieved before initiating anti-allergic drug (6). It is possible to combine DSCG with other oral anti-allergic drugs, and then multiple effects of both drugs can be expected in some cases. Anti-allergic drugs can be changed for another drug if there is no effect. But the latency to demonstrable effectiveness of a drug can occasionally involve long-term therapy. For the judgement of effectiveness of an anti-allergic drug, perennial asthmatic children should take drugs for 2–3 months, and the course of the illness has to stand under constant surveillance. There is no adequate index for the evaluation of most effective drugs for an individual case. There are also no indications of anti-allergic drugs in accordance with the severity of the disease. For seasonal cases the drug should be given for several months, from 2–4 weeks before season and till the end of it. Clinically if asthmatic symptoms are not observed for 2 years, then the patient is said to be cured of the disease (remission), but we consider it necessary to observe the course of disease for another 6 months to 2 years after clear improvement in attacks. However, asthma is a disease which progressively improves and can be become milder throughout the course of illness (13). The benefit derived from anti-allergic drug therapy can be maximized if the patient/parents understand the principles behind this type of therapy.

Recent Trends of Prophylactic Anti-Allergic Drugs

Several prophylactic anti-allergic drugs share common pharmacologic properties, including progressive improvement with a slow onset, similar to the effect of allergen avoidence in children. Recent studies which have biopsied the airways of patients with asthma show persistent airway inflammation, even in individuals with mild disease. Since the degree of bronchial hyperresponsiveness may equate with the severity of the disease and the possibility of death, the use of anti-inflammatory therapy to reduce bronchial injury has immediate appeal. Anti-allergic drugs, such as cromolyn and Ketotifen, etc., are current choices of anti-inflammatory therapy (14). Children with atopic constitution experience one or several atopic diseases early on. Usually gastrointestinal and/or dermal disorders appear first and are later followed by respiratory problems. Such a pattern of problems has been designated as "Allergic March". Baba suggested that the anti-allergic drug is somewhat capable of suppressing the progress of an Allergic March (15). In most countries the number of allergic patients is increasing, including those with bronchial asthma. But, in some countries, asthma deaths have not shown an increasing trend in recent years (16,17). However, it is not so easy to ascribe the reason for this lack of increased mortality rates to the rapid growth in the use of prophylactic anti-allergic medication. Nevertheless, there has been a reduction in asthma attacks since the introduction of prophylactic anti-allergic drugs; this leads to less dependence on bronchodilators and steroids, and it seems reasonable to state that asthmatic patients are comparatively milder in severity than before (8).

Conclusion

Judging from the present status of anti-allergic drugs, it is clear that prophylactic therapy has been well accepted by clinicians and patients, but there are no remarkable improvements yet for the treatment of allergic diseases at the present time. Lately, mechanisms of production and release of chemical mediators in allergic reaction and of inflammatory lesion in target organs have been demonstrated progressively. With this background of immunopharmacological studies, fundamental studies of new anti-allergic drugs have continued. We are expecting the development of new anti-allergic drugs in the near future.

References

1. Altounyan, R.E.C. 1967. Inhibitor of experimental asthma by a new compound, disodium cromoglycate "Intal". Acta Allergologica. 22:487.
2. Altounyan, R.E.C. 1989. Review of clinical activity and mode of action of sodium cromoglycate. Clin. Allergy. 10:481.
3. Jackson, R.T., and Mitchell, E.A. 1983. Trends in hospital admission and drug treatment in New Zealand. N. Z. Med. J. 96:728.
4. Durham,S.R., Lee, T.H., Cromwell, O., Shaw, R.J., Merrett, T.G., Cooper, P., and Kay, A.B. 1984. Immunologic studies in allergen-induced late-phase asthmatic reactions. J. Allergy Clin. Immunol. 74:49.
5. Durham, S.R., Carroll, M., Walsh, G.M., and Kay, A.B. 1984. Leukocyte activation in allergen-induced late phase asthmatic reactions. N. Engl. J. Med. 311:1398.
6. Noche, M.L., Jr. 1990. Prophylaxis in childhood Asthma. Acta Paediat. Jpn. 32:176.
7. MacDonald, G.F. 1990. Chemoprohylaxis in Asthma. J. Asthma. 27:269.
8. Kurosawa, M. 1990. Prophylactic antiasthma drugs in Japan. J. Asthma. 27:299.
9. Shapiro, G.G. and Konig, P. 1985. Cromolyn Sodium: Review. Pharmacology. 5:156.
10. Cavagni, G., and Caffarelli, C. 1989. Sodium Cromoglycate in childhood atopic dermatitis treatment. Allergy. 44 (Suppl 9):124.
11. Kimata, H., and Igarashi, M. 1990. Topical cromolyn (disodium cromoglycate) solution in the treatment of young children with atopic dermatitis. Clin. Experim. Allergy. 20:281.
12. Naspitz,C.K., and Tinkelman, D.G. 1987. Therapeutic approaches to the treatment of chronic asthma. Childhood asthma, pathophysiology & treatment. New York: Dekker, p. 249.

13. Iwasaki, E. 1991. The current status of anti-allergic anaphylactic drugs. J. Pediat. Practice. 54:1115 (in Japanese).
14. Busse, W.W. 1990. Treatment of asthma. A comprehensive approach. J. Asthma. 27:265.
15. Baba, M. 1990. Prevention of allergic disease. Jap. J. Pediatr. 43:768.
16. Sheffer, A.L., Buist, A.S., and Nicklas, A.R. (Eds). 1987. Proceedings of the Asthma Mortality Task Force. J. Allergy Clin. Immunol. 80:361.
17. Mitsui, S. 1986. Death from bronchial asthma in Japan. Sino-Jpn. A. Allergol. Immunol. 3:249.

Aspects of Allergy Prediction and the Importance of Diets and Pollution

Karin Fälth-Magnusson, N.-I. Max Kjellman*

Reliable methods for allergy prediction are prerequisites for an adequate allergy prevention program. So far, the most widely used methods are evaluation of family history and/or assessment of cord blood IgE levels. Although none of these methods are perfect, they are still the best choices. The predictive capacity of CB-IgE for longstanding, serious allergic disease is good. Intervention in the maternal diet during pregnancy and/or lactation has been used in several large-scale allergy prevention studies. In summary, elimination of highly allergenic foods from the maternal diet seems to give a temporary reduction in the incidence of atopic dermatitis in the child, but the development of rhinitis and asthma is not substantially reduced. The beneficial effect seems to be confined to elimination diet during the lactation period, and must be weighted against the inconvenience, costs and possible adverse effects noted with elimination diet to the mother. Polluting agents, such as tobacco smoke, act as adjuvants and enhance the effects of true allergens. This interaction is particularly evident in the genetically susceptible individual.

The possibility to predict the risk for development of allergic disease in a child is of great concern for both the parents and the doctor. Reliable methods for prediction are prerequisites for intervention aiming at prevention of allergic diseases. Environmental factors, like feeding regimens and air pollution, interact with the genetic propensity inherited in each individual. Since the genetics of mankind presumably do not change dramatically in the short run, we must suspect that the increasing incidence of allergic diseases today is caused by environmental changes.

Predictive Aspects

The two most widely used parameters for allergy prediction are the evaluation of the family history (FH) and the assessment of cord blood IgE (CB-IgE).

Family History

The impact of a positive FH was studied in 1,325 Swedish school children (1). A biparental history of atopic disease was found in 3% and a single FH of atopic disease in 22%. The risk for development of allergic disease in the child was 72% if the parents had identical atopic disease. Also without a FH for allergic disease, the risk for the child was 10%.

Cord Blood IgE

In a cohort study of 1,701 consecutively born, non-selected infants the predictive capacity of CB-IgE was evaluated at 18 months (2), 7 years (3) and 11 years (4). In summary, the capacity of CB-IgE to predict allergy was better for individuals who had more serious, multiple and longstanding allergic diseases. Children with a high CB-IgE had a five-fold increased risk to develop asthma. The specificity of a CB-IgE to predict allergic disease up to 11 years was 94%, but the sensitivity only 26%, which makes it unsuitable as a general screening method (4). It may still be of value in selected cases, however, e.g. as an adjunct in evaluating the effect of preventive measures in high risk individuals (4).

Other methods for allergy prediction like measuring IgE-binding factors in CB (5), determination of lymphocyte subsets in CB (6), measuring of eosinophilic counts in CB or metachromatic cells in nasal scrapings (7) have

* Department of Pediatrics, Faculty of Health Sciences, University of Linköping, Linköping, Sweden.
Acknowledgments: This study was supported financially by the Tore Nilson Fund for Medical Research and the Medical Research Fund of the County of Östergötland.

not been assessed in a large scale, and have so far not proved to offer any advantage compared to FH and CB-IgE.

The Importance of Diets

There are several large-scale studies that monitor the effect of intervention in the maternal diet during pregnancy (8–11), during pregnancy and lactation (12–17) or during lactation only (18,19).

Diet During Pregnancy and Lactation

In the complex allergy-prevention program performed by Zeiger et al. (12,15) maternal elimination diet during the last trimester and during breast-feeding was one part, beside reduction of exposure to environmental allergens and tobacco smoke. The dieting mothers totally avoided cow's milk and dairy products, egg and soy, and limited their intake of wheat. The babies were given solid foods after 6 months, and cow's milk after 12 months. The diet babies showed a transient reduction of cutaneous and gastro-intestinal symptoms, compared to the control children, but the prevalence of asthma or rhinitis at 24 months was not affected. The authors also point out some possible disadvantages with maternal diet manipulation: reduced maternal weight gain during pregnancy and a small decrease in infant birth weight in the diet group. In the prevention programs performed by Chandra et al. (13,16) and Businco (14,17) maternal elimination diets during both pregnancy and lactation in allergy risk families were reported to decrease the risk of allergy in the child.

Diet During Pregnancy

The two Swedish studies dealing with maternal diet during pregnancy were both prospective and randomized; they enrolled families at risk for allergy, but set out from different immunological starting-points. In the Stockholm-Uppsala study, enrolling 171 pregnant women, one group of mothers was taking increased amounts of cow's milk and egg. The study design was chosen to evaluate in man the hypothesis that antigen exposure of the offspring *in utero* can induce tolerance (20,21), with the hope that increased exposure would diminish the risk of allergy in the child.

The Linköping study (8,9), enrolling 210 pregnant women, was an allergen-avoidance study. In the diet group, mothers totally abstained from cow's milk and egg during the last trimester. Their food intake was monitored by a dietician, and they took extra calcium and a casein hydrolysate as a supplement. Diet compliance was monitored by mother's reports and by analysis of IgG antibodies to cow's milk and egg. The mothers in the non-diet group took normal food throughout pregnancy. The theoretical starting-point for this study was the observation that human fetal cells have been shown to possess the capacity for IgE production from the 11th gestational week (22), and the rare reports about intra-uterine sensitization, manifested as specific IgE-antibodies already in CB sera (reviewed in 12). In a cooperative report summarizing the two studies (11), the effect of four different maternal regimens, ranging from no intake to increased intake of cow's milk and egg, was evaluated. No significant differences in the CB-IgE were noted in spite of the differences in the maternal diet. No specific IgE antibodies to ovalbumin, ovomucoid or betalactoglobulin were found in any of the CB sera. In the Linköping study, the development of allergic disease in the babies was evaluated when the children were 6 weeks, 3 months, 6 months and 12 months old. A blind examination by one pediatric allergist was performed when the children were 18 months. The prevalence of allergic disease in the groups (diet and non-diet) was similar at that age, and the predominant symptoms were atopic dermatitis and food allergy. A further follow-up when the children were five years (Fälth-Magnusson & Kjellman, submitted) showed that the number of children with rhinitis and asthma had increased, but there were still no significant differences between the groups apart from one observation. Six children were still partially or totally egg intolerant at five years. Their mothers had all been on elimination diet during pregnancy and, due to maternal choice, they had also reduced their intake of cow's milk and egg during early lactation. This observation points to another possible hazard of an elimination diet, namely interference with the normal process of tolerance induction.

Diet During Lactation

The possibility of allergy prevention by maternal elimination during the first three months of lactation was evaluated in 115 high allergy risk infants in two adjacent Swedish communities (18,19). The diet mothers took no cow's milk, egg or fish and their food intake was guided by a dietician. The control group had unrestricted food intake. If breast feeding was unsufficient the babies were fed with a casein hydrolysate. The diet babies had significantly less atopic eczema up to and at 6 months of age, but not at 18 months. The prevalence of rhinitis and asthma was not affected by the maternal dietary regimen at the four-year follow-up, but significantly less eczema was again observed in the diet group (19).

Pollution

Polluting agents such as tobacco smoke and industrial air discharges do not act as antigens but as adjuvants enhancing the effects of allergens on the genetic keyboard (23). In a questionnaire study of 4,990 Swedish children the effects of environmental factors were studied (24). Children living near a paper pulp plant had significantly more often symptoms of bronchial hyperreactivity and allergic asthma, than children living in an unpolluted, rural district. In another recent study (25), reporting both results from questionnaires and skin prick testing, urban living was shown to be a risk factor for atopic sensitization in children. Tobacco smoke is the most important indoor pollutant. Children with smoking mothers have an earlier onset of allergic symptoms, and a higher incidence of wheezy bronchitis (26). In a study using the information from the health reports of 4,331 children it was again confirmed that maternal smoking was associated with higher rates of asthma, increased likelihood of use of asthma medication and an earlier onset of asthma in the children (27). In an animal model it was shown that smoking rats had higher IgE levels and were more easily sensitized to inhaled allergens than the non-smoking control rats (28). This may be one part of the explanation of how tobacco smoke acts as an adjuvant for the development of asthma, although the exact mechanism is not yet known.

References

1. Kjellman, N.-I.M. 1977. Atopic disease in seven-year-old children. Incidence in relation to family history. Acta Paediatr. Scand. 66:465.
2. Croner, S., Kjellman N.-I.M., and Roth, A. 1982. IgE screening in 1701 newborn infants and the development of atopic disease during infancy. Arch. Dis. Childh. 57:364.
3. Kjellman, N.-I.M., and Croner, S. 1984. Cord blood IgE determination for allergy prediction - a follow-up to seven years of age in 1651 children. Ann. Allergy 53:167.
4. Croner, S., and Kjellman, N.-I.M. 1990. Development of atopic disease in relation to family history and cord blood IgE levels. Eleven year follow-up in 1654 children. Pediatr. Allergy Immunol. 1:14.
5. Kim, K.-M., Inoue, Y., et al. 1990. Prediction of the development of atopic symptoms in early childhood by cord IgE-binding factors (soluble FcR2). Immunol. Lett. 24:63.
6. Lilja, G., and Öman, H. 1991. Prediction of atopic disease in infancy by determination of immunological parameters: IgE, IgE- and IgG-antibodies to food allergens, skin prick tests and T lymphocyte subsets. Pediatr. Allergy Immunol. 2:6.
7. Borres, M., Irander, K., and Björkstén, B. Nasal metachromatic cells in infants in relation to allergic disease and family history of atopic disease. Pediatr. Allergy Immunol., in press.
8. Fälth-Magnusson, K., Öman, H., and Kjellman, N.-I.M. 1987. Maternal abstention from cow's milk and egg in allergy risk pregnancies; effect on antibody production in the mother and the newborn. Allergy 42:64.
9. Fälth-Magnusson, K., and Kjellman, N.-I.M. 1987. Development of atopic disease in babies whose mothers were receiving exclusion diet during pregnancy - a randomized study. J. Allergy Clin. Immunol. 80:868.
10. Lilja, G., Dannaeus, A., Fälth-Magnusson, K., et al. 1988. Immune response of the atopic woman and foetus: Effects of high- and low-dose food allergen intake during late pregnancy. Clin. Allergy 18:131.
11. Lilja, G., Dannaeus, A., Foucard, T., et al. 1989. Effects of maternal diets during late pregnancy and lactation on the development of atopic diseases in infants up to 18 months of age – *in vivo* results. Clin. Exp. Allergy 19:473.
12. Zeiger, R.S., Heller, S., Mellon, M. H., et al. 1986. Effectiveness of dietary manipulation in

the prevention of food allergy in infants. J. Allergy Clin. Immunol. 78:224.
13. Chandra, R.K., Puri, S., Suraiya, C., et al. 1986. Influence of maternal food antigen avoidance during pregnancy and lactation on incidence of atopic eczema in infants. Clin. Allergy 16:563.
14. Businco, L., Cantani, A., Meglio, P., et al. 1987. Prevention af atopy: Results of a long-term (7 months to 8 years) follow-up. Ann. Allergy 59 (part II):183.
15. Zeiger, R.S., Heller, S., Mellon, M.H., et al.1989. Effect of combined maternal and infant food-allergen avoidance on development of atopy in early infancy: A randomized study. J. Allergy Clin. Immunol. 84:72.
16. Chandra, R.K, Puri, S., and Hamed, A. 1989. Influence of maternal diet during lactation and use of formula feeds on development of atopic eczema in high risk infants. Br. Med. J. 299:228.
17. Businco, L., and Cantani, A. 1990. Prevention of childhood allergy by dietary manipulation. Clin. Exp. Allergy 20(suppl III):9.
18. Hattevig, G., Kjellman, B., Sigurs, N., et al. 1989. Effect of maternal avoidance of eggs, cow's milk and fish during lactation upon allergic manifestations in infants. Clin. Exp. Allergy 19:27.
19. Sigurs, N., Hattevig, G., and Kjellman, B. 1991. The effect of maternal avoidance of eggs, cow's milk and fish during lactation upon allergic manifestations, skin prick tests and specific IgE antibodies in children at age four. Pediatrics, accepted.
20. Jarrett, E.E., and Hall, E. 1984. The development of IgE-suppressive immunocompetence in young animals: Influence of exposure to antigen in the presence or absence of maternal immunity. Immunology 53:365.
21. Telemo, E., Jakobsson, I., Weström, B.R., et al. 1987. Maternal dietary antigens and the immune response in the offspring of the guineapig. Immunology 62:35.
22. Miller D.L., Hirvonen, T., and Gitlin, D. 1973. Synthesis of IgE by the human conceptus. J. Allergy Clin. Immunol. 52:182.
23. Riedel, F. 1991. Influence of adjuvant factors on development of allergy. Evidence from animal experiments. Pediatr. Allergy Immunol. 2:1.
24. Andrae, S., Axelson, O., Björkstén, B., et al. 1988. Symptoms of bronchial hyperreactivity and asthma in relation to environmental factors. Arch. Dis. Childh. 63:473.
25. Bråbäck, L., and Kälvesten, L. 1991. Urban living as a risk factor for atopic sensitization in Swedish schoolchildren. Pediatr. Allergy Immunol. 2:14.
26. Rantakallio, P. 1978. Relationship of maternal smoking to morbidity and mortality of the child up to the age of five. Acta Paediatr. Scand. 67:621.
27. Weitzman, M., Gortmaker, S., Klein Walker, D., et al. 1990. Maternal smoking and childhood asthma. Pediatrics 85:505.
28. Zetterström, O., Nordvall, S.L., Björkstén, B., et al. 1985. Increased IgE antibody responses in rats exposed to tobacco smoke. J. Allergy Clin. Immunol. 75:594.

How to Prevent Death from Asthma in Children

John A. Anderson*

Deaths from asthma in children account for about 2–3% of all asthma deaths yearly in the USA. Clues to prevention come from studies of the circumstances leading to death. Delay in seeking medical attention may be an important factor. Sudden onset of asthma, leading to death in the home or shortly after reaching medical attention, seems to be an important factor. The profile of the child at risk for dying from asthma is: (a) the severe asthmatic; (b) an adolescent; (c) male; (d) of a minority race; (e) a history of hypoxic seizure; (f) a rapidly changing corticosteroid requirement; (g) a psycho-social problem; (h) a history of noncompliance. Changes in asthma management have affected the risk of asthma deaths in US hospitals where death from asthma is uncommon in children (since 1970). Background factors such as allergy, low birth weight, broncho-pulmonary dysplasia, prior bronchiolitis or chlamydia infection, and negative socio-economic factors affect the likelihood of asthma control and possibly death. The short term strategy to prevent death from asthma involves national education programs. Emphasis is being made on the: (a) use of home peak expiratory flow units; (b) use of crisis plans for asthmatics; (c) early use of corticosteroid bursts; (d) early use of inhaled anti-inflammatory agents; (e) increased reliance upon protocol management; and (f) increased attention to background factors. Longterm strategies include development of newer, safer and simpler medication as well as more studies about the influence of background factors and basic mechanisms of asthma so this disease can be controlled and deaths from asthma can be prevented.

Although death from asthma was recognized as early as the second century B. C. by Aretaeus of Cappadocia and Moses Maimonides (1136–1204 A. D.), many later prominent physicians did not consider the disease, asthma, as a sole cause of death (1). Laennec (1786–1826) believed that asthma "conferred a prospect for a long life". In the later 1800's, Oliver Wendell Holmes called asthma "a slight ailment that promotes longevity" and A. Trousseau stated that asthma is "not fatal". Finally, Sir William Osler is quoted as saying that asthmatics "don't die, they just pant into old age" (2). For many years, we have known that these old myths about asthma are not true. Asthma is now, and always has been, a life-threatening disease, both for children as well as adults! This is in spite of modern therapeutic techniques and therapeutics. Dr. Frank Speizer best summarized it as follows: "One cannot deny that more modern therapies are more effective in improving the lot of patients with asthma: however, the warning must be repeated that *not* all people with asthma wheeze into old age" (2).

Total asthma deaths in the USA have ranged from 2,598 (1979) to 4,080 (1988) (3,4). Deaths from asthma in the USA, in children younger than 15 years of age, represent 2–3% of this total (3). This amounts to 0.2 (whites under 1 year of age) to 0.7 (blacks 5–14 years of age) per 100,000 population (1982) (5). Clues to asthma death prevention in children can be found in the analysis of the death of an asthmatic child or a group of deaths. The analysis in this paper will be divided into four general categories: (a) a study of the circumstances of the immediate events on the day of asthma death; (b) a profile of the child most likely to be at risk of dying from asthma; (c) a critical review of current asthma management trends; and (d) a study of the background of inherited conditions, environmental exposures, and socio-economic factors which may influence the outcome of asthma control measures.

Circumstances of the Immediate Events on the Day of Asthma Death

The outcome of the two New Zealand mortality studies evaluating asthma deaths in that country in 1981–1983, uncovered the following

* Division of Allergy and Clinical Immunology, Department of Medicine, Henry Ford Hospital, Detroit, Michigan, USA.

factors which were felt to directly contribute to the ultimate demise of the asthmatic (6).

1. Delay in seeking medical assistance at the time of the acute asthma attack which led to the death of the patient (38% of cases).
2. Lack of appreciation before it was too late, either by the patient or by the parent/caretaker, of the severity of the specific asthma attack which led to death.
3. Lack of appreciation of the severity of asthma attack by the doctor or doctors who first saw the patient.
4. Over-reliance of the patient or the parent/caretaker of the patient on the use of inhaled bronchodilators (sympathomimetics/beta$_2$ agonists) for the fatal acute attack, the over-reliance, in turn, leading to delay in seeking further medical attention.
5. Lack of corticosteroid use or availability of such drugs for an acute attack of asthma.
6. Lack of a patient's crisis asthma management plan.

"Lack of appreciation of the severity of a specific asthma attack" may be a key issue. A study of 90 patients who died of asthma in the 1970's in England found that 10% died without the disease ever being diagnosed (7). In another 74% of the cases, the patient or the relative did not appreciate the severity of the attack. It is generally understood that asthma is under-diagnosed in children (5,8). In a recent review of 163 deaths from asthma in Victoria, Australia, in 1986–1987, allegedly 13% had a previous history of only "trivial" asthma (9). In a series of 14 inner-city asthmatic children (ages 2–18 years) who died between 1983 and 1990 in Brooklyn, New York, USA, 11/14 died at home or in extremis in the hospital emergency department after "sudden onset" of the fatal attack (10). (Asthma management was felt to be sub-optimal in 12/14 cases.) However, an analysis of the circumstances surrounding the deaths of 15 adolescent asthmatics (9–19 years of age) in Philadelphia, PA, USA, (1969–1985) at home, revealed that although ½ had "mild wheezing" 1–24 hours before the fatal episode, the degree of this attack would not usually have been felt to be significant (13). Eight of the 15 cases died a sudden death. It has been noted before that ¼ of all patients who die of asthma out of the hospital do so within 30 minutes of the attack of asthma. In the Philadelphia series of 15 cases, only one case could be documented as being directly related to a delay in seeking medical help as an incriminating factor (11). In the English studies of deaths (7), 75% of the time when the patient was seen by a primary care physician first, he did not appreciate the severity of the disease and this caused, in 25% of the 90 cases under study, a delay in referral to a hospital.

The over-reliance upon inhaled sympathomimetics such as isoproterenol in the past, and upon inhaled beta$_2$ agonists now, has been considered to directly contribute to the death of asthmatics (12). Today, beta$_2$ agonists, especially by the inhaled route, are the mainstay of acute asthma management, world-wide (4,5). Their ease of use can lead to over-use or abuse by the patient, or by well-meaning parents. This therapy is easily substituted for prophylactic therapy, especially since instantaneous gratification occurs or seems to occur with the relief of symptoms. Inhaled beta$_2$ agonist use tends to keep the patient at home or away from knowledgeable physicians and medical assistance. Easy, over-the-counter availability of potent beta$_2$ agonists MDI's accentuates this problem. Newer studies suggest that regular use of beta$_2$ agonists in MDI's (greater than two canisters per month) increases the risk of death (13). Regular use of beta$_2$ agonists may also increase bronchial reactivity in some but not all patients (14). In spite of these new revelations and assumptions, in only a few cases of children dying from asthma can the over-use of inhaled beta$_2$ agonist be categorically incriminated as a direct cause of death (10,11,12,15,16,17,18).

Profile of the Child Most Likely to be at Risk for Dying from Asthma

Severe Asthma

Most patients who die of asthma have severe disease, whether diagnosed or not or treated appropriately. This is true whether the patient lives in England (7), New Zealand (6), Australia (9), or the USA: Los Angeles (18), Denver (15), Philadelphia (11), or Brooklyn (10). Of the patients who died, 65–71% were felt to have had severe asthma. The assertion that significant numbers of patients who die of asthma may have had only mild disease, needs to be confirmed (9). As a measure of severity, previous hospitalizations are important, especially in the last 3 months (11) and especially when multiple. A history of previous ICU admissions with either pending or actual respiratory failure contributes to the risk of death (63% in the Philadelphia group and 67% in the Denver group of children) (11,15). Another measure of severity has been the necessity to control asthma with corticosteroids on a daily basis. This was the case in 73% of the Philadelphia group of children (11) and 92% of the Denver group (15). Another measure of asthma severity is the assessment of the multiple drugs that the patient must take daily to clinically tolerate asthma. Any one drug type may be taken in excess and may decrease the effectiveness of overall asthma control (e.g., $beta_2$ agonists) (19) or may place the patient at risk of serious side effects such as seizure or even death (e.g., theophylline, $beta_2$ agonists) (13,20). A physiologic measure of asthma severity is consistent abnormal pulmonary function parameters. In the Philadelphia teenagers who died at home, 87% were shown to have consistently abnormal maximal expiratory flow rates ($FEF_{25\text{-}75}$) that failed to improve with $beta_2$ agonist inhalations (11).

Age: Adolescents

The 1981–1983 New Zealand asthma mortality studies established the risky age group as 15–24 years of age (6). The USA mortality studies show the greatest increase in asthma death rates in children to be at the age of 10–14 years (1979–1982) (3). The Philadelphia teenagers who died at home (1969–1985) range from age 9–19 years (11). In Brooklyn, New York, USA, the children who died of asthma (1983–1990) ranged from 2–18 but 8/14 (57%) were in a narrow range of 10–15 years of age (10). In the two groups of severely afflicted asthmatic children who were first institutionalized in Denver, National Jewish Hospital, USA, (1974–1984) and then later, usually within 1 or 2 years, died of asthma in their home community, ages ranged from 5–18 (15). Other investigators have recognized the increase in the risk of death in this age group (16,17).

Sex: Males or Females, But More Likely to be Male

Males outnumber females 2:1 in childhood overall as to those who are afflicted with asthma, but this sex difference in the prevalence of asthma disappears in the late teenage years beyond the age of 15 (21). Still, in the teenage years, asthma deaths are more likely to occur in males (22) (e.g., male to female: Philadelphia group 15:7; Denver groups 29:16; Brooklyn group 11:3) (10,11,15).

Race: Any Race But a Minority is Most at Risk

Especially at risk are: Blacks in the USA (3,10,11,15,17,23,24); Mamoré Polynesian in New Zealand (4,19); and West Indian in England (7).

History of Hypoxic Seizures

This history was present in 9 of 21 in the first group of Denver patients who ultimately died and in 7 of 24 from the second group (15).

Rapid Change in Corticosteroid Requirement to Control Asthma Clinically

A physiologic variable that distinguished asthmatic children who died, versus case control patients, in the two Denver studies, was a rapid change in the corticosteroid requirement to control asthma (15), the "brittle asthmatic" (16).

The Presence of Significant Psychological Problems

Several psychological variables distinguish the child who was at risk during his or her disease in the Denver, Colorado, USA case control studies (15). These included: (a) the child's disregard for his or her own asthma symptoms and an unwillingness to seek help; (b) an unwillingness to take responsibility for management protocols for the patient's own asthma; (c) continued conflict of the patient with the staff including refusal on many occasions to follow medical directions; (d) presence of or tendency to depression; and (e) conflicts with the parents or family of the patient. In the Philadelphia group of teenager asthmatics who died at home, two-thirds had been seen by a psychiatrist because of emotional factors which directly seemed to be influencing the control of their disease (11). The patients with asthma may consciously be non-compliant about taking their medication, following medical advice or seeking help, even though they know that they are having a serious asthma attack (15). This behavior is suggestive of suicide or suicidal gestures.

Non-Compliance

The very nature of being an adolescent is to be non-compliant (16). It is small wonder, therefore, that treating any chronic disease which requires regular prophylactic medication and a regimented life-style plus a great deal of self reliance during the adolescent period is difficult! The severe psychological problems outlined in the Denver studies directly led to non-compliance (24). In 40% of the Philadelphia teenagers who died at home, non-compliance in use of their prescribed medications was documented in the year before death (11).

Critical Review of Current Asthma Management Trends

There is no doubt that asthma management trends have changed over the decades and such trends have affected the mortality rate from asthma in the inpatient-hospital setting. An example of this is the longitudinal 38 year analysis of asthma deaths in Los Angeles, USA, County Hospital, a tertiary care institution (18). The deaths from asthma per year fell from a high of 7.5/year during the period of 1949–1960 to 1.3/year from 1981–1986, with no pediatric deaths from 1971–1986. Asthma deaths in pediatric tertiary care hospitals in the USA are now uncommon (11). This trend is in spite of a nearly three-fold increase in US hospitalizations for asthma between 1970 and 1987 (4), many of these being children (11). Many of the patients now admitted to hospitals for acute asthma in the United States have moderate to severe disease, are followed by knowledgeable physicians and are already on some prophylactic regime of medications, including cromolyn sodium, theophylline and corticosteroids. Their admission often represents "break through disease". In some cases, however, multiple hospital admissions for asthma stabilization are an indication of poorly controlled disease at home (17).

Many of the patients with acute asthma who are hospitalized today are initially placed in an intensive care setting, utilizing techniques which were not available before (18). This new technology could be considered as the reason for better survival of patients in recent years in a hospital setting as suggested by the investigators from Philadelphia Children's Hospital (USA) (11), or it could be an indication of more severe disease as suggested by other investigators (18,25).

The current trend in asthma management targets the airway inflammation in this disease (4,26). Key to pharmacologic management of asthma is the early use of corticosteroids (or cromolyn sodium), especially by inhalation for the moderate or severe disease as primary prophylactic measures (4,14,26). Earlier and more frequent use of systemic "bursts of corticosteroids" have also shown experimentally to better control acute asthma exacerbations (27). The national promotion of the use of these new asthma management principals has been credited with reducing asthma mortality trend rates in New Zealand since 1985 (24), but it remains to be seen if a similar program in asthma education in the USA will also have an effect upon asthma mortality rates in that country (4).

The rekindling of a previous concern in the 1960's that the over-use (and abuse) of inhaled potent sympathomimetics or $beta_2$ agonists may directly contribute to asthma death is very important considering the plight of the adolescent with severe asthma (12,13,14). The adolescent, especially the non-compliant patient, will tend not to use prophylactic medication (26) as directed (11,15,16), and to be more likely to over-use and abuse $beta_2$ agonist MID's. Sudden death at home, or delay (conscious or unconscious) in seeking further medical care at this critical time, may be directly traced to the use of these types of medications, but further studies are needed to confirm this assumption (12).

Background of Inherited Conditions, Environmental Exposures and Socio-Economic Factors

Most children with asthma are atopic (4,5,21). The allergic reaction in the airways may be important in two ways. The allergic asthmatic may react immediately upon exposure to an allergen (e.g., cat induced asthma). Being allergic contributes to airway inflammation, and non-specific bronchial reactivity (4). The more exposure to allergens (e.g., house dust mite) in children born to atopic (asthmatic) parents, the more likely the child is to develop asthma, at an early age (28). A vivid example of allergy contributing to death due to acute asthma was brought out by a study of a cluster of 11 young asthmatics (ages 11–25) who lived in the mid-Western USA and were followed at the Mayo Clinic in Rochester, Minnesota (29). Between 1980 and 1989, these patients (nine females and two males) had 18 episodes of sudden respiratory failure during the summer and fall months and two deaths. A strong correlation was found between allergy to alternaria mold spores and respiratory failure (29). Allergen avoidance (26) and allergen immunotherapy (30) have been shown to decrease asthmatic specific and non-specific bronchial reactivity, to some allergens. Allergen immunotherapy has not been shown to decrease the risk of death from asthma, however.

Certain other inherited or acquired associations relating to the risk of asthma and asthma deaths in children have not been thoroughly investigated. For instance, there seems to be an association with low birth weight and the prevalence of asthma in 17 year old males (3). It is also known that 25% of very low birth weight babies may require prolonged O_2 supplementation and mechanical ventilation during the neonatal period (32). These babies, if they survive, frequently develop chronic lung disease (bronchopulmonary dysplasia) and wheeze for prolonged periods. It is known that bronchiolitis from respiratory syncytial virus may trigger asthma, especially in a baby born to an atopic family (5). A new association has been made between asthma onset and *chlamydia*-pneumonia bacterial infection (33).

The consequences of negative socio-economic factors affecting optimal daily asthma management and increasing the risk of death, are inescapable. A compelling argument in this regard can be made with statistics showing a marked difference in the median household income between Whites and Blacks with lower employment rates for Blacks (23). These rate differences were more marked in regions of the United States where there were higher death rates in Blacks versus Whites from asthma.

Strategies to Prevent Asthma Death in Children

1. Identify the specific individual patients who are at risk and tailor management, based on the knowledge that exists today, so as to optimize care.
2. Educate the physicians as to the optimal management techniques and procedures to control asthma, especially in the patients with moderate to severe disease.
3. Investigate, more fully, the management techniques and the drugs that we are now using to treat and control asthma so that they are used in such a fashion so as not to make asthma control more difficult or contribute to death.
4. Investigate new techniques, procedures and drugs to treat and control asthma that are more efficacious than we are now using and, hopefully, are safer, simpler to use and less expensive.
5. Research more fully the background factors such as the role of race, minority groups who live in new locations, the role of urban environment, allergens, chemical pollutants, and socio-economic, psychologic and cultural issues, all of which are known to affect asthma management outcome, independently or collectively, and possibly death from asthma.
6. Research the fundamental root causes of asthma from a genetic, physiologic, and molecular basis so as to direct new and better therapies and management techniques.

There is nothing new about these strategies. Assertive new education and asthma management programs have been introduced in New

Zealand, and have, apparently, been effective in reducing mortality rates from asthma in that country (6,24). There is new concern relating to the possibility that excessive use of beta$_2$ agonists may be harmful (12,13,14). After much discussion concerning the increase in asthma prevalence, hospitalization and death in the USA (3,22,23), the US government has sponsored a new, nation-wide campaign to educate physicians and the public as to the best way to manage asthma with the resources that we have available to us today (4). The basic tenets from the NIH-NHLBI Expert Panel Report (4) for the US National Asthma Education Program are to promote: (a) the use of home peak expiratory flow monitors to allow the patient/parent to have an objective parameter of airway patency; (b) a crisis plan for all asthmatics; (c) the early use of not only beta$_2$ agonists for acute attacks of asthma, but also corticosteroid bursts, po; (d) the early use, on a regular basis, of inhaled anti-inflammatory agents such as corticosteroids or cromolyn sodium; (e) protocol management of asthma attacks in the home, in the doctor's office, in the emergency department, and in the hospital inpatient unit; and (f) attention to background factors such as allergy, psychosocial and economic issues which may play a negative role and obstruct optimal management.

An asthma management plan utilizing the same basic tenets of the NIH-NHLBI report was studied at a San Diego, California, USA, health maintenance (HMO) setting and was shown to be an improvement over conventional asthma management (34). Hopefully,the NIH-NHLBI National Education Program will not only improve overall asthma control as shown in the San Diego pilot study, but also ultimately decrease death rates from asthma in the USA, including death in children.

From a research perspective, the USA National Institute of Allergy and Infectious Disease has recently launched a new national 5 year (1991–1995), multi-center, inner-city asthma study. This study will target areas of the USA which have excess asthma morbidity and mortality (35), and seek to investigate the root causes (e.g., allergens, health care access/delivery) so that changes can be implemented. Studies relating to the earlier use of corticosteroids to prevent asthma disease will be important to monitor closely, so as to access potential risk versus short-term benefit (4,14,26,32). Future asthma management, world-wide, will undoubtedly change, as new treatments are perfected. Hopefully, newer non-steroidal asthma anti-inflammatory preventative agents and drugs directed against important pharmacologic mediators will enable asthma to be better and more simply managed, and to reduce asthma deaths, including those in children.

References

1. Siegel, S.C. 1987. History of asthma deaths from antiquity. J. Allergy Clin. Immunol. 80(2):458.
2. Speizer, F.S. 1987. Historical perspectives: The epidemic of asthma deaths in the United Kingdom in the 1960's. J. Allergy Clin. Immunol. 80(2):368.
3. Sly, R.M. 1986. Mortality from asthma. NER Allergy Proceeding 7:425.
4. National Heart, Lung, and Blood Institute National Asthma Education Program Expert Panel Report. 1991. Pediatric Asthma Allergy & Immunol. 5:57.
5. Ellis, E. 1988. Asthma in infancy and childhood. In: Allergy principles and practice. E. Middleton, C.E. Reed, E.F. Ellis, N.F. Adkinson, and J.W. Yunginger, eds. St. Louis, MO: C.V. Mosby, p. 1037.
6. Sears, M.R., Rea, H.H. 1987. Patients at risk of dying of asthma: New Zealand experience. J. Allergy Clin. Immunol. 87(2):477.
7. Stabeforth, D.E. 1987. Asthma mortality and physician competence. J. Allergy Clin. Immunol. 80(2):463.
8. Speight, A., Lee, D., and Hey, E. 1983. Underdiagnosis and undertreatment of asthma in childhood. Brit. Med. J. 286:1253.
9. Robertson, C.F., Rubinfeld, A.R., and Bowes, G. 1990. Deaths from asthma in Victoria, a 12 month survey. Med. J. Australia 152:511.
10. Rao, M., Kravath, R.E., Abadco, D., Arden, J., and Steiner, P. 1991. Childhood asthma mortality: The Brooklyn experience and a brief review. J. Assoc. Acad. Minority Physicians 2:127.
11. Kravis, L.P. 1987. An analysis of fifteen childhood asthma fatalities. J. Allergy Clin. Immunol. 80(2):467.
12. Poynter, D. 1987. Fatal asthma: Is treatment incriminated? J. Allergy Clin. Immunol. 80(2):423.

13. Spitzer, W.O., Suissa, S., Ernst, P., Horwitz, R.I., Habbick, B., Cockcroft, D., Boivin, J.-F., McNutt, M., Buist, S.A., and Rebuck, A.S. 1992. The use of β-agonists and the risk of death and near death from asthma. New Eng. J. Med. 326:501. And editorial: Burrows, B., and Lebowitz, M. 1992. Editorial: The β-agonist dilemma. New Eng. J. Med. 326:560.
14. Haahtela, T., Jinen, M., Kava, T., Kiviranta, K., Koskinen, S., Lehtonen, K., Nikander, K., Persson, T., Reinikainen, K., Selroos, O., Soviji, A., Stenius-Aarniala, B., Svahn, T., Tammivaara, R., and Laitinen, L.A. 1991. Comparison of a β_2-agonist, terbutaline, with an inhaled corticosteroid, budesonide, in newly detected asthma. N. Engl. J. Med. 325:388.
15. Strunk, R.C. 1987. Asthma deaths in childhood: Identification of patients at risk and intervention. J. Allergy Clin. Immunol. 80(2):472.
16. Lewiston, J.J., and Rubinstein, S. 1986. Sudden death in adolescent asthma. NER Allergy Proc. 7:448.
17. Attaway, N.J., Birkhead, G.S., Townsend, M.C., and Strunk, R.C. 1988. Investigation of a cluster of asthma deaths in teenagers. J. Allergy Clin. Immunol. 81:306(A).
18. Flora, G.S., Sharma, A.M., and Sharma, O.P. 1991. Asthma mortality in a metropolitan county hospital, a 38 year study. Allergy Proceed. 12:169.
19. Sears, M.D., Taylor, D.R., and Prink, C.G. 1990. Regular inhaled beta-agonist treatment in bronchial asthma. Lancet 336:1391.
20. Kraemer, M., Furukawa, C., and Kaup, J. 1982. Altered theophylline clearance during an *influenza* B outbreak. Pediatrics 62:476.
21. Gergen, P.J., Mullally, D.I., and Evans, R. 1988. National survey of prevalence of asthma among children in the U.S.A., 1976–1980. Pediatrics 81:1.
22. Evans, R. 1987. Recent observations reflecting increases in mortality from asthma. J. Allergy Clin. Immunol. 80(2):377.
23. Sly, R.M., and O'Donnell, R. 1989. Regional distribution of deaths from asthma. Ann . Allergy 62:347.
24. Sears, M.R. 1991. International trends in asthma mortality. Allergy Proceed. 12:155.
25. Sears, M.R., Rea, H.H., and Rothwell, R.P.G. 1986. Asthma mortality comparison between New Zealand and England. Brit. Med. J. 293:342.
26. Crockcroft, D.W. 1991. Therapy for airway inflammation in asthma. J. Allergy Clin. Immunol. 87:914.
27. Chapman, K.R., Verbeek, P.R., White, J.G., and Rebuck, A.S. 1991. Effect of a short course of prednisone in the prevention of early relapse after the emergency room treatment of acute asthma. N. Engl. J. Med. 324:788.
28. Sporik, R., Holgate, S.T., Platts-Mills, T.A.E., and Cogswell, J.J. 1990. Exposure to housedust mite allergen (Der p I) and the development of asthma in childhood. A prospective study. N. Engl. J. Med. 323:502.
29. O'Hallaren, M.T., Yunginger, J.W., Offord, K.P., Somers, M.J., O'Connell, E.J., Ballard, D.J., and Sachs, M.I. 1991. Exposure to an aeroallergen as a possible precipitating factor in respiratory arrest in young patients with asthma. N. Engl. J. Med. 324:359.
30. Hedlin, G., Graff-Lonnevig, V., Heiborn, H. Lilja, G., Norrlind, K., Pegelow, K., Sundin, B., and Lowenstein, H. 1991. Immunotherapy with cat and dog dander extracts. J. Allergy Clin. Immunol. 87:955.
31. Seidman, D.S., Laor, A., Gale, R., Stevenson, D.K., and Dannon, Y.L. 1991. Is low birth weight a risk factor for asthma during adolescence? Archives of Dis. Children 66:584.
32. Collaborative Dexamethasone Trial Group. 1991. Dexamethasone therapy in neonatal chronic lung disease: An international placebo-controlled trial. Pediatrics 88:421.
33. Hahn, D., Dodge, R., and Golubjatnikov, R. 1991. Association of *Chlamydia pneumoniae* (strain TWAR) infection with wheezing, asthmatic bronchitis, and adult-onset asthma. JAMA 266:225.
34. Zeiger, R.S., Heller, S., Mellon, M.H., Wald, J., Falkoff, R., and Schatz, M. 1991. Facilitated referral to asthma specialist reduces relapses in asthma emergency room visits. J. Allergy Clin. Immunol. 87:1160.
35. Weiss, K.B., and Wagener, D.K. 1990. Changing patterns of asthma mortality: Identifying target populations at high risk. JAMA 264:1683.

Section XXI

Physical Allergy

Solar Allergy: A Role of Inhibition Spectrum in Solar Urticaria

Masamitsu Ichihashi, Yoko Funasaka*

Solar urticaria is characterized by an immediate wheal reaction of the skin to solar radiation. Solar urticaria may be induced by both allergic and non-allergic mechanisms. Most solar urticaria cases, however, are possibly induced by Ag-Ab reaction, since positive transfer and/or existence of photoallergens in serum, plasma or skin eluates from the patients, and normal subjects were identified in a number of cases. In some cases, molecular weights of chromophores in serum or plasma have been shown to be in the range of 10^4–10^5 daltons or between 3×10^5 and 10^6 daltons. In some solar urticaria cases with lag time between the onset of wheal reaction and the end of irradiation, an inhibition spectrum suppressing wheal reaction was shown to exist in long visible light. Further, augmentation spectrum enhancing wheal formation was also found to exist in at least one case. The possible allergic mechanisms including a role of inhibition spectrum are discussed in this paper based on findings reported recently.

Solar allergy can be classified into two types, one immediate and one delayed type. The former is represented by solar urticaria and the latter is represented by allergic contact dermatitis, chronic actinic dermatitis and possibly polymorphic light eruption. Solar urticaria was first identified by Merklen in 1904 (1). Thereafter, a number of new cases were studied with their immunological characteristics, and further the action spectrum of the cases were extensively examined. Ive et al·(2) collected data from 17 patients and classified three different categories depending on the deferences of action spectra. Later in 1963, Harber et al.(3) defined six classes according to action spectra and immunological reactions. Solar urticaria usually develops on skin (4) that has not been exposed to the sun for more than a week, such as the extensor surfaces of the forearms, and upper arms, whereas chronically sun-exposed skin, such as the face and the dorsa of the hands are rather resistant to solar radiation, possibly due to exhaustion of mediator reserves consumed by frequent exposure to sunlight, an increase in the mast-cell degranulation threshold (5), or due to a long-term occupation of IgE binding sites by the photoallergens which suppress histamine release from mast cells (6). In the present study, recent advances on the mechanisms of solar urticaria focussing on immunopathological findings and the role of inhibition spectrum are discussed.

Action Spectrum of Solar Urticaria

Solar radiation on the earth surface is composed of ultraviolet B (290–320 nm), ultraviolet A (320–400 nm), visible light (400–720 nm) and infrared (longer than 720 nm) light. Each patient has his or her own action spectrum for wheal formation. Some are reactive to UVB wavebands and others are sensitive to visible light spectrum. Blum et al. (7) divided solar urticaria into two groups: one reactive to wavebands shorter than 370 nm, and positive to passive transfer test by patient's serum, the other reactive to waveband ranging from 400 through 500 nm but non-reactive to passive transfer test. Solar urticaria cases non-classifiable to these two categories, however, have accumulated since Blum's proposal. Other cases hypersensitive to both UVA and visible light or hypersensitive to wavebands ranging from UVA to infared light have been reported. Harber et al. (3) identified six categories in solar urticaria, depending on the action spectrum and immunological reactivities. Since Harber et al.'s proposal of six categories for solar urticaria, the action spectrum of individual cases has been

* Department of Dermatology, Kobe University School of Medicine, 7-5-1 Kusunoki-cho, Chuo-kuu, Kobe, 650 Japan.

clarified during the last 30 years using monochromator or other polychromatic light sources. Porphyrin, however, is the only chromophore identified as a responsible substance of solar urticaria belonging to category VI. Chromosphores in the other five categories have not been identified yet, except molecular weight studies of photoallergen (8) or a precursor of photoallergen (9).

Inhibition Spectrum

A 46-year-old woman who developed urticaria in the sun-exposed areas approximately 10 min after cessation of constant solar radiation was observed by the authors in 1981 (10). As of that time, there were no reports of solar urticaria cases which developed wheal with constant 10 minutes lag time between wheal onset and the end of radiation (Fig. 1). The action spectrum of the patient was fully examined by monochromatic wavebands ranging from 290 nm through 720 nm at 10–50 nm intervals, and also by UVB, UVA and mixed visible light radiation sources. Monochromatic wavebands between 400 nm and 500 nm could induce wheal. In skin exposed to 425 nm visible light for 15 min or 5 min, wheal appeared immediately or 10 min after the end of radiation, respectively. These results indicate that 15 min irradiation at 425 nm monochromatic radiation did not show 10 min lag time between the onset of wheal and the end of radiation. Based on these results, we speculated the existence of a waveband in solar radiation which inhibits or suppresses wheal reaction. An almost complete inhibition of wheal reaction was observed by subsequent radiation of visible light longer than 530 nm or 690 nm immediately following 10 min of whole visible light irradiation. We also confirmed the existence of the inhibition spectrum by a similar study using 425 nm monochromatic light as action spectrum followed by visible light irradiation longer than 590 nm. Since the first report of a solar urticaria case with inhibition spectrum by Hasei and Ichihashi, nearly 20 cases (11,12,13,14) with inhibition spectrum have been documented. Most of the cases have an action spectrum in the range from 400 to 500 nm, and an inhibition spectrum in the visible light usually longer than 530 nm, but a rare case with action spectrum in UVA (13) and a case with inhibition spectrum in UVA (14) were reported recently. Incomplete inhibition of urticaria reaction by inhibition spectrum may induce erythema alone in the skin exposed to elicitation radiation (12). The patient's serum exposed *in vitro* to wheal-eliciting light induced urticaria when injected into the patient's own dermis, but failed to produce urticaria when the serum was re-exposed *in vitro* to long visible light prior to intradermal injection. Therefore, in solar urticaria with inhibition spectrum wheal develops after a short lag time, or erythema alone without wheal develops during or after the end of exposure to sunlight.

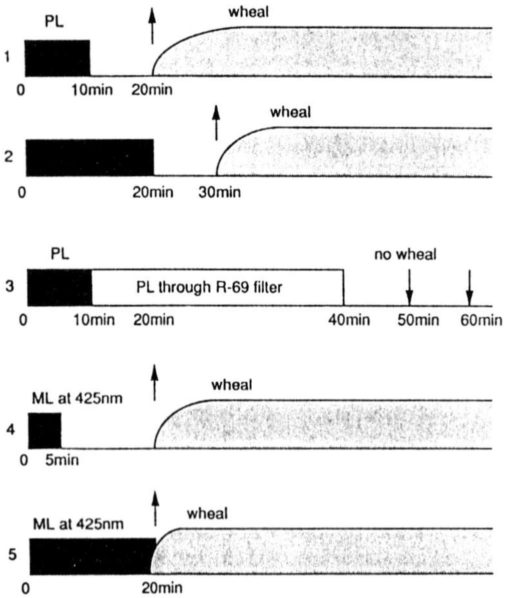

Figure 1. Relationship between exposure time and skin reactions to different radiation sources.
Deep shaded area (PL) indicates period of irradiation with visible light from a projector, black area indicates monochromatic radiation, and faint shaded area indicates wheal induced by light.

Mechanism of Wheal Reaction

Allergic urticaria reactions are apparently similar in every respect whether they are elicited by chemical or physical agents, and it is unlikely that the reactions are induced by basically different mechanisms. There are several findings which strongly indicate that wheal formation in solar urticaria may be produced by allergic mechanisms: (A) The positive passive transfer test by Sulzberger and Bear (15) shows IgE antibody on mast cell surfaces, and further antigen-formation in the healthy subjects' skin exposed to action spectrum radiation. (B) The positive response of the reverse passive transfer test (16) demonstrates the presence of antigen in the skin of the healthy subject. Epstein's observation does not support the IgE mediated allergic mechanism of solar urticaria, since the wheal reaction in the reverse passive transfer test was produced without reasonable incubation time usually required for IgE binding on mast cell surface. Further, as no positive cases have been reported since Epstein's findings, we are not able to evaluate the significance of reverse passive transfer test in solar urticaria. Further, due to ethical reasons, it is not acceptable at present, nor will it be in the future, to perform passive transfer and reverse passive transfer tests for new solar urticaria subjects. And, finally, (C) Production of antigen in serum, plasma or skin eluate by exposure to wheal-eliciting light *in vitro*. Molecular weights (MW) of a serum chromophore and photoallergen responsible for wheal induction were investigated by Horio et al. (9) and Kojima et al. (8). Horio et al. showed that MW of a serum factor was more than 10^5 daltons and not a simple chemical substance. Kojima et al. reported that the moleculer weight of photoallergens was between 3×10^5 and 1.0×10^6 daltons in one patient, and $2.5 \times 10^4 - 4.5 \times 10^4$ daltons in another patient using the gel filtration method. Recently, Leenutaphong et al. (17) reported a case in which a chromophore was not in serum or plasma, but the patient developed urticaria reacting to eluates of *in vitro* irradiated isolated epidermis and irradiated eluates of epidermis. No abnormal reaction was observed with injection of non-irradiated eluates of non-irradiated epidermis. They concluded that in this patient the pre-photoallergen (chromophore) was present in the skin, possibly in the epidermis but not in the circulation. Further investigations are needed to clarify the moleculer size and other characteristics of intrinsic photoallergens in solar urticaria.

Role of Inhibition Spectrum in Allergic Solar Urticaria

Irradiation of the patient's skin with inhibition spectra before and after the injections of histamine and a histamine-releasing agent did not suppress the wheal development. Therefore, mast cell stabilization, unresponsiveness of the vessels to chemical mediators, or inactivation of chemical mediator in the post irradiation of the inhibiting spectra are not the events responsible for the inhibition of urticarial reaction. We speculate that in cases when post-irradiation of inhibition spectra suppresses wheal reaction, an inactivation of photoallergen or inhibition of the binding of photoallergen to mast cell surface may take place in the patient's skin. Further, inhibition of the binding of photoallergen may be caused by the molecular alteration of photoallergen or alteration of antibody receptor sites by the absorption of inhibition spectrum (Fig. 2). In cases when pre-irradiation with inhibiting light suppresses urticaria production, alterations of chromophore or receptor site of antibody could be the cause for the suppression of urticaria formation by subsequent wheal-eliciting light.

Augmentation Spectrum for Solar Urticaria

In one solar urticaria case, Horio and Fujigaki (18) found that the irradiation of visible light before exposure to urticaria-eliciting light enhanced a wheal reaction in an augmentative but not in an additive fashion. The action spectrum was in the range from 320 to 420 nm, whereas the augmentation spectrum ranged from 450 to 500 nm. In this case, they observed the inhibition spectrum in the range from 550 to 660 nm. The augmentation spectrum had no effects on the wheal formation induced by histamine or compound 48/80 in the patient. Although the mechanism of augmentation of UV-A-induced urticaria is not clear yet, they speculated that a pre-photoallergen activated by augmentation light energy may be altered to a state that is more easily reactive to urticaria-eliciting light.

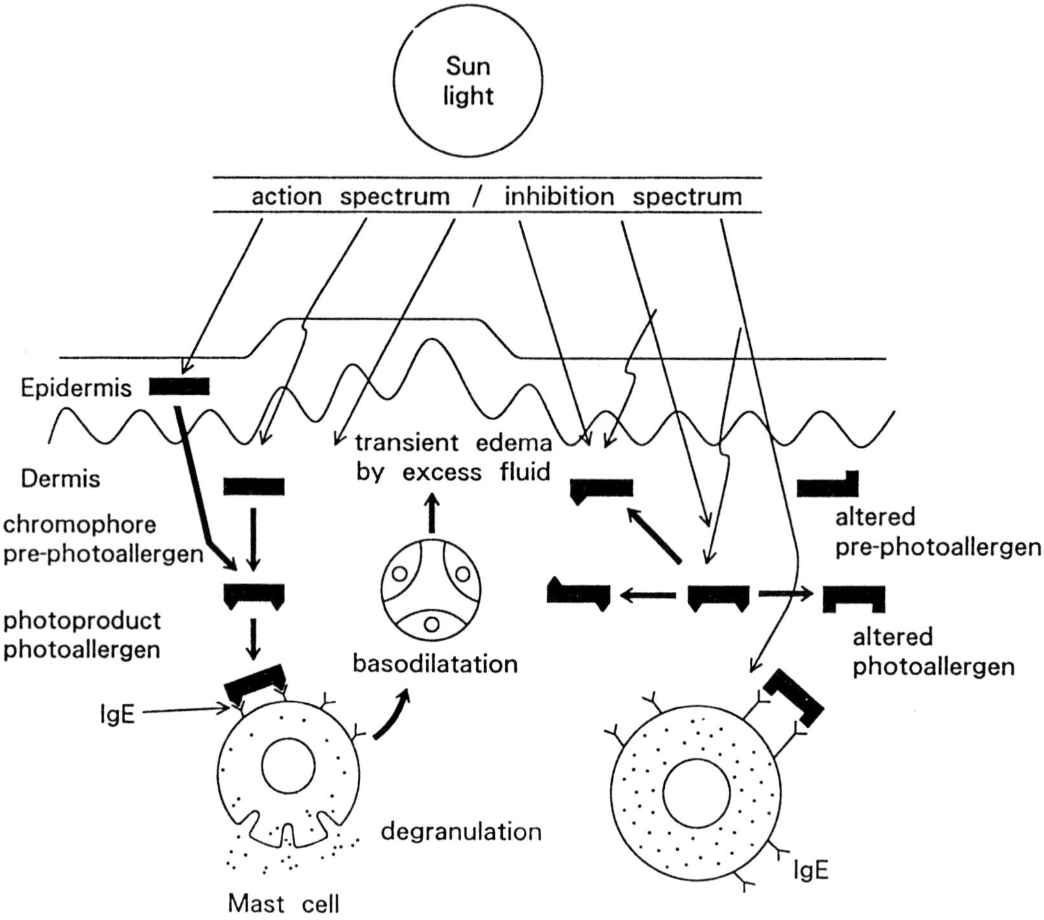

Figure 2. Proposed mechanisms of induction and inhibition of solar urticaria.
Solar radiation has both action and inhibition spectra. Chromophore (pre-photoantigen) in the serum, plasma or epidermis becomes active photoallergen (photoproduct) after absorbing action spectrum. The photoallergens formed bind to the specific IgE on the mast cell surface, and then degranulation of the mast cells leads to vasodilatation by chemical mediators. Inhibition spectrum, on the other hand, alters photoallergen formed or inhibits the binding of photoallergen to the IgE on mast cells or possibly alters a molecular structure of the receptors on mast cells.

Solar Urticaria with Delayed Onset

Two unique cases (19,20) in which wheal began to develop 2–5 h after the end of wheal-eliciting radiation have been reported so far. The injection of *in vitro* irradiated serum did not induce urticaria. Clinical and immunological characteristics suggest that the mechanisms of these cases may not be IgE dependent, immediate allergic reaction, but a reaction involving kinin activation.

Conclusions

Solar urticaria may be caused by both allergic and non-allergic mechanisms. Most solar urticaria cases, however, are possibly induced by

Table 1. Classification of Solar Urticaria

SU Type	Action Spectrum	Passive Transfer	Reverse Passive Transfer	In vitro Irradiation (photoallergen)	Inhibition Spectrum	Augmentation Spectrum	Mechanism
I	285 – 320	+	+	?	–	?	allergic
II	320 – 400	–	–	+∼–	+	+	unknown
III	400 – 500	–	–	–∼+	+	?	allergic
IV	400 – 500	+	–	+∼–	+∼–	?	allergic
V	280 – 600	–	–	? –	? +	?	unknown
VI	400 – 410	–	–	–∼+	–	?	non-allergic

Ag-Ab reaction, since positive passive transfer and/or existence of photoallergen in serum, plasma or skin eluates from the patient and normal subjects were demonstrated in a number of cases. The characteristics of six categories of solar urticaria classified by Harber et al. should be revised with the addition of immunological and photobiological findings after their proposal (Table 1). Inhibition spectrum may suppress the urticaria reaction by the inactivation of photoallergen caused by wheal-eliciting light or by inhibiting the Ag-Ab reaction on mast cell surface, but in some cases in which pre-irradiation of inhibiting spectrum inhibits the reaction, chromophore or IgE receptors on mast cell surfaces may be altered by inhibition light. The precise mechanisms of solar urticaria are not yet clear. Determination of the role of cytokines released from various kinds of infiltrating cells in relevance to action spectra and immunologic characteristics, and an understanding of chemical and physical properties of photoallergen may contribute to the elucidation of the mechanisms of solar urticaria.

References

1. Sams, W.M. 1970. Solar urticaria: Studies of the active serum factor. J. Allergy Clin. Immunol. 45:295.
2. Ive, H., Lloyd, J., and Magnus, I.A. 1965. Action spectra in idiopathic solar urticaria: A study of 17 cases with a monochromator. Br. J. Dermatol. 77:229.
3. Harber, L.C., Holloway, R.M., Wheatley V.R., et al. 1963. Immunologic and biophysical studies in solar urticaria. J. Invest. Dermatol. 41:439.
4. Ramsay, A.C. 1980. Solar Urticaria. Internatl. J. of Dermatol. 19(5):233.
5. Keahey, T.M., Lavker, R.M., Kaidbey, K.H., et al. 1984. Studies on the mechanism of clinical tolerance in solar urticaria. Br. J. Dermatol. 110:327.
6. Leenutaphong, V., Holzle, E., and Plewig, G. 1990. Solar urticaria: Studies on mechanisms of tolerance. Brit. J. of Dermatol. 122:601.
7. Blum, H.F., Allington, H., and West, R. 1935. On urticaria response to light and its photophysiology. J. Clin. Invest. 14:435.

8. Kojima, M., Horiko, T., Nakamura, Y., and Aoki, T. 1986. Solar urticaria. Arch. Dermatol. 122:550.
9. Horio, T. 1978. Photoallergic urticaria induced by visible light: Additional cases and further studies. Arch. Dermatol. 114:1761.
10. Hasei, K., and Ichihashi, M. 1982. Solar urticaria. Arch. Dermatol. 118:346.
11. Torinuki, W., Kumai, N., and Miura, T. 1983. Solar urticaria inhibited by visible light. Dermatologica 166:151.
12. Ichihashi, M., Hasei, K., and Hayashibe, K. 1985. Solar urticaria. Arch. Dermatol. 121:503.
13. Horio, T., Yoshioka, A., and Okamoto, H. 1984. Production and inhibition of solar urticaria by visible light exposure. J. Am. Acad. Dermatol. 11:1094.
14. Leenutaphong, V., Kries, V.R., Holzle, E., and Plewig, G. 1988. Solar urticaria induced by visible light and inhibited by UVA. Photodermatology 5:170.
15. Sulzberger, M.B., and Baer, R.L. 1945. Studies in hypersensitivity to light. I. Preliminary report. J. Invest. Dermatol. 6:345.
16. Epstein, S. 1949. Urticaria pathogenica: Report of two cases, one of them associated with purpura photogenica. Ann. Allergy 7:443.
17. Leenutaphong, V., Holzle, E., and Plewig, G. 1989. Pathogenesis and classification of solar urticaria: A new concept. J. Am. Acad. Dermatol. 21:237.
18. Horio, T., and Fijigaki, K. 1988. Augmentation spectrum in solar urticaria. J. Am. Acad. Dermatol. 18:1189.
19. Ihm, C.W. 1979. Solar urticaria. Report of an unusual case. Cutis. 23:784.
20. Monfrecola, G., Nappa, P., and Pini, D. 1988. Solar urticaria with delayed onset:a case report. Photodermatology 5:103.

Cold Urticaria Syndromes: New Treatment

Leonardo Greiding*

Cold urticaria consists of a group of syndromes characterized by cutaneous lesions like erythema, papules, edema, and itching. Edema of mucosa and systemic reactions such as hypotension and shock can also be present. These syndromes can be triggered by exposure to cold elements such as water, cold wind, or cold food. Symptomatic treatment includes antihistamines such as cyproheptadine (1), doxepine (2), or ketotifen associated with terfenadine, cetirizine or loratidine. Tolerance can be induced during several hours by regular and continuous exposures to cold (3). We carried on a "hyposensitizing" treatment in idiopathic or atypical primary urticaria (according to the classification of Wanderer: Ref. 4). This treatment consisted of biweekly subcutaneous injections of serum obtained from the forearm effluent vein after cold challenge of the skin. The study included a control treatment with placebo. This was performed by inoculating with autologous serum obtained without cooling during 2–3 months. The clinical and cold stimulation time test parameters between the two treatments proved to be statistically significant ($p < 0.002$ and $p < 0.0017$, respectively). We hypothesized that the cold challenge of the skin might release an antigen to the circulation, which could be recognized by the IgE and be passible to hyposensitization.

Cold urticaria designates a group of syndromes characterized by cutaneous lesions such as erythema, papules, edema, and itching; edema of mucosa and systemic reactions including hypotension and shock can also be present. These syndromes can be triggered by exposure to cold elements such as water, cold wind, or cold food. Shock is frequently observed when the patients dive in cold water. The syndrome can be investigated by the cold stimulation test, using ice or refrigerated tubes or plastics (from 0°C to 4°C over the skin. The test is considered positive if erythema followed by a white papule appears conforming to the shape of the cold object after a few minutes of having removed it. According to Wanderer (4), cold urticaria syndromes may be classified by the response to the cold-contact test in two groups: (a) typical with positive cold-contact skin, and (b) atypical with negative cold-contact skin test responses. Typical urticaria may be further classified as primary or secondary. Primary or idiopathic is not associated with other pathologies and shows negative tests for cryoglobulines, cryohemolysines and cryofibrinogenemia. Typical urticaria is secondary when any of the aforementioned serum tests are positive. It could be present in association with several pathologies such as syphilis, chronic lymphocytic leukemia, lymphosarcoma, cytomegalovirus or other viral infections. Atypical cold urticaria not responding to a cold-contact test includes a series of different pathologies such as atypical systemic cold urticaria, cold-dependent dermographism, cold-induced cholinergic urticaria, delayed cold urticaria, and localized cold reflex urticaria. A familial type of cold urticaria has also been described, characterized by autosomal-dominant inheritance with different clinical characteristics. The primary typical cold urticaria is the most frequent type and generally occurs abruptly, affecting a population with a mean age of 18 to 25 years, though it may affect a wider age range varying from 3 months to 74 years. Both sexes are affected, though it is more frequent in women (65%). According to Wanderer (4), the level of atopic individuals in this population group is 30% and the mean duration of the disease ranges from 4.8 to 9.3 years. According to the intensity of the clinical response, a classification can be made into three different groups: (a) localized reaction without generalized manifestations (hypotension or shock); (b) generalized reactions but without hypotension or shock; and (c) generalized reactions with hypotension and shock. The incidence of the different groups are, according to Wanderer (4): 30% for type I, 32% for type II

* Instituto Argentino de Alergia e Inmunologia, Medrano 291, (1178) Buenos Aires, Argentina.
Acknowledgements: The statistical analysis was performed by Dr. E. Roldan. The manuscript was reviewed by Dr. L. Squiquera.

and 38% for type III. The cold-contact test can be quantified in relation to the minimum time necessary to induce a reaction, and a correlation has been established between persons who need less time for a reaction after exposure (3 min or less) and those who suffer from more severe forms of the disease. Vice versa, more prolonged minimum times (5 to 10 min) are observed in those who suffer from less intense forms of the disease.

There is significant evidence that mast cells are involved in the reaction. Light and electron-microscopy have demonstrated the presence of skin mast cells which degranulate after cold challenges (5). This process can be inhibited by cold-induced tolerance with repeated localized or generalized exposures. This tolerance is specific because the skin continues to react to stimuli like substance P and histamine. These findings suggest the participation of mast cells, IgE and the release of chemical mediators during the cold-contact test. The repetitive exposure could probably act by inhibiting the formation of antigens. Research which has obtained serum samples from effluent vein of the limbs after being exposed to cold has shown the presence of histamine (6), neutrophil chemotactic factors (7), eosinophil chemotactic factors (8), as well as PAF (9) and Prostaglandin D2 (10). The participation of platelet is controversial in this phenomenon, although the complement system does not seem to be involved (11,12). The reaction can be transmitted passively with serum of the patient containing IgE to control skin, and this could be determined by (a) warming the serum to 56° for 4 h, which turns the reaction negative; (b) the persistence of the positive reaction from 24 h to 28 days (only the IgE remains active during such prolonged periods due to its specific receptors, type I); (c) the passive transmission that is inhibited by immunoabsorption of IgE; or by (d) treating the serum with 2 mercaptoethanol that reduces disulfide bridges in the IgE (13). The fixation time increases with the titer of IgE, without any relation with the clinical intensity. With another sample of serum with high levels of IgE directed to another antigen (ragweed) (13), it is also possible to block the capacity to transmit passively the response to cold, suggesting that it may interact with the same receptor of IgE. The IgE antibodies can be absorbed by cooled skin (14). It is difficult to perform a passive transmission in monkeys, suggesting that the release of antigen from monkey skin by cold-contact is not present or shows less affinity (15). Kaplan demonstrated (16) that skin, cooled and then warmed, is capable of inducing release of histamine from leukocytes in patients with cold urticaria, and this finding supports the presence of an antigen released by cold-contact of the skin. Occasionally, the response to cold has been transmitted passively by IgG or IgM, thus anti IgE antibodies could be present. These antibodies are not exclusive of cold urticaria and can be found in other types of urticaria like urticaria vasculitis(17).

Hyposensitizing Treatment

Several observations demonstrate the participation of IgE in a group of patients with cold-urticaria. We postulate the probability of an antigen being released by cold contact with the skin, and perhaps mucosa, and we assume that, as in other examples of IgE dependent sensitization, a specific "hyposensitization" can be developed, in case a specific antigen should be available. We think that after applying cold to skin, besides mediators released by mast cells in the effluent veins, a skin derived antigen could be released in the circulation. In an attempt to confirm this possibility, we obtained serum from the forearm effluent vein after a 10 min cold exposure over the mentioned area and tested the same patients with primary typical urticaria by intradermal testing. We observed that the intradermal reaction with post-cold autologous serum produced positive reactions in three out of nine patients. This phenomena was not found in the skin of non-cold urticaria. Based on these data we assume that a substance is present that produces a reaction after 5–10 min of cold and that is not present in the serum from the forelimbs not challenged by cold. This would support the role of chemical mediators in the development of the reaction or the involvement of other unspecific causes. The low frequency of this finding may be understood as the result of the little amount of free antigen in circulation. We believe that, if a free antigen in the circulation does exist, we could use the same serum to try to desensitize the patients. For these reasons, we selected patients with cold primary typical urticaria, with negative serology for HIV, hepatitis virus, syphilis, cold agglutinin, cryoglobulin, cryofibrinogenemias, and antinuclear antibodies.

We classified the patients clinically, as explained above, in groups I, II and III. Additionally, according with the cold test time, the patients were further classified, according to the time of cold exposure needed to produce a papule, in three groups: those who produced a weal after (a) 3 min; (b) 6 min; or (c) 9 min (we assigned the arbitrary value of 10 to the negative cases, so as to facilitate the analysis of the data). The passive transmission was performed in every case, and we only took trial serum from patients if it was capable of producing passive transmission in 24–72 h, if the transmission could be inhibited by warming to 56for 4 h, and if it was negative after the serum absorption by immunoaffinity chromatography with specific antibody anti IgE, lowering to 0 all the IgE values of the serum investigated.

We obtained "hyposensitizing serum" from the forearm effluent veins after applications of a 5 by 10 cm refrigerating plastic during 10 min. We conserved the serum with 0.4% phenol and started the hyposensitization treatment with a serum dilution of 50% in saline, in biweekly subcutaneous injections of 0.05 to 0.40 cc (increasing 0.05 cc in every shot). The next month, we continued the treatment with concentrated serum in applications of 0.05 to 0.40 cc. When the trial could be continued, the following month we used 0.40 cc in the same way twice a week (18). For the "placebo" treatment, we obtained serum under the same conditions but without cooling the skin, and carried on the treatment in the same concentration for 2 months. The treatment was performed during autumn and winter months with a maximum mean temperature of 17°C. Eleven patients were included in the present study (mean age of 23.18 years, four patients being females and seven males). The average duration of the disease at the beginning of the treatment was 32.9 months (ranging from 8 to 48 months). All the patients, except for one, showed a high IgE level over the second standard deviation, with a medium of 200.7 KU/l (range 110/264). Eight patients showed symptoms of atopy, seven were of clinical type II, and four of clinical type III. No patient was of type I.

The time assessment of the cold-contact test was positive up to 3 min in five patients, up to 6 min in six others and no patient needed more than 6 min to positivize the test.

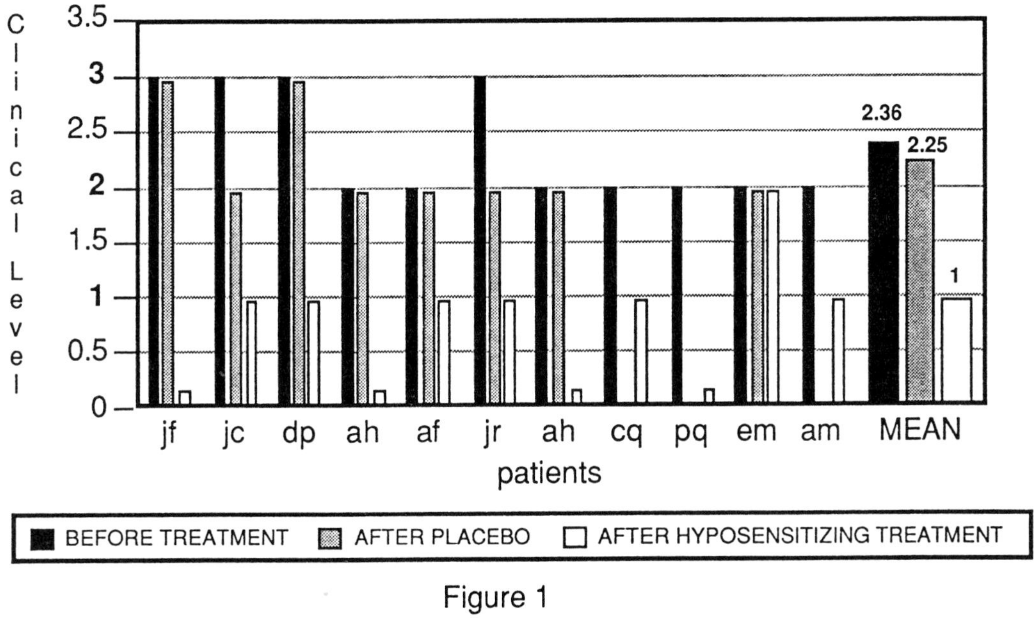

Figure 1. Cold urticaria, clinical evolution.

Results

A "placebo" treatment was performed before the "hyposensitizating" treatment in eight patients. Two of them showed clinical improvement, two changed from type III to type II, and one showed improvement in the test time from 3 to 6 min.

The "hyposensitizing" treatment included eleven patients, during a mean period of treatment of 2.5 months (range 2–3 months). A clinical improvement was noted in ten of eleven patients: One developed from type III to type 0, three patients from type II to type 0, three from type III to type I, and another three from type II to type I. One patient of type II experienced no change. In a total of 11 patients, three improved over one type, six improved over two types and one improved over three types. There was no change in one patient. The statistical analysis was performed using the Kruskal-Wallis test, with a Tadpole statistic program for an IBM PC. A highly favorable relation for the "hyposensitizing" treatment was found against the placebo ($p<0.002$: see Figure 1).

The average test time for the cold-contact test at the beginning of the study was 4.63 min. After the placebo treatment, the mean time was 4.87 min. After the "hyposensitizing" treatment, it was extended to 6.90 min. With the "placebo", one of eight patients improved the time test. With the "hyposensitizing" treatment, the time test changed from 3 to 10 min (negative) in one patient, and from 6 to 10 min in three others, and went from 3 to 6 min in four. Three patients manifested no change in 6 minutes; therefore, eight of eleven patients improved their reaction time with the "hyposensitizing" treatment. This improvement in the experimental group compared to the placebos had a p-value of $p<0.017$ (see Figure 2).

Now that we have demonstrated such a significant improvement with the proposed treatment, we are now looking for a method that would enable us to recognize and then identify the antigen we estimate is released during the exposure of the skin to cold. We know that in case it is available, there should be more specific elements for the study and treatment of this disorder. Meanwhile, we believe that the treatment we propose, due to its lack of toxicity and because of its simplicity, is an interesting alternative to shorten the disease periods.

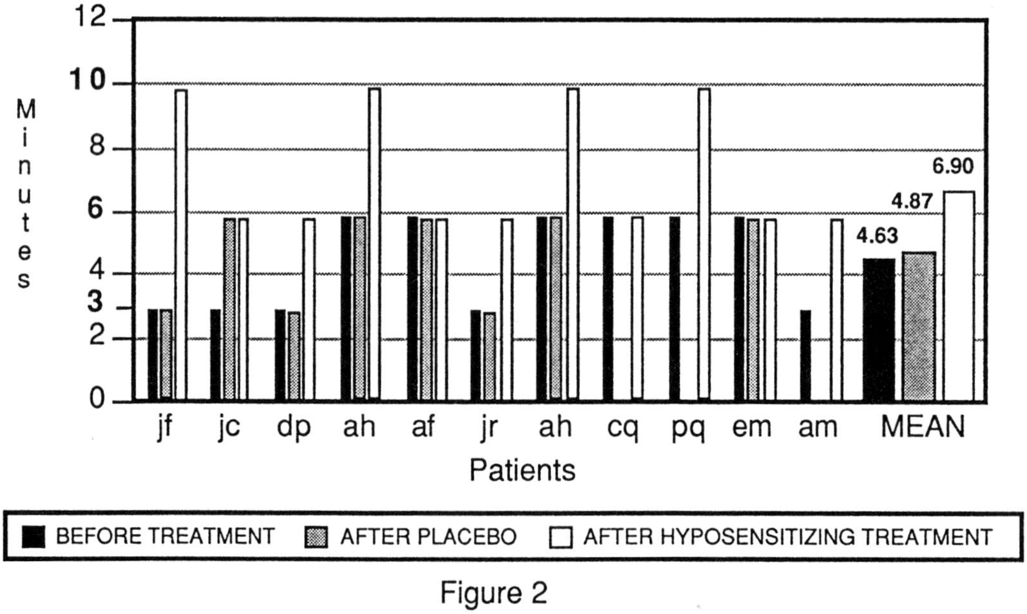

Figure 2. Cold urticaria, cold stimulation time test.

References

1. Wanderer, A.A., St.Pierre, J.P., and Ellis, E.F. 1977. Primary aquired cold urticaria: Double blind comparative study of treatment with cyproheptadine, chlorpheniramine and placebo. Arch. Dermatol. 113:1375.
2. Neittasanmaki, H., Myohanen, T., and Fraki, J.E. 1984. Comparison of cinarizine, cyproheptadine, doxepin, and hydroxyzine in treatment of idiopathic cold urticaria: Usefulness of doxepin. J. Am. Acad. Dermatol. 11:483.
3. Eady, R.A.J., and Greaves, M.W. 1978. Induction of cutaneous vasculitis with repeated cold challenge in cold urticaria. Lancet 2:336.
4. Wanderer, A.A. 1990. Cold urticaria syndromes: Historical background, diagnostic classification, clinical and laboratory characteristics, pathogenesis and management. J. Allergy Clin. Immunol. 85(6):965.
5. Keahey, T.M., Indrisano, J., and Kaliner, M. 1988. A case study on the induction of clinical tolerance in cold urticaria. J. Allergy Clin. Immunol. 82:256.
6. Kaplan, A.P., and Beaven, M.A. 1976. *In vivo* studies of the pathogenesis of cold urticaria, cholinergic urticaria, and vibration induced swelling. J. Invest. Dermatol. 67:326.
7. Wasserman, S.I., Soter, N.A., Center, D.M., and Austen, K.F.1977. Cold urticaria: Recognition and characterization of a neutrophil chemotactic factor which appears in serum during experimental cold challenge. J. Clin. Invest. 60:189.
8. Wasserman, S.I., Austen, K.F., and Soter, N.A. 1982. The functional and physicochemical characterization of three eosinophilotactic activities released into the circulation by cold challenge of patients with cold urticaria. Clin. Exp. Immunol. 47:570.
9. Grandel, K.E., Farr, R.S., Wanderer, A.A., Eisenstadt, T.C., and Wasserman, S.I. 1985. Association of platelet-activating factor with primary acquired cold urticaria. N. Engl. J. Med. 313:405.
10. Heavey, D.J., Kobza-Black, A., Barrow, S.E., Chapell, C.G., Greaves, M.W., and Dolleery, C.T. 1986. Prostaglandin D2 and histamine release in cold urticaria. J. Allergy Clin. Immunol. 78:458.
11. Ormerod, A.D., Kobzda-Black, A., Dawes, J. Murdoch, R.D., Koro, O., Barr, R.M., and Greaves, M.W. 1988. Prostaglandin D2 and histamine release in cold urticaria unaccompanied by evidence of platelet activation. J. Allergy Clin. Immunol. 82:586.
12. Wasserman, S.I., and Ginsberg, M.H. 1984. Release of platelet factor 4 into the blood after cold challenge of patients with cold urticaria. J. Allergy. Clin. Immunol. 74:275.
13. Houser, D.D., Arbesman, C.E., Koji, I., and Wicher, K. 1970. Cold urticaria immunologic studies. Am. J. Med. 49:23.
14. Sherman, W.B., and Seebohm, P.M. 1950. Passive transfer of cold urticaria. J. Allergy 21:414.
15. Mish, K., Kobza-Black, A., Greaves, M., Almosawi, T., and Stanworth, D.R. 1983. Passive transfer of idiopathic cold urticaria to monkeys. Acta Dermatovener. 63:163.
16. Kaplan, A.P., Garofalo, J., Sigler, R., Hauber, T. 1981. Idiophatic cold urticaria: *In vitro* demonstration of histamine release upon challenge of skin biopsies. N. Engl. J. Med. 305:1074.
17. Inoue, S., Teshima, H., Ago, Y., and Nagata, S. 1980. Cold urticaria associated with immunoglobunlin M serum factor. J. Allergy Clin. Immunol. 66(4):299.
18. Greiding, L. (Ed.) 1984: Urticaria al frio. Progresos en Alergia e Inmunologia Pediatrica. Buenos Aires: Celcius, 119.

of moderate severity, electron micrographs and mediator measurements (tryptase, histamine) (27) confirm that mast cell degranulation is ongoing. Taken together, these studies suggest an important role for the mast cell in the pathogenesis of allergen-induced asthma. In contrast, the two studies which have measured levels of mast cell derived mediators in BAL fluid of patients with EIA (21,28) have not noted evidence of mast cell activation. In addition, while recruitment of eosinophils (27,29) and eosinophil degranulation (27) are prominent features of antigen-induced asthma, studies of BAL fluid have not identified recruitment of eosinophils into the airway in subjects with EIA. Thus, the characteristic signs of inflammation associated with allergen-induced asthma, i. e., mast cell degranulation (27), recruitment and degranulation of eosinophils (27), cytokine production by memory T lymphocytes (29) and alveolar macrophages (29), and epithelial desquamation, contrast with cellular findings in studies of the airway inflammatory response to exercise challenge. These studies underscore the heterogeneity of cellular mechanisms that may be associated with the clinical expression of asthma.

If neither the mast cells nor eosinophils are the principal cells important to the pathogenesis of EIA, then what other possible cellular mechanisms might be operative? Although there are no definitive studies at present, theoretical possibilities include vascular hyperemia (30) or activation of the autonomic nervous system (31).

The vascular hyperemia hypothesis is based on the facts that airway cooling during exercise induces vasoconstriction of airway mucosal blood vessels and the resulting rewarming of the airway post-exercise induces a reactive hyperemia of the airway mucosal blood vessels with resultant airway edema and obstruction. This hypothesis is consistent with the observation that maximal bronchoconstriction in patients with EIA occurs after exercise at the time when the airways would be rewarming. Explanations for the refractory period in EIA and why the vascular response would be present only in asthmatic subjects (the increased vascular bed of subjects with asthma is a suggested explanation) require further investigation.

An alternative theory for the pathogenesis of EIA suggesting reflex autonomic nervous system cholinergic bronchoconstriction has not received much recent attention, as earlier studies with anticholinergic (i.v. or inhaled) yielded variable results. Whether vasoconstrictor neuropeptides are released by local nerve endings during episodes of EIA has not yet been explored.

At present, the pathogenesis of EIA remains an enigma. However, the use of fiberoptic bronchoscopy, coupled with the analytic techniques of cellular immunology and molecular biology, provides investigators with the tools to solve the puzzle of the pathogenesis of EIA.

References

1. Adams, F. 1856. The extant works of Aretaeus the Cappadocian. London: Sydenham Society, p. 316.
2. Floyer, J.A. 1698. Treastise of the asthma. London: R. Wilkin.
3. Deal, E.C., McFadden, E.R., Ingram, J.R., Strauss, R.H., and Jaeger, J.J. 1979. Role of respiratory heat exchange in production of exercise-induced asthma. J. Appl. Physiol. 46:467.
4. Deal, E.C., McFadden, E.R., Ingram, J.R., and Jaeger, J.J. 1979. Hyperpnea and heat flux: Initial reaction sequence in exercise-induced asthma. J. Appl. Physiol. 46:476.
5. Anderson, S.D. 1985. Issues in exercise induced asthma. J. Allergy Clin. Immunol. 76:763.
6. Tomioka, M., Ida, S., Yuriko, S., Ishihara, T., and Takishama, T. 1984. Mast cells in bronchoalveolar lumen of patients with bronchial asthma. Am. Rev. Respir. Dis. 129:1000.
7. Eggleston, P.A., Kagey-Sobotka, A., Schleimer, R.B., Lichtenstein, L.M. 1984. Interaction between hyperosmolar and IgE mediated histamine release from basophils and mast cells. Am. Rev. Respir. Dis. 130:86.
8. Togias, A.G., Naclerio, R.M., Proud, D., Fish, J.E., Adkinson, N.F., Kagey-Sobotka, A., Norman, P.S., Lichtenstein, L. 1985. Nasal challenge with cold, dry air results in release of inflammatory mediators: Possible mast cell involvement. J. Clin. Invest. 76:1375.
9. Lee, T.H., Nagy, L., Nagakura, T., Walport, M.J., Kay, A.B. 1982. Identification and partial characterization of an exercise-induced neutrophil chemotactic factor in bronchial asthma. J. Clin. Invest. 69:889.
10. Bierman, C.W., Spiro, S., Petheram, I. 1984. Characterization of the late response in exer-

cise induced asthma. J. Allergy Clin. Immunol. 74:701.
11. Anderson, S.D., Bye, P.T.P., Schoeffel, R.E., Seale, J.P., Taylor, K.M., and Ferris, L.N. 1981. Arterial plasma histamine levels in rest, and during and after exercise in patients with asthma: Effects of terbutaline aerosol. Thorax 36:259.
12. Barnes, P.J., and Brown, M.J. 1982. Venous plasma histamine in exercise- and hyperventilation-induced asthma in man. Clin. Sci. 61:159.
13. Silber, G, Proud, D., Warner, J., Naclerio, R., Kagey-Sobotka, A., Lichtenstein, L., and Eggleston, P. 1988. In-vivo release of inflammatory mediators by hyperosmolar solutions. Am. Rev. Resp. Dis. 137:606.
14. Gilbert, I.A., Fouke, J.M., and McFadden, E.R. 1987. Heat and water flux in the intrathoracic airways and exercise induced asthma. J. Appl. Physiol. 63:1681.
15. Togias, A.G., Proud, D., Lichtenstein, L.M., Adams, III G.K., Norman, P.S., Kagey-Sobotka, A., and Naclerio, R.M. 1988. The osmolality of nasal secretions increases when inflammatory mediators are released in response to inhalation of cold, dry air. Am. Rev. Respir. Dis. 137:625.
16. Zawadski, D.K., Lenner, K.A., and McFadden, E.R. 1988. Reexamination of the late asthmatic response to exercise. Am. Rev. Respir. Dis. 137:837.
17. Rubinstein, I., Levison, H., Slutsky, A., Hak, H, Wells, J., Zamel, N., Rebuck, A.S. 1987. Immediate and delayed bronchoconstriction after exercise in patients with asthma. N. Engl. J. Med. 317:482.
18. Hartley, J.P.R., Charles, T.J., Monie, R.D.H., Seaton, A., Taylor, A., Westwood, A., Williams, J.D. 1981. Arterial plasma histamine after exercise in normal individuals and in patients with exercise-induced asthma. Clin. Sci. 61:151.
19. Deal, E.C., Wasserman, S.I., Soter, N.A., Ingram, R.H., McFadden, E.R. 1980. Evaluation of role played by mediators of immediate hypersensitivity in exercise induced asthma. J. Clin. Invest. 65:659.
20. Howarth, P.H., Pao, G.J., Church, M.K., Holgate, S.T. 1984. Exercise and isocapnic hyperventilation-induced bronchoconstriction in asthma: Relevance of circulating basophils to measurement of plasma histamine. J. Allergy Clin. Immunol. 73:391.
21. Broide, D.H., Eisman, S., Ramsdell, J.W., Ferguson, P., Schwartz, L.B., and Wasserman, S.I. 1990. Airway levels of mast cell derived mediators in exercise induced asthma. Am. Rev. Respir. Dis. 141:563.
22. McNeill, R.S., Nairn, J.R., Millar, J.S., Ingram, C.G. 1966. Exercise-induced asthma. Q. J. Med. 35:55.
23. Ben-Dov, I., Bar-Yishay, E., Godfrey, S. 1982. Refractory period after exercise-induced asthma unexplained by respiratory heat loss. Am. Rev. Respir. Dis. 125:530.
24. Weiler-Ravell, D, Godfrey, S. 1981. Do exercise and antigen induced asthma utilize the same pathways? Antigen provocation in patients rendered refractory to exercise induced asthma. J. Alergy Clin. Immunol. 67:391.
25. Wenzel, S.E., Fowler, A.A., Schwartz, L.B. 1988. Activation of pulmonary mast cells by bronchoalveolar allergen challenge. *in vivo* release of histamine and tryptase in atopic subjects with and without asthma. Am. Rev. Resp. Dis. 137:1002.
26. Murray, J.J., Tonnel, A.B., Brash, A.R., et al. 1986. Release of prostaglandin D2 into human airways during acute antigen challenge. N. Engl. J. Med. 315:800
27. Broide, D.H., Gleich, G.J., Cuomo, A.J., Coburn, D.A., Federman, E.C., Schwartz, L.B., and Wasserman, S.I. 1991. Evidence of ongoing mast cell and eosinophil degranulation in symptomatic asthma airway. J. Allergy. Clin. Imm. 88:637.
28. Jarjour, N., and Calhoun, W. 1992. Exercise induced asthma is not associated with mast cell activation or airway inflammation. J. Allergy Clin. Immunol., in press.
29. Broide, D.H., and Firestein, G.S. 1991. Endobronchial allergen challenge in asthma. Demonstration of cellular source of GM-CSF. J. Clin. Invest. 88:1048.
30. McFadden, E.R., Lenner, K.A.M., Strohl, K.P. 1986. Postexertional airway rewarming and thermally induced asthma: New insights into pathophysiology and possible pathogenesis. J. Clin. Invest. 78:18.
31. Boner, A.L., Vallone, G., De Stefano, G. 1989. Effect of inhaled ipratropium bromide on methacholine and exercise provocation in asthmatic children. Pediatr. Pulmonol. 6:81.

Physical Urticaria and Exercise-Induced Anaphylaxis

Richard F. Horan, Albert L. Sheffer*

The physical allergies comprise a heterogenous group of disorders in which urticaria, angioedema, and/or anaphylaxis may be precipitated by physical stimuli. Precipitants include cold, elevation of core body temperature, pressure, light, vibration, and exercise. Exercise-induced anaphylaxis (EIA) is a unique form of physical allergy now recognized as increasing in frequency as the world population becomes committed to health through exercise. Ingestion of food or medication prior to exercise clearly increases the occurrence of anaphylaxis during exertion. Elevated plasma and/or serum histamine levels and evidence of mast cell degranulation on skin biopsy have been demonstrated in the setting of experimentally induced physical allergies including EIA. Treatment of such disorders consists of avoiding or modifying precipitating factors and use of H1 blocking agents for physical urticaria. Epinephrine is the drug of choice for reversing symptoms of anaphylaxis.

Physical Allergies

In the physical allergies urticaria, angioedema, and occasionally anaphylaxis can be precipitated by physical stimuli such as exercise, cold, increase in core body temperature, pressure, vibration, and/or light. Only exercise-induced anaphylaxis does not occur in a reproducible fashion following the apparent stimulus but, in many cases, appears to require an additional variable.

Urticaria consists of pruritic, edematous, erythematous plaques, blanchable, frequently with serpiginous borders, and generally transient. Angioedema is characterized by diffuse, well-demarcated swelling that is non-pruritic. The skin overlying lesions of angioedema may appear entirely normal. Both urticaria and angioedema result from postcapillary venule leakage. In urticaria, the leakage occurs from vessels more superficial in the dermis, whereas vessels in the deep dermis and subcutis are involved in the development of angioedema (1–3).

Activation of mast cells, and possibly of basophilic leukocytes, with subsequent elaboration of biologically potent substances, appears central to the pathogenesis of urticaria and angioedema. Release of pre-formed and newly-generated mast cell-derived mediators occurs with experimental challenge, with consequent clinical symptoms (4–7). Because of the reproducibility of such reactions, the physical urticarias have been particularly useful for studying mast cell-derived mediators. Thus, an operational classification of urticaria and angioedema has been developed, based upon the physiologic mechanisms presumed to be involved in the genesis of this condition. Clinical entities relegated to this operational classification include IgE-mediated urticaria and angioedema; complement-mediated urticaria and angioedema; urticaria and angioedema secondary to mast cell-releasing agents; urticaria/angioedema secondary to presumptive abnormalities of arachidonic acid metabolism; and idiopathic urticaria/angioedema. A special category, the physical urticarias, appears to represent IgE-mediated phenomena (8).

Cold Urticaria

Cold urticaria is characterized by pruritis, erythema, and swelling, developing within several minutes of cold exposure and often becoming most prominent on rewarming. Clinical findings are confined to the exposed area, although systemic anaphylaxis has been described following cold exposure of a large surface area, presumably resulting in release of large quantities of mast cell-derived mediators (9–13). Clinical findings generally resolve within 1–2 hours after cold exposure. Involvement of the hypopharynx/larynx with upper respiratory obstruction is extremely unusual but has been described. Diagnosis can be established by application of an ice cube to the patient's

* Harvard Medical School, Boston, Massachusetts.

forearm for 5 minutes, with subsequent follow-up observation of the area. Occasionally, passive transfer experiments have suggested an IgE-dependent mechanism (11). Experimental challenge of patients with idiopathic acquired cold urticaria has revealed release of histamine (4–7), eosinophil chemotactic peptides (10), high molecular weight neutrophil chemotactic factor (12), PGD_2 (6,7), and platelet activating factor (13) in effluent venous blood (as compared with the levels of these substances in effluent venous blood from unchallenged contralateral extremities). Ultrastructural evidence of mast cell activation following experimental challenge has also been obtained from patients with cold-induced urticaria (14). In a minority of instances, cold urticaria has been reported to be associated with the presence of an abnormal, cold-dependent protein (19–23). In most instances, the etiology of this condition remains unknown. Most instances of idiopathic cold urticaria are acquired, although familial-delay cold urticaria has also been described (24). Other variants of systemic cold urticaria have included cold-induced cholinergic urticaria, and cold-induced dermatographism (22–28). Acquired idiopathic cold urticaria probably accounts for about 2% of urticaria seen in clinical practice (16).

Cholinergic Urticaria

Cholinergic urticaria is characterized by the development of intensely pruritic, punctate (1–3 mm in diameter) papules surrounded by a prominent erythematous flare. Cholinergic urticaria accounts for about 3.5% to 4% of urticaria seen in clinical practice (3). Precipitating events appear to be related to increases in core body temperature and can include exercise, hot showers and baths, fever, and anxiety. Occasionally, other symptoms suggestive of cholinergic stimulation including lacrimation, salivation and diarrhea, may be associated with the cutaneous lesions. Changes in pulmonary function testing have also been documented (28). A neurogenic reflex may be involved, with efferent cholinergic discharge as the result of a central trigger caused by perceived core body temperature elevation. Methacholine intradermal skin test reproduces the clinical lesion in most patients with cholinergic urticaria (28). Experimental challenge may be performed using immersion in hot baths or by exercise in an occlusive sweat suit. Experimental challenge has been demonstrated to result in elaboration of histamine, eosinophil chemotactic peptides, and high molecular weight neutrophil chemotactic factor (26,27). Variant forms of heat-induced urticaria have been described, including urticaria localized to the point of contact, analogous to cold-induced urticaria, generalized, heat-induced, common urticaria, and a delayed, familial, heat-induced urticaria (28,29).

Dermatographism

In dermatographism, a wheal and flare response develops at the site of firm stroking of the skin. This is the most common form of physical urticaria and can be demonstrated in approximately 5% of the population, although most afflicted individuals are asymptomatic. Dermatographism represents approximately 9% of urticaria seen in clinical practice (30–32). With extensive involvement, elevation of plasma histamine levels has been demonstrated (30). Passive transfer studies have suggested an IgE-mediated reaction in about half of the cases evaluated (31). The diagnostic test is stroking of the skin with a dermatographometer at 3600 gm/cm2. Delayed-pressure urticaria/angioedema differs from dermatographism in that the onset of clinical findings generally occurs 4–6 hours after pressure, with pain being described more commonly than itch. Rarely, fever, malaise, and leukocytosis may accompany delayed-onset urticaria/angioedema (32).

Morphologically distinctive forms of cutaneous mast cell degranulation have been revealed by comparison of skin biopsy specimens from patients with dermatographism and with cold-induced urticaria, subjected to experimental challenge (14). Individuals with cold-induced urticaria demonstrated morphologic changes only following experimental stimulus. Ultrastructural studies have revealed enlargement and uniform disorganization of some but not all granules, fusion of membranes of adjacent granules, fusion of granule membranes with mast cell membranes, and discharge of electron-lucent and disorganized granule contents into the extracellular space. By contrast, mast cells from patients with immediate as well as with delayed dermatographism have demonstrated alterations both prior to experimental challenge and following application of the experimental stimulus. These changes consisted of an enlargement of mast cell granules, nonuniform (zonal) solubilization of granule contents, fusion of granule membranes with mast cell membranes, and extracellular discharge of granule contents. The presence of differential forms of mast cell degranulation might suggest different mechanisms of lesion formation, or, alternatively, differential susceptibility to physical stimuli of specific sub-populations of cutaneous mast cells.

Exercise-Induced Anaphylaxis

Exercise-induced anaphylaxis (EIA) is a unique form of physical allergy, now recognized as having become more frequent during the past 20 years (33–36). Affected individuals have been identified from early adolescence until at least the sixth decade of life (36). Generalized pruritis with a flushing sensation, a feeling of warmth, and the development of urticaria occurring in association with vigorous physical exertion have been the hallmarks of this syndrome. Such cutaneous manifestations often herald the onset of a fully-developed, life-threatening attack, with the angioedema, gastrointestinal colic, and upper respiratory obstruction rarely progressing to vascular collapse. Cessation of exercise at the onset of symptoms may ameliorate further evolution of the episode. While a few patients have been reported to develop punctate papular eruptions reminiscent of cholinergic urticaria, most of them have developed more typical, giant urticarial eruptions. Respiratory symptoms are commonly choking and stridor rather than wheezing, and the gastrointestinal manifestations include nausea, vomiting, colicky abdominal pain, and diarrhea. Headaches, persisting as long as 72 hours, have been a late sequela of the fully-developed attacks.

The setting in which attacks of EIA have occurred has varied among patients (33). Some individuals have experienced attacks with exertion alone. However, other affected individuals have experienced attacks only with exertion in the postprandial state; exertion associated with ingestion of a specific food (in particular, shellfish or celery); or exertion associated with the use of aspirin or nonsteroidal anti-inflammatory drugs. Elevated ambient temperature has appeared to be associated with increased likelihood of attacks. Personal and family history of atopy appear increased in afflicted individuals. The presence of elevated plasma histamine levels during experimentally-induced attacks has been associated with the demonstration of mast cell degranulation on skin biopsy during appropriate exercise challenge (14,34).

Other Physical Urticarias

These are less common and consist of vibratory urticaria, solar urticaria (which can be further subclassified by the precipitating wavelengths eliciting the reaction), and aquagenic urticaria. These are all unusual but definitely described types of physical urticaria.

Therapy and Management of the Physical Urticarias

Therapy requires avoidance of the precipitating factor. Care must be taken to avoid the physical stimulus associated with the development of symptoms. For example, appropriate cold avoidance and thermal protection are important in cold urticaria. For patients with cold urticaria, it is crucial that exposure of a large surface area to cold be vigilantly avoided (as in boating, diving, jumping into pools, and any sudden exposure to cold). Similarly, avoidance of stimuli resulting in elevation of core body temperature may be appropriate in individuals with cholinergic urticaria, and sun screens may be helpful to some individuals with solar urticaria. Patients with exercise-induced anaphylaxis should be cautioned to moderate or discontinue their activity at the slightest suggestion of the onset of symptoms and to avoid ingestion of food for at least 4–6 hours prior to exercise. Similarly, the use of aspirin or nonsteroidal anti-inflammatory agents with cyclooxygenase-inhibiting activity should be avoided in those individuals prior to exercise. Such patients should be advised to exercise with a companion who is apprised of their condition. They should obtain and carry materials for self-administration of subcutaneous epinephrine to be used in the event of any life-threatening reaction such as upper respiratory obstruction and/or feeling of faintness, and they should immediately seek medical care if such occurs. Antihistamines are the mainstay of therapy for patients with chronic idiopathic urticaria and can be used to treat physical urticarias prophylactically. Such has not been helpful, however, in preventing exercise-induced anaphylaxis. Therapy should be instituted with the use of a H_1-antagonist. It is important that treatment be around-the-clock rather than on an as-needed basis. The agent chosen must be individualized. Soporific side effects of antihistamines often represent the most common limiting factor in treatment, although the anticholinergic effects of antihistamines can also limit their utility. The dosage of H_1-antagonist chosen should be increased to tolerance; and if adequate alleviation of symptoms is not achieved at maximum tolerable doses, trials utilizing agents from each of the various pharmacological subclasses are warranted. However, because of the life-threatening potential for several of the physical urticarial reactions, it is critical that most of these patients have a readily-utilizable form of adrenalin such as epinephrine available.

Thus, physical allergy is a unique form of urticaria, angioedema and anaphylaxis. Because of the life-threatening possibilities for many of these entities, it is critical that they be identified and the patient be appropriately instructed about avoiding such exposure. In most instances, patients appropriately forewarned have been able to continue to exist without significant incapacitation.

References

1. Lever, W.F., and Schaumburg-Lever, G. 1990. Histopathology of the skin. Philadelphia: Lippincott.
2. Sheldon, J.M., Matthews, K.P., and Lovell, R.G. 1954. The vexing urticaria problem. Present concepts of etiology and management. J. Allergy 25:525.
3. Champion, R.H., Roberts, S.O.B., Carpenter, R.G., and Roger J. 1969. Urticaria and angiooedema: a review of 554 patients. Br. J. Derm. 81:588.
4. Kaplan, A.P., Gray, L., Shaff, R.E., Horakova, Z., and Beaven, M.A. 1975. *In vivo* studies of mediator release in cold urticaria and cholinergic urticaria. J. Allergy Clin. Immunol. 55:394.
5. Kaplan, A.P., Garofolo, J., Sigler, R., and Hauber, T. 1981. Idiopathic cold urticaria: *In vitro* demonstration of histamine release upon challenge of skin biopsies. N. Engl. J. Med. 305:1074.
6. Heavey, D.J., Kobza-Black, A., Barrow, S.E., Chappell, C.G., Greaves, M.W., and Dollery, C.T. 1986. Prostagladin. D2 and histamine release in cold urticaria. J. Allergy Clin. Immunol. 78:458.
7. Ormerod, A.D., Kobza-Black, A., Dawes, J., Murdock, R.D., Koro, O., Barr, R.M., and Greaves, M.W. 1988. Prostaglandin. D2 and histamine release in cold urticaria unaccompanied by evidence of platelet activation. J. Allergy Clin. Immunol. 82:586.
8. Sheffer, A.L., and Wasserman, S. 1979. Anaphylaxis. In: The science and practice of clinical medicine (Vol. 4). A.S.Cohen, ed. New York: Grune & Stratton.
9. Horton, B.T., Brown, G.E., and Roth, G.M. 1936. Hypersensitivities to cold with local and systemic manifestations of a histamine-like character: Its amenability to treatment. J. Am. Med. Assoc. 107:1263.
10. Soter, N.A., Wasserman, S.I., and Austen, K.F. 1976. Cold urticaria: Release into the circulation of histamine and eosinophil chemotactic factor of anaphylaxis during cold challenge. N. Engl. J. Med. 294:687.
11. Houser, D.D., Arbesmann, C.E., Ito, K., and Wicher, K. 1970. Cold urticaria: Immunologic studies. Am.J. Med. 49:23.
12. Wasserman, S.I., Soter, N.A., Center, D.M., and Austen, K.F. 1977. Cold urticaria. Recognition and characterization of a neutrophil chemotactic factor which appears in serum during experimental cold challenge. J. Clin. Invest. 60:189.

13 Grandel, K.E., Farr, R.S., Wanderer, A.A., Eisenstadt, T.C., and Wasserman, S.I. 1985. Association of a platelet-activating factor with primary acquired cold urticaria. N. Engl. J. Med. 313:405.

14. Murphy, G.F., Austen, K.F., Fonferko, E., and Sheffer A.L. 1987. Morphologically distinctive forms of cutaneous mast cell degranulation induced by cold and mechanical stimuli: An ultrastructural study. J. Allergy Clin. Immunol. 80:603.

15. Sheffer, A.L., Tong, A.K.F., Murphy, G.F., McFadden, E.R., and Austen, K.F. 1985. Exercise-induced anaphylaxis: A serious form of physical allergy associated with mast cell degranulation. J. Allergy Clin. Immunol. 75:479.
16. Costanzi, J.J., and Coltman, C.A., J.r. 1967. Kappa chain cold-precipitated IgG associated with cold urticaria. Clin. Exp. Immunol. 2:167.
17. Harns, K.E., Lewis, T., and Vaughan, J. 1929. Haemoglobinuria and urticaria from cold occurring singly or in combination: Observations referring especially to the mechanism of urticaria with some remarks upon Reynaud's disease. Heart, Lung 14:305.
18. Shafar, J. 1965. Cold hypersensitivity states. Lancet 2:431.
19. Costanzi, J.J., Coltman, C.A., Jr., and Donaldson, V.H. 1969. Activation of complement by a monoclonal cryoglobulin associated with cold urticaria. J. Clin. Med. 74:902.
20. Rawnsley, H.M., and Shelly, W.B. 1968. Cold urticaria with cryoglobulinemia in a patient with chronic lymphocytic leukemia. Arch. Dermatol. 98:12.
21. Soter, N.A., Joski, N.P., Twarog, F.J., et al. 1977. Delayed cold-induced urticaria: A dominantly inherited disorder. J. Allergy Clin. Immunol. 54:294.
22. Kaplan, A.P. 1984. Unusual cold-induced disorders: Cold dependent dermatographism and systemic cold urticaria. J. Allergy Clin. Immunol. 73:453.
23. Kaplan, A.P., and Garofalo, J. 1981. Identification of a new physically induced cholinergic urticaria. J. Allergy Clin. Immunol. 68:438.
24. Grant, R.T., Pearson, R.S.B., and Corneau, W.J. 1935. Observations on urticaria provoked by emotion, by exercise and by warming the body. Clin. Sci. 2:266.
25. Soter, N.A., Wasserman, S.I., Austen, K.F., and McFadden, E.R., Jr. 1980. Release of mast cell mediators and alterations in lung function in patients with cholinergic urticaria. N Engl. J. Med. 302:604.
26. Kaplan, A.P., Natbony, S., Tawal, A.P., and Fruchter, M. 1981. Exercise-induced anaphylaxis as a manifestation of cholinergic urticaria. J. Allergy Clin. Immunol. 68:319.
27. Sigler, R.W., LevinsoN, A.I., Evans, R., et al. 1979. Evaluation of a patient with cold and cholinergic urticaria. J. Allergy Clin. Immunol. 63:35.
28. Harber, L.C., and Baer, R.L. 1978. Reactions to light, heat, and trauma. In: Immunological diseases. M. Samter, et al., eds. Boston (MA): Little, Brown & Company.
29. Michaelsson, G., and Ros, A. 1971. Familial localized heat urticaria of delayed type. Acta Derm Venereol. 51:279.
30. Garofalo, J. and Kaplan, A.P. 1981. Histamine release and therapy of severe dermatographism. J. Allergy Clin. Immunol. 68:103.
31. Newcomb, R.W., and Nelson, H. 1973. Dermographia mediated by immunoglobulin E. Am. J. Med. 54:174.
32. Estes, S.A., and Wang, C.W. 1981. Delayed pressure urticaria: An investigation of some parameters of lesion induction. J. Am. Acad. Dermatol. 5:25.
33. Sheffer, A.L., and Austen, K.F. 1980. Exercise-induced anaphylaxis. J. Allergy Clin. Immunol. 66:106.
34. Sheffer, A.L., Soter, N.A., McFadden, E.R., Jr., and Austen, K.F. 1983. Exercise-induced anaphylaxis: A distinct form of physical allergy. J. Allergy Clin. Immunol. 71:311.
35. Sheffer, A.L. 1984. Exercise-induced anaphylaxis. J. Allergy Clin. Immunol. 73:699.
36. Wade, J..P., Liang, M.H., and Sheffer, A.L. 1989. Exercise-induced anaphylaxis: Epidemiologic observations. Prague Clin. Biol. Res. 297:157.

SUBJECT INDEX*

---

* This index was prepared on the basis of the *key words* supplied by the authors. The page numbers refer to the first page of a chapter referring to the subject.